VOLUME 2

3rd Edition

DIAGNOSIS OF BONE AND JOINT DISORDERS

Donald Resnick, M.D.

Professor of Radiology
University of California, San Diego
Chief of Osteoradiology Section
Veterans Administration Medical Center
San Diego, California

With the Editorial Assistance of Catherine F. Fix
With the Technical Assistance of Debra J. Trudell

W.B. SAUNDERS COMPANY
A Division of Harcourt Brace & Company
Philadelphia   London   Toronto   Montreal   Sydney   Tokyo

W.B. SAUNDERS COMPANY
A Division of
Harcourt Brace & Company

The Curtis Center
Independence Square West
Philadelphia, Pennsylvania 19106

Library of Congress Cataloging-in-Publication Data

Resnick, Donald

Diagnosis of bone and joint disorders / Donald Resnick.—3rd ed.

p.   cm.

Includes bibliographical references and indexes.

ISBN 0–7216–5066–X (set)

1. Musculoskeletal system—Diseases—Diagnosis.   2. Bones—Diseases—
Diagnosis.   3. Joints—Diseases—Diagnosis.   4. Diagnostic
imaging.   I. Title.

[DNLM: 1. Bone Diseases—diagnosis.   2. Joint Diseases—diagnosis.
3. Diagnosis Imaging.   WE 300 R434d 1995]

RC925.7.R47 1995

616.7′1075—dc20

DNLM/DLC   93–48321

Diagnosis of Bone and Joint Disorders, 3rd edition

Volume One	ISBN	0–7216–5067–8
Volume Two	ISBN	0–7216–5068–6
Volume Three	ISBN	0–7216–5069–4
Volume Four	ISBN	0–7216–5070–8
Volume Five	ISBN	0–7216–5071–6
Volume Six	ISBN	0–7216–5072–4
Six Volume Set	ISBN	0–7216–5066–X

Printed in the United States of America.

Last digit is the print number: 9   8   7   6   5   4   3   2   1

CONTENTS

▼

Contents

SECTION

III

Basic Sciences of Musculoskeletal Diseases

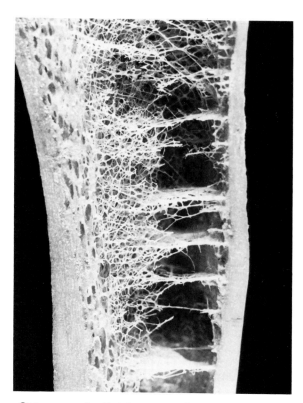

Osteoporosis: Reinforcement lines, or bone bars, extend in a parallel fashion from the posterior surface of the proximal portion of the tibia.

20

Histogenesis, Anatomy, and Physiology of Bone

Donald Resnick, M.D.
Stavros C. Manolagas, M.D., Ph.D.
Gen Niwayama, M.D.
Michael D. Fallon, M.D.

Bone is a remarkable tissue. Although its appearance on the radiograph might be misinterpreted as indicating inactivity, bone constantly is undergoing change, not only in the immature skeleton, in which growth and development are readily apparent, but in the mature skeleton as well, through the constant and balanced processes of bone formation and resorption. It is when these processes are modified such that one or the other dominates that a pathologic state may be created. In some instances, the resulting imbalance between bone formation and resorption is easily detectable on the radiograph. In others, a more subtle imbalance exists that may be identified only at the histologic level.

The initial architecture of bone is characterized by an irregular network of collagen, termed woven-fibered bone, which is a temporary material that is either removed to form a marrow cavity or subsequently replaced by a sheet-like arrangement of osseous tissue, termed parallel-fibered or lamellar bone. As a connective tissue, bone is highly specialized, differing from other connective tissues by its rigidity and hardness that relate primarily to the inorganic salts that are deposited in its matrix. These properties are fundamental to a tissue that must maintain the shape of the human body, protect its vital soft tissues, and allow locomotion, transmitting from one region of the body to another the forces generated by the contractions of various muscles. Bone also serves as a reservoir for ions, principally calcium, that are essential to normal fluid regulation and are made available as a response to stimuli produced by a number of hormones, particularly parathyroid hormone, vitamin D, and calcitonin.

This chapter provides an analysis of the histogenesis, anatomy, and histology of bone and an overview of its physiology and pathophysiology. Additional information on these and related subjects can be found in Chapters 51, 52, and 53.

HISTOGENESIS
Developing Bone

The histogenesis of bone has been well summarized by Jaffe and others.[1, 2, 89, 90] Bone develops by the process of intramembranous bone formation (by transformation of condensed mesenchymal tissue) or endochondral bone formation (by indirect conversion of an intermediate cartilage model), or both. At some locations, such as the bones of the cranial vault (frontal and parietal bones as well as parts of the occipital and temporal bones), the mandible and maxilla, and the midportion of the clavicle, intramembranous (mesenchymal) ossification is detected; in other locations, such as the bones of the extremities, the vertebral column, the pelvis, and the base of the skull, both endochondral and intramembranous ossification can be identified. The actual processes of bone tissue formation essentially are the same in both intramembranous and endochondral ossification, and include the following sequence: (1) osteoblasts differentiate from mesenchymal cells; (2) osteoblasts deposit matrix that subsequently is mineralized; (3) bone initially is deposited as a network of immature (woven) trabeculae, the primary spongiosa; (4) the primary spongiosa is replaced by secondary bone, removed to form bone marrow, or converted into primary cortical bone by filling of spaces between the trabeculae.[3] A variety of congenital disorders, such as cleidocranial dysplasia (Fig. 20–1), may lead to abnormalities in intramembranous or endochondral bone formation, or both.

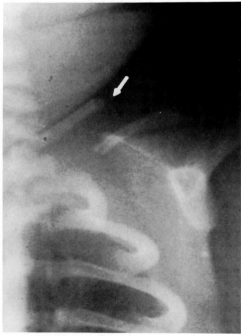

FIGURE 20–1. Defective bone formation: Cleidocranial dysplasia. Observe abnormal clavicular ossification (arrow), a characteristic component of this disorder.

Intramembranous Ossification. Intramembranous ossification is initiated by the proliferation of mesenchymal cells about a network of capillaries. At this site, a transformation of mesenchymal cells is accompanied by the appearance of a meshwork of collagen fibers and amorphous ground substance. The primitive cells change in number, shape, and size. They proliferate, enlarge, and become arranged in groups, which extend in a strandlike configuration into the surrounding tissue. The cells have now become osteoblasts and are intimately involved in the formation of an eosinophilic matrix within the collagenous tissue. This sequence represents the initial stage of the ossification process, which becomes more prominent and more widespread as the osteoid matrix undergoes calcification with the deposition of calcium phosphate. Some of the osteoblasts on the surface of the osteoid and woven-fibered bone become entrapped within the substance of the matrix in a space called a lacuna. The osteoblast then becomes an osteocyte, and although it is isolated in some respects from the neighboring proliferating mesenchymal tissue, it maintains some contact with the precursor cells by sending out elongated processes or projections through canaliculi that extend through the matrix. Embedded osteocytes are devoted primarily to maintaining the integrity of the surrounding matrix and are not directly involved in bone formation. Through the continued transformation of mesenchymal cells into osteoblasts, the elaboration of an osteoid matrix, and the entrapment of osteoblasts within the matrix, the primitive mesenchyme is converted into osseous tissue. The ultimate characteristics of the tissue depend on its location within the bone: In the cancellous areas of the bone, the meshwork of osseous tissue contains intervening vascular connective tissue representing the embryonic precursor of the bone marrow; in the compact areas of the bone, the osseous tissue becomes more condensed, forming cylindrical masses containing a central vascular channel, the haversian system. On the external and internal surfaces of the compact bone, fibrovascular layers develop (periosteum and endosteum) that contain cells which remain osteogenic, giving bone its ever-changing quality. In the process of further development, coarse-fibered nonlamellar primitive, or woven, bone (Fig. 20–2) eventually is converted to fine-fibered lamellar mature bone (Fig. 20–3).

Endochondral Ossification. Endochondral (intracartilaginous) ossification is prominent in the bones of the appendicular skeleton, the axial skeleton, and the base of the skull. In this process, cartilaginous tissue derived from mesenchyme serves as a template and is replaced with bone (Figs. 20–4 and 20–5). The initial sites of bone formation are called centers of ossification, and their precise location within the bone is very much dependent on the specific bone that is being analyzed. In the tubular bones, the primary center of ossification is located in the central portion of the cartilaginous model, whereas later-appearing centers of ossification (secondary centers) are located at the ends of the models within epiphyses and apophyses. Vascular mesenchymal tissue or perichondrium, whose deeper layers contain cells with osteogenic potential, surrounds the cartilaginous model.

The initial changes in the primary center of ossification are hypertrophy of cartilage cells, glycogen accumulation, and reduction of intervening matrix. Subsequently, these cells degenerate, die, and become calcified. Simultaneously,

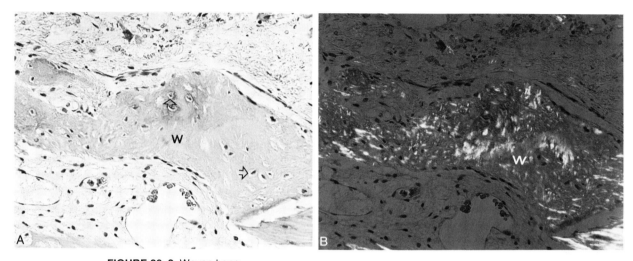

FIGURE 20–2. Woven bone.
A Immature woven bone *(W)*. Note the large osteocytic lacunae (open arrows).
B Same field, viewed by polarized light, showing birefringent pattern of random collagen.

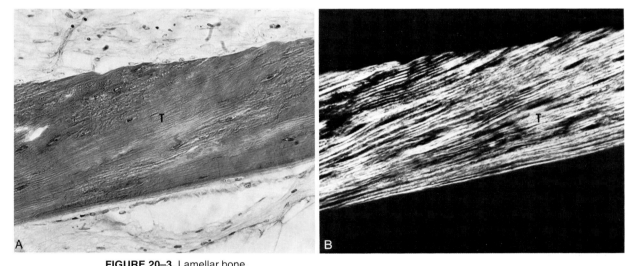

FIGURE 20–3. Lamellar bone.
A Mature lamellar trabecular bone *(T)*.
B Same field, viewed by polarized light, showing birefringent pattern of lamellar collagen.

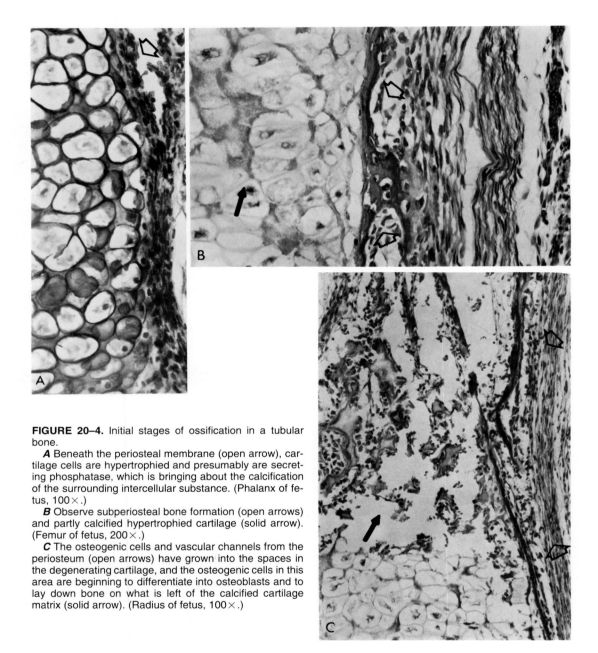

FIGURE 20–4. Initial stages of ossification in a tubular bone.

A Beneath the periosteal membrane (open arrow), cartilage cells are hypertrophied and presumably are secreting phosphatase, which is bringing about the calcification of the surrounding intercellular substance. (Phalanx of fetus, 100×.)

B Observe subperiosteal bone formation (open arrows) and partly calcified hypertrophied cartilage (solid arrow). (Femur of fetus, 200×.)

C The osteogenic cells and vascular channels from the periosteum (open arrows) have grown into the spaces in the degenerating cartilage, and the osteogenic cells in this area are beginning to differentiate into osteoblasts and to lay down bone on what is left of the calcified cartilage matrix (solid arrow). (Radius of fetus, 100×.)

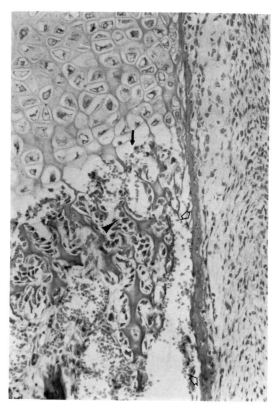

FIGURE 20–5. Endochondral and intramembranous ossification in a tubular bone: Radius of a 4½ month old fetus. The large and confluent cartilage cell lacunae are being penetrated by vascular channels (solid arrow), thus exposing intervening cores of calcified cartilage matrix. The osteoblasts are depositing osseous tissue on these cartilage matrix cores (arrowhead). Observe subperiosteal bone formation (open arrows).

the deeper or subperichondrial cells undergo transformation to osteoblasts and, through a process identical to intramembranous ossification, these osteoblasts produce a subperiosteal collar or cuff of bone, which encloses the central portions of the cartilaginous tissue. Periosteal tissue is converted into vascular channels, and these channels perforate the shell of bone, entering the degenerating cartilaginous foci. The aggressive vascular tissue disrupts the lacunae of the cartilage cells, creating spaces that fill with embryonic bone marrow. Osteoblasts appear, which transform the sites of degenerating and dying cartilage cells into foci of ossification by laying down osteoid tissue in the cartilage matrix. Osteoblasts become trapped within the developing bone as osteocytes in a fashion similar to that occurring in the process of intramembranous ossification. The entire area is highly active as the cartilaginous model gradually is replaced with bone.

From the center of the tubular bone, ossification proceeds toward the ends of the bone as cells in adjoining cartilaginous areas undergo hypertrophy, death, calcification in association with vascular invasion, osteoblast transformation, and conversion to bone. Similarly, the periosteal collar, which is actively participating in intramembranous ossification, spreads toward the ends of the bone, slightly ahead of the band of endochondral ossification. Through a process of resorption of some of the initially formed trabeculae, a

marrow space is created, and through a process of subperiosteal deposition of bone, a cortex becomes evident, grows thicker, and is converted into a system with longitudinally arranged compact bone surrounding vascular channels (haversian system). The frontier of endochondral ossification that is advancing toward the end of the bone becomes better delineated, appearing as a plate of cellular activity. It is this plate that ultimately becomes located between the epiphysis and diaphysis of a tubular bone, forming the growth plate (cartilaginous plate or physis) that is the predominant site of longitudinal growth of the bone. The plate contains clearly demarcated zones: a resting zone of flattened and immature cells on the epiphyseal aspect of the plate, and zones of cell growth and hypertrophy and of transformation with provisional calcification and ossification on the metaphyseal or diaphyseal aspect of the plate.

The size and shape of the most recently formed portion of the metaphysis of a tubular bone is dependent on the effects of an encircling fibrochondro-oseous structure, designated the periphysis, that consists of the zone of Ranvier, the ring of La Croix, and the bone bark they produce (Fig. 20–6).[91] That portion of the periphysis adjacent to the physis is the zone or groove of Ranvier; that portion adjacent to the metaphysis is the ring of La Croix. Together, these portions lay down a continuous thin layer of bone, termed bone bark, through the process of intramembranous ossification.[91] In the first several years of life, that portion of the metaphysis surrounded by the periphysis is flat and longitudinally directed, and it is referred to as a metaphyseal collar.[92] Furthermore, the bone bark appears as a straight linear extension of the metaphysis, occurring at the margins of the physis. This normal projection of bone must be differentiated from the metaphyseal fractures associated with child abuse.[91]

In this setting of progressive ossification of the diaphysis with longitudinal spread toward the ends of the bone, characteristic changes appear within the epiphysis (Fig. 20–7). Epiphyseal invasion by vascular channels is followed later by the initiation of endochondral bone formation, creating secondary centers of ossification. The process again is characterized by cartilage cell hypertrophy and death, followed by calcification. Vascular mesenchyme invades these epiphyseal foci, and osteoblasts appear, which deposit osseous tissue on the calcified matrix. In this fashion, an enlarging ossification nucleus is created whose peripheral margins contain zones of cell hypertrophy, degeneration, calcification, and ossification. The epiphyseal ossification center at first develops rapidly, although later the process slows. The epiphyseal cartilage thus is converted to bone, although a layer on its articular aspect persists, destined to become the articular cartilage of the neighboring joint. With continued maturation of both the epiphysis and diaphysis, the growth plate is thinned still further (Figs. 20–8 and 20–9). Gradually, cellular activity within the plate diminishes and a layer of bone is applied to its diaphyseal surface. Soon, vascular invasion of the plate's remaining cartilage cells is associated with ossification via the process of creeping substitution. In this fashion, the growth plate disappears, allowing fusion of epiphyseal and diaphyseal ossification centers, followed by cessation of endochondral bone formation deep to the articular cartilage of the epiphysis, with formation of a subchondral bone plate. Although the growth plate has now ceased to function, a band of horizontally oriented

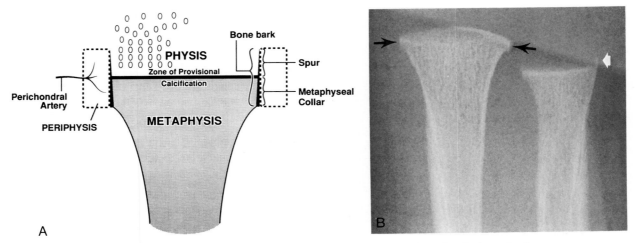

FIGURE 20–6. Endochondral and intramembranous ossification in a tubular bone: Periphysis and metaphyseal collar.
A In this diagram, observe the periphysis (dashed boxes) and metaphyseal collar and spur. The bone bark is indicated.
B In the distal portion of the radius of a normal infant, note the straight metaphyseal margins (black arrows) forming the edges of the metaphyseal collar as well as a well-defined bone bark (white arrow) at the medial margin of the ulnar physis.
(From Oestrich AE, Ahmad BS: Skel Radiol *21*:283, 1992.)

trabeculae may persist, marking the previous location of the plate as a transverse radiopaque fusion line.

Abnormalities of endochondral ossification in the physis are well recognized in a number of disorders and are fundamental to the diagnosis of rickets (Fig. 20–10*A,B*). Transient aberrations of such ossification lead to the development of growth recovery lines (Fig. 20–10*C*).

This process of endochondral ossification has its counterpart in bones other than the tubular ones of the extremities. Enlarging ossification nuclei are recognized in the developing carpus and tarsus, while in the vertebral column, multiple centers of ossification appear in the vertebral body and the neural arches and, through a process of enlargement and fusion, create the vertebral structure that characterizes the mature skeleton (Fig. 20–11).

Developing Joint

An articulation eventually appears in the mesenchyme that exists between the developing ends of the bones. In this interzone, mesenchyme is not converted to cartilage or bone but rather undergoes change that is influenced by the type of joint destined to be formed. In a fibrous joint, the interzonal mesenchyme is modified to form the fibrous tissue that will connect the adjacent bones; in a synchondrosis it is converted into hyaline cartilage; and in a symphysis it is changed into fibrocartilage. At the site of a synovial joint, the central portion of the mesenchyme becomes loose-meshed and is continuous in its periphery with adjacent mesenchyme that is undergoing vascularization (Figs. 20–12 to 20–14). The synovial mesenchyme that is created will later form the synovial membrane as well as some additional intra-articular structures, whereas the central aspect of the mesenchyme undergoes liquefaction and cavitation, creating the joint space. Condensation of the peripheral mesenchyme leads to joint capsule formation.

Modeling and Remodeling of Bone

The term intermediary organization has been used to describe the control and regulation of coordinated cellular events that occur in the living human (or animal) skeleton.[93] Intermediary organization is dependent on a number of bone cells, such as osteoblasts and osteoclasts, whose activity is linked together, or coupled (see later discussion). Thus, the processes of bone formation and bone resorption are intertwined, and it is difficult to consider one without the other. Four discrete functional subdivisions of intermediary organization have been described: growth, modeling, remodeling, and fracture healing.[93] In each of these, the same bone cells are at work to accomplish the function, but the organization of these cells is unique to the task that is required.[89] The following discussion addresses two of these subdivisions, modeling and remodeling of bone.

The gradual conversion in the fetus of immature, spongy, or woven-fibered bone, containing a labyrinth of connecting vascular spaces, into concentric tracts of nonlamellated, parallel-fibered bone, termed atypical haversian systems or primary osteons and, subsequently, into typical haversian systems or secondary osteons composed of lamellae of parallel-fibered bone is well described in a number of publications.[1, 3, 4] This transformation from woven-fibered bone to parallel-fibered bone is readily apparent at the time of birth and continues thereafter throughout life. Although lamellar bone is dominant in the adult, woven bone is prominent in some sites (e.g., lining the tooth sockets) and in some situations (e.g., the repair of fractures). At any age, bone should be regarded as a dynamic tissue, constantly undergoing change. Major adjustments in the size and shape of bone, which are prominent in the immature skeleton of the infant, child, and adolescent, are known as modeling; less obvious alterations in the quality of bone, with the replacement of structurally inferior woven-fibered bone, as is seen in the infant, with stronger, more organized lamellar bone, which predominates in the adult, are termed remodeling.

Modeling. It is the process of modeling that significantly alters the shape and form of bone. Modeling, or sculpting, of the skeleton is responsive to the mechanical forces that are placed on the skeleton. This process occurs continually throughout the growth period at varying rates and involves all bone surfaces. Classic examples of the modeling process

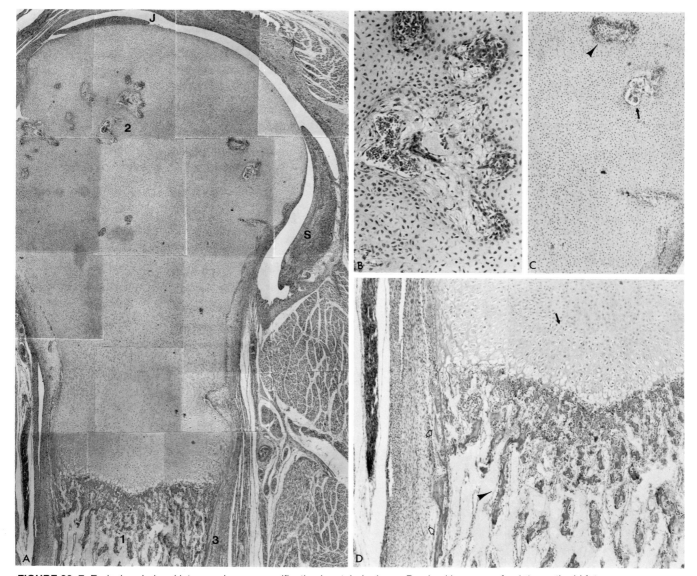

FIGURE 20–7. Endochondral and intramembranous ossification in a tubular bone: Proximal humerus of a 4½ month old fetus.

A A composite photomicrograph (25×). Observe sites of endochondral ossification in the diaphysis *(1)* and several foci in the epiphysis *(2)* and of intramembranous ossification related to the periosteal membrane *(3)*. J, Glenohumeral joint space; S, synovial membrane.

B A high power photomicrograph (215×) shows a developing ossification center of the epiphysis with a vessel-rich focus of developing osteoblasts.

C A high power photomicrograph (86×) of a portion of the proximal humeral epiphysis demonstrates blood vessels (arrow) about a small ossifying focus (arrowhead).

D A high power photomicrograph (86×) demonstrates the features of the band of endochondral ossification that exists between the cartilage (solid arrow) and diaphyseal bone (arrowhead). Observe a layer of bone (open arrows) beneath the periosteal membrane related to intramembranous ossification.

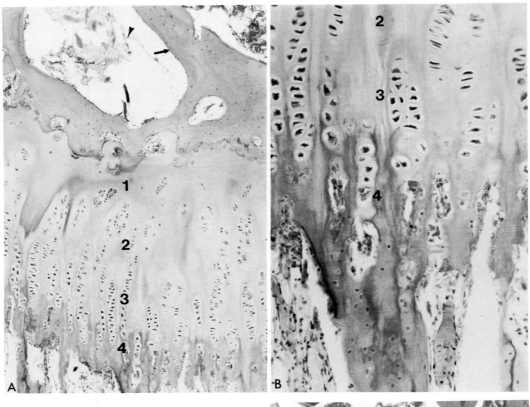

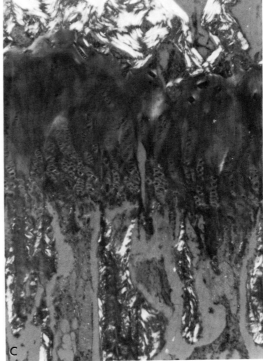

FIGURE 20–8. Cartilaginous growth plate in a 16 year old patient.

A, B Observe the bone (arrow) and marrow (arrowhead) of the epiphysis. The areas of the growth plate include a zone of resting cartilage *(1),* proliferating cartilage *(2),* maturing cartilage *(3),* and calcifying cartilage *(4).* (*A*, 86×; *B*, 215×.)

C In a different patient of similar age, polarized light microscopy reveals lamellated bone in the epiphysis (at top), the cartilaginous zones in the physis (center), and nonlamellated developing trabeculae in the metaphysis (at bottom). (66×.)

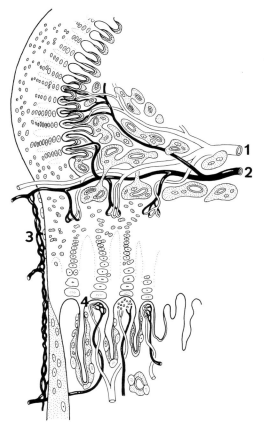

FIGURE 20–9. Cartilage growth plate and adjacent metaphysis and epiphysis. Note the epiphyseal vein *(1)* and artery *(2)*, the perichondrial vascular ring *(3)*, the terminal loops of the nutrient artery *(4)* in the metaphysis, and ongoing endochondral ossification in the physis and epiphysis. (Redrawn from R Warwick, PL Williams [Eds]: Gray's Anatomy. 35th British Ed. Philadelphia, WB Saunders Co, 1973, p 227.)

are (1) drifting of the midshaft of a tubular bone; (2) flaring of the ends of a tubular bone; and (3) enlargement of the cranial vault and modification of cranial curvature.[3] As in the other subdivisions of intermediary organization, proper modeling of bone is dependent on the coordinated activities of the osteoblasts and osteoclasts, but as the process of modeling results in a net increase in the amount of bone tissue, it is the osteoblast that is called upon to do the bulk of the work.[89] Two other characteristics of bone modeling have been emphasized.[89] First, the process is age-dependent; the potential for modeling is greatly reduced in humans after adolescence, and it becomes almost nonexistent by the middle of the third decade of life. Second, the bone gain is predominantly subperiosteal.

Although the expansion and lengthening of a tubular bone are readily apparent to a parent who witnesses the growth of his or her child and to the physician who is able to compare sequential radiographic examinations of the child's limbs, the ability of bone to shift or drift eccentrically in a lateral or medial direction to fulfill changing mechanical demands is less evident. This form of modeling is a prerequisite to the normal development of tubular bones, ribs, and other osseous structures. It is accomplished by resorption, which dominates in one aspect of a bone, and apposition, which dominates in another. In the long tubular bones of the extremity, resorption is more evident on that side of the bone surface that is nearer the body core, and apposition occurs on the opposite surface, accounting for a lateral drift of the entire bone. As a consequence, a point initially present on the periosteal surface may eventually come to lie within the medullary cavity.[5] Studies using sequential radiographs of the long bones and a process of superimposition of osseous landmarks allow the documentation of the precise rate and direction of lateral drift and indicate that the movement generally is parallel to the long axis of the bone and only rarely angular.[5, 6] This modeling phenomenon has been used to explain the configuration and the incomplete nature of persistent growth recovery lines in the child as well as in the adult[7] (see Chapter 76).

The flaring that normally is evident in the end of a long tubular bone is a second example of bone modeling (Fig. 20–15). As the bone grows in length, the wide metaphyseal region, a product of the growth plate, later is occupied by a narrow diaphysis, a change that requires close coordination of bone resorption and apposition.[3] Reduction of the metaphysis, creating a metaphyseal funnel, is accomplished by osteoclastic resorption along its periosteal surface that is coupled with osteoblastic bone formation in the endosteal surface of the metaphyseal cortex. Subsequently, as the metaphysis migrates shaftward, the marrow cavity is enlarged owing to the processes of osteoclastic resorption of trabecular bone and endosteal bone resorption, and the overall diameter of the shaft is increased as a result of periosteal bone formation.[3] A variety of factors, including certain drugs (e.g., diphosphonates) and diseases, may upset this delicate balance of bone resorption and bone formation. Overtubulation, presumably related to a failure of periosteal deposition of bone, is encountered in osteogenesis imperfecta (Fig. 20–16*A*), and lack of tubulation (undertubulation) is seen in craniometaphyseal and craniodiaphyseal dysplasias.[8] The causative events leading to these abnormal changes in osseous shape, however, are complex, and also include disturbances in endochondral bone formation within the physis and alterations in the composition of the bone marrow, as occur in certain anemias and storage diseases (Fig. 20–16*B*)

Some of the constituents of the cranial vault, such as the parietal bone, normally exhibit during growth not only an increase in thickness and surface area but also a decrease in curvature, becoming less convex in shape (Fig. 20–17). The change in convexity requires periosteal resorption along the internal circumference of the bone and periosteal apposition externally, and it is accompanied by growth at the adjacent sutures.

Remodeling. To produce and maintain biomechanically and metabolically competent tissue, the transformation of immature, woven-type bone to more compact lamellar bone is required. This process of remodeling normally is most prominent in the young but continues at reduced rates throughout life; in the abnormal situation at any age, in the presence of a variety of diseases, metabolic stimuli may lead to accentuation of bone remodeling. Remodeling of bone requires the coordinated activity of a group of highly specialized cells, each with a finite life span, which along with the quantum of bone that is altered is referred to as a bone remodeling or basic multicellular unit.[3] These units are active in both the cortical and the spongiosa bone; they

Text continued on page 623

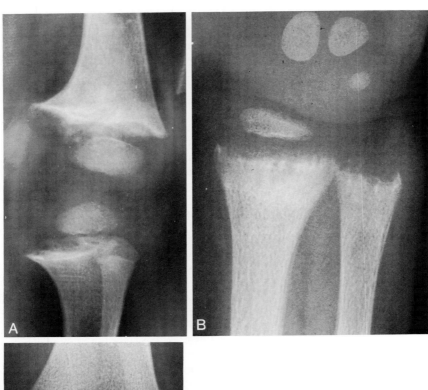

FIGURE 20–10. Abnormalities in endochondral ossification in the growth plate.

A, B Rickets. Widening of the physis and irregularity and enlargement of the metaphysis are among the manifestations of this disease.

C Growth recovery lines. Note multiple, wavy radiodense lines in the metaphyses of the femur and tibia. The configuration of these lines is similar to the shape of the adjacent physis.

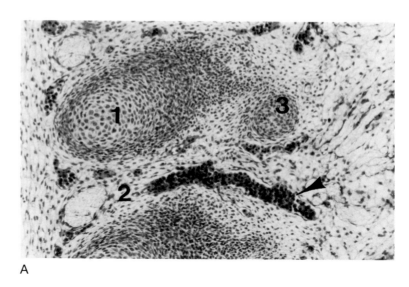

A

FIGURE 20–11. Development of vertebra and intervertebral disc.

A Photomicrograph of a sagittal section of a young embryo. Observe sites of the primitive vertebral body *(1)*, intervertebral disc *(2)*, and posterior elements *(3)*. Blood vessels are evident (arrowhead). (56×.)

B At this stage of chondrification of the mesenchyme of the primitive vertebral column, proliferation of cartilage cells is most evident in the posterior elements *(3)*. *1*, Vertebral body; *2*, intervertebral disc. (56×.)

C Within the intervertebral disc, an aggregate of notocord cells (arrowhead) can be identified. The cells form a syncytial mass separated by clefts in which mucoid material is found. *1*, Vertebral body; *2*, intervertebral disc. (250×.)

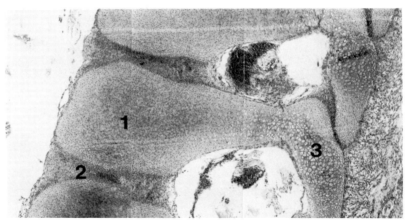

B

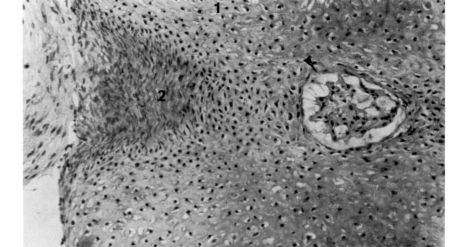

C

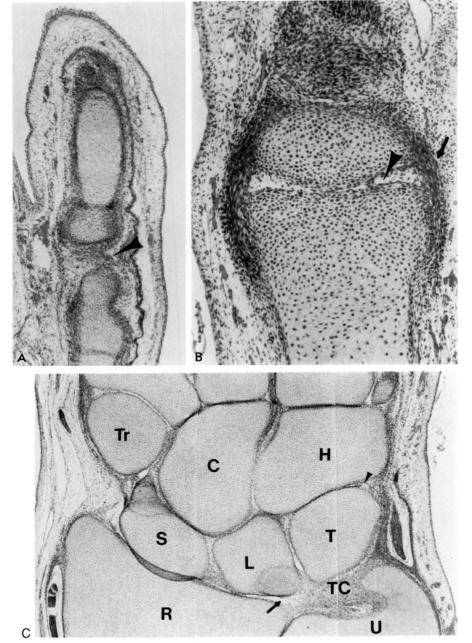

FIGURE 20–12. Development of a synovial joint.

A The site of the primitive joint (arrowhead) can be identified as an interspace between the phalanges of a finger. (56×.)

B At this stage, cavitation (arrowhead) within the interzone has created the primitive joint cavity. (140×.) Condensation at the periphery of the joint (arrow) will lead to capsule formation.

C The developing wrist shows mesenchyme tissue within the various carpal bones (*S,* scaphoid; *L,* lunate; *T,* triquetrum; *H,* hamate; *C,* capitate; *Tr,* trapezoid), cavitation of the radiocarpal (arrow) and midcarpal (arrowhead) joints, and the appearance of a primitive triangular cartilage *(TC). R,* Radius; *U,* ulna. (56×.)

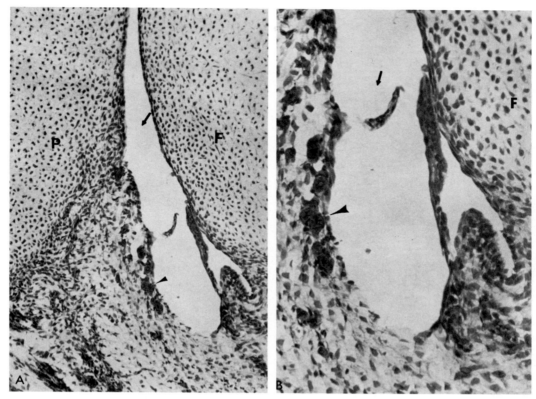

FIGURE 20–13. Development of the synovial membrane. In the knee joint, a space between the femur *(F)* and patella *(P)* can be identified (arrows), which is lined by a synovial membrane. The synovial membrane consists of flat synovial cells and well-formed vascular channels (arrowheads). (*A*, 215×; *B*, 430×.)

FIGURE 20–14. Development of the meniscus in the knee. Even in early fetal life, the undifferentiated mesenchymal tissue that is to become the knee meniscus is semilunar in shape (arrows) (100×.)

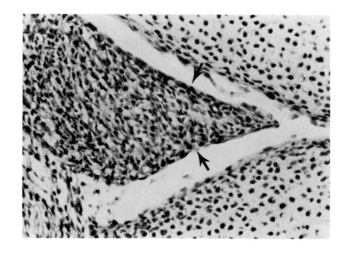

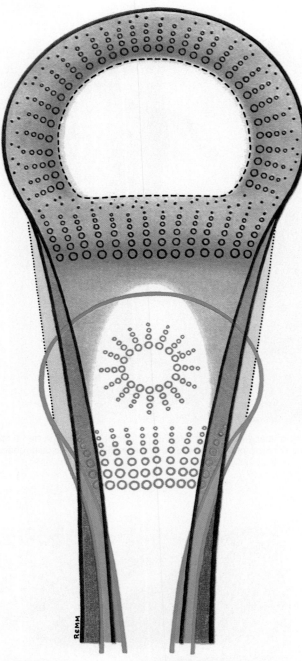

FIGURE 20–15. Modeling of bone: Growth of a tubular bone. Note the changing shape of the epiphyseal ossification center, the altered organization of the growth plate, and the varying zones of bone deposition and resorption (absorption). (From R Warwick, PL Williams [Eds]: Gray's Anatomy. 35th British Ed. Philadelphia, WB Saunders Co, 1973, p 230.)

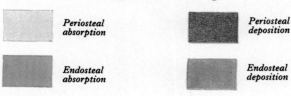

Periosteal absorption

Endosteal absorption

Endochondrial bone

Periosteal deposition

Endosteal deposition

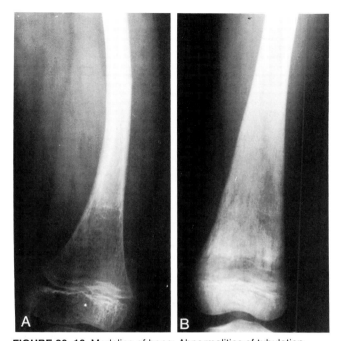

FIGURE 20–16. Modeling of bone: Abnormalities of tubulation.
A Overtubulation. In this child with osteogenesis imperfecta, note the relatively narrow diaphysis compared with the wide appearance of the metaphysis and epiphysis.
B Undertubulation. In this child with Gaucher's disease, the metaphysis is abnormally wide.

rely on cellular events that initially involve the osteoclast and then the osteoblast and that are tightly controlled by metabolic and hormonal stimuli, including those mediated by parathyroid hormone, calcitonin, and 1,25-dihydroxyvitamin D. The general sequence includes, initially, the activation of progenitor (hematopoietic stem) cells that proliferate into osteoclasts and, later, osteoclastic excavation of a volume of old bone, disappearance of the osteoclasts, smoothing of the resorption space with the production of a reversal zone and the laying down of a cement line, and the appearance of osteoblasts, which are involved in producing new bone.[3] The linkage of resorption and formation of bone is very tight; formation follows resorption at the resorption site, not at some other location, and the amount of bone that is formed almost always is very nearly equal to the amount that is removed.[89] The remodeling process replaces aged or injured bone tissue with new bone tissue; repeated strain of skeletal tissue that occurs during ordinary physical activity results, over time, in microdamage that, if not repaired, eventually leads to structural failure.[89]

In the endosteal and periosteal surfaces of the cortex, osteoclastic resorption leads to a tube-shaped tunnel, designated a resorption canal.[4] Initially, this tunnel is oriented approximately perpendicular to the surface of the bone and corresponds in position to a Volkmann canal. Subsequently, in a wormlike fashion, the osteoclasts create longitudinally oriented canals and, by excavating first in one direction and then in the opposite direction, liberate the osteocytes from their lacunae and displace the vascular channels; when these events are followed by osteoblastic apposition, cylinders of bone are formed about linear vascular channels, representing the basic component of a haversian system or osteon.[4] When viewed longitudinally (Fig. 20–18), a mature cortical remodeling unit consists of a cutting zone lined by osteoclasts in which a resorption canal is formed, a reversal zone lined predominantly by osteoprogenitor cells, in which bone resorption is complete and bone formation has not begun, and a closing zone lined by osteoblasts, in which the resorption canal is being refilled by the formation of concentric lamellae of bone.[3] The canal is progressively reduced in diameter owing to the continued deposition of lamellar bone and, eventually, is large enough to accommodate only the blood vessels.[4] The initial osteons, or primary osteons, later are replaced by secondary or tertiary osteons until the creation of the mature haversian system is completed.

In trabecular bone, similar events take place on the osseous surfaces rather than within the interior of the bone, as occurs in the cortex. Thus, the trabecular remodeling unit is characterized by a pit or cavity created by osteoclasts that subsequently is filled in by bone laid down by osteoblasts.

It must be emphasized that bone remodeling is not confined to the immature skeleton but proceeds throughout life and is modified in accordance with alterations in cellular activities that indicate a decrease or increase in the rate of bone turnover. The processes of resorption and formation predominate on bone surfaces, of which four types have been emphasized. Three surfaces are present in the cortical bone: periosteal (outer region of the cortex), haversian or osteonal (within the cortex, along the haversian and Volkmann canals), and endosteal (inner region of the cortex). One surface exists in the trabecular bone, the endosteal surface (at the interface of the marrow and the plates and arches of trabecular bone). At any specific time, these surfaces may be quiescent (free of osteoblasts and osteoclasts),

FIGURE 20–17. Modeling of bone: Normal change in size and shape of the cranial vault. Note changes in the surface area, thickness, and curvature of the bone that occur as part of normal osseous development. (*Vertical hatching,* site of periosteal bone resorption; *horizontal hatching,* remaining portion of original bone; *stippled area,* site of periosteal bone apposition; *white areas,* sites of sutural growth). (Redrawn after R Warwick, PL Williams [Eds]: Gray's Anatomy. 35th British Ed. Philadelphia, WB Saunders Co, 1973, p 229.)

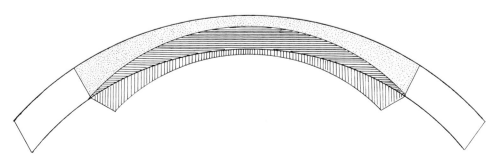

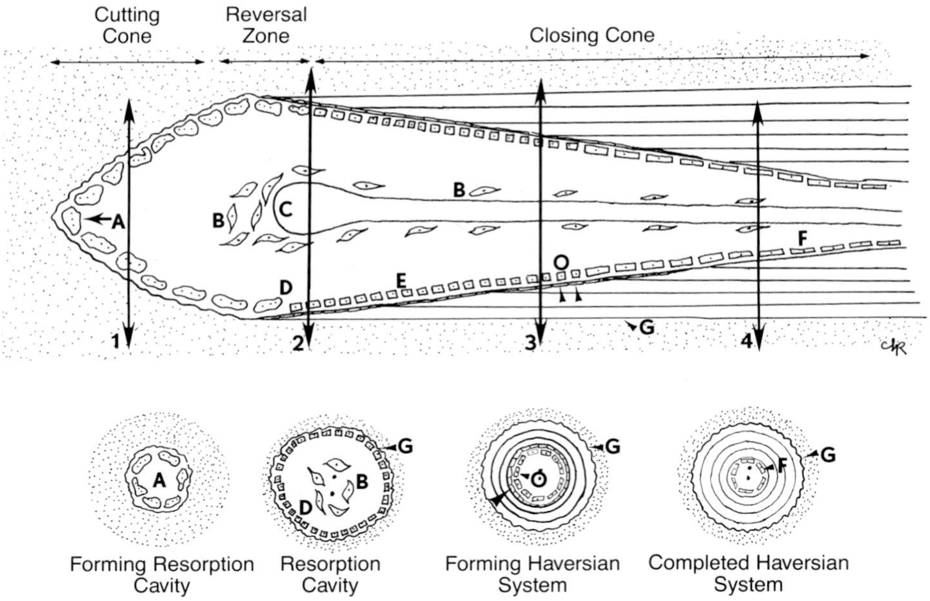

FIGURE 20–18. Remodeling of bone: Cortical remodeling unit. A diagram shows a longitudinal section through a cortical remodeling unit with corresponding transverse sections below (1–4). A, Multinucleated osteoclasts in Howship's lacunae advancing longitudinally from right to left and radially to enlarge a resorption cavity; B, perivascular spindle-shaped precursor cells; C, capillary loops; D, mononuclear cells lining reversal zones; E, osteoblasts depositing new bone centripetally; F, flattened cells lining the haversian canal of a complete haversian system.

Transverse sections at different stages of development: 1, Resorption cavities lined with osteoclasts; 2, completed resorption cavities lined by mononuclear cells, the reversal zone; 3, forming haversian system or osteons lined with osteoblasts that had recently formed three lamellae; 4, completed haversian system with flattened bone cells lining canal. G, Cement line; osteoid (arrowheads) is present between osteoblast (O) and mineralized bone.

(Redrawn after Parfitt AM: The action of parathyroid hormone on bone. Relation of bone remodeling and turnover, calcium homeostasis and metabolic bone disease. I. Metabolism 25:809–844, 1976. By permission of author and Grune and Stratton, Inc, Publisher.)

forming bone (containing osteoid and a covering of osteoblasts), or resorbing bone (containing osteoclasts and scalloped cavities known as Howship's lacunae).[3] The metabolic activity of any particular osseous site depends directly on the surface area of that portion of the bone. Although trabecular bone represents only 20 to 25 per cent of the total skeletal volume, it contributes more than 60 per cent of the total surface area; conversely, cortical bone is characterized by a relatively small amount of surface area[3] (Table 20–1). Routine radiography, even when supplemented with magnification techniques, is far more sensitive in detecting changes in cortical bone in the form of subperiosteal or endosteal resorption or intracortical ''tunneling'' than it is in detecting changes in trabecular bone. It is this inefficiency that has led to the development of supplementary techniques, such as CT scanning, that can be used in evaluating alterations in the more metabolically active trabecular bone (see Chapter 52).

ANATOMY

General Structure of Bone

The prime ingredients of the mature bone are an outer shell of compact bone termed the cortex, which encloses a more loosely appearing meshwork of trabeculae, the cancellous or spongy bone, with its interconnecting spaces containing myeloid or fatty marrow, or both. The cortical bone is clothed by a periosteal membrane, which contains arterioles and capillaries that pierce the cortex, entering the medullary canal (Fig. 20–19).[94] These vessels, along with larger structures that enter one or more nutrient canals, provide the blood supply to the bone. The periosteum is continuous about the bone except for that portion that is intra-articular and covered with synovial membrane or cartilage. At sites of attachment to bone, the fibers of tendons and ligaments blend with the periosteum (entheses) (Fig.

20–20). The structure of the periosteal membrane varies with the age of the person, being thicker, vascular, active, and loosely attached in the infant and child, and thinner, inactive, and more firmly adherent in the adult. For this reason, the periosteal membrane in the immature skeleton contains two relatively well defined layers, an outer fibrous and an inner osteogenic layer, whereas that in the mature skeleton is characterized by a single layer, which has resulted from fusion of the fibrous and osteogenic layers. These structural characteristics underscore the augmented ability of the infant's and child's periosteum to be lifted from the parent bone and to be stimulated to form osseous tissue. Although a layer that may be identified on the inner surface of the cortex sometimes is called an endosteum to emphasize its similarities with the periosteum, this layer is less well defined than the periosteum, may be involved with significant normal bone formation only in the fetus, and may be absent in the adult.

A closer look at the cortex identifies its remarkable structure (Figs. 20–21 and 20–22). Cylindrical units, called haversian systems or osteons, consist of a central haversian canal containing neurovascular supply, which is surrounded

TABLE 20–1. Adult Bone Surfaces (Envelopes)

Surface	Surface Area ($\times 10^6$ sq mm)
Cortical Surfaces	
Periosteal	0.5
Haversian (osteonal)	3.5
Corticoendosteal	0.5
Trabecular Surfaces	
Endosteal	7
Total Surfaces	11.5

Reprinted by permission of the publisher from Jee WSS: The skeletal tissues, in L Weiss, L Lansing (Eds): Histology: Cell and Tissue Biology. 5th Ed, p 221. Copyright 1983 by Elsevier Science Publishing Co, Inc.

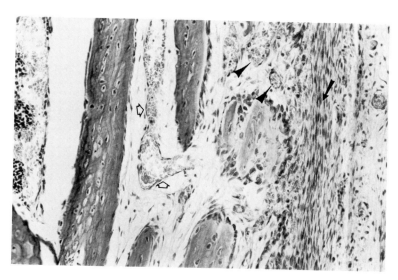

FIGURE 20–19. Development of the periosteum and the process of intramembranous ossification (tibia in a 4½ month old fetus). The periosteum (solid arrow) is a vascular tissue. Its capillaries (arrowheads) enter the vascular channels of the underlying cortex (open arrows). The developing bone is lined by numerous osteoblasts and contains osteocytes. (420×.)

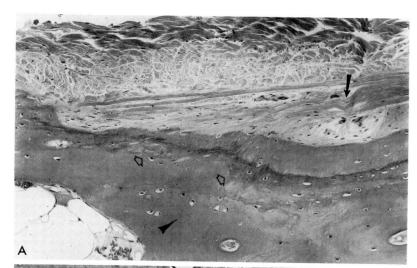

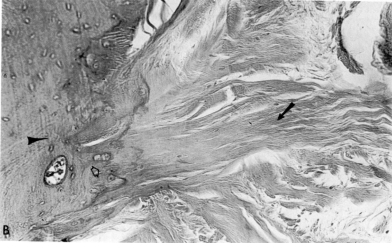

FIGURE 20–20. Sites of ligament attachment to bone (entheses). The ligament (solid arrows) and the bone (arrowheads) can be identified. Note that the fibers of the ligament are incorporated into the osseous tissue (open arrows). (**A**, 210×; **B**, 420×.)

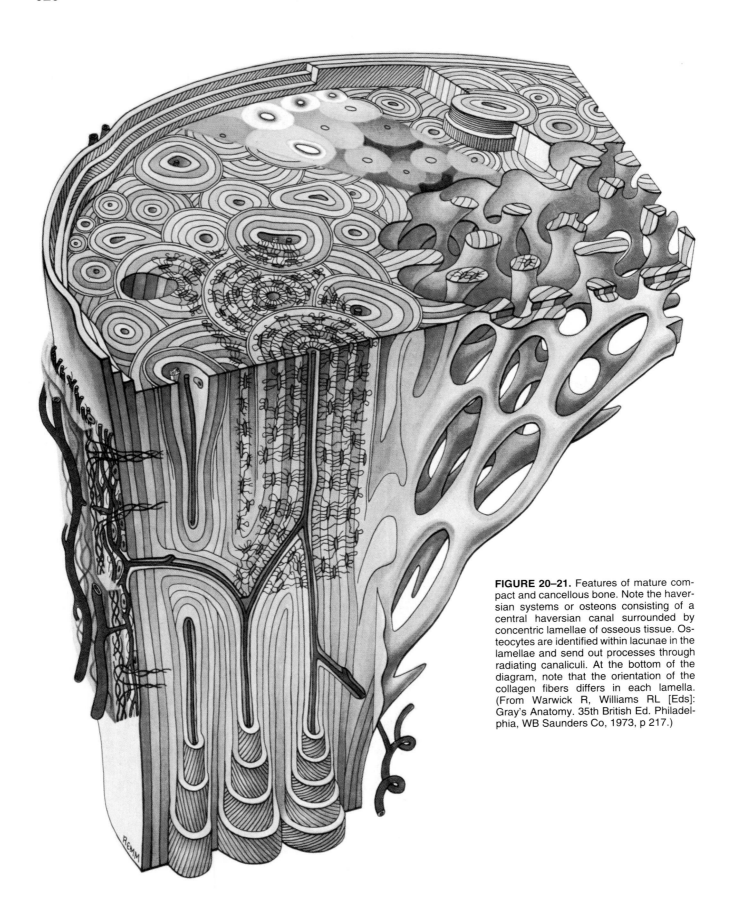

FIGURE 20–21. Features of mature compact and cancellous bone. Note the haversian systems or osteons consisting of a central haversian canal surrounded by concentric lamellae of osseous tissue. Osteocytes are identified within lacunae in the lamellae and send out processes through radiating canaliculi. At the bottom of the diagram, note that the orientation of the collagen fibers differs in each lamella. (From Warwick R, Williams RL [Eds]: Gray's Anatomy. 35th British Ed. Philadelphia, WB Saunders Co, 1973, p 217.)

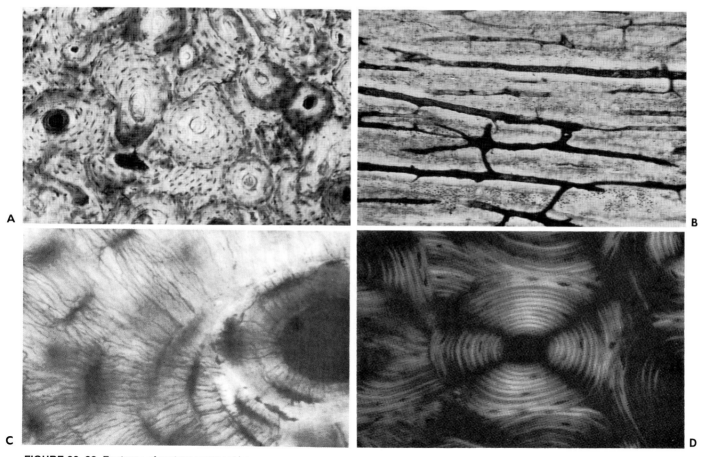

FIGURE 20–22. Features of mature compact bone.

A, B Transverse *(A)* and longitudinal *(B)* ground sections of compact bone from a human femoral shaft. Note the variation in shape and size of the osteons and their canals and in the distribution of lacunae in *A*.

C A high power view of part of an osteon in transverse section as seen with transmitted light. Note the relation of the osteocyte lacunae and their canaliculi to each other and to the central haversian canal.

D A single secondary osteon viewed with high power polarization optics to illustrate its lamellar architecture.

(From R Warwick, PL Williams [Eds]: Gray's Anatomy. 35th British Ed. Philadelphia, WB Saunders Co, 1973, pp 218, 219.)

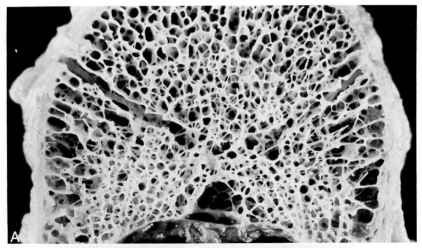

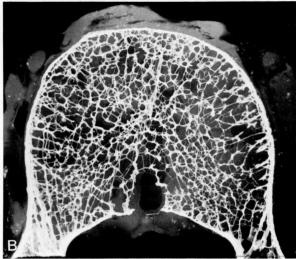

FIGURE 20–23. Features of mature spongy bone. A photograph **(A)** and radiograph **(B)** of a transverse section of the midportion of a macerated vertebral body reveal the delicate, honeycomb appearance of the trabeculae. Note a surrounding, thin rim of compact bone and normal vascular channels.

by concentric lamellae of osseous tissue. The haversian canals run in a more or less longitudinal direction, with branches connecting each system to neighboring haversian canals. These branching vessels are normal findings and should not be confused with Volkmann's canals, which represent additional channels whose formation is provoked by a pathologic state associated with neovascularity and bone resorption. Interstitial lamellae exist in spaces between the haversian systems. The haversian systems and most of the interstitial systems are separated from their neighbors by basophilic smoothly curved or indented lines, called cement lines. About each haversian canal and contained within the individual lamellae are the osteocytes, each in its own lacuna, which are connected to other osteocytes and to the central canal by radiating canaliculi. Within a single lamella, collagen fiber bundles and hydroxyapatite crystals are oriented in a specific and complex fashion, which differs from the orientation of these substances in adjacent lamellae.

The spongiosa bone differs in structure from the cortical bone. Individual trabeculae in a cross-hatched or honeycomb distribution can be identified, which divide the marrow space into communicating compartments (Fig. 20–23). The precise distribution, orientation, and size of the individual trabeculae differ from one skeletal site to another, although the trabeculae often appear most numerous and prominent in areas of normal stress, where they align themselves in the direction of physiologic strain. The major difference, then, between spongy and cortical bone is in the porosity of the osseous tissue. In the compact bone of the cortex, porosity is less striking than in the spongiosa, in which large spaces and a paucity of bone are characteristic.

Cellular Constituents of Bone

Five types of bone cells are found in skeletal tissue: osteoprogenitor cells, osteoblasts, osteocytes, osteoclasts, and bone lining cells.

Osteoprogenitor Cells. Undifferentiated stromal cells have the capacity to proliferate by mitotic division and develop into osteoblasts, or bone-forming cells.[9] The precise stromal origin of the osteoprogenitor cells is a matter of debate; these cells may be related to capillary pericytes, endothelial cells, or reticular cells.[95, 96] It also is not clear if osteogenic, chondrogenic, and fibrogenic cells are the product of one cell line or different cell lines.[97] Osteoprogenitor cells typically are located near the bone surfaces and are thin and elongated, or spindle-shaped, with oval nuclei and

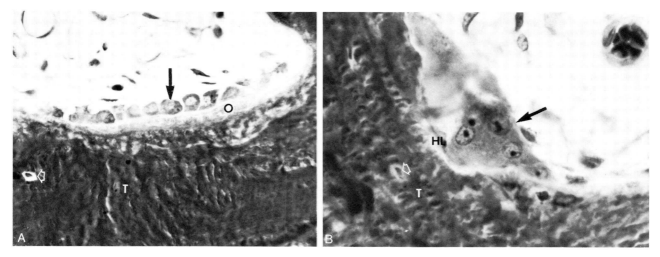

FIGURE 20–24. Cellular constituents of bone: Osteoblasts, osteocytes, and osteoclasts.
A Prominent osteoblasts (arrow) secreting osteoid matrix *(O)*. Note perinuclear clear zone, representing the Golgi apparatus. *T,* Mineralized trabecular bone; open arrow, osteocyte. (Trichrome stain, 340×.)
B Multinucleated osteoclast (arrow) residing in a resorption bay or Howship's lacuna *(HL)*. *T,* Mineralized trabecular bone; open arrow, osteocyte. (Trichrome stain, 340×.)

pale or inconspicuous cytoplasm. Until recently, it generally was believed that similar osteoprogenitor cells also were able to differentiate into osteoclasts by an identical or similar pathway, although considerable debate had existed with regard to the precise steps involved in this cellular transformation.[10–12] It now is known that osteoclasts are derived from a different source, cells of the hematopoietic system, although the precise steps involved in cellular differentiation to osteoclasts are not clear (see later discussion).

Osteoblasts. Osteoblasts are derived from cells that probably are components of the stromal system of bone and marrow.[97] Osteoblasts are intimately involved in the processes of intramembranous and endochondral bone formation (Fig. 20–24). Indeed, any cell that forms bone—whether during growth and modeling, remodeling, or fracture healing—is defined as an osteoblast.[89] The activity of the precursor cells is governed directly by the principle of supply and demand; at times when new bone is required, as during the healing of a fracture, these cells are called to action in the generation of osteoblasts. The osteoblast is a mononuclear cell whose shape depends on its level of activity: When actively involved in the production of bone matrix, the osteoblast is cuboidal or columnar in configuration, whereas in its quiescent phase, the osteoblast is flat and elongated. Although numerous and large in the developing skeleton, osteoblasts decrease in number and size as the skeleton reaches maturity. Despite this decrease in size and number, a dormant osteoblast is capable of responding to the stimulus produced by a pathologic process by demonstrating the same degree of cellular activity that characterizes the osteoblast in the fetus. Osteoblasts are fundamental to the process of collagen and mucopolysaccharide production in bone. The functional life span of an osteoblast is variable; at a remodeling site, it may range from 3 to 4 months to 18 months.[89] The life span of osteoblasts may cease somewhat abruptly with their incorporation into the osseous tissue in the form of a new cell, the osteocyte.

The ultrastructural characteristics of the osteoblast show it to be well suited to its function as a synthesizer and secretor of proteins; these cells have an abundant, widely distributed endoplasmic reticulum and a well-developed Golgi apparatus containing many secretory vacuoles. Numerous mitochondria within the cytoplasm become more prominent with increased cellular activity, indicating their important role in bone mineralization, and the diffusion of calcium from the osteoblast to the matrix potentially is accomplished by bundles of fine filaments that are located in the finger-like processes of the osteoblast.[13] One product of the osteoblast, alkaline phosphatase, is believed to be involved in the synthesis of procollagen and may be important in the process of mineralization.[14] Other specific enzymes histochemically demonstrated in osteoblasts include phosphorylase, glycogen synthetase, and collagenase.[13]

Osteocytes. The osteocytes arise from preosteoblasts and osteoblasts. Initially present at the surface of the bone, some, but not all, of the osteoblasts subsequently become entrapped within the osseous tissue as osteocytes (Fig. 20–24). Here, the osteocyte lies in a lacuna and sends out branches through interconnected canaliculi. Osteocytes are unable to divide, so that only one cell is present in each lacuna. Their life span varies with that of the bone tissue in which they are embedded; they are destroyed when bone is resorbed.[89] Three phases in the life of an osteocyte have been described: formative phase, resorptive phase, and degenerative phase.[15] In the formative phase, the osteocyte acts as an active secretory cell and reveals many of the structural characteristics of an osteoblast, with a sizable nucleus, an extensive endoplasmic reticulum, a large Golgi complex, and numerous mitochondria. In the resorptive phase, the endoplasmic reticulum and mitochondria are less prominent, whereas in the degenerative phase, vacuolization of the cytoplasm, mitochondria, and Golgi apparatus is observed. The osteocyte is concerned with proper maintenance of the bone matrix, a process that is facilitated by the transport of material and fluid via the canaliculi. This exchange usually is confined to the space outlined by the cement lines in the bone. The osteocyte has the ability to synthesize bone matrix, although this ability is less pronounced than that of the osteoblast. It has been proposed that the osteocyte also may be involved in bone resorption, a process called osteocytic osteolysis. This process involves the active participation of the cells, in which surrounding matrix is modified by the extraction of specific ions. Evidence cited to support the ability of an osteocyte to periodically remove and replace minute amounts of perilacunar bone includes the following: the variations in size of lacunae; the presence of osmophilic laminae that resemble reversal lines in perilacunar bone; the incorporation of a fluorescent bone marker, tetracycline, into perilacunar bone; and the ultrastructural morphology reflecting bone-forming and bone-resorbing clastic activities.[3] Conversely, the inability to document osteocytic osteolysis with scanning electron microscopy argues against a role for this cell in the removal and replacement of perilacunar bone and underscores the controversy that surrounds this issue. Of related interest is the considerable effect on osteocyte morphology and adjacent bone matrix that is known to follow the administration of parathyroid hormone,[13] leading to a shortened life span of the osteocyte.

Osteoclasts. Another cell, the osteoclast, has been the subject of much interest and investigation.[16–20, 98] This is a multinucleated cell (2 to 100 nuclei) with a short life span that is intimately related to the process of bone resorption (Fig. 20–24). Osteoclasts vary in size from 20 to 100 μm.

The origin of osteoclasts has been investigated extensively. Initially, it was believed that osteoblasts and osteoclasts were related, derived from a common source.[13] According to this concept, which was supported only by indirect evidence, a mesenchymal cell became transformed into an osteoclast that could dedifferentiate into a mesenchymal cell and become an osteoblast. Later evidence indicated that this concept is incorrect, and that osteoclasts and osteoblasts arise from histogenetically distinct cell lines.[65] Whereas the osteoblasts are derived from cellular components of the stromal system of bone and marrow (stromal stem cell), the osteoclasts appear to be a product of one of the cell lines of the hematopoietic system, being derived from a hematopoietic stem cell (monocyte-phagocyte line).

Osteoclasts engage actively in bone resorption. The exact manner in which bone resorption takes place about the osteoclast is not entirely known, although two different mechanisms may be important: the secretion of lytic enzymes (e.g., collagenase) that lead to modifications of the structure of the collagen and mucopolysaccharide; and the incorporation and digestion of the liberated matrix and mineral components. Measurements of serum and urinary levels of hydroxyproline, an amino acid almost unique to collagen, are useful indicators of the extent of turnover of bone matrix. It generally is agreed that a modification in the ground substance of bone must occur prior to the resorption of the osseous tissue by the osteoclast. This process is associated with the appearance of resorption pits or Howship's lacunae. The osteoclasts within the lacunae have prominent nuclei and cytoplasmic granules, as well as vacuoles that may contain degenerating osteocytes. The active osteoclast often reveals a finely striated brush or ruffled border where it is in contact with the bone. A clear or filamentous zone about the ruffled border appears to represent the site of adhesion of the cell to the bone surface.[3] This site of adhesion, or seal, apparently localizes the highly acidic microenvironment, which is conducive to bone resorption.[89] When the erosive process is terminated and the osteoclast departs from the bone surface, both the clear zone and the ruffled border no longer are seen, and osteoclasts become less numerous and may even disappear entirely. The ultimate fate of these cells, however, is not clear. Their life span may be as long as 7 weeks; the average normal duration of a resorption site in humans is about 4 weeks.[89]

It is well known that bone-regulating hormones have a dramatic effect on the appearance and function of osteoclasts. Administration of exogenous parathyroid hormone (Fig. 20–25) leads to rapid development or enlargement of ruffled borders, whereas that of calcitonin causes an equally rapid disappearance of these borders.[3] Furthermore, 1,25-dihydroxyvitamin D increases the differentiation of precursor cells into osteoclasts, thereby increasing the number of osteoclasts as well as their activity. As multinucleated osteoclasts originate from the fusion of cells of the mononuclear phagocytic system, it is of considerable interest that blood monocytes also can resorb bone either directly or indirectly through the elaboration of potent bone-resorbing factors, such as prostaglandins and interleukin-1.[66] In fact,

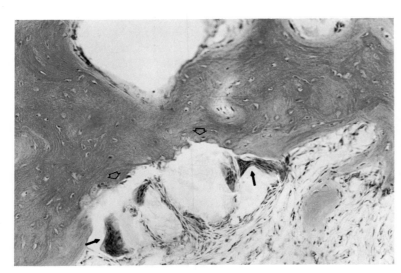

FIGURE 20–25. Chronic renal disease and secondary hyperparathyroidism. Numerous osteoclasts (solid arrows) are evident in Howship's lacunae (open arrows). New bone formation and periosseous fibrosis are seen. (420×.)

interleukin-1β appears to be identical to osteoclast activating factor.

Bone Lining Cells. The precise nature of the commonly identified flat and elongated cells with spindle-shaped nuclei that line the surface of the bone is not clear, although generally they are believed to be derived from osteoblasts that have become inactive.[3] Lining cells communicate with the syncytium of osteocytes through the osteocytic canaliculi.[89] Their function also is unknown but may include maintenance of mineral homeostasis, control of the growth of bone crystals, or the ability to differentiate into other cells, such as osteoblasts.

Noncellular Constituents of Bone

Water is responsible for about 20 per cent of the wet weight of bone tissue. The major cellular components—the osteoblasts, osteocytes, and osteoclasts—account for a very small fraction of the total weight of bone. The other constituents of bone include the remaining organic matrix (collagen and mucopolysaccharides), accounting for approximately 20 to 30 per cent of osseous tissue by dry weight, and the inorganic material, accounting for approximately 70 to 80 per cent of osseous tissue by dry weight. It is these constituents, in physiologic amounts, that create bone tissue that is both dynamic and uniquely capable in providing the support that the body requires.

Organic Matrix. The organic matrix of bone, which surrounds the cellular components,[3] is composed primarily of protein, glycoprotein, and polysaccharide. Collagen is the major constituent (90 per cent) of the organic matrix of bone; the collagen is embedded in a gelatinous mucopolysaccharide material (ground substance). The mucopolysaccharides of bone include chondroitin sulfate A, keratosulfate, and other sulfated and nonsulfated substances; the most important noncollagenous protein of bone is γ-carboxyglutamic acid, also known as BGP, which is produced by the osteoblasts. Although the mucopolysaccharides represent a minor quantitative part of the structure of osseous tissue, they appear to be very important in the process of bone matrix maturation and mineralization. The collagen fiber consists of an aggregate of rod-shaped tropocollagen subunits, each unit being composed of three coiled polypeptide chains wound about each other.[21] The collagen of bone is characterized by the presence of two identical coils and a third coil with a different amino acid composition; important amino acid constituents are hydroxylysine and hydroxyproline. Linked to the amino acid components of collagen are carbohydrates, the principal one being galactosyl-hydroxylysine. A characteristic pattern of overlap or staggering of adjacent collagen molecules creates a pore or hole zone, measuring approximately 40 nm, between the end of one molecule and the beginning of the next; these holes are the sites of earliest deposits of the hydroxyapatite crystals of bone.

Inorganic Mineral. The inorganic mineral of bone exists in a crystalline form that resembles hydroxyapatite—$Ca_{10}(PO_4)_6OH_2$—that is distributed regularly along the length of the collagen fibers, surrounded by ground substance. It appears that structural characteristics of the mineral change somewhat during the processes of bone formation and dissolution, reflected by changing molar ratios of calcium and phosphate.[22] Furthermore, the bone crystals are impure. There are substantial quantities of carbonate, citrate, sodium, and magnesium in bone mineral.[3] The quantity of fluoride is variable. Trace amounts of iron, zinc, copper, lead, manganese, tin, aluminum, strontium, boron, and silicon also are present.[3]

Bone Marrow

Bone marrow is a soft pulpy tissue that lies in the spaces between the trabeculae of all bones and even in the larger haversian canals.[105] It is one of the most extensive organs of the human body, weighing between 2600 and 3000 gm in adults.[106] Its functions include the provision of a continual supply of red cells, white cells, and platelets to meet the body's demand for oxygenation, immunity, and coagulation.[106] A complex vascular supply relies mainly on a nutrient artery that, in the long tubular bones, pierces the diaphyseal cortex at an angle, penetrates the cortex, reaches the medullary bone, and extends toward the ends of the tubular bone, running parallel to its long axis.[107] Branches from the nutrient artery enter the endosteal surface of the cortex as capillaries and coalesce with transosteal vessels of periosteal origin.[106] As they re-exit the endosteum, these vessels widen to form primary and collecting sinusoids.[107] The sinusoidal network forms a very extensive, anastomosing complex among the fat cells of the marrow.[106] A central venous sinus in the medullary bone then receives the blood, which, ultimately, exits through the nutrient foramen in the cortex. The nerve supply of the bone marrow, composed of both sympathetic and afferent nerve fibers, traces a course similar to that of the arterial supply.[108]

Marrow Composition. The basic composition of the bone marrow consists of mineralized osseous matrix, connective tissue, and a variety of cells. As described previously, the trabeculae in the medullary space represent the osseous component of the bone marrow. The marrow itself occupies the spaces between and around the plates and struts of trabecular (cancellous or spongy) bone, and it is held in place by a network of fine fibrous tissue, called a reticulum, which is attached to the inner walls of the cortex and to the trabeculae.[89] The cancellous trabeculae, encased within the outer shell of the cortex, provide architectural support and serve as a mineral depot.[106] The interface between the marrow and the trabecular bone, the endosteal envelope, is very active metabolically in comparison to the other bone envelopes (see previous discussion), with cells such as osteoblasts and osteoclasts that are extremely sensitive to metabolic stimuli.[89]

The cells of the marrow consist of all stages of erythrocytic and leukocytic development, as well as fat cells and reticulum cells. Groups of these cells are separated by the network of vascular channels, or sinusoids. The marrow microenvironment supporting the progenitor and precursor cells must provide for the normal steady state rates of renewal of the cellular elements of blood.[109] The blood cell progenitor cells can be divided into a pool of stem cells and pools of erythroid, myeloid, and megakaryocytic cells.[110] Several hormones, including erythropoietin (produced mainly in the kidney but also in the liver), thrombopoietin, and colony-stimulating activity (a product of macrophages and T lymphocytes), regulate both the amplification and the differentiation of the hematopoietic progenitor cells.[109] Under homeostatic conditions, the production rate of the hematopoietic cells precisely equals the destruction rate. The average life span of a human red cell is approximately 120 days and that of a platelet is 7 to 10 days; the life span of leukocytes is more variable, being relatively short for granulocytes (6 to 12 hours) and long for lymphocytes (months or even years).[109]

Fat cells also are a major component of bone marrow. Although smaller than fat cells from extramedullary sites, the marrow fat cells are active metabolically and respond by changes in size to hematopoietic activity.[106] During periods of decreased hematopoiesis, the fat cells in the bone marrow increase in size and number, whereas during increased hematopoiesis, the fat cells atrophy. Two types of reticulum cells, the phagocytic type and the undifferentiated nonphagocytic type, are found in the bone marrow. Their precise functions are not clear.

Two forms of bone marrow are encountered. Red marrow is hematopoietically active marrow and consists of approximately 40 per cent water, 40 per cent fat, and 20 per cent protein; yellow marrow is hematopoietically inactive and consists of approximately 15 per cent water, 80 per cent fat, and 5 per cent protein.[106] The red marrow consists of a framework of reticular connective tissue with argyrophilic fibers and attached phagocytic cells, containing in its meshes a variety of blood cells and their precursors and a few fat cells.[105] Small nodules of lymphoid tissue also are scattered through the red marrow, but no lymph vessels are present. The yellow marrow consists of connective tissue supporting numerous blood vessels and cells, most of which are fat cells.[105]

Marrow Conversion. The amount of red marrow versus yellow marrow at any given time is dependent on the age of the person, the site that is being sampled, and the health of the individual. At birth, red marrow is present throughout the skeleton, but with increasing age, owing to the normal conversion process of hematopoietic to fatty marrow, the proportion of hematopoietic marrow decreases. Fatty marrow represents approximately 15 per cent of the total marrow volume in the child but 60 per cent of this volume by the age of 80 years. The volume of red marrow in vertebral bodies decreases from a mean of 58 per cent in the first decade of life to 29 per cent by the eighth decade of life.[111] A further rise in the percentage of fatty marrow versus hematopoietic marrow in advanced years of life is attributed to the additional fat cells that are necessary to replace the trabecular bone that is lost as a result of senile and post-

menopausal osteoporosis.[106] Many of the factors that initiate or modulate this conversion of red to yellow marrow are not clear,[106] although temperature, vascularity, and low oxygen tension may be important in this process.[112–114]

The conversion of red to yellow marrow that occurs during growth and development is predictable and orderly, and it has been well summarized by Vogler and Murphy.[106] In the immediate postnatal period, this conversion first becomes evident in the extremities, specifically in the terminal phalanges of the hands and feet.[115] After about the fifth year of life, the red marrow gradually is replaced in the long tubular bones (Fig. 20–26). This replacement commences earlier and is more advanced in the more distal bones of the extremities; furthermore, in each bone, the conversion to yellow marrow proceeds from the distal to the proximal end, although some authors maintain that it commences in the center of the shaft and extends in both directions but more rapidly in the distal segment.[105] Cartilaginous epiphyses and apophyses lack marrow until they ossify. Although such ossified centers initially may contain hematopoietic marrow,[116] rapid conversion to yellow marrow is the rule. Thus, as a general rule, marrow conversion in the epiphyses and apophyses as well as in the diaphyses of tubular bones occurs in the first decade of life, and that in the distal metaphyses of tubular bones occurs in the second decade of life. By the age of 20 to 25 years, marrow conversion usually is complete. At this time, the adult pattern is characterized by the presence of red marrow only in portions of the vertebrae, sternum, ribs, clavicles, scapulae, skull, and innominate bones and in the metaphyses of the femora and humeri. Minor variations in this distribution, however, are encountered. With advanced age, gelatinous degeneration of some of the marrow, such as that in the skull, is seen.[105]

Although the visualized patterns of signal intensity do not correspond precisely to anatomic sites of red and yellow marrow, magnetic resonance (MR) imaging represents an effective, albeit indirect, means to determine the cellular characteristics of the bone marrow.[117–119] The basic constituents of bone marrow that contribute individual signal intensities on MR images are fat, water, and mineral.[106] The last of these contributes in a negative fashion for two reasons: First, the mineral matrix produces little or no signal due to a lack of mobile protons; second, local field gradients are produced as a result of inhomogeneous susceptibility where mineral matrix interfaces with water or fat.[106] Although anatomic correlation with MR imaging findings

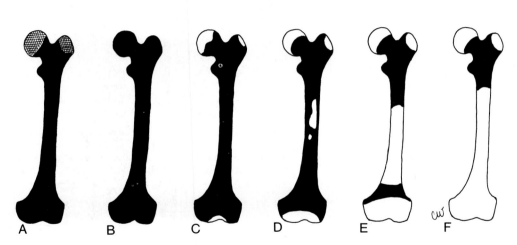

FIGURE 20–26. Marrow conversion: Long tubular bones (femur). The distribution of red marrow (black) and yellow marrow (white) in the femur is shown at birth *(A)* and at the ages of 5 years *(B)*, 10 years *(C)*, 15 years *(D)*, 20 years *(E)*, and 24 years *(F)*. The stippled area in *A* represents cartilage. (From Moore SG, Dawson KL: Radiology *175*:219, 1990.)

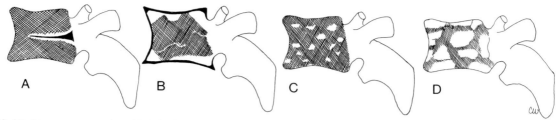

FIGURE 20–27. Marrow conversion: Vertebral bodies. MR imaging appearance on T1-weighted spin echo images. Four patterns are observed. Pattern 1 **(A)** is characterized by the presence of high-signal-intensity fatty marrow confined to linear areas along the basivertebral vein. Pattern 2 **(B)** is characterized by bandlike and triangular areas of fatty marrow in a peripheral location. Pattern 3 **(C)** is characterized by multiple small regions of high-signal-intensity fatty marrow. Pattern 4 **(D)** is characterized by multiple large regions of fatty marrow. Pattern 1 is common in all regions of the spine in the first two or three decades of life and patterns 2, 3, and 4 become more dominant after the age of 30 or 40 years, particularly in the thoracic and lumbar regions. (From Ricci C, et al: Radiology *177*:83, 1990.)

of the bone marrow in normal children and adults generally is lacking,[118] the appearances of red and yellow marrow, owing to their compositional differences, are not the same. Composed predominantly of fat, yellow marrow displays the T1 and T2 relaxation patterns of adipose tissue; containing considerable amounts of water and protein as well as fat, red marrow has T1 and T2 relaxation patterns that differ from those of fatty marrow.[106] Although the major contributor to signal intensity of both types of marrow is fat, the longer T1 and T2 relaxation times of protein and water in red marrow also contribute significantly to its final signal intensity.[106] Therefore, on standard T1-weighted spin echo sequences, red marrow demonstrates lower signal intensity than yellow marrow.

Using such sequences, Ricci and coworkers[117] have reported in great detail the MR imaging characteristics of the normal age-related conversion of red to yellow marrow in the pelvis, proximal portion of the femur, skull, and various portions of the spine. Their findings with regard to the vertebral bodies, pelvis, and femora are illustrated in Figures 20–27 to 20–29 and underscore the variability of the MR imaging findings that characterize the normal, orderly process of conversion from hematopoietic to fatty marrow.

At times at which the body's demand for hematopoiesis increases, a reconversion of yellow marrow to red marrow occurs. The extent of reconversion depends on the severity and duration of the stimulus, and the process may be initiated or modulated by such factors as temperature, low oxygen tension, and elevated levels of erythropoietin.[106] The process of reconversion follows that of conversion but in reverse. Initial changes occur in the axial skeleton and thereafter from a proximal to distal direction in the extremities.

PHYSIOLOGY

Mineralization of Bone

Although certain aspects of the process have been well defined, at present no unified concept exists for the mechanism of bone mineralization. As has been defined with electron microscopy, the initial nucleation or deposition of inorganic calcium and phosphate occurs at regular intervals along the longitudinal axis of the collagen fibril, at specific sites in or on the fibril.[23] It appears likely that these crystals gain access to the substance of the fibril by normal gaps or holes resulting from overlap of linear polymers of collagen.

In fact, it also is likely that the precise structure of the collagen is of fundamental importance in calcium deposition and must be maintained if nucleation is to be initiated, as chemical modifications of collagen in vitro interfere with this process. The axes of the deposited crystals are parallel to the axis of the collagen fibril itself, an orientation that is attributable to the interaction of the mineral with the collagen and some of its associated noncollagenous proteins; the size and arrangement of the crystals are determined by additional interaction with other noncollagenous macromol-

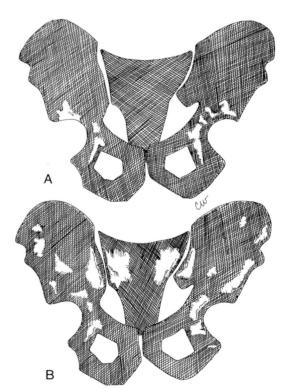

FIGURE 20–28. Marrow conversion: Pelvis. MR imaging appearance on T1-weighted spin echo images. Two patterns are observed. Pattern 1 **(A)** is characterized by small areas of high-signal-intensity fatty marrow in the para-acetabular region. Pattern 2 **(B)** is characterized by more widespread regions of high signal intensity, involving para-acetabular bone, ilii, and subchondral zones about the sacroiliac joints. Pattern 1 is more frequent in the first three decades of life, and pattern 2 thereafter. (From Ricci C, et al: Radiology *177*:83, 1990.)

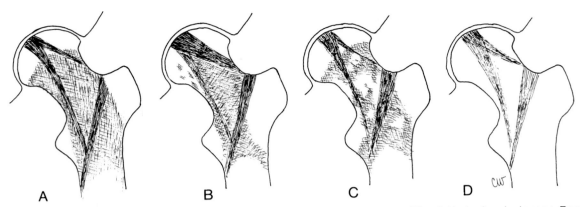

FIGURE 20–29. Marrow conversion: Proximal portion of the femur. MR imaging appearance on T1-weighted spin echo images. Four patterns are observed. Pattern 1 **(A)** is characterized by high-signal-intensity fatty marrow confined to the capital femoral epiphysis and greater and lesser trochanters. Pattern 2 **(B)** resembles pattern 1 with the addition of fatty marrow in the medial portion of the femoral head and in the lateral portion of the intertrochanteric region. Pattern 3 **(C)** resembles pattern 1 with the addition of many small, sometimes confluent, areas of fatty marrow in the intertrochanteric region. Pattern 4 **(D)** is characterized by uniform high-signal-intensity fatty marrow throughout the proximal portion of the femur with the exception of the regions of the major trabecular groups. Patterns 1 and 2 predominate in the first three decades of life, pattern 3 predominates in the fifth and sometimes the fourth decades of life, and pattern 4 predominates after the age of 50 or 60 years. (From Ricci C, et al: Radiology *177*:83, 1990.)

ecules, including the γ-carboxyglutamic acid-containing proteins, phosphoproteins, or glycoproteins.[24, 25] Crystal growth may be inhibited by the presence of carbonate, pyrophosphate, proteoglycans, nucleoside triphosphates, or other crystal poisons.[24] After nucleation has been initiated, further precipitation of calcium and phosphate ions leads to growth of the crystal, which eventually assumes a chemical structure similar to that of hydroxyapatite. The composition of the mineral that is deposited initially, however, is not clear. Some investigators believe that the first mineral deposits are brushite,[26] which may serve as a precursor to hydroxyapatite deposition.[27]

The process of biologic calcification, in which hydroxyapatite or some similar material is deposited within an organic matrix, is complex.[24] The ions essential in the formation of the crystalline unit in bone are calcium (Ca^{+2}) and phosphate (PO_4^{-3}), and initial interpretations of the calcification process emphasized precipitation dynamics in which the unique milieu of the organic matrix of bone provided the specific conditions (e.g., alkaline phosphatase activity increasing the local concentration of phosphate, or elevation of local pH values leading to a reduction in the solubility of the calcium salt) required for the deposition of these ions.[28] It now is known that additional factors are important, including specific activity coefficients that govern the behavior of the ions. In studying the nature of the mineral phase of bone, Neuman and Neuman[29] in 1953 proposed the theory of epitactic nucleation, based upon the concept of epitaxy or seeding. In this view, a nucleus is formed, possessing a crystalline structure similar to that of hydroxyapatite, which causes the initial aggregation of calcium and phosphate ions. Such nucleation, which results in the appearance of the smallest stable combination of ions that can persist in solution, requires considerable energy and is followed by crystal growth, a process that involves lesser degrees of energy.[24] Attempts to identify an initial locus for the process of nucleation led to varying opinions that implicated the collagen fibrils, the ground substance, and the proteoglycans.[28] Subsequently investigators suggested that the initial site of nucleation was within cellular extrusions

of the osteoblasts themselves and that involvement of adjacent collagen fibrils was a secondary phenomenon.[30]

Although no uniform theory yet exists with regard to the sites of nucleation, the general agreement is that certain cellular products, including enzymes such as alkaline phosphatases and inorganic pyrophosphatases, may regulate the process of calcification by removing inhibitors that either compete with the ions in solution for sites on the critical nucleus, combine with the ions in solution, or impede in other ways the nucleation and growth phenomena.[24] Matrix vesicles, consisting of minute membrane-bound spheres, represent products of osteoblasts (as well as chondroblasts and odontoblasts) that are rich in various enzymes that may promote the concentration of calcium and phosphorus ions and hence the process of crystallization.[28] Although additional hypotheses emphasize alternative mechanisms involved in this process, most emphasize the cells themselves as the central or unifying factor that leads to the deposition of the crystalline unit essential to the structure of bone.

Calcium Homeostasis

The skeleton, containing 99 per cent of the body's calcium, serves as the reservoir that is essential in the maintenance of stable plasma levels of calcium. The concentration of calcium in the plasma normally is approximately 10 mg/dl, with minor fluctuations in this value. Approximately 70 per cent of the plasma calcium is believed to be maintained by a continuous exchange of calcium ions between bone tissue and extracellular fluid; this interchange occurs between the hydroxyapatite crystals of all bone surfaces and proceeds independently of any change in bone volume (i.e., formation and resorption).[3] Hypocalcemia stimulates a release of calcium ions from the bone mineral into the extracellular fluid and, conversely, hypercalcemia promotes an inward flux of calcium ions from the extracellular fluid to the bone mineral. The remaining 30 per cent of plasma calcium may be mediated by the actions of parathyroid hormone and other hormones (see later discussion).

The process of calcium exchange, termed blood-bone

transfer or disequilibrium, has been well outlined by Jee[3] and is summarized here. Important in the transfer of calcium ions between the bone and the plasma fluid compartments is the bone fluid compartment that is intimate with available osseous surfaces, being located between the osteoblasts or bone-lining cells, or both, and the endosteal bone surface; and between the osteocytes and their lacunar and canalicular walls. The bone fluid compartment is surrounded by a perivascular fluid compartment that itself surrounds the vascular tissue within the haversian canals, Volkmann canals, bone marrow, and other vascular spaces. The transfer of calcium ions between the immediate environment of the tissue and the plasma apparently is accomplished by events transpiring in the bone fluid and the perivascular fluid compartments, although the precise mechanisms governing these events are not clear; circulation of fluid through these compartments is essential, depending, perhaps, on a pumping mechanism, membrane compartmentalization, pinocytotic calcium transfers, localized acid production, local solubilizers, or a stabilized regulator phase, or any combination of these factors. Undoubtedly, parathyroid hormone represents a key ingredient in the mobilization of calcium from bone and its transfer to the plasma, and its impact is felt not only at the ''pump'' controlling the movement of fluid in the bone fluid and perivascular fluid compartments but also in the cells themselves. As there is little evidence to suggest that osteoclasts possess receptors for parathyroid hormone or that osteoclasts respond directly to this hormone, it has been suggested that bone resorption is mediated by the action of parathyroid hormone on osteoblasts.[67] Parathyroid hormone (as well as prostaglandins) induces a change in shape of the osteoblasts that uncovers the bone matrix, exposing it to osteoclast projections. The resulting matrix digestion may further enhance bone resorption by releasing collagen and osteocalcin, attracting monocytic osteoclast precursors and possibly idle osteoclasts.[67] Products released by the hormonal action on the osteoblasts may activate the osteoclasts directly.

Bone Resorption and Formation

The processes of resorption and formation occur continuously in normal bone (Fig. 20–30). They are prominent in the immature skeleton, in which modeling leads to the major changes in the size and shape of the bone that are required for normal osseous growth and development; in the mature skeleton these processes are less evident but nonetheless essential for the maintenance of biomechanically competent tissue and calcium homeostasis.

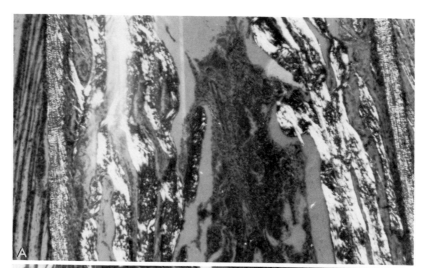
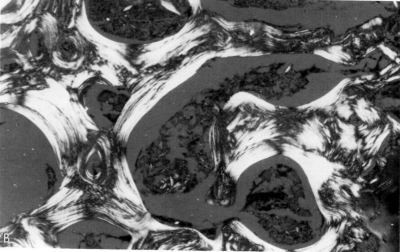

FIGURE 20–30. Changing structure of osseous tissue.
A In a 4½ month old fetus, a polarized photomicrograph (84×) of the femoral shaft indicates the absence of a lamellated cortical structure.
B In the adult skeleton, a polarized photomicrograph (210×) indicates the organized structure of the cortex.

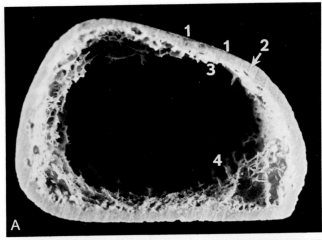

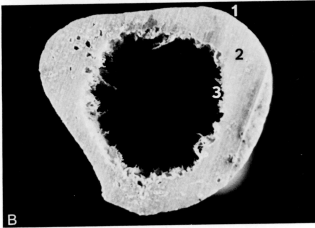

FIGURE 20–31. Bone resorption and formation: Available bone envelopes. Transverse sections of the metaphysis *(A)* and diaphysis *(B)* of a tubular bone reveal the osseous envelopes that are involved in the processes of resorption and apposition. In the cortex, these are the periosteal *(1)*, haversian or osteonal *(2)*, and corticoendosteal *(3)* envelopes; in the spongiosa, an endosteal or transitional *(4)* envelope is present.

As indicated previously, resorption and apposition dominate on the bone surfaces that are present in the cortex and the spongiosa. Four or, perhaps, five broad surface areas exist in the skeleton, each functionally distinct (Fig. 20–31).[89] These areas often are referred to as envelopes. The first of these, related to the outer surface of the cortex, is the *periosteal envelope* (or periosteum), consisting of an outer sheath of fibrous connective tissue and an inner, or cambrian, layer of undifferentiated cells. These two distinct histologic layers are not present everywhere, being absent in intra-articular locations such as the femoral neck, at entheses or sites of tendinous and ligamentous attachments to bone, and about the sesamoid bones. The periosteal envelope is involved primarily in bone formation, although in certain disease states, such as hyperparathyroidism, which are characterized by aggressive bone resorption, the periosteal envelope is involved in bone removal. The *haversian envelope*, the second of the envelopes, lies within the bone cortex and surrounds the individual haversian systems, each containing vessels and a nerve. Although the haversian

envelope is not involved consistently in diseases associated with slow, or low-turnover, bone loss, it may participate in processes accompanied by high-turnover bone loss, resulting in longitudinally oriented striations, or spaces, in the cortex. The *cortico-endosteal envelope* relates to the inner surface of the bone cortex and, therefore, is the outermost boundary of the medullary bone. It is interrupted at sites at which the trabeculae of the medullary cavity are connected to the cortex.[89] This envelope functions primarily as a bone resorptive surface, accounting for the general thinning of the cortex that occurs with advancing age in adults. The fourth envelope is the *endosteal envelope*, representing the interface of medullary bone and marrow. As indicated previously, this envelope is characterized by a very large surface area and is primarily a bone-losing envelope.[89] At its outer portion, a *transitional envelope* has been identified, intimately associated with the inner margin of the cortex and actively involved in bone remodeling.

These bone envelopes, and particularly the endosteal envelope, contain three types of surfaces that have been well described by Recker.[89] *Resting surfaces* are quiescent, not being involved in bone formation or resorption. Such surfaces are smooth and are covered by a very thin layer of bone lining cells. These surfaces are responsive to stimuli associated with bone remodeling that lead to differentiation of bone cells from their precursors, to selection of a specific site of remodeling activity, and to regulation of the extent of remodeling that takes place. *Forming surfaces*, also referred to as osteoid surfaces, are characterized by the presence of unmineralized osteoid, with or without osteoblasts. Active bone formation takes place intermittently at these surfaces. The degree of activity taking place at the forming surfaces can be assessed quantitatively using tetracycline labeling. The final bone surface is referred to as the *resorbing surface*. This surface has a scalloped margin owing to the presence of Howship's lacunae. Active resorbing surfaces are characterized by the presence of osteoclasts; inactive resorbing surfaces, also said to be in a resting or reversal stage, are devoid of osteoclasts.

Thus, at any particular time, such surfaces normally may be quiescent or, less commonly, be actively involved in the synthesis or resorption of bone. Their cellular composition varies according to their functional state; quiescent surfaces generally are free of osteoblasts or osteoclasts, whereas those that are resorbing or forming bone contain osteoclasts or osteoblasts, respectively. Owing to this close relationship between the presence and type of cells and the functional state of the bone surfaces, considerable attention has been given to the cellular mechanisms responsible for the resorption and formation of bone and the effect on these mechanisms produced by such substances as parathyroid hormone, 1,25-dihydroxyvitamin D (calcitriol), calcitonin, prostaglandin E$_2$, interleukin-1, diphosphonate compounds, and mithramycin.

It is the *coupling* of bone resorption to bone formation that controls the volume of bone that is present at any particular time. It appears likely that the mechanisms responsible for coupling are intrinsic to bone (i.e., coupling is a local event). Although such mechanisms are essential to the balance between osteoclastic and osteoblastic activity, the site of production (e.g., osteoclasts, bone matrix) and the precise nature of the coupling factor(s) are not clear. What is clear, however, is that an increase in bone resorption subsequently must be coupled to an increase in bone formation if bone volume is to remain unchanged.

Bone Resorption. Although it has long been held that the osteoclast is the principal cell involved in the degradation of the organic bone matrix and the release of bone mineral, a potential (albeit controversial) role for the osteocyte in removing at least a small amount of perilacunar bone also has been emphasized, and accumulating evidence has indicated that mononuclear phagocytes, including peripheral blood monocytes and tissue macrophages, are involved in bone resorption.[10, 31, 32] As summarized by Coccia,[31] monocytes and tissue macrophages have organelles and enzyme systems similar to those of osteoclasts; furthermore, in vitro, they have been shown to resorb bone and to excrete a variety of substances that stimulate bone resorption. Products released by bone undergoing resorption appear to be chemotactic for monocytes that have specific calcitriol receptors; calcitriol may be important in cellular differentiation into multinucleated macrophage cells that are capable of resorbing bone.

Mast cells, a virtual storehouse of many potent chemical mediators, also exert an influence on bone resorption.[33] Certain products of the mast cell, such as prostaglandin or heparin (which stimulates the release of collagenase), have dramatic effects on bone that can culminate in osseous resorption.[34] Mast cell proliferation is a well-recognized feature of hyperparathyroidism and certain forms of osteoporosis.[35]

It is a histologic and ultrastructural fact that surfaces of bone involved in extensive resorption are sites of accumulation of multinucleated osteoclasts that reside in Howship's lacunae or pits. The finely striated (brush) border of the osteoclast is in contact with the adjacent bone and is in a state of vigorous movement. The surface of the osteoclast contains irregular cell processes or lobopodia, separated by extracellular clefts in which minute crystals of bone mineral and fragments of collagen may be found.[28]

All of the aforementioned features and observations strongly support the active role played by the osteoclast in the resorption of bone. It is the precise mechanisms of the process, including the participation of other cells, that are not clear. Vaes[100] has emphasized three successive steps that are required for bone resorption. The first involves the formation of osteoclast progenitor cells in hematopoietic tissues followed by their vascular dissemination and the generation of resting preosteoclasts and osteoclasts in bone. The second consists of the activation of osteoclasts at their contact with mineralized bone. Osteoblasts may control this second step by exposing the mineral to osteoclasts and preosteoclasts or by releasing a factor that activates these cells, or by both mechanisms. In the third step, activated osteoclasts resorb both the mineral and the organic components of mineralized bone through the action of agents they secrete in the segregated zone underlying their ruffled border. The importance of cells of the osteoblastic lineage in the initiation of bone resorption also has been emphasized by Raisz.[99] The removal of proteins and proteoglycans on the bone surface is thought to be accomplished by the release of procollagenase and plasminogen activator from osteoblastic cells. Plasminogen activator also has been identified in osteoclasts.

Osteoclasts appear to be the major cell responsible for the skeletal contribution to the regulation of serum concentration of calcium[99, 100]; all of the agents that have been shown to increase serum calcium concentration in vivo have been shown also to increase osteoclastic activity, and the hormones and drugs that lower this concentration have been shown to inhibit osteoclastic activity.[99] Among the substances capable of directly or indirectly stimulating existing osteoclasts or increasing the formation of new osteoclasts, or both, are parathyroid hormone, active metabolites of vitamin D, prostaglandin E_2, thyroid hormone, heparin, and interleukin-1; among those substances inhibiting resorption are calcitonin, glucocorticoid, diphosphonates, glucagon, phosphate, and carbonic anhydrase inhibitors.[3] Osteoclastic resorption plays a major role in the pathogenesis of a variety of skeletal disorders, including metabolic processes such as osteoporosis, neoplastic and inflammatory conditions accompanied by bone lysis, Paget's disease, and osteopetrosis.[99]

Bone Formation. The principal cell involved in the formation of bone is the osteoblast. Osteoblasts are derived from mesenchymal osteoprogenitor cells, or preosteoblasts, are involved in the synthesis of bone matrix, and subsequently either become internal osteocytes or become inactive as bone lining cells. New bone formation may result from the activation of bone lining cells or the proliferation and differentiation of preosteoblasts, or both.

The formation of bone occurs in two phases, matrix formation and mineralization: Matrix formation precedes mineralization and occurs at the interface between osteoblasts and existing osteoid; mineralization occurs at the junction of osteoid and newly mineralized bone, a region that is designated the mineralization front.[3] The layer of unmineralized matrix, termed the osteoid seam, is approximately 8 to 10 μm in adults owing to the usual interval of 10 days between matrix production and mineralization.[3] In certain disease states, such as osteomalacia (Fig. 20–32), the thickness of the osteoid seam is increased.

The fact that newly formed matrix is not immediately mineralized supports the concept that a series of changes in the matrix is required initially. As outlined by Jee,[3] these events include (1) an increase in the cross-linking of collagen fibers; (2) the binding of phospholipids to collagen fibers; (3) an increase in the concentration of noncollagenous matrix proteins, especially γ-carboxyglutamic acid (BGP); (4) the binding of calcium to these matrix proteins; (5) the accumulation of silicon and zinc; and (6) an early increase followed by a later decline in glycosaminoglycans.

Once modified, the matrix is suitable to the mineralization process that has been described previously and is incompletely understood. What is clear is that various hormones influence this process directly as well as indirectly by modifying the supply of calcium and phosphate. The major regulators of bone formation can be divided into five groups: (1) calcium-regulating hormones (parathyroid hormone, 1,25-dihydroxyvitamin D, and calcitonin); (2) additional hormones (glucocorticoids, insulin, thyroxine, sex hormones, and growth hormone); (3) growth factors (somatomedin, epidermal growth factor, fibroblast growth factor, platelet-derived growth factor); (4) local factors (prostaglandin E_2, interleukins, and bone-derived growth factors); and (5) ions (calcium and phosphate)[36] (Table 20–2).

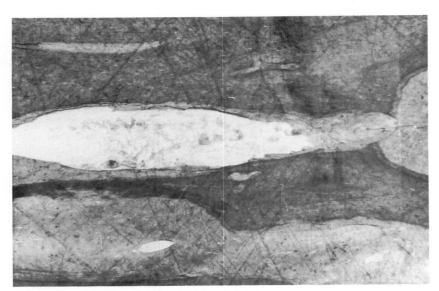

FIGURE 20–32. Increased thickness of osteoid seams: Osteomalacia. A photomicrograph of undecalcified bone that has been stained for calcium shows a thick, superficial layer of unstained osteoid and adjacent, heavily stained bone. (50×.)

Humoral Regulation of Bone Metabolism

Bone metabolism and calcium homeostasis are intimately related to the interactions among the skeleton, intestines, and kidneys and to the presence of many chemical factors, of which three hormones—parathyroid hormone, calcitonin, and 1,25-dihydroxyvitamin D—are most important.

Parathyroid Hormone. An important regulator of skeletal metabolism is parathyroid hormone, whose two main functions are to stimulate and control the rate of bone

Table 20–2. Factors That May Regulate Bone Growth*

Agent	Effect on Bone Formation	
	Direct	Indirect
Calcium Regulatory Hormones		
Parathyroid hormone	↓	↑
1,25-Dihydroxyvitamin D	↓	↑
Calcium	—	? ↑
Systemic Hormones		
Glucocorticoids	↑ ↓ †	↓
Insulin	↑	↑
Thyroxine	?	↑
Sex hormones	—	↑
Growth hormone	—	↑
Growth Factors		
Somatomedin (insulin-like growth factor)	↑	↑
Epidermal growth factor	↓	?
Fibroblast growth factor	↓	?
Platelet-derived growth factor	↑	?
Local Factors		
Prostaglandin E₂	↑ ↓ †	↑
Osteoclast activating factor	↓	?
Bone-derived growth factor(s)	↑	?
Ions		
Calcium	↑	↑
Phosphate	↑	↑

*Agents that have been tested for their direct effects in vitro are listed as increasing (↑), decreasing (↓), or not changing (—) bone formation. Where there is evidence for an important indirect effect, mediated through another factor, the dominant direction is indicated.

†Biphasic or dual response, depending on dose or direction of treatment. Reprinted with permission from Raisz LG, Kream BE: N Engl J Med 309:29, 1983.

remodeling, and to influence mechanisms governing the control of the plasma level of calcium.[3] This hormone, which is produced by the chief cells of the four parathyroid glands, consists of a single chain polypeptide of 84 amino acids; after secretion into the circulation, the hormone is metabolized to smaller, inactive polypeptide fragments. The precise sequence of the 84 amino acids and the critical importance of the amino terminal third of the molecule for biologic activity have been shown.[37–39] The synthesis and secretion of parathyroid hormone are known to be closely regulated by the level of ionized calcium in the extracellular fluid, with elevated levels of serum calcium suppressing parathyroid hormone secretion and depressed levels increasing such secretion, although the specific mechanisms accounting for this regulation are not entirely clear. Cyclic adenosine monophosphate (cAMP) is known to be a major cellular regulator of the action of parathyroid hormone, and the activation and inhibition of cAMP are influenced by additional substances, including intracellular calcium, adrenergic catecholamines, dopamine, secretin, and prostaglandins.[39] Furthermore, magnesium can affect parathyroid hormone secretion; either elevated or depressed levels of magnesium inhibit such secretion.

Parathyroid hormone has a direct effect on the bone (enhancing the mobilization of calcium from the skeleton) and on the kidney (stimulating the absorption of calcium from the glomerular fluid) and an indirect effect on the intestines (influencing the rate of calcium absorption). These actions in concert serve to increase the level of calcium in the extracellular fluid, although the target tissues (bone, kidneys, and intestines) are affected to different degrees and at differing rates: The renal effects are the most rapid; those in the bone occur in phases; and the effects in the intestines are relatively slow and mediated through the action of 1,25-dihydroxyvitamin D.[39]

Osseous Effects. Parathyroid hormone acts directly on bone (Fig. 20–33), and the result of this action may be bone resorption or formation, or both. An immediate action of parathyroid hormone involves the processes of osteoclastic and osteocytic resorption that are fundamental to calcium homeostasis; more prolonged effects of parathyroid hor-

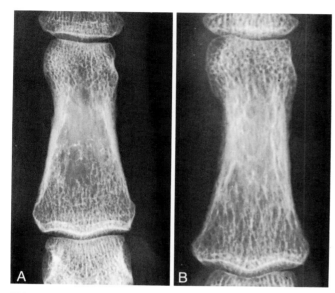

FIGURE 20–33. Osseous effects of parathyroid hormone: Hyperparathyroidism. Magnification radiographs of the phalanges in a normal person **(A)** and a patient with hyperparathyroidism **(B)** reveal the effects of parathyroid hormone on bone. In **B**, note osteopenia, indistinct trabeculae, and prominent subperiosteal bone resorption.

mone are influential on bone remodeling and mediated principally by the action of osteoclasts.[3, 39] Thus, at the cellular level, parathyroid hormone influences osteoclasts, osteoblasts, osteocytes, and bone surface cells. A significant increase in the number of osteoclasts and in the ratio of osteoclasts to osteoblasts may occur within hours after the administration of the hormone.[40] This effect suggests that parathyroid hormone, at least indirectly, activates existing osteoclasts (perhaps related to its direct effects on osteoblasts with exposure of bone surfaces) or increases the recruitment of new osteoclasts (perhaps related to accumulation of migrating extraskeletal progenitor cells to bone). Morphologic changes in the osteoclasts suggesting increased activity of the cells also are noted, including an increase in the number of nuclei within the cell.[41, 42] It also is clear that osteoblasts contain receptors for parathyroid hormone and are influenced directly by circulating levels of this hormone. Osteoblast function is decreased initially, leading to a suppression of bone formation. Shortly after the administration of parathyroid hormone, the closely packed osteoblasts on the surface of the bone become separated and spindle-like, and collagen synthesis begins to decrease.[36] Subsequently, however, stimulation of osteoblasts results in an increase in bone formation, although the precise mechanism of this action is not clear.[43] In response to parathyroid hormone, osteoblasts produce interleukin-6 and insulin-like growth factors, and these substances (and perhaps others) may provide the intercellular stimulus that is recognized by the osteoclast.

These known effects of parathyroid hormone on different bone cells at different times are compatible with the importance of this hormone in maintaining calcium homeostasis. A fall in the serum level of calcium leads to a release of parathyroid hormone and a relatively rapid activation of osteocytes and osteoclasts. These cells promote bone resorption with the mobilization of calcium from the skeleton.

As the initial effect of parathyroid hormone on the osteoblast appears to be inhibitory, the mobilized calcium is made available for cellular metabolism. Later, owing to additional effects of parathyroid hormone that occur in the kidney and indirectly in the intestines, supplementary sources of calcium become available to the body, lessening the need for that derived from the skeleton. Stimulation of osteoblasts at this time results in the incorporation of calcium into the skeleton, manifested as an increase in bone synthesis.

Intestinal Effects. An increase in intestinal absorption of calcium that accompanies hyperparathyroidism represents an indirect effect of this hormone that is mediated through regulation of synthesis of 1,25-dihydroxycholecalciferol, a vitamin D metabolite, in the kidney (see Chapter 53). Furthermore, parathyroid hormone directly stimulates gastrin release and has a relaxant effect on gastrointestinal smooth muscle.

Renal Effects. The renal excretion of calcium, phosphate, bicarbonate, and other ions is regulated directly by parathyroid hormone. Although calcium reabsorption predominates in the proximal tubules of the kidney, it appears that the effect of parathyroid hormone in enhancing reabsorption of calcium from the glomerular fluid occurs more distally in the tubules. The precise sites of calcium resorption in the kidney influenced by parathyroid hormone are the thick ascending limb of the loop of Henle, the distal convoluted tubule, and the early portion of the cortical collecting tubule.[101] An increased level of urinary calcium excretion, however, is a well-recognized manifestation of hyperparathyroidism but one that represents a secondary effect of hypercalcemia. Apparently, owing to the state of hypercalcemia, the amount of calcium filtered at the glomerulus exceeds even the enhanced capacity for calcium conservation by the renal tubules.[101]

The inhibition of phosphate resorption in the kidney, the phosphaturic effect, by parathyroid hormone occurs principally in the proximal tubules but also, to a lesser extent, in the distal tubules. This effect is mediated through cAMP that is formed in response to parathyroid hormone.

Additional renal effects of this hormone include inhibition of bicarbonate reabsorption with alkalinization of the urine and stimulation of the activity of 1-α-hydroxylase enzyme, leading to an increase in the production of 1,25-dihydroxycholecalciferol, the active metabolite of vitamin D.[39]

Calcitonin. Calcitonin is a peptide consisting of 32 amino acids that is secreted by the parafollicular or C cells of the human thyroid gland. Characteristic chemical features of calcitonin include an N-terminal seven membered disulfide ring and a C terminus of prolineamide.[44] The secretion of calcitonin is controlled by the circulating levels of calcium; as the serum level of calcium rises, calcitonin is released from the thyroid gland with an elevation in its plasma concentration and a fall in the content of calcitonin in the gland itself owing to depletion of secretory granules from the parafollicular cells. Experimental studies in animals have revealed significant interrelationships between gastrointestinal and calcitropic hormones and, despite the absence of sufficient data, such interrelationships in humans could be relevant to the manifestations of multiple endocrine neoplasia syndromes.[39] With regard to the metabolism of calcitonin after its release from the thyroid gland, clearance appears to occur in the kidney and, to a lesser extent, in other tissues, including the liver, bones, and thyroid gland.[45]

Calcitonin inhibits bone resorption and may lead to significant hypocalcemia and hypophosphatemia. Data also exist that indicate a stimulatory effect of calcitonin on bone growth in vivo.[46, 47] The importance of calcitonin as a regulator of calcium metabolism in humans, however, is not clear at present. Indeed, in athyrotic persons, skeletal growth may proceed normally if thyroid hormone replacement is provided.[48] Conversely, high levels of calcitonin that are evident in patients with medullary carcinoma of the thyroid gland do not lead to significant inhibition of bone resorption or prominent alterations in calcium homeostasis.[49]

At the cellular level, calcitonin has no direct effect on osteoblasts[36] but rather appears to reduce bone resorption by inactivation of osteoclasts[50] and, perhaps, by decreasing their number.[51] Calcitonin also interferes with the transfer of calcium from bone to extracellular fluid, and its overall effect in producing a decrease in bone resorption is reflected in a reduction in the urinary excretion of hydroxyproline.[48]

Vitamin D. Vitamin D represents one of the most potent humoral factors involved in the regulation of bone metabolism. Although its biochemistry and mechanisms of action are described in detail in Chapter 53, a summary of its biologic effects is appropriate here. The general term vitamin D refers to both vitamin D_2 (ergocalciferol), which originates in plants and is obtained by dietary sources, and vitamin D_3 (cholecalciferol), which occurs naturally in the skin. In humans, these two forms of vitamin D have very similar potency and, hence, considering them separately has little, if any, clinical significance.

The classic biologic role of vitamin D is regulation of intestinal mineral absorption and maintenance of skeletal growth and mineralization.[68] It now is widely accepted that these functions are mediated through the actions of 1,25-dihydroxyvitamin D (1,25[OH]$_2$D) on the intestine, bone, and kidney. The recent discovery, however, of 1,25(OH)$_2$D receptors in a variety of tissues where they were previously not known to exist suggests that this hormone has a biologic role much greater than one related simply to mineral metabolism.

Intestinal Effects. 1,25(OH)$_2$D is the key hormone responsible for the absorption of calcium from the diet. Deficiency of this hormone causes calcium malabsorption and leads to a negative calcium balance. 1,25(OH)$_2$D appears to exert a trophic effect on intestinal growth as well as a stimulatory effect on several functions of this organ.[69] The exact biochemical events by which 1,25(OH)$_2$D regulates calcium absorption, however, remain unclear. 1,25(OH)$_2$D has been found to induce the formation of a high affinity calcium binding protein (CaBP) in the intestine.[70] In addition, the hormone increases the activities of alkaline phosphatase and a calcium-dependent ATPase in the mucosal cells and promotes the phosphorylation of a high molecular weight brush border membrane protein. These effects are manifested a few hours after the administration of 1,25(OH)$_2$D and can be blocked by protein synthesis inhibitors. In view of this, it has been proposed that 1,25(OH)$_2$D is responsible for the control of the active transport component of calcium absorption that involves protein synthesis.[71] Whether the quantitatively less important passive calcium transport that occurs by simple diffusion also can be facilitated by 1,25(OH)$_2$D remains unclear.

In addition to its effect on calcium absorption, 1,25(OH)$_2$D increases active phosphate transport by a mechanism that is not well understood. Phosphate transport appears to be independent of calcium transport and, compared with the latter, is less strictly dependent on 1,25(OH)$_2$D.

Osseous Effects. The vitamin D endocrine system appears essential for normal bone formation and mineralization; states of vitamin D deficiency are manifested by dramatic disturbances in these processes. The understanding of the precise role of vitamin D in bone metabolism, however, is incomplete because of the complexity of the tissue, the presence of several different bone cells, each with unique cellular functions, and the complex interactions that occur between 1,25(OH)$_2$D and other humoral factors that also are involved in bone regulation.

Currently, considerable evidence exists to indicate that 1,25(OH)$_2$D acts directly on the osteoblast to modify its function. Indeed, specific receptors for 1,25(OH)$_2$D have been identified in these cells.[72, 73] The hormone has been shown to induce the synthesis of γ-carboxyglutamic acid containing protein (BGP)[74] and to stimulate the bone specific isoenzyme of alkaline phosphatase[75] as well as the synthesis of collagen in osteoblasts.[76] The precise effects of 1,25(OH)$_2$D on the synthesis of collagen, an essential component of bone matrix, and on alkaline phosphatase, an enzyme apparently linked to the process of mineralization, are not yet clear, as experimental data have been conflicting. Evidence suggests that the response of osteoblasts to this hormone depends on their state of cellular differentiation and that 1,25(OH)$_2$D promotes the conversion of osteoblasts from immature to mature forms.[77, 78]

It is an interesting paradox that although vitamin D is essential for mineralization of bone matrix, it also possesses potent bone resorbing activity. Data derived from biochemical and autoradiographic studies have demonstrated conclusively that osteoclasts, unlike osteoblasts, do not possess receptors for 1,25(OH)$_2$D; thus, a direct effect of this hormone on osteoclasts in the stimulation of bone resorption appears unlikely. Rather, the prominent role of 1,25(OH)$_2$D in osseous resorption may be mediated by its ability to promote the cellular differentiation of hematopoietic precursors to cells capable of resorbing bone. As it has been shown that 1,25(OH)$_2$D interacts with hematolymphatic cells to modify their function,[79] and as cells of the hematolymphatic tissue are known to produce humoral factors that are capable of bone resorption, such as interleukins and prostaglandins, the effects of vitamin D on cells of the hematolymphatic system may be essential to its role in osseous resorption.

Renal Effects. The effects of the vitamin D endocrine system on the kidney are not well understood. Although the administration of vitamin D to rachitic animals increases the renal tubular reabsorption of phosphorus and calcium,[80] renal wasting of calcium and phosphate is not a serious clinical problem in states of vitamin D deficiency. Analysis of the precise manner in which vitamin D affects the kidney is made more difficult owing to differences in the acute and long-term renal effects of 1,25(OH)$_2$D.[81]

Hematolymphopoietic Effects. In recent years, accumulating evidence indicates that 1,25(OH)₂D has important regulatory effects on blood mononuclear cells and on the immune system. Receptors for 1,25(OH)₂D exist in human monocytes as well as other cells (e.g., macrophage precursor cell lines). Monocytes themselves can resorb bone and, furthermore, regulate the production of the osteoclast-activating factor,[82] with properties now known to be identical to those of interleukin-1β. Therefore, it seems likely that the bone-resorbing capacity of vitamin D may be mediated through an effect on monocytes; 1,25(OH)₂D has been shown to promote multinucleation of mononuclear macrophages (cellular precursors of osteoclasts) and to enhance macrophage-mediated bone resorption.[83] Indeed, 1,25(OH)₂D has been used effectively in the treatment of osteopetrosis, a congenital disorder associated with aberrations in bone resorption related to defective osteoclast function.[84]

In addition, some evidence suggests that 1,25(OH)₂D plays a significant role in intrathymic differentiation of lymphocytes. In contrast to human monocytes, resting peripheral T and B lymphocytes do not possess 1,25(OH)₂D receptors. Activation of T and B lymphocytes, however, causes the expression of the 1,25(OH)₂D receptor.[79] Activation of lymphocytes triggers the release of lymphokines, including interleukin-2, as well as the expression of interleukin-2 receptors in T lymphocytes. Under the influence of interleukin-2, the T cells reactive to the initial antigen proliferate and differentiate to cells that mediate effector functions, including cytotoxicity, and aid or suppress antibody production. It has been established that 1,25(OH)₂D is a very potent inhibitor of interleukin-2.[85] Through its effect on interleukin-2 and perhaps through other actions, 1,25(OH)₂D inhibits lymphocyte proliferation as well as antibody production by B cells and generation of cytotoxic lymphocytes.[86] The known effects of 1,25(OH)₂D on hematolymphatic cells and the potential relationship of these cells to the osseous actions of this hormone are illustrated diagramatically in Figure 20–34.

Currently it is unclear what relevance these experimental data regarding the immunoregulatory role of 1,25(OH)₂D have to clinical situations, although vitamin D deficiency commonly is associated with recurrent infections and decreased mobility and impaired phagocytic capacity of leukocytes.

Other Effects. Receptors for 1,25(OH)₂D have been identified in a variety of tissues in animals or humans, or both. It has been suggested that 1,25(OH)₂D may suppress the secretion of parathyroid hormone, promote the secretion of thyroid stimulating hormone, and either inhibit or stimulate prolactin secretion.[87, 88]

Other Humoral Factors. Additional hormones and humoral factors involved in the regulation of bone metabolism have been well summarized by Raisz and Kream.[36, 52]

Glucocorticoids. Glucocorticoids lead to a decrease in intestinal absorption of calcium and phosphate and an increase in their renal excretion,[53] which probably are unrelated to interference in the pathways of vitamin D biosynthesis.[54] As glucocorticoids also inhibit the formation of new bone matrix, wide osteoid seams (osteomalacia) are not apparent.[52] This reduction in bone synthesis may relate

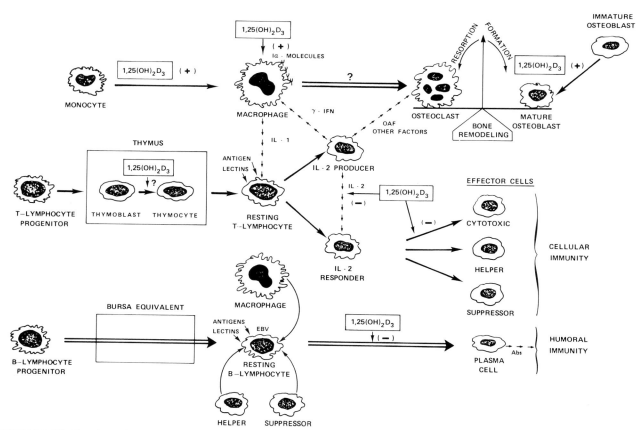

FIGURE 20–34. The sites of the involvement of 1,25(OH)₂D₃ in the differentiation and function of monocytes and T and B lymphocytes are depicted. Plus signs (+) indicate stimulatory effect of the hormone; minus signs (−) indicate inhibitory effects.

to an inhibitory effect on osteoblast precursor cells[55] rather than an interference with the synthesis of collagen[56]; an absence of active osteoblasts on bone-forming surfaces is evident.[57] The interactions of glucocorticoids and various calcium-regulating hormones, such as 1,25-dihydroxyvitamin D, calcitonin, and parathyroid hormone, are not clear.[52] Similarly, the direct stimulation of bone resorption by glucocorticoids is not proved. It is possible that glucocorticoids can enhance transiently the formation or function of osteoclasts, but when the hormone is present for longer periods, bone resorptive activity is reduced as a result of decreased replication of precursor cells.[99]

Insulin. Although osteopenia with a decrease in bone mass is a recognized manifestation of diabetes mellitus, it is not certain if insulin is directly responsible for this finding, as abnormal levels of calcium-regulating hormones also may be evident in this disease.[52] The direct osseous effects of insulin, as defined in a number of investigations,[58-60] have been summarized by Raisz and Kream[52] and include increases in the uptake of amino acids into fetal bone, in the RNA synthesis in isolated bone cells, and in the synthesis of type I collagen and total protein in fetal rat bone. Indirectly, insulin increases somatomedin production in the liver and 1,25-dihydroxyvitamin D synthesis in the kidney.[52]

Thyroid Hormones. The known association of hyperthyroidism with osteopenia (see Chapter 56) has led to considerable interest in the effects of thyroid hormones on skeletal metabolism. Direct effects of these hormones include stimulation of growth in cartilage[61] and of osteoclastic activity.[62] As thyroid hormones are linked physiologically to other humoral substances, such as somatomedin secreted by the liver, it is difficult to define precisely the primary or secondary nature of the skeletal effects of these hormones in patients with hyperthyroidism.

Sex Hormones. The current interest in estrogen as a therapeutic agent in postmenopausal osteoporosis is based primarily on the belief that estrogens, apparently indirectly, inhibit bone resorption, perhaps by increasing the absorption of calcium from the intestines, the synthesis of serum 1,25(OH)$_2$D, the secretion of calcitonin, or various combinations of the three.[63, 64] Estrogens also may have a direct effect on bone, which may involve both inhibition of resorption and stimulation of formation.[99]

Growth Hormone. Growth hormone increases bone turnover, the intestinal absorption of calcium, and vitamin D–dependent intestinal calcium-binding protein; the skeletal effects of growth hormone probably are mediated by somatomedins.[52]

Other Agents. Some of the additional humoral factors that affect the skeleton are indicated in Table 20–2.

Metabolic Bone Disorders

Histologic Techniques. During the last two decades, several technical advances have permitted more precise assessment of bone structure. Biochemical methods were developed to measure circulating hormones and vitamins that influence bone, such as parathyroid hormone, calcitonin, and vitamin D metabolites. New noninvasive radiologic methods, such as single and dual photon absorptiometry, dual energy x-ray absorptiometry, and CT scanning, now allow detection of changes in skeletal mass that are not evident with routine radiography (see Chapter 52). These diagnostic tools, however, are indirect indicators of skeletal morphology. Rather, it is the preparation of histologic sections of bone that has permitted the direct examination of skeletal tissue. Microstructural studies of bone can determine not only the state of skeletal mineralization but also the level of bone remodeling activity (i.e., bone formation and bone resorption).

As the differentiation between the two major metabolic bone diseases, osteoporosis and osteomalacia, is based in part on the quantity and quality of bone mineral, the ability to distinguish between calcified and uncalcified bone matrix (osteoid) is critical. The traditional procedures for processing bone (acid decalcification and paraffin embedding) require the removal of inorganic matrix to facilitate histologic sectioning and therefore prevent the subsequent determination of the degree of skeletal mineralization. Owing to deficiencies in traditional histologic techniques, additional methods including the qualitative and quantitative microscopic assessment of undecalcified specimens and the use of in vivo bone markers, such as tetracycline, have been employed. Typically, the iliac crest is used as the biopsy site from which nondecalcified tissue sections are prepared.

Bone histomorphometry is the quantitative analysis of undecalcified bone in which the parameters of skeletal remodeling are expressed in terms of volumes, surfaces, and cell numbers (Table 20–3). To obtain this information from a two dimensional format, principles of stereology are used to reconstruct a third dimension. This method, described by the French mineralogist Delesse in 1848, is based on the theory that if measurements are made at random on extremely thin sections, a ratio of areas is equal to a ratio of volumes. Areas are measured by counting the number of cross-marks or "hits" that coincide in position with the histologic feature of interest. The array of points is projected onto the tissue section from a grid in the microscope eyepiece (Fig. 20–35). The average number of hits that fall on the component of interest (as a fraction of the total number of possible hits) is equal to the volume of that component within the total unit volume. Measurements of bone surfaces or perimeter lengths are obtained by counting the number of intersections between the bone perimeter and wavy parallel grid lines. The distance between two items of interest, such as the distance between two tetracycline labels, is measured by a calibrated linear reticle. The number of osteoclasts, osteoclast nuclei, or osteocytes may be counted on each field and expressed per square millimeter.

In nondecalcified bone sections, osteomalacia usually is characterized by the accumulation of osteoid owing to a defect in the mineralization process. It must be recognized, however, that excess quantities of osteoid may result not only from a decreased rate of mineralization but also from an accelerated rate of bone matrix synthesis. In routine nondecalcified bone sections, these two forms of osteoid excess will appear identical. Differentiation between these states is based on the determination of mineralization rates, using tetracycline as an in vivo bone marker.

The binding affinity of autofluorescent tetracycline antibiotics for immature mineral deposits, but not for the mature crystal, allows the identification of calcification foci and subsequently permits the determination of the rate of bone mineralization.[102] Bound tetracycline thereby is incorporated into the maturing crystalline lattice of bone and

TABLE 20–3. Histomorphometric Parameters

Determination	Abbreviation	Definition	Calculation	Units
Trabecular bone volume, volumetric bone density	TBV, V_v	Percentage of biopsy tissue occupied by mineralized and unmineralized bone tissue	$\dfrac{\text{Total number of bone hits} + \text{total number of osteoid hits}}{\text{Total number of hits}}$	%
Relative osteoid volume	OV, ROV	Percentage of trabecular bone volume composed of unmineralized matrix	$\dfrac{\text{Total number of osteoid hits}}{\text{Total number of bone hits} + \text{osteoid hits}}$	%
Osteoid surface, total osteoid surface	OS, TOS	Percentage of trabecular surface covered by osteoid seams	$\dfrac{\text{Number of intersects with osteoid seams}}{\text{Total number of intersects}}$	%
Mean osteoid seam width, thickness of osteoid seams	MOSW, S	Thickness of osteoid seams	Measured directly, or $\dfrac{\text{total osteoid volume}}{\text{Osteoid surface}}$	μm
Osteoblastic osteoid surface, active osteoid	OB, AO	Percentage of trabecular surface covered by osteoid, which is lined by cuboidal osteoblasts	$\dfrac{\text{Number of intersects with osteoblasts}}{\text{Total number of intersects with osteoid}}$	%
Osteoclastic resorption surface, active resorption surface	ARS, OCS	Percentage of trabecular surface covered with osteoclasts	$\dfrac{\text{Total number of intersects with osteoclasts}}{\text{Total number of intersects}}$	%
Osteoclasts per square millimeter	OC	Number of osteoclasts per square millimeter of trabecular bone	Measure directly	no/sq mm
Peritrabecular fibrosis	FIB	Percentage of trabecular surface covered by fibrous tissue	$\dfrac{\text{Total number of intersects with fibrosis}}{\text{Total number of intersects}}$	%
Linear extent of bone formation, fractional labeled surfaces	LEBF, fractLAB	Extent of tetracycline labeled trabecular surface	$\dfrac{\text{Tetracycline labeled surface intersects}}{\text{Total trabecular surface intersects}}$	sq μm/sq μm
Mineralization front activity, calcification front	MF, CF	Percentage of mineralized bone-osteoid seam interfaces labeled with tetracycline	$\dfrac{\text{Number of labeled interface hits}}{\text{Total number of interface hits}}$	%
Appositional rate, calcification rate, mineral appositional rate	AR, CR, MAR	Average amount of new matrix deposited and mineralized over the tetracycline labeling period	Mean distance between the midpoints of the double tetracycline labels	μm/day
Bone formation rate—tissue level referent	BFR-tissue	Amount of bone formed per unit surface area of trabecular bone per day	LEBF × AR	cu μm/sq μm/d

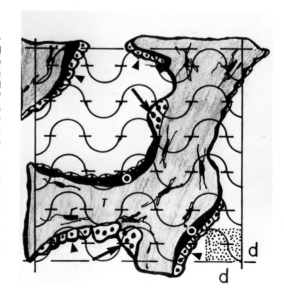

FIGURE 20–35. Histomorphometry. A Merz-Schenk grid in the microscope eyepiece is shown projected onto a field of mineralized bone (shaded areas), osteoid (black areas), and marrow (unshaded areas). Of the 36 cross marks or hits in the grid, 13 are superimposed on mineralized bone, 3 on osteoid, 16 on marrow, 2 on osteoclasts, and 2 on osteoblasts. Therefore, 44.4 per cent of the field is occupied by bone. Because 3 of the 16 hits on bone fall on osteoid, the relative volume of osteoid is 18.8 per cent. The absolute area occupied by the grid therefore is 36 times the square of the distance (d) (dotted square) between the cross marks or hits (area = 36 d^2). When viewed at 250× magnification, d is measured by a calibrated ocular micrometer (the grid covers 0.155 sq mm). Approximately 200 fields (30 sq mm) should be measured for statistically valid results.

The six wavy parallel lines help compensate for nonrandomly oriented trabeculae, and the distance between the lines (d) is the same as that between hits (d). There are 18 intersections between the parallel lines and the trabecular perimeter. Seven intersections are at osteoid surfaces, five are at resting mineralized surfaces, and four are at osteoclast-filled Howship's lacunae. Therefore, the osteoid surface represents 38.9 per cent, the resting surface 27.8 per cent, and the active resorption surface 22.2 per cent of the total number of intersections with the bone perimeter. O, Osteoid; T, trabecular bone; arrow, osteoclast; arrowhead, osteoblasts lining osteoid seam.

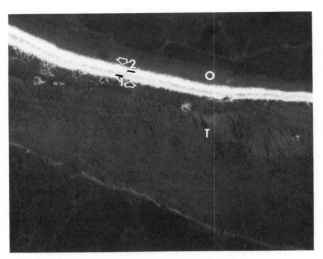

FIGURE 20–36. Normal double fluorescent tetracycline labels (open arrows). The first label *(1)* is located in the mineralized trabecular bone *(T)*. The second *(2),* more recently administered label, is at the current mineralization front, at the osteoid seam *(O)* interface. (Ultraviolet light; unstained; 125×.)

remains as a marker of mineral deposition, unless it is removed by decalcification or osteoclastic resorption (Fig. 20–36). Two discrete, fluorescent tetracycline bands separated by a nonfluorescent, measurable interlabel distance (Table 20–4) are produced. A variety of tetracycline labeling compounds and schedules are available. Dimethylchlortetracycline, oxytetracycline, or demeclocycline (declomycin) are equally satisfactory for this purpose. Most labeling schemes employ a "3–14–3" schedule: During the first labeling course, tetracycline (1 gm/day in divided doses) is administered for 3 days; after a 14 day hiatus, a second course of tetracycline is given over 3 days. The bone biopsy is performed 3 to 4 days after the last dose of tetracycline.

Tetracycline fluorescence is evaluated on unstained, nondecalcified tissue sections by ultraviolet light. The first course of tetracycline (Fig. 20–36) appears as a discrete fluorescent band within the mineralized bone. The second, more recently administered course of tetracycline is located at the current mineralization front (i.e., mineralized bone–

osteoid seam interface). The distance between the two bands represents the amount of new bone synthesized and mineralized over the drug-free interval.

Normal Histologic Appearance. Normally, the contour of the external cortical margins is smooth. Subperiosteal osteoid deposits, as well as eroded surfaces containing osteoclasts, normally are absent. Subperiosteal bone resorption is evidence of activation of osteoclasts, seen in states of high bone turnover or accelerated remodeling, as in hyperparathyroidism.

Loss of cortical bone mass is suggested when the cortical thickness is reduced (Fig. 20–37). The normal mean cortical width is variable, ranging from less than 500 μm to more than 1600 μm. Cortical porosity is determined by the presence of normal or abnormal vascular canals (haversian and Volkmann's canals). The degree of intracortical porosity tends to increase with increasing bone turnover. Activation of osteoclasts leads to increased resorption of bone, enlarging the preexisting vascular canals. The resorption of bone in the longitudinally oriented canals results in the formation of cavities termed cutting cones. The junction between the cortical and medullary trabecular bone, which normally is sharply demarcated, is termed the endosteum. Loss of distinction between the cortex and the medullary cavity occurs with increasing cortical porosity owing to increased cortical osteoclastic resorptive activity, as is seen in severe hyperparathyroidism. Endosteal resorption cavities increase in number and depth until the previously solid cortical bone becomes whittled into what appears to be new thick trabeculae, a process referred to as cancellization or trabecularization of cortical bone (Fig. 20–37).

The total amount and quality of the trabecular bone located between the two cortices reflect the weight-bearing properties of the skeleton. Usually the trabecular bone occupies 15 to 25 per cent of the marrow space. A trabecular bone volume below 15 per cent is histologic evidence of osteopenia. Normally, the individual trabeculae are continuous interconnecting or branching bands; atrophic trabecu-

TABLE 20–4. Tetracycline Labeling Regimen for Bone Biopsy

Day	Regimen
1,2,3	Tetracycline hydrochloride, 250 mg orally four times daily or 500 mg orally twice daily*†
4–17	Hiatus (no tetracycline)‡
18,19,20	Tetracycline hydrochloride, 250 mg orally four times daily or 500 mg orally twice daily†
24	Bone biopsy§

*Tetracycline is given 1 hour before or 2 hours after meals. A larger dose is used if malabsorption or severe osteomalacia is suspected; up to 3 gm/day may be necessary for patients after intestinal bypass.

If the patient has recently received tetracycline hydrochloride, the use of oxytetracycline or demeclocycline in equivalent doses may help to distinguish the new tetracycline bone labels from the old, owing to differences in the fluorescent color produced by the different tetracyclines.

†Avoid all dairy products, antacids, and iron-containing medicines on days 1, 2, 3, 18, 19, and 20.

‡An interval of at least 10 days is required between the two courses of tetracycline.

§Biopsy may be performed several days later, but not sooner.

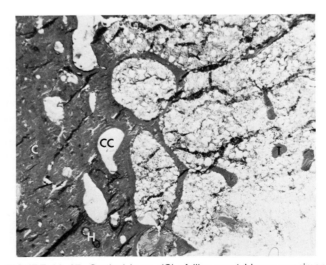

FIGURE 20–37. Cortical bone *(C)* of iliac crest biopsy specimen undergoing remodeling. Osteoclasts within cutting cones *(CC)* resorb endosteal bone, resulting in cortical cancellization (i.e., the formation of cancellous trabecular bone from preexisting cortical bone). A reduction in the cortical width ultimately occurs. H, Normal haversian canal, prior to activation. (Trichrome stain, 25×.)

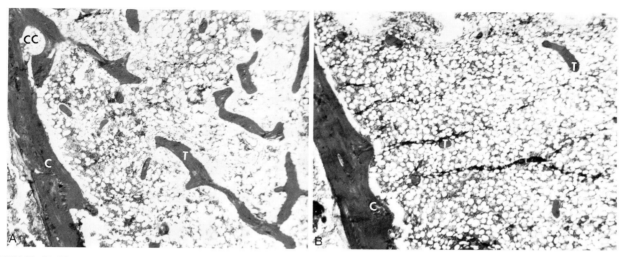

FIGURE 20–38. Normal and abnormal trabecular bone architecture.
   A Low power view of iliac crest biopsy specimen. Cortical thickness is reduced owing to progressive erosion by cortical cutting cones *(CC)*. Trabecular bone *(T)*, however, exhibits a normal platelike connecting architectural pattern. (Trichrome stain, 25×.)
   B Reduction in trabecular *(T)* bone volume. Not only is the volume of bone reduced but also the architecture of trabecular bone now is abnormal owing to the presence of thin, widely spaced, atrophic rods of bone *(T)*. (Trichrome stain, 25×.)

lae appear as struts, bars, or blots (Fig. 20–38) (i.e., a reduction in the mean trabecular plate density).

Relative osteoid volume (expressed as a percentage of trabecular bone) normally ranges from 0.6 to 4.0 per cent, osteoid surface (expressed as a percentage of trabecular surface) from 4 to 20 per cent, and mean osteoid seam width from 8 to 16 μm. Excess osteoid may result from an increase in the percentage of the trabecular bone surface enveloped by osteoid, from an augmentation of the mean osteoid seam width, or from a combination of the two.

Normally, about 35 to 40 per cent of the osteoid surface is lined by plump, cuboidal osteoblasts and is termed the osteoblastic osteoid surface (representing 2 to 8 per cent of the total trabecular surface).

Bone resorption is reflected by measurements of the number of osteoclasts and the extent of the osteoclastic resorptive surface (as a percentage of trabecular surface). The percentage of trabecular surface with resorptive bays however, is tenfold greater than the osteoclastic resorptive surface because 90 per cent of Howship's lacunae normally are devoid of osteoclasts. These empty resorptive bays are referred to as reversal surfaces because they are thought to represent evidence of the intermediate phase between the phases of bone resorption and formation that are characteristic of coupling.

Examination of marrow is required for identification of peritrabecular fibrosis, a feature associated with states of increased bone turnover.

Decalcified sections taken from the bone core should be examined under polarized light for evidence of woven collagen architecture. Woven bone in a transiliac crest specimen is an abnormal finding in the adult patient and reflects accelerated skeletal turnover. Examination of the specimen with fluorescent light also is required. About 80 to 90 per cent of the interfaces between mineralized bone and osteoid will exhibit two parallel tetracycline fluorescence lines, with each band appearing as narrow, discrete linear labels (i.e., the calcification front activity). The percentage of trabecular surface bearing tetracycline labels should be re-

corded individually as it represents the linear extent of bone formation. Finally, the mean distance between the midpoints of the double tetracycline labels is measured with a linear reticle. This distance divided by the number of days between the two courses of tetracycline is the average daily mineral appositional rate and normally ranges from 0.4 μm to 0.9 μm (mean, 0.65 μm). As the rate of bone apposition increases, the distance between the labels grows wider. In contrast, with a reduced rate of mineralization, the parallel bands become narrower and may fuse to produce single labels.

Abnormal patterns of fluorescent label deposition are the hallmark of osteomalacia and represent the morphologic expression of defective mineralization.[103] The amount of tetracycline fluorescence is proportional to the amount of immature amorphous calcium phosphate deposits in the mineralizing foci of the osteoid seam. In some cases, osteoid seams are deficient in mineral and therefore are incapable of binding tetracycline, leading to an absence of fluorescence. As a result, the activity of the mineralization front (percentage of osteoid seams bearing normal tetracycline labels) is reduced (Fig. 20–39). A second common abnormal tetracycline pattern characteristic of osteomalacia is diffuse, irregular fluorescence of an entire osteoid seam. Accumulation of immature bone mineral is thought to reflect a failure of maturation of amorphous calcium phosphate into hydroxyapatite crystals, thus permitting excessive tetracycline binding (Fig. 20–40).

Abnormal Histologic Appearance. The location and extent of bone removal and deposition determine the physical anatomy of the skeleton and the physiologic status of mineral metabolism. Bone remodeling activity is influenced by physical forces, serum levels of endocrine hormones, and nutritional and metabolic factors. Normally, bone resorption and formation are in balance. A net loss of bone tissue may occur from excessive bone resorption or deficient bone formation, or a combination of both, during the coupling process. Bone diseases resulting from an abnormality of remodeling activity are characterized by a failure of the skeleton

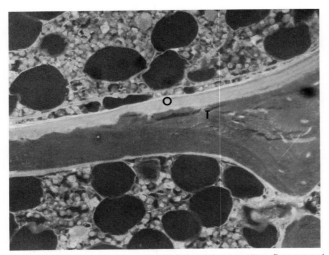

FIGURE 20–39. Osteomalacia: Abnormal tetracycline fluorescent pattern. The mineralization defect is manifested as a failure of the osteoid seams (O) to assimilate tetracycline. Histomorphometrically this is referred to as a subnormal mineralization front index. T, Trabecular bone. (Ultraviolet light; unstained; 98×.)

to provide structural support, generally owing to a deficiency in skeletal mass. When the bone mass can no longer sustain normal forces, a fracture may ensue, leading to pain and deformity. A metabolic bone disease is defined as any generalized disorder of the skeleton, regardless of cause; most metabolic bone diseases result from either an imbalance in remodeling activity or a disorder of matrix mineralization.

Osteopenia refers to the generalized reduction in bone mass that, on radiographic examination, appears as an exaggerated radiolucency of the skeleton. Osteoporosis and osteomalacia are the two major causes of osteopenia. Histologically, osteoporotic diseases may be accompanied by either increased or decreased rates of bone turnover. Osteomalacic syndromes are characterized by histologic evidence of defective mineralization (Table 20–5).

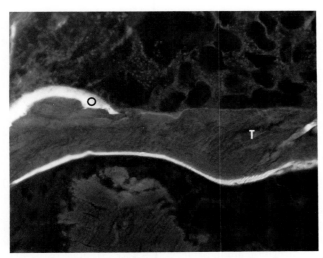

FIGURE 20–40. Osteomalacia: Abnormal tetracycline fluorescent pattern. Osteoid seams (O) exhibit an irregular diffuse fluorescence instead of dual thin, linear bands, also indicating a reduction in the osteoid seam mineralization front activity (see Fig. 20–36). T, Trabecular bone. (Ultraviolet light; unstained; 98×.)

TABLE 20–5. General Morphologic Classification of Metabolic Bone Diseases

Osteoporosis
 High remodeling: Active bone turnover
 Low remodeling: Inactive bone turnover
Osteomalacia
 Low remodeling: Pure osteomalacia
 High remodeling: Mixed osteomalacia and osteitis fibrosa cystica

High bone turnover diseases (Table 20–6) are characterized by evidence of both increased formation and increased resorption of bone (Fig. 20–41). Histologic correlates of increased formation include increased quantities of osteoid, increased osteoid surfaces, moderately increased osteoid seam thickness, and increased osteoblastic surfaces. By tetracycline fluorescence, an increase may be seen in the fraction of trabecular bone surfaces bearing double labels, indicating an increase in the linear extent of bone formation. The linear extent parameter is a function of the activation of additional osteoblasts. The mineralization rate (the distance between the double labels) may be increased, reflecting an augmentation of individual cell activity. Increased resorptive activity is manifested as an increase in the number of osteoclasts and in the fraction of bone surfaces engaged in bone resorption, resulting in Howship's lacunae complete with osteoclasts. In some cases, woven bone deposition may be noted. Deposition of peritrabecular fibrous tissue indicating osteitis fibrosa is a manifestation of general increased mesenchymal cell activity. This feature is not specific for hyperparathyroidism, as it may be associated with any condition resulting in accelerated tissue turnover.

Skeletal mass is reduced in states of accelerated bone turnover, despite the fact that a normal or even excessive rate of bone formation is seen. Because of the coupling of bone formation and bone resorption, bone formation is preceded by an even greater degree of resorptive activity, resulting in a net loss of skeletal mass.

Those states associated with reduced bone turnover (Table 20–6) show little evidence of either bone formation or bone resorption (Fig. 20–42). Consequently, osteoid seams are thin and scanty, osteoblasts are flattened, and osteoclasts are reduced in number. Few tetracycline labels are apparent, consistent with the small amount of osteoid seen by light microscopy. As a result, the activity of the mineralization front (fraction of tetracycline labeled seams) is preserved, but the front is characterized by a reduction in the linear extent of bone formation (fraction of labeled trabecular bone surfaces). Single fluorescent labels predominate, because the rate of bone matrix deposition is so low as to prevent spatial separation of the two courses of tetracycline.

Osteomalacia usually is characterized by excessive quantities of osteoid, owing to a failure of matrix calcification despite continued matrix synthesis by osteoblasts (Table 20–7). Marked increases in the thickness of osteoid seams are characteristic, but osteomalacia may be associated with normal or even reduced quantities of osteoid[104] (Fig. 20–43A,B). The static and dynamic parameters that classically characterize osteomalacia include an increase in the amount of osteoid and a reciprocal decrease in the rate of mineralization, respectively (Fig. 20–43C). These two components permit the distinction between osteomalacia and osteoporotic disorders in which the level of bone remodel-

TABLE 20-6. Bone Morphology Associated with Specific Metabolic Diseases

Increased Bone Remodeling Activity (Accelerated Turnover Osteoporosis)
  Anticonvulsant drug-related
  Calcium deficiency states, chronic (secondary hyperparathyroidism)
  Small intestinal disease (early, compensated mineral malabsorption)
  Postgastrectomy (mineral malabsorption)
  Some forms of postmenopausal or senile osteoporosis
  Erythroid hyperplasia
  Hemochromatosis
  Hyperparathyroidism
  Hyperthyroidism
  Osteoporosis of young men
  Mastocytosis
Decreased Bone Remodeling Activity (Reduced Turnover Osteoporosis)
  Glucocorticoid-associated
  Hepatic disease
    Alcohol related
    Cholestatic
  Hypothyroidism
  Severe systemic disease

  Starvation, malnutrition
  Some forms of postmenopausal or senile osteoporosis
  Total parenteral nutrition (hyperalimentation)
Osteomalacia (Pure)
  X-linked hypophosphatemia (vitamin D-resistant rickets)
  Sporadic hypophosphatemia
  Antacid-induced osteomalacia
  Oncogenic osteomalacia
  Primary vitamin D deficiency
  Chronic pancreatitis
  Chronic extrahepatic obstruction
  Metabolic acidosis
  Renal osteodystrophy (aluminum-associated osteomalacia)
Osteomalacia (Mixed Osteomalacia and Osteitis Fibrosa Cystica)
  Primary vitamin D deficiency (nutritional, lack of exposure to sunlight)
  Small intestinal disease (vitamin D and calcium malabsorption)
  Postgastrectomy (vitamin D and calcium malabsorption)
  Renal osteodystrophy (mixed)
  Calcium deficiency of children
  Vitamin D-dependent rickets

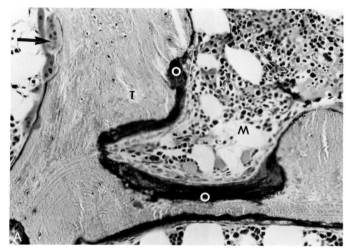 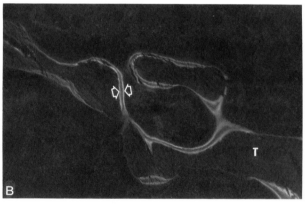

FIGURE 20–41. Accelerated bone turnover.
A Histologic appearance of accelerated bone turnover, or active remodeling, in a nondecalcified bone biopsy specimen. Bone resorption by osteoclasts (arrow) is accompanied by increased osteoid *(O)* deposition by osteoblasts, resulting in an increase in the total osteoid surface and in the amount of osteoblastic osteoid. *T,* Trabecular bone; *M,* marrow. (Trichrome stain, 98×.)
B Although the quantity of osteoid is increased at the light microscopic level, kinetic tetracycline labeling reveals an increased surface extent of double fluorescent labels (open arrows) (i.e., increased linear extent of bone formation), reflecting normal matrix synthesis by a greater number of active modeling units bearing osteoblasts. (Ultraviolet light; unstained; 25×.)

TABLE 20-7. Histologic Features of Osteomalacia

Bone Formation Parameters	Parameter	Pure Osteomalacia (Low Remodeling State)	Mixed Osteomalacia and Osteitis Fibrosa Cystica (High Remodeling State)
Increased osteoid volume	Osteoblastic surface	Reduced	Normal to increased
Increased osteoid surface	Osteoclast number	Normal to decreased	Normal to increased
Markedly increased osteoid seam thickness	Active resorption surface	Normal to decreased	Normal to increased
Subperiosteal osteoid accumulation	Linear extent of bone formation	Reduced (may be 0)	May be reduced; normal; or increased
Cortical bone osteoid deposits	Appositional rate	Reduced (often 0)	Reduced
	Tetracycline labels	Predominantly abnormal (diffuse, unlabeled)	Predominantly abnormal (diffuse, unlabeled)
	Mineralization front activity	Approaches 0	Reduced
	Peritrabecular fibrosis	Absent	Usually present
	Subperiosteal resorption	Absent	May be present
	Cortical cancellization	Absent	May be present

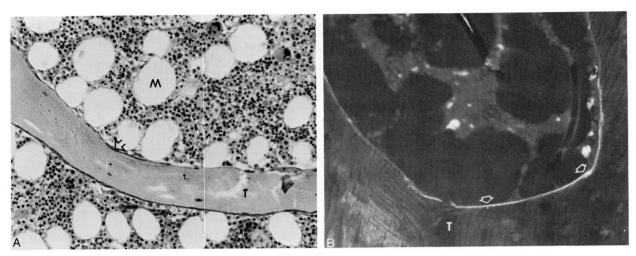

FIGURE 20–42. Reduced bone turnover.

A Trabecular bone *(T)* is lined by thin, inactive osteoid seams (arrow). Bone surfaces are smooth, free of Howship's resorption lacunae. *M,* Marrow. (Trichrome stain, 98×.)

B Because of reduced osteoblastic activity, osteoid seams exhibit only a single discrete linear label (open arrows). The matrix appositional rate was so low that it did not permit the spatial separation of the two previously administered courses of tetracycline. Because osteoid seams, if present, will bear at least one discrete linear label, the mineralization front activity is reduced only modestly, thereby excluding the presence of a mineralization defect. *T,* Trabecular bone. (Ultraviolet light; unstained; 125×.)

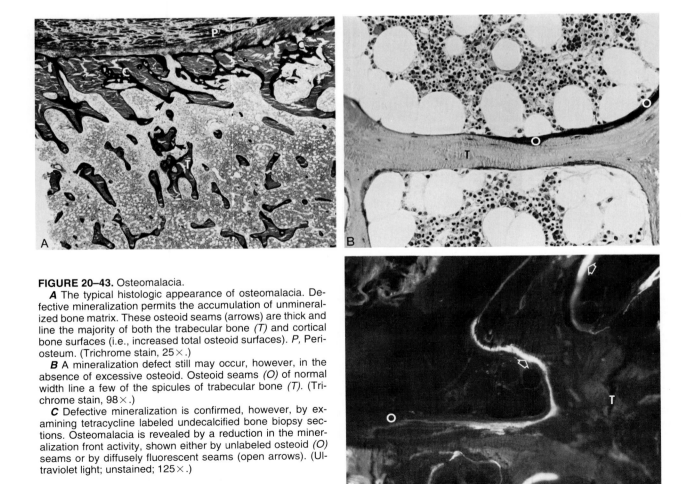

FIGURE 20–43. Osteomalacia.

A The typical histologic appearance of osteomalacia. Defective mineralization permits the accumulation of unmineralized bone matrix. These osteoid seams (arrows) are thick and line the majority of both the trabecular bone *(T)* and cortical bone surfaces (i.e., increased total osteoid surfaces). *P,* Periosteum. (Trichrome stain, 25×.)

B A mineralization defect still may occur, however, in the absence of excessive osteoid. Osteoid seams *(O)* of normal width line a few of the spicules of trabecular bone *(T).* (Trichrome stain, 98×.)

C Defective mineralization is confirmed, however, by examining tetracycline labeled undecalcified bone biopsy sections. Osteomalacia is revealed by a reduction in the mineralization front activity, shown either by unlabeled osteoid *(O)* seams or by diffusely fluorescent seams (open arrows). (Ultraviolet light; unstained; 125×.)

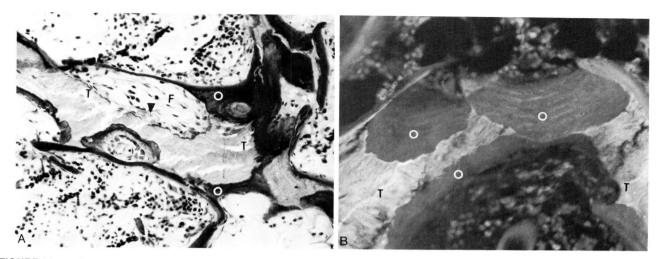

FIGURE 20–44. Osteomalacia with accelerated turnover: Active features.

A Increased quantities of osteoid *(O)* may coexist with features of high turnover disease, including peritrabecular fibrosis *(F)* and increased osteoclastic resorption (arrowhead). This mixed histologic pattern, consisting of features of both defective mineralization and osteitis fibrosa cystica, may superficially mimic the histologic features of active remodeling osteoporosis. *T,* Trabecular bone. (Trichrome stain, 125×.)

B In this condition, presence of defective mineralization can be determined only by examining the pattern of tetracycline fluorescent labels. In this case, osteomalacia is diagnosed by the absence of fluorochrome uptake at the widened osteoid seams *(O)*. *T,* Trabecular bone. (Ultraviolet light; unstained; 125×.)

ing activity influences the quantity of osteoid that is produced. In low turnover states, for example, the mineralization rate may be low, but the quantity of osteoid is appropriately reduced (Fig. 20–42). In high turnover states, when matrix apposition is accelerated, a mineralization defect is unlikely, despite the presence of excessive amounts of osteoid.

Although pure osteomalacia usually is associated with low activity of bone remodeling, features of osteoblast activation, osteoclast proliferation, and peritrabecular fibrosis—all indicative of accelerated turnover—may be present (Table 20–6). Osteomalacia, therefore, may coexist with osteitis fibrosa cystica (hyperparathyroidism) (Fig. 20–44).

SUMMARY

Bone is a remarkable and unique tissue, constantly undergoing change. It develops through the processes of endochondral and intramembranous ossification and subsequently is modified and refined by processes of modeling and remodeling to create a structurally and metabolically competent, highly organized architectural marvel. Its cells, including the osteoblasts, osteocytes, and osteoclasts, reside in organic matrix, primarily collagen, and inorganic material is deposited in a form that resembles hydroxyapatite. The process of mineralization is complex and incompletely understood.

Bone is essential in maintaining calcium homeostasis, stabilizing the plasma level of calcium. Its cells are highly responsive to stimuli provided by a number of humoral agents of which parathyroid hormone, thyrocalcitonin, and 1,25-dihydroxyvitamin D are most important. Synthesis and resorption of bone, which continue normally in a delicate balance throughout life, are mediated by the action of such humoral agents through processes that include stimulation of osteoblasts to form bone and of osteoclasts and, perhaps, osteocytes to remove bone. The presence of a variety of

diseases results in characteristic alterations that are readily detectable on radiographs or by other imaging methods. It is these alterations that are illustrated throughout the pages of this textbook.

References

1. Jaffe HL: Metabolic, Degenerative, and Inflammatory Diseases of Bones and Joints. Philadelphia, Lea & Febiger, 1972, p 1.
2. Warwick R, Williams PL: Gray's Anatomy. 35th British Ed. Philadelphia, WB Saunders Co, 1973, p 207.
3. Jee WSS: The skeletal tissues. *In* L Weiss, L Lansing (Eds): Histology: Cell and Tissue Biology. 5th Ed. New York, Elsevier Biomedical, 1983.
4. Warshawsky H: Embryology and development of the skeletal system. *In* RL Cruess (Ed): The Musculoskeletal System. Embryology, Biochemistry, Physiology. New York, Churchill Livingstone, 1982, p 33.
5. Garn SM: Contributions of the radiographic image to our knowledge of human growth. AJR *137:*231, 1981.
6. Garn SM, Goodspeed G, Hertzog KP: A longitudinal test of angular remodeling in the tibia. Am J Phys Anthropol *30:*311, 1969.
7. Garn SM, Silverman FN, Herzog KP, et al: Lines and bands of increased density. Their implication to growth and development. Med Radiogr Photogr *44:*58, 1968.
8. Kirkpatrick JA Jr: Bone and joint growth—normal and in disease. Clin Rheum Dis *7:*671, 1981.
9. Young RW: Cell proliferation and specialization during endochondral osteogenesis in young rats. J Cell Biol *14:*357, 1962.
10. Teitelbaum SL, Kahn AJ: Mononuclear phagocytes, osteoclasts, and bone resorption. Mineral Electrolyte Metab *3:*2, 1980.
11. Owen M: The origin of bone cells. Int Rev Cytol *28:*213, 1970.
12. Ash P, Loutit JF, Townsend KMS: Osteoclasts derived from haematopoietic stem cells. Nature *283:*669, 1980.
13. Marie PJ: Structure, organization, and healing. *In* RL Cruess (Ed): The Musculoskeletal System. Embryology, Biochemistry, and Physiology. New York, Churchill Livingstone, 1982, p 109.
14. Salomon CD: A fine structural study on the extracellular activity of alkaline phosphatase and its role in calcification. Calcif Tissue Res *15:*201, 1974.
15. Jande SS, Bélanger LF: The life cycle of the osteocyte. Clin Orthop *94:*281, 1973.
16. Hanaoka H: The origin of the osteoclast. Clin Orthop *145:*252, 1979.
17. Göthlin G, Ericsson JLE: The osteoclast. Review of ultrastructure, origin and structure-function relationship. Clin Orthop *120:*201, 1976.
18. Bonucci E: New knowledge on the origin, function and fate of osteoclasts. Clin Orthop *158:*252, 1981.
19. Ash P, Loutit JF, Townsend KMS: Osteoclasts derive from hematopoietic stem cells according to marker, giant lysosomes of beige mice. Clin Orthop *155:*249, 1981.

20. Marks SC Jr: Congenital osteopetrotic mutations as probes of the origin, structure, and function of osteoclasts. Clin Orthop 189:239, 1984.
21. Glimcher MK, Krane SM: Organization and structure of bone and the mechanism of calcification. In BS Gould, GN Ramachandran (Eds): Treatise on Collagen. New York, Academic Press, 1965, p 68.
22. Potts JT Jr, Deftos LJ: Parathyroid hormone, calcitonin, vitamin D, bone and bone mineral metabolism. In PK Bondy, LE Rosenberg (Eds): Duncan's Diseases of Metabolism. 7th Ed. Vol II. Endocrinology. Philadelphia, WB Saunders Co, 1974, p 1225.
23. Glimcher MJ: Composition, structure and organization of bone and other mineralized tissues and the mechanism of calcification. In RO Greep, EB Astwood (Eds): Handbook of Physiology—Endocrinology. Baltimore, Williams & Wilkins, 1976, p 25.
24. Boskey AL: Current concepts of the physiology and biochemistry of calcification. Clin Orthop 157:225, 1981.
25. Posner AS: The mineral of bone. Clin Orthop 200:87, 1985.
26. Roufosse AH, Landis WJ, Sabine WK, et al: Identification of brushite in newly deposited bone mineral from embryonic chicks. J Ultrastruct Res 68:235, 1979.
27. Francis MD, Webb NC: Hydroxyapatite formation from a hydrated calcium monohydrate phosphate precursor. Calcif Tiss Res 6:335, 1971.
28. Williams PL, Warwick R (Eds): Gray's Anatomy. 36th British edition. Philadelphia, WB Saunders Co, 1980, p 259.
29. Neuman WF, Neuman M: The nature of the mineral phase of bone. Chem Rev 53:1, 1953.
30. Bernard GW, Pease DC: An electron microscopic study of intramembranous osteogenesis. Am J Anat 125:271, 1969.
31. Coccia PF: Cells that resorb bone. N Engl J Med 310:456, 1984.
32. Mundy GR: Monocyte-macrophage system and bone resorption. Lab Invest 49:119, 1983.
33. McKenna MJ, Frame B: The mast cell and bone. Clin Orthop 200:226, 1985.
34. Avioli LV: Heparin-induced osteopenia: An appraisal. Adv Exp Med Biol 52:375, 1975.
35. Fallon MD, Whyte MP, Craig RB, et al: Mast-cell proliferation in postmenopausal osteoporosis. Calcif Tissue Int 35:29, 1983.
36. Raisz LG, Kream BE: Regulation of bone formation. N Engl J Med 309:29, 1983.
37. Habener JF, Potts JT Jr: Biosynthesis of parathyroid hormone. Part 1. N Engl J Med 299:580, 1978.
38. Keutmann HT: Chemistry of parathyroid hormone. In LJ Degroot, GF Cahill Jr, L Martini, et al: Endocrinology. New York, Grune & Stratton, 1980, p 593.
39. Aurbach GD, Marx SJ, Spiegel AM: Parathyroid hormone, calcitonin, and the calciferols. In RH Williams (Ed): Textbook of Endocrinology. Sixth Ed. Philadelphia, WB Saunders Co, 1981, p 922.
40. Tatevossian A: Effect of parathyroid extract on blood calcium and osteoclast counts in mice. Calcif Tissue Res 11:251, 1973.
41. Feldman RS, Krieger NS, Tashjian AJ: Effects of parathyroid hormone and calcitonin on osteoclast formation in vitro. Endocrinology 107:1137, 1980.
42. Addison WC: The effect of parathyroid hormone on the number of nuclei in feline osteoclasts in vivo. J Anat 130:479, 1980.
43. Howard GA, Bottemiller BL, Turner RT, et al: Parathyroid hormone stimulates bone formation and resorption in organ culture; evidence for a coupling mechanism. Proc Natl Acad Sci 78:3204, 1981.
44. Deftos LJ: The thyroid gland in skeletal and calcium metabolism. In LV Avioli, S Krane (Eds): Metabolic Bone Diseases. New York, Academic Press, 1978, p 447.
45. Deftos LJ: Calcitonin secretion. In F Bronner, J Coburn (Eds): Disorders of Mineral Metabolism. New York, Academic Press, 1982, p 433.
46. Weiss RE, Singer FR, Gorn AH, et al: Calcitonin stimulates bone formation when administered prior to initiation of osteogenesis. J Clin Invest 68:815, 1981.
47. Raisz LG, Kream BE: Hormonal control of skeletal growth. Annu Rev Physiol 43:225, 1981.
48. Glorieux FH: Hormonal control of mineral homeostasis. In RL Cruess (Ed): The Musculoskeletal System. Embryology, Biochemistry, and Physiology. New York, Churchill Livingstone, 1982, p 171.
49. Melvin KE, Miller MH, Tashjian AH Jr: Early diagnosis of medullary carcinoma of the thyroid gland by means of calcitonin assay. N Engl J Med 285:1115, 1971.
50. Holtrop ME, Raisz LG, Simmons HA: The effect of parathyroid hormone, colchicine and calcitonin on the ultrastructure and the activity of osteoclasts in organ culture. J Cell Biol 60:346, 1974.
51. Deftos LJ: Medullary Thyroid Carcinoma. New York, S Karger, 1983.
52. Raisz LG, Kream BE: Regulation of bone formation. N Engl J Med 309:83, 1983.
53. Bringhurst FR, Potts JT Jr: Calcium and phosphate distribution, turnover and metabolic actions. In LJ De Groot (Ed): Endocrinology. New York, Grune & Stratton, 1979, p 551.
54. Lubert BP, Stanbury SW, Mawer EB: Vitamin D and intestinal transport of calcium: Effects of prednisolone. Endocrinology 93:718, 1973.
55. Jee WSS, Park HZ, Roberts WE, et al: Corticosteroid and bone. Am J Anat 129:477, 1970.
56. Dietrich JW, Canalis EM, Maina DM, et al: Effects of glucocorticoids on fetal rat bone collagen synthesis in vitro. Endocrinology 104:715, 1979.
57. Raisz LG: Effect of corticosteroids on calcium metabolism. Prog Biochem Pharmacol 17:212, 1980.
58. Peck WA, Messinger K: Nucleoside and ribonucleic acid metabolism in isolated bone cells: Effects of insulin and cortisol in vitro. J Biol Chem 245:2722, 1975.
59. Henry HL: Insulin permits parathyroid hormone stimulation of 1,25-dihydroxyvitamin D₃ production in cultured kidney cells. Endocrinology 108:733, 1981.
60. Hahn TJ, Downing SJ, Phang JM: Insulin effect on amino acid transport in bone: Dependence on protein synthesis and Na⁺. Am J Physiol 220:1717, 1971.
61. Burch WM, Lebowitz HE: Triiodothyronine stimulates maturation of porcine growth-plate cartilage in vitro. J Clin Invest 70:496, 1982.
62. Mundy GR, Shapiro JL, Bandelin JG, et al: Direct stimulation of bone resorption by thyroid hormones. J Clin Invest 58:529, 1976.
63. Gallagher JC, Riggs BL, DeLuca HF: Effect of estrogen on calcium absorption and serum vitamin D metabolites in postmenopausal osteoporosis. J Clin Endocrinol Metab 51:1359, 1980.
64. Riggs BL, Jowsey J, Goldsmith RS, et al: Short- and long-term effects of estrogen and synthetic anabolic hormone in postmenopausal osteoporosis. J Clin Invest 51:1659, 1972.
65. Owen M: Lineage of osteogenic cells and their relationship to the stromal system. In WA Peck (Ed): Bone and Mineral Research. New York, Elsevier Science Publishers, 1985, p 1.
66. Provvedini DM, Deftos LJ, Manolagas SC: 1,25-dihydroxyvitamin D₃ promotes in vitro morphologic and enzymatic changes in normal human monocytes consistent with their differentiation into macrophages. Bone 7:23, 1986.
67. Rodan GA, Martin TJ: Role of osteoblasts in hormonal control of bone resorption—a hypothesis. Calcif Tissue Int 33:349, 1981.
68. DeLuca HF: The vitamin D hormonal system: Implications for bone diseases. Hosp Pract 15:57, 1980.
69. Bikle DD, Morrissey RL, Zolock DT: The mechanism of action of vitamin D in the intestine. Am J Clin Nutr 32:2322, 1979.
70. Wasserman RH, Taylor AN: Vitamin D₃-induced calcium binding protein in chick intestinal mucosa. Science 152:791, 1966.
71. Pansu D, Bellaton C, Bronner F: Effect of Ca intake on saturable and nonsaturable component of duodenal Ca transport. Am J Physiol 240:632, 1981.
72. Kream BE, Jose M, Yamada S, et al: A specific high affinity binding macromolecule for 1,25-dihydroxyvitamin D₃ in fetal rat bone. Science 197:1086, 1977.
73. Manolagas SC, Haussler MR, Deftos LJ: 1,25-dihydroxyvitamin D₃ receptor-like macromolecules in rat osteogenic sarcoma cell lines. J Biol Chem 255:4417, 1980.
74. Price PA, Baukol SA: 1,25-dihydroxyvitamin D₃ increases synthesis of the vitamin K-dependent bone protein by osteosarcoma cells. J Biol Chem 255:928, 1981.
75. Manolagas SC, Burton DW, Deftos LJ: 1,25-dihydroxyvitamin D₃ stimulates the alkaline phosphatase activity of osteoblast-like bone tumor cells. J Biol Chem 256:7115, 1981.
76. Rowe DW, Kream BE: Regulation of collagen synthesis in fetal rat calvaria by 1,25-dihydroxyvitamin D₃. J Biol Chem 257:8009, 1982.
77. Rodan GA, Rodan SB: Expression of the osteoblastic phenotype. In WA Peck (Ed): Bone and Mineral Research Annual 2. New York, Elsevier, 1984, p 244.
78. Spiess YH, Price PA, Deftos LJ, et al: Phenotype-associated changes in the effects of 1,25(OH)₂D₃ on alkaline phosphatase and bone GLA-protein of rat osteoblastic cells. Endocrinology 118:1340, 1986.
79. Provvedini DM, Tsoukas CD, Deftos LJ, et al: 1,25-dihydroxyvitamin D₃ receptors in human leukocytes. Science 221:1181, 1983.
80. Bijvoet OLM: Kidney function in calcium and phosphorous metabolism. In LV Avioli, SM Krane (Eds): Metabolic Bone Disease. Vol 1. New York, Academic Press, 1977.
81. Bonjour JP, Preston C, Fleish H: Effect of 1,25-dihydroxyvitamin D₃ on the renal handling of phosphate in thyroparathyroidectomized rats. J Clin Invest 60:1419, 1977.
82. Yoneda T, Mundy GR: Monocytes regulate osteoclast-activating factor production by releasing prostaglandins. J Exp Med 150:338, 1979.
83. Bar-Shavit Z, Teitelbaum SL, Reitsma P, et al: Induction of monocytic differentiation and bone resorption by 1,25-dihydroxyvitamin D₃. Proc Natl Acad Sci USA 80:5907, 1983.
84. Key L, Carnes D, Cole S, et al: Treatment of congenital osteopetrosis with high-dose calcitriol. N Engl J Med 310:409, 1984.
85. Tsoukas CD, Provvedini DM, Manolagas SC: 1,25-dihydroxyvitamin D₃: A novel immunoregulatory hormone. Science 224:1438, 1984.
86. Manolagas SC, Provvedini DM, Tsoukas CD: Interactions of 1,25-dihydroxyvitamin D₃ and the immune system. Molec Cell Endocrinol 43:113, 1985.
87. Haussler MR, Manolagas SC, Deftos LJ: Evidence for a 1,25-dihydroxyvitamin D₃ receptor-like macromolecule in rat pituitary. J Biol Chem 255:5007, 1980.
88. Rose SD, Holick MF: Effects of 1,25-dihydroxyvitamin D₃ on the function of rat anterior pituitary cells in primary culture. In AW Norman et al (Eds): Vitamin D: Chemical, Biochemical and Clinical Update. New York, de Gruyter, 1985, p 253.
89. Recker RR: Embryology, anatomy, and microstructure of bone. In FL Coe, MJ Favus (Eds): Disorders of Bone and Mineral Metabolism. New York, Raven Press, 1992, p 219.
90. Robey PG, Bianco P, Termine JD: The cellular biology and molecular biochemistry of bone formation. In FL Coe, MJ Favus (Eds): Disorders of Bone and Mineral Metabolism. New York, Raven Press, 1992, p 241.
91. Oestrich AE, Ahmad BS: The periphysis and its effect on the metaphysis. I. Definition and normal radiographic pattern. Skel Radiol 21:283, 1992.
92. Laval-Jeantet M, Balmain N, Juster M, et al: Les rapports de la virole périchon-

drate et du cartilage en croissance normale et pathologique. Ann Radiol *11*:327, 1968.

93. Frost HM: Intermediary Organization of the Skeleton. Boca Raton, FL, CRC Press, 1986.

94. Campos FF, Pellico LG, Alias MG, et al: A study of the nutrient foramina in human long bones. Surg Radiol Anat *9*:251, 1987.

95. Diaz-Flores L, Gutierrez R, Lopez-Alfonso A, et al: Pericytes as a supplementary source of osteoblasts in periosteal osteogenesis. Clin Orthop *275*:280, 1992.

96. Brighton CT, Lorich DG, Kupcha R, et al: The pericyte as a possible osteoblast progenitor cell. Clin Orthop *275*:287, 1992.

97. Wlodarski KH: Properties and origin of osteoblasts. Clin Orthop *252*:276, 1990.

98. Hanaoka H, Yabe H, Bun H: The origin of the osteoclast. Clin Orthop *239*:286, 1989.

99. Raisz LG: Mechanisms and regulation of bone resorption by osteoclastic cells. *In* FL Coe, MJ Favus (Eds): Disorders of Bone and Mineral Metabolism. New York, Raven Press, 1992, p 287.

100. Vaes G: Cellular biology and biochemical mechanism of bone resorption. A review of recent developments on the formation, activation and mode of action of osteoclasts. Clin Orthop *231*:239, 1988.

101. Fitzpatrick LA, Coleman DT, Bilezikian JP: The target tissue actions of parathyroid hormone. *In* FL Coe, MJ Favus (Eds): Disorders of Bone and Mineral Metabolism. New York, Raven Press, 1992, p 123.

102. Frost HM: Tetracycline-based histological analysis of bone remodeling. Calcif Tissue Res *3*:211, 1969.

103. Fallon MD, Teitelbaum SL: The interpretation of fluorescent tetracycline markers in the diagnosis of metabolic bone disease. Hum Pathol *13*:416, 1982.

104. Teitelbaum SL: Osteomalacia and rickets. Clin Endocrinol Metab *9*:43, 1980.

105. Warwick R, Williams PL: Gray's Anatomy. 35th British ed. Philadelphia, WB Saunders Co, 1973, p 49.

106. Vogler JB III, Murphy WA: Bone marrow imaging. Radiology *168*:679, 1988.

107. De Bruyn PH, Breen PC, Thomas TB: The microcirculation of the bone marrow. Anat Rec *168*:55, 1970.

108. DePace DM, Webber RH: Electrostimulation and morphologic study of the nerves of the bone marrow of the albino rat. Acta Anat *93*:1, 1975.

109. Nathan DG: Introduction. Hematologic and hematopoietic diseases. *In* JB Wyngaarden, LH Smith Jr (Eds): Cecil Textbook of Medicine. 16th Ed. Philadelphia, WB Saunders Co, 1982, p 824.

110. Erslev AJ: Medullary and extramedullary blood formation. Clin Orthop *52*:25, 1967.

111. Dunnill MS, Anderson JA, Whitehead R: Quantitative histological studies on age changes in bone. J Pathol Bacteriol *94*:275, 1967.

112. Piney A: The anatomy of the bone marrow. Br Med J *2*:792, 1922.

113. Tribukait B: Experimental studies on the regulation of erythropoiesis with special reference to the importance of oxygen. Acta Physiol Scand *58*:1, 1963.

114. Huggins C, Blocksom BH Jr: Changes in outlying bone marrow accompanying a local increase of temperature within physiologic limits. J Exp Med *64*:253, 1936.

115. Emery JL, Follett GF: Regression of bone-marrow haematopoiesis from the terminal digits in the foetus and infant. Br J Haematol *10*:485, 1964.

116. Jaramillo D, Laor T, Hoffer FA, et al: Epiphyseal marrow in infancy: MR imaging. Radiology *180*:809, 1991.

117. Ricci C, Cova M, Kang YS, et al: Normal age-related patterns of cellular and fatty bone marrow distribution in the axial skeleton: MR imaging study. Radiology *177*:83, 1990.

118. Dawson KL, Moore SG, Rowland JM: Age-related changes in the pelvis: MR and anatomic findings. Radiology *183*:47, 1992.

119. Moore SG, Bisset GS III, Siegel MJ, et al: Pediatric musculoskeletal MR imaging. Radiology *179*:345, 1991.

21

Articular Anatomy and Histology

Donald Resnick, M.D., and Gen Niwayama, M.D.

Skeletal structures are connected to each other in a variety of ways; these junctions have been termed articulations, arthroses, juncturae, and joints. Methods used to classify joints have included divisions based on (1) extent of joint motion, and (2) type of articular histology. Neither of these two systems is ideal.

The classification of articulations based on the extent of joint motion is as follows:

Synarthroses: Fixed or rigid joints.
Amphiarthroses: Slightly movable joints.
Diarthroses: Freely movable joints.

This classification fails to disclose the fact that motion between rigid skeletal structures may result from either apposition of two sliding surfaces, as occurs in synovial joints, or changes and deformity of intervening tissue, which may be noted in fibrous or cartilaginous joints. Thus, any classification based solely upon the extent of joint mo-

tion will group together articulations whose histologic components are very dissimilar.

The classification of joints on the basis of histology emphasizes the type of tissue that characterizes the junctional area.[1, 2] The following categories are recognized:

Fibrous articulations: Apposed bony surfaces are fastened together by fibrous connective tissue.
Cartilaginous articulations: Apposed bony surfaces initially or eventually are connected by cartilaginous tissue.
Synovial articulations: Apposed bony surfaces are separated by an articular cavity that is lined by synovial membrane.

This second method of classification leads to difficulty because joints that are similar histologically may differ considerably in function and degree of allowable motion. As an example, certain fibrous joints (sutures) are virtually fixed in position and others (syndesmoses) permit some degree of movement. Furthermore, some articulations contain admixtures of a variety of tissues, such as fibrous and

TABLE 21–1. Types of Articulations

Fibrous	
Suture	Skull
Syndesmosis	Distal tibiofibular interosseous membrane
	Radioulnar interosseous membrane
	Sacroiliac interosseous ligament
Gomphosis	Teeth
Cartilaginous	
Symphysis	Symphysis pubis
	Intervertebral disc
	Manubriosternal joint
	Central mandible
Synchondrosis	Physeal plate (growth plate)
	Neurocentral joint
	Spheno-occipital joint
Synovial	
	Large, small joints of extremities
	Sacroiliac joint
	Apophyseal joint
	Costovertebral joint
	Sternoclavicular joint

cartilaginous tissues, whereas others change their constituency as they develop.

Despite these obvious weaknesses in current classification systems, the following discussion will use one of these methods of classification—that based on joint histology—rather than introduce new problems by deviating from these customary schemes (Table 21–1).

FIBROUS ARTICULATIONS

In this type of joint, apposed bony surfaces are fastened together by intervening fibrous tissue. Fibrous articulations can be further subdivided into three types: sutures, syndesmoses, and gomphoses.

Suture

Limited to the skull, sutures (Fig. 21–1) allow no active motion and exist where broad osseous surfaces are separated only by a zone of connective tissue. This connective tissue, along with two layers of periosteum on the outer and inner surfaces of the articulating bone, is termed the sutural membrane or ligament. The precise structure of a suture has been outlined by Pritchard and associates.[3] Five layers intervene between the ends of the bone: cambial, capsular, middle, capsular, and cambial. The cambial layer, a zone of flattened osteogenic cells, is covered by a capsular layer. The middle layer consists of loose fibrous connective tissue of varying thickness, containing blood vessels that communicate with the diploic vessels of the cranial vault.

Although classically a suture is considered to be a fibrous joint, areas of secondary cartilage formation may be observed during the growth period, and in later life sutures may undergo bony union or synostosis. Bony obliteration of the sutures is somewhat variable in its time of onset and cranial distribution.[4–8] It commences on the inner or deep surface of the suture between the ages of 30 and 40 years and on the outer or superficial surface approximately 10 years later. This obliteration usually occurs at the bregma and subsequently extends into the sagittal, coronal, and lambdoid sutures, in that order. Minor variations also occur in the way in which the two osseous surfaces approach each other and are fitted together. The bony surfaces rarely are smooth. When they possess minimal roughness or irregularities, the articulation is termed a plane suture. Serrated sutures contain irregular projections of bone that interdigitate with similar outgrowths on the adjacent bone, whereas denticulate sutures contain similar bony excrescences that are finer in nature. A squamous suture occurs when the margin of one bone overlaps its neighbor to some degree.

Despite the normal variations in suture development and closure, their assessment is important in the diagnosis of obstructive hydrocephalus as well as of cranial synostosis. Radiographic indices of skull size have been established in children,[41, 42] whereas accurate delineation of sutural width by routine radiography, particularly when applied to the cranial base, is difficult. CT scanning appears to represent a superior technique in this delineation.[43, 44]

Syndesmosis

A syndesmosis (Fig. 21–2) is a fibrous joint in which adjacent bony surfaces are united by an interosseous ligament, as in the distal tibiofibular joint, or an interosseous membrane, as at the diaphyses of radius, ulna, tibia, and fibula. An additional example of a syndesmosis is the interosseous ligament between the superior aspect of sacrum and ilium. In fact, the term syndesmosis could be used for almost all ligaments in the body, as such ligaments are "interosseous" in nature. A syndesmosis may demonstrate minor degrees of motion related to stretching of the interosseous ligament or flexibility of the interosseous membrane.

The conversion of other types of joints to those containing fibrous tissue (and differing little from syndesmoses) is exemplified by the sacroiliac joint, in which a synovium-lined articulation is invaded by fibrous material in the later decades of life.[2]

Gomphosis

This special type of fibrous joint (Fig. 21–3) is located between the teeth and maxilla or mandible. At these sites, the articulation resembles a peg that fits into a fossa or socket. The intervening membrane between tooth and bone is termed the periodontal ligament. This ligament varies in width from 0.1 to 0.3 mm and decreases in thickness with advancing age. The ligament has no elastic fibers, although its structure does allow slight movement of the tooth.

CARTILAGINOUS ARTICULATIONS

There are two types of cartilaginous joints: symphysis and synchondrosis.

Symphysis

In symphyses (Figs. 21–4 and 21–5), adjacent bony surfaces are connected by a cartilaginous disc, which arises from chondrification of intervening mesenchymal tissue. This tissue is composed eventually of fibrocartilaginous or fibrous connective tissue, although a thin layer of hyaline cartilage usually persists, covering the articular surface of the adjacent bone. The hyaline cartilage contributes to the growth of the neighboring osseous tissue. Symphyses, of which typical examples are the symphysis pubis and the intervertebral disc, allow a small amount of motion, which occurs through compression or deformation of the intervening connective tissue.

Some symphyses, such as the symphysis pubis and manubriosternal joint, reveal a small cleftlike central cavity, which contains fluid and which may enlarge with advancing age and be demonstrable radiographically owing to the presence of gas (vacuum phenomenon). This feature is reminiscent of cavities within synovial joints, perhaps indicating an intermediate phase of joint evolution. Furthermore, fibrous ligaments at the peripheral area of a symphysis bear some resemblance to joint capsules about synovial articulations.

Symphyses are located within the midsagittal plane of the human body and are permanent structures, unlike synchondroses, which are temporary joints. Rarely, intra-articular ankylosis or synostosis may obliterate a symphysis, such as occurs at the manubriosternal joint.

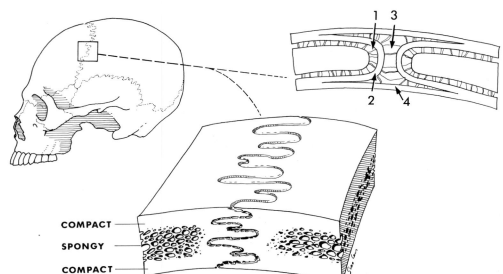

FIGURE 21–1. Fibrous articulation: Suture.

A Schematic drawings indicating structure of typical suture in the skull. Note the interdigitations of the osseous surfaces. The specific layers that intervene between the ends of the bones are indicated at the upper right. These include the cambial *(1)*, capsular *(2)*, and middle *(3)* layers. A uniting *(4)* layer also is indicated. (Reproduced in part from Pritchard JJ, Scott JH, Girgis FG: The structure and development of cranial and facial sutures. J Anat *90:*73, 1956. Courtesy of Cambridge University Press.)

Illustration continued on opposite page

Synchondrosis

Synchondroses (Fig. 21–6) are temporary joints that exist during the growing phase of the skeleton and are composed of hyaline cartilage. Typical synchondroses are the cartilaginous growth plate between the epiphysis and metaphysis of a tubular bone, the neurocentral vertebral articulations, and the unossified cartilage in the chondrocranium, the spheno-occipital synchondrosis. With skeletal maturation, synchondroses become thinner and eventually are obliterated by bony union or synostosis. Two synchondroses that persist into adult life are the first sternocostal and the petrobasilar joints.

SYNOVIAL ARTICULATIONS

A synovial joint is a specialized type of joint that is located primarily in the appendicular skeleton (Fig. 21–7). Synovial articulations generally allow unrestricted motion.[9] The structure of a synovial joint differs fundamentally from that of fibrous and cartilaginous joints; osseous surfaces are bound together by a fibrous capsule, which may be reinforced by accessory ligaments. The inner portion of the articulating surface of the apposing bones is separated by a space, the articular or joint cavity. Articular cartilage covers the ends of both bones; motion between these cartilaginous surfaces is characterized by a low coefficient of friction. The inner aspect of the joint capsule is formed by the synovial membrane, which secretes synovial fluid into the articular cavity. This synovial fluid acts both as a lubricant, encouraging motion, and as a nutritive substance, providing nourishment to the adjacent articular cartilage. In some synovial joints, an intra-articular disc of fibrocartilage partially or completely divides the joint cavity. Additional intra-articular structures, including fat pads and labra, may be noted.

The important constituents of a synovial joint are articular cartilage, subchondral bone plate, articular capsule (fibrous capsule and synovial membrane), intra-articular disc, fat pad and labrum, and synovial fluid. Surrounding structures include tendon sheaths, bursae, and small accessory bones or sesamoids.

Articular Cartilage

The articulating surfaces of the bone are covered by a layer of glistening connective tissue, the articular cartilage (Fig. 21–8). Its unique properties include transmission and distribution of high loads; maintenance of contact stresses at acceptably low levels; movement with little friction; and shock absorption.[45] In most synovial joints, the cartilage is hyaline in type; exceptions include the apophyseal joints of the spine, the acromioclavicular and sternoclavicular joints, and the temporomandibular articulation.[45] The deep layers of the articular cartilage are involved in the growth of the underlying bone via endochondral ossification. At the cessation of growth, a narrow zone of calcification, the calcified zone of articular cartilage, appears and merges with the subjacent subchondral bone plate. At its periphery, articular cartilage merges with joint capsule and periosteum.

Articular cartilage is devoid of lymphatic vessels, blood vessels, and nerves. A large portion of the cartilage derives its nutrition through diffusion of fluid from the synovial cavity. This cartilage-synovial fluid interface indeed is a dynamic area; synovial fluid may be expressed into the joint cavity from articular cartilage during movement and reabsorbed by cartilage when movement ceases.[10] This method of weeping lubrication allows movement with remarkably low friction.[46] A second source of cartilage nourishment is vascular in nature.[11] Small blood vessels pass from the subchondral bone plate only into the deepest stratum of cartilage, providing nutrients to this area of articular cartilage. Additionally, a vascular ring is located within the synovial membrane at the periphery of the cartilage. At this site, larger vessels of the synovium form a vascular circle. The terminal branches of this circle overlie the margin of the cartilage.[12] This latter source of vascularity at the peripheral aspect of the cartilage may explain marginal new bone formation or osteophytes, which are characteristic of such diseases as osteoarthritis.

Articular cartilage is variable in thickness. It may be thicker on one articulating bone than on another. Furthermore, articular cartilage is not necessarily of uniform thickness over the entire osseous surface. In general, it varies from 1 to 7 mm thick, averaging 2 or 3 mm. Jaffe[13] noted

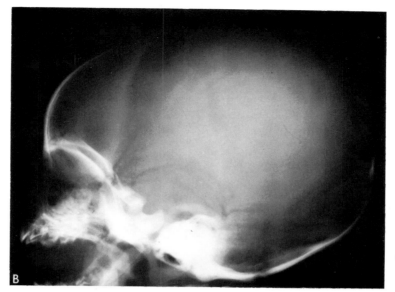

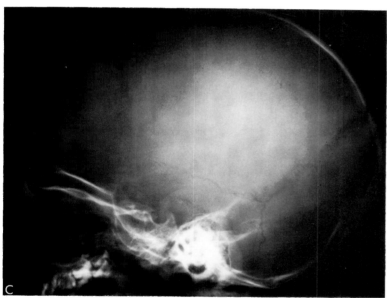

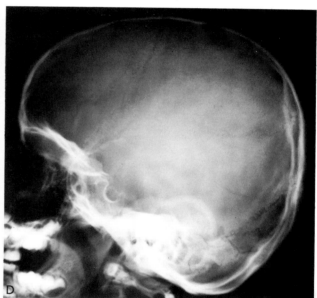

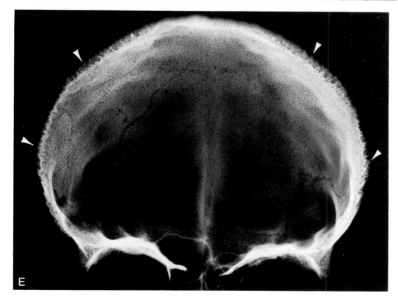

FIGURE 21–1 *Continued*

B–D Appearance of skull sutures in a 4 week old child *(B)*, the somewhat more narrowed sutures of a child aged 14 months *(C)*, and further narrowing of the sutures in a child of 7 years *(D)*.

E A radiograph of the frontal bone in a young child reveals the serrated, irregular nature of the bone (arrowheads) that interdigitates with similar outgrowths in the adjacent bone near the time of sutural closure.

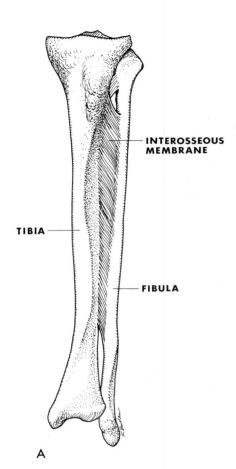

INTEROSSEOUS
MEMBRANE

TIBIA

FIBULA

A

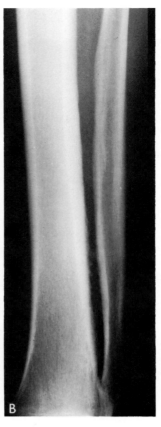

B

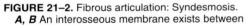

FIGURE 21–2. Fibrous articulation: Syndesmosis.

A, B An interosseous membrane exists between
the lateral border of the tibia and the medial border
of the fibula. Note the orientation of its fibers and
observe the slight irregularity of the apposing osseous surfaces on the radiograph.

C, D The interosseous membrane between the
medial aspect of the radius and the lateral aspect
of the ulna originates approximately 3 cm below the
radial tuberosity and extends to the wrist, containing apertures for various interosseous vessels. The
radiograph reveals an osseous crest on apposing
surfaces of bone.

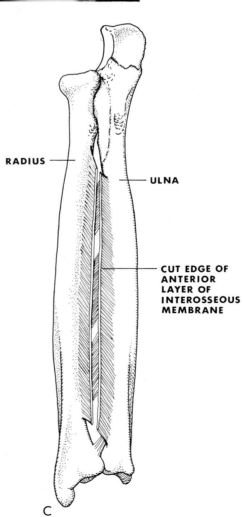

RADIUS

ULNA

CUT EDGE OF
ANTERIOR
LAYER OF
INTEROSSEOUS
MEMBRANE

C

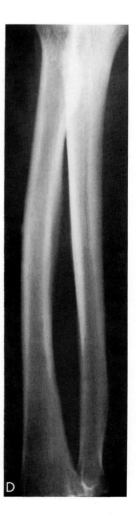

D

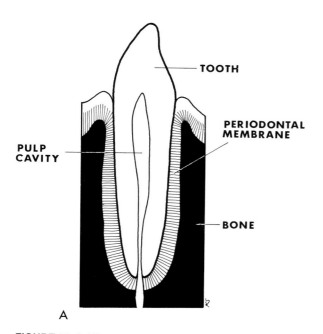

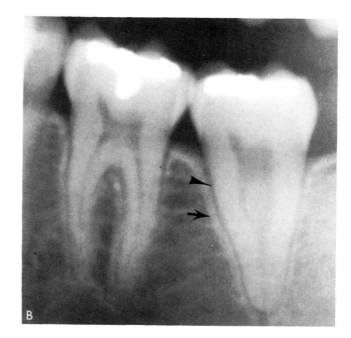

FIGURE 21–3. Fibrous articulation: Gomphosis.
A A diagrammatic representation of this special type of articulation located between the teeth and the maxilla or mandible. Note the location of the periodontal membrane.
B A radiograph reveals the radiolucent periodontal membrane (arrowhead) and the radiopaque lamina dura (arrow).

other principles governing the thickness of articular cartilage; such cartilage is thicker (1) in large joints than in small joints; (2) in joints or areas of joints in which there is considerable functional pressure or stress, such as those in the lower extremity; (3) at sites of extensive frictional or shearing force; (4) in poorly fitted articulations compared with smoothly fitted ones; and (5) in young and middle-aged persons; it is thinner in older people. Nonuse of a joint may lead to cartilage thinning, whereas excessive use during exercise may lead to temporary cartilage swelling related to imbibition of fluid by cartilage cells and matrix.

The color of articular cartilage varies with age; it is white or bluish-white in children, white and glossy in young adults, yellowish-white in middle-aged persons, and yellowish-brown in elderly persons.[13] Although cartilage appears perfectly smooth when viewed by the naked eye, microscopic examination, particularly using electron microscopy, demonstrates minor surface irregularities produced by wear and tear of normal life.[1] These surface undulations may vary between 76.2×10^{-6} cm and 508×10^{-6} cm. With advancing age, the undulating cartilaginous surface may become even more irregular. Synovial fluid may pool between the surface irregularities, accounting for the low coefficient of friction that is characteristic of articular cartilage.[46]

Histologic examination of articular cartilage demonstrates a cellular component (chondrocytes) embedded within an intercellular matrix consisting of collagenous fibrils in a homogeneous ground substance. The ground substance contains water and mucopolysaccharides, particularly chondroitin sulfate. The superficial tangential zone of cartilage consists of densely packed collagen fiber bundles, 20 to 32 nm in diameter.[14] Many of these fibers parallel the articular surface. Beneath the superficial zone, collagen fi-

ber bundles have a more random orientation, and individual collagen fibers have a diameter of approximately 80 nm. A cross-linked latticework of fine fibrils can be noted.

There are differences in the appearance of cells in these various zones of articular cartilage. Cells in the superficial layer generally are smaller in size, flattened in shape, and arranged parallel to the articular surface. In the more deeply situated transitional and radial zones of cartilage, cells appear less flattened and may be arranged in groups or columns.[13] The radial zone is the largest layer, beneath which is the calcified zone of articular cartilage, which connects the hyaline cartilage to the subarticular bone.

Cartilage has a high water content, being approximately 70 to 75 per cent water by weight. The water is distributed within the cells in the matrix.[15, 16] The dry weight composition of hyaline cartilage is approximately one half collagen and one half chondroitin sulfate bound to protein.[9] Chondroitin sulfate occurs in two forms—the A and C types—and is important in regulating the consistency and elasticity of the cartilage matrix.[15, 17, 18] In elderly persons, small amounts of keratosulfate also may be noted.

Subchondral Bone Plate and Tidemark

The bony or subchondral endplate is a layer of osseous tissue of variable thickness that is located beneath the cartilage (Fig. 21–8). Its features have been well delineated by Jaffe.[13] In most articulations the subchondral bone plate consists of trabeculae that curve around the inferior aspect of the cartilage. Occasionally the plate consists of thick trabeculae resembling a subchondral cortex, which is perforated in certain areas by vessels extending from subchondral bone into overlying cartilage.

Immediately superficial to the subchondral bone plate is

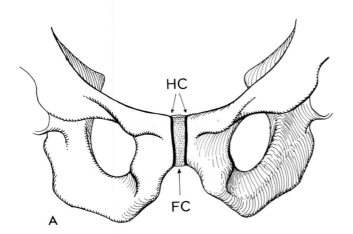

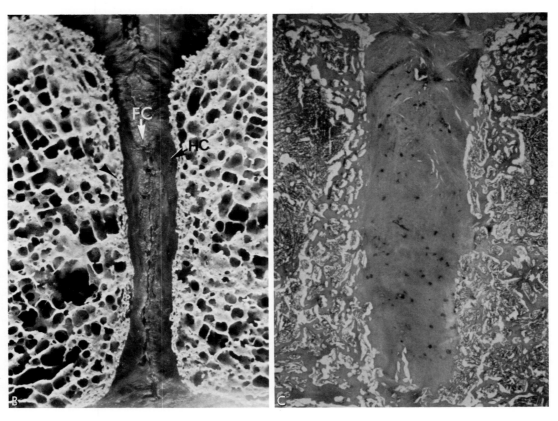

FIGURE 21–4. Cartilaginous articulation: Symphysis (symphysis pubis).

A On the diagram, note the central fibrocartilage *(FC),* with a thin layer of hyaline cartilage *(HC)* adjacent to the osseous surfaces of the pubis.

B A photograph of a partially macerated symphysis pubis better delineates the structure of the central fibrocartilage *(FC),* peripheral hyaline cartilage *(HC),* and subchondral bone (arrowhead).

C A photomicrograph (8×) of a symphysis pubis outlines central fibrocartilage, surrounding hyaline cartilage, and subchondral trabeculae.

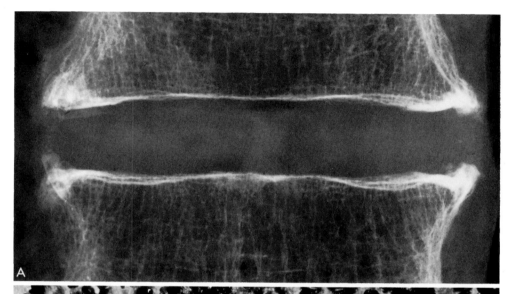

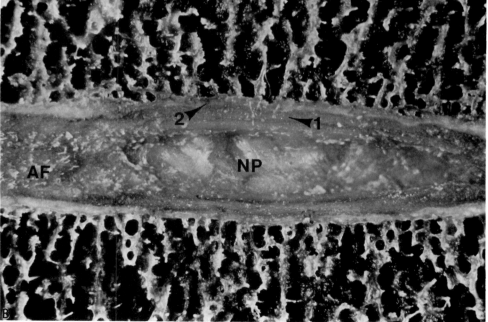

FIGURE 21–5. Cartilaginous articulation: Symphysis (intervertebral disc).

A A magnification radiograph of the discovertebral junction reveals the radiolucent intervertebral disc surrounded by two vertebral bodies. Note the well defined subchondral bone plate of each vertebra.

B A photograph of the discovertebral junction reveals the nucleus pulposus *(NP),* anulus fibrosus *(AF),* cartilaginous endplate *(1),* and subchondral bone plate *(2).*

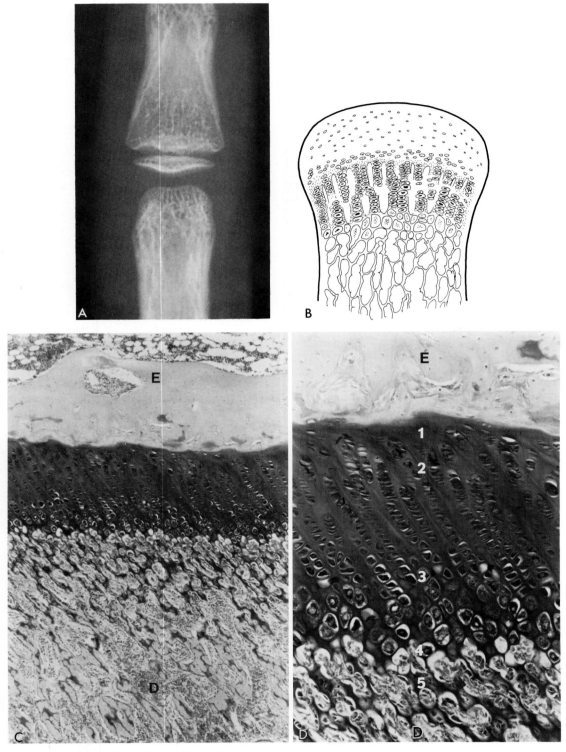

FIGURE 21–6. Cartilaginous articulation: Synchondrosis.

A A radiograph of the phalanges in a growing child demonstrates a typical epiphysis separated from the metaphysis and diaphysis by the radiolucent growth plate.

B A schematic drawing of a growth plate between the cartilaginous epiphysis and the ossified diaphysis of a long bone. Note the transition from hyaline cartilage through various cartilaginous zones, including resting cartilage, cell proliferation, cell hypertrophy, cell calcification, and bone formation.

C, D Photomicrographs of a physeal (growth) plate in a rabbit femur. The lower power (20×) and higher power (50×) photomicrographs reveal the various zones of cartilage in the physeal plate separating the epiphysis *(E)* and diaphysis *(D)*. These zones include resting cartilage *(1),* cell proliferation *(2),* cell hypertrophy *(3),* cell calcification *(4),* and ossification *(5).*

the calcified zone of articular cartilage, termed the tidemark.[19-21] Projections from this zone interdigitate with indentations on the osseous surface and firmly anchor the calcified cartilage to the subchondral bone. Furthermore, fibrils within the deepest part of the noncalcified cartilage are attached to the calcified zone of cartilage. Thus, the tidemark serves a mechanical function; it anchors the collagen fibers of the noncalcified portion of cartilage and, in turn, is anchored to the subchondral bone plate. These strong connections resist disruption by shearing force.

The calcified layer of cartilage may have additional functions. Some investigators believe that this layer limits harmful diffusion of water and solutes between bone and cartilage.[22, 23] In addition, the calcified layer forms an integral part of the enlarging epiphysis[24] and therefore is important in endochondral ossification during growth and remodeling.

Articular Capsule

The articular capsule is connective tissue that envelops the joint cavity. It is composed of a thick, tough outer layer, the fibrous capsule, and a more delicate thin inner layer, the synovial membrane.

Fibrous Capsule. The fibrous capsule consists of parallel and interlacing bundles of dense white fibrous tissue. At each end of the articulation, the fibrous capsule is firmly adherent to the periosteum of the articulating bones. The site of attachment of the capsule to the periosteum is variable; in some articulations, a large segment of bone may be intracapsular whereas in others a short segment of bone is present within the capsule.

The fibrous capsule is not of uniform thickness. Ligaments and tendons may attach to it, producing focal areas of increased thickness. In fact, at some sites the fibrous capsules are replaced by tendons or tendinous expansions from neighboring muscles. Extracapsular accessory ligaments, such as those about the sternoclavicular joint, and intracapsular ligaments, such as the cruciate ligaments of the knee, also may be found. These ligaments are tough strands of connective tissue that resist excessive or abnormal motion. They generally are inelastic, although they may demonstrate small degrees of elasticity.[25]

The fibrous capsule is richly supplied with blood and lymphatic vessels and nerves, which may penetrate the capsule and extend down to the synovial membrane. Capsular blood vessels are particularly prominent and numerous at the margin of the articular cartilage. Additional openings in the capsule may be found that allow the synovial membrane to protrude in the form of a pouch or sac.

Microscopic evaluation of the fibrous capsule reveals tissue of varying cellularity.[13] Areas exist that appear tendinous, being poorly supplied with cells, whereas other areas consist of richly cellular connective tissue.

Synovial Membrane. The synovial membrane is a delicate, highly vascular inner membrane of the articular capsule (Fig. 21–9). It lines the nonarticular portion of the synovial joint and any intra-articular ligaments or tendons. The synovial membrane also covers the intracapsular osseous surfaces, which are clothed by periosteum or perichondrium but are without cartilaginous surfaces. These latter areas occur frequently at the peripheral portion of the joint and are termed ''marginal'' or ''bare'' areas of the joint.

Sleevelike extensions of synovial tissue may extend for short distances between the cartilage-covered bones,[26] but the central cartilaginous tissue and intra-articular discs are free of synovial tissue. Synovial tissue also lines bursae and tendon sheaths.

The synovial membrane generally is pink, moist, and smooth, although small finger-like projections, termed synovial villi, may be apparent on its inner surface.[27, 28] These villi, which are visible microscopically, are vascular, variable in size and shape, and composed of collagenous fibrils. They are found in special areas of the joint—for example, in sites at which the synovial membrane covers loose areolar tissue. Synovial villi may form as a developmental outgrowth of the synovial membrane or by splitting and detachment of the surface tissue, or both.[47] Synovial membrane inflammation or irritation causes excessive villus formation and, in pathologic situations, villous projections may cover the entire inner surface of the synovial membrane.

In addition to synovial villi, the synovial membrane also may reveal thickened folds that extend into the articular cavity (e.g., alar folds and ligamentum mucosum of knee). Furthermore, adipose tissue may accumulate within the synovial membrane, forming articular fat pads. These latter collections act as flexible, compressible cushions extending into irregular areas of the joint cavity. In some joints, such as the elbow, the fat pads occupy a depression on the osseous surface and are displaced during articular motion.

The synovial membrane demonstrates variable structural characteristics in different segments of the joint. In general, there are two synovial layers, a thin cellular surface layer (intima) and a deeper vascular underlying layer (subintima). The subintimal layer merges on its deep surface with the fibrous capsule. In certain locations, the synovial membrane is attenuated and fails to demonstrate two distinct layers. Sites at which the synovial membrane lines intra-articular ligaments or tendons, such as the cruciates and quadriceps, may not possess a distinct subintima, as the fibrous tissue merges imperceptibly with the adjacent capsule or tendon.

Synovial Intima. The synovial intima consists of one to four rows of synovial cells embedded in a granular, fiber-free intercellular matrix.[2] The cells are of variable shape and may appear flattened and elongated or polyhedral.[29] The cells may be closely packed in some areas of the articular cavity and poorly apposed elsewhere, allowing subintimal tissue to be interspersed among the surface cells and to be in direct contact with the synovial cavity. Two types of synovial lining cells have been identified: type A cells resemble macrophages and appear important in phagocytic functions, whereas type B cells, which are less numerous, have a somewhat different appearance and may be responsible for hyaluronate secretion.[9, 48] This classification system should not be applied rigorously as, frequently, cells are identified with characteristics of both types A and B cells.[49] Although it is generally believed that type A cells are derived from macrophages and type B cells from fibroblasts, actually both may arise from a single cell type.

Synovial Subintima. The synovial subintima usually contains areolar tissue. Occasionally it is composed of either loose or more fibrous connective tissue.[30] Cellular constituents include fat cells, fibroblasts, macrophages, and mast cells. An elastic component consisting of elastin fibers paralleling the surface of the membrane prevents the for-

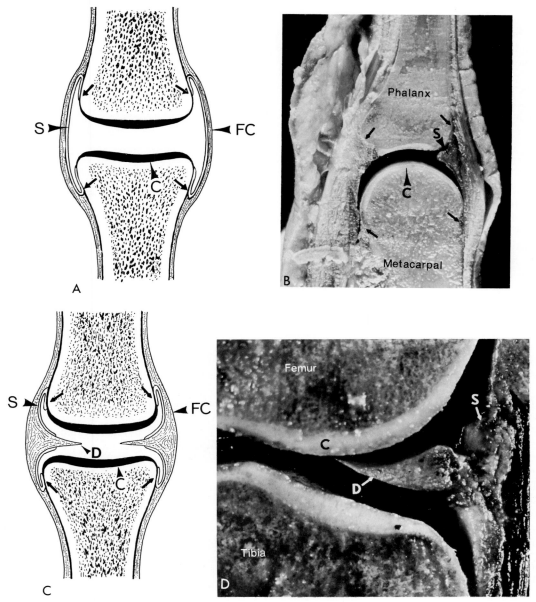

FIGURE 21–7. Synovial articulation: General features.

A, B Typical synovial joint without an intra-articular disc. A diagram and photograph of a section through a metacarpophalangeal joint outline important structures, including fibrous capsule *(FC)*, synovial membrane *(S)*, and articular cartilage *(C)*. Note that there are marginal areas of the articulation where synovial membrane abuts on bone without protective cartilage (arrows).

C, D Typical synovial joint containing an articular disc that partially divides the joint cavity. Diagram and photograph of a section through the knee joint reveal fibrous capsule *(FC)*, synovial membrane *(S)*, articular cartilage *(C)*, and articular disc *(D)*. The marginal areas of the joint again are indicated by arrows.

Illustration continued on opposite page

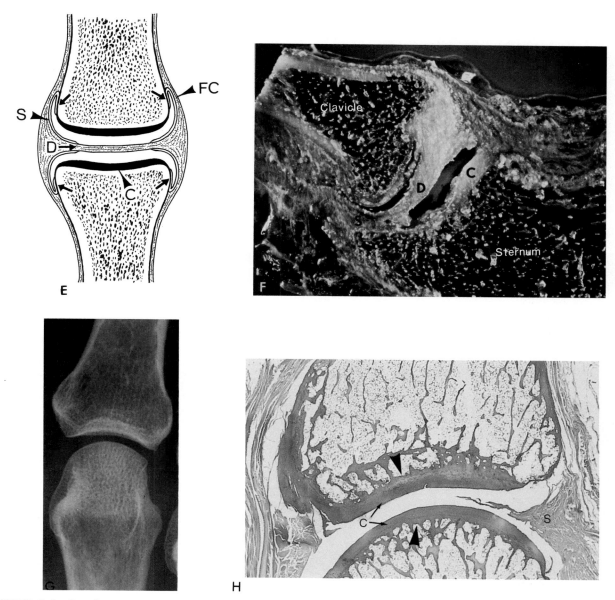

FIGURE 21–7 *Continued*

E, F Typical synovial joint with an articular disc that completely divides the joint cavity. Diagram and photograph of a section through the sternoclavicular joint reveal fibrous capsule *(FC),* articular cartilage *(C),* synovial membrane *(S),* and intra-articular disc *(D).* The marginal areas are indicated by arrows.

G A radiograph of a metacarpophalangeal joint, indicating smooth articular surfaces of the metacarpal head and proximal phalanx separated by a joint cavity.

H A photomicrograph (10×) of a metacarpophalangeal joint. Observe synovium *(S),* articular cartilage *(C),* and subchondral bone plate (arrowheads).

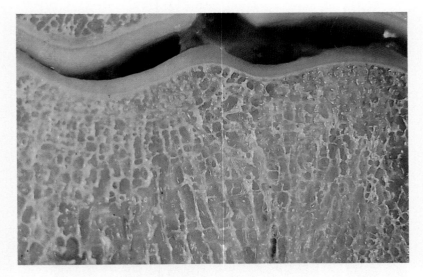

A

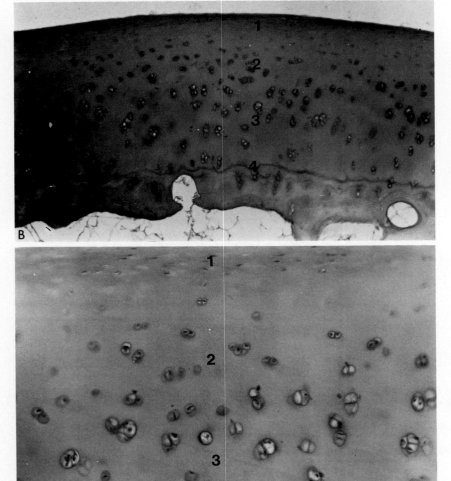

B

C

FIGURE 21–8. Synovial articulation: Articular cartilage and subchondral bone plate.

   A A photograph of a macerated joint demonstrates the articular cartilage, subchondral bone plate, and adjacent trabeculae.

   B, C Photomicrographs at low power (80×) and high power (200×). Observe the tangential zone *(1)* with flattened cartilage cells, the transitional zone *(2)* with numerous irregularly distributed cells, the radial zone *(3)* with columnar arrangement of cells, and the calcified zone *(4)* adjacent to the osseous surface.

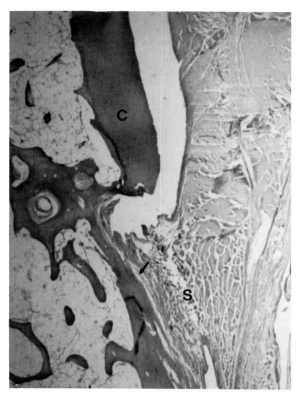

FIGURE 21–9. Synovial articulation: Synovial membrane. Low power (80×) photomicrograph of the chondro-osseous junction about a metacarpophalangeal joint delineates the synovial membrane *(S)* and articular cartilage *(C)*. The marginal area of the joint at which synovial membrane abuts on bone is well demonstrated (arrow).

mation of redundant synovial folds, which might be compromised during articular motion.

The synovial membrane has several functions (Table 21–2). First, it is involved in the secretion of a sticky mucoid substance into the synovial fluid. Second, owing to its inherent flexibility, loose synovial folds, villi, and marginal recesses, the synovium facilitates and accomodates the changing shape of the articular cavity that is required for normal joint motion, an ability that is lost in instances of adhesive capsulitis, which are accompanied by a decrease in synovial flexibility.[49] In addition, the synovial membrane aids the removal of substances from the articular cavity. The route of egress of these intra-articular substances depends on the size of the particles; small particles may traverse the synovial membrane and enter subintimal capillaries and venules directly, whereas larger particles may be removed via lymphatic channels.

TABLE 21–2. Synovial Membrane

Function	Site
Mucin component of synovial fluid	? Type B cells
Dialysate component of synovial fluid	Capillaries
Phagocytosis	Type A cells
Drainage of wastes from cavity	Lymphatics
	Capillaries
Regulation of entry of nutrients	Entire synovial membrane

Intra-articular Disc (Meniscus), Labrum, and Fat Pad

A fibrocartilaginous disc or meniscus may be found in some joints, such as the knee, wrist, and temporomandibular, acromioclavicular, sternoclavicular, and costovertebral joints (Fig. 21–10). The peripheral portion of the disc attaches to the fibrous capsule. Blood vessels and afferent nerves may be noted within this peripheral zone of the disc. Most of the articular disc, however, is avascular. The disc may divide the joint cavity partially or completely; complete discs are found in the sternoclavicular and wrist joints, whereas partial discs are noted in the knee and acromioclavicular articulations. In the temporomandibular joint, the disc may be partial or complete. Even the complete disc may reveal small perforations. Although the tissue of the intra-articular disc generally is referred to as fibrocartilage, it more accurately may represent fibroelastic connective tissue.[13] Collagenous connective tissue is interspersed with elastic fibers. The elastic tissue is particularly prominent in the central portion of a disc. Cellular components also are evident.

The exact function of intra-articular discs is unknown. Suggested functions include shock absorption, distribution of weight over a large surface, facilitation of various motions (such as rotation) and limitation of others (such as translation), and protection of the articular surface.[31] It has been suggested that intra-articular discs play an important role in the effective lubrication of a joint.[32] For example, in the knee joint, interposed menisci separate the synovial fluid into two wedge-shaped collections of lubricant. These collections provide efficient lubrication, which allows one surface to roll over an adjacent one. Further evidence that articular discs play an important role in joint motion is the presence of these structures in joints that display translation movements.[2] In these articulations, such as the temporomandibular joint, intra-articular cartilaginous discs may provide increased congruity of joint surface and even distribution of intervening synovial fluid.

Some joints, such as the hip and glenohumeral articulations, contain circumferential cartilaginous folds termed labra (Fig. 21–10). These lips of cartilage usually are triangular in cross section and are attached to the peripheral portion of an articular surface, thereby acting to enlarge or deepen the joint cavity. They also may help increase contact and congruity of adjacent articular surfaces, particularly at the extremes of joint motion.

Fat pads represent additional structures that may be present within a joint (Fig. 21–10). These structures possess a generous vascular and nerve supply, contain few lymphatic vessels, and are covered by a flattened layer of synovial cells. Fat pads may act as cushions, absorbing forces generated across a joint, thus protecting adjacent bony processes. They also may distribute lubricants in the joint cavity.

Synovial Fluid

Minute amounts of clear, colorless to pale yellow, highly viscous fluid of slightly alkaline pH are present in healthy joints. The exact composition, viscosity, volume, and color vary somewhat from joint to joint. This fluid represents a dialysate of blood plasma to which has been added a mu-

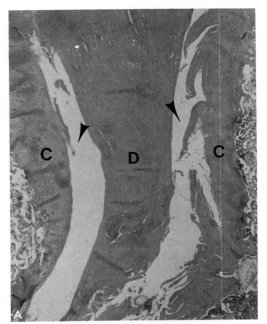

FIGURE 21–10. Synovial articulation: Intra-articular disc, labrum, and fat pad.

A A photomicrograph (10×) reveals the structure of the intra-articular disc *(D)* of the sternoclavicular joint. Note the two joint cavities (arrowheads) and articular cartilage *(C)* of sternum and clavicle.

B A photograph of a coronal section through the superior aspect of the glenohumeral joint demonstrates a cartilaginous labrum (arrowhead) along the superior aspect of the glenoid. Note the adjacent rotator cuff tendons (arrow).

C In a photograph of a sagittal section through the humeroulnar aspect of the elbow joint, note the intra-articular anterior and posterior fat pads (arrowheads), which are elevated by a large amount of intra-articular air.

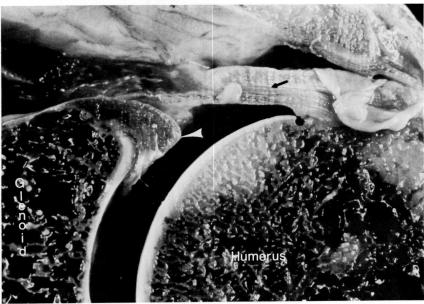

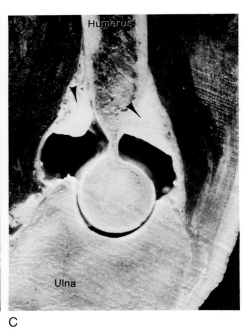

coid substance secreted by the synovial cells. A small number of cells is present within the synovial fluid, consisting of monocytes, lymphocytes, macrophages, polymorphonuclear leukocytes, and free synovial cells.[33] Erythrocytes occasionally are noted in normal synovial fluid, most likely representing contamination of the fluid due to the trauma of joint aspiration. Particles, cell fragments, and fibrous tissue also may be seen in the synovial fluid as a result of wear and tear of the articular surface. Various enzymes, such as alkaline phosphatase, are found in synovial fluid.

Functions of the synovial fluid are nutrition of the adjacent articular cartilage and disc and lubrication of joint surfaces, which decreases friction and increases joint efficiency. The cells within the synovial fluid are important in phagocytosis, removing microorganisms and joint debris.

Synovial Sheaths and Bursae

Synovial tissue also is found about various tendon sheaths and bursae (Fig. 21–11). This tissue is located at sites where closely apposed structures move in relationship to each other. Typical examples include tendons that are reflected or angulated about bony surfaces and bursae that separate skin from subjacent bony protuberances.

Tendon sheaths completely or partially cover a portion of the tendon where it passes through fascial slings, osseofibrous tunnels, and ligamentous bands. They function to promote the gliding of tendons and contribute to the nutri-

tion of the intrasheath portion of the tendons.[50] Tendon sheaths are composed of two coats separated by a thin film of synovial fluid. The inner coat or visceral layer is attached to the surface of the tendon by loose areolar tissue. The outer coat or parietal layer is attached to adjacent connective tissue or periosteum. The invaginated tendon allows apposition of visceral and parietal layers in the form of a mesotendon. This latter structure carries blood vessels and is attached to a longitudinal line or hilus along the nonfrictional surface of the tendon. The tendon sheath also contains nerves and lymphatics. The microscopic structure of the tendon sheath resembles that of a synovial membrane.[13] Some areas are cellular, whereas others are poorly cellular. Small amounts of areolar tissue are focally interposed between the two coats of the tendon sheath.

Bursae represent enclosed flattened sacs consisting of synovial lining and, in some locations, a thin film of synovial fluid, which provides both lubrication and nourishment for the cells of the synovial membrane. Intervening bursae facilitate motion between apposing tissues. Subcutaneous bursae are found between skin and underlying bony prominences, such as the olecranon and patella; subfascial bursae are placed between deep fascia and bone; subtendinous bursae exist where one tendon overlies another tendon; submucosal bursae are located between muscle and bone, tendon, or ligament; interligamentous bursae separate ligaments. When bursae are located near articulations, the synovial membrane of the bursa may be continuous with

FIGURE 21–11. Tendons and tendon sheaths.
A Extensor tendons with surrounding synovial sheaths pass beneath the extensor retinaculum on the dorsum of the wrist.
B A drawing of the fine structure of a tendon and tendon sheath reveals an inner coat or visceral layer adjacent to the tendon surface and an outer coat or parietal layer. Note that the invaginated tendon allows apposition of visceral and parietal layers in the form of a mesotendon. This latter structure provides a passageway for adjacent blood vessels.

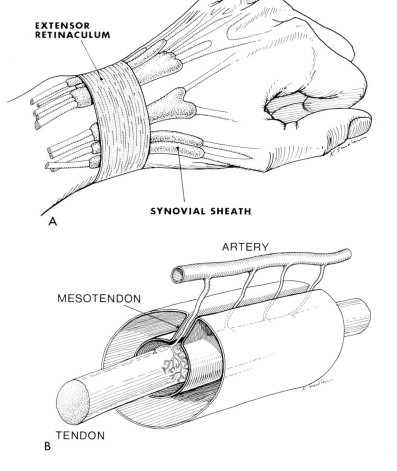

B

that of the joint cavity, producing communicating bursae. This occurs normally about the hip (iliopsoas bursa) and knee (gastrocnemiosemimembranous bursa) and abnormally about the glenohumeral joint (subacromial bursa) owing to defects in the rotator cuff. Distention of communicating bursae may serve to lower intra-articular pressure in cases of joint effusion. At certain sites where skin is subject to pressure and lateral displacement, adventitious bursae may appear, allowing increased freedom of motion. Examples of adventitious bursae include those that may develop over a hallux valgus deformity, those occurring about prominent spinous processes, and bursae located adjacent to exostoses.[50] Deeply situated adventitious bursae may appear in areas of pseudarthrosis and internal fixation devices.[50]

Fluid similar to joint fluid normally is present in deep bursae, but not in such superficial bursae as those in the olecranon and prepatellar regions.[51] In the latter locations, a lubricating film (perhaps hyaluronic acid) may be responsible for the gliding motions that exist between the bursal surfaces.[50, 51]

Sesamoid Bones

Sesamoids generally are ovoid nodules of small size that are embedded in tendons (Fig. 21–12). They are found in two specific situations in the skeleton.

Type A. The sesamoid is located adjacent to a joint, and its tendon is incorporated into the joint capsule. The sesamoid nodule and adjacent bone form an extension of the articulation. Examples of this type are the patella and the hallucis and pollicis sesamoids.

Type B. The sesamoid is located at sites where tendons are angled about bony surfaces. They are separated from the underlying bone by a synovium-lined bursa. An example of this type of sesamoid is the sesamoid of the peroneus longus.

In both type A and type B situations, the arrangement of the sesamoid nodule and surrounding tissue resembles a synovial joint. Osseous surfaces are covered by cartilage and are intimate with the synovium-lined cavity. This type of arrangement has led many investigators to consider sesamoids as primarily articular in nature, their association with tendons representing a secondary phenomenon. In the hand, sesamoid nodules adjacent to joints (type A) are present most frequently on the palmar aspect of the metacarpophalangeal joints, particularly the first.[60] In this location, two sesamoids are found in the tendons of the adductor pollicis and flexor pollicis brevis, articulating with facets on the palmar surface of the metacarpal head. Additional sesamoids are most frequent in the second and fifth metacarpophalangeal joints and adjacent to the interphalangeal joint of the thumb.[34] This distribution of sesamoids in the hand is not constant. Examples of decreased and increased numbers of sesamoids have been described.[35]

Sesamoid distribution in the foot parallels that in the hand. Two sesamoids are located on the plantar aspect of the first metatarsophalangeal joint in the tendons of the flexor hallucis brevis. Sesamoid nodules also may be present at other metatarsophalangeal joints and the interphalangeal joint of the great toe. Sesamoid bones unassociated with synovial joints (type B) are more frequent in the lower extremity than in the upper extremity. In the foot, sesa-

moids of this type are noted in the tendon of the peroneus longus muscle adjacent to a facet on the tuberosity of the cuboid bone, in the tendon of the tibialis anterior muscle in contact with the medial surface of the medial cuneiform bone, and in the tendon of the tibialis posterior muscle adjacent to the medial aspect of the talus.

Alterations of sesamoids include their displacement in instances of joint effusion,[52] fracture and dislocation,[53] participation in various articular disorders,[54, 60] congenital anomalies, and, perhaps, idiopathic inflammation (sesamoiditis).

SUPPORTING STRUCTURES

A variety of supporting structures exist in periarticular locations or in a more general distribution; these structures influence the manifestations of articular disorders. In some disorders, the supporting structures are themselves involved. Rather than review in depth all of these structures, several important ones are identified here.

Tendons

Tendons represent a portion of a muscle and are of constant length, consisting of collagen fibers that transmit muscle tension to a mobile part of the body. They are flexible cords, white in color, smooth in texture, that can be angulated about bony protuberances, changing the direction of pull of the muscle. On the surface of the tendon, areolar connective tissue—the epitendineum—allows passage of vessels and nerves. Synovial sheaths may surround portions of the tendon.

The attachment sites of tendons are of particular interest.[50] At the muscle, tendon collagen fibrils are embedded in invaginations of the muscle cell membrane at the end of each muscle fiber. With regard to the osseous attachment of the tendon (an *enthesis*), four histologic zones can be identified (Fig. 21–13): the tendon itself; unmineralized fibrocartilage, consisting of collagen fibers and chondrocytes; mineralized fibrocartilage in which crystals are apparent between and within the collagen fibrils; and bone, at which site there is no perceptible separation between mineralized fibrocartilage and the collagen fibrils of the osseous matrix.[50, 55] These fibrous connections commonly (though not consistently) are referred to as Sharpey's (perforating) fibers. The enthesis is nourished by anastomosing channels within the peritenon, perichondrium, and periosteum. Entheses are metabolically active, have a prominent nerve supply, and are involved in a number of degenerative, traumatic, and inflammatory processes.[56, 57]

Aponeuroses

Aponeuroses consist of several flat layers or sheets of dense collagen fibers associated with the attachment of a muscle. The fasciculi within one layer of an aponeurosis are parallel and different in direction from fasciculi of an adjacent layer.

Fasciae

Fascia is a general term used to describe a focal collection of connective tissue. Superficial fascia consists of a

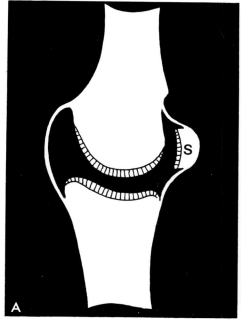

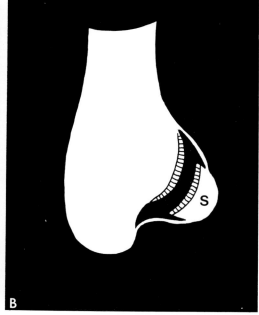

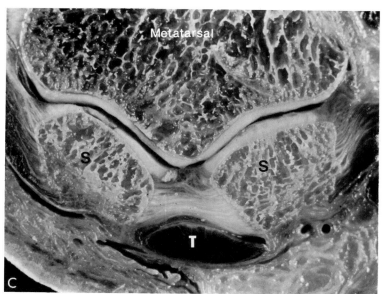

FIGURE 21–12. Sesamoid bones.

A, B There are two types of sesamoids[2]: type A **(A),** in which the sesamoid is located adjacent to an articulation, and type B **(B),** in which the sesamoid is separated from the underlying bone by a bursa. In both types, the sesamoid is intimately associated with a synovial lining and articular cartilage (hatched areas).

C A photograph of the sesamoids *(S)* of the first metatarsophalangeal joint. At this articulation, there are medial and lateral sesamoid bones *(S)* embedded in the plantar part of the capsule of the joint within the tendon of the flexor hallucis brevis *(T)*. Note the articular cartilage on the sesamoids and adjacent metatarsal.

D The sesamoid distribution in the hand and foot is revealed. Type A sesamoids are present most constantly about the metacarpophalangeal joint and interphalangeal joint of the first digit of the hand and the metatarsophalangeal joint and interphalangeal joint of the first digit of the foot. Inconstant sesamoids may be located about any metacarpophalangeal, metatarsophalangeal, or interphalangeal joint.

(**A–D**, From Resnick D, Niwayama G, Feingold ML: Radiology *123*:57, 1977.)

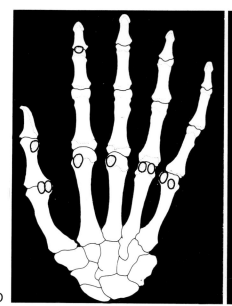

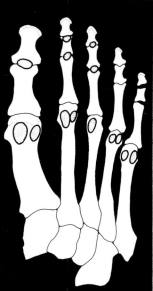

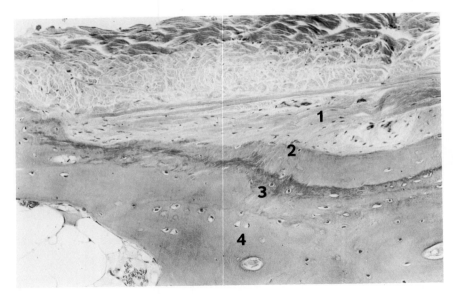

FIGURE 21–13. Tendinous attachment to bone: Enthesis. A photomicrograph outlines the four zones of an enthesis: *1*, tendon; *2*, unmineralized fibrocartilage; *3*, mineralized fibrocartilage; *4*, lamellar bone. (Hematoxylin and eosin stain, 210×).

layer of loose areolar tissue of variable thickness beneath the dermis. It is most distinct over the lower abdomen, perineum, and limbs. Deep fascia resembles an aponeurosis, consisting of regularly arranged, compact collagen fibers. Parallel fibers of one layer are angled with respect to the fibers of an adjacent layer. Deep fascia is particularly prominent in the extremities, and in these sites, muscle may arise from the inner aspect of the deep fascia. At sites where deep fascia contacts bone, the fascia fuses with the periosteum. It is well suited to transmit the pull of adjacent musculature. Intermuscular septa extend from deep fascia between groups of muscles, producing functional compartments. Retinacula are transverse thickenings in the deep fascia that are attached to bony protuberances, creating tunnels through which tendons can pass. An example is the dorsal retinaculum of the wrist, under which extend the extensor tendons and their synovial sheaths.

Ligaments

Ligaments represent fibrous bands that unite bones. They do not transmit muscle action directly but are essential in the control of posture and the maintenance of joint stability.[50] Classification of ligaments according to constituency (collagenous and elastic) or location (articular, extra-articular, and vertebral) is possible.[50] Histologically and biomechanically, ligaments resemble tendons, and their sites of osseous attachment (entheses) are similar to those of tendons.

Ligaments also can be classified into those connecting skeletal elements and those joining other soft tissues.[58] Precise names of ligaments in the former group reflect sites of bone attachment (e.g., coracoacromial), function (e.g., capsular), relationship to joints (e.g., collateral), and shape (e.g., deltoid).[58]

VASCULAR, LYMPHATIC, AND NERVE SUPPLY

The blood supply of joints arises from periarticular arterial plexuses that pierce the capsule, break up in the syno-

vial membrane, and form a rich and intricate network of capillaries. Many of the vessels are located superficially in the synovium, perhaps explaining the frequency of hemorrhage after even relatively insignificant trauma to the joint.[36] A circle of vessels (circulus articuli vasculosus) within the synovial membrane is adjacent to the peripheral margin of articular cartilage.

The lymphatics form a plexus in the subintima of the synovial membrane. Efferent vessels pass toward the flexor aspect of the joint and then along blood vessels to regional deep lymph nodes.

The nerve supply of movable joints generally arises from the same nerves that supply the adjacent musculature.[59] The fibrous capsule and to a lesser extent the synovial membrane are both supplied by nerves. Each nerve supplies a specific segment of the capsule, but a good deal of overlap in innervation exists. Some of the nerves in the fibrous capsule have encapsulated nerve endings; others have free nerve endings. The encapsulated endings are thought to be proprioceptive in nature,[37, 38] whereas the free nerve endings, numerous at the attachments of fibrous capsule and ligaments, are believed to mediate pain sensation.[39] This would explain the extreme pain that is common after injury to joint ligaments. The synovial membrane itself is relatively insensitive to pain.[40]

References

1. Walmsley R.: Joints. *In* GJ Romanes (Ed): Cunningham's Textbook of Anatomy. 11th Ed. London, Oxford University Press, 1972, p 207.
2. Warwick R, Williams PL: Arthrology. *In* Gray's Anatomy. 35th British Ed. Philadelphia, WB Saunders Co, 1973, p 388.
3. Pritchard JJ, Scott JH, Girgis FG: The structure and development of cranial and facial sutures. J Anat 90:73, 1956.
4. Todd TW, Lyon DW Jr: Endocranial suture closure. Its progress and age relationship. Part I. Adult males of white stock. Am J Phys Anthropol 7:325, 1924.
5. Todd TW, Lyon DW Jr: Cranial suture closure. Part II. Ectocranial closure in adult males of white stock. Am J Phys Anthropol 8:23, 1925.
6. Todd TW, Lyon DW Jr: Suture closure. Part III. Endocranial closure in adult males of negro stock. Am J Phys Anthropol 8:47, 1925.
7. Todd TW, Lyon DW Jr: Suture closure. Its progress and age relationship. Part IV. Ectocranial closure in adult males of negro stock. Am J Phys Anthropol 8:149, 1925.
8. Abbie AA: Closure of cranial articulations in the skull of the Australian aborigine. J Anat 84:1, 1950.

9. Hamerman D, Rosenberg LC, Schubert M: Diarthrodial joints revisited. J Bone Joint Surg [Br] 52:725, 1970.

10. Barnett CH, Cobbold AF: Lubrication within living joints. J Bone Joint Surg [Br] 44:662, 1962.

11. Ingelmark BE: The nutritive supply and nutritional value of synovial fluid. Acta Orthop Scand 20:144, 1951.

12. Hunter W: On the structure and diseases of articular cartilage. Phil Trans B 42:514, 1743.

13. Jaffe HL: Metabolic, Degenerative and Inflammatory Diseases of Bones and Joints. Philadelphia, Lea & Febiger, 1972, p 80.

14. Weiss C, Rosenberg L, Helfet AJ: An ultrastructural study of normal young adult human articular cartilage. J Bone Joint Surg [Am] 50:663, 1968.

15. Linn FC, Sokoloff L: Movement and composition of interstitial fluid of cartilage. Arthritis Rheum 8:481, 1965.

16. Eichelberger L, Akeson WH, Roma M: Biochemical studies of articular cartilage. I. Normal values. J Bone Joint Surg [Am] 40:142, 1958.

17. Linn FC, Radin EL: Lubrication of animal joints. III. The effect of certain chemical alterations of the cartilage and lubricant. Arthritis Rheum 11:674, 1968.

18. Sokoloff L: Elasticity of articular cartilage: Effect of ions and viscous solutions. Science 141:1055, 1963.

19. Redler I, Mow VC, Zimny ML, et al: The ultrastructure and biomechanical significance of the tidemark of articular cartilage. Clin Orthop 112:357, 1975.

20. Green WT Jr, Martin GN, Eanes ED, et al: Microradiographic study of the calcified layer of articular cartilage. Arch Pathol 90:151, 1970.

21. Fawns HT, Landells JW: Histochemical studies of rheumatic conditions; observations on the fine structures of the matrix of normal bone and cartilage. Ann Rheum Dis 12:105, 1953.

22. Maroudas A, Bullough P, Swanson SAV, et al: The permeability of articular cartilage. J Bone Joint Surg [Br] 50:166, 1968.

23. Ishido B: Gelenkuntersuchungen. Virchows Arch Pathol Anat 244:424, 1923.

24. Mankin HJ: The calcified zone (basal layer) of articular cartilage of rabbits. Anat Rec 145:73, 1963.

25. Smith JW: The elastic properties of the anterior cruciate ligament of the rabbit. J Anat 88:369, 1954.

26. Grant JCB: Interarticular synovial folds. Br J Surg 18:636, 1931.

27. Palmer DG: Synovial villi: An examination of these structures within the anterior compartment of the knee and metacarpo-phalangeal joints. Arthritis Rheum 10:451, 1967.

28. Sigurdson LA: The structure and function of articular synovial membranes. J Bone Joint Surg 12:603, 1930.

29. Barland P, Novikoff AB, Hamerman D: Electron microscopy of the human synovial membrane. J Cell Biol 14:207, 1962.

30. Davies DV: The structure and functions of the synovial membrane. Br Med J 1:92, 1950.

31. Barnett CH, Davies DV, MacConaill MA: Synovial Joints; Their Structure and Mechanics. Springfield, Ill, Charles C Thomas, 1961.

32. MacConaill MA: The function of intra-articular fibrocartilages, with special reference to the knee and inferior radio-ulnar joints. J Anat 66:210, 1932.

33. Bauer W, Ropes MW, Waine H: The physiology of articular structures. Physiol Rev 20:272, 1940.

34. Gray DJ, Gardner E, O'Rahilly R: The prenatal development of the skeleton and joints of the human hand. Am J Anat 101:169, 1957.

35. Jacobs P: Multiple sesamoid bones of the hand and foot. Clin Radiol 25:267, 1974.

36. Davies DV: Anatomy and physiology of diarthrodial joints. Ann Rheum Dis 5:29, 1945.

37. Stopford JSB: The nerve supply of the interphalangeal and metacarpophalangeal joints. J Anat 56:1, 1921.

38. Mountcastle VB, Powell TPS: Central nervous mechanisms subserving position sense and kinesthesis. Bull Johns Hopkins Hosp 105:173, 1959.

39. Gardner ED: Physiology of movable joints. Physiol Rev 30:127, 1950.

40. Kellgren JH, Samuel EP: The sensitivity and innervation of the articular capsule. J Bone Joint Surg [Br] 32:84, 1950.

41. Cronqvist, S: Roentgenologic evaluation of cranial size in children. Acta Radiol Diagn 7:97, 1968.

42. Austin JHM, Gooding CA: Roentgenographic measurement of skull size in children. Radiology 99:641, 1971.

43. Furuya Y, Edwards MSB, Alpers CE, et al: Computerized tomography of cranial sutures. Part 1. Comparison of suture anatomy in children and adults. J Neurosurg 61:53, 1984.

44. Furuya Y, Edwards MSB, Alpers CE, et al: Computerized tomography of cranial sutures. Part 2. Abnormalities of sutures and skull deformities in craniosynostosis. J Neurosurg 61:59, 1984.

45. Ghadially FN: Structure and function of articular cartilage. Clin Rheum Dis 7:3, 1981.

46. McCutchen CW: Joint lubrication. Clin Rheum Dis 7:241, 1981.

47. Edwards JCW, MacKay AR, Sedgwick AD, et al: Mode of formation of synovial villi. Ann Rheum Dis 42:585, 1983.

48. Edwards JCW, Willoughby DA: Demonstration of bone marrow derived cells in synovial lining by means of giant intracellular granules as genetic markers. Ann Rheum Dis 41:177, 1982.

49. Hasselbacher P: Structure of the synovial membrane. Clin Rheum Dis 7:57, 1981.

50. Canoso JJ: Bursae, tendons and ligaments. Clin Rheum Dis 7:189, 1981.

51. Canoso JJ, Stack MT, Brandt KD: Hyaluronic acid content of deep and subcutaneous bursae of man. Ann Rheum Dis 42:171, 1983.

52. Friedman AC, Naidich TP: The fabella sign: Fabella displacement in synovial effusion and popliteal fossa masses. Normal and abnormal fabello-femoral and fabello-tibial distances. Radiology 127:113, 1978.

53. Feldman F, Pochaczevsky R, Hecht H: The case of the wandering sesamoid and other sesamoid afflictions. Radiology 96:275, 1970.

54. Resnick D, Niwayama G, Feingold ML: The sesamoid bones of the hands and feet: Participators in arthritis. Radiology 123:57, 1977.

55. Cooper RR, Misol S: Tendon and ligament insertion. A light and electron microscopic study. J Bone Joint Surg [Am] 52:1, 1970.

56. Ball J: Enthesopathy of rheumatoid and ankylosing spondylitis. Ann Rheum Dis 30:213, 1970.

57. Resnick D, Niwayama G: Entheses and enthesopathy. Anatomical, pathological, and radiological correlation. Radiology 146:1, 1983.

58. Frank C, Amiel D, Woo S L-Y, et al: Normal ligament properties and ligament healing. Clin Orthop 196:15, 1985.

59. Wyke B: The neurology of joints: A review of general principles. Clin Rheum Dis 7:223, 1981.

60. Goldberg I, Nathan H: Anatomy and pathology of the sesamoid bones. The hand compared to the foot. Int Orthop (SICOT) 11:141, 1987.

22

Anatomy of Individual Joints

Donald Resnick, M.D., and Gen Niwayama, M.D.

Anatomic features related to articular and periarticular soft tissue and osseous structures govern the manner in which disease processes become evident on radiographs. This chapter summarizes important osseous and soft tissue anatomy of individual joints in the body. Anatomic features important to internal derangements of joints are discussed further in Chapter 70.

WRIST

Osseous Anatomy

The bony structures about the wrist are the distal portions of the radius and ulna, the proximal and distal rows of carpal bones, and the metacarpals[1,2] (Figs. 22–1 and 22–2).

The distal aspects of the radius and ulna articulate with the proximal row of carpal bones. On the lateral surface of the radius is the radial styloid process, which extends more distally than the remainder of the bone, and from which arises the radial collateral ligament of the wrist joint. The articular surface of the radius is divided into an ulnar and a radial portion by a faint central ridge of bone. The ulnar portion articulates with the lunate and the radial portion articulates with the scaphoid. The articular surface is continuous medially with that of the triangular fibrocartilage. The medial surface of the distal end of the radius contains the concave ulnar notch, which articulates with the distal end of the ulna. The posterior surface of the distal radius is convex and grooved or irregular in outline to allow passage of tendons and tendon sheaths. A prominent ridge in the middle of this surface is the dorsal tubercle of the radius. The anterior surface of the distal portion of the radius allows attachment of the palmar radiocarpal ligaments.

The distal end of the ulna contains a small round head and a styloid process. The lateral aspect contains an articular surface for contact with the ulnar notch of the radius. The ulna also has a distal articular surface, which is intimate with the triangular fibrocartilage. The ulnar styloid process, which extends distally from the posteromedial aspect of the bone, gives rise to the ulnar collateral ligament. Between the styloid process and inferior articular surface, the ulna has an area for attachment of the triangular fibrocartilage and a dorsal groove for the extensor carpi ulnaris tendon and sheath.

The proximal row of carpal bones consists of the scaphoid, lunate, and triquetrum, as well as the pisiform bone within the tendon of the flexor carpi ulnaris. The distal row of carpal bones contains the trapezium, trapezoid, capitate, and hamate bones. The dorsal surface of the carpus is convex from side to side, and the palmar surface presents a deep concavity, termed the carpal groove or canal. The medial border of this palmar carpal groove contains the pisiform and hook of the hamate. The lateral border of the carpal groove contains the tubercles of the scaphoid and the trapezium. A strong fibrous retinaculum attaches to the palmar surface of the carpus, converting the groove into a carpal tunnel, through which pass the median nerve and flexor tendons. Evaluation of this tunnel in cases of median

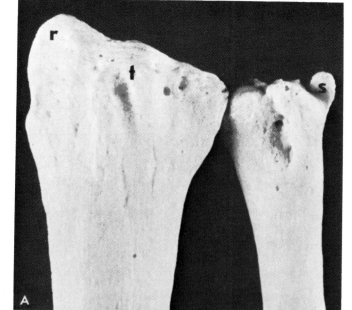

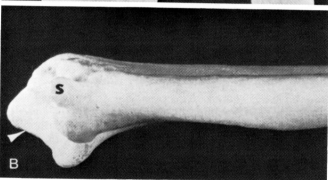

FIGURE 22–1. Distal portions of the radius and ulna: Osseous anatomy.

A Posterior aspect. Note convex surface of the distal end of the radius with radial styloid process *(r)*, dorsal tubercle *(t)* with grooves for passage of various tendons and tendon sheaths, and the surface of the distal end of the ulna with styloid process *(s)* and groove for the extensor carpi ulnaris tendon and tendon sheath.

B Ulnar aspect. Observe ulnar styloid *(s)* and articular surface of distal radius (arrowhead).

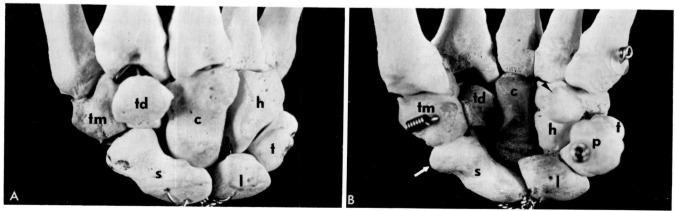

FIGURE 22–2. Carpal bones: Osseous anatomy. Dorsal **(A)** and volar **(B)** aspects. The carpal bones include scaphoid *(s)*, lunate *(l)*, triquetrum *(t)*, pisiform *(p)*, hamate *(h)*, capitate *(c)*, trapezoid *(td)*, and trapezium *(tm)*. Observe the hook of the hamate (arrowhead) and scaphoid tubercle (arrow).

nerve entrapment is best accomplished with CT and MR imaging[230–232] (Chapter 77).

The distal row of carpal bones articulates with the bases of the metacarpals. The trapezium has a saddle-shaped articular surface for the first metacarpal.[233] The trapezoid fits into a deep notch in the second metacarpal. The capitate articulates mainly with the third metacarpal, but also with the second and fourth metacarpals. The hamate articulates with the fourth and fifth metacarpals. The bases of the metacarpals articulate not only with the distal row of carpal bones but also with each other.

The alignment of the bones of the wrist joints varies with wrist position (Fig. 22–3). When the wrist is in neutral position without dorsal or palmar flexion, the distal end of the radius articulates with the scaphoid and approximately 50 per cent of the lunate. The degree of radial shift of the carpus at the radiocarpal joint is determined by comparing the distance between the central axis of the distal end of the radius and the distal aspect of the radial styloid process in the two wrists.[294] Several methods exist for the measurement of ulnar translocation, or ulnarward displacement, of the carpus at the radiocarpal joint.[294] The degree of radial deviation of the radiocarpal compartment can be measured on a posteroanterior radiograph with the wrist in this neutral attitude. A line is drawn through the longitudinal axis of the second metacarpal at its radial cortex.[3] A second line is constructed from the ulnar limit of the distal end of the radius to the tip of the radial styloid process. The second line intersects the first, creating an obtuse angle, which normally averages 112 degrees (range, 92 to 127 degrees).[4] In the neutral position, the spaces between carpal bones are approximately equal in the normal wrist. An abnormal widening of the scapholunate space is termed scapholunate dissociation. On a posteroanterior radiograph of a normal wrist, a line drawn tangentially from the distal tip of the radial styloid through the base of the ulnar styloid process intersects a second line drawn along the midshaft of the radius with an average angle of 83 degrees (72 to 95 degrees).[5]

On a lateral radiograph of a normal wrist in neutral position without palmar flexion or dorsiflexion, a continuous line can be drawn through the longitudinal axes of the radius, lunate, capitate, and third metacarpal.[6] A second line through the longitudinal axis of the scaphoid intersects this first line, creating a scapholunate angle of 30 to 60 degrees. A scapholunate angle of less than 30 degrees or more than 60 degrees suggests carpal instability, which can be classified as (1) dorsiflexion instability, or dorsal intercalated segment instability, in which the lunate is dorsiflexed and displaced in a palmar direction and the scaphoid is displaced vertically, or (2) palmar flexion instability, or volar intercalated segment instability, in which the lunate is flexed in a palmar direction (Chapter 68). On the lateral view, a line drawn tangentially along the distal articular surface of the radius intersects a second line through the midshaft of the radius with an average angle of 86 degrees (79 to 94 degrees).[5]

Radial and ulnar deviation and flexion and extension of the wrist cause changes in the alignment of the carpal bones.[7, 216, 294] In radial deviation, palmar flexion of the proximal carpal bones is noted as the distal end of the scaphoid rotates into the palm. In ulnar deviation, the scaphoid is seen in full profile, the lunate and triquetrum

become more closely apposed, and the pisiform becomes intimate with the tip of the ulnar styloid. Dorsiflexion of the wrist is particularly prominent at the capitate-lunate space, and palmar flexion is pronounced at the lunate-radial space.[7] During wrist flexion, the pisiform tilts on the triquetrum and moves in a volar direction for 2 to 3 mm.[8] During wrist extension, the pisiform slides distally and undergoes some rotation.

The complexity of wrist motion has led to differing concepts of functional osseous anatomy.[234] Some regard the wrist as composed of carpal bones arranged in two rows (proximal and distal) with the scaphoid bridging the two. Others describe a vertical arrangement of the joint as consisting of three columns. A mobile lateral column contains the scaphoid, trapezium, and trapezoid, in which osteoarthritis is most frequent. The central column, containing the lunate and capitate, is concerned with flexion and extension[295] and is primarily implicated in most varieties of carpal instability. The medial column is composed of the triquetrum and hamate, and, on the axis of this column, the rotation of the forearm is extended into the wrist. A third concept considers the wrist as a dynamic ring, with a fixed distal half and a mobile proximal half. Distortion or rupture of the mobile segment with respect to the rigid part explains both instability and dislocation (see Chapter 68).[234]

Soft Tissue Anatomy

The wrist is not a single joint. Rather, it consists of a series of articulations or compartments[1, 2, 9–12] (Figs. 22–4 and 22–5):

1. Radiocarpal compartment.
2. Inferior radioulnar compartment.
3. Midcarpal compartment.
4. Pisiform-triquetral compartment.
5. Common carpometacarpal compartment.
6. First carpometacarpal compartment.
7. Intermetacarpal compartments.

Radiocarpal Compartment. The radiocarpal compartment (Fig. 22–6A, B) is formed proximally by the distal surface of the radius and the triangular fibrocartilage and distally by the proximal row of carpal bones exclusive of the pisiform. In the coronal plane, the radiocarpal compartment is a C-shaped cavity with a smooth, shallow curve, which is concave distally. In the sagittal plane, this compartment also is C-shaped, but the curve is more acute. Interosseous ligaments extend between the carpal bones of the proximal row and prevent communication of this compartment with the midcarpal compartment. A triangular fibrocartilage prevents communication of the radiocarpal and inferior radioulnar compartments, whereas a meniscus may attach to the triquetrum, preventing communication of the radiocarpal and pisiform-triquetral compartments. The triangular fibrocartilage, the meniscus, the dorsal and volar radioulnar ligaments, the ulnar collateral ligament, the ulnocarpal ligaments, and (sometimes) the sheath of the extensor carpi ulnaris tendon have been termed the triangular fibrocartilage complex of the wrist and represent important stabilizers about the inferior radioulnar joint (see Chapter 70).[235]

The radial collateral ligament is located at the radial limit of the radiocarpal compartment, whereas the ulnar limit of

Text continued on page 679

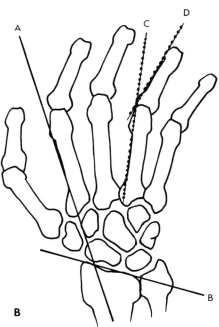

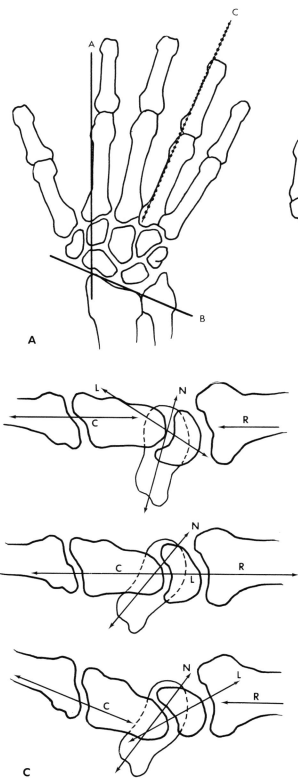

FIGURE 22-3. Hand and wrist: Normal and abnormal alignment.

A, B Frontal projection. The angle of intersection of lines *A* and *B,* measuring radial deviation of the radiocarpal compartment, normally averages 112 degrees **(A)** and is increased in rheumatoid arthritis **(B)**. Lines *C* and *D* measure ulnar deviation at the metacarpophalangeal joints. (From Resnick D: Med Radiogr Photogr *52*:50, 1976.)

C Lateral projection. Line drawings of longitudinal axes of third metacarpal, navicular *(N)* or scaphoid, lunate *(L),* capitate *(C),* and radius *(R)* in dorsiflexion instability (upper drawing), in normal situation (middle drawing), and in palmar flexion instability (lower drawing). When the wrist is normal, a continuous line can be drawn through the longitudinal axes of the capitate, the lunate, and the radius, and this line will intersect a second line through the longitudinal axis of the scaphoid, creating an angle of 30 degrees to 60 degrees. In dorsiflexion instability, the lunate is flexed toward the back of the hand and the scaphoid is displaced vertically. The angle of intersection between the two longitudinal axes is greater than 60 degrees. In palmar flexion instability, the lunate is flexed toward the palm and the angle between the two longitudinal axes is less than 30 degrees. (From Linscheid RL, et al: J Bone Joint Surg [Am] *54*:1612, 1972.)

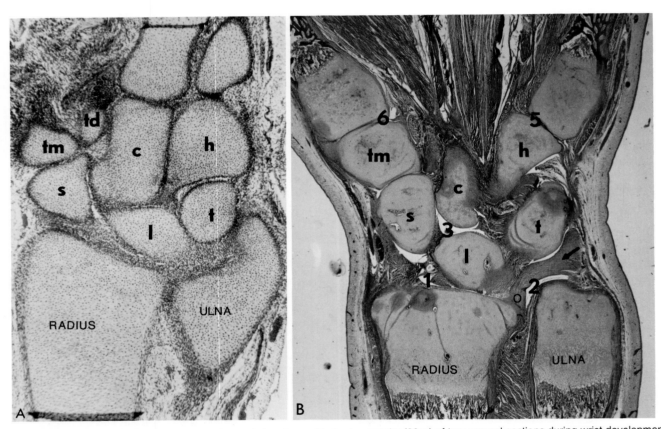

FIGURE 22–4. Articulations of the wrist: Developmental anatomy. Photomicrographs (20×) of two coronal sections during wrist development reveal important structures, including the radiocarpal compartment *(1),* inferior radioulnar compartment *(2),* midcarpal compartment *(3),* common carpometacarpal compartment *(5),* and first carpometacarpal compartment *(6).* Note the triangular fibrocartilage (arrow). *s,* Scaphoid; *l,* lunate; *t,* triquetrum; *h,* hamate; *c,* capitate; *td,* trapezoid; *tm,* trapezium.

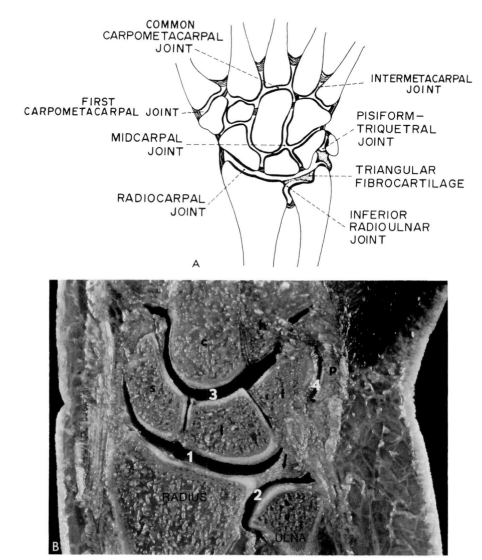

FIGURE 22–5. Articulations of the wrist: General anatomy. Observe the various wrist compartments on a schematic drawing **(A)** and photograph **(B)** of a coronal section. These include the radiocarpal *(1)*, inferior radioulnar *(2)*, midcarpal *(3)*, and pisiform-triquetral *(4)* compartments. Note the triangular fibrocartilage (arrow). *s,* Scaphoid; *l,* lunate; *t,* triquetrum; *p,* pisiform; *h,* hamate; *c,* capitate.

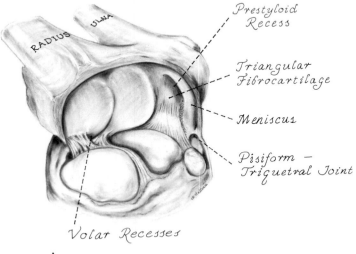

Prestyloid Recess

Triangular Fibrocartilage

Meniscus

Pisiform — Triquetral Joint

Volar Recesses

A

FIGURE 22–6. Articulations of the wrist: Specific compartments.

A Radiocarpal compartment, open and flexed. The prestyloid recess approaches the ulnar styloid process. Observe the palmar (volar) radial recesses and the pisiform-triquetral joint, which communicates with the radiocarpal compartment in this drawing. (From Lewis OJ, et al: The anatomy of the wrist joint. J Anat *106*:539, 1970. Courtesy of Cambridge University Press.)

B Ulnar limit of radiocarpal compartment (coronal section). Note the extent of this compartment *(1)*, its relationship to the inferior radioulnar compartment *(2)*, the intervening triangular fibrocartilage (arrow), and the prestyloid recess (arrowhead), which is intimate with the ulnar styloid *(s)*.

C Inferior radioulnar compartment (coronal section). This L-shaped compartment (2) extends between the distal radius and ulna and is separated from the radiocarpal compartment (1) by the triangular fibrocartilage (arrow). Note the saclike proximal contour of the inferior radioulnar compartment.

Illustration continued on opposite page

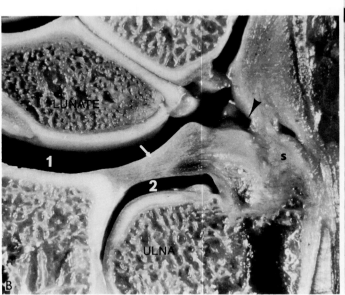

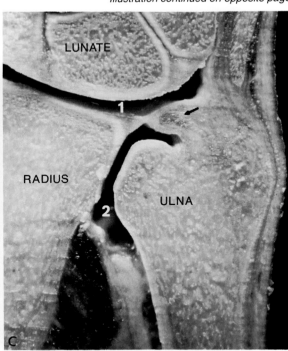

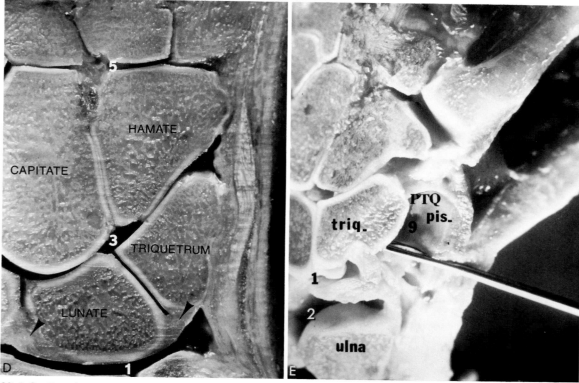

FIGURE 22–6 *Continued*

D Midcarpal compartment (coronal section). The ulnar side of the midcarpal compartment *(3)* is well shown. This compartment is separated from the radiocarpal compartment *(1)* by interosseous ligaments (arrowheads) extending between bones of the proximal carpal row. Observe the common carpometacarpal compartment *(5)* between the distal carpal row and the bases of the four ulnar metacarpals.

E Pisiform-triquetral compartment (coronal section). This compartment (PTQ-9) exists between the triquetrum *(triq.)* and pisiform *(pis.)*. The radiocarpal *(1)* and inferior radioulnar *(2)* compartments also are indicated.

this compartment is the point at which the meniscus is firmly attached to the triquetrum. This ulnar area is Y-shaped; a proximal limb or diverticulum, termed the prestyloid recess, approaches the ulnar styloid[10] and a distal limb is intimate with two thirds of the proximal aspect of the triquetrum.

Palmar radial recesses extend proximally from the radiocarpal compartment beneath the distal articulating surface of the radius.[13] These recesses vary in number and size.

The meniscus occasionally contains ossification, termed the lunula,[10] which produces a circular radiodense shadow of variable size adjacent to the ulnar styloid.

Inferior Radioulnar Compartment. The inferior radioulnar compartment (Fig. 22–6C) is an L-shaped joint whose proximal border is the cartilage-covered head of the ulna and ulnar notch of the radius. Its distal limit is the triangular fibrocartilage. This latter ligament is a band of tough fibrous tissue that extends from the ulnar aspect of the distal part of the radius to the base of the ulnar styloid.[235, 236]

Midcarpal Compartment. The midcarpal compartment (Fig. 22–6D) extends between the proximal and distal carpal rows. On the ulnar aspect of this compartment, the head of the capitate and the hamate articulate with a concavity produced by the scaphoid, lunate, and triquetrum. This ulnar side widens between the triquetrum and hamate. On the radial aspect of the midcarpal compartment, the trapezium and trapezoid articulate with the distal aspect of the scaph-

oid. The radial side of this compartment is termed the trapezioscaphoid space.

Pisiform-Triquetral Compartment. The pisiform-triquetral compartment (Fig. 22–6E) exists between the palmar surface of the triquetrum and the dorsal surface of the pisiform. A large proximal synovial recess can be noted. The pisiform-triquetral compartment is surrounded by a loose fibrous articular capsule. Considerable normal motion between the pisiform and the triquetrum in flexion and extension should not be interpreted as abnormal.

Common Carpometacarpal Compartment. The common carpometacarpal compartment exists between the base of each of the four medial metacarpals and the distal row of carpal bones. This synovial cavity extends proximally between the distal portion of the carpal bones and distally between the bases of the metacarpals, to form three small intermetacarpal joints. Occasionally, the articulation between the hamate and the fourth and fifth metacarpals is a separate synovial cavity, produced by a ligamentous attachment between the hamate and fourth metacarpal (Fig. 22–5A).

First Carpometacarpal Compartment. The carpometacarpal compartment of the thumb is a separate saddle-shaped cavity between the trapezium and base of the first metacarpal.[14] It possesses a loose, fibrous capsule, which is thickest laterally and dorsally.

Intermetacarpal Compartments. Three intermetacarpal

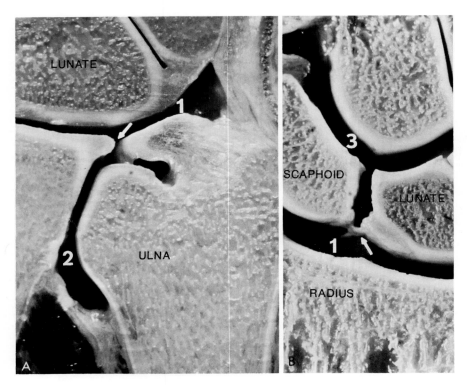

FIGURE 22–7. Compartmental communications.

A In elderly persons, perforation of the triangular fibrocartilage (arrow) will allow communication between the radiocarpal *(1)* and inferior radioulnar *(2)* compartments (coronal section).

B In elderly persons, perforation of the interosseous ligaments (arrow) between bones of the proximal carpal row allows communication between radiocarpal *(1)* and midcarpal *(3)* compartments (coronal section).

compartments extend between the bases of the second and third, the third and fourth, and the fourth and fifth metacarpals. These compartments usually communicate with each other and with the common carpometacarpal compartment.

Although the compartments of the wrist are distinct structures, communication among these compartments has been demonstrated anatomically[10, 15] and arthrographically[13, 16, 17] (Fig. 22–7).

Communication Between Radiocarpal and Inferior Radioulnar Compartments. Direct communication between these compartments has been noted in radiocarpal compartment arthrograms in 7 per cent[16] of living persons and in 16 per cent[17] of cadavers. Dissection of anatomic specimens has outlined similar connections in 30 per cent[15] and 60 per cent[10] of cadavers. This communication results from perforation of the triangular fibrocartilage, a finding seen more frequently in elderly persons, which relates to cartilaginous degeneration. Small defects within this structure may not be revealed during arthrographic examination of the wrist.

Communication Between Radiocarpal and Midcarpal Compartments. Communication between these two compartments results from disruption of the interosseous ligaments that extend between the bones of the proximal carpal row. Anatomic study of elderly cadaveric wrists has revealed disruption of the scapholunate ligament in 40 per cent of cadavers and of the lunotriquetral ligament in 36 per cent of cadavers.[10] Arthrography has demonstrated communication between the radiocarpal and midcarpal compartments in 13 per cent of cadavers.[17]

Communication Between Radiocarpal and Pisiform-Triquetral Compartments. Dissection of cadaveric wrists has outlined communication between these two compartments in 34 per cent of cadavers.[10] This communication may be demonstrated during arthrography.[8, 13, 18, 19]

Communication Among Midcarpal, Carpometacarpal, and Intermetacarpal Compartments. Arthrographic demonstration of communication among the midcarpal, common carpometacarpal, and intermetacarpal compartments is frequent. Such communication with the first carpometacarpal joint is unusual.

Movement of the wrist is complex, related to the associated changes in many of these compartments.[1, 2, 11–14, 20–26, 234, 237] Wrist flexion occurs at both the radiocarpal and midcarpal joints, particularly the former.[295] In wrist extension, movement again occurs at both of these compartments and is greater at the radiocarpal joint.[295] Adduction or ulnar deviation of the hand occurs mainly at the radiocarpal compartment, whereas abduction or radial deviation occurs predominantly at the midcarpal compartment. The movements at the common carpometacarpal and intermetacarpal compartments almost are limited to mild gliding of one articular surface on an adjacent one. This movement is most pronounced in the fourth and fifth digits. Movement at the first carpometacarpal joint includes flexion, extension, abduction, adduction, rotation, and circumduction of the thumb.[14, 22, 23, 233] Pronation and supination of the hand result from movement at the inferior and superior radioulnar joints.

The joint capsule of the wrist compartment is strengthened by various ligaments that extend from the radius and ulna toward the carpal bones.[238] Dorsal and volar radiocarpal and ulnocarpal ligaments have been identified, although a standard nomenclature for these structures currently does not exist (see Chapter 70). Collateral ligaments, particularly the proximal or radioscaphoid portion of the radial collateral ligament and the ulnar collateral ligament, also reinforce the joint capsule. The ulnar collateral ligament extends from the ulnar styloid to the triquetrum and pisiform. The tip of the ulnar styloid is devoid of ligamentous attach-

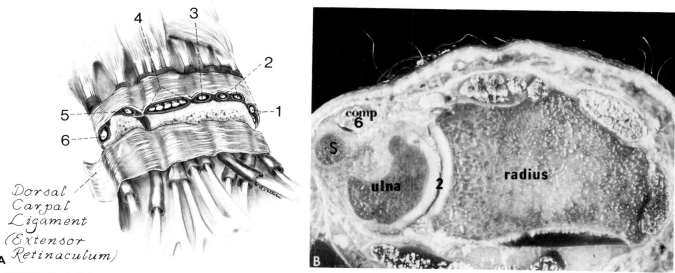

FIGURE 22–8. Extensor tendons and tendon sheaths.

A Drawing showing dorsal carpal ligament and extensor tendons surrounded by synovial sheaths traversing dorsum of wrist within six separate compartments. These compartments are created by the insular attachment of the dorsal carpal ligament on the posterior and lateral surfaces of the radius and ulna. The extensor carpi ulnaris tendon and its sheath are in the medial compartment (6) and are closely applied to the posterior surface of the ulna.

B Cross section through distal end of radius and distal ulna reveals relationship of the extensor carpi ulnaris tendon and tendon sheath (comp 6) and ulnar styloid (S). The inferior radioulnar compartment (2) also is shown.

(From Resnick D: Med Radiogr Photogr *52*:50, 1976.)

ment. Pisohamate and pisometacarpal ligaments connect the pisiform, the hook of the hamate, and the base of the fifth metacarpal.

Extensor tendons traverse the dorsum of the wrist, surrounded by synovial sheaths (Fig. 22–8). The attachment of the dorsal carpal ligament to the adjacent radius and ulna creates six separate compartments or bundles of tendons.

Flexor tendons with surrounding synovial sheaths pass through the carpal tunnel on the palmar aspect of the wrist (Fig. 22–9).

Certain tissue planes about the wrist have received attention in the literature. The navicular (scaphoid) fat pad[27] is a triangular or linear collection of fat between the radial collateral ligament and the synovial sheath of the abductor

FIGURE 22–9. Flexor tendons and tendon sheaths. Photograph of dissected palmar surface of wrist reveals the flexor tendons as they pass beneath the flexor retinaculum within the carpal tunnel (CT). As they approach the metacarpophalangeal joints (2–5), the tendons are surrounded by synovial sheaths (arrows). (From Resnick D: Med Radiogr Photogr *52*:50, 1976.)

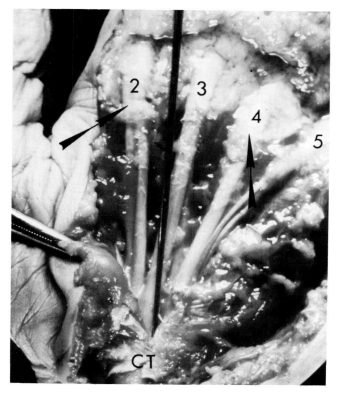

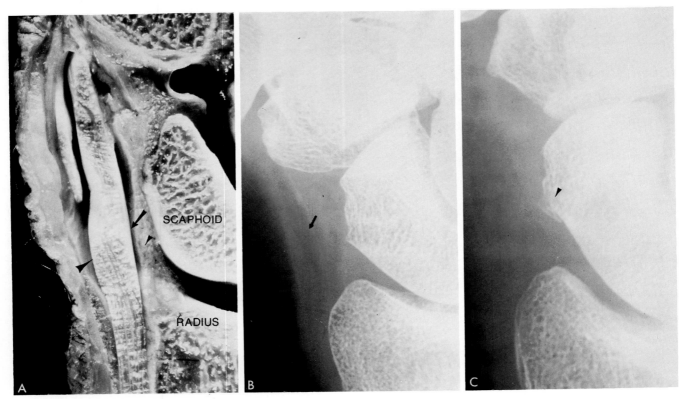

FIGURE 22–10. Navicular (scaphoid) fat pad.

A A coronal section demonstrates the radial aspect of the wrist. Note the location of the fat plane (arrow) between the radial collateral ligament (small arrowhead) and the synovial sheath and tendons of the abductor pollicis longus and extensor pollicis brevis (large arrowhead).

B On a normal radiograph, the navicular fat pad (arrow) produces a triangular or linear radiolucent shadow paralleling the lateral surface of the scaphoid.

C This fat plane may be obscured with acute fractures of the neighboring bones. In this patient, a subtle scaphoid fracture (arrowhead) has resulted in obliteration of the navicular fat pad.

pollicis longus and extensor pollicis brevis (Fig. 22–10). On radiographs, this fat pad may produce a thin radiolucent line or triangle paralleling the lateral surface of the scaphoid. It is more difficult to discern in children less than 11 or 12 years of age. Obliteration, obscuration, or displacement of this fat plane is reported to be common in acute fractures of the scaphoid, the radial styloid process, and the proximal first metacarpal bone.[27, 239]

A second important soft tissue landmark is the fat plane that exists between the pronator quadratus muscle and the tendons of the flexor digitorum profundus[28] (Fig. 22–11). On a lateral radiograph, the fat pad produces a radiolucent region on the volar aspect of the wrist, which appears as a gentle convex curve beneath the distal aspect of the radius and ulna in almost all persons from infancy to advanced age. Displacement, distortion, or obliteration of the pronator quadratus fat pad has been reported in fractures of the distal ends of the radius and ulna, osteomyelitis, and septic arthritis of the wrist.[28, 29]

METACARPOPHALANGEAL JOINTS

Osseous Anatomy

At the metacarpophalangeal joints, the metacarpal heads articulate with the proximal phalanges (Fig. 22–12). The medial four metacarpal bones lie side by side; the first metacarpal lies in a more anterior plane and is rotated medially along its long axis through an angle of 90 degrees.[1] In this fashion, the dorsal surface of the thumb is aligned in a radial direction, whereas its ulnar surface is oriented superiorly. This position allows the thumb to appose the other four metacarpals during flexion and rotation.[22, 23]

The metacarpal heads are smooth and round, extending farther on the palmar than on the dorsal aspect of the bone.[30] On the palmar aspect, the articular surface of the metacarpal head is divided in such a fashion that it resembles condyles. The head of the first metacarpal is less convex than those of the other metacarpals and has two palmar articular eminences, which relate to sesamoid bones. Tubercles are found on the heads of all metacarpals; these tubercles occur at the sides of the metacarpal heads where the dorsal surface of the body of the bone extends onto the head. Collateral ligaments attach to the metacarpal tubercles. The bases of the phalanges contain concave oval surfaces that articulate with the metacarpal heads.

Soft Tissue Anatomy

Articular cartilage covers the osseous surfaces of metacarpals and phalanges,[30] and the synovial membrane is attached to the articular margin of the metacarpal head[31] (Fig.

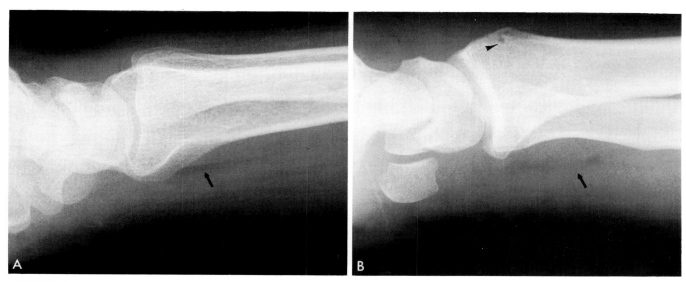

FIGURE 22–11. Pronator fat pad.
   A In normal situations, a fat plane between the pronator quadratus and tendons of the flexor digitorum profundus creates a radiolucent area (arrow) on the volar aspect of the wrist.
   B With fractures, such as a subtle fracture of the distal end of the radius (arrowhead), this fat plane may be obscured or displaced (arrow).

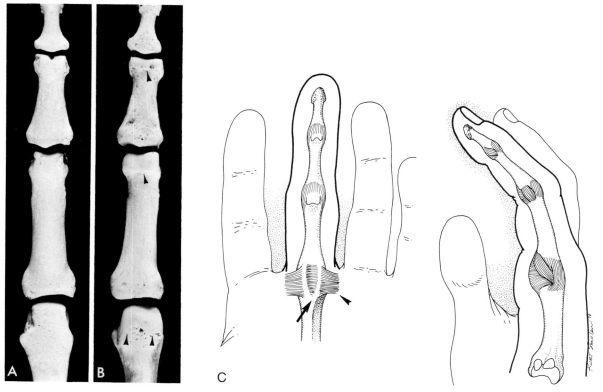

FIGURE 22–12. Metacarpals and phalanges: Osseous anatomy.
   A, B Dorsal **(A)** and ventral **(B)** aspects of third metacarpal and phalanges. Note the more extensive articular surface on the volar aspect of the metacarpal head and phalanges (arrowheads).
   C Drawings of the palmar and medial aspects of the metacarpophalangeal and interphalangeal joints of the fourth digit reveal the deep transverse metacarpal ligament (arrowhead) with its central groove for the flexor tendons (arrow) and the capsule of the interphalangeal joints.

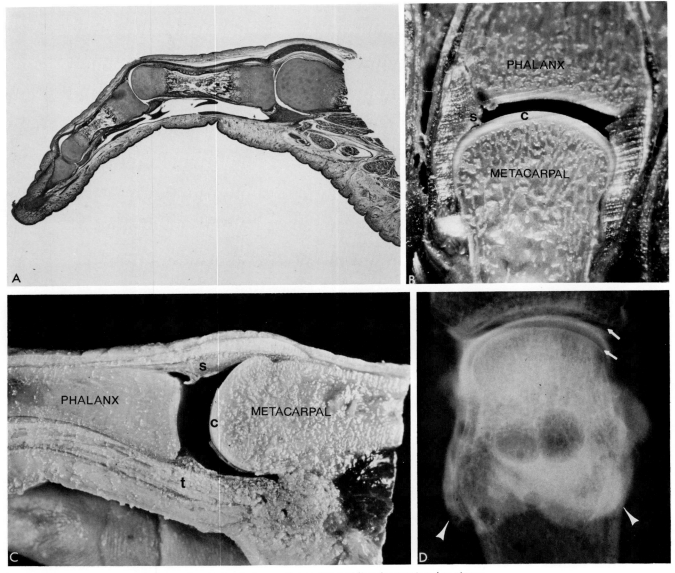

FIGURE 22–13. Metacarpophalangeal and interphalangeal joints: Normal development and anatomy.

A During a stage of development, these articulations are well demonstrated between the unossified epiphyses of the metacarpal and phalanges on this sagittal section of a finger (20×).

B, C Metacarpophalangeal joint. Coronal **(B)** and sagittal **(C)** sections. Observe the articular cavity, cartilage *(c)*, synovial membrane *(s)*, and flexor tendon *(t)*.

D On an arthrogram of a metacarpophalangeal joint, the proximal extent of the contrast-filled articular cavity is well seen (arrowheads). Observe the radiolucent cartilage of the metacarpal head and proximal phalanx (arrows).

22–13). This membrane is particularly prominent on the volar aspect of the metacarpal head and neck. The capsule about the metacarpophalangeal joint is somewhat loose, allowing motion of the proximal phalanx. It attaches to the elevated bony crest surrounding the smooth articular surface of the metacarpal head and to the bony ridge about the articular surface of the base of the phalanx. On the dorsal surface of the metacarpophalangeal joints, the fibrous capsule is thin; in this location, a bursa separates the capsule from the extensor tendon.

Each metacarpophalangeal joint has a palmar ligament and two collateral ligaments.[1, 2, 12] The palmar ligament is located on the volar aspect of the articulation and is firmly attached to the base of the proximal phalanx and loosely united to the metacarpal neck. Laterally the palmar ligament blends with the collateral ligaments, and volarly the palmar ligament blends with the deep transverse metacarpal ligaments, which connect the palmar ligaments of the second through fifth metacarpophalangeal joints. The palmar ligament also is grooved for the passage of the flexor tendons, whose fibrous sheaths are attached to the sides of the groove. The collateral ligaments reinforce the fibrous capsule laterally. These ligaments pass obliquely from the posterior tubercles and depressions on the radial and ulnar aspects of the metacarpal to attach to the base of the proximal phalanx.

Active movements of the metacarpophalangeal articulations include flexion, extension, adduction, abduction, circumduction, and limited rotation. Accessory movements include rotation, gliding, and distraction. The metacarpophalangeal joint of the thumb, in general, has less extensive movement than the others; movement of the thumb occurs in two planes, that parallel to the remainder of the hand and that at right angles to this first plane.[22, 23, 240]

INTERPHALANGEAL JOINTS OF THE HAND

Osseous Anatomy

The interphalangeal joints of the hand consist of four distal interphalangeal joints, four proximal interphalangeal articulations, and an interphalangeal joint of the first digit.

At the proximal interphalangeal joints, the head of the proximal phalanx articulates with the base of the adjacent middle phalanx. The articular surface of the phalangeal head is wide (from side to side), with a central groove and ridges on either side for attachment of the collateral ligaments. The base of the middle phalanx contains a ridge that fits into the groove on the head of the proximal phalanx.

At the distal interphalangeal joints, the head of the middle phalanx articulates with the base of the distal phalanx. This phalangeal head, like that of the proximal phalanx, is pulley-like in configuration and conforms to the base of the adjacent phalanx. This latter structure is relatively large.

The interphalangeal joint of the thumb separates the proximal and distal phalanges of that digit. These phalanges are similar in structure to those of the other digits but in general are shorter and broader.

Soft Tissue Anatomy

Apposing surfaces of bone are covered by articular cartilage. A fibrous capsule surrounds the articulation, and on its inner aspect the capsule is covered by synovial membrane, which extends over intracapsular bone not covered by articular cartilage.[31, 32] At the interphalangeal joints, synovial pouches exist proximally on both dorsal and palmar aspects of the articulation.[32, 33] The interphalangeal articulations have a palmar and two collateral ligaments whose anatomy is similar to those about the metacarpophalangeal joints. Active movements at these joints include flexion and extension, both of which may be accompanied by a small amount of rotation; accessory movements are rotation, abduction, adduction, and gliding.[1, 2, 12, 32, 34]

RADIOULNAR SYNDESMOSIS (MIDDLE RADIOULNAR JOINT)

The diaphyses of radius and ulna are united by an interosseous membrane whose fibers run in an inferior and medial direction from radius to ulna. This membrane originates approximately 3 cm below the radial tuberosity, extends to the wrist, and contains an aperture for various interosseous vessels.[229] A crest can be noted on both bones at the interosseous border.

ELBOW

The articulation about the elbow has three constituents: (1) humeroradial—the area between the capitulum of the humerus and the facet on the radial head; (2) humero-ulnar—the area between the trochlea of the humerus and the trochlear notch of the ulna; and (3) superior (proximal) radioulnar—the area between the head of the radius and radial notch of the ulna and the annular ligament.

Although the superior or proximal radioulnar area generally is considered a separate articulation, it is convenient to discuss all three areas of the elbow region together.

Osseous Anatomy

The osseous structures about the elbow include the proximal end of the ulna and radius and the distal end of the humerus[1, 2] (Fig. 22–14).

The proximal end of the ulna contains two processes, the olecranon and the coronoid. The olecranon process is smooth posteriorly at the site of attachment of the triceps tendon. Its anterior surface provides the site of attachment of the capsule of the elbow joint. The coronoid process contains the radial notch, below which is the ulnar tuberosity.

The proximal end of the radius consists of head, neck, and tuberosity. The radial head is disc-shaped, containing a shallow, cupped articular surface, which is intimate with the capitulum of the humerus. The articular circumference of the head is largest medially, where it articulates with the radial notch of the ulna. The radial neck is the smooth, constricted part of the bone below the radial head. The radial tuberosity is located beneath the medial aspect of the neck.

The distal aspect of the humerus is a wide, flattened structure. The medial third of its articular surface, termed the trochlea, is intimate with the ulna. Lateral to the trochlea is the capitulum, which articulates with the radius. The sulcus is between the trochlea and the capitulum. A hollow area is found on the posterior surface of the humerus above the trochlea, termed the olecranon fossa; the posterior capsular attachment of the humerus is located above this fossa. A smaller fossa, the coronoid fossa, lies above the trochlea on the anterior surface of the humerus, and a radial fossa lies adjacent to it, above the capitulum. The anterior capsular attachment to the humerus is located above these fossae. When the elbow is fully extended, the tip of the olecranon process is located in the olecranon fossa, and when the elbow is flexed, the coronoid process of the ulna is found in the coronoid fossa and the margin of the radial head is located in the radial fossa.

The medial epicondyle is a blunt osseous projection of the distal end of the humerus. The posterior smooth surface of this epicondyle is crossed by the ulnar nerve. The anterior surface of the medial epicondyle is the site of attachment of superficial flexor muscles of the forearm. The lateral epicondyle is located on the lateral surface of the distal portion of the humerus. Its lateral and anterior surface represents the site of origin of the superficial group of extensor muscles of the forearm.

The degree of congruity of apposing articulating surfaces of radius, ulna, and humerus varies in different positions of the elbow joint; the greatest congruity exists when the forearm is in a position midway between full supination and full pronation and the elbow is flexed to a right angle.[2] When the elbow is extended, the inferior and posterior aspects of the trochlea contact the ulna; when the elbow is flexed, the trochlear notch slides forward on the anterior

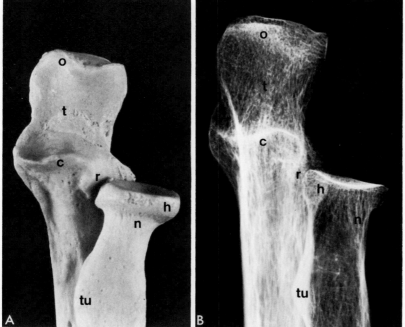

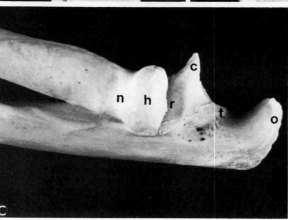

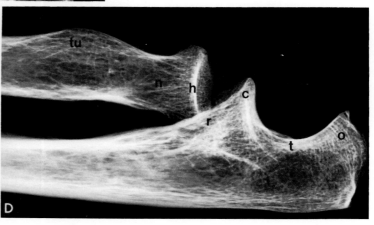

FIGURE 22–14. Elbow joint: Osseous anatomy.
   A, B Radius and ulna, anterior aspect. Note the olecranon *(o)*, coronoid process *(c)*, trochlear notch *(t)*, radial notch *(r)*, radial head *(h)*, radial neck *(n)*, and radial tuberosity *(tu)*.
   C, D Radius and ulna, lateral aspect.
Illustration continued on opposite page

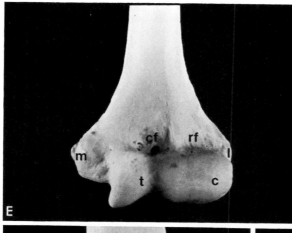

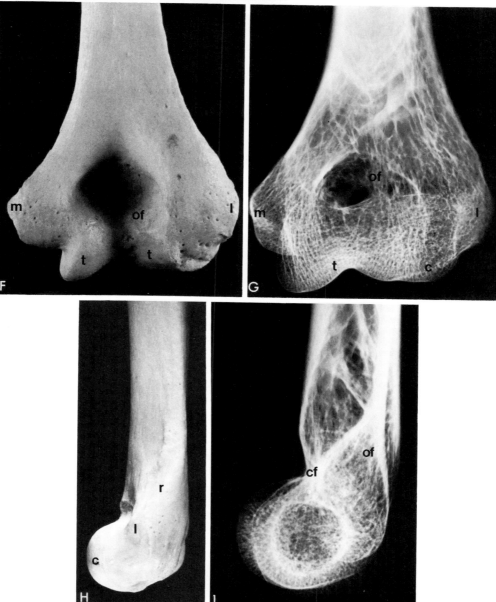

FIGURE 22–14 *Continued*

E–G Distal end of humerus, anterior and posterior aspects. An anterior view **(E)** reveals the trochlea *(t)*, capitulum *(c)*, medial epicondyle *(m)*, lateral epicondyle *(l)*, coronoid fossa *(cf)*, and radial fossa *(rf)*. A posterior view **(F)**, oriented in the same fashion, outlines some of the same structures and, in addition, the olecranon fossa *(of)*. An anteroposterior radiograph **(G)** demonstrates pertinent osseous anatomy.

H, I Distal end of humerus, lateral aspect. Observe the capitulum *(c)*, lateral epicondyle *(l)*, and lateral supracondylar ridge *(r)*. Although there is superimposition of structures on the lateral radiograph, the areas of the coronoid fossa *(cf)* and olecranon fossa *(of)* are indicated.

aspect of the ulna, exposing the posterior aspect of that bone. The capitulum and the radial head are curved reciprocally; in a midprone position, extensive contact occurs between radius and capitulum.

Radiographic anatomy of the axial relationships at the elbow has been described.[5] The carrying angle of the elbow is described as the obtuse angle created by the intersection of the longitudinal axes of the shafts of the humerus and ulna measured on the radial side. In men this angle averages 169 degrees (154 to 178 degrees), and in women it averages 167 degrees (158 to 178 degrees). The humeral angle is formed by the intersection of a line through the longitudinal axis of the humerus with a second line drawn tangentially to the articular surface of the trochlea and capitulum. In men this angle averages 85 degrees (77 to 95 degrees) and in women it averages 83 degrees (72 to 91 degrees). The ulnar angle is formed by the intersection of a line through the longitudinal axis of the ulna with a second line drawn tangentially to the articular surfaces of the trochlea and capitulum. The ulnar angle averages 84 degrees (74 to 99 degrees) in men and 84 degrees (72 to 93 degrees) in women.

Soft Tissue Anatomy

The articular surface of the humerus consists of a grooved trochlea, the spheroidal capitulum, and a sulcus between them[1, 2] (Fig. 22–15). It is covered with a continu-

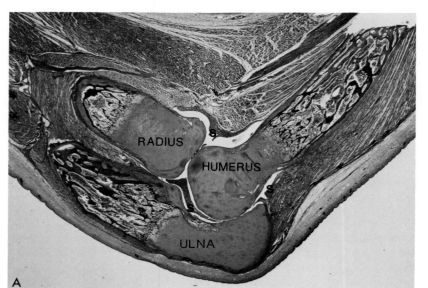

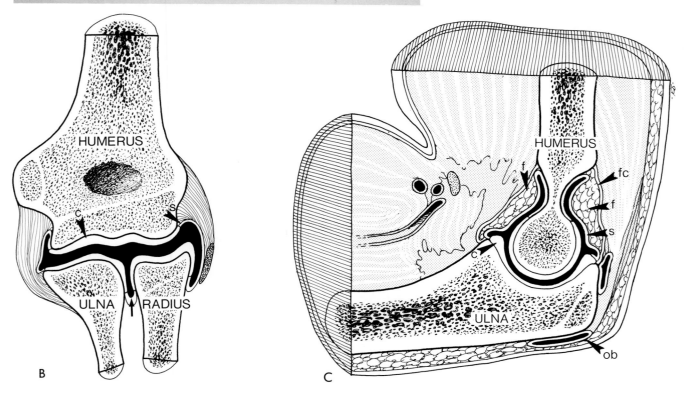

FIGURE 22–15. Elbow joint: Normal development and anatomy.

A A sagittal section of the developing elbow outlines the articular cavity between unossified epiphyses of radius, ulna, and humerus. Synovial tissue *(s)* can be seen (20×).

B, C Drawings of coronal **(B)** and sagittal **(C)** sections. Observe synovium *(s)*, articular cartilage *(c)*, fibrous capsule *(fc)*, anterior and posterior fat pads *(f)*, and olecranon bursa *(ob)*. Note the extension of the elbow joint between radius and ulna as the superior radioulnar joint (arrow).

Illustration continued on opposite page

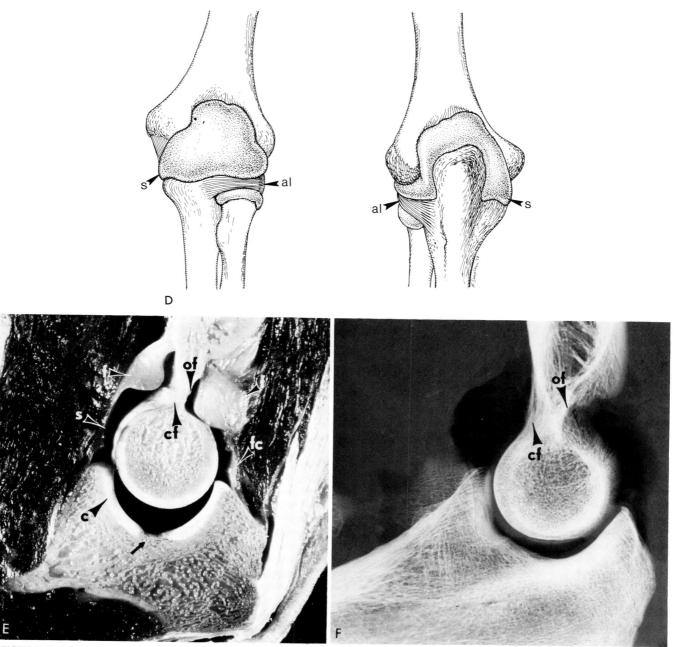

FIGURE 22–15 *Continued*

D A drawing of the anterior (left) and posterior (right) aspects of the distended elbow joint with the fibrous capsule removed. Observe the synovial membrane *(s)* and the annular ligament *(al)* extending around the proximal end of the radius, constricting the joint cavity. (From Warwick R, Williams P: Gray's Anatomy. 15th British Ed. Philadelphia, WB Saunders Co, 1973.)

E, F Photograph and radiograph of a sagittal section through the ulnar aspect of the elbow joint after air arthrography, showing distended articular cavity, fat pads *(f)*, synovium *(s)*, articular cartilage *(c)*, fibrous capsule *(fc)*, olecranon fossa *(of)*, and coronoid fossa *(cf)*. Note the area of the trochlear notch, which normally is devoid of cartilage (arrow).

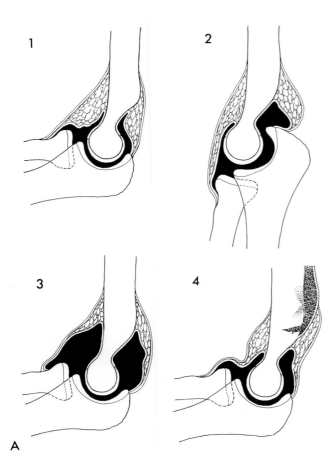

A

FIGURE 22–16. *See legend on opposite page*

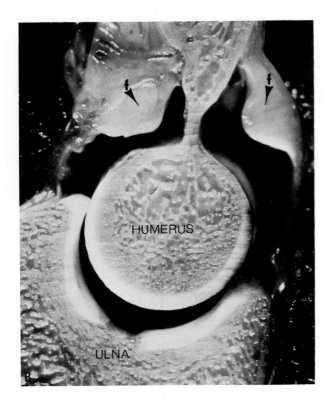

HUMERUS

ULNA

B

ous layer of articular cartilage. The ulnar articulating surface is the trochlear notch. This notch is covered with cartilage, which is interrupted in a transverse fashion across its deepest aspect. The trochlear notch of the ulna and the trochlea of the humerus articulate. The radial articulating area is the radial head, which is covered with articular cartilage. This cartilage is continuous with that along the sides of the radial head, including an area in the superior radioulnar articulation. The radial head articulates with the capitulum and the capitulotrochlear groove.

A fibrous capsule invests the elbow completely. The attachments of its broad, thin, and weak anterior part are the anterior humerus along the medial epicondyle and above the coronoid and radial fossae, the anterior surface of the ulnar coronoid process, and the annular ligament. The superior attachments of its thin, weak posterior part are the posterior surface of the humerus behind the capitulum, the olecranon fossa, and the medial epicondyle. Inferomedially the capsule is attached to the upper and lateral margins of the olecranon. Laterally the capsule is continuous with that about the superior radioulnar joint. The fibrous capsule is strengthened at the sides of the articulation by the radial and ulnar collateral ligaments.

The synovial membrane of the elbow lines the deep surface of the fibrous capsule and annular ligament. It extends from the articular surface of the humerus and contacts the olecranon, radial, and coronoid fossae and the medial surface of the trochlea. A synovial fold projects into the joint between the radius and ulna, partially dividing the articulation into humeroulnar and humeroradial portions.[1]

Several fat pads are located between fibrous capsule and synovial membrane (Fig. 22–16). Fat pads are near the synovial fold between the radius and ulna, and over the olecranon, coronoid, and radial fossae. These fat pads, which are extrasynovial but intracapsular, are of radiographic significance.[35–40] On lateral radiographs, an anterior radiolucent area represents the summation of radial and coronoid fossae fat pads. These fat pads are pressed into their respective fossae by the brachialis muscle during extension of the elbow. A posterior radiolucent region represents the olecranon fossa fat pad. It is pressed into this fossa by the triceps muscle during flexion of the elbow. The anterior fat pad normally assumes a teardrop configuration anterior to the distal end of the humerus on lateral radiographs of the elbow exposed in approximately 90 degrees of joint flexion. The posterior fat pad normally is not visible in radiographs of the elbow exposed in flexion. Its occasional appearance on such films may reflect unusually large fat pads or slightly oblique projections.[37] Any intra-articular process that is associated with a mass or fluid may

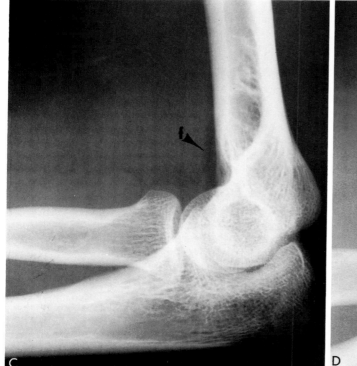 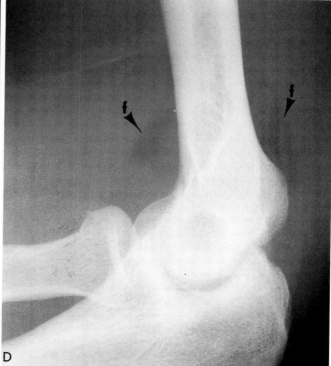

FIGURE 22–16. Elbow joint: Normal and abnormal appearance of fat pads.

    A Schematic drawings of anterior and posterior fat pads in normal and abnormal situations. Normally *(1),* the extrasynovial anterior and posterior fat pads are closely applied to the distal end of the humerus. In extension *(2),* the anterior fat pad is pressed tightly against the humerus, whereas the posterior fat pad may be elevated by contact between the olecranon and humerus. With a joint effusion *(3),* both anterior and posterior fat pads may be elevated by intra-articular fluid. With distal humeral fractures *(4),* a paradoxic elevation of the posterior fat pad may occur. (From Murphy WA, Siegel MJ: Radiology *124*:659, 1977.)

    B A sagittal section of the elbow after marked distention of the joint with air reveals the elevated anterior and posterior fat pads *(f).*

    C On a radiograph of the normal elbow flexed to approximately 90 degrees, the anterior fat pad *(f)* assumes a teardrop configuration and the posterior fat pad is not visible.

    D With a joint effusion, both fat pads *(f)* are elevated. The anterior fat pad assumes a "sail" configuration, whereas the posterior fat pad becomes visible.

produce a ''positive fat-pad sign'' characterized by elevation and displacement of anterior and posterior fat pads. A variety of disease processes can be manifested in this fashion.[40]

Radial and ulnar collateral ligaments reinforce the fibrous capsule.[290] The radial collateral ligament attaches superiorly to the lateral epicondyle of the humerus and inferiorly to the radial notch of the ulna and the annular ligament. The ulnar collateral ligament is composed of three distinct bands that are continuous with each other. The anterior band extends from the anterior aspect of the medial epicondyle of the humerus to the medial edge of the coronoid process; a posterior band passes from the posterior aspect of the medial epicondyle to the medial edge of the olecranon; a thin intermediate band extends from the medial epicondyle to merge via a transverse or oblique band with the anterior and posterior bands on the coronoid process and the olecranon.

The superior radioulnar joint exists between the radial head and the osseous-fibrous ring formed by the annular ligament and the radial notch of the ulna. This notch is lined with articular cartilage that is continuous with that on the lower part of the trochlear notch. The radial head also is covered with cartilage. The annular ligament is attached anteriorly to the anterior margin of the radial notch. It encircles the head of the radius, and posteriorly it contains several bands that attach to the ulna near the posterior margin of the radial notch. The superior portion of the annular ligament is lined with fibrocartilage where it apposes the circumference of the radial head. The inferior portion of the annular ligament is covered with synovial membrane, which extends downward onto the radial neck. The quadrate ligament, a thin, fibrous layer, covers the synovial membrane.[41]

Various extracapsular fat planes can be observed on radiographs of the elbow. Extracapsular fat may be apparent on an anteroposterior projection as a radiolucent line closely applied to the lateral aspect of the capitulum, continuing downward over the lateral aspect of the radial head and neck.[42] Lateral to this fat, a second fat plane may be seen over the supinator muscle in this projection. On a lateral radiograph, the normal fat plane over the supinator muscle can appear as a radiolucent line, 4 to 5 cm in length, paralleling the radial head, neck, and upper shaft.[43] Changes in this latter fat plane have been reported in various elbow disorders.

Along the posterior aspect of the elbow, a subcutaneous bursa, the olecranon bursa, separates the skin from the ulnar olecranon (Fig. 22–17). This synovium-lined sac can be outlined by contrast material, revealing that it is situated like a cap on the olecranon process.[44]

Active movements of the elbow include flexion and extension. Accessory movements are slight rotation, abduction and adduction of the ulna, and forward and backward movement of the radial head on the capitulum. Supination and pronation result, in part, from movement at the superior radioulnar joint.

GLENOHUMERAL JOINT

The glenohumeral joint lies between the roughly hemispheric head of the humerus and the shallow cavity of the glenoid region of the scapula. Stability of this articulation

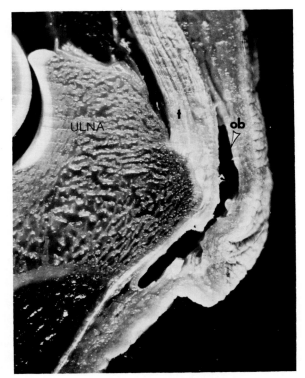

FIGURE 22–17. Olecranon bursa. A sagittal section through the ulna demonstrates the synovium-lined olecranon bursa *(ob)* between the skin and ulnar olecranon. Note the triceps tendon *(t)*.

is limited, for two reasons: the scapular ''socket'' is small compared to the size of the adjacent humeral head, so that apposing osseous surfaces provide little inherent stability; and the joint capsule is quite redundant, providing little additional support.[241] Stability of the glenohumeral joint is supplied by surrounding tendons, muscles, ligaments, and labral tissue (see Chapter 70).[45, 46]

Osseous Anatomy

The upper end of the humerus consists of the head and the greater and lesser tuberosities (tubercles) (Fig. 22–18). With the arm at the side of the body, the humeral head is directed medially, upward, and slightly backward to contact the glenoid cavity of the scapula. Beneath the head is the anatomic neck of the humerus, a slightly constricted area that encircles the bone, separating the head from the tuberosities. The anatomic neck is the site of attachment of the capsular ligament of the glenohumeral joint. The greater tuberosity is located on the lateral aspect of the proximal end of the humerus. The tendons of the supraspinatus and infraspinatus muscles insert on its superior portion, whereas the tendon of the teres minor muscle inserts on its posterior aspect. The lesser tuberosity is located on the anterior portion of the proximal humerus, immediately below the anatomic neck. The subscapularis tendon attaches to the medial aspect of this structure. Between the greater and lesser tuberosities is located the intertubercular sulcus or groove (bicipital groove) through which passes the tendon of the long head of the biceps brachii, surrounded by a synovial sheath and fixed by a transverse ligament extending between the tuberosities.[242] The rough lateral lip of the groove

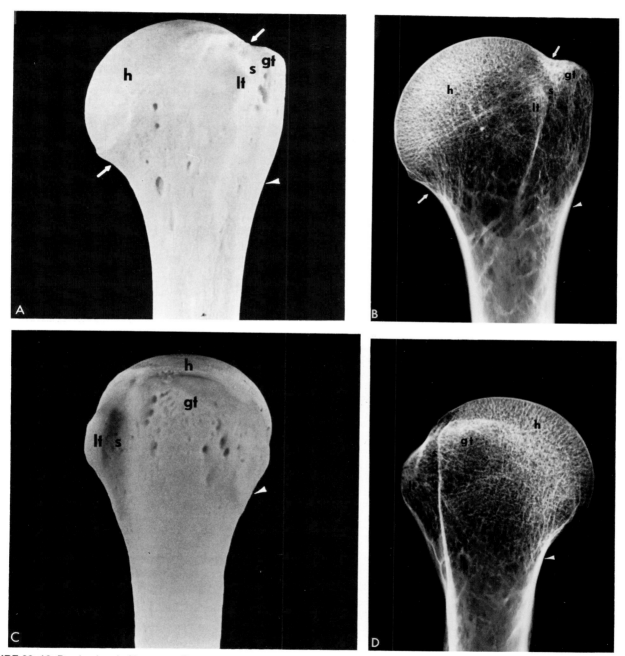

FIGURE 22–18. Proximal end of humerus: Osseous anatomy.

A, B Anterior aspect, external rotation. Observe the articular surface of the humeral head *(h)*, greater tuberosity *(gt)*, lesser tuberosity *(lt)*, intertubercular sulcus *(s)*, anatomic neck (arrows), and surgical neck (arrowheads).

C, D Anterior aspect, internal rotation. The same structures as in **A** and **B** are indicated. The lesser tuberosity is seen in profile on the medial aspect of the humeral head and the greater tuberosity is seen en face.

is the site of attachment of the tendon of the pectoralis major; the floor of the groove gives rise to the attachment of the tendon of the latissimus dorsi; the medial lip of the groove is the site of attachment of the tendon of the teres major.

The shallow glenoid cavity is located on the lateral margin of the scapula (Fig. 22–19). Although there is variation in the osseous depth of the glenoid region,[45] a fibrocartilaginous labrum encircles and slightly deepens the glenoid cavity.[243] The glenoid contour may be almost flat or slightly curved, or it may possess a deep, socket-like appearance. A supraglenoid tubercle is located above the glenoid cavity, to which is attached the long head of the biceps tendon. Below the cavity is a thickened ridge of bone, the infraglenoid tubercle, which is a site of attachment for the long head of the triceps.

Radiographic landmarks about the glenohumeral joint have been described.[47] With the arm in external rotation, the angle of intersection of two lines is calculated. The first line is drawn along the longitudinal axis of the humerus. The second line is drawn between the apex of the greater tuberosity and the junction of the shaft with the distal artic-

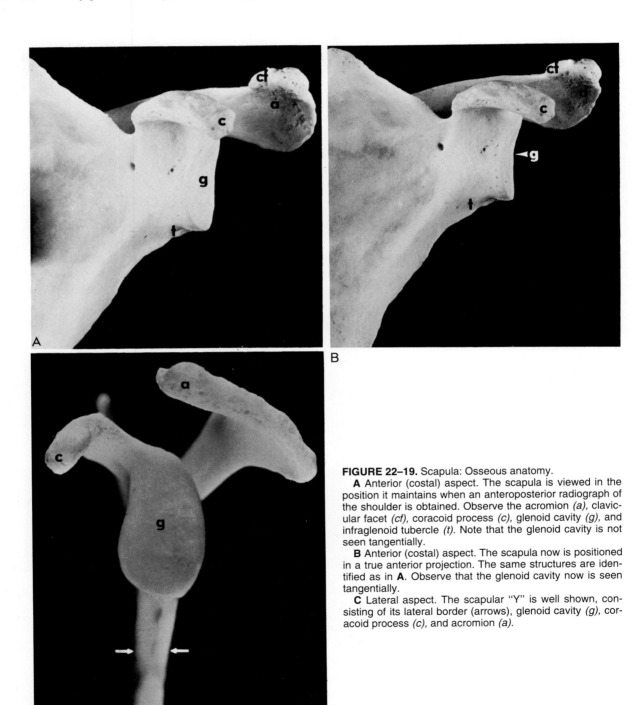

FIGURE 22–19. Scapula: Osseous anatomy.

A Anterior (costal) aspect. The scapula is viewed in the position it maintains when an anteroposterior radiograph of the shoulder is obtained. Observe the acromion *(a)*, clavicular facet *(cf)*, coracoid process *(c)*, glenoid cavity *(g)*, and infraglenoid tubercle *(t)*. Note that the glenoid cavity is not seen tangentially.

B Anterior (costal) aspect. The scapula now is positioned in a true anterior projection. The same structures are identified as in **A**. Observe that the glenoid cavity now is seen tangentially.

C Lateral aspect. The scapular "Y" is well shown, consisting of its lateral border (arrows), glenoid cavity *(g)*, coracoid process *(c)*, and acromion *(a)*.

ular surface of the head. The average angle of intersection of these lines is 60 degrees (52 to 70 degrees) in men and 62 degrees (50 to 70 degrees) in women. The width of the glenohumeral joint surface at the central portion of the glenoid generally is less than 6 mm.[48, 244] The subacromial space, defined as the distance between the head of the humerus and the inferior aspect of the acromion, in adults is approximately 9 or 10 mm; a measurement less than 6 mm in a middle-aged person suggests rotator cuff atrophy or tear.[245] The angle of ''humeral torsion'' is defined as the angle between the upper and lower articulating surfaces of the humerus.[1] This angle equals approximately 164 degrees, being greater in men than in women, and in adults than in children.

Soft Tissue Anatomy

The articular surfaces of the glenoid and the humerus are covered with hyaline cartilage (Fig. 22–20). The cartilage on the humeral head is thickest at its center and thinner peripherally, whereas the reverse is true on the glenoid portion of the joint.[1] A fibrocartilaginous structure, the labrum, attaches to the glenoid rim and adds an element of stability to the glenohumeral articulation (see Chapter 70).[49]

A loose fibrous capsule arises medially from the circumference of the glenoid labrum or, anteriorly, from the neck of the scapula.[241] It inserts distally into the anatomic neck of the humerus and periosteum of the humeral diaphysis. In certain areas the fibrous capsule is strengthened by its intimate association with surrounding ligaments; it is reinforced above by the supraspinatus, below by the long head of the triceps, anteriorly by the subscapularis, and posteriorly by the infraspinatus and teres minor. The tendons of the supraspinatus, infraspinatus, teres minor, and subscapularis form a cuff—the rotator cuff—which blends with and reinforces the fibrous capsule.[246] The coracohumeral ligament strengthens the upper part of the capsule. It arises from the lateral edge of the coracoid process, extends over the humeral head, and attaches to the greater tuberosity. Anteriorly, the capsule may thicken to form the superior, middle, and inferior glenohumeral ligaments.[1, 46] These ligaments and the recesses formed between them are variable in configuration (see Chapter 70). The fibrous capsule is strengthened additionally by extensions from the tendons of the pectoralis major and teres major.

Three openings may be found in the fibrous capsule.[1] An anterior perforation below the coracoid process establishes joint communication with the bursa behind the subscapularis tendon, the subscapular ''recess.'' A second opening between the greater and lesser tuberosities allows passage of the tendon and synovial sheath of the long head of the biceps. A third, inconstant perforation may exist posteriorly, allowing communication of the articular cavity and a bursa under the infraspinatus tendon.

A synovial membrane lines the inner aspect of the fibrous capsule. It covers the anatomic neck of the humerus and extends to the articular cartilage on the humeral head. The synovium passes distally to line the bicipital groove and is reflected over the biceps tendon.

Several bursae are present about the glenohumeral joint:

Subscapular Recess. This bursa lies between the subscapularis tendon and the scapula, communicating with the joint via an opening between the superior and middle gleno-

humeral ligaments. This bursa is readily apparent on shoulder arthrograms as a tongue-shaped collection of contrast material extending medially from the glenohumeral space underneath the coracoid process.[50] It is prominent in internal rotation but is less obvious in external rotation, as the taut subscapularis muscle compresses the bursa.

Bursa About the Infraspinatus Tendon. This inconstant bursa separates the infraspinatus tendon and joint capsule and may communicate with the joint cavity.

Subacromial (Subdeltoid) Bursa. This important bursa lies between the deltoid muscle and joint capsule.[51] It extends underneath the acromion and the coracoacromial ligament. The subacromial bursa is separated from the articular cavity by the rotator cuff and does not communicate with the joint unless there has been a perforation of the cuff. Layers of fat tissue about this bursa have been identified on radiographs of the normal shoulder[52]; a thin, crescentic radiolucent area passes from the inferior aspect of the acromion process and distal end of the clavicle along the outer margin of the upper humerus. This fat layer is designated the peribursal fat plane, and its obliteration when detected with routine radiography, CT, or MR imaging is a secondary sign of a pathologic condition of the shoulder.[296]

Bursa Above the Acromion. This bursa is located on the superior surface of the acromion process of the scapula.

Miscellaneous Bursae. Additional bursae[1] may be found between the coracoid process and the capsule, behind the coracobrachialis, between the teres major and the long head of the triceps, and about the latissimus dorsi.

The mobile glenohumeral joint is active in a variety of movements, including flexion, extension, abduction, adduction, circumduction, and medial and lateral rotation. Accessory movements of this articulation include upward, downward, forward, and backward motions.[1, 46, 53–55]

ACROMIOCLAVICULAR JOINT

The acromioclavicular joint is a synovial articulation between the lateral aspect of the clavicle and the medial aspect of the acromion.[1, 2, 56]

Osseous Anatomy

The lateral or acromial end of the clavicle is a flattened structure with a small, oval articular facet that faces laterally and slightly downward (Fig. 22–21). This facet articulates with the acromial facet of the scapula and is the site of attachment of the joint capsule of the acromioclavicular joint. The inferior surface of the acromial end of the clavicle possesses a rough osseous ridge, termed the trapezoid line. A conoid tubercle is located at the posterior aspect of the lateral clavicle. The trapezoid line and conoid tubercle are the sites of attachment of the trapezoid and conoid parts of the coracoclavicular ligament.

The acromion is a forward protuberance of the lateral aspect of the scapula. An articular facet, the acromial facet, is located on the medial border of the acromion and is small and oval in size and configuration, directed medially and superiorly. The inferior surface of the acromion varies in its slope and configuration, factors that may be important in the pathogenesis of the shoulder impingement syndrome and rotator cuff pathology (see Chapter 70).

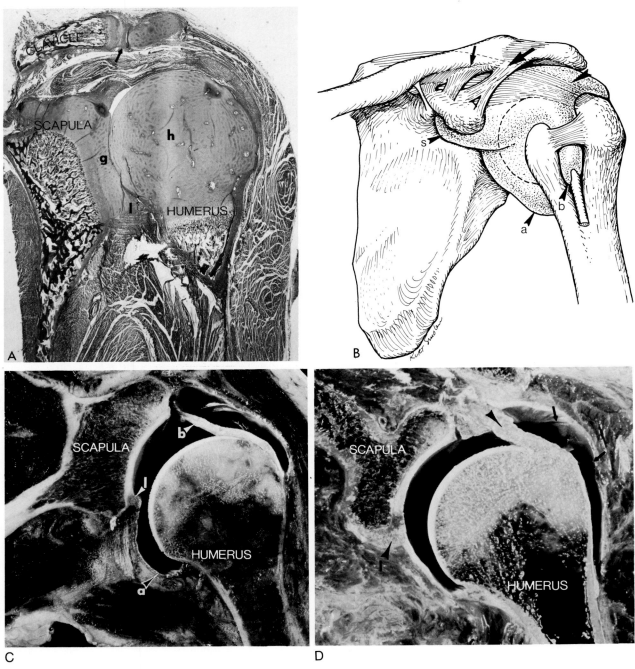

FIGURE 22–20. Glenohumeral joint: Normal development and anatomy.
  A A coronal section of the developing glenohumeral joint (20×) reveals the joint between unossified humeral head *(h)* and glenoid cavity *(g)*. Additional structures are the acromioclavicular joint (arrow) between acromion and distal end of the clavicle and the glenoid labrum *(l)*.
  B A drawing of the anterior aspect of the distended glenohumeral joint depicts axillary pouch *(a)*, subscapular recess *(s)*, and synovial extension over the bicipital tendon *(b)*. Note the rotator cuff (arrowhead), coracoacromial ligament (heavy arrow), and coracoclavicular ligament (light arrow).
  C, D Two coronal sections through different portions of the air-distended glenohumeral joint outline articular cavity, axillary pouch *(a)*, tendon of the long head of the biceps *(b)*, glenoid labrum *(l)*, rotator cuff (arrowhead), and subacromial (subdeltoid) bursa (arrows).

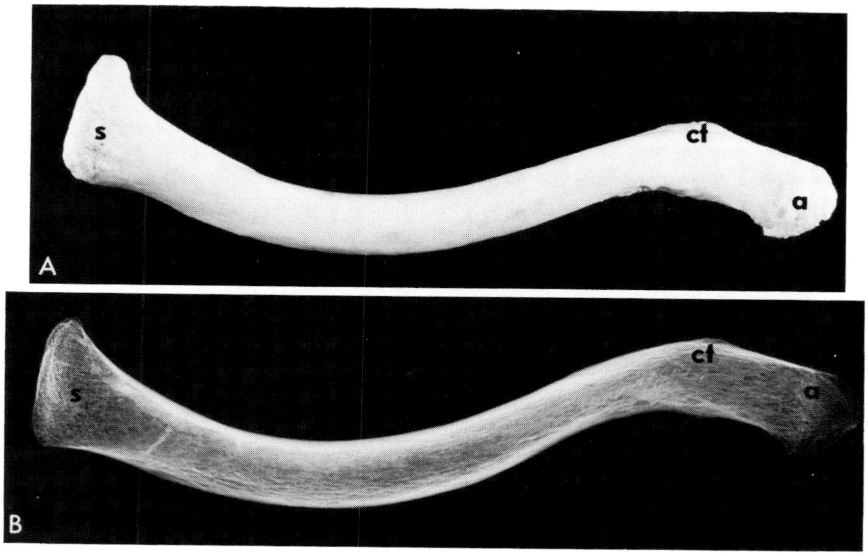

FIGURE 22–21. Clavicle: Osseous anatomy. **A, B** Superior aspect. Photograph and radiograph delineate sternal *(s)* and acromial *(a)* ends of the clavicle. Note the conoid tubercle *(ct)* on the posterior surface of the distal end of the clavicle.

Soft Tissue Anatomy

The articular surfaces about the acromioclavicular joint are covered with fibrocartilage (Fig. 22–22). In the central portion of the joint is an articular disc[56, 57] that partially or, more rarely, completely divides the joint cavity. The fibrous capsule surrounds the articular margin and is reinforced on its superior and inferior surfaces. Surrounding ligaments include the acromioclavicular and coracoclavicular ligaments. The former ligament, which is located at the superior portion of the joint, extends between the clavicle and acromion. The coracoclavicular ligament, which attaches to the coracoid process of the scapula and clavicle, is composed of a trapezoid part and a conoid part. The trapezoid portion extends from the upper surface of the coracoid process to the trapezoid line on the inferior aspect of the clavicle; the conoid portion extends from the coracoid process to the conoid tubercle on the inferior clavicular surface. The trapezoid and conoid parts of the coracoclavicular ligament may be separated by fat or a bursa.

A joint may be noted between the clavicle and coracoid process in 0.1 to 1.2 per cent of people.[220–223, 293] In these cases, a triangular or rectangular outgrowth from the under-surface of the clavicle approaches the dorsomedial surface of the coracoid process (Fig. 22–23). On dissection, the articulation may be found to contain a capsule and synovial membrane as well as a cartilaginous disc.[218]

Normal anteroposterior radiographs of the acromioclavicular joint may reveal a soft tissue plane about the joint related to the aponeurosis associated with the trapezius and deltoid muscles.[58, 59] Contrast opacification of the joint reveals an L-shaped articular cavity with a horizontal limb extending under the inferior surface of the distal end of the clavicle.[59]

The acromioclavicular joint allows the acromion to glide in a forward and backward direction and to rotate on the clavicle. These movements depend on additional movements at the sternoclavicular joint.[1]

STERNOCLAVICULAR JOINT

At the sternoclavicular articulation, the medial end of the clavicle articulates with the clavicular notch of the manubrium sterni and with the cartilage of the first rib[1, 56] (Figs. 22–24 to 22–26).

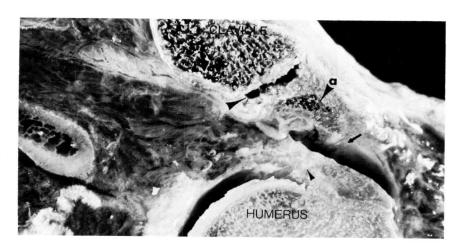

FIGURE 22–22. Acromioclavicular joint: Normal anatomy. Visualized structures on this coronal section are the articular space (large arrowhead) between distal end of the clavicle and acromion *(a)* (an articular disc is not visible), rotator cuff (small arrowhead), and subacromial (subdeltoid) bursa (arrow).

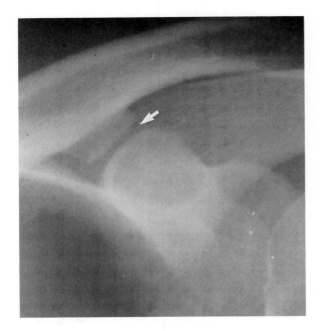

FIGURE 22–23. Accessory coracoclavicular joint. Note the space (arrow) between the coracoid process and an outgrowth from the undersurface of the clavicle.

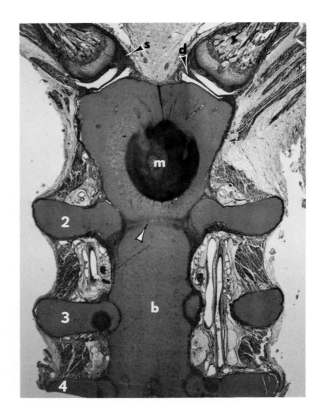

FIGURE 22–24. Sternum and clavicle: Developmental anatomy: A photomicrograph (20×) of a coronal section through the sternum and clavicle outlines the unossified manubrium *(m)* and body *(b)* of the sternum, partially ossified medial clavicle, and costal cartilage of the second *(2)*, third *(3)*, and fourth *(4)* ribs. Observe the sternoclavicular joints with synovium *(s)* and articular disc *(d)* and manubriosternal joint (arrowhead).

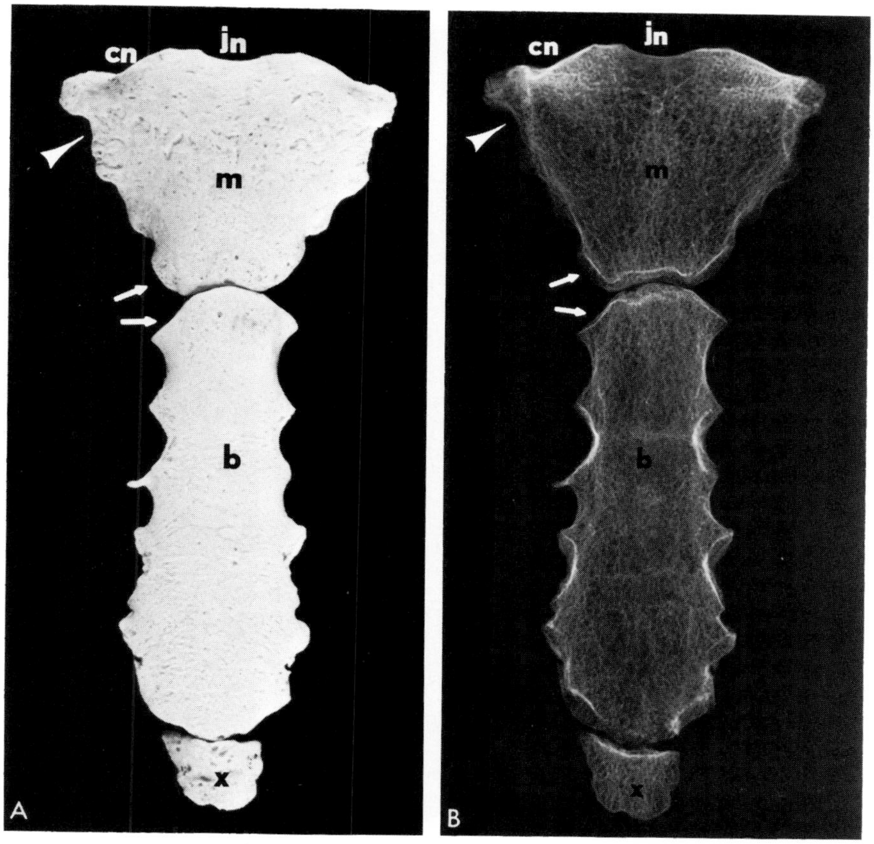

FIGURE 22–25. Sternum: Osseous anatomy. Anterior aspect. The three segments of the sternum are the manubrium *(m)*, body *(b)*, and xiphoid process *(x)*. Additional landmarks are the clavicular notch *(cn)* and jugular notch *(jn)*. A sternal facet for articulation with the first costal cartilage (arrowheads) and hemifacets for articulation with the second costal cartilage (arrows) are indicated. Other articular facets also are apparent on the body of the sternum.

Osseous Anatomy

The enlarged medial or sternal end of the clavicle projects above the upper margin of the manubrium and is directed medially, inferiorly, and anteriorly (Fig. 22–21). The articular surface is smooth except on its superior portion, where a roughened area allows attachment of an articular disc. The inferior portion of the articular surface is extended to allow articulation with the first costal cartilage. The medial portion of the inferior surface of the clavicle has a rough impression for attachment of the costoclavicular ligament.

The superolateral portions of the manubrium contain oval articular surfaces, the clavicular facets or notches, which are directed superiorly, posteriorly, and laterally. Below each clavicular notch is a rough projection, which receives the first costal cartilage.

Soft Tissue Anatomy

The articular end of the clavicle is covered with a layer of fibrocartilage that is thicker than the cartilage on the sternum. A flat, circular disc is located between the articulating surfaces of the clavicle and sternum; it is attached superiorly to the posterior border of the clavicle, inferiorly to the cartilage of the first rib, and, at other sites, to the fibrous capsule, and it divides the joint into two articular cavities.[227] The disc acts as a checkrein against medial displacement of the inner clavicle. Perforations in the disc are frequent in older persons. A fibrous capsule surrounds the joint[60] and is attached to the clavicular and sternomanubrial

articular surfaces. The inferior portion of the capsule is weak as it passes between the clavicle and superior surface of the first costal cartilage. Elsewhere the capsule is strong, reinforced by the anterior and posterior sternoclavicular ligaments and the interclavicular ligament. Nearby, the costoclavicular ligament attaches below to the upper surface of the first rib and adjacent cartilage and above to the inferior surface of the medial end of the clavicle. This ligament consists of anterior and posterior portions, between which is located a bursa.[61] This ligament resists forces that attempt to displace the medial clavicle anteriorly, posteriorly, upward, or laterally.

The sternoclavicular joint is freely mobile. It participates in movements of the upper extremity, including elevation, depression, protraction, retraction, and circumduction.[54, 62]

STERNAL JOINTS

Osseous Anatomy

The sternum consists of three portions, a proximal portion termed the manubrium, a middle portion, the body, and a distal portion, the xiphoid process (Fig. 22–25). The pattern of ossification during the development of the sternum is variable.[63–65, 226] The manubriosternal junction usually remains unossified in the adult. Ossification between segments in the lower portion of the sternal body occurs soon after puberty; ossification between segments in the upper portion of the body occurs between puberty and the twenty-fifth year of life. Ossification between the body and xiphoid process occurs at approximately 40 years of age.

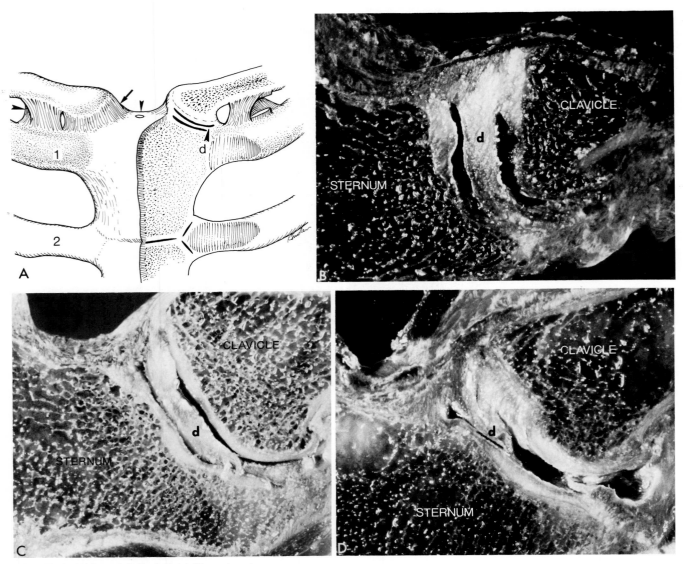

FIGURE 22–26. Sternoclavicular joint: Normal anatomy.

A A diagrammatic depiction of the anterior aspect of the upper sternum and medial clavicles. On the right-hand side, the superficial bone has been removed, exposing the sternoclavicular, manubriosternal, and second sternocostal joints. Identified structures are the anterior sternoclavicular ligament (arrow), costoclavicular ligament (arrowhead on left), interclavicular ligament (arrowhead in center), and articular disc *(d)*. Note the first *(1)* and second *(2)* costal cartilages. (From Warwick R, Williams P: Gray's Anatomy. 35th British Ed. Philadelphia, WB Saunders Co, 1973.)

B–D Photographs of coronal sections through the sternoclavicular joint in three different cadavers reveal characteristics of the intra-articular disc *(d)*. Observe a relatively normal articular disc **(B)**, a slightly irregular disc **(C)**, and a perforated disc **(D)**. In the last-mentioned instance, the two articular cavities communicate.

The manubrium is the widest portion of the sternum and is quadrilateral in shape. The jugular (suprasternal) notch is located at the midportion of the superior border of the manubrium. The body of the sternum is approximately twice as long as the manubrium. Its anterior surface contains three transverse ridges of bone, representing the sites of union between osseous sternal segments. The posterior surface has similar but less marked ridges. The xiphoid process is the smallest part of the sternum and is quite variable in appearance. It may be perforated in its central portion.

Soft Tissue Anatomy

Two articulations exist between segments of the sternum: the manubriosternal joint and the xiphisternal joint (Fig. 22–25).

Manubriosternal Joint. The joint between manubrium and body of the sternum is a symphysis; the apposing osseous surfaces are covered with hyaline cartilage and separated by a fibrocartilaginous disc. In approximately 25 to 30 per cent of persons, the central portion of the disc undergoes cavitation; in approximately 10 to 15 per cent of persons over the age of 30 years, complete ossification produces a synostosis between these two segments of the sternum, a process that increases with advancing age.[66, 67, 217] Synostosis may be related to persistence of a synchondrosis rather than a symphysis at this junction.[68]

Xiphisternal Joint. This articulation is a symphysis that exists between the sternal body and xiphoid. Although it may remain unossified even in elderly persons, it usually becomes a synostosis by the fortieth year of life.[1]

STERNOCOSTAL AND INTERCOSTAL JOINTS

The anterior aspect of each rib is firmly attached to a column of hyaline cartilage, termed the costal cartilage, at the costochondral junction.[69] The first costal cartilage is united with the sternum, the second through seventh costal cartilages articulate with sternal facets, and the lower costal cartilages, except for the eleventh and twelfth, articulate with each other. Costal cartilage calcification proceeds with advancing age, and the pattern of ossification appears different in men and women.[70–74]

Osseous Anatomy

On the manubrium is a rough facet below each clavicular notch, which articulates with the first costal cartilage (Fig. 22–25). At the manubrium-body junction, hemifacets are present that articulate with the second costal cartilage. Additional articular facets occur between the segments of the body for articulation with the third to fifth costal cartilages, on the fourth segment of the body for articulation with the sixth costal cartilage, and at the xiphisternal junction for articulation with the seventh costal cartilage.

Soft Tissue Anatomy

The costal cartilages are involved in two types of joints (Fig. 22–27).

Sternocostal (Sternochondral) Joints. The articulation between the first costal cartilage and the sternum is a synchondrosis.[228, 297] Elsewhere synovial articulations exist at the sternocostal junctions.[298] The synovial cavity in each of these junctions is divided into two by an intra-articular ligament. This cavity persists at the second costal cartilage–sternal junction, but the other synovial cavities usually become obliterated with advancing age as ossification in the fibrocartilage-clothed articular surfaces unites costal cartilage and sternum.[75] Fibrous capsules about the joints are strengthened in front and back by radiating fibers, termed the anterior and posterior radiate ligaments. Slight gliding motions, important in respiration, occur at the sternocostal joints.[1, 76]

Intercostal (Interchondral) Joints. Contiguous borders of certain costal cartilages articulate with each other via facets separated by a synovial cavity, surrounded by a fibrous capsule, and strengthened laterally and medially by interchondral ligaments. This situation occurs most frequently between the sixth and seventh, seventh and eighth, and eighth and ninth costal cartilages. Occasionally a similar situation exists between the fifth and sixth and between the ninth and tenth costal cartilages, although at the latter site a syndesmosis is more common.

COSTOVERTEBRAL JOINTS

The ribs and vertebral column articulate at two areas: between the heads of the ribs and vertebral bodies; and between the necks and tubercles of the ribs and transverse processes of the vertebrae[77–82, 247, 299] (Table 22–1).

Osseous Anatomy

The posterior end of a typical rib contains an enlarged head with two sloping articular facets and an intervening osseous ridge or crest (Fig. 22–28). The neck of a rib is a flattened structure adjacent to the head, which lies anteriorly to the transverse process of the corresponding vertebra. The obliquely oriented neck contains an anterior surface that faces forward and upward. The upper border is the sharp crest of the neck of the rib. The lower border of the neck is round. The tubercle of the rib occurs at its posterior surface at the junction of the neck and body. The tubercle has an articular and a nonarticular portion. The former area contains a small, oval facet that articulates with

---

TABLE 22–1. Articulations of the Spine

Synovial Joints
  Apophyseal (facet) joints
  Atlas—odontoid process
  Odontoid process—transverse ligament
  Costovertebral joints
    Joints of the heads of the ribs
    Costotransverse joints
  Joints of Luschka*

Symphyses
  Intervertebral discs

Syndesmoses
  Ligamentous connections of vertebral bodies
  Ligamentous connections of vertebral arches

*Resemble synovial joints.

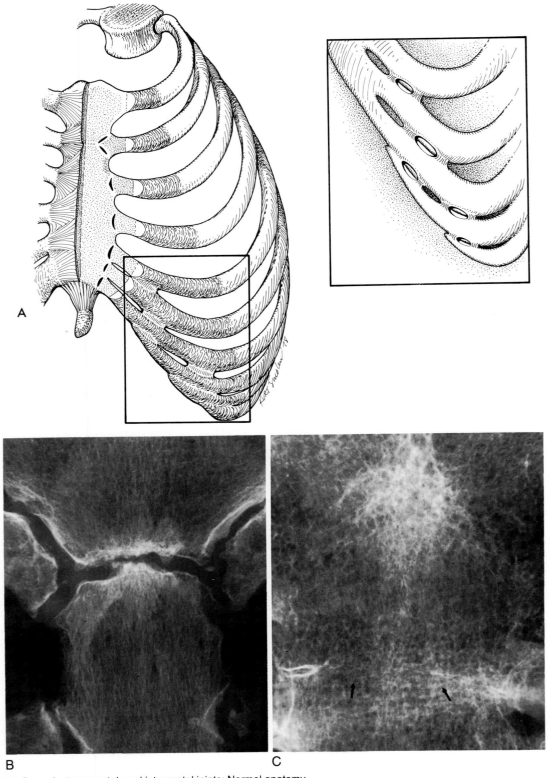

FIGURE 22–27. Sternal, sternocostal, and intercostal joints: Normal anatomy.

A A schematic drawing of the anterior aspect of the chest wall depicts the manubriosternal and sternocostal joints. At the manubriosternal joint, hemifacets on the sternum articulate with the second costal cartilage. A synchondrosis exists at the articulation between the first costal cartilage and the sternum. The third through seventh costal cartilages also articulate with the sternum. A close-up of the intercostal joints (inset) demonstrates facets separated by synovial cavities. (From Warwick R, Williams P: Gray's Anatomy. 35th British Ed. Philadelphia, WB Saunders Co, 1973.)

B, C Frontal radiographs of the manubriosternal joint in two different cadavers outline sequential stages of ossification resulting in a synostosis (arrows) between manubrium and body of the sternum.

Illustration continued on opposite page

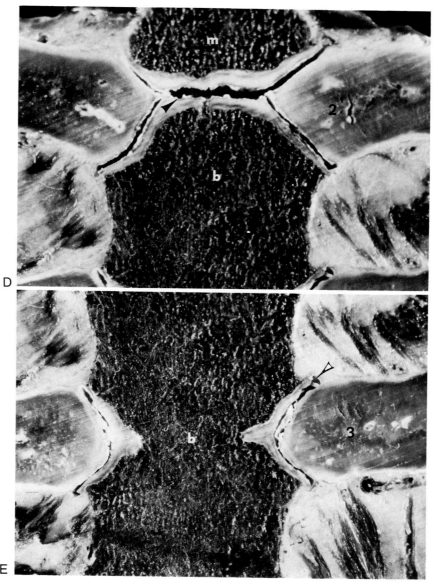

FIGURE 22–27 *Continued*

   D Manubriosternal and second sternocostal articulations (coronal section). In this cadaver, the manubriosternal joint has undergone cavitation (arrowhead). This articulation is communicating with the sternocostal joint (*m*, manubrium; *b*, body; *2*, second costal cartilage).

   E Third sternocostal articulation (coronal section). Observe sternal body *(b)*, third costal cartilage *(3)*, and intervening synovial articulation (arrowhead).

Illustration continued on following page

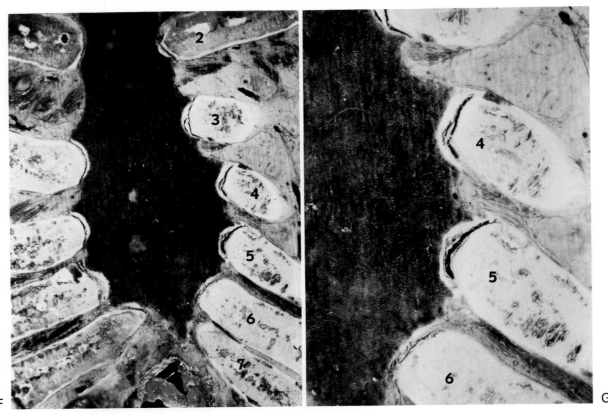

FIGURE 22–27 *Continued*
F, G Sternocostal articulations. A coronal section of a cadaveric sternum, demonstrating second through seventh *(2–7)* sternocostal joints.

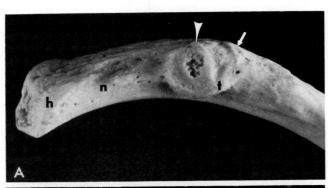

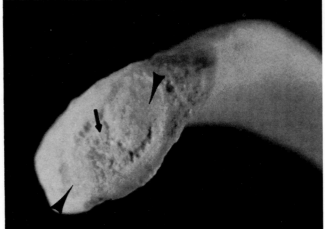

FIGURE 22–28. Posterior rib: Osseous anatomy.
   A Inferior aspect of typical rib. Note the head *(h)*, neck *(n)*, and tubercle *(t)*. The last consists of an articular (arrowhead) and nonarticular (arrow) portion.
   B Medial aspect. A photograph of the head of a typical rib outlining two articular facets (arrowheads) with intervening osseous crest (arrow).

the transverse process of the vertebra, and the latter area, which is roughened, represents the site of attachment of the lateral costotransverse ligament.

The first rib contains a small head with a single articular facet. It also possesses a long narrow neck and a large tubercle, which has a medial oval facet for articulation with the transverse process of the first thoracic vertebra. The tenth rib has a single articular facet on its head. The eleventh and twelfth ribs also have articular facets on their heads but have no necks or tubercles.

A typical thoracic vertebra contains two costal facets on each side of the body. The larger upper facet is located at the superior margin of the vertebral body in front of the pedicle. The smaller inferior facet is apparent at the inferior margin of the vertebral body, anterior to the vertebral notch. Additionally, an oval facet is located at the tip of the transverse process. This facet articulates with the tubercle of the numerically corresponding rib.

The upper costal facets on the body of the first thoracic vertebra are circular in appearance, as they articulate with the entire facet of the first pair of ribs. The ninth thoracic vertebral body may not articulate with the joints of the tenth rib; in these cases, inferior facets are absent on this vertebra. Similarly, its transverse process may or may not have an articular facet. The transverse processes of the eleventh and twelfth vertebrae likewise do not have articular facets.

Soft Tissue Anatomy

Joints of the Heads of Ribs (Fig. 22–29). A short, thick intra-articular ligament extends from the bony crest of the second through ninth ribs to the adjacent intervertebral disc, separating the articular cavity into two parts, each containing a synovial membrane. The first, tenth, eleventh, and twelfth ribs articulate with a single vertebral body and hence create a single synovial joint. The articulations are surrounded by a fibrous capsule whose thickened anterior portion is termed the radiate ligament of the head of the rib.

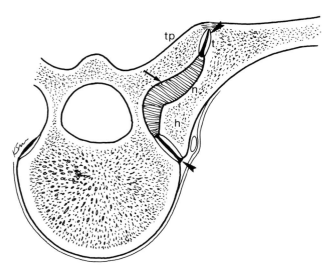

FIGURE 22–29. Costovertebral joints: Normal anatomy (transverse section). There are two synovial cavities (arrowheads) separated by costotransverse ligaments (arrow). The head *(h),* neck *(n),* and tubercle *(t)* of the rib are indicated. The head articulates with the vertebral body and the tubercle articulates with the transverse process *(tp)* of the vertebra.

Costotransverse Joints (Fig. 22–29). The costotransverse joint is a synovial articulation surrounded by a fibrous capsule. The lateral costotransverse ligament strengthens the posterolateral aspect of the joint. The costotransverse ligament also binds the rib and adjacent transverse process, whereas the superior costotransverse ligament attaches the rib to the transverse process of the vertebra above. The costotransverse ligaments of the lowest two ribs are poorly defined or absent, and synovial joints between tubercles of rib and transverse processes of these vertebrae are not present.

At the costotransverse and rib head joints, minimal gliding movements between articular surfaces are possible. Movements at these two sets of joints occur simultaneously. The direction of movement varies between upper and lower ribs as the shape of the tubercle facets on these ribs is different.[1] The facets on the upper six ribs are oval and convex from above downward; they fit into concavities on the anterior portion of the transverse processes, allowing upward and downward movement of the tubercle and rotation of the neck of the rib on its longitudinal axis. The facets on the tubercles of the seventh through tenth ribs are relatively flat, facing downward, backward, and medially. They articulate with the superior aspects of the transverse processes. In these joints, the rib and neck move upward, backward, and medially, or downward, forward, and laterally.

JOINTS OF THE VERTEBRAL BODIES

Osseous and Soft Tissue Anatomy

Joints separating vertebral bodies are of two types: articulations between vertebral bodies that consist of intervertebral discs are symphyses; those between vertebral bodies that consist of anterior and posterior longitudinal ligaments are syndesmoses[1, 2, 83, 84] (Fig. 22–30).

Intervertebral Discs (Fig. 22–30). Intervertebral discs separate the vertebral bodies from the axis to the sacrum. The attachments of the discs include the anterior and posterior longitudinal ligaments and the intra-articular ligaments, which extend to some of the heads of the ribs. The intervertebral discs differ in shape and thickness at various levels of the vertebral column. Discs are thickest in the lumbar region and thinnest in the upper thoracic area. In the cervical and lumbar regions, they are thicker anteriorly than posteriorly, whereas in the thoracic region, they are of uniform thickness.

The intervertebral discs between the cervical vertebrae do not extend to the lateral edges of the vertebral bodies (Fig. 22–31). In this area, articular modifications are found on both sides of the intervertebral discs as cleftlike cavities between the superior surface of the uncinate process of one vertebra and the lateral lips of the inferior articulating surface of the vertebra above. These modifications, called the joints of Luschka, are a source of controversy.[2, 83–86, 248] The fetus has no joints of Luschka. These joints, which form postnatally by fibrillation and fissuring in the marginal fibers of the anulus fibrosus or by slow absorption of loose fibrous tissue, usually are apparent by 4 years of age and well established by 14 years of age.[85] They may not be present in all persons or at all cervical spine levels. Rarely they are observed at the first thoracic level as well but not

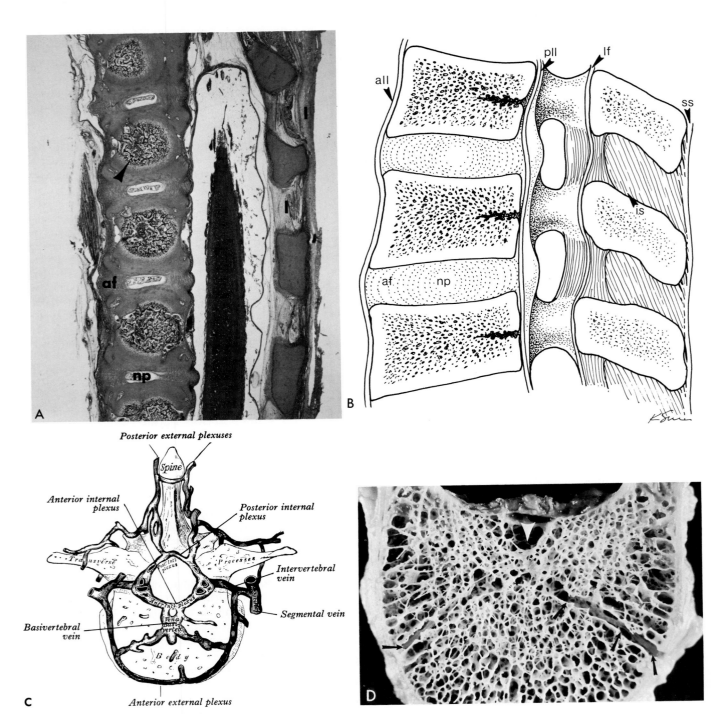

FIGURE 22–30. Vertebral column. Normal development and anatomy.

A Sagittal section (20×) of fetal spine. Ossification (arrowhead) within the vertebral bodies can be identified. Observe the developing intervertebral disc, consisting of anulus fibrosus *(af)* and nucleus pulposus *(np)*, spinal cord, and interspinous and supraspinous ligaments *(l)*.

B Drawing of a sagittal section of adult spine depicts vertebral bodies separated by intervertebral discs, consisting of anulus fibrosus *(af)* and nucleus pulposus *(np)*. The anterior longitudinal ligament *(all)*, posterior longitudinal ligament *(pll)*, ligamentum flavum *(lf)*, and interspinous *(is)* and supraspinous *(ss)* ligaments are indicated.

C A transverse section through the body of a thoracic vertebra, showing the vertebral venous plexuses and basivertebral veins. (From Warwick R, Williams P: Gray's Anatomy. 35th British Edition. Philadelphia, WB Saunders Co, 1973.)

D Photograph of a transverse section through a macerated vertebral body showing the osseous grooves (arrows) and large posterior fenestration (arrowhead) marking the position of the basivertebral veins.

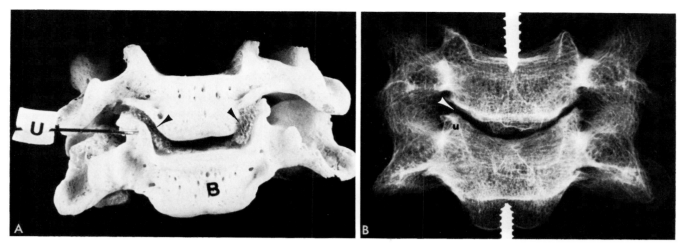

FIGURE 22–31. Cervical spine: Joints of Luschka.
  A On a photograph of the anterior aspect of the cervical spine, the joints of Luschka (arrowheads) are seen between the superior surface of the uncinate process *(U)* of one vertebra *(B)* and the lateral lips of the inferior articulating surface of the vertebra above.
  B A radiograph of the specimen in **A** indicates the structure of the joints of Luschka (arrowhead) and the uncinate processes *(u)*.

caudal to that vertebra. The lining of the Luschka joint is provided by the cartilaginous endplate of the vertebral body. A serum transudate usually is present within the cleft, and the arrangement simulates that of a synovial joint. A true synovial lining is not apparent, however.

The individual discs are adherent to hyaline cartilaginous endplates, which cover the central depressions of the upper and lower aspects of the vertebral bodies (Fig. 22–32). The deep surface of the cartilaginous endplate contains calcified cartilage. The subchondral bone of the vertebral body is variable in appearance. In some areas, a thick layer of subchondral bone and calcified cartilage can be identified; elsewhere, the bony surface may be thin, with numerous perforations allowing direct contact of bone marrow and nonmineralized cartilage.[87] Complete perforations of the chondro-osseous junction by blood vessels may be noted at the discovertebral junction.[87] Vascular channels embedded within the cartilaginous endplates are particularly prominent in very young children. They allow diffusion of fluid from bone marrow to intervertebral disc.[88]

Each disc consists of an inner portion, the nucleus pulposus, surrounded by a peripheral portion, the anulus fibrosus. The nucleus pulposus is particularly well developed in the cervical and lumbar segments of the spine. It is located eccentrically, related more closely to the posterior surface of the disc. The nucleus pulposus is soft and gelatinous in young persons, but it gradually becomes replaced by fibrocartilage with increasing age. In older persons, the nucleus pulposus becomes amorphous, discolored, and dehydrated, and it is difficult to differentiate it from the remainder of the intervertebral disc.[89–92]

The anulus fibrosus encircles the nucleus pulposus and unites the vertebral bodies firmly. This structure consists of a peripheral zone of collagenous fibers and an inner zone of fibrocartilage. The lamellae of the anulus fibrosus are thinner and more closely packed between the nucleus and dorsal aspect of the intervertebral disc. Anteriorly, the lamellae are stronger and more distinct. The direction in which they are oriented varies with their relative position in the intervertebral disc.[83] In central areas, lamellae of the

anulus fibrosus curve inward with their convexity facing the nuclear substance. More peripherally, the bands of fibers are vertical. At the extreme periphery of the intervertebral disc, the lamellae again may become curved, with their convexity facing the periphery of the intervertebral disc.

The anulus fibrosus is attached to the adjacent vertebral bodies in two ways. At sites of endochondral ossification, such as the cartilaginous endplates and marginal osseous rims, the attachment consists essentially of fibers that penetrate the cartilaginous endplate and subchondral bony trabeculae. A stronger attachment between anulus fibrosus and vertebral body is apparent at sites of intramembranous ossification such as the anterior vertebral surface. Here, the fibers of the stoutest external lamellar bands, termed Sharpey's fibers, enter the bone at different angles and extend beyond the confines of the intervertebral disc, blending with the periosteum of the vertebral body and longitudinal ligaments.

The two components of the intervertebral disc, the anulus fibrosus and nucleus pulposus, are avascular except for the most peripheral fibers of the anulus, which receive a blood supply from adjacent vessels.[93] These penetrating vessels are more prominent in children than in adults,[87] although a secondary ingrowth of vessels may be associated with disc degeneration in older persons.[87, 94] The nutrition of the intervertebral disc is dependent on (1) diffusion of fluid from the marrow of the vertebral bodies through the porous upper and lower vertebral endplates in the central portion of the plate, and (2) diffusion of fluid through the anulus fibrosus from the surrounding vessels.[95]

Both external and internal venous plexuses are associated with the vertebral column[95] (Fig. 22–30). The external plexus consists of an anterior and a posterior set of veins. The internal plexus is a series of irregular valveless epidural sinuses that extend from coccyx to foramen magnum. The internal plexus consists of anterior and posterior cross-connected collecting vessels. The anterior channels extend along the posterior surface of the vertebral body just medial to the pedicles and connect to a large, unpaired basiverte-

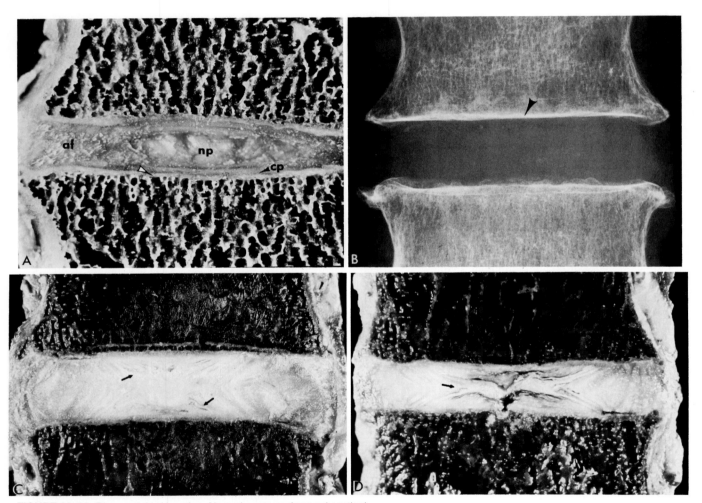

FIGURE 22–32. Discovertebral junction: Normal anatomy (coronal section).
   A, B Labeled structures are the nucleus pulposus *(np),* anulus fibrosus *(af),* cartilaginous endplate *(cp),* and subchondral bone (arrowheads).
   C, D Nucleus pulposus. Progressive changes of dehydration and degeneration in two cadavers (coronal sections). Discoloration and fragmentation (arrows) are apparent.

bral sinus that arises within the spongiosa and drains the intraosseous labyrinth of sinusoids. As the internal plexus is valveless, blood can pass in any direction according to shifts in intra-abdominal and intrathoracic pressure. Batson[96] has emphasized that retrograde flow from venous connections to pelvic organs provides an important route for metastasis to both the spine and the trunk areas (see Chapter 85).

Anterior and Posterior Longitudinal Ligaments. The anterior longitudinal ligament is a strong band of fibers that descends along the anterior surface of the vertebral column. It is relatively narrow in the cervical region and expands in width in the thoracic and lumbar regions, and in the latter regions it covers most of the anterolateral surface of the vertebral bodies and discs. The anterior longitudinal ligament consists of three sets of fibers: deep fibers span only one intervertebral joint; intermediate fibers unite two or three vertebrae; the superficial layer connects four or five vertebrae.[83] The anterior longitudinal ligament is fixed to the intervertebral discs and vertebral bodies. It is particularly adherent to the articular lip at the edge of each vertebral body but loosely attached at intermediate levels of the bodies. The anterior longitudinal ligament is separated or elevated most readily at the midportion of the intervertebral disc, at which site it is loosely attached to the anulus.

The posterior longitudinal ligament extends along the posterior surface of the vertebral bodies and discs from skull to sacrum, within the vertebral canal. Its fibers are attached only to the intervertebral discs and margins of the vertebral bodies and not to the midposterior surface of the bone. In this latter area, the ligament is strung like a bow across the concavity of the posterior osseous surface, allowing venous structures to enter and leave the medullary sinus beneath its fibers. In the cervical and upper thoracic regions, the posterior longitudinal ligament is broad and uniform in width; in the lower thoracic and lumbar regions, it is narrow at the level of the vertebral bodies and broad at the level of the intervertebral discs.

Normal osseous and soft tissue radiography of the anterior vertebral column has received considerable attention. Normal values for the vertical and sagittal diameters of thoracic and lumbar vertebrae and intervertebral discs have been established.[97, 98] Additionally, a cervical prevertebral fat stripe has been described as a radiolucent line that parallels the anterior surface of the cervical vertebral bodies,[99] which may be a more reliable indicator of disease than other cervical prevertebral soft tissue changes.[100] This lucent line, which corresponds to areolar tissue in retropharyngeal and retroesophageal spaces, slants anteriorly at the level of the sixth cervical vertebral body, becoming continuous with areolar tissue behind the scalenus muscles. It is identifiable more readily on adult than on pediatric radiographs. Displacement or blurring of this fat plane may be associated with fracture, inflammation, or neoplasm.

JOINTS OF THE VERTEBRAL ARCHES

Articulations between vertebral arches consist of synovial joints (between articular processes of vertebrae) and syndesmoses (ligamentum flavum; interspinous, supraspinous, and intertransverse ligaments; and ligamentum nuchae).

Osseous Anatomy

The vertebral arch contains two pedicles and two laminae, the latter joining posteriorly to become the spinous process. The transverse process and two articular facets originate from a mass of bone at the junction of lamina and pedicle. One articular facet passes superiorly and a second one inferiorly, to articulate with a facet from the vertebrae above and below, respectively.

The orientation and appearance of the articular processes of the vertebrae vary, depending on the region of the vertebral column. In the cervical spine (C3-C7) the articular processes are large, forming part of a pillar of bone termed the articular mass (Fig. 22–33A). The flat, oval facets on these articular processes lie in an oblique coronal plane. The inferior articular facets of the axis (C2) have the same general orientation. In the thoracic spine, the superior articular processes, which face backward, slightly upward, and laterally, appose inferior articular processes, which face in the opposite direction (Fig. 22–33B). In the lumbar spine, superior processes face medially and posteriorly, whereas inferior processes face laterally and anteriorly (Fig. 22–34). These regional differences in the orientation of articular processes require that different projections be used for their demonstration on radiographs.[101–104] The articulations of the cervical and thoracic portions of the spine are best demonstrated on lateral radiographs, whereas oblique projections are necessary for the lumbar spine. Conventional tomography or CT scanning frequently is required.

The transverse processes of the vertebrae also demonstrate regional differences. In a typical cervical vertebra, the transverse processes have an anterior and a posterior tubercle, connected by a costotransverse lamella. The adjacent foramen transversarium transmits the vertebral artery, veins, and nerves. The transverse process of the axis (C2) is small and contains no anterior tubercle; that of the atlas (C1) resembles that of the axis closely. In the seventh cervical vertebra, the transverse process may extend anteriorly as a cervical rib. The transverse processes of the thoracic vertebrae have a tubercle for articulation with the corresponding rib tubercle. Transverse processes in the lumbar spine are flat, and the processes of the third lumbar vertebra may be the longest.

In the cervical spine, the spinous processes of the second to fifth vertebrae frequently are bifid. The atlas has no spinous process. In the thoracic spine, spinous processes are long and sloping, whereas in the lumbar spine, these processes are broad and horizontal.

Soft Tissue Anatomy

Synovial joints and syndesmoses exist at the joints of the vertebral arches.

Articular Processes (Synovial Joints). The superior articulating process of one vertebra is separated from the inferior articulating process of the vertebra above by a synovial joint, termed the apophyseal joint. This articulation is surrounded by a loose, thin articular capsule, which is attached to the bones of the adjacent articulating processes. The fibers of the articular capsule are longer and looser in the cervical region and are more taut as they proceed downward in the vertebral column. Within the

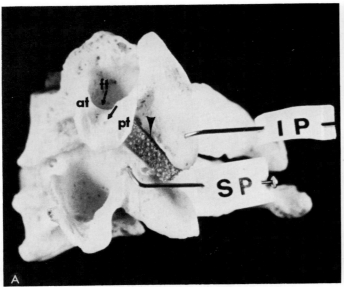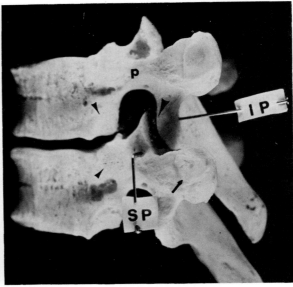

FIGURE 22–33. Articular processes: Cervical and thoracic spine.

 A A photograph of the lateral aspect of two cervical vertebrae reveals the inferior articular process *(ip)* and superior articular process *(sp)*, separated by a synovial joint (arrowhead). Observe the anterior tubercle *(at)* and posterior tubercle *(pt)* of the transverse process, sulcus for the ventral ramus of spinal nerve (arrow), and foramen transversarium *(ft)*.

 B A photograph of the lateral aspect of two thoracic vertebrae demonstrates the inferior articular process *(ip)* and superior articular process *(sp)*, separated by a synovial joint (large arrowhead). Note the pedicle *(p)*, hemifacets for the head of the rib (small arrowheads), and facet for the rib tubercle (arrow).

joint, meniscoid structures consisting of rudimentary fibrous invaginations of the dorsal and ventral capsule and synovial reflections filled with fat and fibrous tissue are seen.[249, 250, 300]

 Ligamentous Articulations (Syndesmoses). The syndesmoses between the vertebral arches are formed by the paired sets of ligamenta flava, intertransverse ligaments, and interspinous ligaments, and the unpaired supraspinous ligament.[1, 2, 83]

 The ligamenta flava connect the laminae of adjacent vertebrae from the second cervical to the lumbosacral levels. The attachment of the ligamenta flava extends from the articular capsule of the apophyseal joint to the area where the laminae fuse to form the spinous process. A small space or cleft between the two ligaments at this site allows passage of veins from the internal to the external venous plexuses. The ligamentum flavum, which consists predominantly of yellow elastic fibers extending in a perpendicular fashion, is thin and broad in the cervical region and thicker in the thoracic and lumbar areas. It is the most prominent elastic ligament in the human body; it permits separation of the laminae with flexion of the vertebral column and does not form redundant folds, which might otherwise compromise adjacent nervous tissue when the spine resumes an erect posture.

 Intertransverse ligaments extend between transverse processes. Their appearance varies at different levels of the spine: in the cervical spine, they are absent or consist of a few irregular, scattered fibers; in the thoracic spine they are cords of tissue associated with the deep musculature of the back; and in the lumbar spine, they are thin and membranous.

 Interspinous ligaments connect adjoining spinous proc-

esses, where their attachment extends from the root to apex of the process. These ligaments, which are placed between the ligamentum flavum in front and the supraspinous ligament behind, are longest and strongest in the lumbar spine. Contrast examination of these ligaments has been described.[105]

 The supraspinous ligament extends along the tips of the spinous processes from the seventh cervical vertebra to the sacrum. It is fused with the posterior edges of the interspinous ligaments. The most superficial fibers of the supraspinous ligament extend over three to four vertebrae. More deeply situated fibers extend over two to three vertebrae. The supraspinous ligament is broader and thicker in the lumbar spine than in the thoracic spine. In the cervical spine, the supraspinous ligament merges with the triangular ligamentum nuchae, the latter passing from the external occipital protuberance to the seventh cervical vertebra. Deep fibers of the ligamentum nuchae extend to the cervical spinous processes and the posterior tubercle of the atlas. Its role or function may be to assist in head position and control.[106] Ossicles resembling sesamoid bones are common in the ligamentum nuchae.

MOVEMENTS OF THE VERTEBRAL COLUMN

 The erect adult vertebral column has four anteroposterior curves, two of which are regarded as primary. An elongated curve, concave ventrally, extends throughout the thoracic spine. A second primary curve, also concave ventrally, is located in the sacral and coccygeal region. Secondary curves include a cervical curve, concave posteriorly, and a lumbar curve, also concave posteriorly.

 The range of motion is slight between any two adjacent

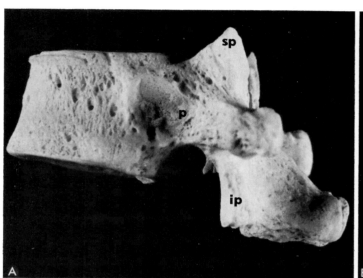

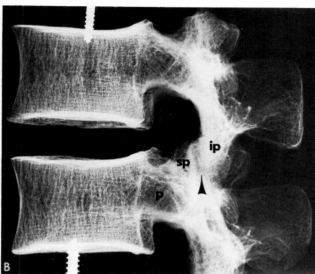

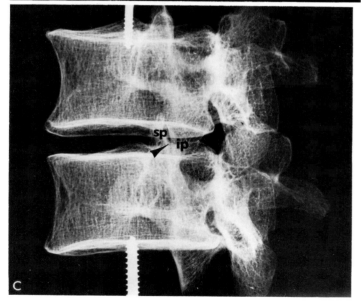

FIGURE 22–34. Articular processes: Lumbar spine.

A, B A photograph and radiograph of the lateral aspect of the lumbar vertebrae outline the superior articular process *(sp)* and inferior articular process *(ip),* separated by a synovial joint (arrowhead). Also observe the pedicles *(p).*

C On a radiograph of the lumbar vertebrae in an oblique projection, the synovial joint (arrowhead) between superior articular process *(sp)* and inferior articular process *(ip)* is better shown.

vertebrae owing to the limited degree of deformation of the intervertebral disc, but the total vertebral movement is considerable.[1, 2, 83] Movements include flexion, extension, lateral bending, rotation, and circumduction. In flexion, the anterior longitudinal ligament is lax and the anterior aspect of the intervertebral disc is compressed. The posterior fibers of the intervertebral discs, posterior longitudinal ligament, and posterior spinal ligaments (ligamenta flava, interspinous and supraspinous ligaments) are stretched, although the fundamental limiting factor to flexion is the tension of the posterior vertebral muscles. During flexion, the space between adjacent laminae is widened, and the inferior articulating process of one vertebra moves superiorly on the superior articulating process of the vertebra below.

In extension, the vertebrae move backward on each other, particularly in the cervical and lumbar segments. During this movement, the anterior longitudinal ligament becomes taut, whereas the other ligaments of the vertebral column are relaxed. In lateral bending, which involves predominantly the cervical and lumbar segments, compression of the lateral aspects of the intervertebral discs is apparent.

Rotation, most prominent in the upper thoracic region, results in twisting of one vertebra in relation to the others, with torsional deformation of intervening intervertebral discs.

Regional differences exist in the degree and type of spinal movement. In the cervical spine, the upper inclination of the superior articulating facets allows considerable flexion and extension. This freedom of motion is accentuated by the relatively large size of the intervertebral discs compared to the length of the bony cervical column. Lateral flexion and rotation in the cervical spine occur simultaneously. In the thoracic spine, motion is limited because the intervertebral discs are relatively thin, the superior articulating facets lack an upward inclination, and adjacent bony structures such as ribs and sternum produce additional stability. Rotation is free, as the articular processes lie in an arc of a circle with its center at or near the center of the vertebral bodies.[107] In the lumbar spine, the intervertebral discs are prominent, allowing considerable flexion and extension. Rotation is somewhat restricted by the articular processes.

ATLANTOAXIAL JOINTS

Osseous Anatomy

The ringlike first cervical vertebra, the atlas, does not possess a vertebral body or a spinous process (Fig. 22–35). It contains a small anterior arch, with a tubercle, a larger posterior arch with a corresponding tubercle, and two bulky lateral masses. The inferior surface of each lateral mass possesses a circular facet that is flat or slightly concave. This facet articulates with a corresponding facet on the superior articular process of the axis. The articular facet of the atlas is oriented inferiorly, medially, and slightly posteriorly. The medial portion of the lateral mass is roughened for the attachment of the transverse ligament of the atlas. The transverse processes of the atlas are long.

The second cervical vertebra, the axis, contains a superior peg of bone, the dens or odontoid process, which possesses a small oval facet for articulation with a facet on the posterior surface of the anterior arch of the atlas. On the

posterior surface of the odontoid process is a groove for the transverse ligament of the atlas. The odontoid process is approximately 1.3 to 1.5 cm long, with flat sides and a pointed apex. The axis also possesses two slightly convex superior articular facets, facing superiorly and laterally, which are intimate with similar facets on the atlas. Posterior to the superior facets are inferior facets, which articulate with the third cervical vertebra. The transverse processes of the axis are small, with a single tubercle.

On lateral radiographs of the cervical spine, the normal space between the anterior arch of the atlas and the odontoid process of the axis in the adult is $1.238 - (0.0074 \times$ age in years), $\pm$ 0.90 mm in women, and $2.052 - (0.0192 \times$ age in years), $\pm$ 1.00 mm in men.[108] A useful rule is that this distance should not be greater than 2.5 mm in adults. In children the average distance between the anterior arch of the atlas and the odontoid process is 2.0 to 2.5 mm in extension and 2.0 to 3.0 mm in flexion.[109] This distance should not exceed 4.5 mm in children. Evaluation of the distance between the anterior arch of the atlas and the odontoid process is more difficult in children below the age of 9 years owing to the rudimentary radiographic appearance of the dens.[301] An increase in distance between the anterior arch of the first cervical vertebra and the odontoid process is common in a variety of diseases, including articular and inflammatory disorders.

Soft Tissue Anatomy

Four synovial articulations occur between the atlas and axis: two lateral atlantoaxial joints, one on each side, between the inferior facet of the lateral mass of the atlas and the superior facet of the axis; and two median synovial joints, one between the anterior arch of the atlas and the odontoid process of the axis and a second between the odontoid process and the transverse ligament of the atlas (Fig. 22–36). In addition to these synovial articulations, syndesmoses between the atlas and axis include continuations of the anterior longitudinal ligament anteriorly and the ligamenta flava posteriorly.

Lateral Atlantoaxial Joints. These synovial joints exist on either side between the reciprocally curved cartilage-covered lateral masses of the atlas and axis and are surrounded by thin, loose fibrous capsules. Each capsule is strengthened posteromedially by an accessory ligament, which extends from the body of the axis to the lateral mass of the atlas.

Median Atlantoaxial Joints. Two synovial joints exist between the odontoid process of the axis and a ring formed by the anterior arch and transverse ligament of the atlas. The smaller of these two joints is located between a facet on the anterior surface of the odontoid and a second facet on the posterior surface of the anterior arch of the atlas. A weak, loose fibrous capsule surrounds this articulation. A second, larger joint lies between the cartilage-covered anterior surface of the transverse ligament of the atlas and the grooved posterior surface of the odontoid process. This joint, which also is surrounded by a loose fibrous capsule, may be continuous with the articular cavity of one or both atlanto-occipital joints.[1, 110]

Movement at the atlantoaxial articulations occurs at all locations simultaneously. This movement results in rotation of the skull and atlas with respect to the axis. The lateral

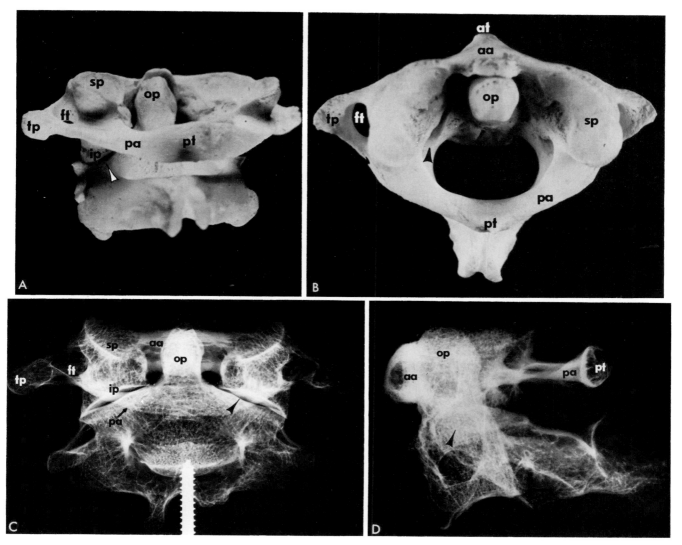

FIGURE 22–35. Atlas and axis: Osseous anatomy.
Posterior **(A)** and superior **(B)** views. Observe the anterior arch *(aa),* posterior arch *(pa),* anterior tubercle *(at),* posterior tubercle *(pt),* superior articular process *(sp),* inferior articular process *(ip),* transverse process *(tp),* and foramen transversarium *(ft)* of the atlas, and the odontoid process *(op)* and superior articular process (arrowheads) of the axis.
Frontal **(C)** and lateral **(D)** radiographs of atlas and axis with same structures indicated.

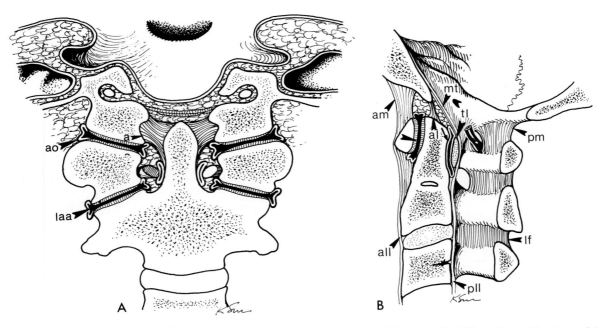

FIGURE 22–36. Atlantoaxial and atlanto-occipital joints: Anatomy. Drawing of coronal **(A)** and sagittal **(B)** sections of the base of the skull and upper cervical spine. Note the lateral atlantoaxial joints *(laa)*, atlanto-occipital synovial joints *(ao)*, anterior median joint (arrowhead) between the odontoid process and anterior arch of the atlas and the posterior median joint (arrow) between the odontoid process and transverse ligament *(tl)* of the atlas. Additional structures are the anterior longitudinal ligament *(all)*, posterior longitudinal ligament *(pll)*, membrana tectoria *(mt)*, anterior atlanto-occipital membrane *(am)*, posterior atlanto-occipital membrane *(pm)*, apical ligament of odontoid process *(al)*, alar ligament *(a)*, and ligamentum flavum *(lf)*.

masses of the atlas glide on the upper articular facets of the axis. This rotation is accompanied by a slight vertical descent of the head related to the oblique character of the articular surfaces. Excessive rotation is limited by the alar ligaments (extending from the odontoid process to the occipital condyles) and, to a lesser extent, by the accessory atlantoaxial ligaments.

ATLANTO-OCCIPITAL JOINTS

Osseous Anatomy

The superior surface of each lateral mass of the atlas has a concave, kidney-shaped facet that articulates with the corresponding occipital condyle. This atlantal facet is oriented medially and superiorly. The occipital condyles are oval, located on the anterolateral aspect of the foramen magnum.

Soft Tissue Anatomy

The atlanto-occipital joints consist of a pair of synovial joints, between the articular facets of the atlas and the condyles of the occiput, and syndesmoses formed by the anterior and posterior atlanto-occipital membranes (Fig. 22–36).

Atlanto-Occipital Synovial Joints. Reciprocally curved superior articular facets of the lateral mass of the atlas[111] and condyle of the occipital bone are separated by a synovial joint surrounded by a fibrous capsule.[112] The capsule is particularly thick on its posterior and lateral surfaces but deficient medially, where it may allow communication of

these joints with the synovial joint between the odontoid process and the transverse ligament.[110]

Atlanto-Occipital Membranes. The anterior atlanto-occipital membrane is attached above to the anterior margin of the foramen magnum and below to the anterior arch of the atlas. Its central portion contains fibers continuous with those of the anterior longitudinal ligament. The posterior atlanto-occipital membrane is attached above to the posterior margin of the foramen magnum and below to the posterior arch of the atlas. The free border of this membrane arches over the vertebral artery and first cervical spinal nerve. This border occasionally may ossify.

Movement at the atlanto-occipital joints occurs as flexion, extension, and lateral bending and may produce changes elsewhere in the cervical spine.[113–115] No significant rotation is present between the occiput and the atlas.

OCCIPITOAXIAL SYNDESMOSES

Ligamentous structures connecting the axis and the occiput are the membrana tectoria, paired alar ligaments, and an apical ligament. The membrana tectoria appears as an upward continuation of the posterior longitudinal ligament and extends from the axis to the occiput. The alar ligaments pass from the upper surface of the odontoid on each side to the medial sides of the occipital condyles. The apical ligament of the odontoid lies between the alar ligaments and runs from the tip of the process to the anterior margin of the foramen magnum. It blends both with the anterior atlanto-occipital membrane and with the cruciform ligament of the atlas.

OSSEOUS RELATIONSHIPS OF CERVICOBASILAR JUNCTION

The osseous relationships at the cervicobasilar junction have received considerable attention (Fig. 22–37). Chamberlain's line[219] can be drawn on a lateral radiograph from the posterior margin of the hard palate to the posterior border of the foramen magnum. In normal situations, the odontoid process should not extend more than 5 mm above this line. A modification of this line, McGregor's line,[224] uses the inferior surface of the occiput rather than the margin of the foramen magnum. In normal persons, the odontoid tip does not extend more than 7 mm above this line. On frontal radiographs, a line connecting the mastoid tips is within 2 mm of the tip of the odontoid,[225] whereas a line connecting the digastric muscle fossae is located at the approximate level of the foramen magnum and above the odontoid process. Additional methods used for the assessment of the relationship between the base of the skull and the upper cervical spine include those described by Ranawat and coworkers[302] and by Redlund-Johnell and Petersson.[303] The first of these methods is based on the distance between the pedicles of the axis and a line connecting the centers of the anterior and posterior arches of the atlas as seen on a lateral radiograph of the cervical spine. In men, this distance normally is 15 mm or greater, and in women, 13 mm or greater. The second method is based on a determination of the distance between McGregor's line and the midpoint of the inferior margin of the body of the axis, again determined on a lateral radiograph of the cervical spine. This distance normally is 34 mm or greater in men and 29 mm or greater in women.[304]

The basilar angle is the angle of intersection of two lines, one drawn from the nasion to the tuberculum sellae and a

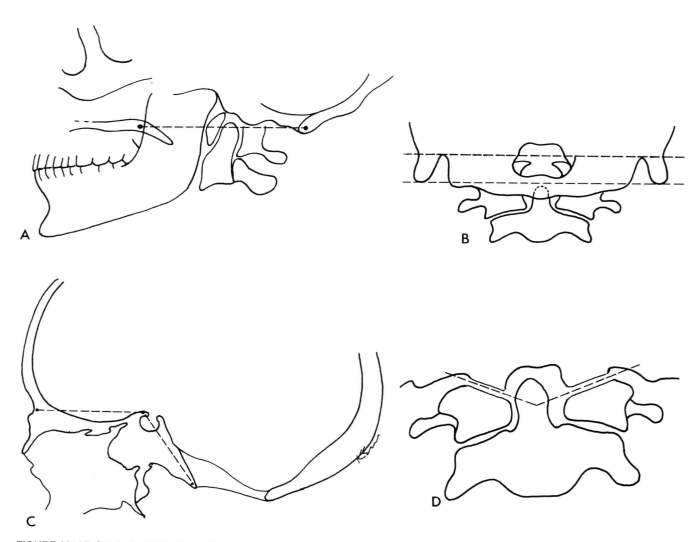

FIGURE 22–37. Cervicobasilar junction: Normal osseous relationships.

A Chamberlain's line is drawn from the posterior margin of the hard palate to the posterior border of the foramen magnum. The odontoid process normally does not extend more than 5 mm above this line.

B The bimastoid line (lower line) connecting the tips of the mastoids normally is within 2 mm of the odontoid tip. The digastric line (upper line) connecting the digastric muscle fossae normally is located above the odontoid process.

C The basilar angle, which normally exceeds 140 degrees, is formed by the angle of intersection of two lines, one drawn from the nasion to the tuberculum sellae and a second from the tuberculum sellae to the anterior edge of the foramen magnum.

D An atlanto-occipital joint angle, constructed on frontal tomograms by the intersection of two lines drawn along the axes of these articulations, normally is not greater than 150 degrees.

second from the tuberculum to the anterior edge of the foramen magnum. This angle normally does not exceed 140 degrees. An atlanto-occipital joint angle is constructed on frontal tomograms by drawing a line along this articulation on either side. The angle formed by the intersection of these two lines normally should not exceed 150 degrees.

JOINTS OF THE SACRUM AND COCCYX

Included here are the lumbosacral, sacrococcygeal, and intercoccygeal joints. The sacroiliac joints will be discussed separately.

Osseous Anatomy

The fifth lumbar vertebra resembles the other lumbar vertebrae, although it has a larger transverse process and body and a smaller spinous process (Fig. 22–38). Although the superior articular processes are wider than the inferior articular processes in the upper lumbar region, these processes are of approximately equal size in the fifth lumbar vertebra.

The sacrum is a large triangular bone (Fig. 22–38). It contains foramina that decrease in size as they proceed caudally. Each foramen is Y-shaped, with the base or stem

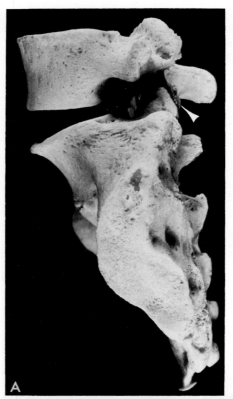

FIGURE 22–38. Sacrum: Osseous anatomy.

A Lumbosacral junction. Note the synovial joint (arrowhead) between the inferior articular process of the fifth lumbar vertebra and the superior articular process of the sacrum.

B, C Sacrum: Anterior and posterior aspects. The anterior view **(B)** demonstrates the promontory *(p)* and pelvic sacral foramina *(f)*. The posterior view **(C)** outlines the superior articular process *(sp)* and sacral foramina *(f)*. Observe an incidental finding, incomplete ossification of sacral spinous processes (arrowhead).

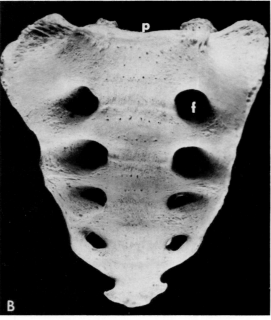

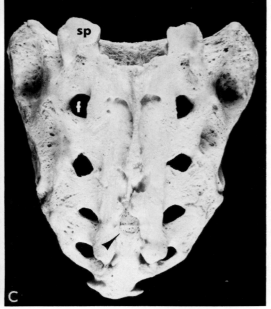

of the letter representing the anterior portion of the foramen and the limbs representing the posterior and intervertebral foramina.[251] The superiorly located base of the sacrum articulates with the fifth lumbar vertebra, creating the sacrovertebral angle. This angle represents the most abrupt change of alignment in the vertebral column and, as such, is subject to shearing forces. This angle has been measured in both normal and abnormal situations. In a lateral projection with the spine parallel to the table, the angle of intersection of two lines, one drawn along the inclination of the first sacral surface, and a second line representing the horizontal, normally is less than 34 degrees.[116]

The concave superior articular processes of the sacrum project upward to articulate with the inferior articular processes of the fifth lumbar vertebra. These sacral processes face posteriorly and medially.

Transitional type vertebrae are not infrequent at the lumbosacral junction. Expanded transverse processes of the fifth lumbar vertebra articulate with the top of the sacrum in either a unilateral or a bilateral distribution, or the entire vertebra may be incorporated into the sacrum. This process is termed sacralization of the fifth lumbar vertebra. Similarly, lumbarization represents elevation of the first sacral segment above the sacral mass so that it assumes the shape of a lumbar vertebra. As the radiographic appearance of sacralization and lumbarization is similar, an accurate diagnosis may require investigation of the entire vertebral column. The reported prevalence of transitional type situations at the lumbosacral junction has varied from 0.6 to 25 per cent of persons.[84] When the transverse processes of the transitional vertebra are connected to the lateral mass of the sacrum by means of an articulation, true joints with cartilaginous surfaces, articular capsules, supporting ligaments, and even bursae are present.

The apex of the sacrum represents the inferior surface of the body of the fifth sacral vertebrae. An oval facet that articulates with the coccyx is apparent. The coccyx consists of three to five rudimentary vertebrae. Its upper surface or base contains an oval facet that articulates with the sacrum. Lateral to this facet are two processes, the coccygeal cornua, which are analogous to superior articular processes and pedicles of the more cephalad vertebrae. These cornua extend superiorly to articulate with the sacral cornua.

Soft Tissue Anatomy

Lumbosacral Joints. The fifth lumbar vertebra and the first sacral segment are united by a series of joints that resemble those present at other levels of the vertebral column. These joints include a symphysis (intervertebral disc), syndesmoses (anterior and posterior longitudinal ligaments, ligamenta flava, interspinous and supraspinous ligaments), and synovial joints (articular processes). One additional syndesmosis peculiar to this region is the iliolumbar ligament.[291] This strong ligament extends from its medial attachment to the fifth lumbar transverse process (and occasionally to the fourth lumbar transverse process) to the pelvis. Two pelvic attachments are apparent. An upper band attaches to the iliac crest and a lower band attaches to the anterosuperior aspect of the sacrum, which blends with the ventral sacroiliac ligament.

The synovial joints at the lumbosacral junction, consisting of articular facets on the fifth lumbar vertebra and

sacrum, are suited for some degree of rotatory movement, although the iliolumbar ligaments certainly inhibit this motion. These synovial articulations must resist forward and downward displacement of the fifth lumbar vertebra in relation to the sacrum.

Sacrococcygeal Joint. The sacrococcygeal joint contains a symphysis, between the apex of the sacrum and the base of the coccyx, surrounded by ventral, dorsal, and lateral sacrococcygeal ligaments. The central fibrocartilaginous disc is thicker anteriorly and posteriorly and thinner laterally. The sacrococcygeal joint may become obliterated partially or completely in advanced age, a finding that has been correlated with coccygeal pain.[252] Rarely, a freely movable coccyx articulates with the sacrum by a synovial joint.[1]

Intercoccygeal Joints. In young persons, symphyses consisting of thin fibrocartilaginous discs exist between the coccygeal segments. In men these symphyses may become obliterated at a younger age than in women. Rarely, the articulation between the first and second coccygeal segments is synovial in type. Throughout life, the coccygeal segments also are connected by ventral and dorsal sacrococcygeal ligaments. Varying degrees of angulation are noted between the coccygeal segments and, when prominent, such angulation may predispose to coccygodynia.[252]

SACROILIAC JOINTS
Osseous Anatomy

The apposing osseous surfaces of the sacrum and the ilium are irregular in character and allow interdigitation of sacrum and ilium, which contributes to the strength of the joint and to its restricted motion (Fig. 22–39).[305] The laterally located L-shaped auricular surface of the sacrum articulates with the ilium. Irregular osseous pits, which are the sites of attachment of various ligaments, are located posterior to the auricular surface. The auricular surface of the ilium is located on the medial aspect of the bone, inferior and anterior to the iliac tuberosity. The sharp anterior portion of the auricular surface is the site of attachment of the ventral sacroiliac ligament. This ligament also attaches to the preauricular sulcus, a groove at the inferior pelvic surface of the ilium, which is more prominent in women.

Soft Tissue Anatomy

The articulation between auricular surfaces of sacrum and ilium is synovial in type (Fig. 22–40). The auricular surface of the sacrum is covered with a thick layer of hyaline cartilage and that on the ilium is clothed by a thinner layer of fibrocartilage.[117, 118, 253] The morphology of the collagen fibrils also differs on the two sides of the joint.[254] This joint has a complete fibrous capsule, which is attached close to the margins of the adjacent surfaces of sacrum and ilium and is lined with synovial membrane. A joint cavity is apparent in younger persons but with advancing age, fibrous and fibrocartilaginous adhesions may obliterate this cavity.[119–122, 255, 256]

A thin and broad band of tissue, the ventral sacroiliac ligament, is noted in front of the joint. Posteriorly, a deep, thick interosseous sacroiliac ligament extends above the articular surface to fill the superior cleft between the sacrum

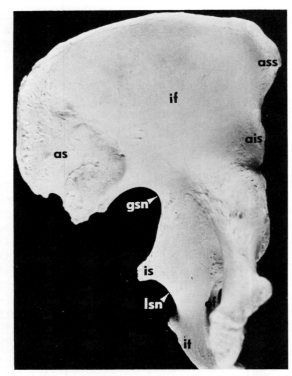

FIGURE 22–39. Innominate bone: Osseous anatomy—internal (medial) aspect. Labeled structures are the auricular surface of ilium *(as)*, iliac fossa *(if)*, anterior superior iliac spine *(ass)*, anterior inferior iliac spine *(ais)*, ischial spine *(is)*, lesser sciatic notch *(lsn)*, greater sciatic notch *(gsn)*, ischial tuberosity *(it)*, and obturator foramen *(of)*.

and the ilium. The dorsal sacroiliac ligament courses superficially to the interosseous ligament, extending medially and inferiorly, some fibers running from the posterior superior iliac spine to the third and fourth sacral segments. These fibers may merge with a portion of the sacrotuberous ligament.[123]

Accessory synovial joints are not uncommon between the lateral sacral crest and the posterior or superior iliac spine and ilial tuberosity.[124, 257, 306]

Movement at the sacroiliac joint is limited, restricted by the undulating articular surfaces and thick dorsal sacroiliac ligaments.[125, 126, 258, 305] A slight degree of anterior and posterior rotatory movement may occur.[123] This movement may be accentuated during pregnancy as hormonal influences result in softening and relaxation of the sacroiliac ligaments and symphysis pubis.[127, 128]

Radiographic evaluation of the sacroiliac joint is difficult.[129, 130] It is important to realize that only the lower one half to two thirds of the space between the sacrum and the ilium represents the synovial joint; the superior aspect of this space is ligamentous. In young adults, the interosseous joint space is 2 to 5 mm, reflecting the combined thickness of sacral and ilial cartilage.[122, 131] Diminution of joint space is common in persons over 40 years of age and increases in frequency thereafter.[117] Bony ankylosis of the articulation has been reported in older persons.[117, 120, 122]

PELVIC-VERTEBRAL LIGAMENTS

In addition to the iliolumbar ligaments, other important ligaments connecting the pelvis and the vertebral column

are the sacrotuberous and sacrospinous ligaments (Fig. 22–41). The sacrotuberous ligament extends from the posterior iliac spine, sacrum, and coccyx to the ischial tuberosity with some fibers running along the ischial ramus. The sacrospinous ligament runs from the ischial spine to the sacrum and the coccyx, where it merges with the fibers of the sacrotuberous ligament. These ligaments stabilize the lower portion of the sacrum and convert the sciatic notches into greater and lesser sciatic foramina.

SYMPHYSIS PUBIS

Osseous Anatomy

The medial aspect of the pubis, the symphyseal surface, articulates with its counterpart on the opposite side (Fig. 22–42). This surface generally is oval, and the apposing bony margins are somewhat irregular.[132, 133]

Soft Tissue Anatomy

The symphysis pubis is a median cartilaginous joint between the pubic bones (Fig. 22–42). Each pubic articular surface is clothed with a thin layer of hyaline cartilage united to its counterpart by a thick fibrocartilaginous disc, the interpubic disc.[292] This disc may contain a cavity, probably related to softening and deformation of the cartilage. This cavity, which begins in the posterosuperior aspect of the disc rarely before the tenth year of life, eventually may extend throughout the cartilage.[1, 2] The cavity is more prominent in women and is not lined by synovial membrane. It may account for vacuum phenomena on radiographs in which radiolucent streaks of gas within the cavity become apparent.[134, 135]

A superior pubic ligament attached to the pubic crest and tubercles on each side strengthens the anterior aspect of the symphysis pubis. The arcuate pubic ligament connects the lower portion of the pubic bones.

Radiographic evaluation of the adult symphysis pubis reveals a mean transverse width of approximately 6 mm in men and 5 mm in women.[136] The width of the symphysis pubis may increase in pregnancy, averaging 7 mm.[135] This apparent increase in joint size during pregnancy probably relates to softening and relaxation of pelvic ligaments, accounting for increased movement at various pelvic joints,[127, 128] perhaps providing minor aid during childbirth.[137] There are several additional factors that allow greater movement of the pelvis in women and thereby assist in childbirth: less interlocking by reciprocal irregularities of bone about the sacroiliac joints, less fibrous ankylosis of the sacroiliac joints, and decreased prevalence of synostosis of coccygeal segments.[2]

HIP

Osseous Anatomy

At the hip, the globular head of the femur articulates with the cup-shaped fossa of the acetabulum. This latter structure develops in fetal life from ossification of the ilium, ischium, and pubis. At birth, the acetabulum is cartilaginous, with a triradiate stem extending medially from its deep aspect, producing a Y-shaped physeal plate between

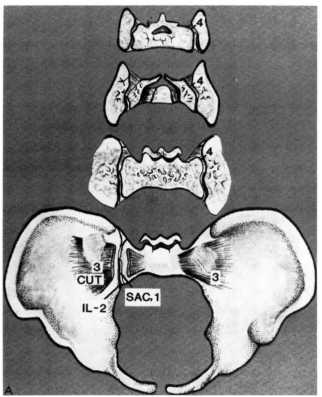

FIGURE 22–40. Sacroiliac joint: Anatomy.

   A Drawing of anterior aspect and coronal sections of articulation. Observe the ventral sacroiliac ligament *(3)* and interosseous ligament *(4)*. When the ventral ligament is cut, thick sacral cartilage *(1)* and thinner iliac cartilage *(2)* are apparent. (From Resnick D, Niwayama G, Goergen TG: Invest Radiol *10*:608, 1975.)

   B, C Coronal section. Photograph and radiograph of two similar specimens reveal extent of synovial articulation (between large arrowheads), thick sacral cartilage (small arrowhead), and thinner iliac cartilage (arrow). Note the interosseous ligament *(il)* above the synovial joint.

   D A photomicrograph (2×) of a coronal section demonstrating synovial joint (between large arrowheads), thick sacral cartilage (small arrowhead), thinner iliac cartilage (arrow), and interosseous ligament *(il)*.

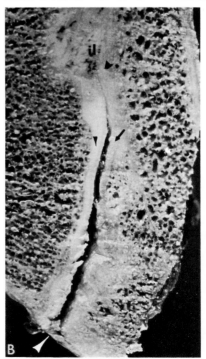

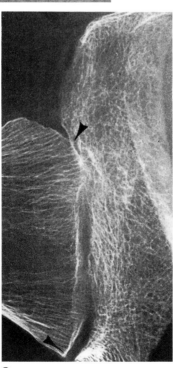

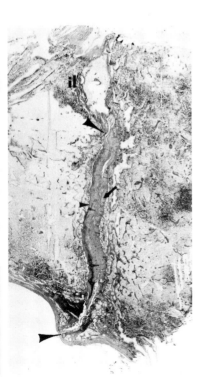

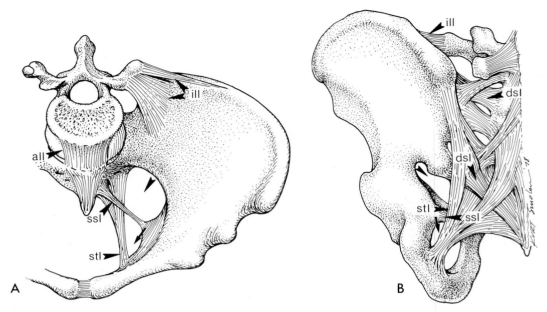

FIGURE 22–41. Pelvic-vertebral ligaments: Anatomy.

    A Anterior aspect. Visualized structures are the iliolumbar ligament *(ill)* with two pelvic attachments, sacrospinous ligament *(ssl),* sacrotuberous ligament *(stl),* anterior longitudinal ligament *(all),* and greater (arrowhead) and lesser (arrow) sciatic foramina.

    B Posterior aspect. Observe the iliolumbar ligament *(ill),* short and long dorsal sacroiliac ligaments *(dsl),* sacrotuberous ligament *(stl),* sacrospinous ligament *(ssl),* and greater (arrowhead) and lesser (arrow) sciatic foramina.

    (From Warwick R, Williams P: Gray's Anatomy. 35th British Ed. Philadelphia, WB Saunders Co, 1973.)

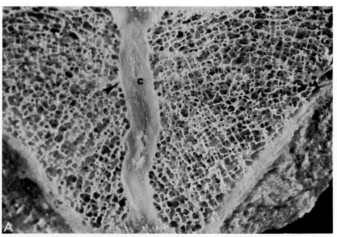

FIGURE 22–42. Symphysis pubis: Anatomy.

    A Coronal section. Observe the central cartilage *(c)* and the well-defined subchondral bone plate (arrowhead).

    B–D Coronal section. On a radiograph **(B)** a curvilinear radiolucent area (vacuum phenomenon) is apparent over the superior aspect of the central cartilaginous disc (arrow). The photograph of the gross specimen **(C)** reveals a cavity or cleft (arrow), which accounts for the vacuum phenomenon. On the photomicrograph (20×) **(D)** the cleft (arrow) in the fibrocartilage is well shown. It does not have a synovial lining.

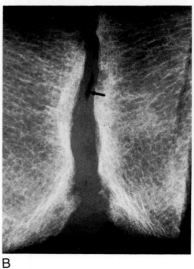

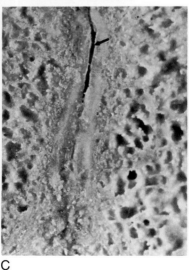

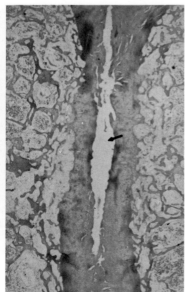

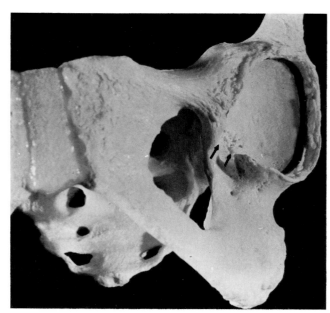

FIGURE 22–43. Acetabular cavity: Osseous anatomy (anterior view). A metal marker (black strip) identifies the posterior acetabular rim. This rim is continuous except at the area of the acetabular notch inferiorly (arrows). (From Armbuster TG, et al: Radiology *128*:1, 1978.)

ilium, ischium, and pubis.[1] Continued ossification results in eventual fusion of these three bones.

The fully developed acetabular cavity is hemispheric in shape and possesses an elevated bony rim (Fig. 22–43). This rim is absent inferiorly, the defect being termed the acetabular notch. A fibrocartilaginous labrum is attached to the bony rim, deepening the acetabular cavity. The acetabular floor above the notch, the acetabular fossa, is depressed and irregular. Between the rim and fossa is a smooth horseshoe-shaped articular lunate surface. A discontinuity in the medial aspect of the acetabular roof, termed the superior acetabular notch, appears to represent an accessory fossa in the apex of the acetabulum.[259]

The hemispheric head of the femur extends superiorly, medially, and anteriorly (Fig. 22–44). It is smooth except for a central roughened pit, the fovea, to which is attached the ligament of the head of the femur. The anterior surface of the femoral neck is intracapsular, as the capsular line extends to the intertrochanteric line; only the medial half of the posterior surface of the femoral neck is intracapsular, as the posterior attachment of the hip capsule does not extend to the intertrochanteric crest. The greater trochanter projects from the posterosuperior aspect of the femoral neck–shaft junction and is the site of attachment of numerous muscles, including the gluteus minimus, gluteus medius, and piriformis. The lesser trochanter is located at the posteromedial portion of the femoral neck–shaft junction. The psoas major and iliacus muscles attach to it.

Radiographic examination of normal osseous structures about the hip has received great attention, and various measurements have been determined. The acetabular angle, iliac angle, and angle of anteversion of the femoral neck are useful measurements, particularly in the young skeleton.[138–142, 307] The center-edge (CE) angle of Wiberg[143] is an indication of acetabular depth (Fig. 22–45). It is the angle

formed by a perpendicular line through the midportion of the femoral head and a line from the femoral head center to the upper outer acetabular margin. The normal CE angle is reported to be 20 to 40 degrees, with an average of 36 degrees.[144] This angle may be slightly larger in women and in older persons.[145]

The pelvic radiograph also is useful in outlining certain normal lines and structures[145, 146] (Fig. 22–46). The acetabular rim appears as an osseous ring surrounding the outer aspect of the acetabulum. The posterior acetabular rim can be identified on radiographs exposed in various obliquities, but the 15 to 30 degree anterior oblique projection offers optimal visualization. The anterior acetabular rim is visualized optimally in the 30 to 45 degree posterior oblique projection. The ilioischial line is formed by that portion of the quadrilateral surface of the ilium that is tangent to the x-ray beam; the iliopubic line is simply the inner margin of the ilium, which forms a continuous line with the inner superior aspect of the pubis. Two columns of bone produce an arch, with the acetabulum located in the concavity of the arch. The ilioischial or posterior column is a thick structure that includes a portion of the ilium and extends to the ischial tuberosity. The iliopubic or anterior column consists of a portion of ilium and pubis and extends superolaterally to the anterior inferior iliac spine.

The "teardrop" is a U-shaped shadow medial to the hip joint that has been utilized to detect abnormalities of acetabular depth,[308] thereby establishing a diagnosis of acetabular protrusion (Fig. 22–47). It has been compared to a pedicle of a vertebra in that its disappearance establishes that significant bone destruction has occurred.[260] The lateral aspect of the teardrop is the wall of the acetabular fossa, and the medial aspect is the anteroinferior margin of the quadrilateral surface. In the usual anteroposterior radiograph of the pelvis, the latter surface is parallel to the x-ray beam and is thereby projected as a typical "teardrop." The configuration of the teardrop varies in normal persons, however. Furthermore, it is affected significantly by positioning the patient in oblique projections[145]; in a slight anterior oblique projection the teardrop is situated anterior to the ilioischial line, creating a "crossed" appearance rather than the more usual "open" or "closed" position. With further anterior obliquity, the teardrop is situated medially to the ilioischial line, creating a "reversed" appearance. In the posterior oblique projection, the teardrop is located lateral to the ilioischial line.

Differentiation of normal acetabular depth and acetabular protrusion (protrusio acetabuli) can be accomplished by careful analysis of plain films in adults.[145] In the past, several different definitions of protrusio acetabuli have been used (Table 22–2): (1) a bony bulge on the inner aspect of the acetabulum; (2) the femoral head reaching the ilioischial line; (3) a CE angle of greater than 40 to 45 degrees; (4) "crossing" of the teardrop; (5) the acetabular line touching or crossing the ilioischial line.

The previous observations have certain limitations:

1. When protrusio acetabuli progresses to frank bulge of the acetabulum into the pelvis, the diagnosis is readily apparent. This certainly is not a reliable indicator of mild protrusio acetabuli.

2. The relationship of the femoral head to the ilioischial line is not adequate as a measurement of protrusio acetabuli

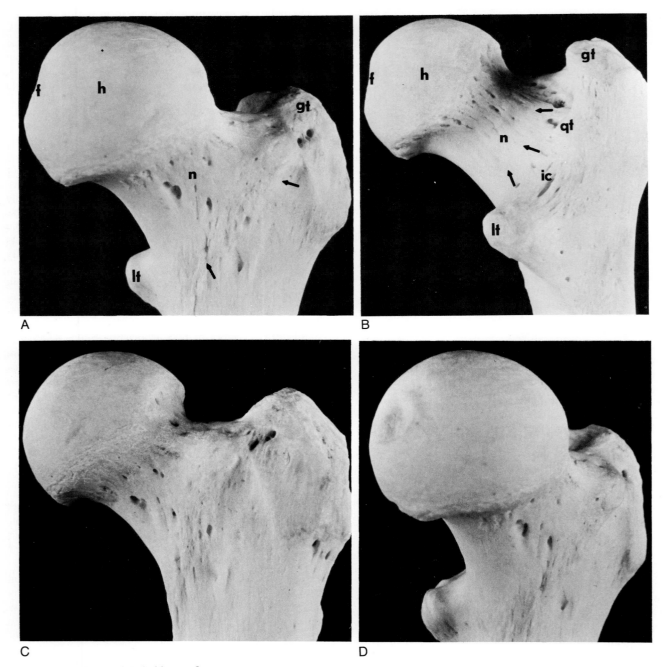

FIGURE 22–44. Proximal end of femur: Osseous anatomy.

A Anterior aspect, neutral position. Observe the smooth femoral head *(h)*, fovea *(f)*, neck *(n)*, greater trochanter *(gt)*, and lesser trochanter *(lt)*. The hip capsule attaches anteriorly to the intertrochanteric line (arrows).

B Posterior aspect, neutral position. The same structures as in **A** are identified. The intertrochanteric crest *(ic)* and quadrate tubercle *(qt)* also are indicated. Arrows point to the site of capsular attachment.

C Anterior aspect, internal rotation. The femoral neck is elongated.

D Anterior aspect, external rotation. The femoral neck is foreshortened.

TABLE 22–2. Protrusio Acetabuli

Date	Author	Criterion
1932	Pomeranz[147]	Dome-shaped mass projecting into pelvis
1935	Overgaard[148]	Acetabular line touching or crossing ilioischial line
1953	Friedenberg[149]	CE angle between 40 and 70 degrees
1965	Alexander[150]	Teardrop crossed on a well-centered film; femoral head reaching ilioischial line; bulge above pelvic brim
1969	Hubbard[151]	Acetabular line medial to ilioischial line
1971	Hooper and Jones[144]	Crossing of the teardrop
1971	MacDonald[152]	CE angle greater than 45 degrees

because it introduces another variable, that is, the integrity of the joint space. If the joint space is decreased, the femoral head will reach the ilioischial line at an earlier stage than if the joint space is "normal."

3. The CE angle, originally described to evaluate congenital and dysplastic hips[143] subsequently was applied to the measurement of protrusio acetabuli, with varying degrees of enthusiasm and success.[144, 149–152] Our analysis has revealed wide ranges in the value of the CE angle.[145] Although 40 degrees had previously been considered to be the upper limit of normal,[144] women over 40 years of age may have an average CE angle of greater than 40 degrees.[145] The authors also have made an attempt to correlate the CE angle with other parameters used in the diagnosis of protrusio acetabuli and have found no significant relationship between the CE angle and the configuration of the teardrop or between the CE angle and the relative position of the acetabular and ilioischial lines.[145] This has led to the conclusion that the CE angle is not a good indicator of protrusio acetabuli.

4. Most authors do not give a definition of a crossed teardrop but simply state that this is an indicator of protrusio acetabuli. We have defined a crossed teardrop as one that is crossed by the ilioischial line. As the teardrop configuration is affected by minimal amounts of rotation, slight anterior oblique projections can lead to crossing of the teardrop. Increasing the degree of anterior obliquity even can lead to a reversed teardrop. In addition, in normal situations on nonrotated pelvic radiographs, such crossing may be apparent; in 15 per cent of normal adult hips, radiographs reveal an acetabular line medial to the ilioischial line in association with an open or closed teardrop.[145] Therefore, the teardrop configuration is not a good index of protrusio acetabuli. Furthermore, the unqualified use of the term crossed teardrop potentially is misleading and unnecessary.

It is more appropriate to use the relationship of the acetabular line to the ilioischial line as the index of protrusio acetabuli (Fig. 22–48). The acetabular line, which is the medial wall of the acetabulum, and the ilioischial line, which is a portion of the quadrilateral surface, are central structures whose relationships are little affected by minimal degrees of rotation. In examining and measuring these central structures, any artifact caused by minor rotation in an anteroposterior pelvic radiograph is minimized. In fact, slight degrees of pelvic obliquity will create a crossed teardrop while the relationship between the acetabular line and the ilioischial line remains normal. In addition, as protrusio acetabuli involves the central structures, it would seem appropriate to use their relative positions to establish the diagnosis.

Although acetabular depth is a continuum from "shallow" to "normal" to "deep" to "protrusio acetabuli," the authors' data[145] have led to the following conclusions:

1. Protrusio acetabuli is diagnosed when the acetabular line projects medial to the ilioischial line by 3 mm or more in men or by 6 mm or more in women. In children, 1 mm in boys and 3 mm in girls are the corresponding values.[309]

2. The teardrop configuration is affected by minor degrees of rotation and therefore cannot be used as an indicator of protrusio acetabuli.

3. Measurement of the CE angle of Wiberg adds little to the diagnosis of protrusio acetabuli.

The normal joint space on frontal radiographs can be analyzed in adults by dividing it into three segments: the superior, axial, and medial joint spaces[145] (Fig. 22–49). The superior and axial joint space measurements usually are quite similar, but the medial joint space measurement normally is greater because it includes the acetabular fossa,[262, 263] which adds synovium and fat to the joint space. Nevertheless, the medial measurement is meaningful because the same situation exists in all hips. The average medial joint space is 9 mm in men and 8 mm in women. The average axial and superior joint spaces are 4 mm in both men and women.[261] Minor modifications of these measurements occur with advancing age of the person.[310] In normal situations, the superior and axial spaces should be equal and approximately one half the medial joint space

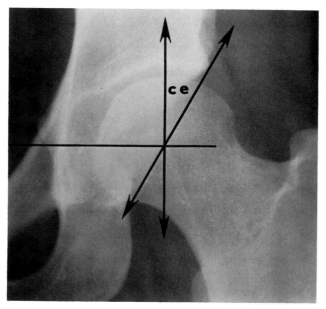

FIGURE 22–45. CE, angle of Wiberg. This is the angle formed by the intersection of a perpendicular line through the midpoint of the femoral head and a line from the femoral head center to the upper outer acetabular margin. The normal value for this angle is reported to be 20 to 40 degrees, with an average of 36 degrees. (From Armbuster TG, et al: Radiology *128*:1, 1978.)

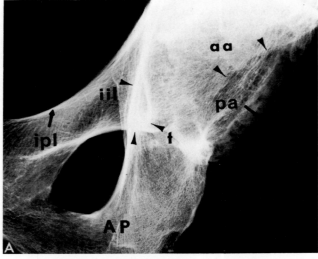

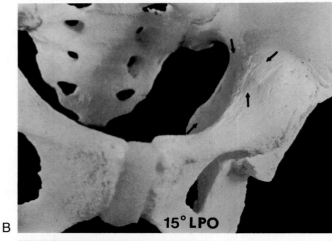

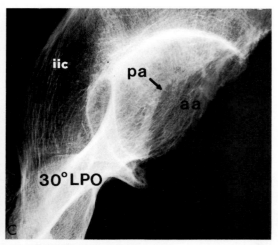

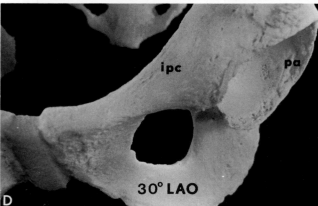

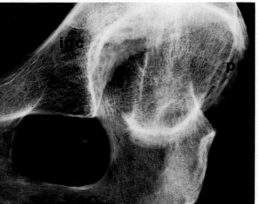

FIGURE 22–46. Normal osseous landmarks of the pelvis.

A, Anteroposterior (AP) view. The posterior acetabular rim *(pa)* is more lateral than the anterior acetabular rim *(aa)*. The ilioischial line *(iil)* is formed by that portion of the quadrilateral surface of the ilium that is tangent to the x-ray beam. The iliopubic line *(ipl)* is the inner margin of the ilium, which forms a continuous line with the inner superior surface of the pubis. The "teardrop" *(t)* also is labeled.

B Fifteen degree left posterior oblique (LPO) view. The quadrilateral surface (arrows) is observed.

C Thirty degree left posterior oblique (LPO) view. The 30 to 45 degree posterior oblique projection best delineates the ilioischial column (iic) and anterior acetabular rim *(aa)*. The posterior acetabular rim *(pa)* is noted.

D, E Thirty degree left anterior oblique (LAO) view. Well delineated are the iliopubic column *(ipc)* and posterior acetabular rim *(pa)*.

(From Armbuster TG, et al: Radiology *128*:1, 1978.)

measurement. In pathologic situations, selective loss or gain of superior, axial, or medial joint space may aid in specific diagnoses.

Soft Tissue Anatomy

The femoral head is covered with articular cartilage, although a small area exists on its surface that is devoid of cartilage, to which attaches the ligament of the head of the femur (Fig. 22–50). The lunate surface is covered with articular cartilage; the floor of the acetabular fossa within this surface does not contain cartilage but has a fibroelastic fat pad covered with synovial membrane.

A fibrous capsule encircles the joint and much of the femoral neck. The capsule attaches proximally to the acetabulum, labrum, and transverse ligament of the acetabulum. Distally it surrounds the femoral neck; in front, it is attached to the trochanteric line at the junction of the femoral neck and shaft; above and below, it is attached to the femoral neck close to the junction with the trochanters; behind, the capsule extends over the medial two thirds of the neck. Because of these capsular attachments, the physeal plate of the femur is intracapsular and the physeal plates of the trochanters are extracapsular. The fibers of the fibrous capsule, although oriented longitudinally from pelvis to femur, also consist of a deeply situated circular group of fibers termed the zona orbicularis. The fibrous capsule is strengthened by surrounding ligaments, including the iliofemoral, pubofemoral, and ischiofemoral ligaments. The external surface of the capsule is covered by musculature and separated anteriorly from the psoas major and iliacus by a bursa. In this area, the joint may communicate with the subtendinous iliac bursa (iliopsoas bursa) beneath the psoas major tendon through an aperture between the pubofemoral and iliofemoral ligaments.[1, 2]

The extensive synovial membrane of the hip extends from the cartilaginous margins of the femoral head over intracapsular portions of the femoral neck. It is reflected beneath the fibrous capsule and covers the acetabular labrum, the ligament of the head of the femur, and the fat pad in the acetabular fossa.

Important ligaments include the iliofemoral, pubofemoral, and ischiofemoral ligaments, the ligament of the head of the femur, the transverse ligament of the acetabulum, and acetabular labrum. The strong iliofemoral ligament attaches proximally to the anterior inferior iliac spine and the adjoining part of the acetabular rim and distally to the intertrochanteric line on the femur. This ligament becomes taut in full extension of the hip. The pubofemoral ligament extends from the pubic part of the acetabular rim and the superior pubic ramus to the undersurface of the femoral neck, some of its fibers blending with the fibrous capsule. This ligament also becomes taut on hip extension. The ischiofemoral ligament is attached to the ischium below and behind the acetabulum and extends in a superolateral direction across the back of the femoral neck. Its fibers are continuous with those of the zona orbicularis or attach to the greater trochanter. This ligament, as the others, becomes taut in extension of the hip. The ligament of the head of the femur is a weak intra-articular ligament, which is attached to the margin of the acetabular fossa and the transverse ligament of the acetabulum. It extends to a pit on the femoral head. Between these areas of attachment, this ligament

is clothed by a synovial sheath. In some persons, the sheath alone is present, without the ligament, and in others, neither sheath nor ligament can be identified. The ligament is stretched when the thigh is flexed, adducted, and rotated laterally. The transverse ligament of the acetabulum is a portion of the acetabular labrum whose fibers extend across the acetabular notch. The acetabular labrum, the fibrocartilaginous rim about the acetabulum, is attached firmly to the bony rim and transverse ligament, is triangular on cross section, and has a free edge or apex that forms a smaller circle that closely embraces the femoral head.

Active movements of the hip are flexion, extension, adduction, abduction, circumduction, and medial and lateral rotation. Because of a close fit between acetabulum and femur and the intimacy of the acetabular labrum, the movements of the hip are restricted in comparison to those of the glenohumeral joint. No accessory movements occur in the hip.

Soft tissue anatomy about the hip has received great attention. A number of periarticular fat planes have been described that can be recognized on radiographs and which, when disturbed, reportedly may indicate significant intra-articular disease[153–158] (Fig. 22–51). Reichmann[159] reviewed the soft tissue anatomy about the hip joint. Four fatty layers were described, which could be identified on anteroposterior radiographs (Fig. 22–52):

Fat plane 1: On the pelvic surface of the acetabulum and pubis.
Fat plane 2: Medial to the femoral neck, extending to the lesser trochanter.
Fat plane 3: Lateral to the hip and extending to the greater trochanter.
Fat plane 4: Lateral to the hip and medial to fat plane 3, extending to the region of the greater trochanter.

Anatomic studies have revealed that fat plane 1 is medial to the obturator internus muscle[153, 160] and fat plane 2 is medial to the iliopsoas muscle.[160, 161] Fat plane 3 is between the gluteus medius (lateral) and the gluteus minimus (medial).[159–161] Fat plane 4 has been termed the "capsular" fat plane,[161] although more recent evidence suggests that this fat pad is not related to the joint capsule.[159] Our investigation of adult hips[160] has supported the concept that this last fat pad indeed is not true capsular fat. The bulk of this fat plane is intermuscular, lying between the rectus femoris and tensor fasciae latae muscles. This region is quite anterior to the hip capsule and it is here that this fat pad is widest. This fat plane has an oblique orientation, and it becomes thinner dorsally as it changes from its intermuscular part to its pericapsular part between the superolateral aspect of the hip joint capsule and the medial aspect of the gluteus minimus muscle. The pericapsular portion of this fat plane is not discernible on routine hip radiography and, therefore, the "capsular" fat plane that frequently is seen on anteroposterior radiography is the intermuscular part of this fat plane and has no intimate relationship to the hip capsule. Although this plane does have a pericapsular extension, this latter extension is strongly reinforced by surrounding ligaments. Thus, intra-articular fluid would not be expected to create a noticeable change in this fat plane.

Our close evaluation of fat plane 2, the iliopsoas fat plane, has documented its periarticular course.[160] It is medial to the tendinous portion of the iliopsoas muscle. Ante-

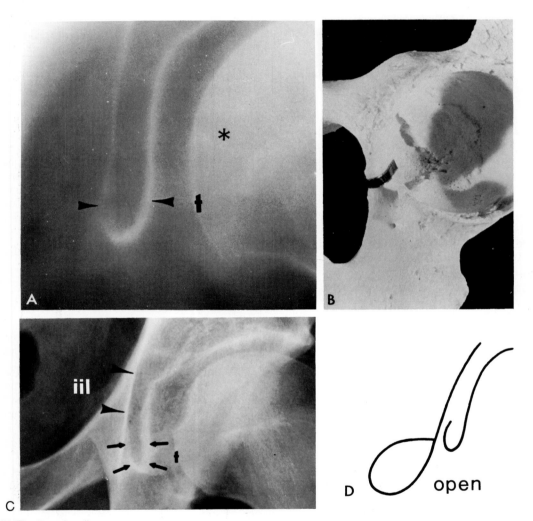

FIGURE 22–47. The "teardrop."

A Anteroposterior tomogram. The teardrop *(t)* and femoral head (asterisk) are seen. The lateral wall of the teardrop is the wall of the acetabular fossa. The medial wall is the anteroinferior margin of the quadrilateral surface.

B On a cadaveric specimen, a metal marker has been placed on the teardrop. The quadrilateral surface is not visualized in this projection.

C–J The different radiographic appearances of the teardrop *(t)* (arrows and small arrowheads) are illustrated. In the open type **(C, D),** the entire teardrop is located lateral to the ilioischial line *(iil)* (large arrowheads). In the closed type **(E, F),** the medial aspect of the teardrop touches the ilioischial line. In the crossed type **(G, H)** the teardrop is crossed by the ilioischial line. In the reversed type **(I, J)** the teardrop is entirely medial to the ilioischial line. In normal persons, minor degrees of rotation of the pelvis significantly influence the radiographic appearance of the teardrop.

(From Armbuster TG, et al: Radiology *128*:1, 1978.)

Illustration continued on opposite page

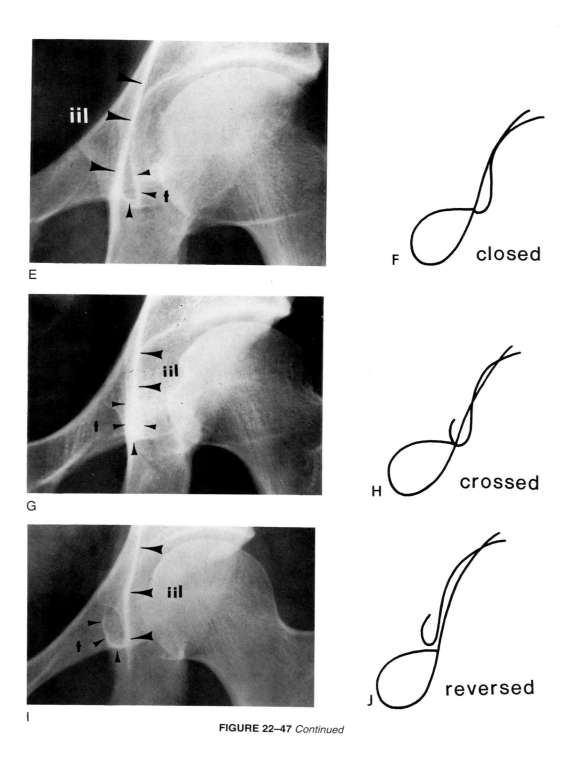

FIGURE 22–47 *Continued*

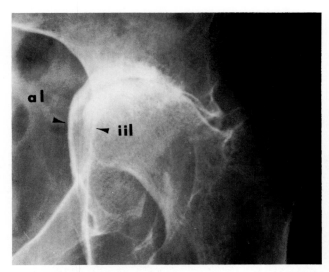

FIGURE 22–48. Acetabular protrusion. A protrusio acetabuli deformity is present when the acetabular line *(al)* projects medial to the ilioischial line *(iil)* by 3 mm or more in men and by 6 mm or more in women. (From Armbuster TG, et al: Radiology *128*:1, 1978.)

riorly it blends with the fat of the femoral triangle just lateral to the femoral vessels. Posteriorly it reaches the superomedial portion of the hip capsule and inferomedial lip of the acetabulum. In its posterior course, it sends a fat plane laterally, posterior to the iliopsoas tendon. Here it makes intimate contact with the medial portion of the hip capsule adjacent to the femoral neck. This represents a point of weakness between the iliofemoral and iliopubic ligaments of the hip capsule. It is here that the iliopsoas bursa originates, a space that potentially could allow decompression of a joint in cases of elevated intra-articular pressure.[160] On radiographs, only the widest portion of the iliopsoas fat plane is seen on anteroposterior projections, a portion that is anterior to the medial aspect of the hip joint. Therefore, a small to moderate amount of intra-articular fluid should not displace the iliopsoas fat plane, although large amounts of fluid may alter it.

The iliopsoas and "capsular" fat planes (fat planes 2 and 4) are visible in a great percentage of hip radiographs, but measurements of the distance of these fat planes to bony landmarks in the pelvis vary.[160] The obturator internus fat plane (fat plane 1) is visualized infrequently and is variable in its distance from the bony pelvis. The gluteal fat plane (fat plane 3) is neither visualized frequently nor constant in position. Additional characteristics of these fat planes are the following:

1. When one obturator internus fat plane is seen, the contralateral fat plane also is seen and has a similar appearance.

2. The iliopsoas fat plane frequently is well defined on one side and indistinct on the other and may have either a neutral or "bulgy" appearance.

3. The "capsular" and gluteal fat planes vary in appearance when compared to their counterparts on the opposite side.

These factors diminish the reliability of radiographically discernible fat plane alterations in predicting hip disease, particularly in adults. In children, intra-articular fluid may produce an increase in width of joint space between the femoral head and the medial acetabular wall. This sign may be more valuable than changes in the position and appearance of periarticular fat planes.

The iliopsoas bursa represents the largest and most important bursa about the hip. It is present in 98 per cent of hips and is located anterior to the joint capsule.[162] It may extend proximally and communicates with the joint space in approximately 15 per cent of normal hips[163, 164] through a gap between the iliofemoral and pubofemoral ligaments.[1, 2, 165] Extension of hip disease into this bursa has been recognized in a variety of articular diseases, occasionally producing a mass in the ilioinguinal region[166] with possible obstruction of the femoral vein (Fig. 22–53). One additional site that represents an inherent weak part of the hip capsule occurs at the crossing of the iliofemoral and iliopubic ligaments. At this site, fluid may extravasate into the fat plane of the obturator externus muscle.[160]

Bursae about the gluteus muscles also may be demonstrated anatomically and radiographically.[167] The bursa deep to the gluteus medius is larger than that deep to the gluteus minimus. Both bursae are intimate with the greater trochanter, and bursitis can lead to pain and soft tissue calcifications in this region.

KNEE

The knee joint is the largest and most complicated articulation in the human body.[1, 2, 168] In this joint, three functional spaces exist: the medial femorotibial space, the lateral femorotibial space, and the patellofemoral space.

Osseous and Soft Tissue Anatomy

The lower end of the femur contains a medial and lateral condyle, separated posteriorly by an intercondylar fossa or notch (Fig. 22–54). The medial condyle is larger than the lateral condyle and possesses a superior prominence called the adductor tubercle for attachment of the tendon of the adductor magnus. Below this tubercle is a ridge, the medial epicondyle. The lateral condyle possesses a similar protuberance, the lateral epicondyle. The intercondylar fossa, between the condyles, stretches from the intercondylar line posteriorly to the lower border of the patellar surface anteriorly. The patella, the largest sesamoid bone of the body, is embedded within the tendon of the quadriceps femoris. It is oval in outline, with a pointed apex on its inferior surface. The ligamentum patellae, a continuation of the quadriceps tendon, is attached to the apex and adjacent bone of the patella.

Articular surfaces of the femur, tibia, and patella are not congruent. The articular surface of the femur comprises the condylar areas (femorotibial spaces) and the patellar surface (patellofemoral space). A shallow groove is present between each condylar surface and the patellar surface. As viewed from below, the outline of the femoral condylar surfaces generally conforms to that of the tibial articular surfaces. The surface on the lateral femoral condyle appears circular, whereas that on the medial femoral condyle is large and oval, elongated in an anteroposterior direction, with concavity extending laterally.

The tibial articular surfaces are the cartilage-clothed condyles, each with a central hollow and peripheral flattened

Text continued on page 733

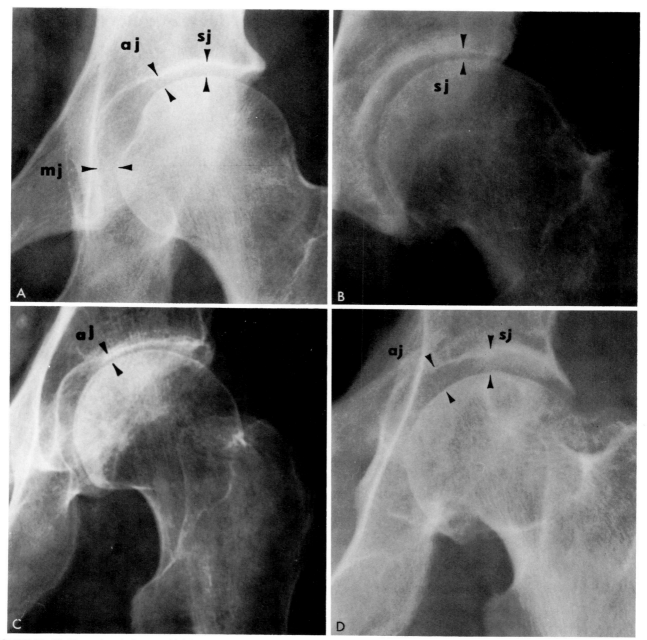

FIGURE 22–49. Normal and abnormal joint space.
    A The joint space measurement includes the intra-articular space and the thickness of the acetabular and femoral head cartilage. The axial joint space *(aj)* and superior joint space *(sj)* should be approximately one half the medial joint space *(mj)*.
    B Superior joint space *(sj)* loss is frequent in degenerative joint disease.
    C Axial joint space *(aj)* loss may be apparent in disuse cartilage atrophy following paralysis.
    D Increase of axial joint space *(aj)* and superior joint space *(sj)* can occur in acromegaly.
    (From Armbuster TG, et al: Radiology, *128*:1, 1978.)

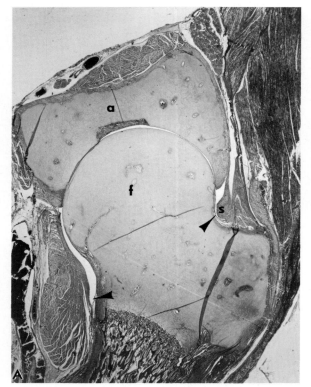

FIGURE 22–50. Hip joint: Normal development and anatomy.

A Photomicrograph (20×) of a coronal section through the hip reveals unossified acetabulum *(a)* and femoral head *(f)*, synovium *(s)*, and distal extent of articular cavity (arrowheads).

B Drawing of a coronal section through the hip.

Illustration continued on opposite page

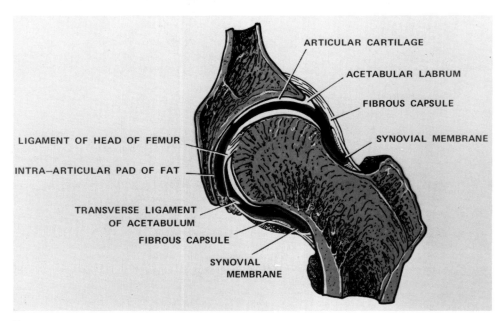

ARTICULAR CARTILAGE

ACETABULAR LABRUM

FIBROUS CAPSULE

SYNOVIAL MEMBRANE

LIGAMENT OF HEAD OF FEMUR

INTRA–ARTICULAR PAD OF FAT

TRANSVERSE LIGAMENT OF ACETABULUM

FIBROUS CAPSULE

SYNOVIAL MEMBRANE

B

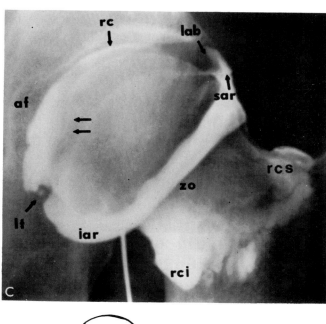

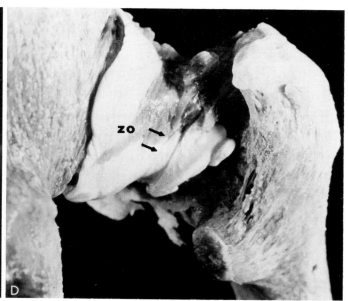

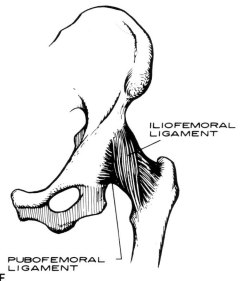

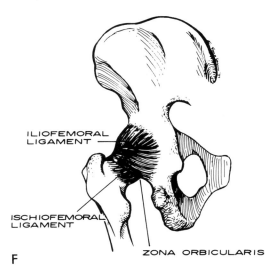

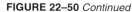

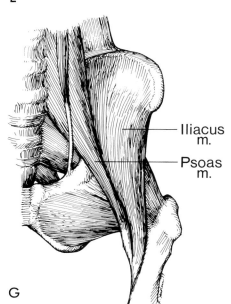

FIGURE 22–50 *Continued*

C Normal left hip arthrogram. The recess capitus *(rc)* is a thin, smooth collection of contrast medium between apposing articular surfaces and is interrupted only where the ligamentum teres (double arrows) enters the fovea centralis of the femoral head. The ligamentum transversum *(lt)* is seen as a radiolucent defect adjacent to the inferior rim of the acetabulum. The ligamentum teres bridges the acetabular notch and effectively deepens the acetabulum. The inferior articular recess *(iar)* forms a pouch at the inferior base of the femoral head below the acetabular notch and ligamentum transversum *(lt)*. The superior articular recess *(sar)* extends cephalad around the acetabular labrum *(lab)*. The acetabular labrum is seen as a triangular radiolucent region adjacent to the superolateral lip of the acetabulum. The zona orbicularis *(zo)* is a circumferential lucent band around the femoral neck, which changes configuration with rotation of the femur. The recess colli superior *(rcs)* and recess colli inferior *(rci)* are poolings of contrast material at the apex and base of the intertrochanteric line and are the most caudad extensions of the synovial membrane.

D Macerated specimen (posterior view) with prior barium-impregnated methylmethacrylate injection demonstrating the zona orbicularis *(zo)* as an impression made by the iliofemoral and ischiofemoral ligaments on the hip capsule.

E Capsular ligaments of hip, anterior view. The iliofemoral ligament extends anterior to the pubofemoral ligament. A gap may persist at this crossing, which allows communication between the iliopsoas bursa and the hip joint.

F Capsular ligaments of hip, posterior view. The iliofemoral and ischiofemoral ligaments are thick posteriorly and without inherent areas of weakness. The zona orbicularis is created by the crossing of the hip ligaments.

G Musculature, anterior aspect of hip. Observe the course of the iliacus and psoas muscles.

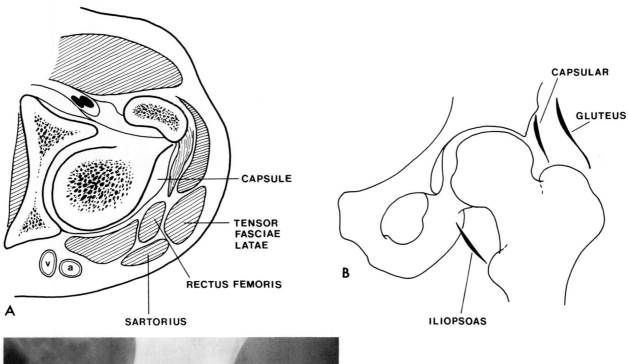

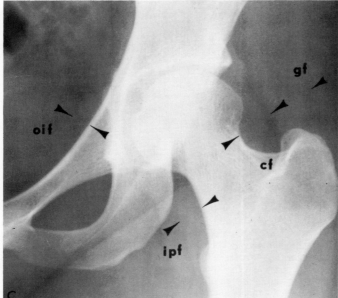

FIGURE 22–51. Periarticular fat planes.

A A simplified schematic representation of a transverse section through the hip.

B A drawing of three of the four fat planes that have been described.

C The fat planes include fat plane 1 (obturator internus fat plane, *oif*), fat plane 2 (iliopsoas fat plane, *ipf*), fat plane 3 (gluteus fat plane, *gf*), and fat plane 4 ("capsular" fat plane, *cf*). In each instance, arrowheads indicate distances of fat plane to adjacent osseous structures. (**C**, From Guerra J Jr, et al: Radiology *128*:11, 1978.)

area (Fig. 22–55). Between the condyles is the intercondylar area. The articular surface of the medial tibial condyle is oval, with its long axis in the sagittal plane, whereas the articular surface of the lateral tibial condyle is circular and smaller than the medial condyle.

The adjacent articular surfaces of the tibia and femur are fitted together more closely by the presence of the medial and lateral menisci (Fig. 22–56). The medial meniscus is nearly semicircular, with a broadened or widened posterior horn. The anterior end of the medial meniscus is attached to the intercondylar area of the tibia anterior to the attachment of the anterior cruciate ligament. The posterior end of the medial meniscus is attached to the intercondylar area of the tibia between the attachments of the posterior cruciate ligament and lateral meniscus. The peripheral aspect of the medial meniscus is attached to the fibrous capsule and tibial collateral ligament. The lateral meniscus, which is of relatively uniform width throughout, resembles a ring. Its anterior aspect is attached to the intercondylar eminence of the tibia behind and lateral to the anterior cruciate ligament. Its posterior portion is attached to the intercondylar eminence of the tibia just anterior to the attachment of the medial meniscus. The lateral meniscus is grooved posteriorly by the popliteus tendon and its accompanying tendon sheath. Meniscofemoral ligaments, both anterior and posterior, represent attachments of the posterior horn of the lateral meniscus. A transverse ligament connects the convex anterior portions of both menisci.

The articular surface of the patella is oval and contains an osseous vertical ridge that divides it into a smaller medial area and a larger lateral area[169] (Fig. 22–57). This patellar ridge fits into a corresponding groove on the anterior surface of the femur. The patellar articulating surface is subdivided still further by two poorly defined horizontal ridges of bone into three facets on either side. One additional vertical ridge of bone separates a narrow elongated facet on the medial border of the articular surface. Contact between these various patellar articular facets and the femur varies, depending on the position of the knee. In full flexion, the most medial facet of the patella contacts the lateral portion of the medial femoral condyle, and the superior aspect of the lateral patellar facet contacts the anterior part of the lateral condyle. With extension of the knee, the middle facet of the patella becomes intimate with the lower portion of the femoral patellar surface, and in full extension, only the lowest patellar articular facets contact the femur.[1] During forced extension of the joint, the patella tends to be displaced laterally, a tendency that is prevented by the action of adjacent musculature and the prominence of the lateral patellar surface of the femur.

The fibrous capsule of the knee joint is not a complete structure. Rather, the knee is surrounded by tendinous expansions, which reinforce the capsule. Between the capsule or tendinous expansions and synovial lining are various intra-articular structures, including ligaments and fat pads.

Anteriorly, the fibrous capsule is absent above and over the patellar surface. The ligamentous sheath in this area is composed mainly of a tendinous expansion from the rectus femoris and the vasti musculature, which descends to attach around the superior half of the bone. Superficial fibers continue to descend onto the strong ligamentum patellae. This structure, which represents the continuation of the quadriceps muscle, is attached above to the apex of the patella

and below to the tibial tuberosity. Adjacent fibers, the medial and lateral patellar retinacula, pass from the osseous margins of the patella to the tibial condyles. Superficial to these tendinous structures are the expansions of the fascia lata. Above the patella, deficiency of the fibrous capsule creates a suprapatellar bursa, which communicates freely with the articular cavity.

Posteriorly, capsular fibers extend from the femoral surface above the condyles and the intercondylar line to the posterior border of the tibia. This portion of the capsule is strengthened by the oblique popliteal ligament, which is derived from the semimembranosus tendon. Additional posterior reinforcement relates to the arcuate popliteal ligament, which emerges from the fibular head to blend with the capsular fibers.

Laterally, capsular fibers run from the femoral to the tibial condyles. In this area, the fibular collateral ligament is found, which is attached above to the lateral epicondyle of the femur and below to the fibular head. It is intimate with the tendon of the biceps femoris muscle. Space exists between capsular fibers and the fibular collateral ligament through which extend genicular vessels and nerves.

Medially, the capsule is strengthened by tendinous expansions from sartorius and semimembranosus muscles. These fibers pass upward to the tibial collateral ligament, which is attached above to the medial epicondyle of the femur and below to the medial tibial condyle and shaft. One or more bursae may separate the tibial collateral ligament from the fibrous capsule.[170] On its deep surface, the fibrous capsule connects the menisci and adjacent tibia, a connection termed the coronary ligament.

The tibial and fibular collateral ligaments reinforce the medial and lateral sides of the joint. They are taut in joint extension, and in this position, they prevent rotation of the knee.

The synovial membrane of the knee joint is the most extensive in the body and can be divided conveniently into several parts[2] (Fig. 22–58).

Central Portion. The central portion extends between the patella and the patellar surface of the femur to the cruciate ligaments. This portion lies between femoral and tibial condyles and, in addition, above and below the menisci. An infrapatellar fat pad below the patella, located deep to the patellar ligament, presses the synovial membrane posteriorly. In this area, a vertical infrapatellar synovial fold runs from the synovial surface of the fat pad to the intercondylar fossa. Horizontal alar synovial folds run from each side of the infrapatellar synovial fold.

Suprapatellar Synovial Pouch. This cavity, which develops separately from the knee joint but eventually communicates with it, extends vertically above the patella between the quadriceps muscle anteriorly and the femur posteriorly.

Posterior Femoral Recesses. The posterior femoral recesses lie behind the posterior portion of each femoral condyle, deep to the lateral and medial heads of the gastrocnemius muscle. Single or multiple bursae may be located between the muscular portions and the fibrous capsule and may communicate with the articular cavity.[171–173, 267] The medial and lateral posterior femoral recesses are separated by a thick central septum formed by a broad synovial fold around the cruciate ligaments, which may be continuous with the infrapatellar synovial fold.[174]

Text continued on page 741

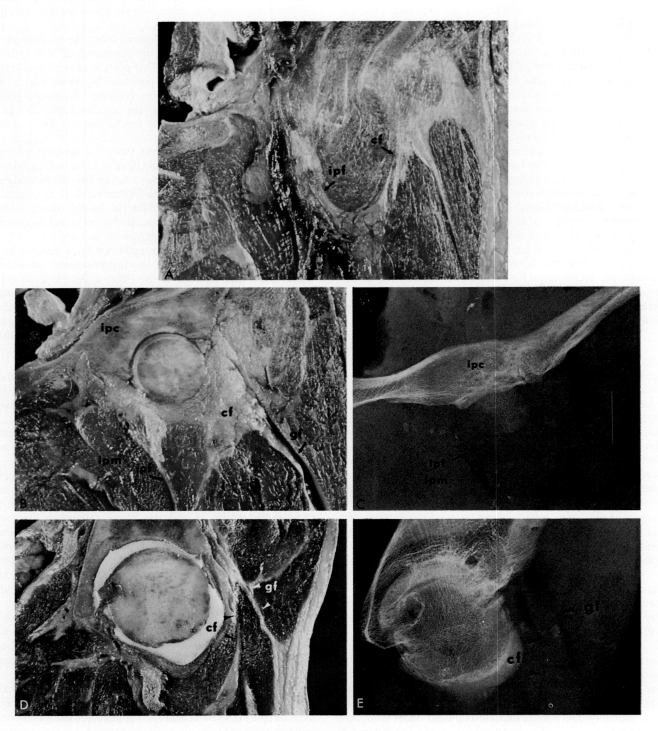

FIGURE 22–52 *See legend on opposite page*

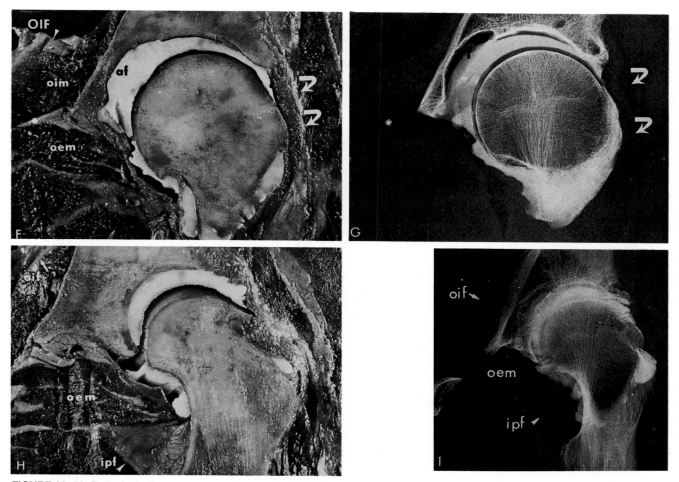

FIGURE 22–52. Periarticular fat planes: cadaveric study. *ipf,* Iliopsoas fat; *cf,* capsular fat; *ipm,* iliopsoas muscle; *gf,* gluteal fat; *ipc,* iliopubic column; *oif,* obturator internus fat; *oim,* obturator internus muscle; *oem,* obturator externus muscle; *af,* acetabular fossa; *gme,* gluteus medius muscle; *gmi,* gluteus minimus muscle.

A–I Corresponding photographs and radiographs of 1 cm thick coronal sections through the hip with prior intra-articular injection of barium-impregnated methylmethacrylate. The sections from **A** to **I** proceed in an anterior to posterior direction. The obturator internus fat *(oif)* is medial to the obturator internus muscle *(oim)* in the pelvis **(F, G, H, I)**. The obturator internus muscle *(oim)* is separated from the hip joint by the acetabulum and from the obturator externus muscle *(oem)* by the obturator membrane (asterisk) **(F, G)**. The iliopsoas fat *(ipf)* **(B, C)** and iliopsoas muscle *(ipm)* are identified. Anteriorly the iliopsoas blends with the fat of the femoral triangle **(A)** (arrow) lateral to the femoral vessels. In its posterior course it sends a fat plane laterally to make contact with the hip capsule adjacent to the medial aspect of the femoral neck **(H, I)**. This is the point of inherent weakness between the iliofemoral and pubofemoral ligaments, which may allow the iliopsoas bursa to communicate with the hip joint. Only the widest portion of the iliopsoas fat *(ipf)* **(B, C)** is seen on an anteroposterior radiograph, and this is anterior to the hip capsule. The most lateral fat plane is the gluteus fat *(gf)*. It lies between the gluteus minimus and gluteus medius muscles and is most prominent in coronal sections through the femoral head **(B through E)**. Its orientation is predominantly sagittal and it becomes thinner and less prominent as it proceeds dorsally. It has no definite connection with the immediate pericapsular region. The "capsular" fat *(cf)* is the more medial of the two lateral fat planes and is related indirectly to the hip capsule. The bulk of this fat plane is intermuscular and between the rectus femoris and tensor fasciae latae muscles anterior to the hip capsule **(A through C)**. It is in this location that the fat plane is at its widest. It takes an oblique course similar to that seen on a routine anteroposterior radiograph of the hip. This fatty layer grows thinner dorsally as it changes from an intermuscular part to a pericapsular part between the superolateral aspect of the hip joint capsule and the medial aspect of the gluteus minimus muscle *(gmi)* **(F, G)**. This true pericapsular fat (curved arrows) is visible on these coronal sections, but it is imperceptible on a routine anteroposterior radiograph of the hip. Furthermore, its orientation is dissimilar to that of the capsular fat plane.

(From Guerra J Jr, et al: Radiology *128*:11, 1978.)

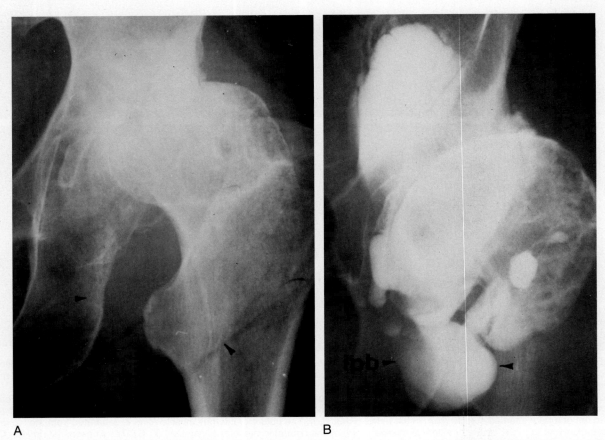

A   B

FIGURE 22–53. Osteoarthritis with enlarged iliopsoas bursa *(ipb)*. The initial film **(A)** demonstrates displacement of the iliopsoas fat (arrow-heads). Arthrography **(B)** reveals communication of the iliopsoas bursa *(ipb)* with the hip joint. (From Warren R, et al: J Bone Joint Surg [Am] *57*:413, 1975.)

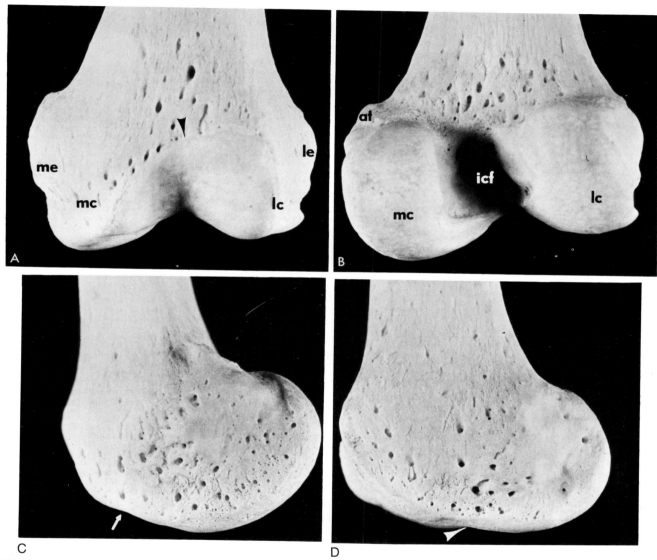

FIGURE 22–54. Distal end of femur: Osseous anatomy.

A, B Anterior **(A)** and posterior **(B)** aspects. Observe the medial *(mc)* and lateral *(lc)* condyles, medial *(me)* and lateral *(le)* epicondyles, adductor tubercle *(at)*, patellar surface (arrowhead), and intercondylar fossa *(icf)*.

C, D Medial **(C)** and lateral **(D)** aspects. On the medial aspect, observe the groove (arrow) that separates the anterior and middle thirds of the distal end of the femur. On the lateral aspect, a groove (arrowhead) divides the femoral surface approximately in half.

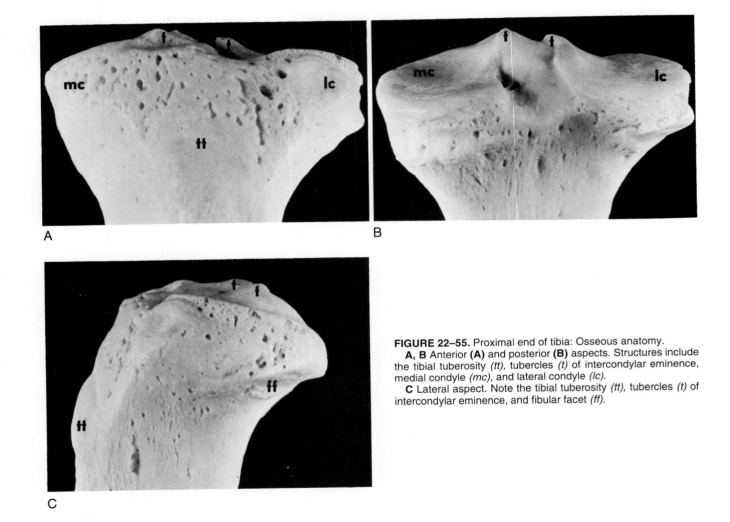

FIGURE 22–55. Proximal end of tibia: Osseous anatomy.

A, B Anterior **(A)** and posterior **(B)** aspects. Structures include the tibial tuberosity *(tt)*, tubercles *(t)* of intercondylar eminence, medial condyle *(mc)*, and lateral condyle *(lc)*.

C Lateral aspect. Note the tibial tuberosity *(tt)*, tubercles *(t)* of intercondylar eminence, and fibular facet *(ff)*.

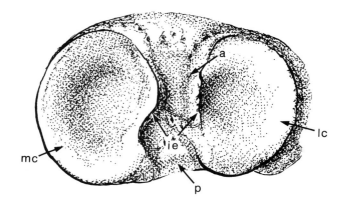

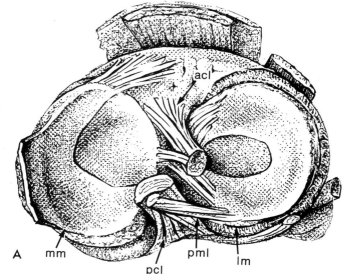

FIGURE 22–56. Meniscal anatomy.

A Drawings of tibial articular surfaces without (upper) and with (below) the addition of soft tissue structures. Note the medial condyle *(mc)*, lateral condyle *(lc)*, intercondylar eminences *(ie)*, anterior intercondylar area *(a)*, and posterior intercondylar area *(p)*. Soft tissue structures are the medial meniscus *(mm)*, lateral meniscus *(lm)*, posterior cruciate ligament *(pcl)*, posterior meniscofemoral ligament *(pml)*, and anterior cruciate ligament *(acl)*.

B On a coronal section, the medial meniscus *(mm)* and lateral meniscus *(lm)* are identified between femur and tibia.

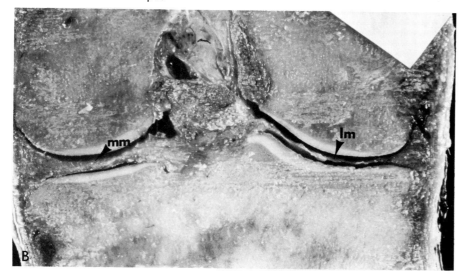

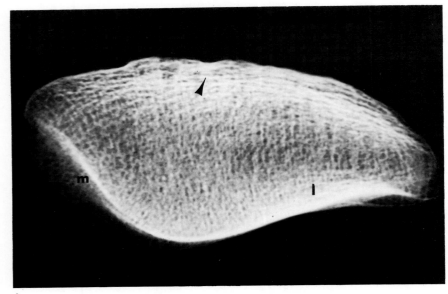

A

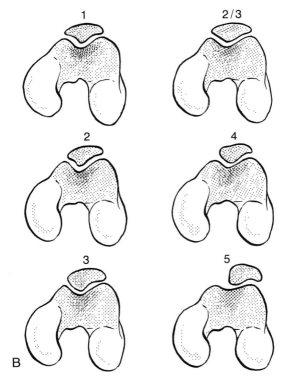

B

FIGURE 22–57. Patella: Osseous anatomy.

A Axial radiograph of the patella showing thick anterior cortex (arrowhead) and smooth articular surface. Observe the medial *(m)* and lateral *(l)* facets.

B Patellar configurations have been delineated by Wiberg, Baumgarten, and other investigators and are summarized in this drawing. For each image, the medial condyle is depicted on the left and the lateral condyle is depicted on the right. Type 1 patellae have equal facets, which are slightly concave. Type 2 patellae are similar, with concave surfaces and a smaller medial facet. Type 3 patellae possess a small medial facet with a convex surface. Type 2/3 patellae have a flat medial facet. Type 4 patellae possess a small or absent medial facet. Type 5 (Jagerhut) patellae demonstrate no medial facet, no central ridge, and lateral subluxation.

Subpopliteal Recess. A small synovial cul-de-sac lies between the lateral meniscus and the tendon of the popliteus, which may communicate with the superior tibiofibular joint in 10 per cent of adults.[175]

Additional Bursae. Numerous additional bursae may be found about the knee.[2, 172, 176–178] These include the subcutaneous prepatellar and subfascial prepatellar bursae anterior to the patella; deep infrapatellar bursa between the upper tibia and ligamentum patellae; anserine bursa between the tibial collateral ligament and tendons of the sartorius, gracilis, and semitendinosus muscles; and bursae between the semimembranosus tendon and tibial collateral ligament, and those between the biceps tendon and fibular collateral ligament.

Intra-articular ligaments can be noted in the knee.[179–181] The anterior and posterior cruciate ligaments extend between the femur and the tibia. The anterior cruciate ligament attaches below to the anterior intercondylar area of the tibia and above to the medial side of the lateral femoral condyle. The posterior cruciate ligament extends from the posterior intercondylar area of the tibia to the lateral side of the medial femoral condyle. These ligaments prevent excessive posterior displacement (anterior cruciate ligament) or anterior displacement (posterior cruciate ligament) of the femur on the tibia.

The radiographic anatomy of the osseous structures about the knee has been reviewed. On anteroposterior radiographs, a line drawn along the midaxis of the femoral shaft intersects a second line drawn tangent to the femoral articular surface with an average angle of 81 degrees (75 to 85 degrees) (femoral angle).[5] Similarly, a line drawn along the midaxis of the tibial shaft intersects a second line drawn tangent to the tibial plateau with an average angle of 93 degrees (85 to 100 degrees) (tibial angle).[5] A variety of additional lines can be used to assess the axial alignment of the lower extremity.[311]

The shallow grooves in the distal articular surface of the femur can be recognized.[182–184, 264] The groove on the medial condyle appears as a sulcus at the junction of the anterior and middle thirds of the articular surface on lateral radiographs. In the same projection, the groove on the lateral condyle is located at the center of the articular surface and generally is more prominent. Deepening of the groove on the lateral condyle has been emphasized as a sign of insufficiency or disruption of the anterior cruciate ligament (see Chapter 70). Landmarks allowing identification of each of the tibial condyles on lateral radiographs also have been summarized.[183]

Trabecular architecture about the knee has been studied,[185] and Blumensaat's line is identified as a condensed linear shadow on the lateral radiograph representing tangential bone in the intercondylar fossa.[186, 187] The location and appearance of Blumensaat's line is extremely sensitive to changes in knee position.[183] In the past, Blumensaat's line has been used to provide an indication of the relative position of the patella in lateral projections. Elevation of the distal pole of the patella above this line with the knee flexed 30 degrees has been used as an indicator of patella alta (an elevated position of the patella). More recently, other measurements on lateral radiographs have been suggested as more reliable indicators of patellar position (Fig. 22–59).[265]

Determination of the ratio of patellar tendon length to greatest diagonal length of the patella has revealed that in the normal situation, both measurements are approximately equal, with a variation of about 20 per cent.[188, 189] A modification of this technique uses the ratio of the distance between the inferior articular surface of the patella and patellar tendon insertion to the length of the articular surface of the patella; a value greater than 2 is considered evidence of patella alta.[312] Another method involves determining the distance between the lower articular surface of the patella and the tibial plateau line. The ratio of this value over the length of the patellar articular surface in normal persons has been reported to be approximately 0.8.[190] Variations of this last method of measurement also exist.[313] The diagnosis of patella alta may have clinical significance, as an abnormally high position of the patella has been recorded in chondromalacia patellae and patellar subluxation or dislocation, whereas a high or low position of the patella has been noted in Osgood-Schlatter's disease.[191, 314]

The normal relationships of the anterior surface of the femur and the patella have been studied using axial radiographs (Fig. 22–59) and CT.[266] Various radiographic projections and measurements have been suggested.

The radiographic anatomy of the knee related to soft tissue shadows also has been described. In the lateral projection of a mildly flexed knee, the collapsed suprapatellar pouch creates a sharp vertical radiodense line between an anterior fat pad superior to the patella (anterior suprapatellar fat) and a posterior fat pad in front of the distal supracondylar region of the femur (prefemoral fat pad) (Fig. 22–60). This line generally is less than 5 mm wide but may be between 5 and 10 mm. Shadows of increased thickness suggest the presence of intra-articular fluid.[192, 268, 269] Distortion of soft tissue planes[192, 193] with the production of a piriform mass[194] in this projection and displacement of fat planes about the suprapatellar pouch on frontal projections[195] are additional but less sensitive signs of knee effusions. Axial radiographs reveal abnormal radiodensity in the medial patellofemoral compartment in such cases.[269] Intra-articular fluid in the knee also may cause displacement of the ossified fabella.[196]

In lateral projections, a thin layer of extrasynovial fat hugs the femoral condyles posteriorly.[177] This fat plane extends from the femoral condyles to the posterior aspect of the lateral tibial condyle, forming a double curve resembling the numeral 3. A fat plane about the posterior cruciate ligament also may be visible. These fat planes become distorted in the presence of intra-articular fluid.

Active movements of the knee are flexion, extension, and medial and lateral rotation. Accessory movements are increased rotation, backward and forward gliding, abduction, adduction, and separation of tibia and femur.

TIBIOFIBULAR JOINTS

Osseous and Soft Tissue Anatomy

Articulations uniting the tibia and the fibula are the proximal (superior) tibiofibular joint (synovial), the crural interosseous membrane (syndesmosis), and the distal tibiofibular joint (syndesmosis). These joints allow limited movement of the fibula with respect to the tibia. As an example, on

Text continued on page 746

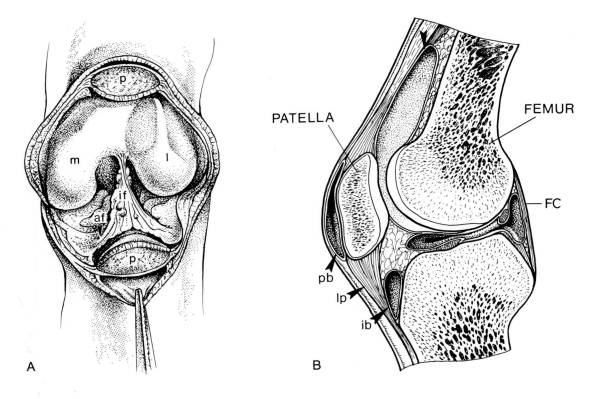

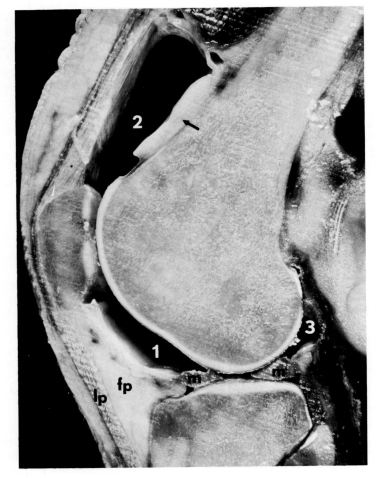

FIGURE 22–58. Knee joint: Normal anatomy.

A Anterior aspect. The patella *(p)* has been divided to expose the joint interior. Observe the medial *(m)* and lateral *(l)* femoral condyles and alar folds *(af)* of synovium, which converge to form the infrapatellar fold *(if)* or ligamentum mucosum.

B Sagittal section. Drawing indicates femur, patella, tibia, fibrous capsule *(FC)*, prepatellar bursa *(pb)*, deep infrapatellar bursa *(ib)*, ligamentum patellae *(lp)*, and suprapatellar pouch (arrowhead).

C Sagittal section. Photograph of an air-distended knee joint outlining ligamentum patellae *(lp)*, infrapatellar fat pad *(fp)*, and lateral meniscus *(m)*. The articulation can be divided into a central portion *(1)*, suprapatellar pouch *(2)*, and posterior femoral recesses *(3)*. Note fatty tissue (arrow), which is pressed against the anterior aspect of the femur.

Illustration continued on opposite page

FIGURE 22–58 *Continued*

D Lateral aspect. Distended joint is indicated in black. Observe the central portion *(1)*, suprapatellar pouch *(2)*, and posterior femoral recesses *(3)*. The prepatellar bursa *(pb)*, ligamentum patellae *(lp)*, fibular collateral ligament *(fcl)*, and popliteus tendon *(pt)* are indicated. The lateral head of the gastrocnemius muscle has been turned up, exposing a communicating bursa (arrow).

E Posterior aspect. The distended joint is indicated in black. The medial *(m)* and lateral *(l)* heads of the gastrocnemius muscle have been sectioned. Note the bursa (arrow) beneath the lifted medial head, medial meniscus *(mm)*, lateral meniscus *(lm)*, popliteus tendon *(pt)*, fibular collateral ligament *(fcl)*, and subpopliteal recess *(4)*.

F, G Photograph and radiograph of a sagittal section through the posterior aspect of the knee, revealing gastrocnemiosemimembranosus bursa (arrows) with communication with the knee joint.

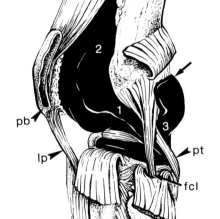

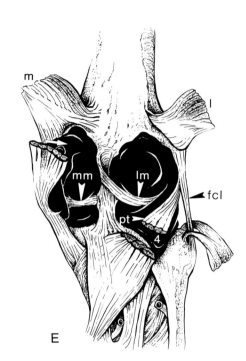

D

E

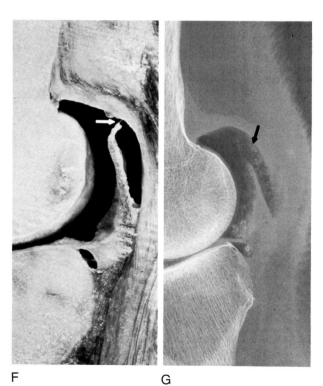

F   G

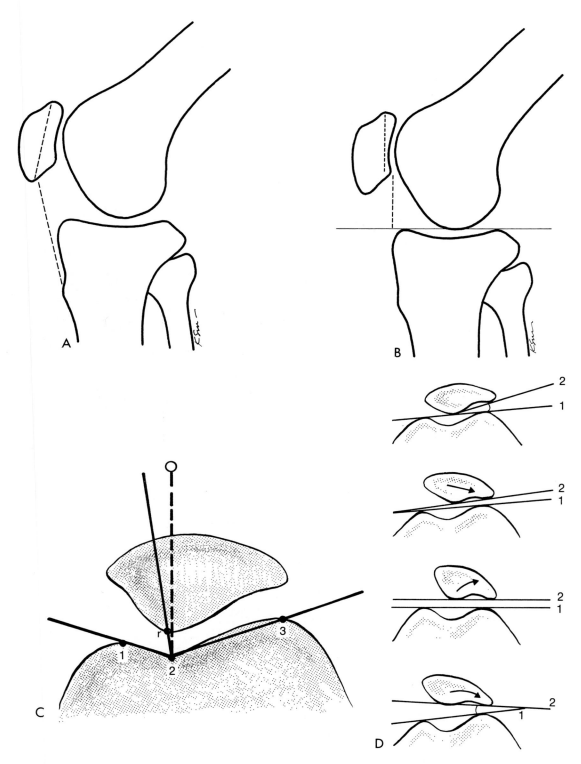

FIGURE 22–59. Patellar position.

A The ratio of patellar tendon length to the greatest diagonal length of the patella may be used to diagnose patella alta.

B The ratio of the distance between the lower articular surface of the patella and the tibial plateau line to the length of the patellar articular surface also has been used for this purpose.

C Merchant and coworkers (Merchant AC, et al: J Bone Joint Surg [Am] *56*:1391, 1974) have suggested that on an axial radiograph, the line connecting the median ridge of the patella *(r)* and trochlear depth *(2)* should fall medial to or slightly lateral to a line *(O)* bisecting angle *1–2–3*. Here the first line lies medial to line O, a normal finding.

D Laurin and coworkers have indicated other measurements that might be appropriate. The upper two diagrams reveal the normal situation; the lower two diagrams indicate the abnormal situation. On axial radiographs, normally an angle formed between a line connecting the anterior aspect of the femoral condyles *(1)* and a second line along the lateral facet of the patella *(2)* opens laterally. In patients with subluxation or abnormal tilting of the patella, these lines are parallel or the angle of intersection opens medially.

(**D**, From Laurin CA, et al: J Bone Joint Surg [Am] *60*:55, 1978.)

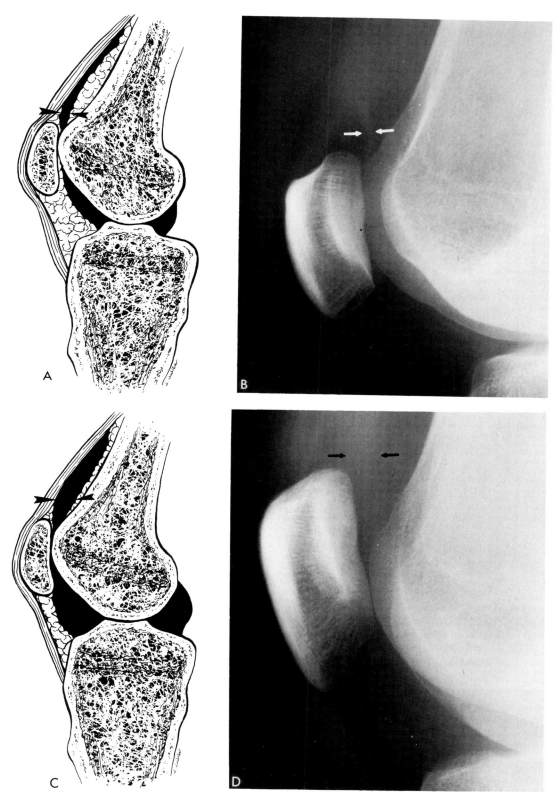

FIGURE 22–60. Diagnosis of a synovial effusion in the knee.
   A, B In normal situations, the collapsed suprapatellar pouch (arrowheads) creates a radiodense area (arrows) that generally is less than 5 mm in width but may be between 5 and 10 mm in width.
   C, D In the presence of intra-articular fluid, distention of the pouch (arrowheads) creates a radiodense region of increased thickness with blurred margins (arrows).

weight-bearing, the fibula descends, providing increased stability to the ankle mortise[271–273]; the weight-bearing function of the fibula is debated, although the fibula is estimated to receive approximately 6 to 16 per cent of the weight, depending on the position of the ankle.[271, 272] A small amount of lateral rotation of the fibula is apparent during dorsiflexion of the ankle.[200]

Proximal Tibiofibular Joint. The head of the fibula contains a circular facet that faces superiorly, anteriorly, and medially. The styloid process of the fibular head is an upward protuberance on the lateral aspect of the posterior portion of the bone. The fibular facet on the lateral condyle of the tibia is directed downward, posteriorly, and laterally. The popliteus tendon creates a groove on the fibula superiorly and medially to the articular facet.

The normal radiographic anatomy of the proximal tibiofibular joint has been outlined[175] (Fig. 22–61). Either of two types of articulations may be apparent[197]: a horizontal articulation (less than 20 degrees of joint inclination) and an oblique articulation (greater than 20 degrees of joint inclination), although intermediate variations also are noted. The horizontal type is associated with increased rotatory mobility and more joint surface area than the oblique type of articulation. The major functions of the proximal tibiofibular joint are dissipating torsional stresses applied at the ankle and providing tensile rather than significant weight-bearing strength.[197]

On an anteroposterior radiograph the medial aspect of the fibular head, which is the actual articulating surface, crosses the lateral border of the tibia. On the lateral radiograph the fibular head overlies the posterior border of the tibia. Its proper position in this projection can be confirmed by identifying its relationship to the lateral tibial condyle. An important landmark on the lateral knee radiograph for locating the exact position of the fibular head is formed by the posteromedial portion of the lateral tibial condyle.[183] If a line is drawn in an anterior to posterior direction along the lateral tibial spine and continued inferiorly along the posterior aspect of the tibia, this line will identify a groove that separates the midportion of the tibial shaft from the bulk of the bone forming the supporting structure of the lateral tibial condyle posteriorly. The sloping radiodense line observed on the lateral knee radiograph proceeds first posteriorly and inferiorly to form an acute angle posteriorly, which identifies the most posteromedial portion of the lateral tibial condyle. The radiodense line then extends inferiorly and anteriorly from this point in the groove described previously. Knowledge of the exact location of this line greatly assists in the interpretation of lateral knee radiographs in tibiofibular joint dislocations (Fig. 22–62).[270]

The optimal view for visualizing the proximal tibiofibular joint is a radiograph exposed with the knee in 45 to 60 degrees of internal rotation[175] (Fig. 22–63). In this projection, the articulation is seen in profile, generally free of overlying osseous structures, and the width of the articular space and appearance of subchondral bone can be evaluated.

Before 12 weeks of fetal age, the proximal tibiofibular joint does not possess a cavity[198] (Fig. 22–64). Subsequently, narrow cavities are apparent, which may be separated from the lateral femorotibial joint by a small amount of loose fibrous or areolar tissue. Communication between the knee joint and proximal tibiofibular joint may be iden-

tified in some fetuses and exists in approximately 10 per cent of adult joints. Subsequent development of the proximal tibiofibular joint includes the formation of articular cartilage, synovial tissue, synovial recesses, and fibrous capsule.

The fully developed articulation is approximately a plane joint, between the lateral condyle of the tibia and the head of the fibula (Fig. 22–65). Apposing bony facets are covered with articular cartilage, and the bones are connected by a fibrous capsule and anterior and posterior ligaments. The fibrous capsule, which is attached to the margins of the tibial and fibular articular facets, is much thicker anteriorly than posteriorly. The anterior ligament passes obliquely upward from the front of the fibular head to the front of the lateral condyle of the tibia; the posterior ligament passes obliquely upward from the back of the fibular head to the back of the lateral condyle of the tibia. The posterior ligament is covered by the popliteus tendon. Superior support is provided by the fibular collateral ligament, extending from the lateral aspect of the fibular head to the lateral femoral epicondyle.

Crural Interosseous Membrane. The crural interosseous membrane is tightly stretched between the interosseous borders of tibia and fibula.[199] Its upper limit is just inferior to the proximal tibiofibular joint, and its lower limit contains fibers that blend with those about the distal tibiofibular joint. The oblique fibers in the crural interosseous membrane extend inferiorly and laterally from tibia to fibula. A large oval opening in the superior aspect of the membrane allows passage of the anterior tibial vessels; a smaller distal opening allows passage of the perforating branch of the peroneal artery.

Distal Tibiofibular Joint. This fibrous joint consists of a strong interosseous ligament that unites the convex surface of the medial distal fibula and the concave surface of the adjacent fibular notch of the tibia. Additionally, the anterior and posterior tibiofibular ligaments reinforce this articulation.[274] Below this ligamentous joint, an upward prolongation of the synovial membrane of the ankle (talocrural joint) can extend 3 to 5 mm. This synovial recess may be associated with cartilaginous surfaces on tibia and fibula.

ANKLE (TALOCRURAL JOINT)

This synovial articulation exists where the talus relates to the lower ends of the tibia and fibula and the inferior transverse tibiofibular ligament.

Osseous Anatomy

The distal end of the tibia contains the medial malleolus and articular surface (Fig. 22–66). The broad malleolus has an articular facet on its lateral surface, which is comma-shaped. On the posterior surface of the distal end of the tibia is a groove, just lateral to the medial malleolus, related to the tendon of the tibialis posterior. The inferior surface of the tibia represents the articular area for the talus. It is smooth, wider anteriorly than posteriorly, concave anteriorly to posteriorly, and minimally convex medially to laterally. The articular surface on the inferior tibia is continuous with that on the medial malleolus. The triangular fib-

Text continued on page 751

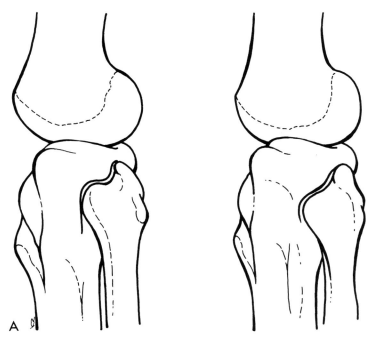

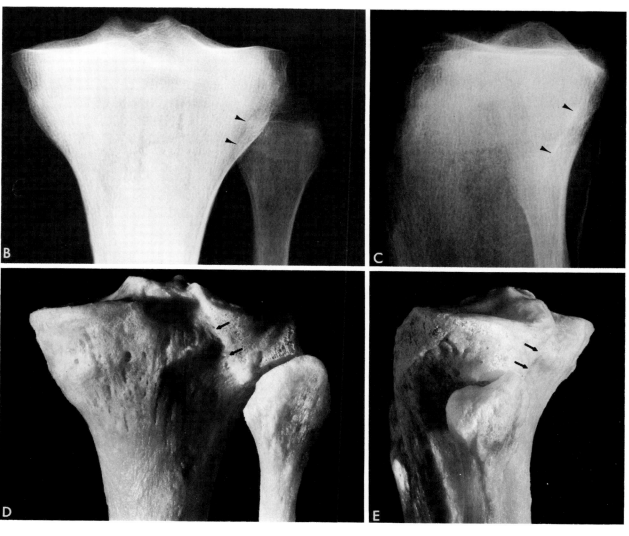

FIGURE 22–61. Proximal tibiofibular joint: Osseous anatomy.

A Types of articulations. A horizontal (left) or oblique (right) type of articulation may be present.

B Anteroposterior radiograph outlining normal relationship of proximal ends of tibia and fibula. Medial aspect of fibular head crosses lateral border of tibia (arrowheads).

C Lateral radiograph showing fibular head overlying posterior border of tibia. Note linear sloping radiodensity (arrowheads), which identifies the most posteromedial portion of lateral tibial condyle. This radiodense line is projected over the midportion of the fibular head.

D Posterior aspect of proximal portions of tibia and fibula showing relationship of fibular head to posterior margin of tibia. Note groove (arrows) that separates midportion of tibial shaft from bulk of the bone forming the supporting structure of the lateral tibial condyle. This groove produces the linear sloping radiodense shadow on lateral knee radiographs.

E Steep oblique view showing relationship of proximal ends of fibula and tibia. Again note groove (arrows).

(**B–E**, From Resnick D, et al: AJR *131*:133, 1978. Copyright 1978, American Roentgen Ray Society.)

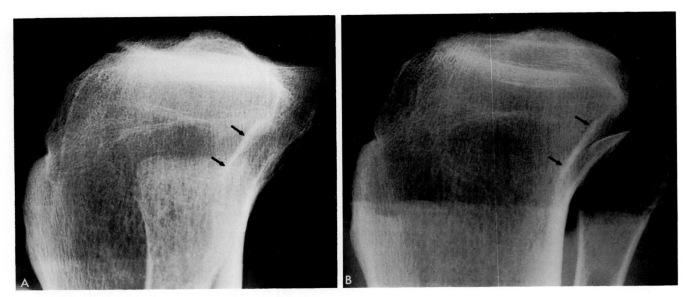

FIGURE 22–62. Dislocation at proximal tibiofibular joint in cadaver.
  A Anterolateral dislocation. Almost the entire fibular head is projected in front of sloping radiodense line (arrows).
  B Posteromedial dislocation. Little overlap is seen between proximal ends of the tibia and fibula. The fibular head is projected entirely posterior to sloping radiodense line (arrows).
  (From Resnick D, et al: AJR *131*:133, 1978. Copyright 1978, American Roentgen Ray Society.)

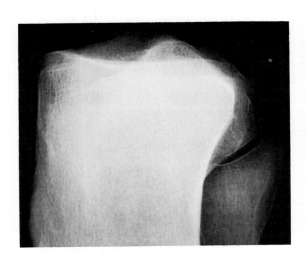

FIGURE 22–63. The optimal view for visualizing proximal tibiofibular joint in profile. Radiograph is exposed in 45 to 60 degrees of internal rotation. (From Resnick D, et al: AJR *131*:133, 1978. Copyright 1978, American Roentgen Ray Society.)

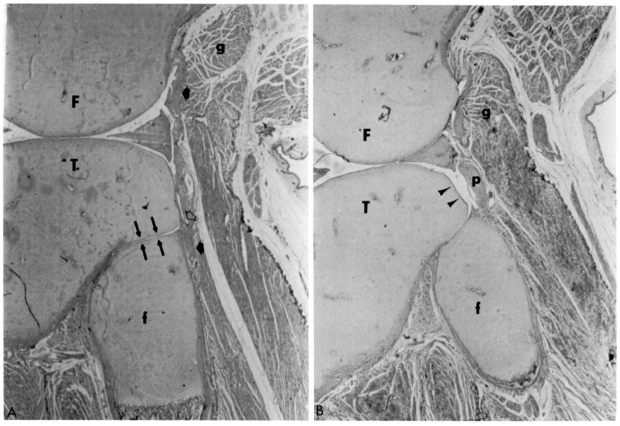

FIGURE 22–64. Proximal tibiofibular joint: Normal developmental anatomy. Sagittal sections through articulation in embryos. *f,* Fibula; *T,* tibia; *F,* femur.

A Tibiofibular joint space (double arrows) is seen as a thin white line 1 mm wide. No articular recesses are present. Posterior horn of lateral meniscus is well developed. The posterior aspect of the knee joint capsule inserts on the fibula and femur (heavy arrows). The insertion of the lateral head of the gastrocnemius muscle *(g)* is noted at the posterior aspect of the lateral femoral condyle. A thin zone of fibrous tissue separates the femorotibial space from the proximal tibiofibular joint (open arrow).

B No central cavity is present within the proximal tibiofibular joint. Note prominent inferior recess beneath lateral meniscus (arrowheads) and direct communication between femorotibial and tibiofibular joints. Popliteus muscle *(p)* is cut in cross section. Lateral head of gastrocnemius muscle *(g)* again is noted.

(From Resnick D, et al: AJR *131*:133, 1978. Copyright 1978, American Roentgen Ray Society.)

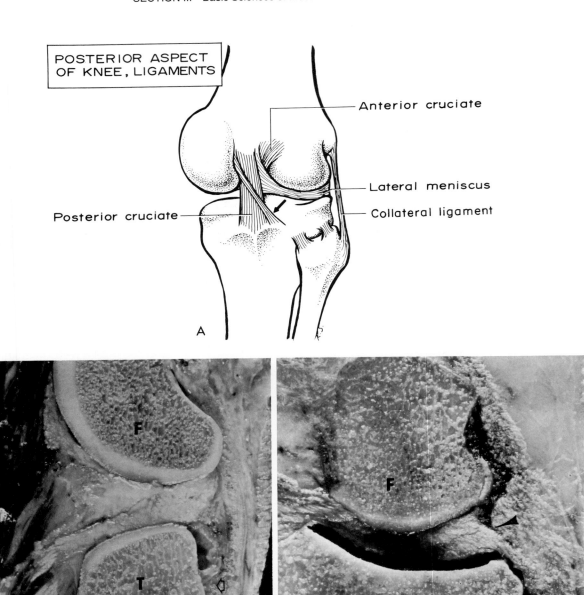

FIGURE 22–65. Proximal tibiofibular joint: Articular anatomy.

A Anatomic features of fully developed proximal tibiofibular articulation. On posterior aspect of femur and tibia, two thick ligamentous bands pass obliquely from fibular head to posterior aspect of the lateral tibial condyle. Similar ligaments strengthen the anterior aspect of the tibiofibular joint (not shown). The fibular collateral ligament extends from the fibular head to the lateral femoral epicondyle. Posterior and anterior cruciate ligaments and the lateral meniscus also are indicated. Also note the posterior meniscofemoral ligament (ligament of Wrisberg, arrow).

B, C Coronal sections through two adult tibiofibular joints. *F,* Femur; *T,* tibia; *f,* fibula. Horizontal articulation **(B)** contains well-developed articular cartilage and joint space. The lateral recess (heavy arrows) is especially well developed, as is the joint capsule. The medial synovial recess is partially obliterated (arrowheads). Bands of fibrous and areolar tissue (open arrow) separate femorotibial and proximal tibiofibular articulations. The obliquely inclining joint is shown in **C** (arrows). An incidental finding is degeneration of the lateral meniscus (arrowhead).

(**B, C**, From Resnick D, et al: AJR *131*:133, 1978. Copyright 1978, American Roentgen Ray Society.)

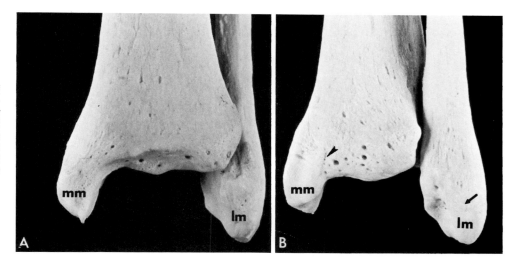

FIGURE 22–66. Distal ends of tibia and fibula: Osseous anatomy. Anterior **(A)** and posterior **(B)** aspects. Observe the medial malleolus *(mm)*, lateral malleolus *(lm)*, groove for the tendon of the tibialis posterior (arrowhead), and groove for the peroneal tendons (arrow).

ular notch is on the lateral side of the tibia. This notch represents the site of attachment of various ligaments that connect the distal portions of the tibia and fibula.

The distal end of the fibula contains the lateral malleolus (Fig. 22–66). This structure projects more inferiorly than the medial malleolus and contains a triangular facet on its medial surface for articulation with the talus and an irregular surface above this facet for the interosseous ligament. Posterior to the convex articular facet is a depression, the malleolar fossa.

The dorsal surface of the talus contains the trochlear articular surface (Fig. 22–67). This surface is convex anteriorly to posteriorly and concave from side to side. The medial surface of the talar body possesses a facet that articulates with the medial malleolus. The lateral surface of the body contains a triangular articular facet that is intimate with the lateral malleolus.

Assessment of alignment of the ankle on radiographs is important in the evaluation of this joint after trauma. Small degrees of lateral displacement of the talus on the tibia may result in the rapid development of secondary degenerative arthritis. It has been shown that even 1 mm of lateral displacement of the talus reduces the tibiotalar contact areas by 42 per cent.[201] Incomplete ligament tears may result in relatively small amounts of displacement, which may be difficult to detect radiographically. This has stimulated investigators to propose radiographic criteria for assessment of tibiotalar alignment.[202]

A short, concave cortical line representing the posteromedial surface of the talus was used by some investigators to determine tibiotalar displacement[203] (Fig. 22–67). This line actually delineates the insertion of the deep deltoid fibers, however, and does not represent the true medial articular surface. In addition, this line cannot be identified accurately with moderate internal or external rotation of the talus, precluding accurate measurements on rotation radiographs. Our attempts to use these inconstant radiographic features to determine tibiotalar shift either by measurement of the so-called medial clear space or by determination of the central weight-bearing line of the talus[202, 203] using ankle specimens with 0 to 3 mm of displacement have yielded markedly inconsistent results. The main pitfalls of these previously reported measurement techniques include (1) in-

ability to identify accurately the posteromedial border of the talus with extreme degrees of rotation, (2) lack of an identifiable posterolateral talar landmark, and (3) variations in the weight-bearing line of the tibia with rotation, because this bone is not a true cylinder even above the metaphysis.

In the adult, the coronal plane of the ankle is oriented in about 15 to 20 degrees of external rotation with reference to the coronal plane of the knee[204] and therefore the lateral malleolus is slightly posterior to the medial malleolus. To obtain a true anteroposterior film of the tibiotalar articulation, the ankle must be positioned with the medial and lateral malleoli parallel to the tabletop—that is, in about 15 to 20 degrees of internal rotation, or the mortise view[205] (Fig. 22–68). This positioning places the medial articular surface tangent to the x-ray beam, and the short concave line representing the posteromedial surface of the talus falls slightly lateral to the medial articular surface. With this view, the radiographic medial clear space represents the actual width of the medial joint space. In adults, the normal interosseous space is about 2.5 to 3.5 mm.[275]

The axial relationships of the ankle have been described.[5] The longitudinal axis of the tibia is perpendicular to the horizontal plane of the ankle joint and continuous with the longitudinal axis of the talus. The tibial angle, the angle formed by the intersection of one line drawn tangentially to the articular surface of the medial malleolus and a second drawn along the articular surface of the talus, averages 53 degrees (45 to 61 degrees). The fibular angle drawn in a corresponding way using the lateral malleolus rather than the medial malleolus averages 52 degrees (45 to 63 degrees).

Soft Tissue Anatomy

The articular surfaces are cartilage-covered and the bones are connected by a fibrous capsule and by the deltoid, the anterior and posterior talofibular, and the calcaneofibular ligaments (Figs. 22–69 and 22–70). The fibrous capsule is attached superiorly to the medial and lateral malleoli and tibia and inferiorly to the talus. The talar attachment of the capsule is close to the margins of the trochlear surface except anteriorly, where the attachment to the neck of the talus is located at some distance from the articular margin.

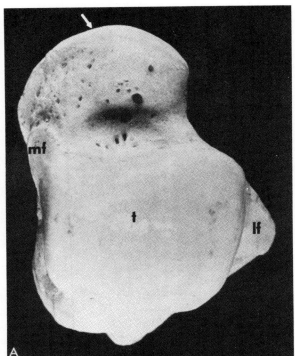

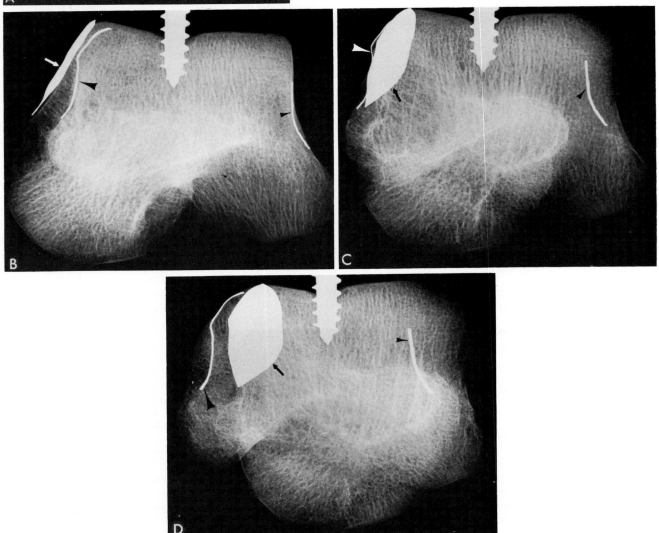

FIGURE 22–67. Talus: Osseous anatomy.

A Dorsal aspect. Structures include the trochlear surface *(t)*, medial facet *(mf)* for articulation with the medial malleolus, and lateral facet *(lf)* for articulation with the lateral malleolus. The distal surface (arrow) of the talus articulates with the tarsal navicular surface.

B–D Anteroposterior radiographs of the talus in 20 degrees of internal rotation **(B)**, 0 degrees of rotation **(C)**, and 15 degrees of external rotation **(D)**. With 20 degrees of internal rotation **(B)**, the medial articular surface, covered with lead foil, is seen in tangent (arrow). Lead strips cover the concave posteromedial surface (large arrowhead) and the posterolateral surface (small arrowhead). In 0 degrees of rotation **(C)**, the posteromedial surface is tangent and forms a border, the medial articular surface is not tangent and obscures the posteromedial surface, and the posterolateral surface is not tangent. In external rotation **(D)**, none of the identified structures is tangent.

(**B–D**, From Goergen TG, et al: J Bone Joint Surg [Am] *59*:874, 1977.)

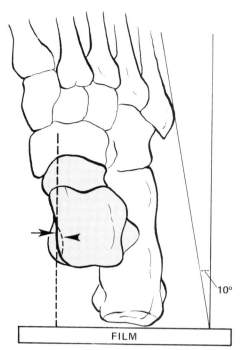

FIGURE 22–68. Mortise radiograph of ankle. By obtaining a radiograph in 10 to 15 degrees of internal rotation of the femur with respect to the fifth metatarsal, the medial articular surface of the talus (arrow) is tangential to the x-ray beam and the concave line representing the insertion of the deep deltoid ligament (arrowhead) falls slightly lateral to the articular surface. (From Goergen TG, et al: J Bone Joint Surg [Am] *59*:874, 1977.)

The capsule is weak both anteriorly and posteriorly, but it is reinforced medially and laterally by various ligaments. A synovial membrane lines the inner aspect of the capsule and extends for a short vertical distance between the tibia and fibula. In this latter area, cartilage may be found on the osseous surfaces, continuous with that in the ankle joint.

Surrounding ligaments[206] include the deltoid, anterior and posterior talofibular, and calcaneofibular ligaments.

The soft tissue anatomy of the talocrural joint governs the radiographic manifestations of an articular effusion. On lateral radiographs, an ankle effusion produces a teardrop-shaped dense shadow anterior to the joint, extending along the neck of the talus,[276] a finding that is accentuated when the ankle is dorsiflexed.[277] A similar radiodense area in the posterior aspect of the joint or a lobulated mass (indicative of articular communication with the posterior subtalar joint) in this region is an additional, although less reliable, sign of an ankle effusion.

Deltoid Ligament. This medial ligament is triangular and is attached above to the apex and the posterior and anterior borders of the medial malleolus. It contains superficial, middle, and deep fibers. Superficial fibers run anteriorly to the tuberosity of the tarsal navicular bone and blend with the plantar calcaneonavicular ligament. Middle fibers attach to the sustentaculum tali of the calcaneus, and posterior fibers pass to the medial talar surface, including its tubercle.

Anterior Talofibular Ligament. The anterior talofibular ligament extends from the anterior margin of the lateral

malleolus to the lateral articular facet on the neck of the talus.

Posterior Talofibular Ligament. The posterior talofibular ligament attaches to the lateral malleolar fossa and extends horizontally to the lateral tubercle of the talus and medial malleolus.

Calcaneofibular Ligament. The calcaneofibular ligament extends from the lateral malleolus to the lateral surface of the calcaneus. It is crossed by the peroneus longus and peroneus brevis tendons.

Active movements of the ankle are dorsiflexion and plantar flexion. Accessory movements are a side to side gliding motion, rotation, abduction, and adduction.

TENDON SHEATHS AND BURSAE ABOUT THE ANKLE AND CALCANEUS

Tendons with accompanying tendon sheaths are intimate with the ankle joint.[207, 278–280] Anteriorly, there are sheaths about the tibialis anterior, extensor hallucis longus, extensor digitorum longus, and peroneus tertius muscles. Medially, sheaths are present about the tibialis posterior, flexor digitorum longus, and flexor hallucis longus muscles. Laterally, the common sheath of the peroneus longus and peroneus brevis muscles may be appreciated.[208]

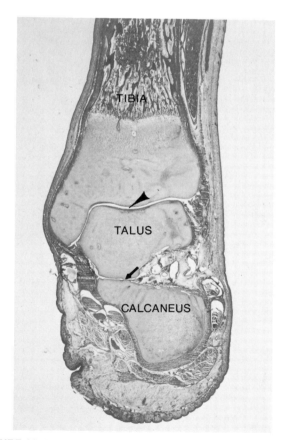

FIGURE 22–69. Ankle joint: Developmental anatomy (coronal section). Photomicrograph (20×) reveals the ankle joint (arrowhead) between the unossified portion of distal ends of the tibia and talus and a portion of the talocalcaneonavicular joint (arrow) between the talus and sustentaculum tali of the calcaneus.

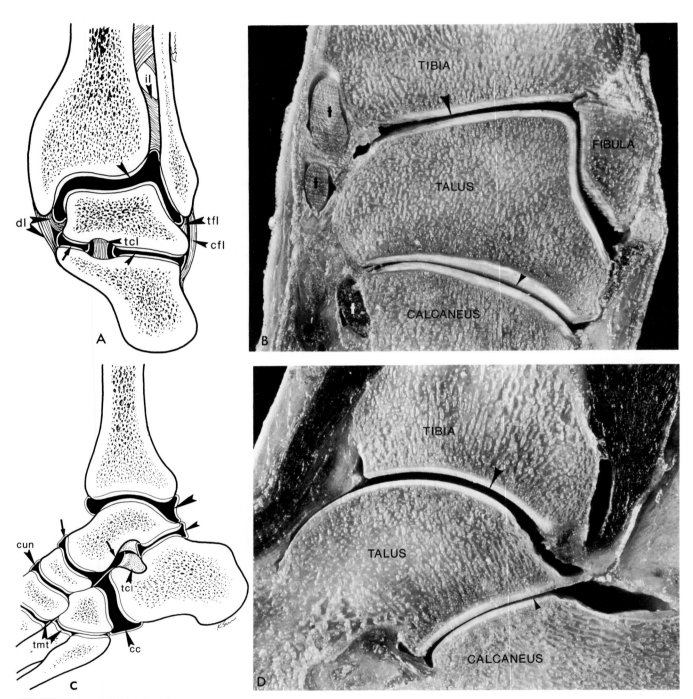

FIGURE 22–70. Ankle joint anatomy.

A, B A drawing and photograph of a coronal section through the distal ends of tibia, fibula, and talus, outlining the ankle joint (large arrowheads), interosseous ligament *(il)* of tibiofibular syndesmosis, interosseous talocalcaneal ligament *(tcl),* portions of the deltoid ligament *(dl),* posterior talofibular ligament *(tfl),* calcaneofibular ligament *(cfl),* surrounding tendons *(t),* subtalar joint (small arrowheads), and talocalcaneonavicular joint (arrow).

C, D Some of the same structures as in **A** and **B** can be identified in a drawing and photograph of a sagittal section of the ankle. Additional articulations that can be seen are the calcaneocuboid *(cc),* cuneonavicular *(cun),* and tarsometatarsal *(tmt)* joints.

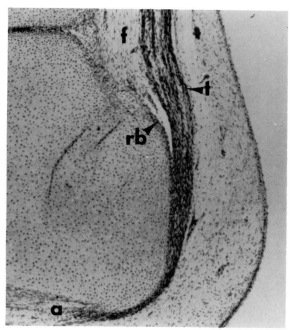

FIGURE 22-71. Soft tissues about the calcaneus: Developmental anatomy. A photomicrograph (20×) of a sagittal section through the calcaneus reveals the preachilles fat pad *(f)*, Achilles tendon *(t)*, retrocalcaneal bursa *(rb)*, and plantar aponeurosis *(a)*.

Important tendons, aponeuroses, and bursae are located about the calcaneus (Fig. 22-71). The plantar aponeurosis contains strong fibers that adhere to the posteroinferior surface of the bone. The Achilles tendon, which is the thickest and strongest human tendon, attaches to the posterior surface of the calcaneus approximately 2 cm below the upper surface of the bone. The retrocalcaneal bursa exists between the Achilles tendon and the posterosuperior surface of the calcaneus[209-212] (Fig. 22-72). This bursal space is lined with synovium, which extends over both the Achilles tendon and the inferior limit of the preachilles fat pad. The posterior surface of the calcaneus is covered with cartilage.

The normal radiographic features of these soft tissue landmarks about the calcaneus include the following[209]:

1. The Achilles tendon has a thickness of 4 to 8 mm at the level of the calcaneus or 1 to 2 cm above the top of the calcaneus (Fig. 22-73).

2. A vertical radiolucent area, the retrocalcaneal recess, of 2 mm or more in length, extends from the posterior aspect of the calcaneus behind the posterior portion of the bone, reflecting fat around the normal retrocalcaneal bursa (Fig. 22-74). The appearance of the retrocalcaneal recess can be influenced by severe dorsiflexion or plantar flexion of the foot.

Articular disorders may produce increased thickness and blurring of the Achilles tendon and obscuration of the retrocalcaneal recess (Fig. 22-75).

A triangular radiolucent area, the posterior triangle or preachilles fat pad, is observed normally on lateral radiographs of the ankle. The posterior margin of the triangle is the Achilles tendon and the anterior border is the flexor hallucis longus.[281] Obscuration of portions of the preachilles fat pad occurs in instances of tendinous rupture,[282] but sim-

ilar findings may indicate accessory or anomalous muscles of the lower calf (see Chapter 70).[283, 284]

INTERTARSAL JOINTS

Osseous and Soft Tissue Anatomy

Numerous synovial joints exist between the tarsal bones (Fig. 22-76).

Talocalcaneal Joints[213, 285] (Figs. 22-77 to 22-79). The talocalcaneal joints are two in number: the subtalar (posterior talocalcaneal or posterior subtalar) joint and the talocalcaneonavicular (anterior subtalar) joint. These joints are separated by the tarsal canal and sinus and their contents.

The subtalar joint exists between the posterior talar facet of the calcaneus and the posterior calcaneal facet of the talus. The talar facet is oval and concave and extends distally and laterally at an angle of approximately 45 degrees with the sagittal plane.[1] The posterior calcaneal facet is oval and convex anteroposteriorly. This synovium-lined joint, which may communicate with the talocrural or ankle joint in approximately 10 to 20 per cent of persons,[213-215] contains a capsule that contributes to the interosseous talocalcaneal ligament, the major bond between talus and calcaneus (Figs. 22-79 and 22-80). Additional structures binding talus and calcaneus are the anterior talocalcaneal ligament (extending from the lateral talar tubercle to the proximal medial calcaneus), the medial talocalcaneal ligament (extending from the medial talar tubercle to the sustentaculum tali), and the lateral talocalcaneal ligament (extending from the lateral surface of the talus to that of the calcaneus).

The talocalcaneonavicular joint also is a synovium-lined articulation, which exists between the head of the talus, the posterior surface of the navicular bone, the anterior articular surface of the calcaneus, and the proximal surface of the plantar calcaneonavicular ligament or ''spring'' ligament. The distal surface of the head of the talus is oval and convex, directed inferiorly and medially to articulate with the oval, concave proximal surface of the navicular bone. The plantar surface of the talar head has three articular areas separated by indistinct osseous ridges: the posterior area is large and oval, convex, and articulates with the sustentaculum tali of the calcaneus; the second area, anterolateral to the posterior area, is flattened, articulating with the superior surface of the calcaneus; and the navicular area, directed distally, is oval and convex, articulating with the tarsal navicular bone. The anterior articular surface of the talus also contacts the plantar calcaneonavicular ligament. This ligament has a central area that consists of fibrocartilage and bridges the triangular space between the anterior and middle talar facets of the calcaneus and navicular bone. The posterior surface of the joint capsule contributes to the interosseous ligament. On its medial side, this articulation is enlarged or deepened by a portion of the deltoid ligament, which is attached to the plantar calcaneonavicular ligament. Movements are coordinated between the talocalcaneonavicular and subtalar articulations and include inversion and eversion of the foot.

Calcaneocuboid Joint (Fig. 22-81). The calcaneocuboid joint is formed between apposing quadrilateral facets on the calcaneus and cuboid bones, and its capsule is reinforced

Text continued on page 763

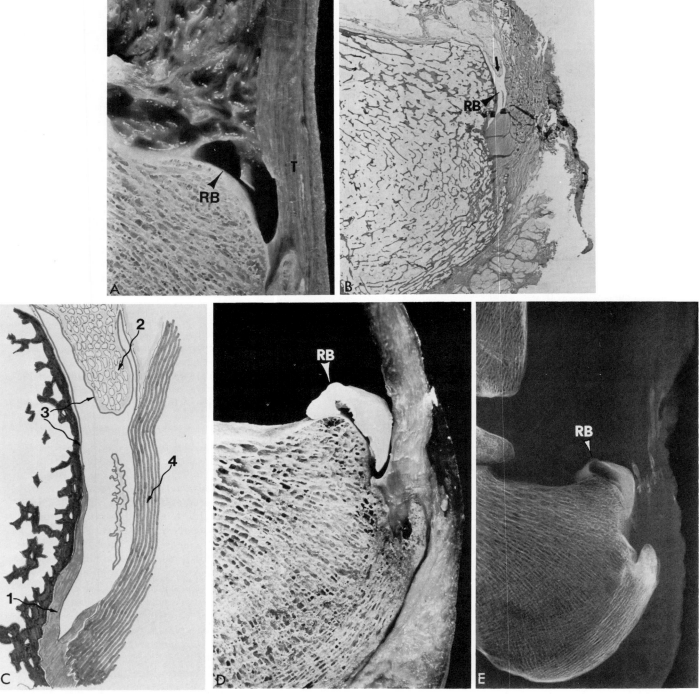

FIGURE 22–72. Retrocalcaneal bursa: Anatomy.

    A In this sagittal section, observe the retrocalcaneal bursa *(RB),* which is located between the Achilles tendon *(T)* and upper border of the calcaneus. Above the bursa, the preachilles fat pad can be identified.

    B On this photomicrograph (4×) the retrocalcaneal bursa *(RB)* is enveloped in a synovial membrane that extends over the inferior limit of the preachilles fat pad (arrow).

    C This drawing of the photomicrograph reveals calcaneal cartilage *(1),* the tip of the preachilles fat pad *(2),* synovium *(3)* lining the bursa, and the Achilles tendon *(4).*

    D, E A photograph and radiograph of a sagittal section through the retrocalcaneal bursa *(RB),* which has been injected percutaneously with barium-impregnated methylmethacrylate, outline the intimate relationship between the bursa and calcaneus.

    (From Resnick D, et al: Radiology *125*:355, 1977.)

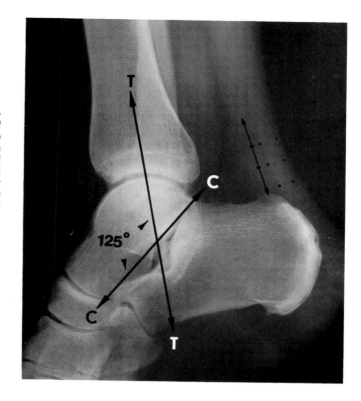

FIGURE 22–73. Achilles tendon: Normal radiographic measurements. The thickness of the Achilles tendon is noted at the level of the calcaneus and at 1 and 2 cm above it. The determination of the calcaneal-talar angle guarantees that the radiograph has been taken in a "neutral" position. This angle is formed by the intersection of two lines, one drawn along the longitudinal axis of the tibia *(T)* and the second drawn along the top of the calcaneus *(C)*. With proper positioning in normal persons, this angle varies from approximately 90 degrees to 140 degrees. (From Resnick D, et al: Radiology *125*:355, 1977.)

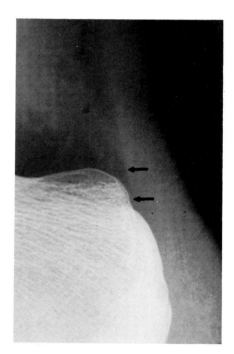

FIGURE 22–74. Retrocalcaneal recess: Normal appearance. This recess appears as a triangular radiolucent area between the Achilles tendon and calcaneus. It normally is 2 mm or more long (between arrows). (From Resnick D, et al: Radiology *125*:355, 1977.)

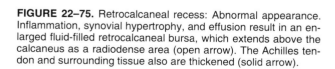

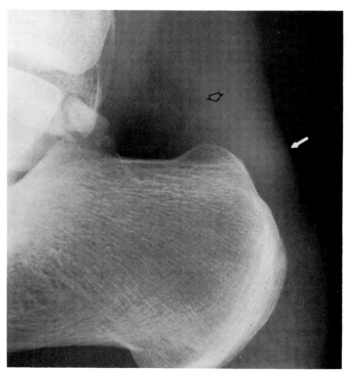

FIGURE 22–75. Retrocalcaneal recess: Abnormal appearance. Inflammation, synovial hypertrophy, and effusion result in an enlarged fluid-filled retrocalcaneal bursa, which extends above the calcaneus as a radiodense area (open arrow). The Achilles tendon and surrounding tissue also are thickened (solid arrow).

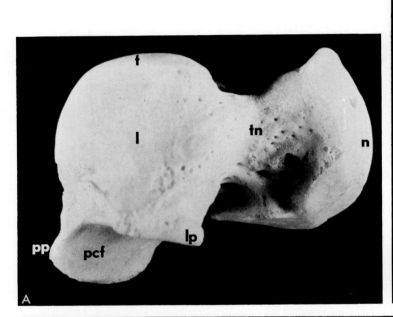

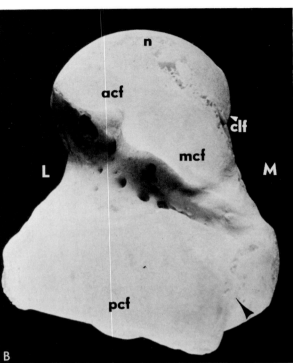

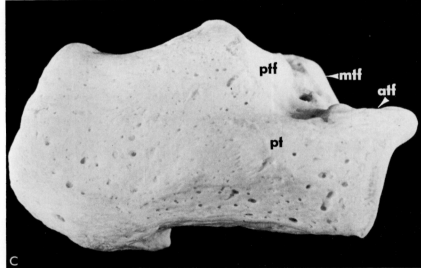

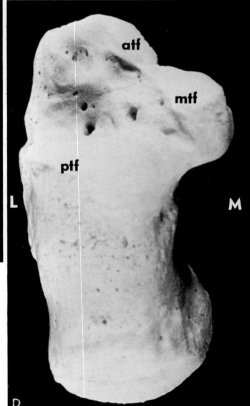

FIGURE 22–76. Talus and calcaneus: Osseous anatomy.

    A Talus: Lateral aspect. Structures include trochlear surface for tibia *(t)*, articular surface for lateral malleolus *(l)*, posterior process *(pp)*, lateral process *(lp)*, talar neck *(tn)*, articular surface for navicular bone *(n)*, and posterior calcaneal facet *(pcf)*.

    B Talus: Plantar aspect. *M,* Medial; *L,* lateral. Observe the posterior calcaneal facet *(pcf)*, middle calcaneal facet *(mcf)*, facet for the plantar calcaneonavicular ligament *(clf)*, anterior calcaneal facet *(acf)*, and facet for the navicular bone *(n)*. Note the groove (arrowhead) for the flexor hallucis longus muscle.

    C Calcaneus: Lateral aspect. Structures are the posterior talar facet *(ptf)*, peroneal trochlea *(pt)*, middle talar facet *(mtf)*, and anterior talar facet *(atf)*.

    D Calcaneus: Superior aspect. *M,* Medial; *L,* lateral. The same structures as in **C** are identified.

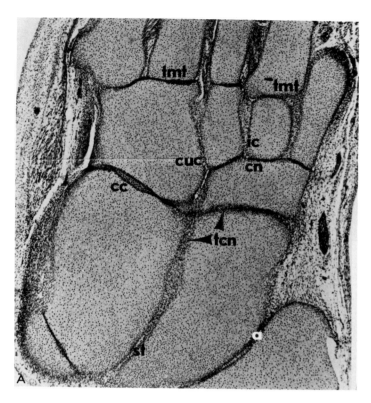

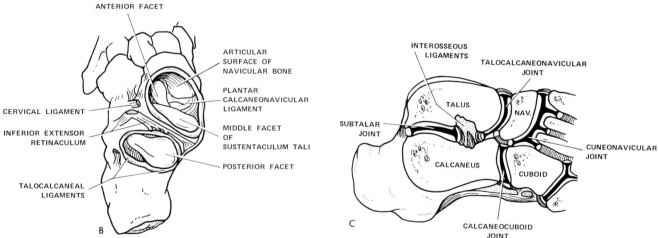

FIGURE 22–77. Talocalcaneal joints: Normal development and anatomy.

A On this photomicrograph (20×) of an oblique section through the hindfoot and midfoot, developing articulations include the ankle *(a),* subtalar *(st),* talocalcaneonavicular *(tcn),* calcaneocuboid *(cc),* cuneonavicular *(cn),* cuneocuboid *(cuc),* intercuneiform *(ic),* and tarsometatarsal *(tmt)* joints.

B Superior surface of calcaneus. Note the broad convex posterior talar facet separated from the anterior and middle talar facets by the tarsal canal and its ligamentous structures. Two completely independent synovium-lined articulations are formed.

C Oblique section of the foot. The interosseous ligaments between the talus and calcaneus are well shown, and the two separate talocalcaneal articulations are indicated. Note the independent calcaneocuboid and cuneonavicular joint cavities.

(B, C, From Resnick D: Radiology *111*:581, 1974.)

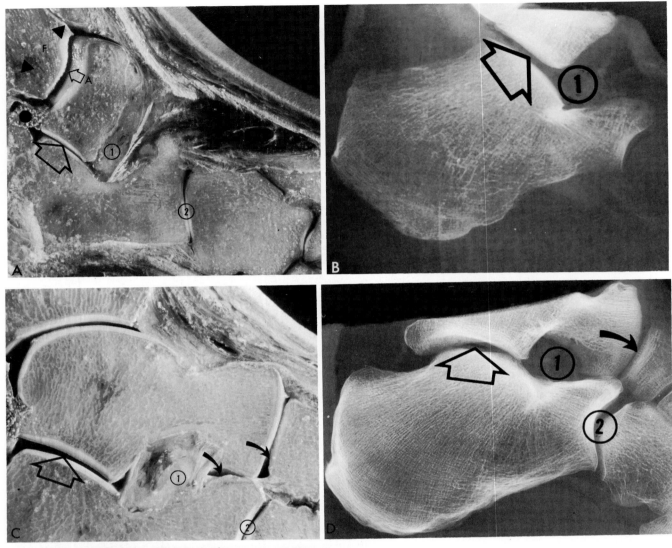

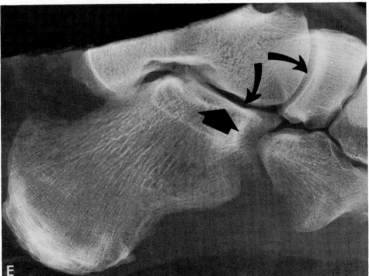

FIGURE 22–78. Talocalcaneal joints: Sagittal cross-sectional anatomy and radiography.

A A lateral sagittal section through the fibula *(F)* and ankle *(A)* demonstrates the subtalar articulation (open arrow) between the posterior facets of the talus and calcaneus. The tarsal sinus *(1)* and posterior talofibular ligament (black dot) are indicated. A separate calcaneocuboid joint *(2)* is evident.

B A radiograph of the section in **A** better reveals the posterior facets, subtalar joint (open arrow), and tarsal sinus *(1)*.

C, D A more medial sagittal section and radiograph outline the talocalcaneonavicular (curved arrows) and subtalar (open arrows) joint cavities completely separated by the contents of the tarsal sinus *(1)*. The calcaneocuboid articulation *(2)* again is indicated.

E A radiograph through a more medial section delineates the sustentaculum tali (heavy arrow) and anterior subtalar joint (curved arrows).

(From Resnick D: Radiology *111*:581, 1974.)

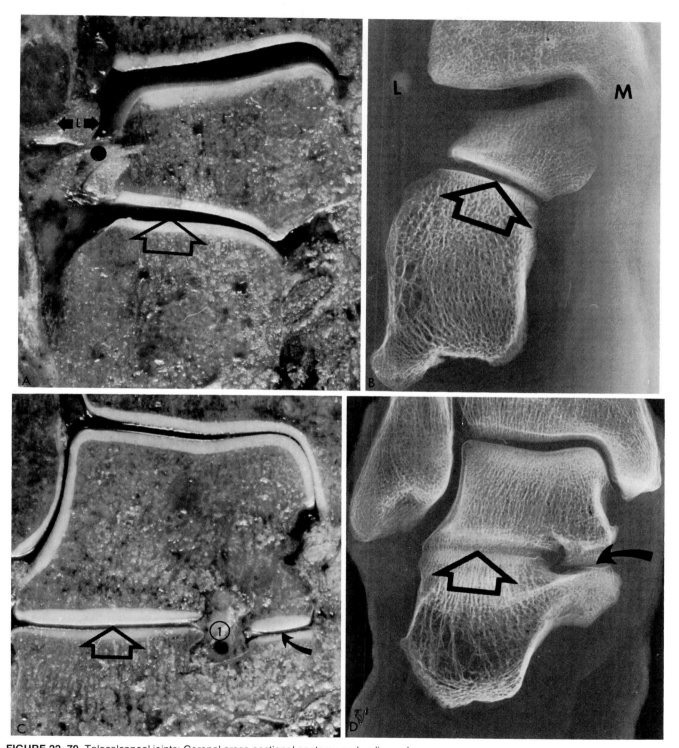

FIGURE 22–79. Talocalcaneal joints: Coronal cross-sectional anatomy and radiography.

A, B A section and radiograph through the subtalar articulation (open arrows) are shown. The lateral *(L)* and medial *(M)* malleoli and posterior talofibular ligament (black dot) are indicated.

C, D A more anterior section and radiograph outline separate subtalar (open arrows) and talocalcaneonavicular (curved arrows) joints. The interosseous ligaments *(1)* are labeled.

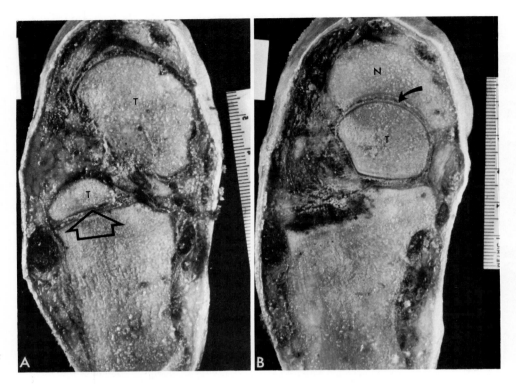

FIGURE 22–80. Talocalcaneal joints: Transverse cross-sectional anatomy.

A A dorsal section taken through the tarsal canal and sinus. Note how the latter is the expanded anterolateral section of the canal. The talus *(T)* has been cut twice, and its posterior aspect is separated from the calcaneus by the subtalar articulation (open arrow).

B A more plantar section outlines the anterior aspect of the talus *(T)* and navicular bone *(N)*, with the intervening talonavicular portion of the talocalcaneonavicular joint (curved arrow).

(From Resnick D: Radiology *111*:581, 1974.)

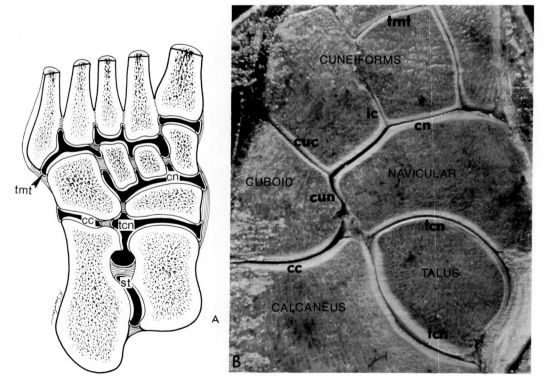

FIGURE 22–81. Joints of the midfoot: Anatomy.

A, B Drawing and photograph of an oblique transverse section through the midfoot, outlining the following joints: subtalar *(st)*, talocalcaneonavicular *(tcn)*, cuneonavicular *(cn)*, calcaneocuboid *(cc)*, cuboideonavicular *(cun)*, cuneocuboid *(cuc)*, intercuneiform *(ic)*, and tarsometatarsal *(tmt)* joints.

by surrounding ligaments, including the long plantar ligament (extending from the plantar surface of the calcaneus to the cuboid and third through fifth metatarsals) and the plantar calcaneocuboid ligament (extending from calcaneus to cuboid). The calcaneocuboid and talocalcaneonavicular joints often are referred to collectively as the transverse tarsal joint. Movements at the calcaneocuboid articulation are limited to gliding and rotation.

Cuneonavicular, Intercuneiform, Cuneocuboid, and Cuboideonavicular Joints (Fig. 22–81). The cuneonavicular joint is formed between the concave articular surfaces of the posterior portion of the three cuneiforms and the convex distal surface of the navicular. The articular capsule of this joint is continuous with two intercuneiform joints (small joint cavities between the proximal portions of the cuneiform bones), cuneocuboid joint (articulation between apposing facets on the cuboid bone and lateral cuneiform), and cuboideonavicular joint (inconstant cavity between cuboid and navicular bones). Movements at all of these joints occur simultaneously and include slight amounts of gliding and rotation of one bone on another.

TARSOMETATARSAL AND INTERMETATARSAL JOINTS

Osseous and Soft Tissue Anatomy

The medial cuneiform and first metatarsal bones possess an independent medial tarsometatarsal joint (Fig. 22–81). The intermediate tarsometatarsal joint is located between

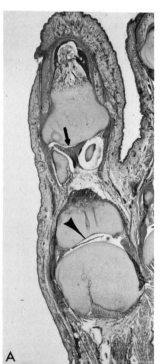
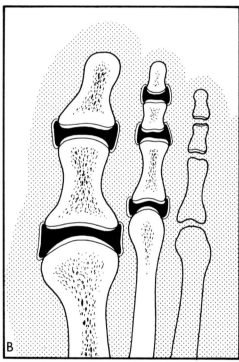
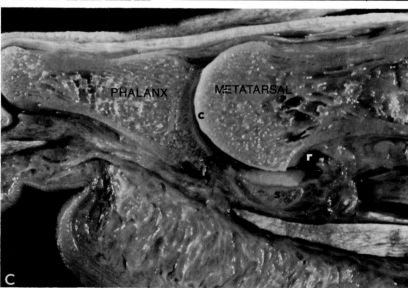

FIGURE 22–82. Metatarsophalangeal and interphalangeal joints: Normal development and anatomy.

A A photomicrograph (20×) of the first digit reveals the first metatarsophalangeal joint (arrowhead) developing between the metatarsal head and proximal phalanx. Portions of the interphalangeal joint of the great toe (arrow) also are observed.

B A drawing of a transverse section of the foot outlining the capsular attachments of the metatarsophalangeal and interphalangeal articulations.

C A sagittal section through the first metatarsophalangeal joint revealing articular cartilage (c), proximal recesses (r), and a plantar sesamoid (s) bone.

the second and third metatarsal bones and the intermediate and lateral cuneiforms. This joint may communicate with the intercuneiform and cuneonavicular joints. The lateral tarsometatarsal joint exists between the distal aspect of the cuboid and the base of the fourth and fifth metatarsal bones. A limited amount of gliding motion may occur between tarsals and metatarsal bones, the motion being accentuated at the medial tarsometatarsal joint. The tarsometatarsal joints extend distally between the metatarsal bases as intermetatarsal joints. Slight gliding motion can occur at these latter articulations.[286]

Osseous landmarks about the tarsometatarsal joints have been established, allowing accurate identification of subluxations and dislocations in this region (see Chapter 68).

METATARSOPHALANGEAL JOINTS

Osseous and Soft Tissue Anatomy

The metatarsophalangeal joints, which are synovial articulations, exist where the rounded heads of the metatarsal bones approximate the cupped surfaces of the proximal phalanges (Fig. 22–82). The articular portions of the metatarsal heads include the distal and plantar aspects of the bone but do not include the dorsal surface. The plantar aspect of the first metatarsal bone is unique, containing two longitudinal grooves separated by a ridge. Each groove may articulate with a sesamoid bone.[287–289] Fibrous capsules surround these articulations. The thin dorsal portion of these capsules frequently is intimate with small bursae that separate the capsule from the extensor tendons. Ligaments about these joints include the plantar ligaments, the deep transverse metatarsal ligaments (which connect the plantar ligaments of adjacent metatarsophalangeal joints), and the collateral ligaments (which are located at each side of the joint and extend from the dorsal tubercle of the metatarsal head to the phalangeal base). Active movements at the metatarsophalangeal joints include extension, flexion, abduction, and adduction. Accessory movements are gliding and rotation of the phalanges.

INTERPHALANGEAL JOINTS OF THE FOOT

Osseous and Soft Tissue Anatomy

In each foot, the nine interphalangeal joints (two in each of the four lateral digits and one interphalangeal joint of the great toe) separate phalanges and are surrounded by a capsule and two collateral ligaments (Fig. 22–82). The plantar ligament represents a fibrous plate on the plantar surface of the capsule. Active movements at the interphalangeal joints are flexion and extension. Accessory movements are rotation, abduction, and adduction.

References

1. Warwick R, Williams PL: Gray's Anatomy. 35th British Ed. Philadelphia, WB Saunders Co, 1973, p 407.
2. Walmsley R: Joints. *In* GJ Romanes (Ed): Cunningham's Textbook of Anatomy. 11th Ed. London, Oxford University Press, 1972, p 214.
3. Shapiro JS: A new factor in the etiology of ulnar drift. Clin Orthop 68:32, 1970.
4. Resnick D: Inter-relationship between radiocarpal and metacarpophalangeal joint deformities in rheumatoid arthritis. J Can Assoc Radiol 27:29, 1976.
5. Lusted LB, Keats TE: Atlas of Roentgenographic Measurement. 2nd Ed. Chicago, Year Book Medical Publishers, 1967, p 122.
6. Linscheid RL, Dobyns JH, Beabout JW, et al: Traumatic instability of the wrist. Diagnosis, classification and pathomechanics. J Bone Joint Surg [Am] 54:1612, 1972.
7. Arkless R: Cineradiography in normal and abnormal wrists. AJR 96:837, 1966.
8. Weston WJ, Kelsey CK: Functional anatomy of the pisi-cuneiform joint. Br J Radiol 46:692, 1973.
9. Lewis OJ: The development of the human wrist joint during the fetal period. Anat Rec 166:499, 1970.
10. Lewis OJ, Hamshere RJ, Bucknill TM: The anatomy of the wrist joint. J Anat 106:539, 1970.
11. Vesely DG: The distal radio-ulnar joint. Clin Orthop 51:75, 1967.
12. Kaplan EB: Functional and Surgical Anatomy of the Hand. 2nd Ed. Philadelphia, JB Lippincott Co, 1965, p 114.
13. Resnick D: Arthrography in the evaluation of arthritic disorders of the wrist. Radiology 113:331, 1974.
14. Kuczynski K: Carpometacarpal joint of the human thumb. J Anat 118:119, 1974.
15. Liebolt FL: Surgical fusion of the wrist joint. Surg Gynecol Obstet 66:1008, 1938.
16. Kessler I, Silberman Z: An experimental study of the radiocarpal joint by arthrography. Surg Gynecol Obstet 112:33, 1961.
17. Harrison MO, Freiberger RH, Ranawat CS: Arthrography of the rheumatoid wrist joint. AJR 112:480, 1971.
18. Resnick D: Rheumatoid arthritis of the wrist. The compartmental approach. Med Radiogr Photogr 52:50, 1976.
19. Resnick D: Early abnormalities of the pisiform and triquetrum in rheumatoid arthritis. Ann Rheum Dis 35:46, 1976.
20. Backdahl M: The caput ulnae syndrome in rheumatoid arthritis. A study of morphology, abnormal anatomy, and clinical picture. Acta Rheumatol Scand (Suppl) 5:1, 1963.
21. MacConaill MA: The mechanical anatomy of the carpus and its bearings on some surgical problems. J Anat 75:166, 1941.
22. Duparc J, De la Caffinière JY: A propos des mouvements du premier métacarpien. Presse Med 78:833, 1970.
23. Harris H, Joseph J: Variation in extension of the metacarpophalangeal and interphalangeal joints of the thumb. J Bone Joint Surg [Br] 31:547, 1949.
24. Johnston HM: Varying positions of the carpal bones in the different movements of the wrist. Part I. J Anat Physiol 41:109, 1907.
25. Johnston HM: Varying positions of the carpal bones in the different movements of the wrist. Part II. J Anat Physiol 41:280, 1907.
26. Arkless R: Rheumatoid wrists. Cineradiography. Radiology 88:543, 1967.
27. Terry DW Jr, Ramin JE: The navicular fat stripe. A useful roentgen feature for evaluating wrist trauma. AJR 124:25, 1975.
28. MacEwan DW: Changes due to trauma in fat plane overlying pronator quadratus muscle: Radiologic sign. Radiology 82:879, 1964.
29. MacEwan DW, Dunbar JS: Early radiologic recognition of pus in joints of children. J Can Assoc Radiol 12:72, 1961.
30. Yeh HC, Wolf BS: Radiographic anatomical landmarks of the metacarpophalangeal joint. Radiology 122:353, 1977.
31. Gad P: The anatomy of the volar part of the capsules of the finger joints. J Bone Joint Surg [Br] 49:362, 1967.
32. Kuczynski K: The proximal interphalangeal joint. Anatomy and causes of stiffness in the fingers. J Bone Joint Surg [Br] 50:656, 1968.
33. Weston WJ, Palmer DG: Soft Tissues of the Extremities. New York, Springer-Verlag, 1978, p 61.
34. Smith RJ: Balance and kinetics of the fingers under normal and pathological conditions. Clin Orthop 104:92, 1974.
35. Bledsoe RC, Izenstark JL: Displacement of fat pads in diseases and injury of the elbow. Radiology 73:717, 1959.
36. Bohrer SP: The fat pad sign following elbow trauma. Its usefulness and reliability in suspecting ''invisible'' fractures. Clin Radiol 21:90, 1970.
37. Kohn AM: Soft tissue alterations in elbow trauma. AJR 82:867, 1959.
38. Jackman RJ, Pugh DG: The positive elbow fat pad sign in rheumatoid arthritis. AJR 108:812, 1970.
39. Norell HG: Roentgenologic visualization of the extracapsular fat: Its importance in the diagnosis of traumatic injuries to the elbow. Acta Radiol 42:205, 1954.
40. Murphy WA, Siegel MJ: Elbow fat pads with new signs and extended differential diagnosis. Radiology 124:659, 1977.
41. Martin BF: The annular ligament of the superior radio-ulnar joint. J Anat 92:473, 1958.
42. Weston WJ: The synovial changes at the elbow in rheumatoid arthritis. Australas Radiol 15:170, 1971.
43. Rogers SL, MacEwan DW: Changes due to trauma in the fat plane overlying the supinator muscle. A radiologic sign. Radiology 92:954, 1969.
44. Weston WJ: The olecranon bursa. Australas Radiol 14:323, 1970.
45. Saha AK: Dynamic stability of the glenohumeral joint. Acta Orthop Scand 42:491, 1971.
46. Rothman RH, Marvel JP Jr, Heppenstall RB: Anatomic considerations in the glenohumeral joint. Orthop Clin North Am 6:341, 1975.
47. Keats TE, Teeslink R, Diamond AE, et al: Normal axial relationships of the major joints. Radiology 87:904, 1966.
48. Arndt JH, Sears AD: Posterior dislocation of the shoulder. AJR 94:639, 1965.
49. Moseley HF, Overgaard B: The anterior capsular mechanisms in recurrent anterior dislocation of the shoulder. J Bone Joint Surg [Br] 44:913, 1962.
50. Killoran PJ, Marcove RC, Freiberger RH: Shoulder arthrography. AJR 103:658, 1968.

51. Weston WJ: Subdeltoid bursa. Australas Radiol *17*:214, 1973.
52. Weston WJ: The enlarged subdeltoid bursa in rheumatoid arthritis. Br J Radiol *42*:481, 1969.
53. Freedman L, Munro R: Abduction of the arm in the scapula plane: Scapular and glenohumeral movements. J Bone Joint Surg [Am] *48*:1503, 1966.
54. Inman VT, Saunders JB, Abbott LC: Observations on function of the shoulder joint. J Bone Joint Surg *26*:1, 1944.
55. Lucas DB: Biomechanics of the shoulder joint. Arch Surg *107*:425, 1973.
56. DePalma AF: Surgical anatomy of acromioclavicular and sternoclavicular joints. Surg Clin North Am *43*:1541, 1963.
57. DePalma AF: Degenerative Changes in the Sternoclavicular and Acromioclavicular Joints in Various Decades. Springfield, Ill, Charles C Thomas, 1957.
58. Weston WJ: Soft tissue signs in recent subluxation and dislocation of the acromioclavicular joint. Br J Radiol *45*:832, 1972.
59. Weston WJ: Arthrography of the acromioclavicular joint. Australas Radiol *18*:213, 1974.
60. Bearn JG: Direct observations on the function of the capsule of the sternoclavicular joint in clavicular support. J Anat *101*:159, 1967.
61. Cave AJE: The nature and morphology of the costoclavicular ligament. J Anat *95*:170, 1961.
62. Moseley HF: Shoulder Lesions. 3rd Ed. Edinburgh, E & S Livingstone Ltd, 1969, p 207.
63. Klima M: Early development of the human sternum and the problem of homologization of the so-called suprasternal structures. Acta Anat *69*:473, 1968.
64. Kozielec T: A roentgenometric study of the process of ossification of the human sternum. Folia Morphol *32*:125, 1973.
65. Spencer RP: Radiographically determined sternal ossification. An approach to skeletal maturity. Biol Neonat *14*:341, 1969.
66. Cameron HU, Fornasier VL: The manubriosternal joint—an anatomicoradiological survey. Thorax *29*:472, 1974.
67. Trotter M: Synostosis between manubrium and body of the sternum in whites and negroes. Am J Phys Anthropol *18*:439, 1934.
68. Ashley GT: The morphological and pathological significance of synostosis at the manubrio-sternal joint. Thorax *9*:159, 1954.
69. Jones DR, Bahn RC, Randall RV, et al: The human costochondral junction. I. Patients without primary growth disturbances. Mayo Clin Proc *44*:324, 1969.
70. Semine AA, Damon A: Costochondral ossification and aging in five populations. Hum Biol *47*:101, 1975.
71. Sanders CF: Sexing by costal cartilage calcification. Letter to the editor. Br J Radiol *39*:233, 1966.
72. King JB: Calcification of costal cartilages. Br J Radiol *12*:2, 1939.
73. Elkeles A: Sex differences in calcification of costal cartilages. J Am Geriatr Soc *14*:456, 1966.
74. Navani S, Shah JR, Levy PS: Determination of sex by costal cartilage calcification. AJR *108*:771, 1970.
75. Gray DJ, Gardner ED: The human sternochondral joints. Anat Rec *87*:235, 1943.
76. Haines RW: Movements of the first rib. J Anat *80*:94, 1946.
77. Meyer PR: Contribution à l'étude des cavités articulaires costo-vertebrales. Arch Anat Histol Embryol Norm Exp *55*:283, 1972.
78. Gloobe H, Nathan H: The costovertebral joint. Anatomical observation in various mammals. Anat Anz *127*:22, 1970.
79. Nathan H, Weinberg H, Robin GC, et al: The costovertebral joints. Anatomical-clinical observations in arthritis. Arthritis Rheum *7*:228, 1964.
80. Goldthwait JE: The rib joints. N Engl J Med *223*:568, 1940.
81. Jones MD: Limitation of hypertrophic spur formation by the costovertebral articulations. Radiology *75*:584, 1960.
82. Hohmann D, Gasteiger W: Zur röntgendiagnostik der Costotransversalgelenke. ROFO *112*:783, 1970.
83. Rothman RH, Simeone FA: The Spine. Philadelphia, WB Saunders Co, 1975, p 19.
84. Schmorl G, Junghanns H: *In* EF Besemann (Ed): The Human Spine in Health and Disease. 2nd Ed. New York, Grune & Stratton, 1971.
85. Hall MC: Luschka's Joint. Springfield, Ill, Charles C Thomas, 1965.
86. Compere EL, Tachdjian MO, Kernahan WT: The Luschka joints. Their anatomy, physiology and pathology. Orthopedics *1*:159, 1959.
87. François RJ, Dhem A: Microradiographic study of the normal human vertebral body. Acta Anat *89*:251, 1974.
88. Nachemson A, Lewin T, Maroudas A, et al: In vitro diffusion of dye through the end-plates and the annulus fibrosus of human lumbar inter-vertebral discs. Acta Orthop Scand *41*:589, 1970.
89. Peacock A: Observations on the postnatal structure of the intervertebral disc in man. J Anat *86*:162, 1952.
90. Walmsley R: The development and growth of the intervertebral disc. Edinburgh Med J *60*:341, 1953.
91. Inman VT, Saunders JB de CM: Anatomicophysiological aspects of injuries to the intervertebral disc. J Bone Joint Surg [Am] *29*:461, 1947.
92. Hendry NGC: Hydration of nucleus pulposus and its relation to intervertebral disc derangement. J Bone Joint Surg [Br] *40*:132, 1958.
93. Walmsley R: The development and growth of the intervertebral disc. Edinburgh Med J *60*:341, 1953.
94. Coventry MB: Anatomy of the intervertebral disc. Clin Orthop *67*:9, 1969.
95. Crock HV, Yoshizawa H, Kame SK: Observations on the venous drainage of the human vertebral body. J Bone Joint Surg [Br] *55*:528, 1973.
96. Batson OV: The function of the vertebral veins and their role in the spread of metastases. Ann Surg *112*:138, 1940.
97. Brandner ME: Normal values of the vertebral body and intervertebral disk index in adults. AJR *114*:411, 1972.
98. Brandner ME: Normal values of the vertebral body and intervertebral disk index during growth. AJR *110*:618, 1970.
99. Whalen JP, Woodruff CL: The cervical prevertebral fat stripe. A new aid in evaluating the cervical prevertebral soft tissue space. AJR *109*:445, 1970.
100. Wholey MH, Bruwer AT, Baker HL Jr: Lateral roentgenogram of the neck. Radiology *78*:350, 1958.
101. Reichmann S: Tomography of the lumbar intervertebral joints. Acta Radiol *12*:641, 1972.
102. Hadley LA: Anatomico-roentgenographic studies of the posterior spinal articulations. AJR *86*:270, 1961.
103. Morton SA: Value of the oblique view in the radiographic examination of the lumbar spine. Radiology *29*:568, 1937.
104. Reichmann S: The postnatal development of form and orientation of the lumbar intervertebral joint surfaces. Z Anat Entwicklungsgesch *133*:102, 1971.
105. Kohler R: Contrast examination of the lumbar interspinous ligaments. Preliminary report. Acta Radiol *52*:21, 1959.
106. Fielding JW, Burstein AH, Frankel VH: The nuchal ligament. Spine *1*:3, 1976.
107. Davis PR: The medial inclination of the human thoracic intervertebral articular facets. J Anat *93*:68, 1959.
108. Hinck VC, Hopkins CE: Measurement of the atlanto-dental interval in the adult. AJR *84*:945, 1960.
109. Jackson H: The diagnosis of minimal atlanto-axial subluxation. Br J Radiol *23*:672, 1950.
110. Cave AJE: Anatomical Notes: On the occipito-atlanto-axial articulations. J Anat *68*:416, 1934.
111. Singh S: Variations of the superior articular facets of atlas vertebrae. J Anat *99*:565, 1965.
112. Dirheimer V, Ramsheyi A, Reolon M: Positive arthrography of the craniocervical joints. Neuroradiology *12*:257, 1977.
113. Jirout J: The dynamic dependence of the lower cervical vertebrae on the atlanto-occipital joints. Neuroradiology *7*:249, 1974.
114. Jirout J: Patterns of changes in the cervical spine on lateroflexion. Neuroradiology *2*:164, 1971.
115. Jirout J: The motility of the cervical vertebrae in lateral flexion of the head and neck. Acta Radiol *13*:919, 1972.
116. Ferguson AB: Roentgen Diagnosis of Extremities and Spine. New York, Paul B Hoeber Inc, 1939.
117. Resnick D, Niwayama G, Goergen TG: Degenerative disease of the sacro-iliac joint. Invest Radiol *10*:608, 1975.
118. Schunke GB: Anatomy and development of sacro-iliac joint in man. Anat Rec *72*:313, 1938.
119. Brooke R: The sacro-iliac joint. J Anat *58*:299, 1924.
120. Sashin D: A critical analysis of the anatomy and the pathologic changes in the sacro-iliac joints. J Bone Joint Surg *12*:891, 1930.
121. Carter ME, Loewi G: Anatomical changes in normal sacro-iliac joints during childhood and comparison with the changes in Still's disease. Ann Rheum Dis *21*:121, 1962.
122. Macdonald GR, Hunt TE: Sacro-iliac joints. Observations on the gross and histological changes in the various age groups. Can Med Assoc J *66*:157, 1952.
123. Weisl H: The articular surfaces of the sacro-iliac joint and their relation to the movements of the sacrum. Acta Anat *22*:1, 1954.
124. Trotter M: Accessory sacro-iliac articulations. Am J Phys Anthropol *22*:247, 1937.
125. Colachis SC Jr, Worden RE, Bechtol CO, et al: Movement of the sacro-iliac joint in the adult male: A preliminary report. Arch Phys Med *44*:490, 1963.
126. Frigerio NA, Stowe RR, Howe JW: Movement of the sacro-iliac joint. Clin Orthop *100*:370, 1974.
127. Abramson D, Roberts SM, Wilson PD: Relaxation of the pelvic joints in pregnancy. Surg Gynecol Obstet *58*:595, 1934.
128. Thorp DJ, Fray WE: The pelvic joints during pregnancy and labor. JAMA *111*:1162, 1938.
129. Cohen AS, McNeill JM, Calkins E, et al: The "normal" sacro-iliac joint. Analysis of 88 sacro-iliac roentgenograms. AJR *100*:559, 1967.
130. Wilkinson M, Meikle JAK: Tomography of the sacro-iliac joints. Ann Rheum Dis *25*:433, 1966.
131. Casuccio C: Studio anatomico e radiografico sull'articolazione sacroiliaco normale nell'adulto. Chir Organi Mov *20*:353, 1934.
132. Todd TW: Age changes in the pubic bone. Am J Phys Anthropol *4*:1, 333, 1921.
133. Brooks ST: Skeletal age at death: The reliability of cranial and pubic age indicators. Am J Phys Anthropol *13*:567, 1955.
134. Camiel MR, Aaron JB: Gas or vacuum phenomenon in pubic symphysis during pregnancy. Radiology *66*:548, 1956.
135. Williams JL: Gas in symphysis pubis during and following pregnancy. AJR *73*:403, 1955.
136. Vix VA, Ryu CY: The adult symphysis pubis: Normal and abnormal. AJR *112*:517, 1971.
137. Young J: Relaxation of the pelvic joints in pregnancy: Pelvic arthropathy of pregnancy. J Obstet Gynaecol Br Emp *47*:493, 1940.
138. Caffey J, Ames R, Silverman WA, et al: Contradiction of the congenital dysplasia-predislocation hypothesis of congenital dislocation of the hip through a study of the normal variation in acetabular angles at successive periods in infancy. Pediatrics *17*:632, 1956.
139. Caffey J, Ross S: Pelvic bones in infantile mongoloidism. AJR *80*:458, 1958.

140. Astley R: Chromosomal abnormalities in childhood, with particular reference to Turner's syndrome and mongolism. Br J Radiol 36:2, 1963.

141. Budin E, Chandler E: Measurement of femoral neck anteversion by a direct method. Radiology 69:209, 1957.

142. Billing L: Roentgen examination of the proximal femur end in children and adolescents. Acta Radiol Suppl 110:5, 1954.

143. Wiberg G: Studies on dysplastic acetabula and congenital subluxation of the hip joint—with special reference to the complication of osteoarthritis. Acta Chir Scand Suppl 58:1, 1939.

144. Hooper JC, Jones EW: Primary protrusion of the acetabulum. J Bone Joint Surg [Br] 53:23, 1971.

145. Armbuster TG, Guerra J Jr, Resnick D, et al: The adult hip: An anatomic study. Part I. The bony landmarks. Radiology 128:1, 1978.

146. Judet R, Judet J, Letournal E: Fractures of the acetabulum: Classification and surgical approaches for open reduction—preliminary report. J Bone Joint Surg [Am] 46:1615, 1964.

147. Pomeranz MM: Intrapelvic protrusion of the acetabulum (Otto pelvis). J Bone Joint Surg 14:663, 1932.

148. Overgaard K: Otto's disease and other forms of protrusio acetabuli. Acta Radiol 16:390, 1935.

149. Friedenberg ZB: Protrusio acetabuli. Am J Surg 85:764, 1953.

150. Alexander C: The aetiology of primary protrusio acetabuli. Br J Radiol 38:567, 1965.

151. Hubbard MJS: The measurement of progression in protrusio acetabuli. AJR 106:506, 1969.

152. MacDonald D: Primary protrusio acetabuli: Report of an affected family. J Bone Joint Surg [Br] 53:30, 1971.

153. Hefke HW, Turner VC: The obturator sign as the earliest roentgenographic sign in the diagnosis of septic arthritis and tuberculosis of the hip. J Bone Joint Surg 24:857, 1942.

154. Jorup S, Kjellberg SR: The early diagnosis of acute septic osteomyelitis, periostitis and arthritis and its importance in the treatment. Acta Radiol (Diagn) 30:316, 1948.

155. Drey L: A roentgenographic study of transitory synovitis of the hip joint. Radiology 60:588, 1953.

156. Bartley O, Chidekel N: Roentgenologic changes in postoperative septic osteoarthritis of the hip joint. Acta Radiol (Diagn) 4:113, 1966.

157. Lewis MS, Norman A: The earliest signs of postoperative hip infection. Radiology 104:309, 1972.

158. Brown I: A study of the "capsular" shadow in disorders of the hip in children. J Bone Joint Surg [Br] 57:175, 1975.

159. Reichmann S: Roentgenologic soft tissue appearances in hip disease. Acta Radiol (Diagn) 6:167, 1967.

160. Guerra J Jr, Armbuster TG, Resnick D, et al: The adult hip: An anatomic study. Part II. The soft-tissue landmarks. Radiology 128:11, 1978.

161. Lange M: Die Erleichterung der Frühdiagnose der Koxitis durch bisher wenig beachtete Veränderungen im Röntgenbild. Z Orthop Chir 48:90, 1927.

162. Armstrong P, Saxton H: Iliopsoas bursa. Br J Radiol 45:493, 1972.

163. Chandler SB: The iliopsoas bursa in man. Anat Rec 58:235, 1934.

164. Staple TW: Arthrographic demonstration of the iliopsoas bursa extension of the hip joint. Radiology 102:515, 1972.

165. Last RJ: Anatomy. Regional and Applied. 5th Ed. London, Churchill Livingstone, 1972, p 211.

166. Warren R, Kaye JJ, Salvati EA: Arthrographic demonstration of an enlarged iliopsoas bursa complicating osteoarthritis of the hip—a case report. J Bone Joint Surg [Am] 57:413, 1975.

167. Weston WJ: The bursae deep to gluteus medius and minimus. Australas Radiol 14:325, 1970.

168. Smillie IS: Injuries of the Knee Joint. 4th Ed. Baltimore, Williams & Wilkins, 1970, p 23.

169. Ficat RP, Hungerford D: Disorders of the Patello-Femoral Joint. Baltimore, Williams & Wilkins, 1977, p 3.

170. Brantigan OC, Voshell AF: The tibial collateral ligament: Its function, its bursae, and its relation to the medial meniscus. J Bone Joint Surg 25:121, 1943.

171. Doppman JL: Baker's cyst and the normal gastrocnemiosemimembranosus bursa. AJR 94:646, 1965.

172. Wilson PD, Eyre-Brook AL, Francis JD: A clinical and anatomical study of the semimembranosus bursa in relation to popliteal cyst. J Bone Joint Surg 20:963, 1938.

173. Wolfe RD, Colloff B: Popliteal cysts. An arthrographic study and review of the literature. J Bone Joint Surg [Am] 54:1057, 1972.

174. Dalinka MK, Garofola J: The infrapatellar synovial fold: A cause for confusion in the evaluation of the anterior cruciate ligament. AJR 127:589, 1976.

175. Resnick D, Newell JD, Guerra J Jr, et al: Proximal tibiofibular joint: Anatomic-pathologic-radiographic correlation. AJR 131:133, 1978.

176. Weston WJ: The deep infrapatellar bursa. Australas Rad 17:212, 1973.

177. Weston WJ: The extrasynovial and capsular fat pads on the posterior aspect of the knee joint. Skel Radiol 2:87, 1977.

178. Lindgren PG, Willén R: Gastrocnemio-semimembranosus bursa and its relation to the knee joint. Acta Radiol 18:497, 1977.

179. Kennedy JC, Weinberg HW, Wilson AS: The anatomy and function of the anterior cruciate ligament. J Bone Joint Surg [Am] 56:223, 1974.

180. Brantigan OC, Voshell AF: The mechanics of the ligaments and menisci of the knee joint. J Bone Joint Surg 23:44, 1941.

181. Robichon J, Romero C: The functional anatomy of the knee joint with special reference to the medial collateral and anterior cruciate ligaments. Can J Surg 11:36, 1968.

182. Harrison RB, Wood MB, Keats TE: The grooves of the distal articular surface of the femur—a normal variant. AJR 126:751, 1976.

183. Jacobsen K: Landmarks of the knee joint on the lateral radiograph during rotation. ROFO 125:399, 1976.

184. Ravelli A: Zum Roentgenbild des menschlichen Kniegelenkes. ROFO 71:614, 1949.

185. Takechi H: Trabecular architecture of the knee joint. Acta Orthop Scand 48:673, 1977.

186. Blumensaat C: Die Lageabweichungen und Verrenkungen der Kniescheibe. Ergebn Chir Orthop 31:149, 1938.

187. Jacobsen K, Bertheussen K, Gjerloff CC: Characteristics of the line of Blumensaat. Acta Orthop Scand 45:764, 1974.

188. Insall J, Salvati E: Patella position in the normal knee joint. Radiology 101:101, 1971.

189. Jacobsen K, Bertheussen K: The vertical location of the patella. Fundamental views on the concept of patella alta, using a normal sample. Acta Orthop Scand 45:436, 1974.

190. Blackburne JS, Peel TE: A new method of measuring patellar height. J Bone Joint Surg [Br] 59:241, 1977.

191. Lancourt JE, Cristini JA: Patella alta and patella infera. J Bone Joint Surg [Am] 57:1112, 1975.

192. Hall FM: Radiographic diagnosis and accuracy in knee joint effusions. Radiology 115:49, 1975.

193. Lewis RW: Roentgenographic study of soft tissue pathology in and about the knee joint. AJR 65:200, 1951.

194. Bachman AL: Roentgen diagnosis of knee-joint effusion. Radiology 46:462, 1946.

195. Harris RD, Hecht HL: Suprapatellar effusions. A new diagnostic sign. Radiology 97:1, 1970.

196. Friedman AC, Naidich TP: The fabella sign: Fabella displacement in synovial effusion and popliteal fossa masses. Radiology 127:113, 1978.

197. Ogden JA: The anatomy and function of the proximal tibiofibular joint. Clin Orthop 101:186, 1974.

198. Gray DJ, Gardner E: Prenatal development of the human knee and superior tibiofibular joints. Am J Anat 86:23, 1950.

199. Minns RJ, Hunter JAA: The mechanical and structural characteristics of the tibiofibular interosseous membrane. Acta Orthop Scand 47:236, 1976.

200. Barnett CH, Napier JR: The axis of rotation at the ankle joint in man. Its influence upon the form of the talus and the mobility of the fibula. J Anat 86:1, 1952.

201. Ramsey PL, Hamilton W: Changes in tibiotalar area of contact caused by lateral talar shift. J Bone Joint Surg [Am] 58:356, 1976.

202. Skinner EH: The mathematical calculation of progress in fractures at the ankle and wrist. Surg Gynecol Obstet 18:238, 1914.

203. Joy G, Patzakis MJ, Harvey JP Jr: Precise evaluation of the reduction of severe ankle fractures. Technique and correlation with end results. J Bone Joint Surg [Am] 56:979, 1974.

204. Hunter CG Jr, Scott W: Tibial torsion. J Bone Joint Surg [Am] 31:511, 1949.

205. Goergen TG, Danzig LA, Resnick D, et al: Roentgenographic evaluation of the tibiotalar joint. J Bone Joint Surg 59:874, 1977.

206. Kaye JJ, Bohne WHO: A radiographic study of the ligamentous anatomy of the ankle. Radiology 125:659, 1977.

207. Palmer DG: Tendon sheaths and bursae involved by rheumatoid disease at the foot and ankle. Australas Radiol 14:419, 1970.

208. Resnick D, Goergen TG: Peroneal tenography in previous calcaneal fractures. Radiology 115:211, 1975.

209. Resnick D, Feingold ML, Curd J, et al: Calcaneal abnormalities in articular disorders. Rheumatoid arthritis, ankylosing spondylitis, psoriatic arthritis and Reiter syndrome. Radiology 125:355, 1977.

210. Bywaters EG: Heel lesions of rheumatoid arthritis. Ann Rheum Dis 13:42, 1954.

211. Sutro CJ: The os calcis, the tendo-achillis and the local bursae. Bull Hosp Joint Dis 27:76, 1966.

212. Weston WJ: The bursa deep to the tendo achillis. Australas Radiol 14:327, 1970.

213. Resnick D: Radiology of the talocalcaneal articulations. Anatomic considerations and arthrography. Radiology 111:581, 1974.

214. Mehrez M, el-Geneidy S: Arthrography of the ankle. J Bone Joint Surg [Br] 52:308, 1970.

215. Olson RW: Arthrography of the ankle: Its use in the evaluation of ankle sprains. Radiology 92:1439, 1969.

216. Youm Y, McMurthy RY, Flatt AE, et al: Kinematics of the wrist. I. An experimental study of radial-ulnar deviation and flexion-extension. J Bone Joint Surg [Am] 60:423, 1978.

217. Candardjis G, DeBosset PH, Saudan Y: L'articulation manubriosternale normale. Technique d'examen et étude des variantes. J Radiol Electrol 59:89, 1978.

218. Cockshott WP: The coracoclavicular joint. Radiology 131:313, 1979.

219. Chamberlain WE: Basilar impression (platybasia). Yale J Biol Med 11:487, 1939.

220. Gradoyevitch B: Coracoclavicular joint. J Bone Joint Surg 21:918, 1939.

221. Nutter PD: Coracoclavicular articulations. J Bone Joint Surg 23:177, 1941.

222. Liberson F: The role of the coracoclavicular ligaments in affections of the shoulder girdle. Am J Surg 44:145, 1939.

223. Wertheimer LG: Coracoclavicular joint. J Bone Joint Surg [Am] *30*:570, 1948.

224. McGregor M: The significance of certain measurements of the skull in the diagnosis of basilar impression. Br J Radiol *21*:171, 1948.

225. Eischgold H, Metzger J: Etude radiotomographique de l'impression basilaire. Rev Rhum Mal Osteoartic *19*:261, 1952.

226. Ogden JA, Conlogue GJ, Bronson ML, et al: Radiology of postnatal skeletal development. II. The manubrium and sternum. Skel Radiol *4*:189, 1979.

227. Ogden JA, Conlogue GJ, Bronson ML: Radiology of postnatal skeletal development. III. The clavicle. Skel Radiol *4*:196, 1979.

228. Brower AC, Woodlief RM: Pseudarthrosis at the first sternocostal synchondrosis. AJR *135*:1276, 1980.

229. Küsswetter W: Die membrana interossea antebrachii—das gemeinsame gelenkband der radioulnargelenke. Z Orthop *117*:767, 1979.

230. Robbins H: Anatomical study of the median nerve in the carpal tunnel and etiologies of the carpal tunnel syndrome. J Bone Joint Surg [Am] *45*:953, 1963.

231. Zucker-Pinchoff B, Hermann G, Srinivasan R: Computed tomography of the carpal tunnel: A radioanatomical study. J Comput Assist Tomogr *5*:525, 1981.

232. Cone RO, Szabo R, Resnick D, et al: Computed tomography of the normal soft tissues of the wrist. Invest Radiol *18*:546, 1983.

233. Cooney WP III, Lucca MJ, Chao EYS, et al: The kinesiology of the thumb trapeziometacarpal joint. J Bone Joint Surg [Am] *63*:1371, 1981.

234. Fisk GR: The wrist. J Bone Joint Surg [Br] *66*:396, 1984.

235. Palmer AK, Werner FW, Eng MM: The triangular fibrocartilage complex of the wrist—anatomy and function. J Hand Surg *6*:153, 1981.

236. Palmer AK: The distal radioulnar joint. Orthop Clin North Am *15*:321, 1984.

237. Berger RA, Crowninshield RD, Flatt AE: The three-dimensional rotational behaviors of the carpal bones. Clin Orthop *167*:303, 1982.

238. Taliesnik J: The ligaments of the wrist. J Hand Surg *1*:110, 1976.

239. Curtis DJ, Downey EF Jr, Brower AC, et al: Importance of soft-tissue evaluation in hand and wrist trauma: statistical evaluation. AJR *142*:781, 1984.

240. Kapandji A: Anatomic funtionnelle et biomecanique de la metacarpophalangienne du pouce. Ann Chir *35*:261, 1981.

241. Uhthoff HK, Piscopo M: Anterior capsular redundancy of the shoulder: Congenital or traumatic? An embryological study. J Bone Joint Surg [Br] *67*:363, 1985.

242. Cone RO, Danzig L, Resnick D, et al: The bicipital groove; a radiographic, anatomic and pathologic study. AJR *141*:781, 1983.

243. Sarrafian SK: Gross and functional anatomy of the shoulder. Clin Orthop *173*:11, 1983.

244. Petersson CJ, Redlund-Johnell I: Joint space in normal glenohumeral radiographs. Acta Orthop Scand *54*:274, 1983.

245. Petersson CJ, Redlund-Johnell I: The subacromial space in normal shoulder radiographs. Acta Orthop Scand *55*:57, 1984.

246. Greenway GD, Danzig LA, Resnick D, et al: The painful shoulder. Med Radiogr Photogr *58*:22, 1982.

247. Sutro DJ, Sutro WH: Articulations of the ribs: A pictorial review. Bull Hosp Joint Dis *41*:1, 1981.

248. Hayashi K, Yabuki T: Origin of the uncus and of Luschka's joint in the cervical spine. J Bone Joint Surg [Am] *67*:788, 1985.

249. Bogduk N, Engel R: The menisci of the lumbar zygapophyseal joints. A review of their anatomy and clinical significance. Spine *9*:454, 1984.

250. Giles LGF, Taylor JR: Intra-articular synovial protrusions in the lower lumbar apophyseal joints. Bull Hosp Joint Dis *42*:248, 1982.

251. Jackson H, Burke JT: The sacral foramina. Skel Radiol *11*:282, 1984.

252. Postacchini F, Massobrio M: Idiopathic coccygodynia. Analysis of fifty-one operative cases and a radiographic study of the normal coccyx. J Bone Joint Surg [Am] *65*:1116, 1983.

253. Bellamy N, Park W, Rooney PJ: What do we know about the sacroiliac joint? Semin Arthritis Rheum *12*:282, 1983.

254. Paquin JD, Van der Rest M, Marie PJ, et al: Biochemical and morphologic studies of cartilage from the adult human sacroiliac joint. Arthritis Rheum *26*:887, 1983.

255. Bowen V, Cassidy JD: Macroscopic and microscopic anatomy of the sacroiliac joint from embryonic life until the eighth decade. Spine *6*:620, 1981.

256. Stewart TD: Pathologic changes in aging sacroiliac joints. A study of dissecting-room skeletons. Clin Orthop *183*:188, 1984.

257. Bakland O, Hansen JH: The "axial sacroiliac joint." Anat Clin *6*:29, 1984.

258. Wilder DG, Pope MH, Frymoyer JW: The functional topography of the sacroiliac joint. Spine *5*:575, 1980.

259. Johnstone WH, Keats TE, Lee ME: The anatomic basis for the superior acetabular roof notch. "Superior acetabular notch." Skel Radiol *8*:25, 1982.

260. Bowerman JW, Sena JM, Chang R: The teardrop shadow of the pelvis: Anatomy and clinical significance. Radiology *143*:659, 1982.

261. Pogrund H, Bloom R, Mogle P: The normal width of the adult hip joint: The relationship to age, sex, and obesity. Skel Radiol *10*:10, 1983.

262. Stein MG, Barmeir E, Levin J, et al: The medial acetabular wall. Normal measurements in different population groups. Invest Radiol *17*:476, 1982.

263. Rubenstein J, Kellam J, McGonigal D: Cross-sectional anatomy of the adult bony acetabulum. J Can Assoc Radiol *33*:137, 1982.

264. Danzig LA, Newell JD, Guerra J Jr, et al: Osseous landmarks of the normal knee. Clin Orthop *156*:201, 1981.

265. Norman O, Egund N, Ekelund L, et al: The vertical position of the patella. Acta Orthop Scand *54*:908, 1983.

266. Martinez S, Korobkin M, Fondren FB, et al: Computed tomography of the normal patellofemoral joint. Invest Radiol *18*:249, 1983.

267. Guerra J Jr, Newell JD, Resnick D, et al: Gastrocnemio-semimembranosus bursal region of the knee. AJR *136*:593, 1981.

268. Butt WP, Lederman H, Chuang S: Radiology of the suprapatellar region. Clin Radiol *34*:511, 1983.

269. Engelstad BL, Friedman EM, Murphy WA: Diagnosis of joint effusion on lateral and axial projections of the knee. Invest Radiol *3*:188, 1981.

270. Veth RPH, Kingma LM, Nielsen HKL: The abnormal proximal tibiofibular joint. Arch Orthop Trauma Surg *102*:167, 1984.

271. Lambert KL: The weight-bearing function of the fibula. A strain gauge study. J Bone Joint Surg [Am] *53*:507, 1971.

272. Takebe K, Nakagawa A, Minami H, et al: Role of fibula in weight-bearing. Clin Orthop *184*:289, 1984.

273. Sutro CJ, Sutro WH: The clinical importance of articulations of the fibula. Bull Hosp Joint Dis *42*:68, 1982.

274. Rasmussen O, Tovborg-Jensen I, Boe S: Distal tibiofibular ligaments. Analysis of function. Acta Orthop Scand *53*:681, 1982.

275. Jonsson K, Fredin HO, Cederlund CG, et al: Width of the normal ankle joint. Acta Radiol Diagn *25*:147, 1984.

276. Towbin R, Dunbar JS, Towbin J, et al: Teardrop sign: Plain film recognition of ankle effusion. AJR *134*:985, 1980.

277. Hall FM: Pitfalls in the diagnosis of ankle joint effusion. AJR *136*:637, 1981.

278. Teng MMH, Destouet JM, Gilula LA, et al: Ankle tenography: A key to unexplained symptomatology. Part I. Normal tenographic anatomy. Radiology *151*:575, 1984.

279. Gilula LA, Oloff L, Caputi R, et al: Ankle tenography: A key to unexplained symptomatology. Part II. Diagnosis of chronic tendon disabilities. Radiology *151*:581, 1984.

280. Meurman KOA: Bursa tendinis musculi flexoris hallucis longi. ROFO *136*:27, 1982.

281. Lieber GA, Lemont H: The posterior triangle of the ankle. Determination of its true anatomical boundary. J Am Podiatr Assoc *72*:363, 1982.

282. Goodman LR, Shanser JD: The pre-Achilles fat pad: An aid to early diagnosis of local systemic disease. Skel Radiol *2*:81, 1977.

283. Nidecker AC, von Hochstetter A, Fredenhagen H: Accessory muscles of the lower calf. Radiology *151*:47, 1984.

284. Percy EC, Telep GN: Anomalous muscle in the leg: Soleus accessorium. Am J Sports Med *12*:447, 1984.

285. Rhea JT, De Luca SA, Sheehan J: Radiographic anatomy of the tarsal bones. Med Radiogr Photogr *59*:2, 1983.

286. Faure C: The skeleton of the anterior foot. Anatomia Clin *3*:49, 1981.

287. de Britto SR: The first metatarso-sesamoid joint. Int Orthop (SICOT) *6*:61, 1982.

288. Scranton PE Jr, Rutkowski R: Anatomic variations in the first ray. Part II. Disorders of the sesamoids. Clin Orthop *151*:256, 1980.

289. McCarthy DJ: The surgical anatomy of the first ray. Part I. The distal segment. J Am Podiatr Assoc *73*:111, 1983.

290. Morrey BF, An K-N: Functional anatomy of the ligaments of the elbow. Clin Orthop *201*:84, 1985.

291. Luk KDK, Ho HC, Leong JCY: The iliolumbar ligament. A study of its anatomy, development and clinical significance. J Bone Joint Surg [Br] *68*:197, 1986.

292. Gamble JG, Simmons SC, Freedman M: The symphysis pubis. Anatomic and pathologic considerations. Clin Orthop *203*:261, 1986.

293. Redlund-Johnell I: The costoclavicular joint. Skel Radiol *15*:25, 1986.

294. Mann FA, Wilson AJ, Gilula LA: Radiographic evaluation of the wrist: What does the hand surgeon want to know? Radiology *184*:15, 1992.

295. Gellman H, Kauffman D, Lenihan M, et al: An in vitro analysis of wrist motion: The effect of limited intercarpal arthrodesis and the contributions of the radiocarpal and midcarpal joints. J Hand Surg [Am] *13*:378, 1988.

296. Mitchell MJ, Causey G, Berthoty DP, et al: Peribursal fat plane of the shoulder: Anatomic study and clinical experience. Radiology *168*:699, 1988.

297. Taddei A, Sick H: Contribution a l'etude des articulations antérieures de la cage thoracique. Arch Anat Hist Embr Norm Exp *66*:3, 1983.

298. Schills JP, Resnick D, Haghighi P, et al: Sternocostal joints. Anatomic, radiographic and pathologic features in adult cadavers. Invest Radiol *24*:596, 1989.

299. Burguet JL, Sick H, Wackenheim A: CT-anatomic correlations of the normal capsulo-ligamentous bands of the extrinsic joints of the thoracic spine. Surg Radiol Anat *9*:217, 1987.

300. Taylor JR, McCormick CC: Lumbar facet joint fat pads: their normal anatomy and their appearance when enlarged. Neuroradiology *33*:38, 1991.

301. Elliott S: The odontoid process in children—is it hypoplastic? Clin Radiol *39*:391, 1988.

302. Ranawat CS, O'Leary P, Pellicci P, et al: Cervical spine fusion in rheumatoid arthritis. J Bone Joint Surg [Am] *61*:1003, 1979.

303. Redlund-Johnell I, Petersson H: Radiographic measurements of the craniovertebral region, designed for evaluation of abnormalities in rheumatoid arthritis. Acta Radiol Diagn *25*:23, 1984.

304. Kawaida H, Sakou T, Morizono Y: Vertical settling in rheumatoid arthritis. Diagnostic value of the Ranawat and Redlund-Johnell methods. Clin Orthop *239*:128, 1989.

305. Vleeming A, Volkers ACW, Snijders CJ, et al: Relation between form and function in the sacroiliac joint. P II. Biomechanical aspects. Spine *15*:133, 1990.

306. Ehara S, El-Khoury GY, Bergman RA: The accessory sacroiliac joint: A common anatomic variant. AJR *150*:857, 1988.

307. Broughton NS, Brougham DI, Cole WG, et al: Reliability of radiological

measurements in the assessment of the child's hip. J Bone Joint Surg [Br] *71*:6, 1989.

308. Goodman SB, Adler SJ, Fyhrie DP, et al: The acetabular teardrop and its relevance to acetabular migration. Clin Orthop *236*:199, 1988.

309. Gusis SE, Babini JC, Garay SM, et al: Evaluation of the measurement methods for protrusio acetabuli in normal children. Skel Radiol *19*:279, 1990.

310. Gregorczyk A, Pospula W, Golda W: Radiological and computed tomographic studies of the width of the normal hip joint in men aged 30–60 years. Röntgenblatter *43*:141, 1990.

311. Moreland JR, Bassett LW, Hanker GJ: Radiographic analysis of the axial alignment of the lower extremity. J Bone Joint Surg [Am] *69*:745, 1987.

312. Grelsamer RP, Meadows S: The modified Insall-Salvati ratio for assessment of patellar height. Clin Orthop *282*:170, 1992.

313. Egund N, Lundin A, Wallengren NO: The vertical position of the patella. A new radiographic method for routine use. Acta Radiol *29*:555, 1988.

314. Kannus PA: Long patellar tendon: Radiographic sign of patellofemoral pain syndrome—a prospective study. Radiology *185*:859, 1992.

23

Articular Cartilage Physiology and Metabolism

Wayne H. Akeson, M.D., David Amiel, Ph.D., and David H. Gershuni, M.D., F.R.C.S.

The purpose of this chapter is to summarize existing knowledge of the composition, metabolism, and function of articular cartilage. When possible, the relationships among these factors in health and disease will be described.

Articular cartilage is a unique tissue in many respects, but especially with regard to its structural, metabolic, and functional interactions. Articular cartilage possesses unparalleled functional efficiency. This efficiency is derived from design features that are marveled at by physicians and engineers attempting to design substitutes for diseased joints. For example, the articular cartilage lubrication efficiency is significantly superior to the best bearing surfaces known to modern engineering. Such efficiencies are achieved in spite of stringent limitations imposed on the tissue, such as the lack of blood supply and a tissue thickness that measures only a few millimeters at the most. Couple these points with a limited repair capability and the consequent requirement that the tissue survive a lifetime of use, and the ques-

tion is "How can synovial joints survive as long as they do?" rather than "Why do these joints fail?" The first task of this chapter will be to describe the morphologic, biochemical, and physiologic interactions of the cartilage matrix to gain insight into the answer to the first question.

OVERVIEW OF CARTILAGE FUNCTION

Before considering details of morphology and biochemistry of articular cartilage matrix it will be helpful for those who are learning joint physiology for the first time, or who are coming back to it after a period of disuse, to consider a simple scheme describing the interrelationship of these elements. A useful analogy for articular cartilage is the air tent seen in parts of the country as a cover for recreational areas such as swimming pools and tennis courts or as a temporary cover for exhibitions (Fig. 23–1). The requirements for the

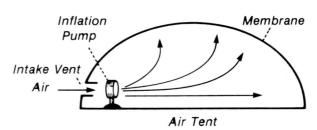

FIGURE 23–1. Air tent articular cartilage analogy. It is conceptually useful to think of cartilage as a pressurized structure such as exemplified by an air tent. The system requires a pump, which must be working constantly to maintain inflation of the system because of leaks through the fabric. In the case of cartilage, the surface membrane is the fine collagen fibril network concentrated at the surface. The inflation pump is the proteoglycan molecules, and the inflation medium is an ultrafiltrate of synovial fluid. In cartilage, of course, there is no single intake vent for the inflation medium to enter: rather, the fluid that inflates the tissue enters through the same fabric pores at the surface from which it exits when compressed (see text).

tent are a membrane (fabric cover), an inflation medium (air), and an energy source to keep the tent inflated (fan). These elements are interrelated, and a deficiency in any of them will result in failure of the system, with collapse of the tent. If the fabric has a tear, an air leak occurs, for which the pump may not be able to compensate, and the tent will collapse. Or, if the pump fails, the tent will collapse gradually as pressurized air leaks through the pores of the fabric. The tent obviously could not work in an environment such as the moon, which has no atmosphere to permit inflation of the space under the fabric.

Articular cartilage is analogous to the air tent in a number of respects. There is a fabric-like structure at the cartilage surface, which consists of fine collagen fibrils packed tightly in a matted pattern, much different from that seen in the deeper layers, where fibers become thicker, the orientation becomes vertical, and the spaces between the fibers increase. The surface "fabric" of cartilage has tiny pores that permit fluid and small molecules access to and egress from the tissue but block movement of large molecules. The inflation medium in articular cartilage is, of course, fluid, not air. The cartilage fluid is in equilibrium with the synovial fluid, which in turn is essentially an ultrafiltrate of plasma. The fluid in articular cartilage is significantly pressurized. Calculations by Ogston[1] led him to conclude that articular cartilage is inflated to "motor tire pressure." The pump for this pressurized system is not intuitively obvious, but its presence has been established without doubt by modern techniques of rheology and biophysics.

The pump for the articular cartilage system is chiefly the proteoglycan (PG) and the proteoglycan aggregate molecules (aggrecan), large macromolecules fixed within the articular cartilage fibrillar matrix as a result of their large size and volume. They are much too large to move between the fibrils of collagen and much, much too large to exit through the small pores in the matted capsule-like surface of the articular cartilage. Side-arm branches of these molecules contain many negative surface charges that repel each other, causing the molecules to attempt to unwind and enlarge their domain within the cartilage. In addition, the protein polysaccharides have a large number of hydroxyl groups, which attract water molecules by a phenomenon called hydrogen bonding. These reactions collectively cause fluid to be pulled into articular cartilage through the matrix pores and cause the collagen matrix of the system to be expanded. This tendency to imbibe water creates a swelling pressure within the enclosed cartilage space. The collagen fibers therefore are placed under tension as the fluid pressure rises. In this manner the cartilage is pressurized and the collagen "fabric" is inflated. The equilibrium state reached is a balance that can be upset by external applied pressure. If the external pressure exceeds the internal pressure, fluid will be caused to flow outward until a new equilibrium is reached. The theoretical analysis of these flow patterns and viscoelastic properties under various loading configurations[133] and studies of the influence of the charge of the proteoglycan molecules on the mechanical behavior of cartilage[134] have been carried out. This fluid movement is of great interest, as it explains the mechanism of several indispensible elements of the articular cartilage system, such as lubrication, load-bearing, and nutrition.

The collagen matrix of cartilage, the proteoglycan and proteoglycan aggregate, and the movement of fluid within cartilage are described in greater detail in the following sections with respect to morphologic, biochemical, metabolic, and functional aspects.

COLLAGEN

Morphology of the Collagen Framework

The pattern of collagen fibrils within articular cartilage is well suited to the functional requirements of the tissue. The air tent analogy described earlier requires that a pressurized internal medium be constrained from expansion by a membrane. A matted surface layer of collagen fibrils provides this membrane-like function.

The collagen pattern at the cartilage surface is morphologically quite different from the pattern in deeper layers. Benninghoff[2] described an arcade pattern of articular cartilage collagen organization in 1925 (Fig. 23–2). This pattern subsequently has been challenged with respect to the precise accuracy of the proposed scheme.[3] With respect to functional understanding, however, the concept is useful and at least partially correct. Certainly the characteristics of surface fibers differ from those of fibers in deeper layers. The surface collagen fibrils are smaller (30 to 32 nm in diameter) and more closely packed than in the middle and deeper layers.[4] The heterogeneity of concentration of the principal cartilage constituents—collagen and proteoglycan—by dry weight is seen in Figure 23–3. The collagen concentration is greatest at the surface, where the small fibrils are compacted tangentially to the surface. This arrangement creates an effective pore size, which has been

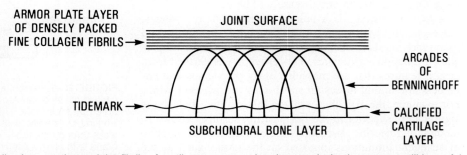

FIGURE 23–2. Schematic diagram of the collagen fibril orientation within articular cartilage. The fibrils are tightly packed near the articular surface in a tangential layer that has been termed the "armor plate" layer. Fibrils in the deeper layers become progressively larger as they progress toward the subchondral bone layer. The fibrils also are more widely spaced in the deeper layers of cartilage. The change in orientation from tangential to perpendicular in the deeper layers creates a pattern that Benninghoff[2] termed an arcade. Although this is an idealized conception and the fibrils of cartilage are not ordered so precisely, the concept still is useful in visualizing the fundamental interaction of fibrils with other constituents of cartilage. The collagen fibrils anchor into the subchondral bone layer after traversing the calcified cartilage, which is demarcated by a change in staining properties termed the "tidemark line." The anchoring of these fibrils into bone is analogous to the continuation of ligamentous attachments into bone termed Sharpey's fibrils.

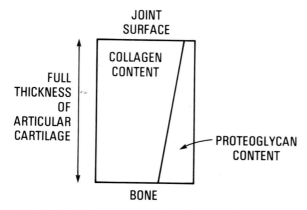

FIGURE 23–3. Relative amounts of collagen and proteoglycan in cartilage. Collagen is the predominant organic constituent by weight in articular cartilage and is most concentrated at the surface layer. In contrast, proteoglycan is most concentrated in the deeper layers. The functional importance of the two constituents is more equal than these percentages might suggest, both constituents being essential for normal cartilage function.

calculated by McCutchen[5] to be about 6 nm. The largest molecule that can traverse a pore of this dimension is hemoglobin. Therefore, the surface pores readily admit most of the synovial fluid molecules. Small ions and glucose, for example, easily traverse these pores, but larger molecules such as proteins and hyaluronan (hyaluronic acid) do not enter cartilage in significant amounts under normal conditions.

Collagen fibers in the intermediate layers no longer are oriented principally tangentially to the surface but are directed obliquely or randomly. They are larger than the surface fibrils, most ranging between 40 and 100 nm.[4] The deepest fibrils are the largest in cartilage. They are disposed perpendicularly relative to the joint surface. They perforate the calcified basal layers of cartilage through the tidemark regions and eventually enter the subchondral bone layer, where they are attached firmly, much as in the case of Sharpey's fibers of cortical bone.

This anatomic arrangement is the key to the secure structural anchorage of cartilage to the bone that it overlies. The surface collagen fibrils possess characteristics that create the necessary functional barrier to fluid movement. This movement is rate-limited by the small pore size of the collagen meshwork of the cartilage surface, however, an important factor that prevents all the fluid from being expressed, as, for example, when an individual stands for hours at a time.

The surface pattern of the collagen framework described has been recognized implicitly for decades by the term "armor plate layer," referring to the tough resilient cartilage surface. It has been well demonstrated clinically that loss of the densely packed collagen mat at the surface of cartilage in weight-bearing regions is the prelude to fibrillation, thinning, and ensuing degenerative arthritis. This seems completely logical, as the coarse, widely spaced fibrils in deeper layers that are oriented principally vertically are poorly suited to constraining the swelling forces generated by the matrix proteoglycans. The term "fibrillation" describes the tendency of these fibrils to be split vertically all the way to their subchondral attachment, much as wood splits along the grain of its fibers. The villus-like strands so

exposed collectively resemble a shag rug, and the individual strands are prone to tear off at the base when mechanically loaded and exposed to shear stresses. It is clear that the "armor plate" term applies well to the normal surface mat of collagen fibrils, and that loss of this layer no longer permits the cartilage to function as a pressurized unit suited to weight-bearing.

Evidence of the fibril pattern of collagen derives from several types of observation, including routine histology, transmission electron microscopy, scanning electron microscopy, and the demonstration of Hultkrantz lines.[6] Hultkrantz lines are typically observed on the surface of cartilage and are analogous to the Langer's lines of skin.[7] These lines become visible when the surface of cartilage is pricked with a pin that is circular in cross section. The defect so created is emphasized by coating the cartilage with India ink and then wiping it dry. Hultkrantz noted many years ago that the puncture holes appeared as slits rather than round holes. Furthermore, the slits have an axis that generally is perpendicular to the principal axis of movement of the joint. Hultkrantz lines are therefore different for each joint of the body. Mechanical tensile tests have shown that the Hultkrantz lines indicate the preferred orientation of the collagen fibrils at the surface of the joint because the specimens are found to be strongest when the long axis of the specimen is parallel to the Hultkrantz lines. Bullough and Goodfellow[8] have shown this characteristic of joint surfaces in experiments illustrated in Figures 23–4 and 23–5. Notice

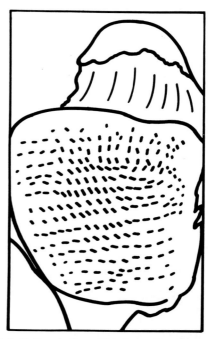

FIGURE 23–4. Hultkrantz lines. This figure illustrates the pattern of slit lines on the surface of the human talus. The slit lines are created by a pin pushed through the surface in a perpendicular direction. The lines typically are made more obvious by coating the surface with India ink and subsequently wiping it dry. The pattern of the defect is a slit rather than a circle because of the predominant orientation of the underlying collagen fibrils of the surface layers. The slit line phenomenon is similar to that seen in skin (Langer's lines). Hultkrantz lines run predominantly perpendicular to the main axis of motion of the particular joint. (Redrawn after Bullough P, Goodfellow J: J Bone Joint Surg [Br] *50*:852, 1968.)

CORONAL SECTION OF JOINT SURFACE

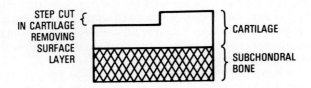

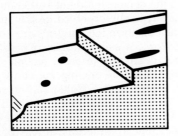

FIGURE 23–5. Hultkrantz lines. This figure shows the change in pattern of the Hultkrantz slit lines in deeper layers of cartilage compared with the surface. If a step cut is made in cartilage, removing the surface layer after the Hultkrantz lines have been established, a different pattern is seen in the deeper layers. A circle rather than a slit is the typical pattern made by a penetrating pin. The reason for the difference is that in the deeper layers there is no preference of direction of fibrils in the tangential plane. (Redrawn after Bullough P, Goodfellow J: J Bone Joint Surg [Br] *50*:852, 1968.)

that in deeper layers the slits disappear, indicating that the fibril orientation is more random or more vertical, or both. Electron microscopy also has been used to show a preferred orientation of these fibrils at the surface and to characterize the dimensions of the fibrils at different depths from the surface,[4, 8] as well as to provide further support to the Benninghoff concept of fiber orientation.[9]

Routine histologic techniques do not show the collagen fibrils of cartilage well because they tend to be masked by the abundant proteoglycan that is intertwined within the fibril network. The proteoglycan contains dense electronegative charges that are responsible for many of the observed staining characteristics of cartilage, such as metachromasia.

The collagen fibril pattern can be inferred by viewing sections with polarized light, however, because a fibrillar pattern of preferred orientation will alter the polarized light characteristically. Examples of cartilage sections viewed with polarized light are given in Figures 23–6 and 23–7. A paper by Bullough and Goodfellow on cartilage fibril patterns describes the interpretation of this type of photomicrograph.[8]

Collagen Chemistry

The molecular structure of collagen has been of considerable interest for over a century, because it is the principal structural protein by mass for all mammals. It constitutes 65 to 80 per cent of the mass by dry weight of such specialized connective tissues as tendons, ligaments, skin, joint capsules, and cartilage. It is the only protein with significant tensile force–resisting properties with the exception of elastin, whose functional role is insignificant in comparison. Therefore, collagen is the key protein in musculoskeletal stability: It provides the mechanical properties imparting the ''connect'' ability in connective tissue.

The tensile force–resisting properties of cartilage derive from the precise molecular configuration of the collagen macromolecule. This molecule is one of the largest in the body, forming a rodlike structure whose dimensions are 300 nm in length and 1.5 nm in diameter. These rods are termed tropocollagen. They are assembled in a three-dimensional array in the extracellular environment, being somehow influenced by environmental stresses and additional biologic factors, the details of whose nature are as yet unclear. The sum of the extracellular influences somehow affects the orientation and size of fibrils that are assembled from the tropocollagen units. The assembly is typically patterned in a quarter stagger (Fig. 23–8), which is seen as a 64 nm subbonding on transmission electron micrographs. A small gap that exists between the head to tail linear assembly of the tropocollagen units may be of functional importance in bone with respect to nucleation of apatite crystals in the process of matrix mineralization of osteoid.[10]

The individual tropocollagen units are made up of three chains that are synthesized independently intracellularly in the manner of other proteins (Fig. 23–8). The length of the

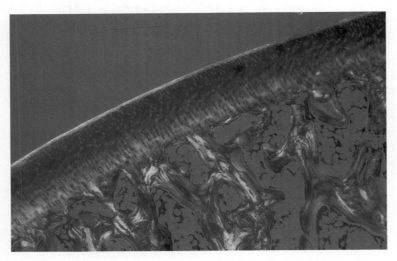

FIGURE 23–6. This photograph of an articular cartilage surface under polarized light shows differences in refractility of the surface layer compared with deeper layers of articular cartilage. The preferred tangential orientation of the collagen fibrils at the surface creates the refractile difference seen as a bright line (45×). (Compare with Fig. 23–7.)

FIGURE 23–7. The articular cartilage surface (same section as in Figure 23–6 with polarizing filter rotated 90 degrees). If the polarizing filter is rotated 90 degrees, a marked change is observed in the refractile pattern. The surface now is dark rather than bright because of the predominant orientation of the tangential layer of fibrils. The "arcade" pattern in the deeper layers also can be perceived with the filter in this rotation, in contrast to Figure 23–6. The polarized light technique used in this way identifies areas in the tissue where a predominant orientation exists, in comparison with a random pattern of fibrils.

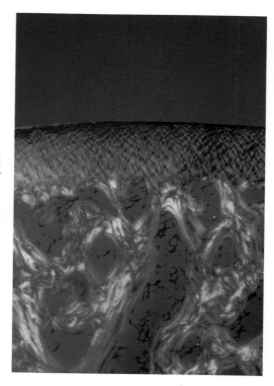

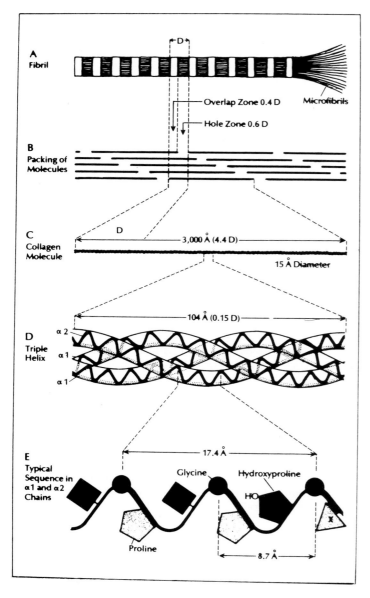

FIGURE 23–8. The relationship between the single strand protein of the alpha chain to the triple helix, the collagen molecule, and the fully developed fibril. The characteristic feature of the collagen molecule is its rigid, very long, narrow, rodlike structure, which is created by the tight winding of three alpha chains into a triple helix termed tropocollagen. (Reprinted by permission from Prockop DJ, et al: N Engl J Med *301*:13, 1979.)

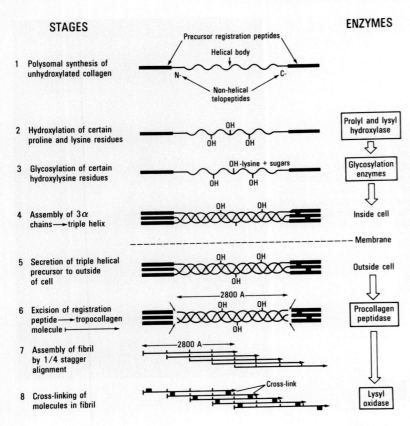

STAGES

1. Polysomal synthesis of unhydroxylated collagen
2. Hydroxylation of certain proline and lysine residues
3. Glycosylation of certain hydroxylysine residues
4. Assembly of 3α chains → triple helix
5. Secretion of triple helical precursor to outside of cell
6. Excision of registration peptide → tropocollagen molecule
7. Assembly of fibril by 1/4 stagger alignment
8. Cross-linking of molecules in fibril

ENZYMES

Prolyl and lysyl hydroxylase

Glycosylation enzymes

Inside cell

— Membrane

Outside cell

Procollagen peptidase

Lysyl oxidase

FIGURE 23–9. Several enzymatic steps are necessary for creation of the final collagen molecule and its maturation into a collagen fibril. These enzymatic steps take place partly within the cell and partly outside the cell. Even those steps that occur inside the cell are posttranslational, that is, they are not directly under genetic control. However, they are very essential for the proper development of the final structure. Defects in many of the steps have been identified in a variety of heritable disorders of connective tissues. The final aggregation of collagen into a structure that becomes cross linked is essential to produce the requisite tensile stress-resistant properties characteristic of mature connective tissue. (From Levene CI: J Clin Pathol Suppl *12*:82, 1978.)

messenger RNA molecule required for the synthesis is extraordinary, as each chain contains about 1000 amino acids. Most of the chains (called alpha chains) are precisely ordered with a general sequence of glycine-proline-hydroxyproline, glycine-proline-x-, or glycine-x-proline-, where x is another amino acid.[11] The higher percentages of the amino acids glycine, proline, and hydroxyproline are unique to collagen. Glycine is the smallest amino acid and permits the close packing necessary for the assembly of the three alpha chains into tropocollagen. Proline and hydroxyproline are cyclic amino acids, whose structure presumably imparts rigidity to the final triple helix configuration. Further details of the collagen molecular arrangement are presented in several reviews.[12–14] Collagen undergoes numerous modifications after ribosomal assembly, which are initiated by intracellular or extracellular enzymes. Examples of these processes include hydroxylation of proline or lysine and glycosylation of lysine. These modifications are termed "secondary features," as distinguished from the direct-coded structure (Fig. 23–9).

The assembly of the three alpha chains into tropocollagen is facilitated by a group of amino acids at the end of each alpha chain called registration peptides. The triple helix plus its registration peptide is larger than the tropocollagen molecule and is called procollagen. Once the assembly of the triple helix is completed, the registration peptides are no longer of utility and are cleaved by an enzyme, procollagen peptidase, as the procollagen passes through the cellular membrane into the extracellular space.

The alpha chains are not identical among species or within a single species. Early data on mammalian skin collagen showed two types of alpha chain, $\alpha1$ and $\alpha2$, present in a ratio of 2 to 1. Three types of alpha chains were identified in codfish skin collagen, $\alpha1$, $\alpha2$, and $\alpha3$.[15] Many studies on typing of collagen soon followed. Miller and Matukas[16] were the first to show that cartilage possesses a collagen different in composition from that in most fibrous connective tissue. This collagen contains a different type of $\alpha1$ chain, which they termed $\alpha1$, type II. The collagen in most cartilages consists of three such identical chains and the abbreviated nomenclature now used is ($\alpha1$ [II])$_3$ or type II collagen.

Fifteen different types of collagen have been described in vertebrates. The collagens can be divided into two major classes on the basis of their primary structure and supramolecular assembly: the fibril-forming collagens and the non–fibril-forming collagens. The fibril-forming collagens include types I, II, III, V, and XI; all of these types have a long central triple helical domain without any interruptions in the glycine-x-y sequence, where x and y are amino acids. The rest of the collagens belong to the non–fibril-forming class. Although they vary in size, they share the feature of having imperfections in the glycine-x-y sequence. Within this class, types IX, XII, and XIV collagens form a subgroup called the fibril-associated collagens with interrupted triple helices (FACIT). They are associated with type I or II collagen fibrils and play a role in the interaction of these fibrils with other matrix components. Although their sizes and primary structures vary, they share several common structural features. Type XVI collagen appears to

TABLE 23–1. Structurally and Genetically Distinct Collagens

Type	Tissue Distribution	Molecular Form	Chemical Characterization
I	Bone, tendon, skin, dentin, ligament, uterus, and artery	$[\alpha_1(I)]_2\,\alpha_2(I)$	Hybrid composed of two kinds of chains; low in hydroxylysine and glycosylated hydroxylysine; small 67 nm banded fibril; increased content of 3- and 4-hydroxyproline and hydroxylysine as compared to the heteropolymer
	Fetal tissues, inflammatory and neoplastic states	$[\alpha_1(I)]_3$	
II	Hyaline cartilage, vitreous body	$[\alpha_1(II)]_3$	Relatively high in hydroxylysine and glycosylated hydroxylysine; small 67 nm banded fibril
III	Skin, artery, and uterus	$[\alpha_1(III)]_3$	High in hydroxyproline and low in hydroxylysine; contains interchain disulfide bonds, associated with type I; small 67 nm banded fibril
IV	Basement membranes Glomerular basement membrane	$[\alpha_1(IV)]_2\,\alpha_2(IV)$ Molecular form of $\alpha_3(IV)$, $\alpha_4(IV)$, $\alpha_5(IV)$ unknown	NF; high in hydroxylysine and glycosylated hydroxylysine; may contain large globular regions
V	Hamster lung cell culture Skin, bone, fetal membranes Synovial membrane, placenta Most interstitial tissues	$[\alpha_1(V)]_3$ $[\alpha_1(V)]_2\,\alpha_2(V)$ $\alpha_1(V)\,\alpha_2(V)\,\alpha_3(V)$	Associated with type I; small fibers; small 67 nm banded fibril; similar to type IV
VI	Intervertebral disc, skin, vessels Most interstitial tissues	$\alpha_1(VI)\,\alpha_2(VI)\,\alpha_3(VI)$	NF; microfibrils; 100 nm banded fibrils; disulfide bonds between tetramers; arginine-glycine-aspartic acid sequences
VII	Dermoepidermal junction Anchoring fibrils	$[\alpha_1(VII)]_3$	NF; long chain
VIII	Descemet's membrane, endothelial cells	Unknown (?)	NF; small helices linked in tandem
IX	Hyaline cartilage, vitreous humor	$\alpha_1(IX)\,\alpha_2(IX)\,\alpha_3(IX)$	Associated with type II; minor cartilage protein; contains attached glycosaminoglycan; NF and FACIT member; FACIT collagen 1 domain
X	Growth plate Chick embryo chondrocytes Hypertrophic mineralizing cartilage	$[\alpha_1(X)]_3$	NF; short chain; high in hydroxyproline and hydroxylysine, 25% amino acids high in aromatic residues in noncollagenous regions
XI	Hyaline cartilage associated with type II	$\alpha_1(XI)\,\alpha_2(XI)\,\alpha_3(XI)$	67 nm banded fibril
XII	Embryonic tendon and skin, periodontal ligament	$[\alpha_1(XII)]_3$	Associated with type I; NF and FACIT member; FACIT collagen 1 domain with similarities to type IX
XIII	Endothelial cells mRNA in skin, intestine, bone (intertrabecular), striated muscle, mesenchyme cartilage	(?) unknown	NF; 1 to 2 short interruptions of glycine-x-y repeat
XIV	Fetal tendon and skin	$[\alpha_1(XIV)]_3$	NF and FACIT member; FACIT col 1 domain similar to that of type IX
XVI	Skin fibroblast Epidermal keratinocytes (?)		Recently found with $\alpha_3(VI)$ complementary DNA probe; approximately 65% of molecules composed of repeating glycine-x-y sequences; 10 separate collagen domains, noncollagen domains contain numerous cystines and often are found in the sequence of cystine-x-y cystine, where x and y are any amino acids; similar to FACIT

NF, nonfibrillar; FACIT, fibril-associated collagens with interrupted triple helices.
Derived from several sources.[12–14, 17–19]

be a member of this group.[17] A summary of the makeup and distribution of the collagen types accepted at present is given in Table 23–1.

Collagen Cross Links

Stabilization of collagen occurs extracellularly after assembly into the quarter-stagger arrays that make up filaments, fibrils, and fibers. The stabilization and ultimate tensile strength of the structure are thought to result mainly from the development of intramolecular and intermolecular cross links. The former occur between alpha chains of the same tropocollagen molecule, the latter between adjacent tropocollagen molecules. The cross links result from enzyme-mediated reactions involving mainly lysine and hydroxylysine. The lysine and hydroxylysine molecules have secondary amine groups on terminal projections extending laterally from the alpha chain, which are available for the cross-linking reaction. The initial reaction in this process is the oxidative deamination of the terminal amine to an aldehyde by the enzyme lysyl oxidase (Fig. 23–10). These reactions have general similarity to the reactions that stabilize elastin. The resulting allysyl residues condense with one another to form an aldol condensation product[19] char-

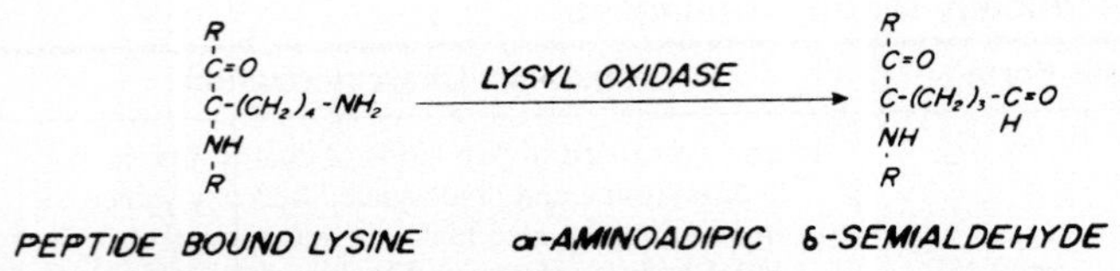

$$R - C = O$$
$$C - (CH_2)_4 - NH_2 \quad \xrightarrow{\text{LYSYL OXIDASE}} \quad C - (CH_2)_3 - C = O$$
$$NH \qquad\qquad\qquad\qquad NH \qquad\quad H$$
$$R \qquad\qquad\qquad\qquad\quad R$$

PEPTIDE BOUND LYSINE α-AMINOADIPIC δ-SEMIALDEHYDE

FIGURE 23–10. The reaction that precedes formation of the collagen cross links illustrated in Figure 23–9 is given here in more detail. The enzyme lysyl oxidase is required for the cleavage of the terminal (secondary) amino group of lysine and the formation of an aldehyde. The aldehyde, in turn, reacts with another lysine or lysine-derived aldehyde to form a cross link (see Fig. 23–11).

acteristic of intramolecular cross links[20, 21] (Fig. 23–11). Intermolecular cross links subsequently form from the reaction of allysine with lysine or hydroxylysine to form a Schiff base (delta semialdehyde) (Fig. 23–11). These aldol condensation and Schiff base reaction products possess double bonds that apparently are reduced to more stable forms in vivo with the passage of time. Most studies on cross linking of collagen in the past 15 years have used the presence of the double bond of the unsaturated compound to label the "reducible" cross links with tritium. Typically this has been done by reducing the aldol condensation product or delta-semialdehyde with tritium-labeled sodium borohydride. The reduced product thereby is labeled with tritium and can be detected after acid hydrolysis and column chromatography using separation systems similar to those used in amino acid analysis. The details of the bifunctional, trifunctional, or quadrifunctional cross links so detected are beyond the scope of this chapter but are presented in several reviews.[22, 23]

The significance of the type II collagen to cartilage is not yet known. The principal differences between this collagen and the more common type I found in fibrous connective tissue consist in the number of hydroxylysine molecules present and the presence of a small number of residues of cysteine. Table 23–1 summarizes the principal differences between type I and type II collagens.

The principal cross-linking residues in mature type II collagen fibrils are hydroxylysyl pyridinoline residues. The fibrils increase in size from less than 20 nm in diameter in fetal tissue to a range of 50 to 100 nm in mature tissue. The fibrils are thinner near the articular surface or the tangential zone. Evidence is being accumulated that type IX collagen, and possibly type XI, makes critical contributions to the organization and mechanical stability of the type II collagen fibrillar network.[13, 24]

Type IX makes up approximately 10 per cent of the collagen protein in fetal mammalian articular cartilage but the amount decreases to about 1 per cent in adult tissue. The molecule also is a proteoglycan. In chicks a single site for attachment of chondroitin sulfate exists. However, it has not been determined whether mammalian type IX collagens attach in this manner in all cases.

In bovine articular cartilage, type IX collagen appears to be linked covalently to at least one molecule of type II collagen. It is found on the surface of type II. The cross-link sites are in the type IX collagen 2 domain, which attach to the telopeptides of type II by covalent bonding via hydroxylysine residues. The two types of collagen appear to be antiparallel. The cross links are similar to those between type II collagen molecules, with the ketoamines that can

mature into hydroxypyridinium residues. From this evidence, it is believed that type IX provides a covalent interface between the surface of type II collagen fibril and the interfibrillar proteoglycan domain. Another theory is that type IX collagen provides interfibrillar links between different type II fibrils and, therefore, would enhance the mechanical stability of the fibrillar network.[13]

Type XI collagen makes up about 3 per cent of mature articular cartilage collagen. During the maturation of cartilage a substitution of $\alpha_1(XI)$ chains with $\alpha_1(V)$ chains appears to take place.[13] In the mature tissue, the cross links seem to be immature, with divalent ketoamines and no significant amount of pyridinoline being formed.[25] The intermolecular links appear to be between N-telopeptide and C-helix sites only.

Other collagens found in articular cartilage are type VI and type X. Both have a short helix (see Table 23–1). Type VI is unique in that it has no aldehyde cross link and has arginine-glycine-aspartic acid (RGD) sequences in each α chain. Thus, it may play a role in cell attachment. Type X is found only in hypertrophic zones of growth plates.

The fundamental process of formation of collagen by the chondroblasts and chondrocytes apparently is nearly identical to the process of synthesis by the fibroblast and fibrocyte. The steps in synthesis are outlined in Figure 23–9. The several posttranslational transformations are notable. The collagen turnover in cartilage proceeds at a rate not unlike that seen in connective tissue of the fibrous type.

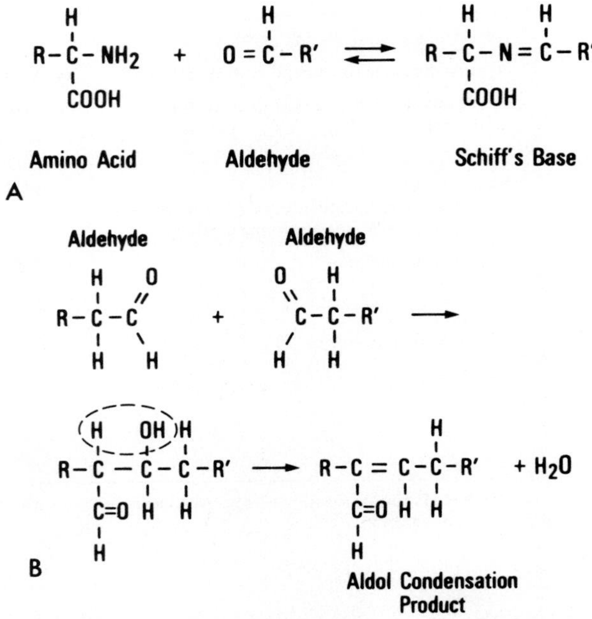

$$\begin{array}{ccc} H & H & H \quad H \\ R-C-NH_2 & + \quad O=C-R' & \rightleftharpoons \quad R-C-N=C-R' \\ COOH & & COOH \end{array}$$

Amino Acid   **Aldehyde**   **Schiff's Base**

A

FIGURE 23–11. **A,** The reaction of lysine with a lysine aldehyde to form a Schiff's base by splitting out water and creating a double bond between the secondary amine of lysine and the terminal carbon of the aldehyde. This is the principal reaction between adjacent tropocollagen molecules, which produces intermolecular cross links. **B,** The complement to the reaction in **A.** In this case, two aldehydes derived from lysine react with each other in such a way as to split out water and create (through an intermediate step) an aldol condensation product. A double bond configuration results between the terminal carbon of one molecule and the carbon adjacent to the terminal carbon on the second molecule. This is the principal intramolecular cross link between alpha chains within a tropocollagen molecule. The reactions shown in **A** and **B** also can participate in more complex tri- and tetramolecular cross links, as catalogued by Tanzer.[23]

Because significant synthesis occurs in adult cartilage, it is clear that control processes for spatial orientation of the product are crucial.

It is a source of frustration to surgeons and their patients that attempts to achieve cartilage repair, as in surgical arthroplasty, seldom are completely satisfactory clinically. This is probably because the collagen architecture of the arthroplasty surface is disordered, and the surface of the arthroplasty lacks the membrane-like characteristics of the surface layer of articular cartilage. Details of the repair process are described later in this chapter.

PROTEOGLYCANS OF ARTICULAR CARTILAGE

The extraordinary size of the proteoglycan aggregate molecules (aggrecan) of articular cartilage is achieved by supra-assembly of three different types of linear chain molecular species: (1) sulfated glycosaminoglycans, (2) the core protein, and (3) hyaluronan (a nonsulfated glycosaminoglycan). The proteoglycans of articular cartilage serve as the "pump" of the highly pressurized cartilage system. The characteristics of the proteoglycan molecules that permit this crucial function include their very large size and hence their immobility within the collagen fibril meshwork, their densely concentrated, fixed, negative charges, and their large number of hydroxyl groups. These characteristics collectively serve to attract water and small ions into the cartilage. The sum of this attraction is termed the swelling pressure and consists of osmotic forces, ionic forces, and Donnan forces. The purpose of this section is to describe briefly the chemical structure of the functionally vital proteoglycan and its aggregate and to illustrate the manner in which the functional role derives from the chemical structure.

Glycosaminoglycans

The terminology for the class of molecules called glycosaminoglycans has undergone complete change in recent years. An earlier review of the modifications in terminology was offered by Mathews.[26] The original term applied to this group of molecules was acid mucopolysaccharides. The more precise chemical term "glycosaminoglycans" has been accepted as preferable, although references are still occasionally found to the older term. Furthermore, there is not complete unanimity with respect to this terminology, and the term "polyanionic glycans" also is applied to these molecules.[2] The "acid" part of the earlier term refers to the large number of carboxyl and sulfate groups, which posses negative charges and which confer many predictable characteristics in chemical and staining reactions to the tissue. The prefix "muco-" refers to the gross physical characteristics of this molecular class, members of which are typically quite viscous and gel-like. Finally, the "polysaccharide" part of the term refers to the chemical structure of the molecule—it is made of many hexose units assembled linearly into long chains in a manner roughly analogous to the assembly of glucose into glycogen, but in this case the chains are unbranched. Further terminology changes continue. The preferred term for hyaluronic acid is now hyaluronan.

In most of the glycosaminoglycan molecules, hexos-

amine alternates with another sugar polymerized in a repeating disaccharide pattern. The predominance of the amine group in this configuration is the reason for the occurrence of "amino-" in the term glycosaminoglycan. Figure 23–12 shows the disaccharide repeating unit for the glycosaminoglycans of articular cartilage: chondroitin-4-sulfate, chondroitin-6-sulfate, hyaluronan, and keratan sulfate. The common features of the group are obvious at first glance. In particular, the location of the N-acetylamine

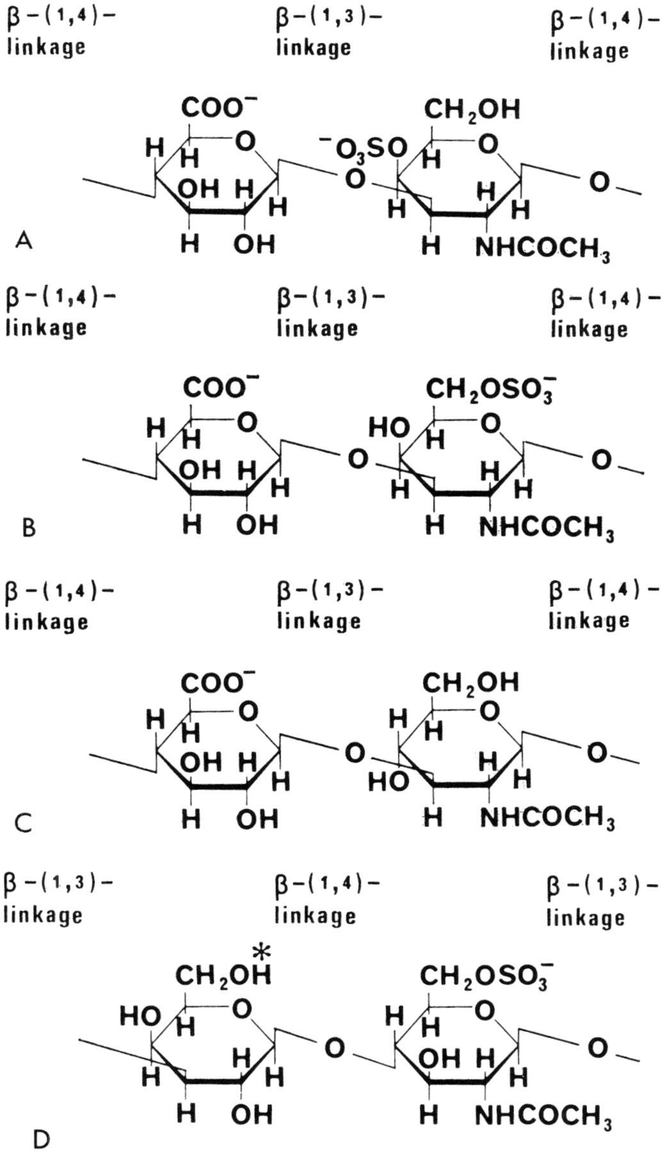

FIGURE 23–12. The disaccharide configuration of the principal glycosaminoglycans of the proteoglycan constituents of articular cartilage.

A The molecular configuration of chondroitin-4-sulfate. This differs from chondroitin-6-sulfate (**B**) only in the location of the sulfate group on the hexosamine molecule. Both contain alternating glucuronic acid and galactosamine sugars.

B Chondroitin-6-sulfate.

C Hyaluronan contains alternating molecules of glucosamine and glucuronic acid but lacks a sulfate group.

D Keratan sulfate contains galactose rather than a uronic acid moiety in the disaccharide. The hexosamine is glucosamine, which is sulfated in the C6 position.

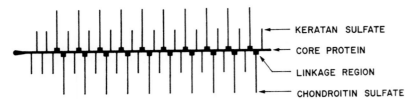

FIGURE 23–13. Proteoglycan. This diagram of the proteoglycan molecule demonstrates the method of aggregation of chondroitin-4-sulfate, chondroitin-6-sulfate, and keratan sulfate to the core protein. The linkage regions indicated are composed of highly specific molecular configurations (see text). The attachment site of the core protein to hyaluronan at which an aggregate is created is seen at the far left of the diagram. There is typically a high concentration of keratan sulfate, a shorter chain glycosaminoglycan, near the attachment site of the core protein to hyaluronan, symbolized by the shorter side arms in that location. (From Rosenberg L: Structure of cartilage proteoglycan. In WH Simon [Ed]: The Human Joint in Health and Disease. Philadelphia, University of Pennsylvania Press, 1978.)

group at the number two carbon (C2) of the hexosamine is common to all the disaccharides shown. The hexosamine is galactosamine in three of the four cases; keratan sulfate possesses glucosamine as the alternating hexosamine. All except hyaluronan are sulfated at the C4 or C6 position of the hexosamine. Each disaccharide contains at least three hydroxyl groups. All except keratan sulfate contain uronic acid as the second element of the disaccharide, with a carboxyl terminal at C6. Keratan sulfate possesses galactose rather than uronic acid as the second half of the disaccharide.

The glycosaminoglycans are covalently bound to core protein in a pattern that locates keratan sulfate side arms preferentially close to the linkage region to hyaluronan. Therefore, a keratan sulfate–rich region exists in the protein polysaccharide, as illustrated in Figure 23–13, which therefore contains little chondroitin sulfate. The keratan sulfate molecules characteristically are of lower molecular weight than the chondroitin sulfate chains, as indicated by the diagrammatic representation in Figure 23–13.

Phosphorylation of the core protein occurs adjacent to the chondroitin sulfate–containing peptides.[27] The phosphorylation involves the serine residues of the core protein. Furthermore, dermatan sulfate has been isolated from mature bovine articular cartilage.[28] The functional significance of these observations in the complex story of articular cartilage proteoglycan remains to be resolved.

Aggrecan

The ability of proteoglycan to aggregate further by combining with hyaluronan was originally described by Hardingham and Muir,[29] who elaborated on the dissociation and association experiments of Sajdera and Hascall[30] to establish the mechanism of formation of aggregate (now called aggrecan) (Fig. 23–14). It has since been demonstrated that the formation of aggrecan is facilitated and stabilized by small proteins termed *link proteins*.[30–33] Much attention has been given to the degree of aggrecan formation in various tissues and in various pathologic conditions. Clearly, the ability of the proteoglycan molecule to form aggregates of even greater molecular size amplifies its physiologic functional properties as the ''pump'' of the system. This is true because the aggregate formed will create even greater fixation of the proteoglycan molecules, locking them more securely within the interstices of the collagen framework of the tissue, ensuring fixation of the negative charges and assuring the cartilage of an adequate swelling pressure to maintain expansion of that matrix.

Nature of the Aggregate Linkage

In distinction to the covalent linkage of glycosaminoglycans to core protein in proteoglycan subunit (PGS), the linkage of PGS to hyaluronan is noncovalent. The linkage is facilitated and strengthened by low molecular weight proteins termed link proteins. Three link proteins have been identified in canine and human articular cartilage, with molecular weights of 41,500, 44,000, and 48,000, respectively.[34, 35] Link proteins also have been identified in synovial cell culture extracts, raising questions about their broader biologic importance in connective tissues other than articular cartilage.[34] The linkage can occur without the presence of a link protein, but such proteins have been found in all cartilages so far examined.[36] The noncovalent linkage of PGS and hyaluronan can be dissociated by concentrated solutions of guanidinium hydrochloride, calcium chloride, or magnesium chloride.[30] The dissociated components can be reassociated by the reduction of the concentration of the dissociative solvents. This process has been the key technique in unraveling the chemical structure of PGS and aggregate and in understanding the nature of their association as well as the role of link proteins. A diagrammatic representation of the experiments of Sajdera and Hascall[30] and of Hardingham and Muir[29] is shown in Figures 23–15 and 23–16. As is illustrated in these figures, a high concentration (approximately 4 molar) of guanidinium hydrochloride cancels the attraction charges of proteoglycan to hyaluronic acid. Under these conditions, density gradient centrifugation results in separation of the higher and lower molecular weight constituents. This step permits a characterization of the molecular species of differing molecular weights. Under conditions of about 0.5 M guanidinium hydrochloride, the three elements hyaluronan, link protein, and proteoglycan reassociate to form the aggrecan once again. Cartilages from different sources possess differing percentages of aggregation of proteoglycan, but factors controlling this process are not yet fully understood.

FLUID OF ARTICULAR CARTILAGE

As was noted in the air tent analogy described earlier, the inflation medium of articular cartilage is synovial fluid. This is essentially an ultrafiltrate of plasma plus hyaluronan. The hyaluronan molecules are too large to enter cartilage through its 6 nm diameter surface pores, but most of the remaining ions and molecules of normal synovial fluid, such as water, sodium, potassium, and glucose, are sufficiently small to pass through these pores easily. Move-

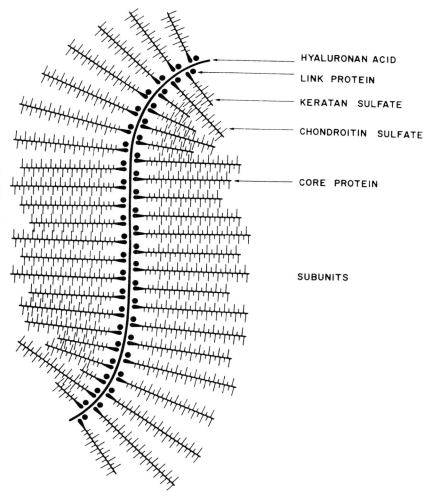

HYALURONAN ACID

LINK PROTEIN

KERATAN SULFATE

CHONDROITIN SULFATE

CORE PROTEIN

SUBUNITS

FIGURE 23–14. Pattern of aggrecan formed by a complex of proteoglycan and hyaluronan. The aggrecan is stabilized in part by a glycopeptide called link protein at the junction site. The spectacular augmentation in molecular weight from the original glycosaminoglycan weight of approximately 50,000 to that of proteoglycan, reaching millions of daltons, and further increase to a structure with molecular weight of many millions of daltons by aggregate formation with hyaluronan is well illustrated by this diagram. (From Rosenberg L: Structure of cartilage proteoglycan. In WH Simon [Ed]: The Human Joint in Health and Disease. Philadelphia, University of Pennsylvania Press, 1978.)

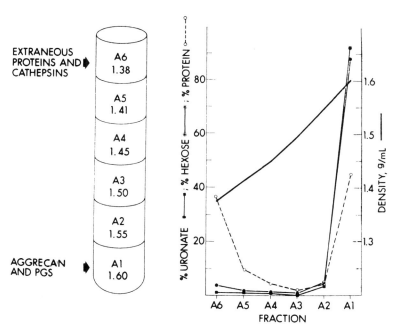

EXTRANEOUS PROTEINS AND CATHEPSINS

AGGRECAN AND PGS

FIGURE 23–15. The separation of components of aggrecan extracted from cartilage with guanidinium hydrochloride. When placed in an ultracentrifuge in a cesium chloride solution, the heavier molecules such as aggrecan and the proteoglycan subunit (PGS) are forced to the bottom of the tube, whereas the lighter molecules, including extraneous proteins and cathepsins, remain in the upper layers. The contents of the tube then can be separated into several fractions, as illustrated at the right of the figure. It can be seen that the uronate-containing material making up the glycosaminoglycans, which is part of the proteoglycan and aggrecan, is located almost entirely in the A1 fraction. Similarly, hexose (the galactose moiety of keratan sulfate) also is in the A1 fraction. (From Rosenberg L: Structure of cartilage proteoglycan. In WH Simon [Ed]: The Human Joint in Health and Disease. Philadelphia, University of Pennsylvania Press, 1978.)

DISSOCIATIVE CONDITIONS   ASSOCIATIVE CONDITIONS

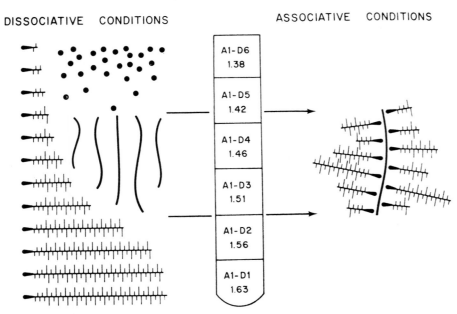

FIGURE 23–16. If the A1 fraction (see Fig. 23–15) is separated into its components using dissociative techniques, these constituents can be separated further arbitrarily into six fractions, as seen on the left. In the uppermost layers are found very short fragments consisting of proteoglycans along with link protein. In the middle layers are hyaluronan and the intermediate-sized fragments of proteoglycan. At the bottom of the gradient are found the heaviest fragments of proteoglycan. The conditions for this separation of aggrecan (dissociative conditions) are achieved with high concentrations of guanidinium hydrochloride or magnesium chloride. Under associative conditions, in which the salt concentrations of guanidinium hydrochloride or magnesium chloride are reduced, the proteoglycan and hyaluronan reaggregate, as seen on the right side of this figure. (From Rosenberg L: Structure of cartilage proteoglycan. In WH Simon [Ed]: The Human Joint in Health and Disease. Philadelphia, University of Pennsylvania Press, 1978.)

ment of fluid into and out of cartilage occurs to some extent by diffusion, but, as will be noted in the discussion on cartilage nutrition, diffusion does not seem adequate in and of itself to provide for cartilage health. Most of the fluid of articular cartilage is water. The percentage of water in cartilage ranges from over 60 to nearly 80 per cent.[37–39] The water is bound by a variety of weak forces, such as hydrogen bonding to proteoglycan and collagen or simple hydration shell formation, but it is sufficiently mobile that clearance studies indicate essential equivalence in behavior between labeled water and urea.[40] Urea is uncharged and is not subject to hydrogen bonding, so that equivalence of movement of the water and urea molecules suggests that the binding forces holding water are extremely weak, and molecular exchange occurs readily.

Mankin and Thrasher[39] performed additional experiments that appeared to demonstrate that a small fraction, about 6 per cent, of water of articular cartilage is not easily exchangeable. After equilibration with tritiated water for 20 days, a small percentage of water remained in cartilage after drying. Net flow into and out of cartilage is induced by the normal weight-bearing function of synovial joints. Maroudas[41] has calculated that for normal articular cartilage the sum of swelling pressures is greatly exceeded (10 times) by loading conditions such as walking. The implications would seem to be that under loading conditions cartilage would be compressed rapidly and completely, much as a wet sponge is compressed by a weight. The rate of fluid movement permitted by the small surface pore size and the cartilage microarchitecture, however, is sufficiently slow that cartilage is compressed only partially even after loading for hours. The experiments of Linn and Sokoloff illustrate this point well.[42] These authors used an apparatus designed to fit into a centrifuge capable of forcing fluid out of cartilage into a receptacle[34] (Fig. 23–17). The cartilage fits into a porous basket-like container into which a plunger rests. The unit is placed into a centrifuge and the faster the centrifuge revolves, the greater the pressure on the cartilage in the basket. In this way the effect of varying loads over varying

periods of time on the rate of fluid expression from cartilage can be evaluated. These experiments showed that the amount of fluid that can be expressed (30 per cent) is extremely small in relation to the total water content (Fig. 23–18). Subsequent experiments by Linn using an animal joint demonstrated the processes of fluid movement in cartilage more directly.[43] The device constructed for this experiment was termed an arthrotripsometer (Fig. 23–19). By developing the necessary design criteria it was possible to

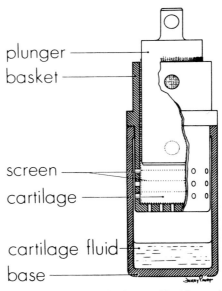

FIGURE 23–17. Illustration of a device used by Linn and Sokoloff to express fluid from articular cartilage. The device consists of a perforated basket within a centrifuge collecting system. A plunger within the basket effectively compresses cartilage at the bottom of the basket when the system is spun in the centrifuge. Time and pressure can be controlled by the duration and speed of the centrifuge operation. This technique permits the amount and composition of cartilage fluid expressed to be analyzed (see Fig. 23–18). (From Linn FC, Sokoloff LH: Arthritis Rheum 8:481, 1965.)

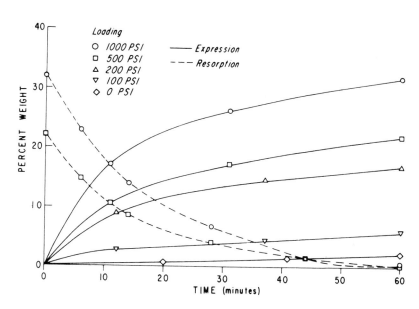

FIGURE 23–18. The rate of expression and resorption of fluid from costal cartilage. It is notable that even at the highest pressure for 60 min, only slightly more than 30 per cent of the weight of the tissue can be expressed. This is approximately half of the water content of tissue. At lower pressures and shorter times the amount of fluid shift is a very small fraction of the total water content of cartilage. This small movement of fluid has great functional importance to articular cartilage, however. (From Linn FC, Sokoloff LH: Arthritis Rheum *8*:481, 1965.)

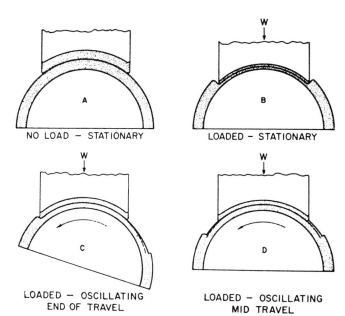

NO LOAD — STATIONARY

LOADED — STATIONARY

LOADED — OSCILLATING
END OF TRAVEL

LOADED — OSCILLATING
MID TRAVEL

FIGURE 23–19. The effect of loading on articular cartilage. A stationary load, as illustrated in example **B,** shows significant cartilage compression after a period of time. When oscillation occurs using the same loading condition, however, the compressive effect for a given time is considerably less. Because the cartilage is unloaded a portion of the time, it resorbs some of the fluid that had been expressed during loading. (From Linn FC: J Bone Joint Surg [Am] *49*:1079, 1967.)

vary loading conditions with respect to amplitude of load and to stationary versus cyclic conditions. The joint was immersed in synovial fluid during testing. Deformation versus time is seen to be greater for stationary than for cyclic loads. The explanation for this observation is that in the cyclic condition, partial recovery occurs, owing to the effect of swelling pressure in pulling fluid back into cartilage during the phase of the cycle when the cartilage is unloaded. This unparalleled system of load bearing by articular cartilage depends for its effectiveness on functional integrity and detailed interaction of each of the architectural, biomechanical, and biochemical elements within the system.

The fluid movement that occurs during the loading process described appears to be important for lubrication of the joint surfaces as well as for load carriage. On the basis of calculations obtained from complex mathematical models, Mow and coworkers have proposed that fluid is expressed out of cartilage in front of the advancing contact surfaces of cartilage.[44] This process provides a fluid film that minimizes cartilage-cartilage contact, thus also minimizing wear. Indeed, if this analysis is correct, we walk on water! Further discussion of the lubrication mechanism of articular cartilage is presented in Chapters 24 and 77.

NUTRITION

Fluid movement is necessary not only for load carriage and lubrication but also for nutrition of the chondrocytes. Students of articular cartilage generally agree that in the adult very little of the chondrocytic nutritional requirement is satisfied from subchondral vessels of bone. Rather, cartilage nutrition derives almost entirely from synovial fluid.[45] The pumping action of fluid into and out of cartilage during loading and unloading appears to be a key to this process. Joints that are immobilized suffer relatively quickly in a number of important respects. The metabolic activity of cells appears affected, as loss of proteoglycan and an increase in water content soon are observed.[46] The normal white, glistening appearance of the cartilage changes to a dull, bluish color, and the cartilage thickness is reduced. How much of this process is due to nutritional deficiency and how much is due to an upset in the stress-dependent metabolic homeostasis is not yet clear. The process is of sufficient significance, in any case, that it adds weight to the arguments for early remobilization of injured extremities.

Experiments on metabolism of cartilage segments subjected to pressure gradients have provided better insight into the quantitative relationships between load and metabolism. Lippiello and colleagues[47] showed that hydrostatic pressure between 75 and 300 psi resulted in 50 per cent reduction in incorporation of labeled substrates, whereas a pressure of 375 psi resulted in a 10 to 15 per cent increase in synthetic activity over normal. Intermittent compressive forces are shown by some investigators to stimulate synthetic activity of high density chick embryonic chondrocyte cultures.[48]

METABOLISM OF ARTICULAR CARTILAGE

It should come as no surprise that articular cartilage, a highly specialized, functionally complex tissue, should be active metabolically. The specialized functional structures of cartilage, the collagen fabric and the proteoglycan pump, require constant maintenance and renewal. The protein synthesis necessary to maintain these elements requires much the same complex synthetic apparatus as that present in other cells of the body. Indeed, the metabolic similarities of chondrocytes are more striking than the dissimilarities compared with other mammalian cell types.

Early anatomists and physiologists, however, tended to the view that articular cartilage had an insignificant metabolic rate. This was reinforced by histologic studies showing the avascular nature of the tissue and its sparse cellular population. In addition, early metabolic experiments seemed to support this concept.[49] Corrections for cell density expressing metabolic activity in relation to cellular volume altered that perception,[50] however. By most measures of cellular activity, cartilage cells are nearly equally active metabolically to other cell types from relatively avascular tissue sources.[51]

Some distinctive metabolic features of chondrocytes can be discerned with modern metabolic pathway analysis. Chondrocytes use anaerobic pathways for the most part,[49, 52] a choice well suited to the relative isolation of the cells, their lack of cell-to-cell contact, and their remote situation from capillary beds. Mankin[51] used autoradiographic techniques to demonstrate that ^{3}H-cytidine is incorporated into cells and that the messenger RNA inhibitor actinomycin D inhibited this incorporation dramatically. This evidence was adduced to show another similarity of chrondrocytes to the general pattern of mammalian cellular metabolism.

Proteoglycan aggregation and collagen cross linking both occur outside the cell. In this respect the chondrocyte is able to avoid a very troublesome problem, that of exporting and properly locating molecules much too large to diffuse through cartilage matrix. As it is, proteoglycan and procollagen are among the largest molecules mammalian cells are called on to synthesize. Each chain of procollagen has over 1000 amino acids, for example. The messenger RNA therefore is necessarily one of the largest in the cellular protein synthetic apparatus. The schemata for synthesis of collagen and proteoglycan are summarized in Figures 23–9 and 23–20. Each of these pathways is intricate. The general mode of synthesis for the proteoglycans involves primary formation of the protein core followed by addition of polysaccharide elements. This is thought to result from a stepwise glycosyl transfer from nucleotide sugars, beginning with transfer to a specific monosaccharide, xylose, to a specific amino acid sequence of the protein. Usually this sequence includes serine or threonine. Chain growth of the polysaccharide then occurs through a series of glycosyl transfer steps in which sugars are transferred to the nonreducing terminal monosaccharide of the lengthening polysaccharide side chain. Studies of the subcellular localization of biosynthesis of cartilage proteoglycans show that the enzymes catalyzing the transfer of the three sugars adjacent to the carbohydrate-protein linkage are found in highest concentration in the rough endoplasmic reticulum. Polymerizing enzymes necessary for the formation of disaccharide repeating units are distributed more uniformly between rough and smooth subcellular membrane fractions. It is as yet uncertain whether the monosaccharide transfers occur exclusively one by one to the growing polysaccharide chain, or whether part of the process might take place by assembly

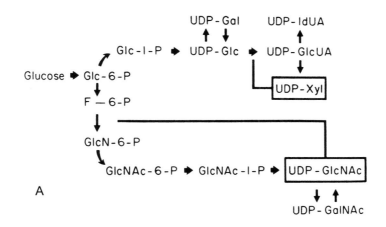

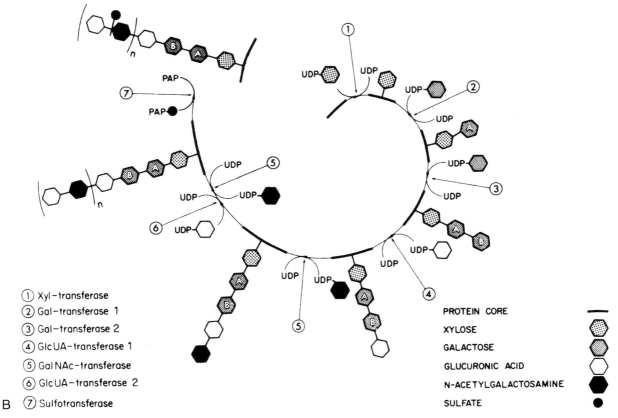

FIGURE 23–20. Proteoglycan synthesis. **A,** The pathways taken by uridine nucleotide sugars involved in mucopolysaccharide synthesis. **B,** The pathway of biosynthesis of a typical glycosaminoglycan, chondroitin-4-sulfate. (From Dorfman A, Matlon R: The mucopolysaccharidoses. In JB Stanbury, et al: The Metabolic Basis of Inherited Disease. 3rd Ed. New York, McGraw-Hill Book Co. 1972.)

of an oligosaccharide chain on a lipid intermediate prior to transfer to the proteoglycan molecule in a manner analogous to certain synthetic steps that occur in glycoprotein synthesis. What is clear is that the enzymes involved in these steps are highly specific. For example, the steps involved in assembly of chondroitin sulfate are shown in Figure 23–20 and require six specific enzymes. Further details of collagen and proteoglycan synthesis are beyond the scope of this chapter, and the interested reader is referred to more detailed reviews on the subject.[53-56]

ENZYMES OF ARTICULAR CARTILAGE

The continuation of normal function of articular cartilage depends on the special properties of the cartilage matrix constituents and maintenance of their normal concentration within the matrix. Thus, a constant turnover of the components of the matrix occurs. If the normal rate of degradation is increased or if synthesis of new matrix is interfered with, the concentration of the various articular cartilage components will change, and this is manifested by a particular disease process. The production, release, and actions of the various enzymes affecting articular cartilage are of primary importance in most articular cartilage diseases. Naturally occurring inhibitors exist in the synovial fluid or serum that can modify the actions of the matrix-degrading enzymes. The inhibitors, however, are mostly relatively large molecules and cannot reach the enzymes in the matrix unless the latter diffuse out of the matrix or until degradation of the matrix has caused an increase in its normal impermeability to molecules with molecular weights of above approximately 50,000, into which group the inhibitors fall. However, a much smaller polypeptide proteinase inhibitor with a molecular weight of 7000 has been isolated from human articular cartilage.[57] It is primarily a serine proteinase inhibitor, but it also can inhibit bacterial collagenase and pepsin. This inhibitor may localize at specific sites on proteoglycan complexes in the cartilage matrix and attenuate degradation by matrix proteinases. Investigators have described collagenase inhibitors isolated from bovine cartilage[58] and human articular cartilage[59] that also are believed to have a role in the regulation of extracellular matrix degradation.

The enzymes active on articular cartilage matrix may be divided into endogenous enzymes peculiar to the cartilage itself and exogenous enzymes arising in the synovium, polymorphonuclear leukocytes, macrophages, or blood serum.

Endogenous Enzymes

Lysosomes are intracytoplasmic vacuoles enclosed by a lipoprotein membrane that contain a number of enzymes responsible for the digestion of the proteoglycan and collagen molecules of articular cartilage matrix.[60] Chondrocytes may be stimulated to release the lysosomal enzymes to the exterior of the cell, where initial degradation of the macromolecules occurs. Subsequent diffusion of products from the matrix for intracellular digestion in the secondary or digestive lysosomes then occurs.[60] In this group of enzymes are the cathepsins, which have maximal activity at acid pH and little or no activity at the neutral pH of the cartilage matrix.[61-64] Only the cathepsins occurring in human articular cartilage are described here.

Cathepsin D is capable of degrading proteoglycan at pH 4.5 to 5.0. It has been shown by electrophoresis to exist in six multiple forms.[65] Extracellular cathepsin D is found mainly in the immediate pericellular region of the chondrocytes,[66] which may in fact have a lower pH than the remainder of cartilage matrix. Cathepsin D splits the polypeptide backbone of proteoglycan without attacking the polysaccharide side chain. The products of this cleavage, the peptide fragments with polysaccharide chains attached, then are able to diffuse into the cells for completion of degradation. Although it is incapable of degrading collagen even at acid pH, cathepsin D is, quantitatively, the most important autolytic enzyme in articular cartilage. Cathepsin D activity in the chondrocytes of guinea pig articular cartilage was found to decrease during growth and midlife and to increase during the later part of life.[67] The range of this activity over the life span of the animals was narrow, which suggests that the process of degradation influenced by cathepsin D proceeds at a relatively uniform rate throughout life in normal cartilage.

Cathepsin B_1 has a maximal activity at pH 6, at which it can degrade both proteoglycans[68] and collagen.[69] Unlike cathepsin D, it is still active at neutral pH[70] and thus may be more important in the normal physiologic turnover of proteoglycans. Both cathepsins B_1 and D show greater activity in the surface layers of articular cartilage than in progressively deeper layers,[68] and a progressive decrease of cathepsin B_1 activity appears to occur with increasing age.

Cathepsin F also is present in cartilage, but its function is not well known.[71, 72]

Pepstatin has been found to inhibit the action of cathepsin D, and this action has been used to demonstrate that other acid and neutral proteases are capable of degrading proteoglycan.[65] Thus, one neutral and two acid metalloproteases have been isolated from human articular cartilage and have been shown to degrade purified nasal septum proteoglycan.[73] The neutral metalloprotease is optimally active at pH 7.25. Overall, cathepsins B_1 and D should have maximum activity at pericellular pH, which normally is acid. This would leave the neutral metalloproteinases to degrade the interterritorial proteoglycan matrix. The acid metalloproteases are distinct from cathepsins B, D, and F and digest proteoglycan subunit at pH 4.5 and 5.5. Neutral proteases may be implicated as mediators of physiologic turnover of ground substance and in pathologic processes such as osteoarthritis.

Arylsulfatase also is capable of initiating the degradation of proteoglycan,[74] and levels of this enzyme have been shown to be elevated in experimental degenerative articular disease[75] and in the synovial fluid of patients with rheumatoid arthritis or osteoarthritis.[76] In addition, vitamin E appears to inhibit arylsulfatase in chondrocyte cultures.[77]

Acid and alkaline phosphatases also are found in the lysosomes,[78, 79] and alkaline phosphatase is present in extracellular matrix vesicles. Alkaline phosphatase is found only in the deeper cells of articular cartilage[80, 81] and may be related to a continuous process of remodeling at the osteochondral junction. Aging changes of enzyme activity have been examined in guinea pigs.[82] The activity of alkaline phosphatase was found to have declined steadily over 2 weeks to 5¾ years, whereas the activity of the glycolytic enzymes in individual chondrocytes increased with advancing age. Acid phosphatase activity showed no consistent pattern of change with aging.

Collagenases are capable of degrading native collagen at physiologic pH and cleaving the helical part of the molecule into an amino terminal 75 per cent fragment and a carboxy terminal 25 per cent fragment.[83] The two smaller fragments denature spontaneously and in their uncoiled state are susceptible to digestion by extracellular proteases. Type II collagen (which is the normally occurring type in articular cartilage) is less susceptible to collagenase than is interstitial type I collagen.[84–86] Cross-linked collagen is very much less sensitive to specific collagenase than it is to non–cross-linked collagenase,[87, 88] and this helps to explain why recently synthesized collagen is especially susceptible to degradation.[89] Conversely, as articular cartilage ages, the formation of intermolecular cross links of the collagen may make the tissue more resistant to breakdown by enzymes.[90, 91] Collagenase has been demonstrated in human osteoarthritic cartilage[92] and is produced by normal rabbit articular chondrocytes.[93] It appears likely, although it has not yet been proved, that a collagenase also is a necessary mediator in the normal slow turnover of human cartilage collagen.

Cathepsin D and collagenase have been shown to affect the hydraulic permeability of articular cartilage.[94] Thus, the enzymes, by altering the flow of essential metabolites from the matrix, or the exposure of chondrocytes to toxins and immunoglobulins normally excluded from the cell, may further aid in degradation of the articular cartilage.

Lysozyme, first described by Fleming and Allison in 1922,[95] belongs to the glycosidase group of enzymes capable of carbohydrate hydrolysis. It is found in numerous locations in the human body, articular cartilage being one site of them. It is synthesized in the chondrocytes and then is released immediately into the territorial matrix, without prior storage in the lysosomes.[96, 97] Lysozyme is found mainly in the deepest layer of articular cartilage.[98] It may be of importance in the final stages of polymer breakdown. Beta-glucuronidase[99] and β-N-acetylglucosaminidase[100] also have been demonstrated histochemically in cartilage and are considered to be involved in polysaccharide depolymerization. Hyaluronidase, which theoretically could attack the hyaluronic acid core of the proteoglycan molecule, has not been found in normal or diseased articular cartilage.[101, 102]

Exogenous Enzymes

The exogenous enzymes affecting articular cartilage matrix may arise from the synovium of the joint and then be secreted into the synovial fluid from lysosomes of both type A and type B lining cells. Enzymes in this category include protease, collagenase, and hyaluronidase.[65, 103] In addition, in pathologic situations, when polymorphonucleocytes and macrophages reach the joint cavity, they may secrete a collagenase,[104] lysozyme,[60] or neutral protease,[105–108] the last being distinguished from the proteases occurring in the synovial membrane. Some studies indicate further that polymorphonuclear leukocytes contain three enzymes, β-glucuronidase, β-N-acetylgalactosaminidase, and a sulfatase, which act synergistically to degrade cartilage-derived chondroitin sulfate further into monosaccharides and inorganic sulfate.[109]

Collagenases have been implicated in several types of arthritis and have been detected in the synovium in rheumatoid arthritis and nonspecific inflammatory synovial conditions. All synovial tissues have the capacity to produce collagenase; however, it is likely that only in states of chronic proliferative synovitis and inflammation is collagenase produced in sufficient quantities to bring about the destruction of articular tissue. Although type II collagen is a poorer substrate for collagenase than interstitial type I collagen, cleavage of the triple helix of collagen can be augmented significantly by raising the temperature above the normal range of 33° to 36°C. Thus, in the inflamed joint affected by rheumatoid arthritis in which the joint temperature is raised,[110] the rate of cartilage degradation by collagenase would be increased.

In this group of exogenous enzymes is plasmin, a proteolytic enzyme derived from the blood. Plasmin is activated from plasminogen by several factors, including the kinases of streptococci and staphylococci. It normally acts as a fibrinolytic agent but when present in excess could theoretically attack the protein of cartilage matrix.[111, 112] Cartilage degradation caused by this enzyme has not been substantiated as occurring in vivo, however.[75, 113, 114]

Finally, mention should be made of the cytokines such as interleukin and tumor necrosis factor that can stimulate and modulate the activities of various enzymes, which in turn can affect the metabolism of articular cartilage directly. Thus, increased destruction of the extracellular matrix of human articular cartilage occurred in organ culture in the presence of interleukin-1β. Concomitantly with the cartilage destruction, increased release of metalloproteinases was measured. The metalloproteinase precursors therefore are thought to be stimulated by interleukin-1 with the final result being cartilage matrix degradation.[115] In turn, the cytokines may be modulated by local wound hormones; thus, platelet-derived growth factor may enhance the interleukin-1 α effects of metalloproteinase activity.[116] A complex interaction between local tissue hormones influencing cartilage metabolism through their effects on cytokines and subsequently through the cytokine effect on enzymatic digestion of the cartilage thus can be visualized.

ENZYMES IN ARTICULAR CARTILAGE DISEASE PROCESSES

The avascular nature of adult cartilage has a bearing on its limited capacity to respond to various insults, whether inflammatory, mechanical, or biomechanical. Thus, although adult joint cartilage has some potential for repair, a given insult usually will result in a degenerative lesion mediated by endogenous or exogenous enzymes.

Osteoarthritis

The cause of articular cartilage destruction in osteoarthritis certainly may be mechanical, but part of the matrix degradation most likely is due to enzymatic action. An increase may occur in the activity of enzymes involved in the normal turnover of the matrix, or the degradation may be due to production and release of special enzymes. The fact that secondary lysosomes are rare in normal articular cartilage but are found readily in the chondrocytes of osteoarthritic cartilage[117, 118] adds weight to this theory. The degradation process is mainly extracellular, but it may be completed within the cell.[119]

Several of the endogenous enzymes mentioned previously have been implicated in osteoarthritis. Cathepsin D was thought to be important in the process,[62–64, 120] but because its greatest activity is at pH 4.5 to 5, this enzyme is difficult to accept as a significant factor in the neutral pH environment of the matrix of articular cartilage. Indeed, Hembry and colleagues[121] present strong experimental evidence that cathepsin D is not responsible for the degradation of articular cartilage. Nevertheless, cathepsin D levels are elevated in intracellular and extracellular situations in osteoarthritic cartilage, although this may be explained to some extent by the increased cellularity of osteoarthritic cartilage.[64, 68, 122] It may be that the microenvironment around the chondrocyte cell is more acid than the rest of the cartilage matrix, and it is mainly in this situation that cathepsin D is found and acts.[60] Because osteoarthritic synovial fluid contains only one fiftieth as much cathepsin D activity as cartilage, it is thought that the chondrocytes are the major or only source of this enzyme.[64] The focal nature of the increased cathepsin D activity in articular cartilage also has been demonstrated.[122]

The importance and possible mechanism of action of cathepsin B in causing a more severe osteoarthritic lesion has been described. Thus, in osteoarthritic cartilaginous tissue an imbalance between cathepsin B levels and its inhibitor was found. Therefore, if additional cathepsin B is released into the extracellular tissue, the capacity of the specific inhibitor to neutralize the enzyme is overcome and degradation of the extracellular matrix occurs.[123]

The discovery of neutral proteases in human osteoarthritic articular cartilage provides an explanation for the initiation of cartilage degradation at neutral pH.[65, 124, 125] Arylsulfatases A and B are lysosomal enzymes that also may be incriminated in the degradation of proteoglycan in osteoarthritic cartilage.[74, 126] Their activity helps to explain the increased sulfate levels in the joint fluid and loss of chondroitin sulfate from the affected cartilage of patients with osteoarthritis. Levels of both arylsulfatases A and B are elevated in osteoarthritic cartilage but that of arylsulfatase B to a greater extent. The role of arylsulfatase B in chondroitin sulfate degradation possibly is substantiated by the increased activity of this enzyme in Hurler's disease.[127]

Although a collagenase capable of splitting the collagen molecule has not been found in normal cartilage, it is present in osteoarthritic human cartilage and is believed to be extralysosomal in origin. It probably is present in minute quantities and its demonstration necessitated prior removal of an inhibitor.[92] Collagenase does occur in the synovial tissue of joints affected by osteoarthritis[128] and has been produced by synovial explants from joints affected by osteoarthritis but in lesser amounts than in rheumatoid arthritis.[129] Neither the hydroxyproline content nor the extractability of collagen is affected in osteoarthritis.[101] In severe osteoarthritis, however, total loss of articular cartilage occurs.

In osteoarthritic cartilage, an elevation in the levels of acid and alkaline phosphatase activities has been found.[122] In addition, a direct relationship between acid phosphatase levels and the severity of the osteoarthritic process has been noted.[78] The same workers demonstrated an even higher level of phosphatase activity in the cartilage of marginal

osteophytes than in that of more central lesions,[78] and the level of acid phosphatase in chondrocyte cultures derived from osteoarthritic cartilage was observed to be elevated in comparison with normal chondrocytes grown under identical conditions.[130] High alkaline phosphatase levels also have been found to occur in association with increased levels of 5'-adenosine monophosphatase and adenosine triphosphate pyrophosphohydrolase in osteoarthritic cartilage and may have significance in the calcification sometimes developing in such cartilage[131] as well as in the cartilage of pyrophosphate deposition disease.

Bollett and Nance[132] reported a decrease in glycosaminoglycan chain length in osteoarthritic articular cartilage and suggested the presence of an hyaluronidase-like enzyme as part of the degenerative process. This logical theory has not been substantiated by finding hyaluronidase in normal or arthritic articular cartilage.[133] Lack and Rogers[111] suggested that plasmin activated by joint damage could attack cartilage proteoglycan and therefore be a factor in degenerative arthritis. This theory could not be substantiated in an experiment in which the intra-articular injection of large doses of plasmin was not followed by articular cartilage damage. This result may be explained by the normal presence of antiplasmin in synovial fluid.[134, 135]

Lysozyme also has been implicated in the osteoarthritic lesion by the finding of significant elevations of the enzyme in hip and knee joint cartilage affected by osteoarthritis.[136] The lysozymal levels were higher in early than in late lesions. It was thought that lysozyme had a hyaluronidase-like activity and could affect link protein.

Various cytokines likewise are of importance in the development of osteoarthritis. Thus, several studies have shown that interleukin-1[137–140] has an effect on proteoglycan metabolism. Also, in an animal model of osteoarthritis produced in the canine knee by sectioning the anterior cruciate ligament, a very high level of interleukin-6 was measured in the knee synovial fluid in the early stages of the experimental arthritis. The high levels of interleukin-6 in the synovial fluid could act directly on articular cartilage chondrocytes and play a role in mediating their responses to cartilage injury.[141] The cytokines tumor necrosis factor,[138, 139, 164] stromelysin,[142] and fibronectin[143] also are involved in the development of osteoarthritis.

One additional aspect of enzyme effects in the osteoarthritic process is the nature of the matrix synthesis response of chondrocytes to lysosomal enzymes. Thus, although the collagen content of osteoarthritic cartilage does not change, the cartilage synthesizes type I collagen in addition to the usual type II collagen. Deshmukh and Nimni[144] demonstrated that lysosomal enzymes could produce the same effect on articular cartilage in vivo. Thus, the enzymes altered the function of chondrocytes, causing them to synthesize nonspecific collagen molecules, which might lead to weakening of the mechanical structure of the cartilage and its subsequent mechanical destruction.

Rheumatoid Arthritis

Rheumatoid arthritis is characterized by destruction of articular cartilage. An as yet unknown stimulus to the synovial lining cells is involved in this disease and causes hyperplasia and hypertrophy of the cells. The resulting inflammatory rheumatoid tissue, or pannus, growing over and under the articular cartilage is thought to release greatly increased amounts of intracellular lysosomal enzymes, which irreversibly destroy proteoglycan and collagen to produce the erosive focal lesion in the cartilage.[66, 145–147] A considerable increase in activity of many of the lysosomal enzymes, such as acid phosphatase, β-glucuronidase, β-acetylglucosaminidase, cathepsin D, and collagenase, has been found in the synovium and synovial fluid of patients with rheumatoid arthritis and provides evidence for their role in the cartilage erosion that occurs in this disease.[108, 128, 147–150]

Woolley and coworkers[147] showed, by an immunofluorescent technique, the specific localization of collagenase to a 20 to 60 per cent length of the cartilage-pannus interface and only minimal distribution of collagenase to areas remote from the erosion front. Harris and McCroskery[85] have explained how synovial collagenase, once in contact with the cartilage, can degrade articular cartilage collagen in rheumatoid arthritic joints. Another cathepsin-type enzyme, leucine aminopeptidase, has been demonstrated in synovial lining cells, in pannus, and in cartilage in rheumatoid arthritis; it may be a significant factor in cartilage damage.[151]

The levels of β-acetylglucosaminidase and cathepsin D also were found to be raised in rheumatoid articular cartilage, but these levels did not correlate with the levels of these same enzymes in the synovial membrane.[152] Poole and associates,[66] although not ruling out the possibility that chondrocytes secrete the enzyme, thought that cathepsin D essentially was restricted to synovial and pannus tissue. Activity of the rheumatoid process was found not to be correlated with enzyme levels by Collins and Cosh.[153] although, conversely, Granda and associates[154] found close correlation between cathepsin D activity and an increased severity of the rheumatoid process. Other cellular sources for lysosomal enzyme release are the polymorphonuclear leukocytes and lymphocyte clusters that are present in large numbers in the inflamed synovial cavity and in the synovium, respectively, in rheumatoid arthritis.[108, 155] In addition, the levels of lysozyme in serum and synovial fluid are increased in rheumatoid arthritis and may accompany the loss of cartilage glycosaminoglycans seen in this disease.[97] In contradistinction, in the arthritis of systemic lupus erythematosus, in which usually no cartilage destruction occurs, normal serum lysozyme levels are seen.[156] The fact that continued inflammation hastens cartilage lysis implies that, in treatment, inflammation should be suppressed to reduce lysosomal protease accumulation and synovial collagenase production.

Although not an enzyme, catabolin, which may be implicated in the pathologic sequence in rheumatoid arthritis, has been identified in porcine synovial culture medium, and a similar substance has been isolated from cultures of rheumatoid synovium. The substance stimulates chondrocyte-mediated cartilage matrix breakdown, although the mechanism of this stimulation is at present unknown.

Enzymatic destruction is only one of several potential mechanisms of articular cartilage destruction in rheumatoid arthritis. Thus, immune complex formation, activation of complement, formation of free radicals, and cytokine production also may be important. The cytokine interleukin-1 produced by monocytes under the influence of T lymphokines is believed to induce glycosaminoglycan release from articular cartilage. Interleukin-1 may in fact be the major cartilage catabolic factor in rheumatoid arthritis.[157]

Pyogenic Arthritis

The result of untreated pyogenic arthritis is a severe and rapid destruction of joint cartilage,[103] which invariably evolves into an osteoarthritic process and possibly leads to fibrous or bony ankylosis. The extensive proteoglycan degradation of cartilage is due to the action of several proteinases, which may be derived from neutrophil leukocytes. The leukocytes can release their lysosomal enzymes on encountering bacteria or after eventual death of the leukocytes.[108] The proteinases incriminated are elastase, cathepsin G, and collagenase, all of which are active at neutral pH.[106, 158, 159] The proteinases elastase and cathepsin G could attack first the proteoglycan molecule and subsequently the collagen molecule.[106] Lazarus and colleagues[160] described how the collagenase and a proteinase found in polymorphonuclear leukocytes can act synergistically to achieve maximal collagen breakdown. Final confirmation of this mode of cartilage destruction in vivo is awaited. In the body, various inhibitors are secreted into the synovial fluid that can prevent the extracellular activity of these above-mentioned enzymes. It does, however, seem logical that in the treatment of septic joints removal of polymorphonuclear leukocytes by operation or aspiration is essential to minimize cartilage destruction.[161]

The fibrinolytic enzyme plasmin is produced in synovial fluid by the action of staphylococcal and streptococcal kinases and disrupted leukocytes on plasminogen. Plasmin could then degrade the proteoglycan of articular cartilage matrix.[111, 112, 162] Plasmin then may be an additional factor in cartilage destruction in pyogenic arthritis, but not in tuberculosis, because the tubercle bacillus does not produce an activator of plasminogen similar to the kinases of staphylococci and streptococci.

The cartilage degradation occurring in an environment of chronic inflammation may particularly involve the metalloproteinase gelatinase. Thus, one study in which cartilage was implanted into a murine air pouch, producing granulation tissue, showed that gelatinase was by far the most important degradative enzyme, although collagenase and stromelysin activities also were detected.[163]

SUMMARY

This chapter reviews the structure of articular cartilage in relation to its special functions. The components of the matrix in which the chondrocytes are dispersed are described in detail with regard to their chemistry, synthesis, maturation, and unique interactions that allow articular cartilage to fulfill those special functions. The mechanisms for load carriage, lubrication, and nutrition and their interrelationships are explained. Some of the distinctive metabolic activities relating to chondrocyte function in the maintenance of the cartilage matrix are described. Finally, the endogenous and exogenous enzymes of articular cartilage and their role, together with that of the cytokines, in maintaining tissue health and in provoking disease are discussed.

References

1. Ogston AG: The biological functions of the glycosaminoglycans. *In* EA Balazs (Ed): Chemistry and Molecular Biology of the Intercellular Matrix. Vol 3. London, Academic Press, 1970, p 1231.
2. Benninghoff A: Form und Bau der Gelenkknorpel in ihren Beziehungen zur Funktion. Z Anat Entwicklungsgesch *76:*43, 1925.
3. Little K, Pimm LH, Trueta J: Osteoarthritis of the hip: An electron microscope study. J Bone Joint Surg [Br] *40:*123, 1958.
4. Weiss C, Rosenberg L, Helfet AJ: An ultrastructural study of normal young adult human articular cartilage. J Bone Joint Surg [Am] *50:*663, 1968.
5. McCutchen CW: The frictional properties of animal joints. Wear *5:*1, 1962.
6. Hultkrantz W: Über die Spaltrichtungen der Gelenkknorpel. Verhandlungen der Anatomischen Gesellschaft *12:*248, 1898.
7. Langer C: Zur Anatomie und Physiologie der Haut. Sitzungsb d k Acad Wissensch *45:*223, 1861.
8. Bullough P, Goodfellow J: The significance of the fine structure of articular cartilage. J Bone Joint Surg [Br] *50:*852, 1968.
9. Clark JM: The organization of collagen in cryofractured rabbit articular cartilage: A scanning electron microscopic study. J Orthop Res *3:*17, 1985.
10. Glimcher MJ, Krane SM: The organization and structure of bone, and the mechanism of calcification. *In* BS Gould (Ed): Treatise on Collagen. Vol 2. Biology of Collagen. New York, Academic Press, 1968, p 67.
11. Mathews MB: Collagen. *In* Connective Tissue: Macromolecular Structure and Evolution. New York, Springer-Verlag, 1975, p 15.
12. Amiel D, Billings E Jr, Akeson WH: Ligament structure, chemistry, and physiology. *In* D Daniel, WH Akeson, J O'Connor (Eds): Knee Ligaments: Structure, Function, Injury, and Repair. New York, Raven Press, 1990, p 77.
13. Eyre DR, Wu JJ, Woods P: Cartilage-specific collagens: Structural studies. *In* K Kuettner et al (Eds): Articular Cartilage and Osteoarthritis. New York, Raven Press, 1992, p 119.
14. Mayne R, Burgeson RE: Structure and Function of Collagen Types. Orlando, Fla, Academic Press, 1987.
15. Piez KA: Characterization of a collagen from codfish skin containing three chromatographically different α chains. Biochemistry *4:*2590, 1965.
16. Miller EG, Matukas VJ: Chick cartilage collagen. A new type of α1 chain not present in bone or skin of the species. Proc Natl Acad Sci USA *64:*1264, 1969.
17. Pan T-C, Zhang RZ, Mattei MG, et al: Cloning and chromosomal location of human α₁(XVI) collagen. Proc Natl Acad Sci USA *89:*6565, 1992.
18. Van der Rest M, Garrone R: Collagen family of proteins, FASEB *5:*2814, 1991.
19. Piez KA: Cross-linking of collagen and elastin. Ann Rev Biochem *37:*547, 1968.
20. Franzblau C: Elastin. *In* M Florkin, EH Stotz (Eds): Comprehensive Biochemistry. Vol 13. Amsterdam, Elsevier, 1971, p 659.
21. Kang AH, Gross J: Relationship between the intra- and intermolecular crosslinks of collagen. Proc Natl Acad Sci USA *67:*1307, 1970.
22. Gallop PM, Blumenfeld OO, Seifter S: Structure and metabolism of connective tissue proteins. Ann Rev Biochem *41:*617, 1972.
23. Tanzer ML: Cross-linking of collagen (endogenous aldehydes in collagen react in several ways to form a variety of unique covalent cross-links). Science *180:*561, 1973.
24. Vuorio E, deCrombruggle B: The family of collagen genes. Annu Rev Biochem *59:*837, 1990.
25. Wu JJ, Eyre DR: Cartilage type IX collagen is cross-linked by hydroxypyridinium residues, Biochem Biophys Res Commun *123:*1033, 1984.
26. Mathews MB: Polyanionic proteoglycans. *In* Molecular Biology, Biochemistry, and Biophysics Series, Vol. 19. Connective Tissue: Macromolecular Structure and Evolution. New York, Springer-Verlag, 1975, p 93.
27. Anderson RS, Schwartz ER: Phosphorylation of proteoglycans. Identification of phosphorphylation sites in chondroitin sulfate-rich region of core protein. Arthritis Rheum *28:*804, 1985.
28. Rosenberg LC, Choi HU, Tang LH, et al: Isolation of dermatan sulfate proteoglycans from mature bovine articular cartilages. J Biol Chem *260:*6304, 1985.
29. Hardingham TE, Muir H: The specific interaction of hyaluronic acid with cartilage proteoglycans. Biochim Biophys Acta *279:*401, 1972.
30. Sajdera SW, Hascall VC: Protein-polysaccharide complex from bovine nasal cartilage. A comparison of low and high shear extraction procedures. J Biol Chem *244:*77, 1969.
31. Gregory JD: Multiple aggregation factors in cartilage proteoglycan. Biochem J *133:*383, 1973.
32. Heinegaard D, Hascall VC: Aggregation of cartilage proteoglycans. III. Characteristics of the proteins isolated from trypsin digests of aggregates. J Biol Chem *249:*4250, 1974.
33. Hascall VC, Sajdera SW: Protein polysaccharide complex from bovine nasal cartilage: The function of glycoprotein in the formation of aggregates. J Biol Chem *244:*2384, 1969.
34. Fife RS, Caterson B, Meyers SL: Identification of link proteins in canine synovial cell cultures and canine articular cartilage. J Cell Biol *100:*1050, 1985.
35. Freshchenko SP, Krasnopol'skaia KD, Shiskin SS: Components of proteoglycan aggregates in human hyaline cartilage. Biokhimiia *49:*1679, 1984.
36. Rosenberg L: Structure of cartilage proteoglycans. *In* WH Simon (Ed): The Human Joint in Health and Disease. Philadelphia. University of Pennsylvania Press, 1978.
37. Campo RD, Tourtellotte CD: The composition of bovine cartilage and bone. Biochim Biophys Acta *141:*614, 1967.
38. Eichelberger L, Akeson WH, Roma M: Biochemical studies of articular cartilage. I. Normal values. J Bone Joint Surg [Am] *40:*142, 1958.
39. Mankin HJ, Thrasher AZ: Water content and binding in normal and osteoarthritic human cartilage. J Bone Joint Surg [Am] *57:*76, 1975.
40. Jaffe FF, Mankin HJ, Weiss C, et al: Water binding in the articular cartilage of rabbits. J Bone Joint Surg [Am] *56:*1031, 1974.
41. Maroudas A: Physicochemical properties of articular cartilage. *In* MAR Freeman (Ed): Adult Articular Cartilage. London, Pitman, 1973.
42. Linn FC, Sokoloff LH: Movement and composition of interstitial fluid of cartilage. Arthritis Rheum *8:*481, 1965.
43. Linn FC: Lubrication of animal joints. I. The Arthrotripsometer. J. Bone Joint Surg [Am] *49:*1079, 1967.
44. Mow VC, Mansour JM, Redler I: The movement of interstitial fluid through normal and pathological cartilage during articulation. *In* JA Brighton, S Goldman (Eds): Advances in Bioengineering: Transactions of the American Society of Mechanical Engineers, p 177, 1974.
45. Lotke PA: Diffusion in cartilage. *In* WH Simon (Ed): The Human Joint in Health and Disease. Philadelphia, University of Pennsylvania Press, 1978.
46. Akeson WH, Eichelberger L, Roma M: Biochemical studies of articular cartilage. II. Values following denervation of an extremity. J Bone Joint Surg [Am] *40:*153, 1958.
47. Lippiello L, Kaye C, Neumata T, et al: In vitro metabolic response of articular cartilage segments to low levels of hydrostatic pressure. Connect Tissue Res *13:*99, 1985.
48. van Kampen GP, Veldhuijzen JP, Kuijer R, et al: Cartilage response to mechanical force in high-density chondrocyte cultures. Arthritis Rheum *28:*419, 1985.
49. Bywaters ECL: The metabolism of joint tissues. J Pathol Bacteriol *44:*247, 1937.
50. Rosenthal O, Bowie MA, Wagoner G: Studies on the metabolism of articular cartilage. I. Respiration and glycolysis of cartilage in relation to its age. J Cell Comp Physiol *17:*221, 1941.
51. Mankin HJ: The metabolism of articular cartilage in health and disease. *In* PMC Burleigh, AR Poole (Eds): Dynamics of Connective Tissue Macromolecules. New York, American Elsevier, 1975, p 327.
52. Tushan FS, Rodnan GP, Altman M, et al: Aerobic glycolysis and lactate dehydrogenase (LDH) isoenzymes in articular cartilage. J Lab Clin Med *73:*649, 1969.
53. Roden L, Schwartz NB: Biosynthesis of connective tissue proteoglycans. *In* WJ Whelan (Ed): MTP International Review of Science: Biochemistry Section. Biochemistry of Carbohydrates. Baltimore, University Park Press, 1975.
54. Muir H: Structure and function of proteoglycan of cartilage and cell-matrix interactions. *In* JW Lash, MM Burger (Eds): Cell and Tissue Interactions. New York, Raven Press, 1977.
55. Prockop DJ, Kivirikko KI, Tuderman L, et al: Biosynthesis of collagen and its disorders. Part I. N Engl J Med *301:*13, 1979.
56. Prockop DJ, Kivirikko KI, Tuderman L, et al: Biosynthesis of collagen and its disorders. Part II. N Engl J Med *301:*77, 1979.
57. Lesjak MS, Ghosh P: Polypeptide proteinase inhibitor from human articular cartilage. Biochim Biophys Acta *789:*166, 1984.
58. Bunning RAD, Murphy G, Kumar S, et al: Metalloproteinase inhibitors from bovine cartilage and body fluids. Eur J Biochem *139:*75, 1984.
59. Dean DD, Woessner JF Jr: extracts of human articular cartilage contain an inhibitor of tissue metalloproteinases. Biochem J *218:*277, 1984.
60. Dingle, JT: The role of lysosomal enzymes in skeletal tissues. J Bone Joint Surg [Br] *55:*87, 1973.
61. Fessel JM, Chrisman OD: Enzymatic degradation of chondromucoprotein by cell free extracts of human cartilage. Arthritis Rheum *7:*398, 1964.
62. Ali SY, Evans L, Stainthorpe E, et al: Characterization of cathepsins in cartilage. Biochem J *105:*549, 1967.
63. Woessner JF: Cartilage cathepsin D and its action on matrix components. Fed Proc *32:*1485, 1973.
64. Sapolsky AI, Altman RD, Howell DS: Cathepsin D activity in normal and osteoarthritis human cartilage. Fed Proc *32:*1489, 1973.
65. Sapolsky AI, Howell DS, Woessner JF: Neutral proteases and cathepsin D in human articular cartilage. J Clin Invest *53:*1044, 1974.
66. Poole AR, Hembry RM, Dingle JT, et al: Secretion and localization of cathepsin D in synovial tissues removed from rheumatoid and traumatized joints. Arthritis Rheum *19:*1295, 1976.
67. Silberberg R, Lesker PA: Enzyme activity in aging articular cartilage. Experientia *27:*133, 1971.
68. Bayliss MT, Ali SY: Studies on cathepsin B in human articular cartilage. Biochem J *171:*149, 1978.
69. Burleigh MC, Barrett AJ, Lazarus GS: A lysosomal enzyme that degrades native collagen. Biochem J *137:*387, 1974.
70. Morrison RIG, Barrett AJ, Dingle JT, et al: Cathepsins B₁ and D: Action on human cartilage proteoglycans. Biochim Biophys Acta *302:*411, 1973.
71. Barrett AJ: The enzymic degradation of cartilage matrix. *In* PMC Burleigh, AR Poole (Eds): Dynamics of Connective Tissue Macromolecules. New York, American Elsevier, 1975, p 189.
72. Blow AMJ: Detection and characterization of cathepsin F, a cartilage enzyme that degrades proteoglycan. Ital J Biochem *24:*13, 1975.
73. Sapolsky AI, Keiser H, Howell DS, et al: Metalloproteases of human articular cartilage that digest cartilage proteoglycan at neutral and acid pH. J Clin Invest *58:*1030, 1976.
74. Schwartz ER, Ogle RC, Thompson RC: Aryl sulfatase activities in normal and pathologic human articular cartilage. Arthritis Rheum *17:*455, 1974.

75. Thompson RC, Clark I: Acid hydrolases in slices of articular cartilage and synovium from normal and abnormal joints. Proc Soc Exp Biol Med *133:*1102, 1970.

76. Peltonen L, Puranen J, Korhonen LK: Lysosomal hydrolases in different compartments of rheumatoid and osteoarthritic joints. Scand J Rheum *10:*97, 1981.

77. Schwartz ER: Action of vitamin E on enzymes and sulfated proteoglycans in human articular cartilage. Transactions of the 25th Annual Meeting, Orthopaedic Research Society, San Francisco, California, Feb 20–22, 1979, p 43.

78. Ehrlich MG, Mankin HJ, Treadwell BV: Acid hydrolase activity in osteoarthritic and normal human cartilage. J Bone Joint Surg [Am] *55:*1068, 1973.

79. Ali SY, Bayliss MT: Enzymic changes in human osteoarthritic cartilage. *In* SY Ali, MW Elves, DH Leaback (Eds): Normal and Osteoarthrotic Articular Cartilage. London, Institute of Orthopaedics, 1974, p 189.

80. Zorzoli A: The histochemical localization of alkaline phosphatase in demineralized bones of mice of different ages. Anat Rec *102:*445, 1948.

81. Shaw NE, Martin BF: Histological and histochemical studies on mammalian knee joint tissues. J Anat *96:*359, 1962.

82. Silberberg R, Stamp WG, Lesker PA, et al: Aging changes in ultrastructure and enzymatic activity of articular cartilage of guinea pigs. J Gerontol *25:*184, 1970.

83. Gross J, Nagai Y: Specific degradation of the collagen molecule by tadpole collagenolytic enzyme. Proc Natl Acad Sci USA *54:*1197, 1965.

84. Woolley DE, Glanville RW, Lindberg KA, et al: Action of human skin collagenase on cartilage collagen. FEBS Lett *34:*267, 1973.

85. Harris ED Jr, McCroskery PA: The influence of temperature and fibril stability on degradation of cartilage collagen by rheumatoid synovial collagenase. N Engl J Med *290:*1, 1974.

86. Woolley DE, Lindberg KA, Glanville RW, et al: Action of rheumatoid synovial collagenase on cartilage collagen. Eur J Biochem *50:*437, 1975.

87. Harris ED Jr, Farrell ME: Resistance to collagenase: A characteristic of collagen fibrils cross-linked with formaldehyde. Biochim Biophys Acta *278:*133, 1972.

88. Steven FS: Observations on the different substrate behaviour of tropocollagen molecules in solution and intermolecularly cross-linked tropocollagen within insoluble polymeric collagen fibrils. Biochem J *155:*391, 1976.

89. Gross J, Bruschi AB: The pattern of collagen degradation in cultured tadpole tissues. Dev Biol *26:*36, 1971.

90. Jolma VH, Hruza Z: Differences in properties of newly formed collagen during aging and parabiosis. J Gerontol *27:*178, 1972.

91. Lust G, Pronsky W: Glycosaminoglycan metabolism in normal and arthritic cartilage. Fed Proc *31:*883A, 1972.

92. Ehrlich MG, Mankin HJ, Jones H, et al: Collagenase and collagenase inhibitors in osteoarthritic and normal human cartilage. J Clin Invest *59:*226, 1977.

93. Malemud CJ, Norby DP, Sapolsky AI, et al: Neutral proteinases from articular chondrocytes in cultures. I. A latent collagenase that degrades human cartilage type II collagen. Biochim Biophys Acta *657:*517, 1981.

94. Lotke PA, Granda JL: Alterations in the permeability of articular cartilage by proteolytic enzymes. Arthritis Rheum *15:*302, 1972.

95. Fleming A, Allison VD: Observations on a bacteriolytic substance (lysozyme) found in secretions and tissues. Br J Exp Pathol *3:*252, 1922.

96. Kuettner KE, Eisenstein R, Soble LW, et al: Lysozyme in epiphyseal cartilage: IV. Embryonic chick cartilage lysozyme—its localization and partial characterization. J Cell Biol *49:*450, 1971.

97. Greenwald RA, Josephson AS, Diamond HS, et al: Human cartilage lysozyme. J Clin Invest *51:*2264, 1972.

98. Kuettner KE, Guenther HL, Ray RD, et al: Lysozyme in preosseous cartilage. Calcif Tissue Res *1:*298, 1968.

99. Gubisch W, Schlager F: Fermente im Knochen- und Knorpel-gewebe. III. Mitteilung: β-D-Glucuronidase. Acta Histochem *12:*69, 1961.

100. Pugh D, Walker PG: Localization of N-acetyl-β-glucosaminidase in tissues. J Histochem Cytochem *9:*242, 1961.

101. Bollett AJ, Bonner WM, Nance JL: The presence of hyaluronidase in various mammalian tissues. J Biol Chem *238:*3522, 1963.

102. Wasteson A, Amado R, Ingmar B, Heldin CH: Degradation of chondroitin sulfate by lysosomal enzymes from embryonic chick cartilage. *In* H Peeters (Ed): Protides of the Biological Fluids. New York, Pergamon Press, 1975, p 431.

103. Weissmann G, Spilberg I: Breakdown of cartilage proteinpolysaccharide by lysosomes. Arthritis Rheum *11:*162, 1968.

104. Lazarus GS, Daniels JR, Brown RS, Bladen HA, Fullmer HM: Degradation of collagen by a human granulocyte collagenolytic system. J Clin Invest *47:*2622, 1968.

105. Ziff M, Gribetz HJ, Lospalluto J: Effect of leukocyte and synovial membrane extracts on cartilage mucoprotein. J Clin Invest *39:*405, 1960.

106. Barrett AJ: The possible role of neutrophil proteinases in damage to articular cartilage. Agents Actions *8:*11, 1978.

107. Janoff A, Blondin J: Depletion of cartilage matrix by a neutral protease fraction of human leukocyte lysosomes. Proc Soc Exp Biol Med *135:*302, 1970.

108. Weissmann G: Lysosomal mechanisms of tissue injury in arthritis. Seminars in Medicine of the Beth Israel Hospital. Boston *286:*141, 1972.

109. Buermann CW, Horowitz MI, Oronsky AL: Degradation of chondroitin-4-sulfate by human polymorphonuclear leukocyte enzymes. Transactions of the 25th Annual Meeting. Orthopedic Research Society, San Francisco, California, Feb 20–22, 1979, p 44.

110. Horvath SM, Hollander JL: Intra-articular temperature as a measure of joint reaction. J Clin Invest *28:*469, 1949.

111. Lack CH, Rogers HJ: Action of plasmin on cartilage. Nature *182:*948, 1958.

112. Lack CH: Chondrolysis in arthritis. J Bone Joint Surg [Br] *41:*384, 1959.

113. Chrisman OD, Southwick WO, Fessel JM: Plasmin and articular cartilage. Yale J Biol Med *34:*524, 1962.

114. Mochan E, Keler T: Plasmin degradation of cartilage proteoglycan. Biochim Biophys Acta *800:*312, 1984.

115. Mort JS, Dodge GR, Roughley PJ, et al: Direct evidence for active metalloproteinases mediating matrix degradation in interleukin-1 stimulated human articular cartilage. Matrix *13:*95, 1993.

116. Harvey AK, Stack ST, Chandrasekhar S: Differential modulation of degradative and repair responses of interleukin-1 treated chondrocytes by platelet-derived-growth factor. Biochem J *15:*129, 1993.

117. Roy S, Meachim G: Chondrocyte ultrastructure in adult human articular cartilage. Ann Rheum Dis *27:*544, 1968.

118. Zimny ML, Redler I: An ultrastructural study of patellar chondromalacia in humans. J Bone Joint Surg. [Am] *51:*1179, 1969.

119. Fell HB: Role of biological membranes in some skeletal reactions. Ann Rheum Dis *28:*213, 1969.

120. Barrett AJ: Cathepsin D: Purification of isoenzymes from human and chicken liver. Biochem J *117:*601, 1970.

121. Hembry RM, Knight CG, Dingle JT, et al: Evidence that extracellular cathepsin D is not responsible for the resorption of cartilage matrix in culture. Biochim Biophys Acta *714:*307, 1982.

122. Ali SY, Evans L: Enzymic degradation of cartilage in osteoarthritis. Fed Proc *32:*1494, 1973.

123. Martel-Pelletier J, Cloutier JM, Pelletier JP: Cathepsin B and cysteine protease inhibitors in human osteoarthritis. J Orthop Res *8:*336, 1990.

124. Nagase H, Woessner JF Jr: Neutral protease from bovine nasal cartilage that digests proteoglycan. Arthritis Rheum *20:*77, 1977.

125. Martel-Pelletier J, Pelletier JP, Cloutier JM, et al: Neutral proteases capable of proteoglycan digesting activity in osteoarthritic and normal human articular cartilage. Arthritis Rheum *27:*305, 1984.

126. Gold EW, Anderson LB, Miller CW, et al: Effect of salicylate on the surgical inducement of joint degeneration in rabbit knees. J Bone Joint Surg [Am] *58:*1012, 1976.

127. Austin J, McAfee D, Armstrong D, et al: Abnormal sulfatase activities in two human diseases (metachromatic leucodystrophy and gargoylism). Biochem J *93:*15C, 1964.

128. Evanson JM, Jeffrey JJ, Krane SM: Human collagenase: Identification and characterization of an enzyme from rheumatoid synovium in culture. Science *158:*499, 1967.

129. Harris ED Jr, Cohen GL, Krane SM: Synovial collagenase: Its presence in culture from joint disease of diverse etiology. Arthritis Rheum *12:*92, 1969.

130. Schwartz ER, Adamy L: Effect of ascorbic acid on arylsulfatase activities and sulfated proteoglycan metabolism in chondrocyte cultures, J Clin Invest *60:*96, 1977.

131. Einhorn TA, Gordon SL, Siegel SA, et al: Matrix vesicle enzymes in human osteoarthritis. J Orthop Res *3:*160, 1985.

132. Bollett AJ, Nance JL: Biochemical findings in normal and osteoarthritic articular cartilage. II. Chondroitin sulfate concentration and chain length, water and ash content. J Clin Invest *45:*1170, 1966.

133. Lust G, Pronsky W, Sherman DM: Biochemical studies on developing canine hip joints. J Bone Joint Surg [Am] *54:*986, 1972.

134. Chrisman OD, Southwick WO: Sulfate metabolism in cartilage. III. The effects of various adjuvants of sulfate exchange in cartilage slices. J Bone Joint Surg [Am] *44:*464, 1962.

135. Curtiss PH Jr, Klein L: Destruction of articular cartilage in septic arthritis. J Bone Joint Surg [Am] *47:*1595, 1965.

136. Howell DS, Pita JC, Sorgente N, et al: Possible role of lysozyme in degradation of osteoarthritic cartilage. Trans Assoc Am Physicians *87:*169, 1974.

137. Hickery MS, Vilim V, Bayliss MT, et al: Effect of interleukin-1 and tumour necrosis factor-alpha on the turnover of proteoglycans in human articular cartilage. Biochem Soc Trans *18:*953, 1990.

138. Lefebvre V, Peeters-Joris C, Vaes G: Modulation by interleukin 1 and tumor necrosis factor alpha of production of collagenase, tissue inhibitor of metalloproteinases and collagen types indifferentiated and dedifferentiated articular chondrocytes. Biochim Biophys Acta *1052:*366, 1990.

139. Pratta MA, Di Meo TM, Ruhl DM, et al: Effect of interleukin-1-beta and tumor necrosis factor-alpha on cartilage proteoglycan metabolism in vitro. Agents Actions *27:*250, 1989.

140. Shinmei M, Masuda K, Kikuchi T, et al: Production of cytokines by chondrocytes and its role in proteoglycan degradation. J Rheumatol *18*(Suppl 27):89, 1991.

141. Venn G, Nietfeld JJ, Duits AJ, et al: Elevated synovial fluid levels of interleukin-6 and tumor necrosis factor associated with early experimental canine osteoarthritis. Arthritis Rheum *36:*819, 1993.

142. Hasty KA, Reife RA, Kang AH, et al: The role of stromelysin in the cartilage destruction that accompanies inflammatory arthritis. Arthritis Rheum *33:*388, 1990.

143. Burton-Wurster N, Horn VJ, Lust G: Immunohistochemical localization of fibronectin and chondronectin in canine articular cartilage. J Histochem Cytochem *36:*581, 1988.

144. Deshmukh K, Nimni ME: Effects of lysosomal enzymes on the type of collagen synthesized by bovine articular cartilage. Biochem Biophys Res Comm *53:*424, 1973.

145. Krane SM: Joint erosion in rheumatoid arthritis. Arthritis Rheum *17:*306, 1974.

146. Kobayashi I, Ziff M: Electron microscopic studies on the cartilagepannus junction in rheumatoid arthritis. Arthritis Rheum *18:*475, 1975.

147. Woolley DE, Crossley MJ, Evanson JM: Collagenase at sites of cartilage erosion in the rheumatoid joint. Arthritis Rheum *20:*1231, 1977.

148. Luscombe M: Acid phosphatase and catheptic activity in rheumatoid synovial tissue. Nature *197:*1010, 1963.

149. Wegelius O, Klockars M, Vainio K: Acid phosphatase activity in rheumatoid synovia. Acta Med Scand *183:*549, 1968.

150. Harris ED Jr, Evanson JM, DiBona DR, et al: Collagenase and rheumatoid arthritis. Arthritis Rheum *13:*83, 1970.

151. Vainio U: Leucine aminopeptidase in rheumatoid arthritis. Ann Rheum Dis *29:*434, 1970.

152. Muirden KD, Deutschmann P, Phillips M: Articular cartilage in rheumatoid arthritis: Ultrastructure and enzymology. J Rheumatol *1:*24, 1974.

153. Collins AJ, Cosh JA: Temperature and biochemical studies of joint inflammation. Ann Rheum Dis *29:*386, 1970.

154. Granda JL, Ranawat CS, Posner AS: Levels of three hydrolases in rheumatoid and regenerated synovium. Arthritis Rheum *14:*223, 1971.

155. Wood GC, Pryce-Jones RH, White DD, et al: Chondromucoprotein degrading neutral protease activity in rheumatoid synovial fluid. Ann Rheum Dis *30:*73, 1971.

156. Josephson AS, Greenwald RA, Gerber DA: Serum lysozyme and histidine in rheumatoid arthritis (Abstr). Clin Res *19:*444, 1971.

157. Keller K, Shortkroff S, Sledge CB, et al: Effects of rheumatoid synovial cells on cartilage degradation in vitro. J Orth Res *8:*345, 1990.

158. Lazarus GS, Daniels JR, Brown RS, et al: Degradation of collagen by a human granulocyte collagenolytic system. J Clin Invest *47:*2622, 1968.

159. Murphy G, Reynolds JJ, Bretz U, et al: Collagenase is a component of the specific granules of human neutrophil leucocytes. Biochem J *162:*195, 1977.

160. Lazarus GS, Daniels JR, Lian J, et al: Role of granulocyte collagenase in collagen degradation. Am J Pathol *68:*565, 1972.

161. Harris ED Jr, Faulkner CS II, Brown FE: Collagenolytic systems in rheumatoid arthritis. Clin Orthop *110:*303, 1975.

162. Curtiss PH Jr, Klein L: Destruction of articular cartilage in septic arthritis. J Bone Joint Surg [Am] *45:*797, 1963.

163. Trancart MM, Chalmeigne N, Girardot C, et al: Gelatinase is the main matrix metalloproteinase involved in granuloma-induced cartilage degradation. Int J Tissue React *14:*287, 1992.

164. Shinmei M, Masuda K, Kikuchi T, et al: Interleukin 1, tumor necrosis factor, and interleukin 6 as mediators of cartilage destruction. Semin Arthritis Rheum *18*(Suppl 1):27, 1989.

24

Basic Biomechanics

Robert G. Volz, M.D.

This chapter is intended to provide basic biomechanical concepts relating to the musculoskeletal system. By definition, biomechanics is the science of how the musculoskeletal system works. Such information should prove to be as valuable to the diagnostic radiologist and orthopedic surgeon as a basic knowledge of physiology is to the internist.

During the past two decades, a considerable amount of research has been devoted to the biomechanics of the musculoskeletal system.[1-7] In great part, this has been stimulated by the rapidly expanding field of total joint replacement. Prior to this time, orthopedic surgeons needed an understanding of only a few basic principles of fracture healing. The rapid evolution of more sophisticated reconstructive orthopedic procedures has made it mandatory that those physicians involved in the performance of such procedures possess a greater appreciation of the mechanical working of the musculoskeletal system. Because of the highly technologic nature of many reconstructive procedures, the potential for significant rates of complications and failures also exists. Fortunately or unfortunately, the radiologist often is at the crossroads where crucial choices are made. The basic biomechanical principles described in this chapter will aid both the radiologist and the orthopedic surgeon in the analysis of problems related to the musculoskeletal system. First the basic concepts are defined, after which their application to the joints of the upper and lower extremities is illustrated. Specific situations are described to coordinate the principles with actual clinical problems.

STRESS, STRAIN, AND MODULUS OF ELASTICITY

Any basic knowledge of biomechanics must begin with an understanding of the terms stress, strain, and modulus of elasticity because the principles underlying these terms relate critically to such areas as fracture mechanics, the internal fixation of fractures, and the entire field of total joint replacement.

Stress

By definition, stress is the condition that results from the application of a force to the surface of an object when the effects of the force are confined totally to the interior of the object. This situation is to be distinguished from one in which a force applied to an object produces external effects. As an example, when a baseball bat strikes a pitched ball, the impact imparts an external effect, which is observed as acceleration of the ball as it passes through the air. At the moment of impact of the bat with the ball, however, the internal effects of the force give rise to sufficient stress within the ball to produce a temporary deformation of its surface. Because stress is a quality that is confined internally to an object, its quantification is possible only when it effects a discernible change in the shape of the object being stressed.

Strain

Strain is the measurable change in the shape of an object being stressed. It therefore is a quantifiable phenomenon.

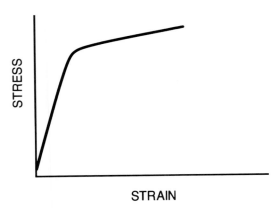

FIGURE 24–1. A graph shows the stress-strain curve for a stiff material such as cortical bone. (From Volz RG: Orthop Rev *14*:718, 1985.)

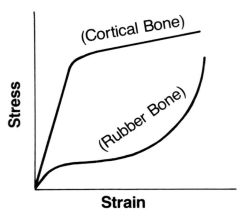

FIGURE 24–2. A more elastic material, such as a synthetic bone fabricated of rubber, exhibits a much greater deformation for any given amount of stress than does a stiffer material, such as cortical bone. (From Volz RG: Orthop Rev *14*:718, 1985.)

Strain, or the change in the original shape of a material, can be expressed in two very different forms: an elastic type and a plastic type. For instance, if, after the removal of the stressing force that produced the material deformation, the object returns to its original shape, the object is said to have undergone elastic strain or to exhibit elastic qualities. A classic example of elastic strain is the stretching of a rubber band without reaching its breaking point. If, however, sufficient stress has been created within the substance of the material to produce a permanent change in the shape of the object, the object has exhibited plastic strain, or plastic deformation. An example of plastic strain is the bending of a metal coat hanger.

Most people have certain preconceptions about how much stress would be required to produce a strain or change in the shape of any particular object or material. This relationship between stress and strain also can be identified precisely in the laboratory and expressed in a mathematical fashion. For instance, a graph of the relationship of stress and strain of healthy cortical bone would appear as shown in Figure 24–1. If the response of an identically shaped object that was fabricated totally of rubber were compared with cortical bone, the graph might appear as noted in Figure 24–2. From these two graphs, it can be observed that material referred to as elastic requires very little stress to produce a significant amount of strain, whereas materials referred to as brittle or rigid require an appreciable amount of stress to produce only a very small amount of strain.

Stress-Strain Ratio

The relationship of stress to strain also can be expressed as a ratio, as shown in the following formula:

$$\Sigma = \frac{\text{stress}}{\text{strain}}$$

where Σ equals Young's modulus of elasticity, a value determined by dividing a measured amount of stress by an identifiable degree of strain. Various materials, of course, may exhibit various moduli of elasticity. Thus, bone, which is quite rigid, is said to have a high modulus of elasticity, whereas rubber objects have a low modulus of elasticity.

It is possible not only to express the relationship of stress and strain within the areas of elastic and plastic deformation

but also to determine the ultimate strength or breaking point of any given material. Figure 24–3 identifies the relationship between these various physical properties of material substances on a graph. For many materials, by the time plastic deformation has occurred very little additional stress is required to produce complete failure (i.e., breakage). This is particularly pertinent to various types of metallic implants, which have lost the great majority of their intrinsic strength by the time they begin to exhibit plastic deformation.

Modulus of Elasticity

Let us now compare the modulus of elasticity of three very different materials, such as metal, bone, and acrylic cement (Fig. 24–4). The graph in Figure 24–4 shows that a considerable discrepancy exists in the physical responses of these various materials to stress. If a composite of bone, cement, and prosthetic material is fabricated that possesses such dissimilar moduli of elasticity, and if stress then is applied to the composite, varying degrees of strain will appear at the interfaces of the materials, with eventual

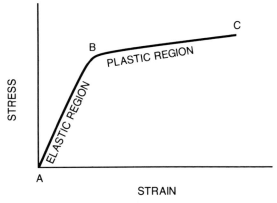

FIGURE 24–3. A stress-strain curve indicates the elastic and plastic regions of a material's physical properties. Point B represents the yield point at which the elastic qualities of the material begin to show plastic or permanent change. Point C represents the ultimate breaking point of the material. (From Volz RG: Orthop Rev *14*:718, 1985.)

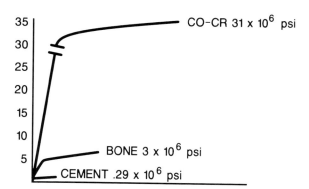

FIGURE 24–4. A stress-strain curve is shown for three different materials: a cobalt-chromium (CO-CR) alloy metal, cortical bone, and acrylic cement. The graph illustrates the great variation in their respective moduli of elasticity. (From Volz RG: Orthop Rev *14*:718, 1985.)

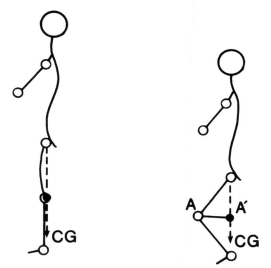

FIGURE 24–6. Significant moment forces (torque) are generated at the knee with varying arcs of flexion. In the act of arising from a chair, forces exceeding three times body weight are generated. CG, Center of gravity; A, A', lever arm of force.

breakdown at these locations (Fig. 24–5). This is precisely what occurs when cemented prosthetic devices become loosened mechanically.

INSTANT CENTER OF MOTION

The term instant center of motion refers to the locus, or axis, around which motion is taking place. Because motion is a prime function of the musculoskeletal system, each joint has its own unique instant center or clustered centers of motion. Objects that are almost entirely round, such as the femoral head, will possess only a single axis or instant center of motion. Articulating surfaces that are complex or elliptical in configuration will have constantly changing centers of motion. Knowledge of the location of the instant center of motion is important to an understanding of the potential forces that can be placed on a given joint by adjacent musculotendinous forces and the static and dynamic effects of the body weight.

LEVER ARM AND TORQUE

The term lever arm refers to the distance between the point of application of a given force and the instant center of motion. Torque is merely the product of the magnitude of the force and the lever arm. The relationship can be

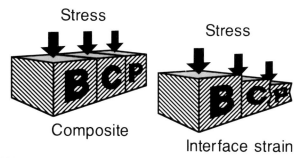

FIGURE 24–5. Schematic diagram of events that occur at the interfaces of three materials with widely varying moduli of elasticity: bone (B), cement (C), and a metallic prosthesis (P). When stress is applied, breakdown occurs at the interfaces owing to the varying degree of strain produced by the given load. (From Volz RG: Orthop Rev *14*:718, 1985.)

expressed by the equation $T = F \times L$, where T = torque, F = force, and L = lever arm. By defining the location of the instant center of motion for the knee and the lever arm of action of the force of the body's weight when a patient attempts to arise from a chair, the physician easily can calculate the force acting on the knee joint (Fig. 24–6). Such calculations have obvious clinical applications, as in cases in which a patient needs to assist himself or herself in arising from a chair when such increased forces may be harmful to a healing fracture about a knee or in cases in which an artificial knee implant is imperfectly secured to the underlying supporting bone.

JOINT REACTIVE FORCE

The magnitude of forces to which bone and joint cartilage are subjected is critical to the maintenance of a physiologically healthy state of these tissues. If excessive stresses are imposed, fracture or failure of tissues follows, whereas if stresses are insufficient, resorption or atrophy of tissue will be noted. These observations follow Wolff's law, which states that the pattern and the quantity of osseous response correlate with the degree of stress placed on that bone.

The term joint reactive force refers to the magnitude of force or stress observed in a particular joint. The definition does not identify the distribution of such force or stress over the articular surface but merely refers to a quantification of the total load. With certain activities, appreciable joint forces arise at articular surfaces, particularly those in the lower extremity. It has been estimated that with vigorous running activities, joint loads placed on the hip joint may approach seven to eight times body weight. In ordinary walking activities, the loads are approximately three times body weight.[8] Similarly, when handheld objects are lifted against gravity, joint reactive forces approaching several hundred pounds easily are generated on the elbow (Volz et al, unpublished data). A calculation of the varying joint reactive forces observed with two-legged and single-legged

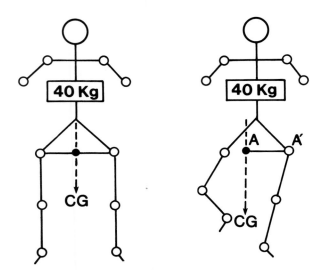

FIGURE 24–7. The sizeable increase in stress placed on a hip as a person progresses from a two-legged stance to single-leg support is explained as follows: A person weighing 60 kg will have approximately two thirds of the the weight distributed to the torso, upper extremities, and head (40 kg). Each leg represents approximately one sixth of the total body weight (10 kg). When weight is borne evenly on both legs, one half of weight of the torso, upper extremity, and head (40 kg) is borne on each hip. As the body weight then is shifted to a single leg of support, several significant changes occur. First, the unsupported body mass is increased to 50 kg owing to the addition of the unsupporting leg. Second, the center of gravity of the body mass is shifted from the centrally located symphysis pubis to a position more toward the unsupported side. This increases the lever arm of action of the body mass with a significant augmentation in the load borne by the supporting hip, amounting to more than three times body weight—a ninefold increase from that observed for a two-legged stance. CG, Center of gravity; A, A′, lever arm of force.

support of the torso is given in Figure 24–7. The tremendous increase in the joint reactive force associated with a single-legged stance explains the protective benefit derived from the use of crutches or a cane when limited weight-bearing is indicated.[7]

FORCES ACTING ON THE MUSCULOSKELETAL SYSTEM

An appreciation of the varying modes of force applied to the musculoskeletal system is essential to understanding the mechanics of fractures, soft tissue injuries, and total joint failure. In essence, only two modes exist by which molecular disruption (tissue failure) can occur: through forces of compression and through forces of tension. Compressive forces tend to compress or drive closer together the molecular material of any structure. Tensile forces distract or pull apart the molecular composition. As a general rule, most materials are more efficient in resisting compressive forces than in resisting tensile forces.

Bending

A common mode of skeletal and soft tissue disruption is by bending forces. Bending forces may be cantilever, three point, or four point in terms of application (Fig. 24–8). When a bending force is applied to a tubular bone such as the femur, a predictable pattern of molecular disruption may follow. Permanent areas of failure (strain) will begin

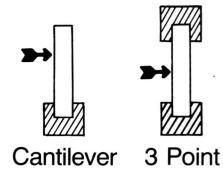

Cantilever   3 Point

FIGURE 24–8. An example of a cantilever bending force is the situation in which a femoral prosthesis is fixed rigidly distally within the medullary canal but has lost all support proximally. Under such loading conditions, the prosthetic stem is in jeopardy of fatigue fracture. Three point bending forces frequently are the cause of transverse fractures involving tubular bones of the upper and lower extremities.

to appear within the substance of the bone as it is loaded beyond its elastic limit of approximately 2 per cent.[9] Because bone is more prone to failure under tensile stress than under a compressive load, fracture disruption appears first on the convex side of the deformed segment. The direction of the fracture line will follow one of two common patterns, transverse or oblique (Fig. 24–9). An oblique fracture line will give rise to the butterfly fragment, which is observed commonly in the fracture disruption of tubular bones. Bending forces are much more disruptive of adjacent soft tissue structures, such as ligaments, periosteum, and neurovascular structures, and these elements also are prone to failure under tensile loading. Thus, bending forces are capable of producing significant disruption not only of bony structures but also of adjacent soft tissue elements. Signifi-

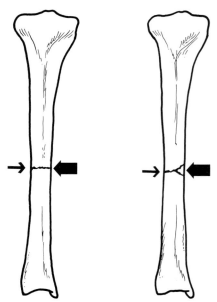

FIGURE 24–9. Bending forces (large arrows) applied to appendicular skeletal structures predictably produce transverse fracture lines. The initiation of the fracture occurs on the tensile (convex) side (small arrows). The presence of a butterfly fragment on the compressive side of the fracture is a sine qua non of a bending type of force application.

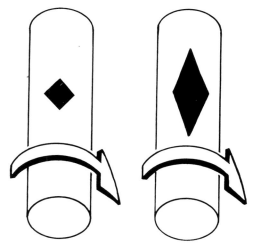

FIGURE 24–10. The application of rotational or torque types of force produces a combination of compression and tension within the substance of the material being loaded. An imaginary diamond drawn on the surface of a tubular bone subjected to rotational moment forces shows the pattern of deformation of such a diamond with the creation of both compressive and tensile strain.

cantly displaced bending force type fractures potentially are more unstable, more difficult to manage by a closed reduction, and, therefore, more suitable to open reduction and internal fixation.

Rotation or Torque

Another common mode of musculoskeletal failure is through rotational or torque force. As with bending forces, the mode of molecular disruption is through a combination of compressive and tensile forces (Fig. 24–10). As a rule, rotationally applied forces do not have as high a potential for disruption of adjacent soft tissue structures as bending forces. Thus, there is less likelihood of associated soft tissue injury. A satisfactory closed reduction generally is easier to achieve and maintain. Rotationally produced fractures are identifiable readily by their pattern of disruption. Fracture lines are more oblique, with an angle of inclination of 30 or 60 degrees to the long axis of the bone, whereas fractures produced by bending forces are either transverse or at a 45 degree angle to the long axis (Fig. 24–11).

Shearing

A third mechanism of bony failure is by shearing force. With this type of force, stress occurs parallel to the surface of the bone, causing body planes to slide by one another. If sufficient distortion of the surface occurs, bending forces are generated and failure will occur.

STRESS RISERS AND STRESS SHIELDING

Stress Risers

A stress riser represents an area at which stress will tend to be concentrated as a result of some peculiar shape or consistency of a material. Classic examples of a stress riser are a fold in a piece of paper placed to facilitate tearing of the material and a sharp edge on an object that is being

compressed into another material, such as a cheese cutter designed with a thin wire. Sharp edges on prosthetic devices that are cemented into place also may act as stress risers, thereby carrying a high potential for producing fracture of adjacent supporting cement or bone. Another example of a stress riser is a drill hole placed within an area of cortical bone. Such a defect, even if quite small, can act as a significant focus for stress concentration and, thus, represents a vulnerable, weakened area of bone.[10] The physiologic response to the placement of a hole in a bone is corticalization of the circumference of the hole (Fig. 24–12). Corticalization is the living bone's attempt to restore the area of weakened bone to its normal strength. This reparative process requires 6 to 8 weeks to complete.[10] Filling in of small drill holes and often larger defects with bone does not take place because insufficient stress occurs within the hole to stimulate new bone formation.

Subsidence

Subsidence is a descriptive term for sinkage of a material within its supporting structure or framework. The term is used most frequently in describing the settling of a prosthetic device, especially in the region of the proximal end of the femur. Because aseptic loosening of cemented devices is the most common mode of prosthetic implant failure today, the possibility of subsidence or a change in position of a prosthetic device should be carefully evaluated in any follow-up radiograph when an artificial joint has been implanted. As bone is a dynamic tissue, the potential for a change in the position of any prosthesis would appear to increase with the passage of time. The recognition of a small degree of subsidence demands a very precise duplication of prior radiographic projections.[11]

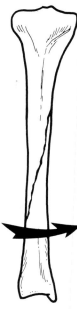

FIGURE 24–11. Fractures arising as a result of torque or rotational forces display a more longitudinal pattern than that observed for bending forces. Fracture lines are oblique, with an angle of inclination of 30 degrees with the long axis of a tubular bone or 60 degrees with its transverse axis.

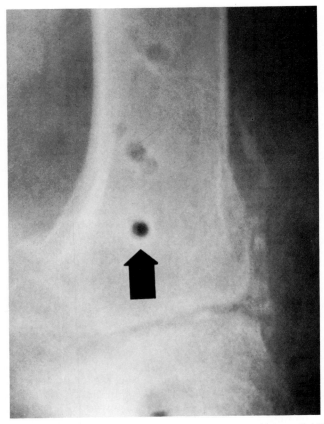

FIGURE 24–12. Cortical defects such as those created by small drill points (arrow) represent significant areas of stress concentration and potential sites for fracture initiation. The body's response to such an area of weakening is to produce a small peripheral rim of denser cortical bone. Because stress is not generated within the substance of the defect, such defects fail to fill in with new bone with the passage of time.

Fatigue Failure

The concept of fatigue failure is an important one, for many if not most metallic implants fail by this mode. The concept of fatigue failure can be defined as the repeated, closely sequenced application of a load that eventually produces failure (breakage of a material). As a general rule, the amount of force required to produce fatigue failure by repeated loading of a metallic implant is approximately 50 per cent of the load required to cause breakage with a single application. Any metallic device that exhibits plastic deformation is extremely prone to further failure through fatigue. This is because of the small component of strength remaining in the implant once it becomes deformed (Fig. 24–13).

Stress Shielding

Bone requires a certain degree of stress for the maintenance of its mineral and protein content. When the amounts of stress over a given period of time are insufficient, varying degrees of bone resorption, or osteopenia, can be observed. Similarly, when excessive amounts of stress are applied to bone, depending on their magnitude, abrupt failure or fatigue failure (fracture) may occur. Because metallic implants are stiffer (have a higher modulus of elasticity) than bone, their attachment to a skeletal part, either by

intramedullary or by cortical fixation, definitely compromises the eventual strength of the bone. As the metallic device assumes some of the load that normally would be carried by the bone, the bone has undergone stress shielding by the implant. In some situations, the degree of stress shielding is of such a magnitude that fatigue failure of the adjacent bone is a very real problem.

BIOMECHANICS OF SPECIFIC JOINTS

Hip

Studies to date have documented differing rates of clinical loosening of femoral and acetabular components[12, 13] of hip prostheses (Fig. 24–14). To appreciate the mechanics of how these devices fail, it is necessary to understand the pattern of stress distributed across the hip joint on weight-bearing. The estimates of forces across a weight-bearing hip vary from three to eight times body weight, depending on whether the subject is doing ordinary walking or sprinting. Figure 24–7 demonstrates the sizeable change in the joint reactive force when a 60 kg person advances from a two-legged stance to a single-legged stance, such as in the act of walking. Forces of these magnitudes are not distributed evenly across the acetabular surface but rather are concentrated in the superior and superolateral areas.[7, 8] If the acetabulum is divided into three equal zones, the majority of the weight-bearing compressive stresses will be found in the two most proximal zones (Fig. 24–15). An assessment of the apparent density of the subchondral bone surrounding the acetabulum in a normal hip will confirm this observation. The area of greatest bony condensation will be found superior to the femoral head. Because of its eyebrow-like configuration, this zone often has been referred to as the sourcil (French for "eyebrow").[8]

The width of the sourcil narrows when the surface area of contact between the femoral head and the acetabulum becomes diminished as a result of injury or arthritic change. Under such conditions, the joint reactive force now is apportioned over a smaller surface area, thereby further en-

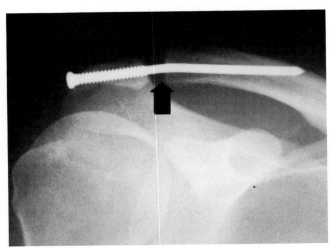

FIGURE 24–13. Radiograph showing a screw transfixing a previously dislocated acromioclavicular joint. The bent configuration of the screw (arrow) suggests that little remaining strength exists within the implant because of the presence of plastic deformation. Fatigue failure of the implant may follow if the patient is not cautioned against overactivity.

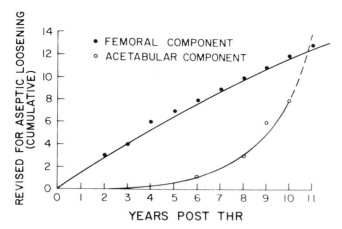

FIGURE 24–14. Aseptic loosening of cemented femoral and acetabular components follows a fairly predictable pattern. Clinical studies have revealed that the likelihood that the femoral component will loosen follows a linear pattern, whereas the likelihood that the acetabular component will loosen appears to accelerate dramatically from the fifth to tenth year postoperatively. THR, Total hip replacement.

hancing the mechanical breakdown of cartilage and subchondral bone (Fig. 24–16).[7, 8] As articular cartilage is lost and the stabilizing effect of the lateral rim of the acetabulum is compromised, lateral subluxation of the femoral head is observed (Figs. 24–16 and 24–17).[8]

Patterns of failure of cemented acetabular cups show that the development of radiolucent lines nearly always begins in zones 1 and 3 (see Figure 24–15). This is because of the sizeable compressive stresses that are present in zone 1 and the negligible stresses observed in zone 3. Loss of rigid fixation of a prosthetic implant occurs where stresses are excessive or minimal. Additionally, the shape of the prosthetic cup offers less resistance to elastic and plastic deformation at its rim than at its apex (Fig. 24–18).

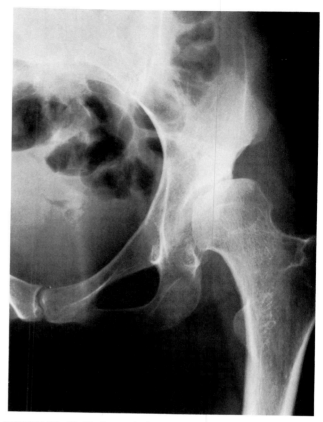

FIGURE 24–16. Radiograph depicting a dysplastic hip with lateral subluxation of the femoral head. The narrowed area of contact between the femoral head and acetabulum has given rise to a greater amount of stress per unit area. This is evidenced by the narrowed sourcil and the presence of increased bone sclerosis about the lateral lip of the acetabulum.

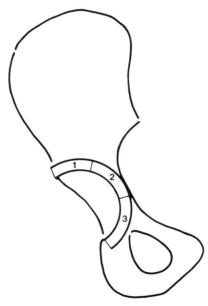

FIGURE 24–15. If the acetabulum is divided into three equal zones, the majority of the weight-bearing stresses will be concentrated in zones 1 and 2.

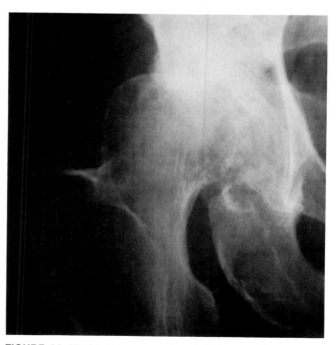

FIGURE 24–17. As stress per unit area is increased across any joint, deterioration of articular cartilage follows. The result frequently is the development of severe osteoarthritis.

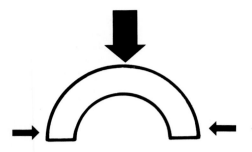

Deformability of Hemisphere

FIGURE 24–18. A hemispherically shaped structure is more susceptible to deformation when a load is applied at its rim than at its apex.
This observation may account for the rapid development of radiolucent lines about some acetabular prosthetic components that possess very thin layers of polyethylene material.

Let us now examine the normal pattern of stress that is
observed in the proximal portion of the femur with weight-
bearing. Because of the offset of the femoral head in relation to the femoral shaft, significant bending forces are
generated in the proximal area of the femur (i.e., the femoral neck and intertrochanteric regions). Bending forces give
rise to a combination of tensile and compressive patterns of
stress (Fig. 24–19). Because bone is weaker in its resistance
to tensile than to compressive stresses, fractures of the
femoral neck and some types of intertrochanteric fractures
begin in the areas of tensile stress (Fig. 24–20).

When a femoral prosthesis is inserted into the proximal
portion of the femur, such as in total hip arthroplasty, a
significant alteration in the stress patterns of the upper part
of the femur arises because the prosthesis now is carrying
a portion of the body's weight. This generally will be manifested on the radiograph by areas of stress shielding to the
cortical and cancellous bone (i.e., a loss of bone density

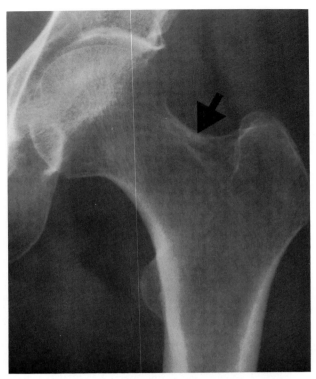

FIGURE 24–20. Because bone is more susceptible to failure by
tensile forces than by compressive forces, fracture lines through the
femoral neck often commence on the lateral or tensile side (arrow).

and areas of stress increase, as shown by areas of increased
cortical thickness). The degree of stress shielding is related
to numerous factors, the predominant ones being the patient's weight and activity level, the transverse diameter of
the femoral medullary canal, the diameter of the femoral
prosthetic stem, and the modulus of elasticity of the implant
material. The following examples further explain these parameters and their effect on stress shielding of the proximal
portion of the femur with its resultant loss of bone.

Let us assume that two patients have femoral shafts of
identical outside diameters of 30 mm but the intramedullary
canal diameters are 12 and 15 mm, respectively. In each
case, a press-fitted stem that matches the medullary canal
dimension has been inserted in the performance of a total
hip arthroplasty. Given the known modulus of elasticity for
bone and the cross-sectional diameter of the femur, the
stiffness of each patient's femur can be computed. Similarly, given the cross-sectional diameter of the implant and
the known modulus of elasticity of the material, the degree
of stiffness of the implant stem likewise can be computed.
Because the implant stem shares load with the cortical
bone, the degree of stress shielding then can be estimated
roughly.

The calculated stiffness of the bone implant composite is
determined by the following equation:

$S = (EI)_{f12} + (EI)_{c12}$, where $(EI)_{f12}$ equals the stiffness
of a cobalt-chrome 12 mm stem and $(EI)_{c12}$ is the stiffness
of a femoral shaft 30 mm in diameter with a 12 mm medullary canal.

$(EI)_{f12} = 220 \ Nm^2$, while $(EI)_{c12} = 697 \ Nm^2$

Load

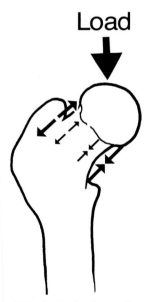

FIGURE 24–19. Loads applied to the femoral head create significant
bending forces through the femoral neck (arrows). These give rise
to a combination of tensile forces laterally and compressive forces
about the calcar.

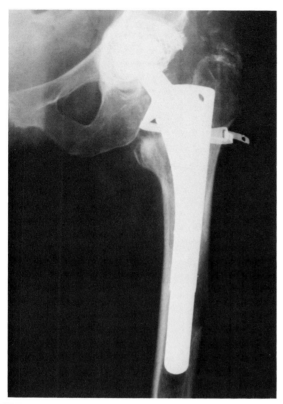

FIGURE 24–21. An anteroposterior radiograph showing a widened intramedullary canal with a 15 mm in diameter pressfitted femoral stem. Because the stiffness of a circle is a function of the fourth power of the diameter, the 15 mm stem is 150 per cent stiffer than the 12 mm stem. This predictably will lead to greater stress shielding of bone and associated pain on weight-bearing activities.

Thus, the composite bone implant stiffness S is 220 Nm^2 + 697 Nm^2 = 917 Nm^2.

In Figure 24–21, a different set of circumstances exists. In this example, the patient is much older with the anticipated greater loss of cortical bone thickness and resultant increase in the diameter of the medullary canal. This situation requires the surgeon to use a stemmed implant with a larger diameter (15 mm) to fill the medullary canal adequately. Because the stiffness of a sphere (the configuration of most femoral stems) is related to the fourth power of its diameter and because the metals presently used in the fabrication of femoral implants are between 7 and 15 times stiffer than cortical bone, the potential now exists for a much greater degree of stress shielding than observed in the patient with the smaller, 12 mm canal. Furthermore, as bone is lost through the process of stress shielding, altered patterns of stress to the remaining bone arise, frequently associated with pain on weight-bearing activities.

Using the same methods of calculating the stiffness of the patient's bone and the implant, the following values are found:

$$\text{bone stiffness} = (EI)_{c15} = 675 \text{ Nm}^2:$$

$$15 \text{ mm implant stiffness} = (EI)_{f15} = 548 \text{ Nm}^2$$

$$\text{with a composite stiffness S of } 1223 \text{ Nm}^2$$

Obviously, the much greater stiffness of the 15 mm stem (220 Nm^2 versus 548 Nm^2) will give rise to greater areas of

stress shielding to the proximal end of the femur with a predictable thinning of proximal diaphyseal bone.

To further understand the clinical effects of these altered stresses on bone, let us examine the stresses that are applied to femoral stemmed implants and the effects they may have on adjacent supporting bone. These stresses are a combination of bending, shear, and moment forces. As a result of the offset of the femoral neck of the implant, significant bending forces are placed on the stem of the prosthesis. Because of the greater stiffness of the stem in comparison to the bone, the situation is a bit analogous to the insertion of a steel rod into a garden hose. When bending forces are applied in this situation, stress occurs in high concentration at the tip of the rod, which, in the case of a femoral prosthesis, translates to the increased bending stresses observed at the tip of the stem and also the concentration of stress in the region of the femoral calcar (Fig. 24–22).

Bone, as with all living tissue, has a certain tolerance to stress. If stresses become excessive, failure (i.e., fracture) of the material may occur. Figure 24–23 demonstrates the effect of the loss of support proximally to a femoral implant with the implant's resultant shift into varus position with an associated increase in the lever arm generated by the body's moment force. Additionally, cortical hypertrophy about the tip of the stem may be observed when stresses are excessive at the tip of a femoral prosthesis. Such radiographic findings often are associated with midthigh pain on weight-bearing activities.

Femoral implants also are subjected to significant moment forces as weight is borne on the femoral prosthesis. These forces frequently play a dominant role in initiating

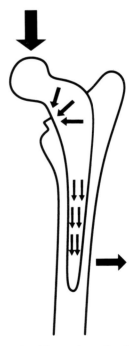

FIGURE 24–22. A proximal femoral prosthesis that is subjected to significant load exhibits an uneven pattern of stress distribution along the stem. Proximally significant compressive forces are observed about the calcar owing to the level arm of the prosthetic implant. Along the stem of the prosthesis, shear forces are generated between the stem and supporting medullary canal. At the tip of the prosthesis, significant compressive loads are observed against the lateral and endosteal surfaces.

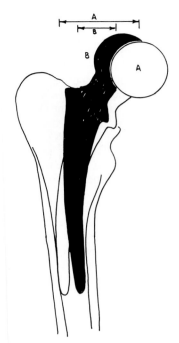

FIGURE 24–23. Loss of support to a cemented or pressfitted proximal femoral prosthesis (B) generally occurs first in the region of the calcar. This permits the prosthesis to tip into a greater degree of varus alignment (A). With this increase in varus position, an increase in the lever arm of action of the body weight acting through the femoral head is observed. Increasing stresses are generated on the prosthetic stem. Prosthetic loosening, thus, becomes a progressive phenomenon.

loosening of the implant from the surrounding bone. The earliest signs of aseptic loosening of a femoral implant are best observed on a lateral projection of the upper femur, where radiolucent lines most commonly are first observed (Fig. 24–24).

Knee

Basic to an understanding of the biomechanics of the knee joint is an appreciation of the weight-bearing axis of the lower extremity. This can be determined by drawing a straight line from the instant center of motion of the hip joint (a point located in the center of the femoral head) to the midportion of the ankle joint. In a normally aligned leg, this axis of weight-bearing force will transect the intercondylar notch of the femur (Fig. 24–25). Thus, the normal alignment of the knee offers optimal sharing of the joint reactive force across both the medial and the lateral tibial plateaus. When varying degrees of malalignment exist, such as in varus or valgus deformity, a significant shift in the joint load to one side of the articulation occurs. Corrective osteotomies about the knees attempt to reestablish a more normal weight-bearing distribution across the joint surface of the knee. A significant increase in the joint reactive force also is observed with varying degrees of knee flexion. At 45 degrees of knee flexion, the lever arm of action of the body mass is maximized, with an increase in the joint reactive force (estimated to approach three to four times body weight). As flexion of the knee takes place and with contracture of the quadriceps muscles, significant bending forces are generated within the patella (Fig. 24–26). These

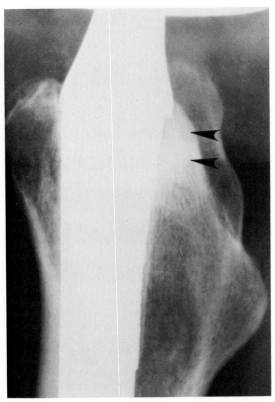

FIGURE 24–24. A lateral view frequently will reveal the earliest evidence of loosening of a cemented or noncemented femoral component (arrowheads). This probably relates to the high moment forces that are generated with normal walking activities.

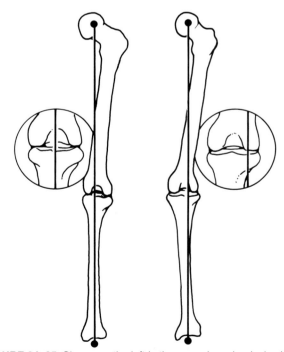

FIGURE 24–25. Shown on the left is the normal mechanical axis for the lower extremity, defined by drawing a line from the instant center of motion of the femoral head to a point transecting the tibial plafond. This line should transect the intercondylar notch of the knee. When malalignment occurs at the knee (right), this mechanical weight-bearing axis is shifted toward the medial or lateral tibial plateau. For every 5 degrees of angulation observed at the knee, the load carried by the joint is doubled.

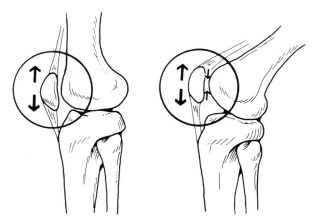

FIGURE 24–26. When the knee is in full extension and the quadriceps mechanism is contracted, only tensile forces are observed within the substance of the patella (left). As the knee assumes an increasing arc of flexion, bending forces are observed within the patella, thus giving rise to a combination of tensile and compressive loads (right). This pattern of loading can lead to aseptic loosening of patellar prostheses.

bending forces are replaced by purely tensile forces when the knee is placed in full extension, because the patella then loses any contact with the underlying intercondylar notch of the femur.

As at the hip joint, the most commonly observed mode of failure of an artificial knee joint is aseptic loosening. This complication can involve all three components of an artificial knee (patellar, femoral, and tibial portions), although by far the highest frequency of loosening is observed on the tibial side. The biomechanical explanation for the higher rate of tibial loosening is that constantly shifting forces are placed on the tibia by the femoral condyles, a situation that is associated with normal walking activities (Fig. 24–27). Thus, loosening of a tibial component usually is observed first at the most medial and most lateral margins of the horizontally oriented portion. Radiolucent shadows will be seen later about the tibial component stem, if such a design has been used (Fig. 24–28). The fixation of the femoral component has been maximized by the complex surface geometry of the distal portion of the femur so that stresses are dissipated more evenly. The identification of loosening of a femoral component requires that a perfect lateral radiograph of the bone-cement interface be obtained. Loosening of the patellar prosthesis also can arise as a result of the significant bending forces that are generated with flexion activities. A fatigue fracture of the supporting bone of the patella likewise is observed occasionally and must be included in the differential diagnosis of knee pain occurring after joint replacement.

Wrist

The complexities of the multiple joints making up the wrist result in some interesting biomechanical observations. The carpus is supported by the pedestal provided by the distal radial articular surface and the confluent surface of the adjacent triangular fibrocartilage. The manner in which the joint reactive force is shared by these two surfaces depends on the relative lengths of the radius and the ulna. Studies have shown that, if at the distal end the ulnar length

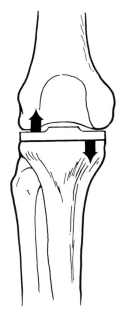

FIGURE 24–27. In the normal act of walking, body load transmitted across the knee joint is distributed unevenly. In most persons, the majority of the body load is borne by the medial femorotibial compartment of the knee. A change in the load distribution across the knee creates significant problems after total knee replacement because rocking forces (arrows) are generated that act on the tibial component-bone junction.

is identical to the radial length, (the zero position), 65 per cent of the joint reactive force is transmitted across the distal radial plate and 35 per cent is transmitted across the triangular fibrocartilage (Fig. 24–29).[14] When the ulna is shorter than the radius (ulnar minus variant), an increased load is borne by the distal radial plate, which is estimated

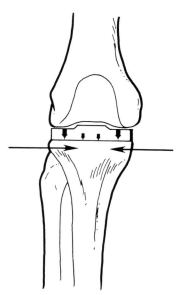

FIGURE 24–28. The uneven distribution of body loads (vertical arrows) placed across an artificial tibial component enhances the appearance of radiolucent lines at the bone-cement interface. The appearance of these radiolucent shadows generally commences toward the periphery of the horizontal portion of the tibial component, progressing toward the intercondylar area (horizontal arrows).

Load

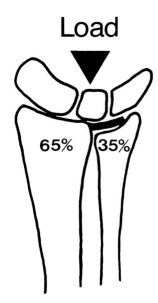

65% 35%

FIGURE 24–29. If the distal end of the ulna approximates the distal end of the radius, approximately 65 per cent of the load placed across the radiocarpal joint is borne by the radius and 35 per cent is borne by the triangular fibrocartilage and distal portion of the ulna. In cases in which the distal portion of the ulna does not reach the level of the distal extent of the radius (ulnar minus variant), an increased percentage of the load (as high as 95 per cent) is borne by the radius.

to be as high as 95 per cent.[14] A careful appraisal of the space between the radius and lunate discloses that only a portion of the lunate is supported by the distal portion of the radius.[14] The observed association of an increased frequency of Kienböck's disease (ischemic necrosis of the lunate) in the presence of an ulnar minus variant suggests that abnormally high joint reactive forces over the lunate provoke a fatigue failure of the cancellous bone.[15] Dramatic resolution of clinical symptoms and reversal of early radiographic changes have been noted after surgical lengthening of the ulna, a procedure aimed at establishing a more physiologic transmission of joint forces at the wrist. Attritional changes of the triangular fibrocartilage as demonstrated by arthrography also have been associated with a relatively long ulna, a condition referred to as ulnar plus variant.[16]

The second important role of the triangular fibrocartilage is that of stabilization of the distal radioulnar joint. The tethering effect of the triangular fibrocartilage is constant throughout the entire arc of pronation and supination of the forearm. Only with extreme positions of pronation and supination do the dorsal and volar aspects of the distal radioulnar capsule offer any appreciable support to joint stability. If the triangular fibrocartilage becomes disrupted, the distal radioulnar joint subluxes as the arc of pronation is increased. Reduction of the distal radioulnar joint is facilitated by a position of supination. It can be presumed that, in isolated fractures of the radius that exhibit more than 1 cm of shortening, disruption of the triangular fibrocartilage has occurred. If normal forearm rotation and stability of the distal radioulnar joint are to be regained, open reduction and internal fixation of the radius are mandatory, with immobilization of the forearm in supination.

The loss of the normal support offered by the triangular fibrocartilage and the distal end of the ulna when both

structures have been excised surgically, as in the treatment of rheumatoid arthritis, can lead to significant translocations of the carpus on the radius (Fig. 24–30). The disparity that is created between the articulating joint surfaces then may lead to significant arthrosis.

BIOMECHANICAL PRINCIPLES OF FRACTURE FIXATION WITH PLATES AND SCREWS

The application of a rigid plate to the cortex of a fractured tubular bone has given rise to several biomechanical considerations. Because the plate must be of sufficient cross-sectional dimension to resist bending or breakage until the fracture has achieved some degree of healing, the metal plate mechanically is quite rigid (i.e., it possesses a high modulus of elasticity). Once the plate is applied securely to the fracture site, all micromotion that might otherwise stimulate periosteal healing is eliminated. It therefore is imperative that precise bony contact be achieved at the time of open reduction if union is to occur. To minimize the stress placed on any single screw as load is being carried by the plate during the course of fracture healing, three screws should be employed on either side of the area of the fracture. As the screws are tightened surgically to the supporting plate, the plate becomes compressed against the cortex while the screw is subjected to increasing tensile forces. Overtightening of the screw may compromise the final fixation through the loss of cortical bone purchase or

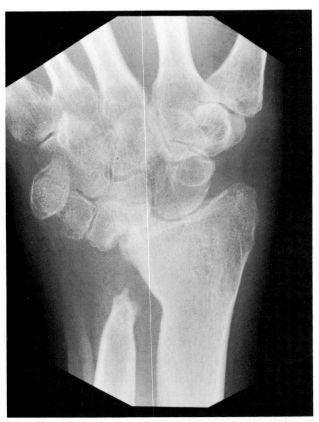

FIGURE 24–30. The important support of the proximal carpal row is provided by the distal portion of the ulna and the triangular fibrocartilage. After resection of the distal end of the ulna, translocation of the carpus, as shown here, frequently is observed.

stripping of the screw thread. Because most tubular bones of the appendicular skeleton are subjected to bending forces in a dominant plane, the plate should be applied to the side of the bone that is subjected to the greatest tensile force. Postoperatively, as repetitive loads are placed on the plate-screw fixation by adjacent muscle forces and gravity, bending forces threaten the integrity of the plate-screw fixation. The ability of the compressive plate to resist these forces and shear forces depends on the degree of friction generated between the plate and the surface of the cortical bone. If micromotion of the plate occurs owing to such shear forces, fatigue fracture of the screw will occur adjacent to the screw head, where the junction of the threaded portion creates a stress riser. Once failure of the screw has occurred, compromise in fixation of the fracture follows.

SUMMARY

The past decade has produced a wealth of new knowledge concerning the biomechanics of the musculoskeletal system. This is fortunate for both the radiologist and the orthopedist, for such knowledge provides a sound scientific basis for understanding and treating many of today's complex musculoskeletal problems. Although experience and empirical judgments often prove adequate in decision-making in medicine, there is no substitute for theoretic knowledge of why something has occurred, or—perhaps more importantly—what the outcome might be.

Most assuredly, in the near future the complexities of treatment of many musculoskeletal problems, such as the surgical treatment of fractures and the artificial replacement of worn and damaged joints, will demand an even greater understanding if accurate diagnoses and prognoses are to be offered by radiologists and orthopedic surgeons.

References

1. Frankel VH, Burstein A: Orthopedic Biomechanics. Philadelphia, Lea & Febiger, 1970.
2. Frankel VH, Nordin M: Basic Biomechanics of the Skeletal System. Philadelphia, Lea & Febiger, 1980.
3. Swanson SAV, Freeman MAR: The Scientific Basis of Joint Replacement. New York, John Wiley & Sons, 1977.
4. Schaldach M, Holman D (Eds): Advances in Artificial Hip and Knee Joint Technology. New York, Springer-Verlag, 1976.
5. Walker PS: Human Joints and Their Artificial Replacements. Springfield, IL, Charles C Thomas, 1977.
6. Cochran GV: A Primer of Orthopedic Biomechanics. New York, Churchill-Livingstone, 1982.
7. Pauwels F: Biomechanics of the Locomotor Apparatus. New York, Springer-Verlag, 1980.
8. Schatzker J (Ed): The Intertrochanteric Osteotomy. New York, Springer-Verlag, 1984.
9. Burstein AH, Curry JD, Frankel VH, et al: The ultimate properties of bone tissue: The effects of yielding. J Biomech 5:35, 1972.
10. Burstein AH, Curry J, Frankel VH, et al: Bone strength: The effects of screw holes. J Bone Joint Surg [Am] 54:1143, 1972.
11. Lippert FG III, Harrington RM, Veress SA, et al: A comparison of convergent and bi-plane x-ray photogrammetry systems used to detect total joint loosening. J Biomech 15:677, 1982.
12. Sutherland CJ, Wilde A, Borden L, et al: A ten-year follow-up of 100 consecutive Muller curved stem total hip replacement arthroplasties. J Bone Joint Surg [Am] 64:970, 1982.
13. Stauffer R: Ten-year follow-up study of total hip replacement with particular reference to roentgenographic loosening of the components. J Bone Joint Surg [Am] 64:983, 1982.
14. Palmer AK, Werner FW: Biomechanics of the distal radioulnar joint. Clin Orthop 187:26, 1984.
15. Sundberg SB, Linscheid RL: Kienböck's disease. Results of treatment with ulnar lengthening. Clin Orthop 187:43, 1984.
16. Epner RA, Bowers WH, Guilford WB: Ulnar variance: The effect of wrist positioning and roentgen filming technique. J Hand Surg 7:298, 1982.

SECTION

IV

Rheumatoid Arthritis and Related Diseases

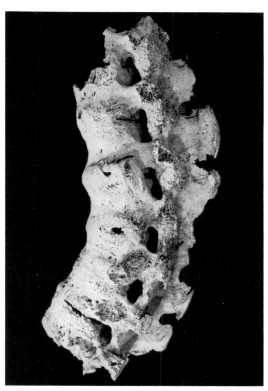

Ankylosing spondylitis: Syndesmophytes and bone ankylosis of apophyseal joints are evident.

25

Rheumatoid Arthritis and the Seronegative Spondyloarthropathies: Radiographic and Pathologic Concepts

Donald Resnick, M.D., and Gen Niwayama, M.D.

An understanding of the radiographic findings of rheumatoid arthritis and the seronegative spondyloarthropathies requires, at the very least, familiarity with the anatomy and the pathology of the involved structures. Armed with such an understanding, the physician need not memorize a long list of radiographic abnormalities that are encountered in each articular disorder. Rather, the radiograph can be viewed as a mirror and the abnormalities it reveals as a reflection of underlying pathologic aberrations. The physician can interpret such alterations as osteoporosis, joint space diminution, osseous erosions, and cysts in terms of the pathogenesis of the articular disorder, thus allowing early and accurate diagnosis to be made.

This chapter summarizes the radiographic and pathologic characteristics of rheumatoid arthritis and the seronegative spondyloarthropathies. Later chapters (Chapters 26 to 32) discuss each of these disorders in greater detail.

RHEUMATOID ARTHRITIS

Overview

The major abnormalities of rheumatoid arthritis appear in synovial articulations of the appendicular skeleton, particularly the small joints of the hand and foot, the wrist, the knee, the elbow, and the glenohumeral and acromioclavicular joints. The synovial articulations of the axial skeleton also may be affected, especially the apophyseal and atlantoaxial joints of the cervical spine. In most of these synovium-lined cavities, changes are distributed symmetrically in both the right and the left sides of the body and consist of fusiform soft tissue swelling, regional osteoporosis, diffuse loss of joint space, marginal and central erosions, and fibrous ankylosis. The synovium of bursae and tendon sheaths also is affected. Abnormalities of cartilaginous articulations and entheses are less frequent and extensive,

Rheumatoid arthritis and the seronegative spondyloarthropathies (ankylosing spondylitis, psoriasis, and Reiter's syndrome) have in common many radiographic and pathologic characteristics. They affect synovium-lined joints, bursae, and tendon sheaths; cartilaginous articulations; entheses or sites of ligamentous and tendinous attachment to bone; soft tissues; and bones. They lead to inflammation in a variety of tissues and, although the distribution and the extent of abnormalities at specific "target" areas in the body vary among the disorders, the musculoskeletal effects of this inflammation are fundamentally similar.

TABLE 25–1. Abnormalities of Synovial Joints in Rheumatoid Arthritis

Pathologic	Radiologic
Synovial inflammation and production of fluid	Soft tissue swelling and widening of joint space
Hyperemia	Osteoporosis
Pannus destruction of cartilage	Narrowing of joint space
Pannus destruction of "unprotected" bone at margin of joint	Marginal bony erosions
Pannus destruction of subchondral bone	Bony erosions and formation of subchondral cysts
Fibrous and bony ankylosis	Bony ankylosis
Laxity of capsule and ligaments and muscular contraction and spasm	Deformity, subluxation, dislocation, fracture, fragmentation, and sclerosis

with the exception of the discovertebral joints of the cervical spine, at which site characteristic and significant findings may be encountered. Alterations in tendons, ligaments, soft tissues, and vessels complete the radiographic and pathologic picture of musculoskeletal involvement in rheumatoid arthritis.

Synovial Joints (Table 25–1) (Figs. 25–1 to 25–5)

General Enzymatic Factors. The fundamental target area in this disease is the synovium, which lines the articulation. Rheumatoid synovitis is the result of a cellular immune response to an antigen present in the synovial membrane; this response sets in motion a series of cytokine mediated reactions which lead to the mobilization of T and B cell lymphocytes.[344] The precise identity of this antigen is not clear; however, the response to it includes the production of inflammatory cytokines and proteolytic enzymes

by monocytes, the transformation and proliferation of fibroblasts with the formation of an erosive pannus, and the generation by B cells of immunoglobulin for immune complexes, factors which together act to injure the joint.[345] Although the earliest histologic events within a joint involved in rheumatoid arthritis are not easily documented, the first lesions appear to be microvascular injury and proliferation of synovial cells.[234] In the presence of infiltration with polymorphonuclear leukocytes and foci of plasma cells in the superficial layers of the synovium, vascular lesions—including the obliteration of small blood vessels and organized thrombi—seem prominent and suggest that etiologic factors responsible for the disease are carried to the joint by the circulation.[234] As rheumatoid arthritis becomes more established, the inflammation within the synovial membrane is characterized by edema, hypertrophy of lining cells, and villous transformation. Further inflammation results in proliferative granulation tissue or pannus, which then extends across the joint, producing cartilaginous and osseous damage. An intimate relationship between the advancing pannus and the site of cartilaginous destruction is evident on light and electron microscopy.[1–3, 235–238, 342] The type of cells participating in the chondral destruction has received a great deal of attention. Fibroblast-like and macrophage-like cells, polymorphonuclear leukocytes, lymphocytes, and mast cells have, in turn, been considered most important in this regard.[235–237, 239, 302–307, 331, 338–341] A tumor-like quality of the pannus has been suggested,[240] and a tumor necrosis factor has been identified in the lining and deeper layers of the synovium, perhaps produced by cells of the monocyte and macrophage lineage.[343] Loss of collagen fibrils is seen in cartilage located within a few micrometers from the edge of the inflammatory cells, whereas in more distant cartilage, much of the structural integrity is maintained. This morphologic evidence, coupled with the

Text continued on page 815

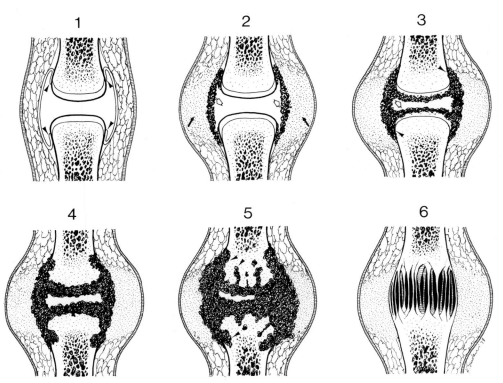

FIGURE 25–1. Rheumatoid arthritis: Abnormalities of synovial joints. Pathologic overview. In the normal joint (1), observe the articular cartilage and synovial membrane. At the edges of the articulation (arrowheads), synovium abuts on bone that does not possess protective cartilage. The very early abnormalities of rheumatoid arthritis (2) consist of synovial proliferation (open arrows), soft tissue edema (solid arrows), and osteoporosis. At a slightly later stage (3), the inflamed synovial tissue or pannus (open arrow) has extended across the cartilaginous surface, leading to chondral erosion. Capsular distention, soft tissue edema, and osteoporosis are seen. Small osseous erosions at the margins of the joint are appearing (arrowheads). In more advanced stages (4,5), large marginal and central erosions and "cysts" are noted (arrowheads). In advanced rheumatoid arthritis (6), fibrous ankylosis of the joint is typical.

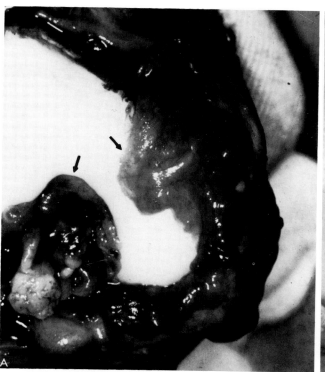

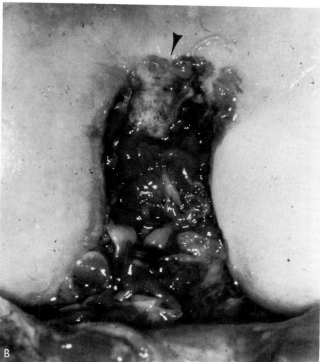

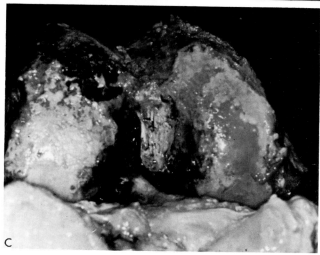

FIGURE 25–2. Rheumatoid arthritis: Abnormalities of synovial joints. Sequential gross pathologic changes.

A, B Photographs of the knee joint in two patients with rheumatoid arthritis reveal a hypertrophied, edematous synovial membrane extending over the femoral condyles (arrows) and into the intercondylar notch (arrowhead).

C. In advanced rheumatoid arthritis, a photograph of the articular surface of the distal end of the femur outlines extensive cartilaginous and osseous erosion and synovial fibrosis.

(Courtesy of R. Convery, M.D., San Diego, California.)

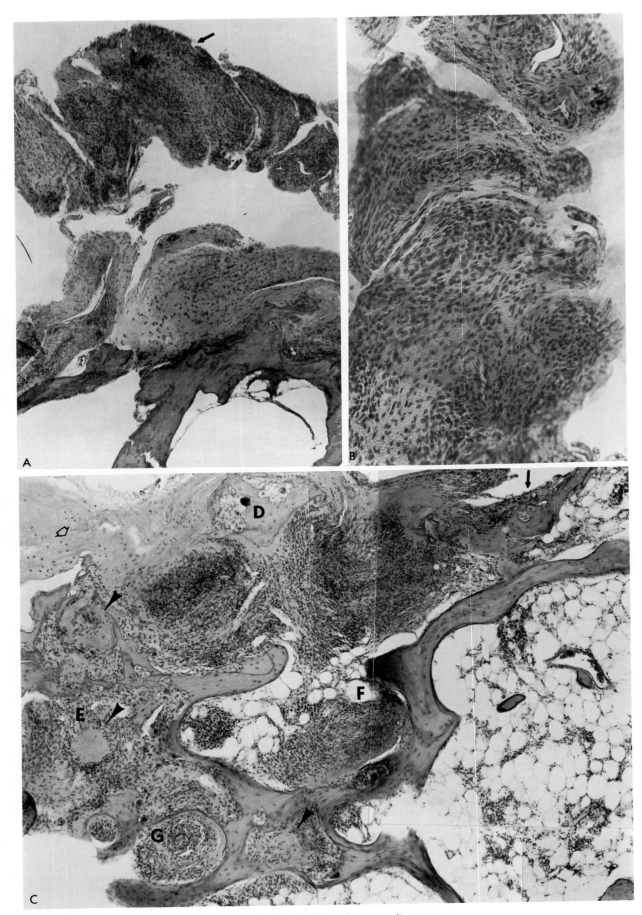

FIGURE 25–3. *See legend on opposite page*

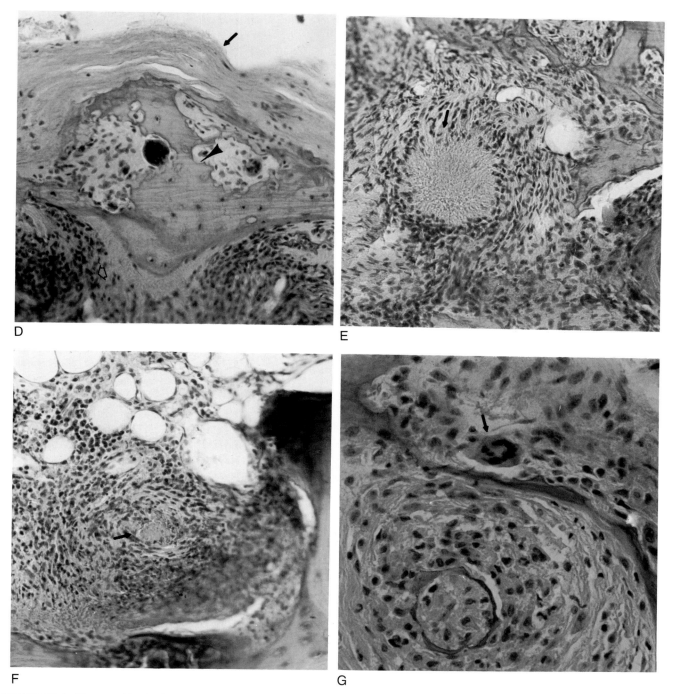

FIGURE 25–3. Rheumatoid arthritis: Abnormalities of synovial joints. Sequential histologic changes.

 A Synovial abnormalities. Papillary and villous hypertrophy of vascular synovial tissue is evident (arrow). There are many plasma cells and lymphocytes associated with proliferation of synovial stromal tissue (86×).

 B Synovial abnormalities. The synovium is vascular, with proliferating stromal cells, many plasma cells, and lymphocytes (215×).

 C Composite abnormalities. Findings include inflamed synovial tissue (solid arrow) extending over the fibrous cartilaginous surface (open arrow). Necrotic lesions are present within the bone marrow (arrowheads) (86×).

 D In this higher power view (215×) of the area marked D in **C**, fibrous tissue (solid arrow) is applied to irregular osseous spicules (arrowhead). Numerous plasma cells and lymphocytes are evident (open arrow).

 E High power photomicrograph (215×) of the area marked E in **C**; note a typical palisading lesion (arrow). The cells are ovoid or spindle-shaped, and central necrosis is evident. Osteoclastic resorption of neighboring trabeculae is apparent.

 F High power photomicrograph (215×) of the area marked *F* in **C**, showing a focal deposit of fibrin exudate (arrow) surrounded by cellular debris with a background of numerous plasma cells and lymphocytes.

 G The area shown in this photomicrograph (215×) is similar to that marked G in **C**. It reveals resorption of bone about multiple osteoclasts (arrow).

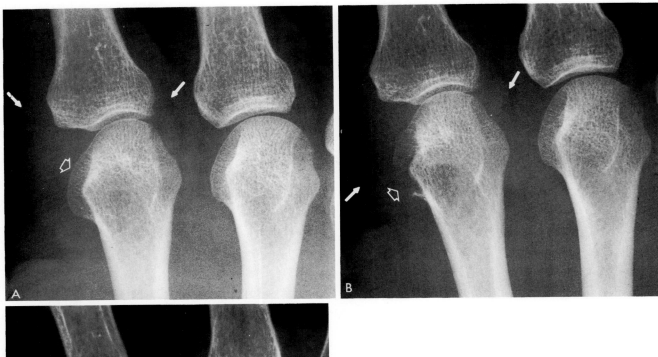

FIGURE 25–4. Rheumatoid arthritis: Abnormalities of synovial joints. Sequential radiographic changes in metacarpophalangeal joints.

A The earliest abnormalities consist of soft tissue swelling (solid arrows), periarticular osteoporosis, loss of a portion of the subchondral bone plate on the metacarpal head (open arrow), and minimal joint space narrowing.

B With progression, increases in soft tissue swelling (arrows) and osteoporosis are associated with marginal erosions of the metacarpal heads (open arrow).

C The later stages of rheumatoid arthritis are characterized by complete obliteration of the articular space and large central and marginal osseous erosions (open arrows).

Illustration continued on opposite page

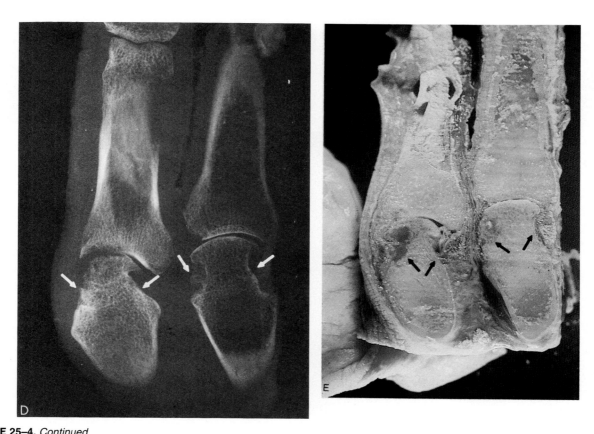

FIGURE 25–4. *Continued*

D, E. A radiograph (**D**) and corresponding photograph (**E**) of a coronal section of the second and third metacarpophalangeal joints in a cadaver with severe rheumatoid arthritis indicate pannus-related erosions of the metacarpal heads (arrows), cartilage destruction, and ulnar deviation of the digits.

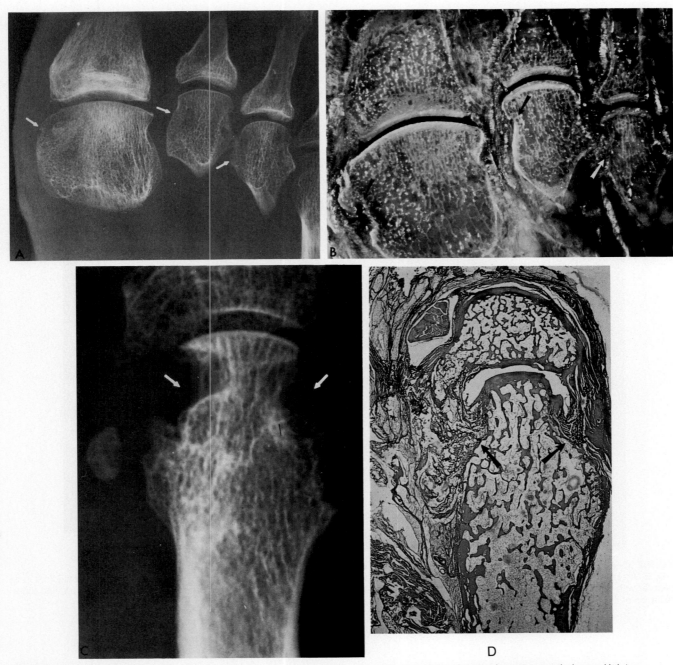

FIGURE 25–5. Rheumatoid arthritis: Abnormalities of synovial joints. Sequential radiographic changes in metatarsophalangeal joints.

A, B On a radiograph and corresponding photograph of a transverse section through the metatarsophalangeal joints in a cadaver with rheumatoid arthritis, observe superficial erosion along the medial aspect of multiple metatarsal heads (arrows) related to pannus erosion of bone. The cartilage is remarkably well preserved, reflected in the normal interosseous spaces noted on the radiograph.

C A magnification radiograph of a metatarsophalangeal joint reveals striking erosions of the metatarsal head (arrows).

D On a photomicrograph (10×) of a metatarsophalangeal joint in a cadaver with rheumatoid arthritis, observe pannus erosion of bone at the margins of the metatarsal head (arrows). The cartilage is partially destroyed.

observation that collagenase produced by the synovial membrane can cause cartilaginous damage,[4–6] suggests that enzymatic degradation of collagen fibers is an initial step in structural damage of the joint. Other types of lytic enzymes, such as lysosomal neutral protease extractable from leukocytes[7–9] and from the synovial membrane,[7] and cathepsin D, released from lysosomes,[10–12] also may participate in cartilaginous erosion.[13] Release of lytic enzymes by chondrocytes also occurs,[14] but this is probably not as significant as enzymatic production by inflamed synovial tissue.[13] Cartilaginous destruction also may be related to interference with proper nutrition by the overlying dense acellular fibrous pannus.[13, 15] In some cases, the pannus-free surface of the cartilage is eroded,[238] a fact that may relate to the presence in the synovial fluid of lysosomal enzymes or to diffuse softening and degradation of cartilage owing to local hyperthermia.[241]

Although histologic examination of synovial articulations in rheumatoid arthritis confirms the presence of osseous erosion in relation to inflammatory cells in synovial tissue,[2] collagen in mineralized bone is relatively resistant to enzymatic degradation.[16] Thus it appears likely that the osseous tissue must first be demineralized before it can be attacked by collagenolytic and other enzymatic agents. In this regard, one study has demonstrated that cultured synovium from patients with rheumatoid arthritis secretes some unidentified factor that is able to stimulate mineral release from bones.[16] Although prostaglandins, which are released by rheumatoid synovium in culture,[17] can accelerate bone resorption in other systems,[18] their role in the pathogenesis of bone destruction in rheumatoid arthritis is not clear.[2]

Synovial Membrane. The earliest recognizable pathologic abnormality in rheumatoid arthritis is acute synovitis,[19–23] which is associated with congestion and edema of the synovial membrane. Capillary proliferation and abnormal permeability are accompanied by exudation of plasma, which penetrates the loose stroma of the synovial layer, reaching the joint cavity.[24] Fibrin is precipitated on the surface of the membrane. It is especially prominent in synovial recesses, is of variable thickness, and adheres firmly to the subjacent synovial tissue.

This exudative phase of rheumatoid arthritis merges into an infiltrative phase.[19] Accumulation of erythrocytes results from altered capillary permeability. Phagocytosis of these cells leads to hemosiderin deposition, with the production of large quantities of synovial iron.[25, 219] Polymorphonuclear leukocytes appear in the acute inflammatory phase. The predominant cells, however, are small lymphocytes. In the superficial portions of the synovium, cellular infiltration occurs diffusely or in small nodular aggregates (Allison-Ghormley nodules). With chronicity, plasma cells and true lymphoid follicles with germinal centers are evident. Distinctive multinucleated giant cells also are found in the synovial membrane in rheumatoid arthritis[26, 27] but are not entirely specific for this disease.[28, 29] These cells may originate from the phagocytic type A synovial lining cells as a reaction to chronic injury, leading to hyperplasia and giant cell transformation. Some investigators have proposed that the presence in significant amounts of one type of giant cell, termed the synovial giant cell, characterized by an ovoid or round shape and multinucleation, at some distance from the synovial surface is somewhat suggestive of rheumatoid arthritis, but most investigators express caution

when interpreting the diagnostic significance of these giant cells.[26]

Enlargement and multiplication of synovial lining cells are additional features of acute synovitis; the hypertrophied cells reach to a depth of six to 10 layers, whereas normally only one to three cell layers are observed.[234] A papillary configuration may result. Associated cellular proliferation in the subjacent stroma of the synovial membrane obliterates its interface with the synovial lining. Metaplasia of connective tissue to fibrocartilage, hyaline cartilage, and even bone can be noted,[20] which must be differentiated from cartilaginous and osseous debris arising from the disintegrating articular surface in more advanced cases of rheumatoid arthritis.[30]

These microscopic abnormalities result in a macroscopically evident thickened and injected synovial membrane. Villous hypertrophy produces papillary fronds 1 to 2 mm in diameter. The irregularity of the synovial tissue is most marked near the edges of the articular cartilage.

Increased amounts of turbid yellow-green synovial fluid of decreased viscosity are produced. The fluid contains relatively large amounts of globulins, so that the ratio of the albumin to globulin fraction of the fluid (which normally is approximately 2 to 1) becomes approximately 1 to 1.[20] The content of gamma globulin is especially prominent owing to the infiltration of numerous plasma cells in the inflamed synovial membrane. The cell content in the synovial fluid frequently is markedly elevated.

The pathologic findings described previously occur in the "synovial" stage of rheumatoid arthritis and are accompanied by characteristic radiographic abnormalities.[31–33] Accumulation of synovial inflammatory tissue within the joint, increase in intra-articular fluid, capsular distention, and surrounding soft tissue edema lead to one early radiographic finding of the disease, soft tissue swelling. The periarticular soft tissue prominence generally is distributed symmetrically or is fusiform in configuration (although eccentric swelling can relate to inflammation of bursae and tendon sheaths, or to adjacent rheumatoid nodules). A homogeneous increase in radiodensity in and around the distended joint and obliteration of adjacent soft tissue planes are detected, especially with xeroradiography or low KV radiography. A more direct appraisal of the degree of synovial membrane irregularity is afforded by arthrography, in which injected contrast material reveals a typical nodular or corrugated appearance and opacification of neighboring lymphatic channels is observed; or by MR imaging, especially after the intravenous injection of a gadolinium contrast agent, in which the altered synovial membrane is enhanced, manifesting increased signal intensity when compared with that of joint fluid.[346, 347]

In response to hyperemia provoked by synovial inflammation, regional or periarticular osteoporosis—the second early radiographic sign of rheumatoid arthritis—can be demonstrated. This finding, which is not invariable and which may be less prominent in men and in persons who are physically active, produces thinning and small areas of discontinuity or gaps (dot-dash pattern) in the subchondral bone plate, abnormalities that are more evident when magnification techniques are employed.

Articular Cartilage. After an acute inflammatory episode, the hypertrophied synovial tissue may recede without producing cartilaginous damage. Exacerbations of disease

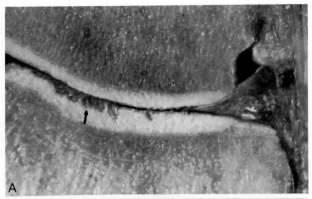
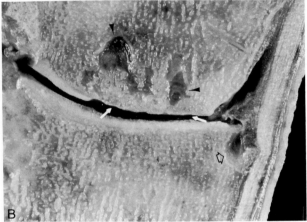

FIGURE 25–6. Cartilaginous abnormalities in rheumatoid arthritis: Knee.

A Superficial erosion of cartilage in the tibia is evident (arrow) on a coronal section. Incidental chondrocalcinosis involving the meniscus is apparent.

B In a different cadaver, a coronal section reveals extensive destruction of cartilage in the femur (solid arrows) with lesser involvement in the tibia. Subchondral cysts (arrowheads) are present in the femur, and the meniscus is irregular. Observe a marginal bone erosion in the tibia (open arrow).

are associated with eventual abnormalities in other articular structures, however, including the cartilage and the bone. The inflamed synovium soon spills from the peripheral portion and marginal pockets of the joint and grows toward the cartilaginous tissue. It forms an enlarging transparent layer of varying thickness across the surface of the cartilage or extends from the articular recesses through adjacent compact bone into the marrow spaces.[21] The synovial tissue applied to the cartilaginous surface causes morphologic changes owing to enzymatic destruction of cartilage or interference with proper cartilaginous nutrition, or both (Fig. 25–6). In a similar fashion, the synovial tissue within the bone marrow erodes the cartilage from beneath. The primary change within the hyaline articular cartilage is a disorganization and loss of intercellular matrix associated with decreased metachromasia.[19] Slight loss of matrix can stimulate new synthesis by chondrocytes, although severe matrix loss is an irreversible tissue injury that provokes replacement fibrosis. Cartilage destruction promoted by components in the rheumatoid synovial fluids[19] may ultimately become widespread and severe; when the cartilagi-

nous surface on two apposing bones is significantly compromised, granulation tissue may bridge the articular cavity. Inflammatory pannus also may extend onto such intra-articular structures as ligaments, menisci, and tendons.[20]

The radiographic counterpart of this "cartilaginous" stage of rheumatoid arthritis is loss of articular space. Classically, joint space diminution is a relatively early finding in the disease, and it may appear within a period of weeks or months in some patients with significant acute synovial inflammation. Along with soft tissue swelling and periarticular osteoporosis, joint space narrowing is one of three early radiographic characteristics of rheumatoid arthritis (the fourth finding, marginal osseous erosions, is discussed later in this chapter). Loss of the articular space usually is diffuse or widespread, related to the generalized nature of the cartilaginous destruction. This pattern of articular space diminution differs from the focal, segmental, or asymmetric type of joint space loss that occurs in osteoarthritis.

With continuing synovial inflammation and cartilage damage, the articular cavity is partially or completely obliterated by fibrous ankylosis, while the cellularity of the bridging tissue progressively decreases.[19] The superficially located pannus also may penetrate the entire cartilaginous coat, reaching the subchondral bone plate. Although dystrophic calcification and secondary ossification may develop within the inflammatory tissue that fills the articular cavity, producing osseous fusion, these findings are observed less frequently in rheumatoid arthritis than in the seronegative spondyloarthropathies. It has been suggested that the presence of large effusions in rheumatoid joints may prevent or delay intra-articular bony ankylosis[19] and that such ankylosis may be a marker of disease that is more severe and of greater duration.[348]

Subchondral Bone. Two alterations in the subchondral bone that occur in the early stages of rheumatoid arthritis are osteoporosis and marginal erosion. In association with active inflammation of the synovial membrane, the subchondral bone marrow may be converted into a loose fiber marrow containing scattered or agglomerated lymphocytes.[20] Subsequently, smooth atrophy of spongy trabeculae leads to the appearance of periarticular osteoporosis on the radiographs. This bony atrophy, which can progress with time and eventually extend along the adjacent diaphyses, is related to a combination of disuse of the articulation, osteoclastic resorption of the subchondral spongy trabeculae (discussed later in this chapter), and steroid-induced osteoporosis. On pathologic examination, a diminution of thickness and perforation of longitudinal trabeculae and a complete loss of many transverse trabeculae that may antedate any significant damage to the articular surface are seen.[243] The alterations extend 1 or 2 cm beneath the joint surface.

The presence of joint inflammation also influences the cell populations in bone, initially at the margins or unprotected areas of the articulation, where pannus is intimate with osseous tissue that does not possess protective cartilage.[34] Intra-articular bone biopsy specimens, which are obtained at the time of early synovectomy from sites distant from the location of inflamed synovial tissue, reveal erosion of bone with scalloped indentations that resemble Howship's lacunae; these lacunae contain mononuclear cells alone[35] or are associated with multinucleated osteoclasts.[36, 337] On the endosteal side of the cortex, inflammatory foci with adjacent bone marrow fibrosis and increase in bone turnover are seen.

The cellular characteristics of bone erosion accompanying rheumatoid arthritis have been outlined in detail by Duncan and coworkers.[37] Three patterns of demineralization and erosion have been identified.

1. Osteoclasts are prominent at many different sites in involved articulations. It is not clear whether these cells provoke demineralization alone, leaving the nonmineralized matrix intact,[38, 39] or whether the osteoclasts themselves complete the entire erosion process.[38] The possibility that the osteoclast's purpose is one of demineralization, exposing the surface to other cells such as the mononuclear macrophage, is strengthened by the close association of osteoclasts and mononuclear cells.[37, 337] Electron microscopy of the junction between the synovial membrane and the bone has indicated large numbers of mononuclear inflammatory cells.[280]

2. Mononuclear cells occupy Howship's lacunae. These cells may remove exposed matrix that has already been demineralized by preexisting osteoclasts or may themselves actively demineralize the subjacent bone.[40, 41]

3. Osteocytic osteolysis and periosteocytic demineralization are identified by enlargement of the osteocytic lacunae and increasing permeability to stain adjacent to these lacunae. Such effects could be related to the metabolic processes of the osteocyte itself or to a demineralizing process effected by the bone fluid, which passes through the canaliculi in and around the osteocytes buried in the bone. Osseous tissue so affected could be more susceptible to destructive enzymes produced by the rheumatoid synovium.

Although analysis of cellular function in damaged bone indicates the complexity of the erosion process and the presence of multiple factors, the radiographic characteristics of this process are well established. The location of the initial marginal erosions in rheumatoid arthritis corresponds to sites of synovial pockets and bare areas that do not possess protective cartilaginous coats (Fig. 25–7).[42] Symmetrically distributed defects appear on both the proximal and the distal bones that constitute the articulation and usually but not invariably are accompanied by soft tissue swelling, periarticular osteoporosis, and joint space narrowing. Such erosions may be a very early manifestation of the disease, occurring within 1 or 2 years of the onset of joint symptoms.[43] Depending on the extent and severity of the joint inflammation, they may remain static for long periods of time or enlarge as more widespread osseous damage becomes manifest.[231, 232]

The radiographic appearance of multiple subchondral lucent areas throughout the articulation in patients with more advanced rheumatoid arthritis is well recognized (Fig. 25–8). These lesions may develop in several different fashions. Transchondral extension of superficial pannus or direct extension of subchondral pannus into bone can lead to osseous destruction.[44–47] Conversely, Soila,[48] using stereoradiography, described enclosed pseudocystic defects within the bone without evidence of articular communication. He emphasized the importance of nutritional and metabolic injury of bone in rheumatoid arthritis and distinguished the peculiar pattern of rheumatoid trabecular disintegration from osteoporosis. Kersley and associates[49] suggested that enclosed cystic defects could be related to true intraosseous

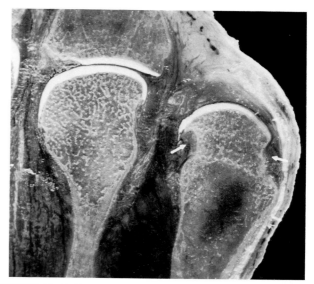

FIGURE 25–7. Marginal erosions of bone in rheumatoid arthritis: Metacarpophalangeal joint. In a coronal section of the fourth and fifth metacarpophalangeal articulations, marginal erosions of bone are evident on the radial and ulnar aspects of the fifth metacarpal head (arrows). Compare with the relatively normal fourth metacarpal head.

rheumatoid nodules (Fig. 25–9). Other authors have reported similar nodules in the spongy bone of vertebrae in rheumatoid arthritis.[50] Barrie[244] emphasized the existence of a reparative response in the subchondral bone, a rheumatoid osteitis characterized by proliferation of fibrovascular connective tissue, cartilage formation, accumulation of macrophages, and osseous deposition, a concept supported by Wyllie.[245]

Castillo and coworkers[51] emphasized the occurrence of large radiolucent cystic areas in rheumatoid arthritis patients who maintained a high level of physical activity. In this peculiar cystic pattern, which subsequently has been termed rheumatoid arthritis of the robust reaction type,[52] lesions were attributed to the effect of elevated intra-articular pressure forcing synovial fluid or granulation tissue into the bone. Investigation has indicated that the application of stress can accelerate the movement of pannus on the chondral surface into the cartilage or even the bone and suggests that joint movement, especially in patients who remain physically active, could encourage the development of finger-like extensions of synovial granulation tissue, which could eventually reach the bone marrow.[242, 350, 351] In support of this concept are the findings of Jayson and colleagues,[53] who measured intra-articular and intraosseous pressures in two patients and demonstrated that alterations in intra-articular pressure were communicated directly to two typical rheumatoid cysts. These results suggested that hydrostatic continuity exists between the cysts and articular space and perhaps explains the occurrence of large cysts in rheumatoid patients who continue to be physically active. Furthermore, Arnoldi and coworkers[285] have demonstrated that an elevation in intra-articular pressure related to an effusion or joint flexion is followed by a rise, albeit slower, in intraosseous pressure, results that are consistent with hydrostatic continuity between articulation and bone or with blockage of draining vessels from the bone marrow produced by the fluid.

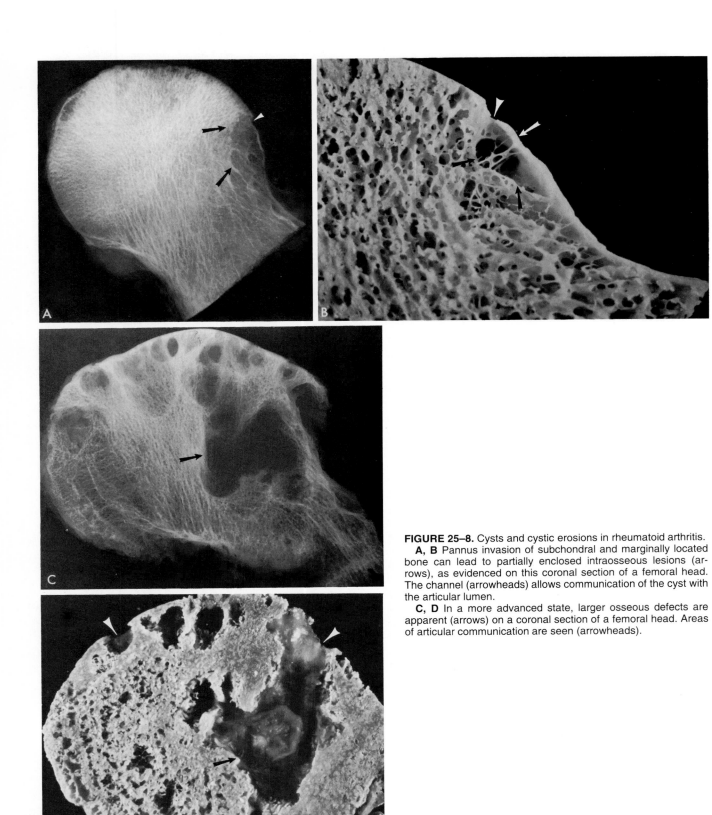

FIGURE 25–8. Cysts and cystic erosions in rheumatoid arthritis.

A, B Pannus invasion of subchondral and marginally located bone can lead to partially enclosed intraosseous lesions (arrows), as evidenced on this coronal section of a femoral head. The channel (arrowheads) allows communication of the cyst with the articular lumen.

C, D In a more advanced state, larger osseous defects are apparent (arrows) on a coronal section of a femoral head. Areas of articular communication are seen (arrowheads).

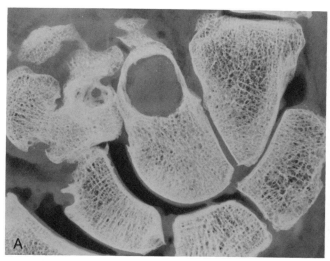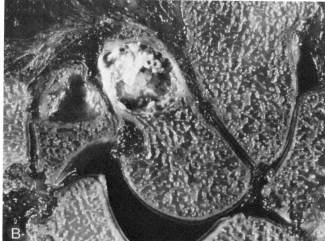

FIGURE 25–9. Intraosseous rheumatoid nodules in rheumatoid arthritis. Coronal sectional radiograph (**A**) and photograph (**B**) show a cystic lesion in the capitate that histologically represented a rheumatoid nodule. No obvious communication of the lesion with the surrounding joints could be found.

Magyar and coworkers[54] examined bone tissue from 21 rheumatoid arthritis patients. In all cases, a communication was demonstrated between the cysts and the articular cavity. The lesions contained granulation tissue resembling pannus, which led the authors to suggest a fundamental role of synovial inflammation in the development of subchondral cysts.

More recent studies using MR imaging have indicated that the subchondral cystlike lesions may contain fluid, inflamed synovia, or both; and that they may[351] or may not[352] reveal obvious communications with the joint.

In view of the previously reported association of cystic rheumatoid arthritis with increasing levels of physical activity and the observation of obvious continuity between the articular cavity and cyst, with transchondral extension of pannus, it is interesting to speculate that cyst formation represents one mechanism of joint decompression (Table 25–2). Intra-articular pressure is dependent on a variety of factors, including age of the person, the specific joint, the presence or absence of an effusion, the volume and rate of change of volume of the fluid, and muscle action.[246] Abnormal elevation of intra-articular pressure can lead to interference of synovial blood flow, impaired synovial nutrition, muscle weakness, and joint instability. Because the rise of intra-articular pressure during use of a joint is related directly to the volume of effusion within that joint,[55] joint decompression might result from any process allowing fluid to escape from the articulation.[44] Three potential pathways exist for such egress: subchondral cysts, synovial cysts, and fistulae or sinus tracts (Fig. 25–10). An inverse relationship between synovial cysts (e.g., popliteal cysts) and subchondral cysts has been noted; knees with large subchondral cysts have been associated with small synovial cysts,

whereas those with smaller or absent subchondral cysts have been associated with synovial cysts of variable size.[56] These observations strengthen the hypothesis that synovial cysts may protect the joint against damage produced by elevated intra-articular pressure. Furthermore, sinus tracts between the articulation and skin are known manifestations of rheumatoid arthritis[57, 58] (see discussion later in this chapter). The possibility that these tracts represent one addi-

TABLE 25–2. Mechanisms of Synovial Joint "Decompression" in Rheumatoid Arthritis

Subchondral cyst formation
Synovial cyst formation
Sinus tract formation

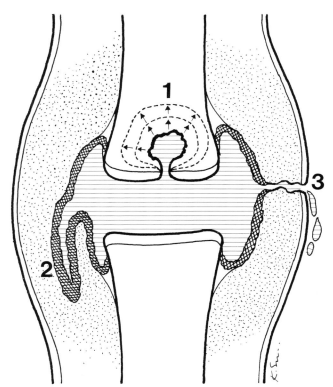

FIGURE 25–10. Mechanism of decompression of joints with raised intra-articular pressure. The three potential pathways are subchondral cystic lesions (1), synovial cysts (2), and fistulae or sinus tracts (3).

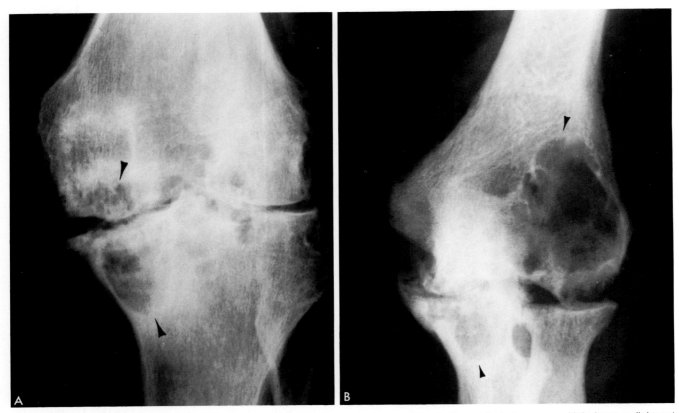

FIGURE 25–11. Pseudocystic rheumatoid arthritis. In some patients with rheumatoid arthritis, particularly men, multiple large radiolucent lesions (arrowheads) about involved articulations can simulate the appearance of gout or neoplasm.

tional mechanism of joint decompression is an intriguing concept.

Whatever their pathogenesis, subchondral lucent areas are an important radiographic manifestation in rheumatoid arthritis[59–62, 350, 351] (Fig. 25–11). Pathologically, these structures do not possess a true epithelial cystic lining, a fact that accounts for the variety of terms that have been applied to these lesions, including cysts, pseudocysts, granulomas, and geodes. They usually are multiple, distributed symmetrically, of small size, and without sclerotic margins. Although joint space narrowing and osteoporosis are encountered frequently as additional findings, subchondral cysts sometimes are observed in the absence of classic marginal bone erosions, articular space loss, and osteopenia.[351] In these instances, the radiographic manifestations resemble those of gout[63, 64]; this goutlike phenomenon is more common in men than in women and more common in those persons who are physically active. In rare instances, the subchondral cystic lesions of rheumatoid arthritis may calcify.[353]

Fibrous Capsule. The fibrous capsule of the synovial joint reveals only minor alterations in rheumatoid arthritis. Focal collections of lymphocytes and plasma cells appear about vessels, and arteries and veins may undergo progressive sclerosis.[21] Rarely, necrotic foci analogous to those of subcutaneous rheumatoid nodules are encountered in the capsular connective tissue.

After prolonged inflammation, capsular contraction can occur. This can aggravate the malalignment and subluxation that are provoked by changes in supporting structures, such

as tendons and ligaments, and in periarticular soft tissues (see later discussion). Capsular fibrosis and contraction can be associated with further cartilaginous injury owing to altered mechanical forces across the joint. In almost all cases, capsular abnormalities are combined with typical inflammatory changes in other intra-articular structures, particularly the synovial membrane, allowing differentiation of rheumatoid arthritis from other disorders, such as Jaccoud's arthropathy and the arthropathy of systemic lupus erythematosus (see Chapters 33 and 38).

Synovial Membrane, Cartilage, and Bone in Advanced Rheumatoid Arthritis. The pathologic and radiographic changes in the synovial joints of patients with rheumatoid arthritis do not always progress relentlessly. Rather, in the early phases of the disease, nearly complete regression of the abnormalities may occur. Even in later phases, after irreversible damage has been accomplished, the changes may remain static for indefinite periods of time. In fact, at any one time in the course of the disease, the synovial membrane can show a mixed picture of acute and chronic changes combined with signs of tissue repair and fibrosis.[65] Furthermore, close correlation does not always exist between the synovial histopathologic changes and the activity of the clinical disease,[66, 67] although active villus formation, subsynovial lymphocyte infiltration, and reduced synovial fluid complement levels have been associated with a severe clinical course and increased joint damage.[68, 69]

In the late stage of rheumatoid arthritis, the total synovial surface area is dramatically increased by the proliferation and hypertrophy of synovial villi during the course of articular inflammation.[21] Once the villi have appeared, they persist even when the synovitis has subsided. Increasing fibrosis of the stroma and accumulations of fibrin within the villous structures are seen. As a terminal event, very elongated villi may become detached, appearing in the joint cavity as "rice bodies."[220] The precise mechanism of formation of rice bodies, however, remains controversial.[251] Their name is derived from the resemblance to grains of polished rice, and these bodies are apparent not only in

rheumatoid arthritis but also in other types of articular disease, including tuberculosis.[256] Rice bodies are variable in size, shape, and consistency, and with maturity contain tissue resembling coarse collagenous fibers, reticulin, and elastin.[21] Through stimulating further fibrogenesis they contribute to the chronicity of the articular process.

In addition to collections of fibrin, fragments of cartilage and bone are found embedded in the synovial tissue (Figs. 25–12 to 25–14). Muirden[30] noted cartilaginous and bony

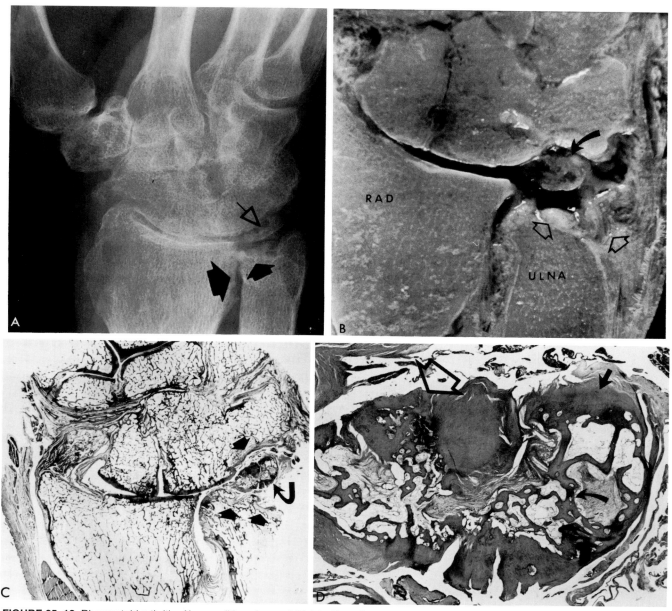

FIGURE 25–12. Rheumatoid arthritis: Abnormalities of synovial joints. Bony fragmentation in a cadaver.

A An oblique projection of the wrist demonstrates erosions of the distal radius and ulna (solid arrows). Carpal fusion, scaphoid erosions with bone production, osteoporosis, and an elongated bony spicule (open arrow) overlying the radiocarpal joint are observed.

B A coronal section through the wrist reveals the fragment (curved arrow) adjacent to the carpal mass. Abnormal synovium (open arrows) extends across the eroded ulna. The scalloped erosive changes of adjacent portions of the radius (RAD) and ulna are evident.

C Histologic evaluation (2×) of the fragment (curved arrow) demonstrates synovial proliferation with subjacent bony erosions of the ulna and carpal bones (arrows).

D The completely sequestered osteocartilaginous fragment is surrounded almost entirely by pannus (15×). Cartilage (straight arrow) and bone (curved arrow) are present. Increased radiodensity suggests endochondral bone formation (open arrow), which was more evident on higher magnification.

(From Resnick D, Gmelich J: Radiology *114*:315, 1975.)

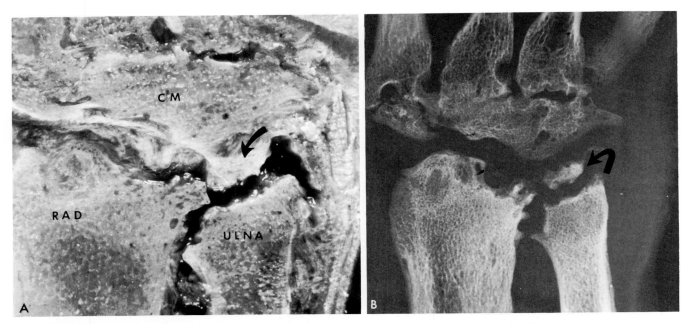

FIGURE 25–13. Rheumatoid arthritis: Abnormalities of synovial joints. Bony fragmentation in an additional cadaver.

A A coronal section through an eroded radius (RAD) and ulna delineates the fragment (curved arrow) adjacent to an irregular carpal mass (CM).

B Radiograph of the section in **A** better outlines the separated bone (curved arrow) within the joint space. Note the extent of osseous destruction of the distal radius and ulna.

(From Resnick D, Gmelich J: Radiology *114*:315, 1975.)

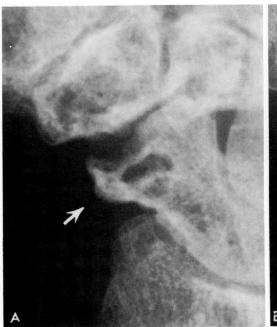

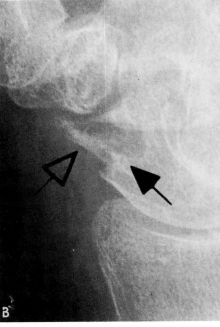

FIGURE 25–14. Rheumatoid arthritis: Abnormalities of synovial joints. Prefragmentation changes in two patients.

A An elongated spicule (arrow) is attached to an eroded scaphoid by several bony bridges.

B Radiograph of another rheumatoid arthritis patient with a similar spicule (open arrow) adjacent to an eroded scaphoid (solid arrow).

(From Resnick D, Gmelich J: Radiology *114*:315, 1975.)

debris in 56 of 100 biopsy specimens of rheumatoid synovium, particularly in association with severe radiographic abnormalities. Although the exact pathogenesis of such fragments is unclear, it is probable that they arise from the erosive process that destroys cartilage and bone within the articulation.[70] Subchondral pannus and osseous destruction and proliferation can result in uneven undermining of the bony surface, creating peninsulas of bone that might either remain attached by fibrovascular tissue or become detached, thus forming free cartilaginous and osseous bodies within the joint. Parasitic implantation with adherence to the synovial membrane could occur at a distant site. The fragmentation process can be accentuated by osseous compression, impaction, and fracture produced by the altered mechanics in the involved articulation, and it can be stimulated further by the presence of osteoporotic bone and the absence of a protective cartilaginous coat.[71, 72, 221] The proximity of sites of bone fragmentation to capsular and ligamentous attachment may indicate that small pieces of bone could be dislodged by stretching of the supporting structures with osseous traction.[70] The separated fragments can be a combination of pannus with both bone and cartilage or pannus with either bone or cartilage. Although metaplastic bone formation also can produce osseous and cartilaginous foci in the synovial membrane,[30] the lack of bone formation in the attached pannus and the sharp demarcation among pannus, cartilage, and bone discount this mechanism in many cases.[70]

The fate of the detached spicules is variable. Observations suggest that degenerated cartilaginous debris within a joint is removed less effectively than healthy cartilage introduced experimentally.[73] This reflects either increased resistance to resorption of degenerative cartilage and bone or decreased efficiency of diseased synovium as a scavenger. Furthermore, the pieces of cartilage and bone are too large to be removed unchanged from beneath the synovial lining; they may remain permanently, demonstrating increased growth, or become digested. Pathologically, foreign body giant cell reaction within the synovial membrane may be noted surrounding the particles.

In some situations, necrotic bone fragments occurring in rheumatoid joints, if numerous and large, may be extruded through the skin.[57, 58] This sequence of events results in fistulous rheumatism (more properly called sinus tract rheumatism) and is reminiscent of that associated with fistulae and sinus tracts in osteomyelitis (see later discussion).

The radiographic appearance associated with bone fragmentation in rheumatoid arthritis is characterized by prefragmentation abnormalities consisting of partially separated small cortical spicules and postfragmentation abnormalities consisting of well-defined separated osseous densities. The last-mentioned findings resemble those in neuropathic osteoarthropathy, osteoarthritis, gout, osteochondritis dissecans, osteonecrosis, and idiopathic synovial osteochondromatosis, although the number of fragmented bony particles in rheumatoid arthritis generally is limited. Typical sites include the wrist and elbow. Although relatively unapparent on plain film radiography, bone fragments are better visualized with conventional or computed tomography.

Osteoarthritis can be a prominent secondary phenomenon in the synovial joints of patients with rheumatoid arthritis. The prerequisites for the development of osteoarthritis in

this setting are the subsidence of the inflammation in the synovial membrane, the occurrence of damage to the articular cartilage, and the continued functional use of the joint, leading to alteration of the articular ends by friction.[20] The pathologic aberrations of osteoarthritis, such as erosion of articular cartilage, thickening of subchondral trabeculae, cyst formation, and osteophytosis, have their typical radiographic counterparts. When prominent, osteoarthritic abnormalities can obscure the underlying rheumatoid process on both pathologic and radiographic examinations. The possibility of underlying rheumatoid arthritis (or other processes characterized by synovial inflammation) should be considered whenever radiographs reveal osteoarthritis with unusual features or in unusual sites. Owing to the superimpo-

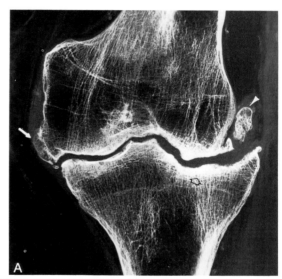

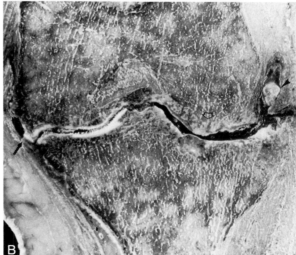

FIGURE 25–15. Rheumatoid arthritis: Abnormalities of synovial joints. Productive changes of bone. Knee. On a radiograph (**A**) and corresponding photograph (**B**) of a coronal section of the knee, observe abnormalities related to bone production in the form of osteophytes (solid arrows) and subchondral sclerosis (open arrows). These findings should not be regarded as evidence supporting a diagnosis other than rheumatoid arthritis. In this case, involvement of both the medial femorotibial space and lateral femorotibial space, with predominant involvement of the latter area, aids in the accurate diagnosis of rheumatoid arthritis. Fragmentation of the articular surface with the formation of a large intra-articular body (arrowheads) is seen.

sition of osteoarthritis on rheumatoid arthritis, the diagnosis of the latter disease cannot be eliminated when radiographs demonstrate productive changes of bone. Furthermore, as subchondral bony eburnation is not uncommon in weight-bearing articulations (such as the hip and the knee) in patients with rheumatoid arthritis, this finding too should not be regarded as radiologic evidence supporting a diagnosis other than rheumatoid arthritis (Fig. 25–15).

Bursae and Tendon Sheaths (Table 25–3)

Synovial inflammation in rheumatoid arthritis is not confined to intra-articular structures; similar inflammation occurs in the synovial lining of tendon sheaths and bursae but usually is of lesser extent.[22] Bursal involvement in this disease may occur in over 5 per cent of patients,[74] particularly in the popliteal region of the knee and in the olecranon,

TABLE 25–3. Abnormalities of Bursae and Tendon Sheaths in Rheumatoid Arthritis

Pathologic	Radiologic
Synovial inflammation and production of fluid	Soft tissue swelling
Hyperemia	Osteoporosis
Pannus destruction of subjacent bone	Surface resorption of bone

subacromial (subdeltoid), and retrocalcaneal bursae,[75–79, 308] as well as about the wrist and the foot[80, 81] (Fig. 25–16). Tenosynovitis is especially prominent on the dorsum of the hand, the fingers, and the foot[81–86] (Fig. 25–17). Bursitis and tenosynovitis can be coupled with typical involvement of adjacent articulations, although they can occur as isolated or predominant manifestations of the disor-

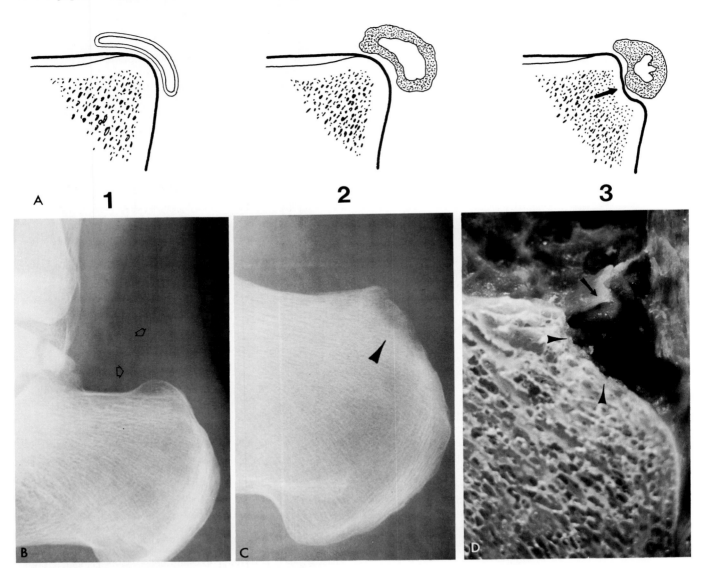

FIGURE 25–16. Rheumatoid arthritis: Abnormalities of bursae.
A Diagram depicting the changes associated with bursal inflammation. In the normal situation (1), a collapsed, noninflamed synovial sac is evident. With progressive inflammation (2, 3), hypertrophy of the synovial lining, increased intrabursal fluid, distention, and possible erosion of subjacent bone (arrow) can be seen.
B–D Retrocalcaneal bursitis. Soft tissue swelling (open arrows) represents a fluid-filled, distended retrocalcaneal bursa. Subjacent osseous erosion (arrowhead, **C**) subsequently can be seen. A photograph of a sagittal section of the posterosuperior aspect of the calcaneus (**D**) demonstrates the irregular synovial lining of the bursa (arrow) and the adjacent bony erosion (arrowheads).

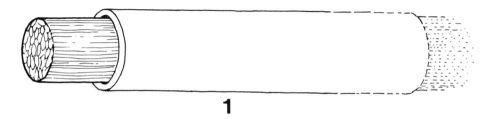

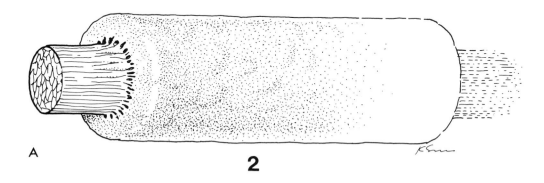

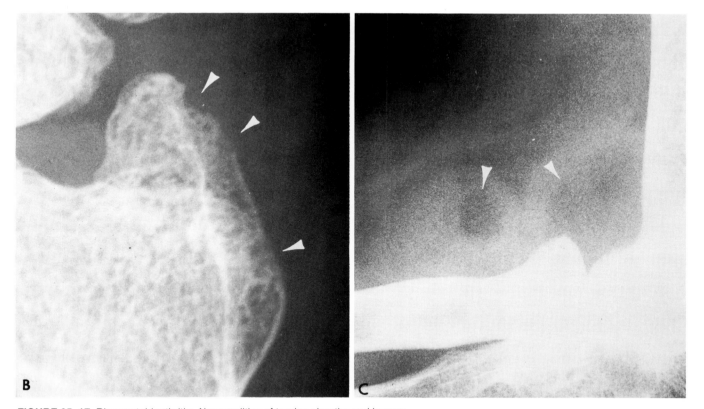

FIGURE 25–17. Rheumatoid arthritis: Abnormalities of tendon sheaths and bursae.

A In the normal situation (1), a smooth synovial lining is reflected over the tendon sheath. In tenosynovitis (2), the tendon sheath fills with fluid. Adhesions exist between it and the subjacent tendon.

B Surface resorption of bone beneath an inflamed extensor carpi ulnaris tendon sheath produces typical defects along the outer aspect of the ulnar styloid (arrowheads).

C With distention of inflamed bursae (or articulations) intrasynovial fatty deposits may create radiolucent areas (arrowheads) within the soft tissue prominence. (Courtesy of John Weston, M.D., Lower Hutt, New Zealand.)

der. In fact, bursae and joints frequently communicate, and a process initially evident in the articulation may subsequently spread to the extra-articular synovial structures (see later discussion).

When inflamed, tendon sheaths and bursae fill with exudate, enlarge, and form clinically detectable soft tissue masses. Histologically, the synovial abnormalities within the bursa or tendon sheath are identical to those that are evident in the joint. Acute and chronic inflammatory changes and necrotic foci surrounded by typical palisading cells can be observed.[21] In association with tenosynovitis, the tendon itself may become affected, leading to a variety of complications, including weakening, subluxation, entrapment, and rupture.

The most common radiographic finding associated with tenosynovitis and bursitis is soft tissue swelling. The soft tissue prominence may be of homogeneous density, although enclosed radiolucent areas can indicate intrasynovial fatty deposits (Fig. 25–17).[87] The swelling frequently is lobulated or nodular in outline, simulating the appearance of a gouty tophus. Adjacent soft tissue planes are displaced or obscured by the inflamed mass. Erosion of subjacent bone can be observed, particularly in the posterosuperior aspect of the calcaneus (in relation to retrocalcaneal bursitis), the olecranon process (in relation to olecranon bursitis), and the inferior surface of the acromion and distal end of the clavicle (in relation to subacromial bursitis).[88] In addition, surface resorption of bone beneath inflamed tendon sheaths is characteristic, particularly in the outer aspect of the distal portion of the ulna (extensor carpi ulnaris tenosynovitis) (Fig. 25–17).

Arthrography, bursography, tenography, and MR imaging (Fig. 25–18) can be used to directly delineate the nature of the soft tissue swelling and the extent of synovial inflammation (see Chapters 10 and 13).

Cartilaginous Joints and Entheses

Although involvement of cartilaginous joints, such as the symphysis pubis and manubriosternal and discovertebral articulations, and of entheses (sites of tendon and ligament attachment to bone), such as those related to the spinous processes of the vertebrae, the inferior surface of the calcanei, the iliac wings, the ischial tuberosities, and the femoral trochanters, is observed in rheumatoid arthritis, the frequency and severity of such involvement are far less striking than in the seronegative spondyloarthropathies.[89-90] Furthermore, the pathogenesis of rheumatoid involvement at some cartilaginous and ligamentous sites, such as the discovertebral junction and spinous processes, is controversial and may be unrelated to primary inflammatory changes of these nonsynovial articulations.

Occasionally a patient with rheumatoid arthritis develops joint space narrowing, bone sclerosis, and soft tissue swelling about the manubriosternal articulations and symphysis pubis. Histologic examination of affected tissue, obtained primarily from patients with ankylosing spondylitis, indicates that osteitis of subchondral bone is associated with infiltration by chronic inflammatory cells and vascular fibrous tissue and with osteoclastic activity.[89] Additional findings are osseous replacement with granulation tissue and fibrocartilage, trabecular thickening, and progressive intra-articular ossification. Similarly, occasionally a patient

TABLE 25–4. Abnormalities of Discovertebral Cartilaginous Joints in Rheumatoid Arthritis

Potential Mechanism	Pathogenesis
Synovial Inflammation	"Pannus" is derived from joints of Luschka (cervical region) and costovertebral articulations (thoracic region)
Trauma	Apophyseal joint instability leads to traumatic disruption of discovertebral junction with cartilaginous node formation
Enthesopathy	Inflammation at ligamentous and capsular attachments leads to adjacent osseous erosion

with rheumatoid arthritis reveals erosion and bony proliferation at tendinous and ligamentous attachments to bone (Fig. 25–19). Histologic evaluation of material, again gathered mainly from patients with ankylosing spondylitis, reveals focal inflammatory lesions at the tendo-osseous junctions.[90]

In certain cartilaginous joints, such as the manubriosternal joint, the pathogenesis of the radiographic features of rheumatoid arthritis may relate to the development of a synovial cavity, lined with synovium-like cells, and to subsequent inflammation similar to that occurring in the peripheral joints in this disease. Schils and colleagues,[354] in a review of cadaveric material, noted fibrinoid necrosis and peripherally located palisading histiocytes in a rheumatoid manubriosternal articulation, entirely consistent with known histologic changes of rheumatoid arthritis. At this site, it also is possible that abnormal synovial tissue may have extended from the adjacent second sternocostal joints (Fig. 25–20).

It is the alterations of the discovertebral junction in rheumatoid arthritis that have sparked a most heated debate (Table 25–4) (Figs. 25–21 and 25–22). Undeniably, significant destruction of these osteochondral junctions, particularly in the cervical region, is a feature of rheumatoid arthritis.[91-94] The controversy centers on the pathogenesis of these alterations. Various schools of thought have advanced the following suggestions: (1) discovertebral abnormalities occur as a secondary manifestation of synovial inflammation in the adjacent neurocentral articulations (joints of Luschka) in the cervical spine and the neighboring costovertebral articulations in the thoracic spine (the synovial school); (2) discovertebral alterations relate to traumatic insults produced by instability of the posterior elements of the spine (the traumatic school); or (3) discovertebral alterations in rheumatoid arthritis, as in ankylosing spondylitis, are produced by a primary enthesopathy (the enthesopathic school).

The synovial school is adequately represented by the investigations of Ball[90, 95] and Bywaters.[96, 97, 264] A pathologic evaluation of 14 rheumatoid cervical spines revealed small macroscopic lesions, most pronounced on the lateral margin of the discs, which were intimately related to the neurocentral articulations.[95] These findings suggested that granulation tissue arising in these latter "synovial" joints spreads across the intervertebral disc–bone border, gradually replacing the anulus fibrosus from its posterior aspect. The synovial theory also could explain alterations in the intervertebral disc of the thoracic spine (considering the

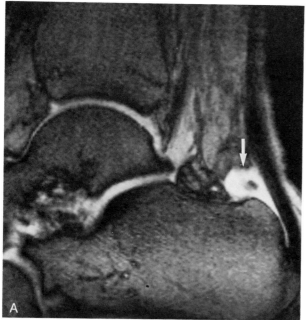

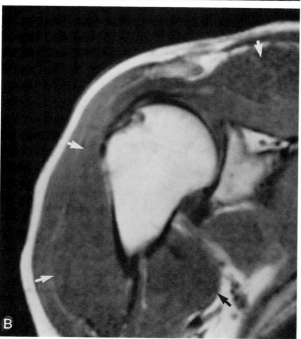

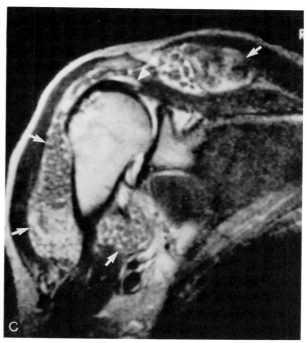

FIGURE 25–18. Rheumatoid arthritis: Abnormalities of bursae. Role of MR imaging.

A Retrocalcaneal bursitis. A sagittal gradient echo MR sequence (MPGR) (TR/TE, 500/20; flip angle, 25 degrees) reveals distention of the retrocalcaneal bursa with fluid, the latter appearing of increased signal intensity (arrow). No subjacent calcaneal erosion is apparent. Elsewhere, it is difficult to differentiate between articular cartilage and joint fluid in the ankle and intertarsal articulations.

B, C Subdeltoid-subacromial bursitis. In a 45 year old woman with rheumatoid arthritis, T1-weighted (TR/TE, 505/20) (**B**) and T2-weighted (TR/TE, 2000/80) (**C**) coronal oblique spin echo MR images reveal a markedly distended bursa (arrows). In **C**, note increase in signal intensity of fluid in the joint and in the bursa; however, regions of low signal density remain in the bursa. At surgery, these areas were found to represent small fibrous nodules, or rice bodies. Also note the tear of the supraspinatus tendon (arrowhead in **C**), which may represent a complication of rheumatoid arthritis.

(**B, C**, Courtesy of J. Hodler, M.D., Zurich, Switzerland.)

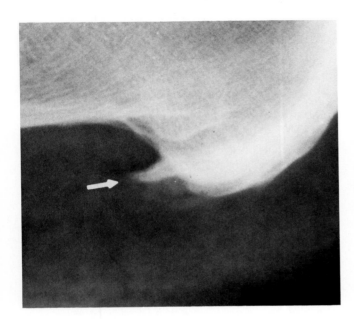

FIGURE 25–19. Rheumatoid arthritis: Abnormalities of attachment sites of ligaments or tendons (entheses). Bony proliferation can occur where the plantar ligaments attach to the undersurface of the calcaneus (arrow). The excrescences usually are well defined in outline in this disease.

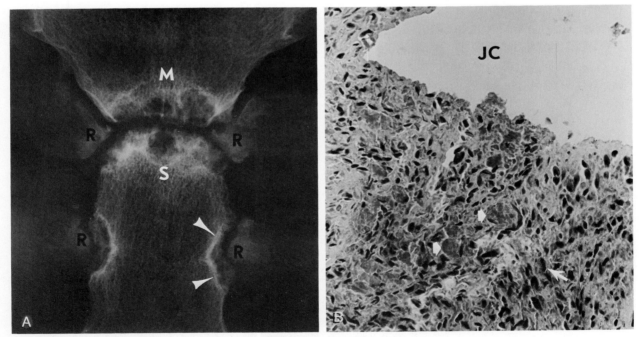

FIGURE 25–20. Rheumatoid arthritis: Abnormalities of the manubriosternal and sternocostal joints.

A A radiograph of a sternum derived from a cadaver with rheumatoid arthritis shows large erosions of the articular surface of both the manubrium (M) and the body of the sternum (S). Subtle irregularities of the second and third sternocostal joints are evident, being most prominent in the sternal facet of the left third sternocostal joint (arrowheads). R, Ossified costal cartilage.

B Histologic examination of tissue derived from a third sternocostal articulation shows a joint cavity (JC). Nearby, a rheumatoid arthritis–type lesion with scattered necrotic foci is seen (short arrows). Palisading of cells is evident in at least one area (long arrow). The sternal body region is located to the left side of the photograph.

(From Schils JP, et al: Invest Radiol 24:596, 1989.)

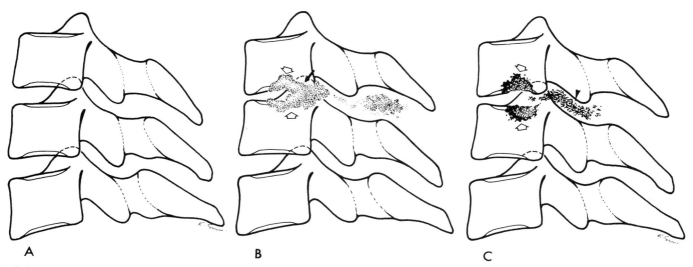

FIGURE 25–21. Rheumatoid arthritis: Abnormalities of the discovertebral junctions of the cervical spine. The normal situation is depicted in **A**. The proponents of the synovial school of thought suggest that inflammatory tissue in the neurocentral joints of Luschka (solid arrow) spreads across the discovertebral junction (**B**), leading to osseous erosion (open arrows). The proponents of the traumatic school of thought believe that instability of the apophyseal joints due to synovial inflammation (arrowhead) produces recurrent discovertebral trauma, leading to cartilaginous nodes with surrounding sclerosis (**C**) (open arrows).

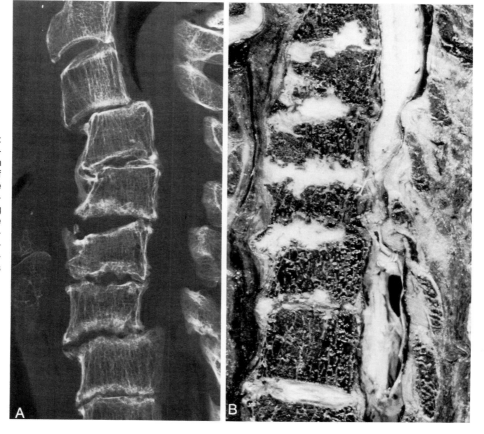

FIGURE 25–22. Rheumatoid arthritis: Abnormalities of the discovertebral junctions of the cervical spine. A radiograph (**A**) and corresponding photograph (**B**) of a sagittal section of the cervical spine reveal widespread alterations of the discovertebral junctions. Observe narrowing of the intervertebral discs, erosion of the vertebral endplates with intraosseous extension of discal material, multiple subluxations, and only mild osteophyte formation. Spinal cord compression is evident.

intimacy of the neighboring synovium-lined costovertebral articulations), although discal changes in the lumbar spine would require a different pathogenesis. A radiographic and pathologic study of the thoracic spine in cadavers with rheumatoid arthritis indicated that the origin of the inflammatory tissue in the discovertebral junction appeared to be the costovertebral articulations.[264] In this investigation, the rheumatoid process initially involved the cartilaginous surfaces of the vertebral facet and head of the rib, and it subsequently extended to the disc as well as beneath the cartilaginous endplate. Pathologic alterations included loss of red marrow, increased vascularity, fibrosis, new bone formation, and, in the disc itself, formation of fibrocartilage and ingrowth of bone. Although pleuritis was occasionally observed, it appeared unlikely that the rheumatoid inflammatory tissue within the costovertebral joint had originated in the pleural lining.

The traumatic school has its main proponent in Martel.[91, 98] His concept that destruction of the cervical discovertebral junctions in rheumatoid arthritis is related to trauma produced by chronic cervical instability is based on several observations: (1) gross vertebral endplate destruction often is preceded by a cartilaginous node–like erosion and disc space narrowing; (2) intervertebral disc destruction frequently is preceded by apophyseal joint destruction and vertebral malalignment at the same level; (3) vertebral endplate destruction occurs where the intervening cartilage is destroyed and where the contiguous vertebrae impinge on one another, whereas nonapposed vertebrae are relatively spared; (4) microscopic examination of the intervertebral disc and adjacent vertebrae shows focal necrosis and degeneration of cartilage with reactive fibrosis but virtually no inflammation, findings that are similar to those described in the thoracolumbar spine in non–rheumatoid arthritis patients[99]; (5) similar lesions occasionally are observed in the

thoracolumbar spine, where there are no neurocentral joints (Fig. 25–23); and (6) bony ankylosis of the cervical apophyseal joints, which is frequent in children and occasionally seen in adults, appears to protect the discovertebral joints from this type of destruction. Martel supports the following sequence of events: apophyseal joint destruction; cervical spine instability; fractures of the endplates of the vertebral bodies; intravertebral disc displacement; degeneration of the intervertebral disc cartilage; and further erosion and sclerosis of vertebral bodies. He also stresses that some previous pathologic descriptions of destructive lesions in rheumatoid arthritis contain findings compatible with this traumatic pathogenesis.[100, 101] Further support for a prominent role of trauma in the development of lesions in the discovertebral junction may come from the observations of Lorber and coworkers[102] and Pearson and colleagues[355] that granulomatous nodular lesions may develop in the vertebrae of patients with rheumatoid arthritis. These lesions, combined with osteoporosis related to the disease itself or to steroid medication, may contribute to osseous weakening and discal displacement.

The enthesopathic school—which believes that inflammatory changes at spinal entheses, well-known manifestations of ankylosing spondylitis, also can be prominent in rheumatoid arthritis—is relatively small. Occasional reports describe spondylitis in rheumatoid arthritis, primarily in the thoracic and lumbar spine, resulting from spread of inflammatory tissue from paraspinal ligamentous, areolar, and connective tissue.[103] The predilection for involvement of the cervical spine, the preponderance of posterior discal lesions, and the absence of syndesmophytes, osteitis, and squaring of vertebral bodies in rheumatoid arthritis, however, suggest that the discovertebral abnormalities in this disease differ in pathogenesis from those in ankylosing spondylitis. Furthermore, the increasing number of well-

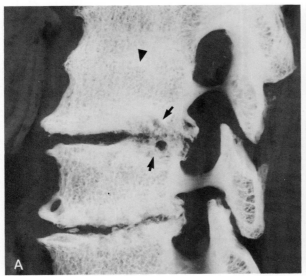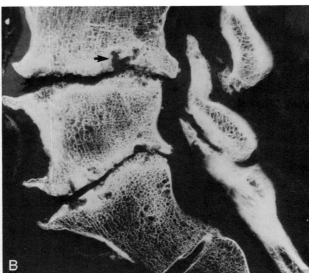

FIGURE 25–23. Rheumatoid arthritis: Similarity of discovertebral lesions in the cervical spine and lumbar spine.

A Cervical spine. Sagittal sectional radiograph reveals, at one discovertebral level, prominent erosions about the neurocentral joints (arrows). At a lower level, widespread discovertebral erosions and disc space loss are apparent. Above, bone ankylosis (arrowhead) has led to obliteration of an intervertebral disc. The apophyseal joints are not well evaluated in this radiograph.

B Lumbar spine. Sagittal sectional radiograph shows extensive erosions of the discovertebral junctions between the fourth lumbar vertebra and the sacrum. Most of the erosions are superficial, but one large osseous defect is apparent (arrow). Moderate osteophyte formation is noted.

documented cases of both rheumatoid arthritis and ankylosing spondylitis occurring in the same person further complicates the interpretation of ''spondylitis-like'' changes in rheumatoid disease (see Chapter 28).

The final word on the pathogenesis of discovertebral joint lesions in rheumatoid arthritis has yet to be written. The similarity of vertebral abnormalities in cervical, thoracic, and lumbar segments of rheumatoid spines to those associated with cartilaginous (Schmorl's) nodes in nonrheumatoid spines[104] cannot, however, be ignored.[354] It does appear that disruption of the cartilaginous endplate and subchondral bone plate of the vertebral bodies, allowing discal displacement, is important in rheumatoid arthritis. Whether this disruption is attributable to trauma alone, to synovitis alone, or to both trauma and synovitis is not known.

Erosion and reactive sclerosis of the spinous processes of the cervical vertebrae appear to be related to two mechanisms.[96] First, an inflammatory process at the sites of ligament attachment to bone is consistent with the enthesopathy that also is recognized in ankylosing spondylitis and other seronegative spondyloarthropathies. Second, synovial inflammation in interspinous bursae may contribute to the destructive process in the neighboring bone. In a pathologic and radiologic study, Bywaters[265] observed the formation of bursae between the spinous processes of the cervical vertebrae in two of nine cadavers with rheumatoid arthritis and, further, the presence of major rheumatoid lesions in the bursae in one cadaver. In this latter instance, the bursal spaces were lined by granulation tissue and the spinous processes were eroded. Although this investigation documented the occurrence of bursal alterations in other articular diseases, the abnormal mobility of the cervical spine due to discal destruction and subluxation in rheumatoid arthritis appeared to be a factor that favored the initiation of bursal inflammation.

Tendons and Ligaments

Significant abnormalities of tendons and ligaments occur in rheumatoid arthritis. Inflammatory changes and laxity resulting from distortion of these structures by the intra-articular process are seen, contributing to the typical joint deformities that accompany long-standing rheumatoid arthritis.

Pathologic studies of tendon abnormalities in rheumatoid arthritis have concentrated predominantly on the hand and the fingers.[105, 106] Enlargement of the tendon may be associated with the appearance of granulation tissue in the peritenon and mesotenon. Fibrin, fibroblasts, polymorphonuclear leukocytes, and lymphocytes characterize the ''tendinitis.'' Focal necrotic areas within the tendon resemble subcutaneous rheumatoid nodules. An edematous granular tendon mass eventually may be produced, which is ineffectual in its role of providing support to adjacent joints.

''Spontaneous'' tendon ruptures are a known manifestation of rheumatoid arthritis (Figs. 25–24 and 25–25). They are encountered most frequently in the hand and the wrist, although ruptures of other tendons can occur, including the Achilles, infrapatellar, tibialis posterior, and rotator cuff tendons.[107–115] Tendon rupture, which can be provoked by local corticosteroid injection,[114] may be attributable to collagenolysis by abnormal production of proteolytic enzymes, such as lysozyme, cathepsin B, and neutral protease.[4–6, 116]

These enzymes can originate from diseased synovium in adjacent structures, such as the retrocalcaneal bursa (which is intimate with the Achilles tendon), the glenohumeral joint (which is intimate with the rotator cuff tendons), and the flexor and extensor tendon sheaths (which are intimate with the tendons of the hand and the wrist). Tendon inflammation itself may further enhance the disruption process. Additional potential factors in tendon rupture in the rheumatoid arthritis patient include abnormal stress produced by malalignment and subluxation, attrition from adjacent irregular osseous spicules, and tissue insult produced by vascular lesions.

Joint subluxation, malalignment, and deformity in rheumatoid arthritis can be attributed to numerous factors (Fig. 25–26). Inflammatory destruction of intra-articular structures leading to surface incongruity, capsular and ligamentous weakening leading to laxity, tendinitis and tenosynovitis leading to contracture and rupture, and muscular contraction are all influential in this regard.[117–124] Articular deformity can become evident in many different sites but is most characteristic at the wrist, the metacarpophalangeal, metatarsophalangeal, and interphalangeal articulations of the hand and the foot, and the atlantoaxial region. In most instances, the deformities allow an accurate clinical diagnosis of rheumatoid arthritis, although other disorders occasionally may produce similar abnormalities.[125] On roentgenographic examination, subluxation is combined almost invariably with typical intra-articular alterations, such as joint space narrowing and osseous erosion. Rarely, a deforming, nonerosive joint disease is apparent, which must be distinguished from the arthropathy of Jaccoud or systemic lupus erythematosus.

Soft Tissues

Edema. In patients with rheumatoid arthritis, widespread peripheral edema can relate to generalized factors such as anemia, fluid retention, and hypoalbuminemia. Localized factors, including obstruction of venous and lymphatic channels, reduced numbers of lymphatic vessels, and increased capillary permeability, also have been implicated.[260, 261, 356, 357] Lymphangiography has been used to delineate sites and patterns of lymphatic obstruction.[262] Positive findings include dermal backflow, lymph stasis, and perivenous extravasation of the contrast material. Although the precise cause of the lymphatic involvement in rheumatoid arthritis is not clear, it may relate to extension of inflammation from a joint to the surrounding soft tissue. Of note, lymphatic channel visualization is not an uncommon finding during arthrography in patients with rheumatoid arthritis, and lymphadenopathy has been observed in this disease.[263]

The appearance of lymphedema in rheumatoid arthritis assumes diagnostic significance owing to the recent identification of a syndrome in elderly patients consisting of peripheral seronegative inflammatory polyarthritis with pitting edema.[358] This condition, which has an excellent prognosis, is discussed in more detail in Chapter 26.

Rheumatoid Nodules. The most frequent soft tissue lesion in rheumatoid arthritis is the subcutaneous nodule. These nodules were first described by Wells[126] early in the nineteenth century in association with rheumatic heart disease and subsequently by Hillier[127] in 1868 and Jaccoud in

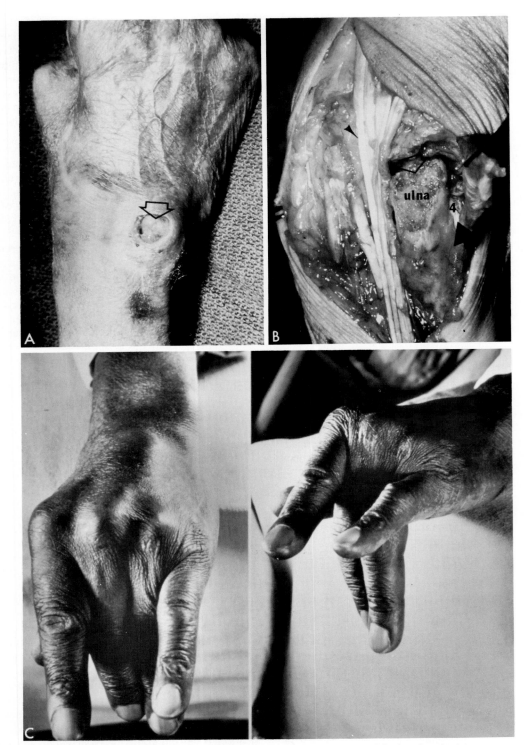

FIGURE 25–24. Rheumatoid arthritis: Spontaneous tendon rupture of the extensor tendons of the hand and wrist.

A A dorsally subluxed ulna (open arrow) may occasionally erode the skin on the dorsum of the rheumatoid wrist.

B A surgical photograph of the same wrist confirms the dorsal position (open arrow) of the eroded ulna, the jeopardy of the neighboring extensor tendons (arrowhead), and the volar displacement of the extensor carpi ulnaris tendon (4) (arrow).

C Two views of the hand and wrist of a different patient with rheumatoid arthritis demonstrate spontaneous rupture of the extensor tendons of the third and fourth digits.

(**A, B**, Courtesy of R. Convery, M.D., San Diego, California; **C**, courtesy of N. Zvaifler, M.D., San Diego, California.)

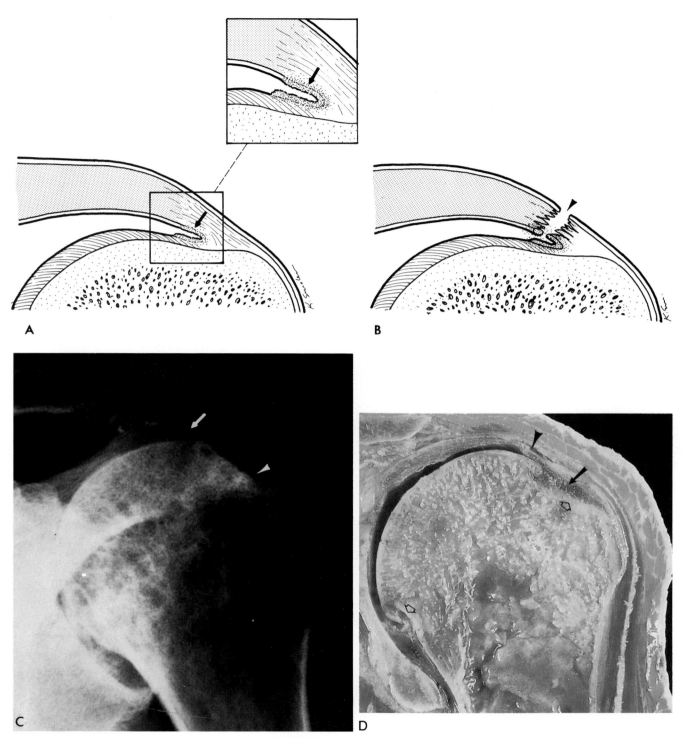

FIGURE 25–25. Rheumatoid arthritis: Spontaneous tendon weakening and rupture of the rotator cuff.

A, B Diagrams illustrate the manner in which inflamed synovial tissue (arrows) on the undersurface of the rotator cuff can erode and disrupt this structure (arrowhead).

C A radiograph of a patient with rheumatoid arthritis delineates the elevated position of the humeral head with respect to the glenoid cavity and the diminished distance between the humerus and acromion (arrow), which are characteristic of rotator cuff atrophy or tear. Note the erosion of the humeral head (arrowhead) and narrowing of the glenohumeral joint space.

D A photograph of a coronal section of the glenohumeral joint in a cadaver with rheumatoid arthritis indicates attrition of the rotator cuff tendons (arrowhead) related to synovial inflammation (solid arrow). Osseous erosions also are apparent (open arrows).

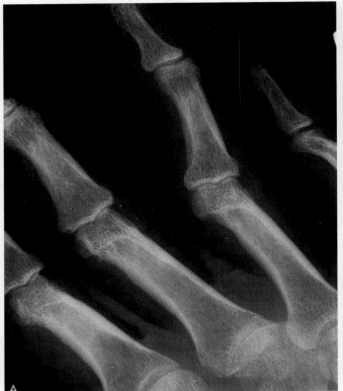
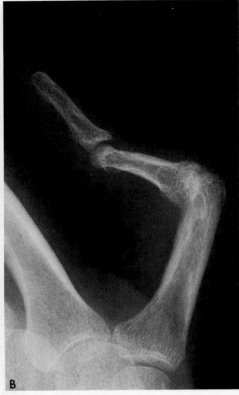
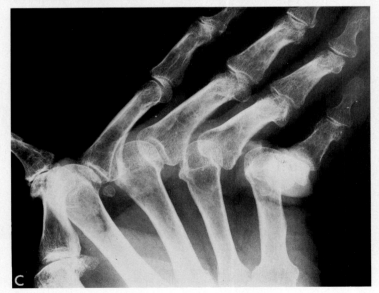

FIGURE 25–26. Rheumatoid arthritis: Joint malalignment.

A, B Typical digital deformities of the hand in rheumatoid arthritis include the swan-neck deformity (hyperextension at proximal interphalangeal joint and flexion at distal interphalangeal joint) (**A**) and boutonnière deformity (flexion at proximal interphalangeal joint and hyperextension at distal interphalangeal joint) (**B**).

C Rarely, severe subluxation of the hand in rheumatoid arthritis is associated with only minor intra-articular abnormality. Note ulnar deviation and flexion at the metacarpophalangeal joints with swan-neck deformities. Minor degrees of joint space narrowing are evident, but erosions are not prominent.

Illustration continued on opposite page

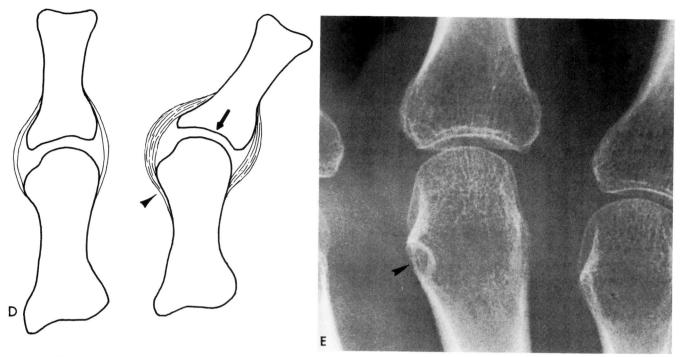

FIGURE 25–26. *Continued*

D, E In some patients (**D**), joint space diminution may relate not to synovial destruction of cartilage but to pressure erosion (arrow) at sites of subluxation; osseous erosion relates not to synovial destruction of bone but to capsular traction (arrowhead). The resulting radiographic picture is identical to that seen in various collagen vascular disorders, including systemic lupus erythematosus, and in Jaccoud's arthropathy. The site of bony erosion (arrowhead) is periarticular, as in this person with scleroderma (**E**), differing in location from the typical marginal intra-articular erosions that usually are encountered in rheumatoid arthritis.

1874.[128] The first detailed analysis was that of Meynet[129] in 1875 in a child of 14 years of age. In 1890, Garrod[130] differentiated the two conditions, rheumatoid arthritis and rheumatic fever, indicating that subcutaneous nodules could be evident in either disease. Despite the clear clinical distinction between rheumatoid arthritis and rheumatic fever, debate continued as to whether the nodules in the two disorders were identical histologically or at least were similar enough to imply a common causation.[128, 131–133] Although the subcutaneous nodule was considered virtually diagnostic of rheumatoid arthritis for a period of time, it now is recognized that these or similar nodules are associated with a wide variety of disorders.[128, 134–136, 309, 310] In addition to rheumatoid arthritis and rheumatic fever, subcutaneous nodules may appear in collagen vascular disorders, sarcoidosis, Weber-Christian disease, gout, dermatologic processes, xanthomatosis, and various infectious disorders, as well as other conditions.[310]

One or more subcutaneous nodules are detectable in approximately 20 to 25 per cent of patients with rheumatoid arthritis,[359] and may develop rapidly in some patients who are being treated with methotrexate.[360, 361] They are located most commonly between the skin and an underlying bony prominence, a site that may be subjected to pressure or mechanical stress. Typical locations include the olecranon, the proximal portion of the ulna (Fig. 25–27), the lateral aspects of the fingers, the gluteal and Achilles tendon regions, and the areas about the femoral trochanters and ischial tuberosities. In the bedridden person, nodules are encountered over the scapula, thoracic spine, sacrum, and occiput. Similar lesions are encountered in noncutaneous structures, such as the synovium, the dura mater, the sclera, the retropharyngeal tissue, the lungs, and the heart.[19, 137–144, 362] Rheumatoid nodules even may occur at the cement-bone interface after arthroplasty in patients with rheumatoid arthritis.[252] Almost invariably, rheumatoid nodules are associated with seropositivity for rheumatoid factor. Their presence also suggests a likelihood for severe erosive disease and vasculitis. They may be identified before the clinical onset of arthritis.[145]

Subcutaneous nodules vary in size from a few millimeters to over 5 cm. They usually are firm and nontender. Nodules frequently are attached to the deep fascia or the periosteum but can be freely movable. They usually are asymptomatic. Nodules exposed to prolonged pressure can ulcerate, becoming sites of secondary infection.

Three distinct zones constitute the histologic picture of a rheumatoid nodule.[128] The central necrotic area of the nodule contains a meshwork of fibrin, cellular fragments, and residue of partly degraded mature collagen fibrils.[19] Fibrin is particularly prominent in early active nodules; liquefaction with cyst formation can be demonstrated in older nodules. Polymorphonuclear granulocytes also have been observed in the necrotic areas of rheumatoid nodules.[247] The area of central necrosis is surrounded by a zone of palisading, elongated cells. These cells appear to be histiocytic in origin as they have lysosome activity and serve as macrophages.[128] The outer layer contains granulation tissue, which initially is vascular but later may become fibrotic. Perivascular plasma cells and lymphocytes can be encountered in this region.

The pathogenesis of rheumatoid nodules is controversial.

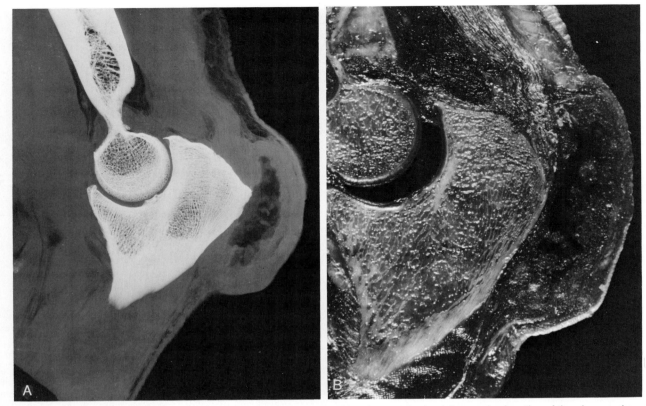

FIGURE 25–27. Rheumatoid arthritis: Soft tissue nodules. A typical site of involvement is about the proximal portion of the ulna, as shown in this sagittal sectional radiograph (**A**) and photograph (**B**). The olecranon bursa also is inflamed.

A vasculitic process has been advocated, leading to proliferation of fibroblasts and capillaries.[146] Coalescence of secondary necrotic foci may produce the necrotic central core of the nodule. The initiation of the vasculitis in the rheumatoid nodule may be related to the presence of immune complexes, a concept that is strengthened by the close association of this lesion with demonstrable rheumatoid factor in the serum and in the nodules themselves.[147]

Radiographically, subcutaneous rheumatoid nodules are associated with lobulated, eccentric soft tissue masses (Fig. 25–28). These masses rarely calcify, a diagnostic point that may be helpful in distinguishing them from gouty tophi, which can, indeed, contain calcification. In unusual instances, rheumatoid nodules can lead to erosion of subjacent bone.[148–150] In this regard, scalloped defects in the cortex of the proximal portion of the ulna, metacarpals, metatarsals, or other bones in rheumatoid arthritis can simulate the appearance of a variety of benign soft tissue neoplasms as well as gout, giant cell tumor of a tendon sheath, ganglia, and xanthoma. Rheumatoid nodules may also be examined with CT and MR imaging (Fig. 25–29).

An atypical variant of rheumatoid disease, rheumatoid nodulosis, is characterized by the presence of multiple subcutaneous nodules and the absence of significant synovitis or systemic manifestations.[151–156, 218, 222, 230, 257, 332, 363] Men usually are affected. In addition to nodular soft tissue masses, roentgenograms may detect intra-articular cystic osseous defects with or without joint space narrowing or osteoporosis. Serologic tests for rheumatoid factor commonly are positive in these persons, and biopsy of the nodules and synovium[152] reveals typical histologic changes of rheumatoid arthritis. In some patients, subsequent and severe articular symptoms and signs appear,[156] whereas other patients reveal abnormalities of additional organ systems.[153] As histologically similar or identical nodules have been observed in other diseases, such as systemic lupus erythematosus, ankylosing spondylitis, Jaccoud's arthropathy, and agammaglobulinemia, the designation of rheumatoid nodulosis as a form of rheumatoid arthritis in certain patients, especially those without any clinical or laboratory evidence of disease, is open to question.[258] In otherwise healthy children, a designation of "benign rheumatoid nodules" or "pseudorheumatoid nodules" has been used.[311]

Calcification. Soft tissue calcification is rare in rheumatoid arthritis. Calcific deposits within rheumatoid nodules and within periarticular subcutaneous tissue have been described occasionally in persons with this disease.[150] In all such cases, the possibility of mixed connective tissue disease or overlap collagen vascular syndromes must be considered (see Chapter 37).

Synovial Cysts. Synovial cysts are a well-known manifestation of rheumatoid arthritis[157] (Fig. 25–30). Their exact pathogenesis is controversial; although some investigators believe synovial cysts arise as rupture of the joint capsule with extravasation of fluid and secondary encapsulation, or as herniation of the synovial membrane, most now consider that these lesions represent abnormal distention of various bursae that communicate with the adjacent articulation.[158–160, 224] These communicating channels have been well documented in the knee[289] (see Chapter 22) and frequently

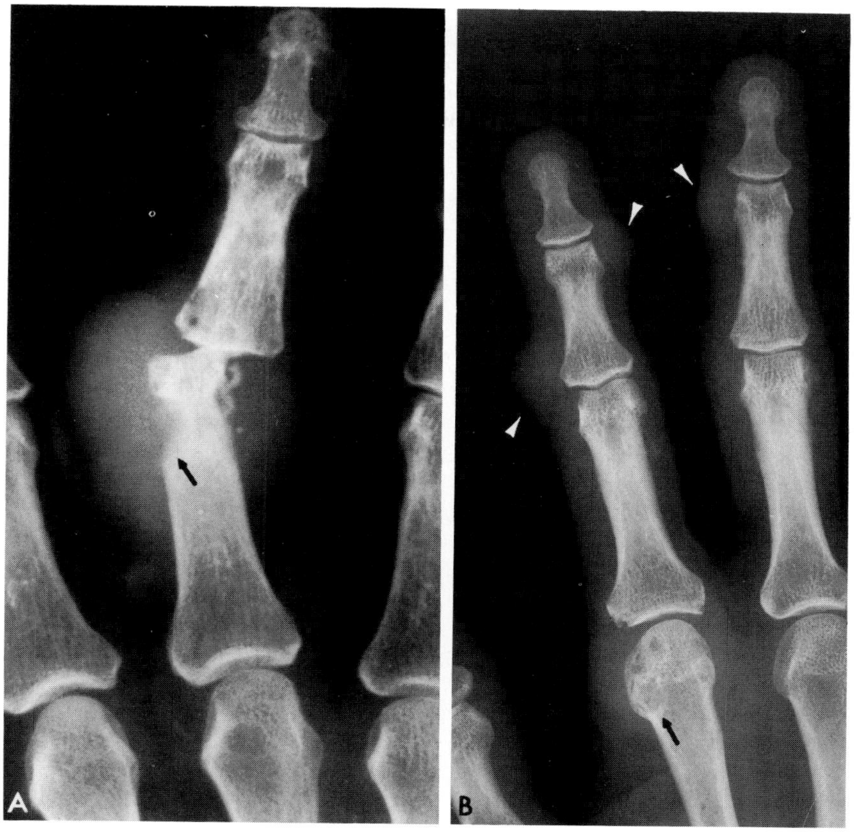

FIGURE 25–28. Rheumatoid arthritis: Soft tissue nodules.

A In unusual circumstances, rheumatoid nodules can erode subjacent bone (arrow) and produce deformity or subluxation. In these cases, the combination of asymmetric soft tissue swelling and eccentric erosions simulates the findings of gout. (Courtesy of J. Smith, M.D., New York, New York.)

B In this patient with rheumatoid nodulosis, multiple lobulated soft tissue nodules (arrowheads) and cystic osseous defects (arrow) are apparent.

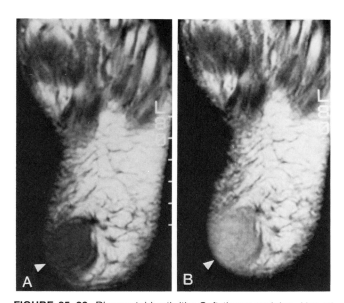

FIGURE 25–29. Rheumatoid arthritis: Soft tissue nodules. Use of MR imaging. This 65 year old woman with rheumatoid arthritis had multiple subcutaneous nodules including one in the plantar aspect of the left heel.

A T1-weighted (TR/TE, 600/20) transverse MR image reveals the soft tissue nodule (arrowhead) surrounded by fat, involving the left heel.

B After the intravenous injection of gadolinium, observe diffuse enhancement of the nodule (arrowhead) in an identical T1-weighted MR image.

(Courtesy of S. Moreland, M.D., San Diego, California.)

possess a valvular mechanism allowing the flow of synovial fluid to proceed in one direction only (from the articulation to the cyst and not from the cyst to the articulation).[283, 288, 290] It is this mechanism that mandates that the optimal way to visualize the cystic mass and its communication with the joint is to inject contrast material directly into the articulation. The contrast-opacified cyst may be smooth or irregular in outline, and, in some cases, free extravasation of contrast material into the adjacent soft tissue planes indicates cyst rupture. Such rupture may be associated with a decrease in a previously recognized soft tissue mass and a rapid increase in pain. Clinical differentiation of signs and symptoms related to synovial cysts about the knee from those due to thrombophlebitis can be difficult.[161, 162] This clinical difficulty is further complicated by the coexistence of both synovial cysts and thrombophlebitis.[284] Although the precise reason for this association is not known, rupture of a synovial cyst is accompanied by swelling and edema that may lead to stasis, inflammation of the wall of the vein, and thrombophlebitis; or, alternatively, soft tissue swelling accompanying thrombophlebitis may produce an increase in the pressure within a synovial cyst and predispose to its rupture.

Although the use of various imaging techniques in the diagnosis of synovial cysts is discussed elsewhere in this book, a few comments are appropriate here. Arthrography has been employed for this purpose,[294] and its accuracy commonly has been compared to that of ultrasonography,[295–298] with variable results, which are dependent on

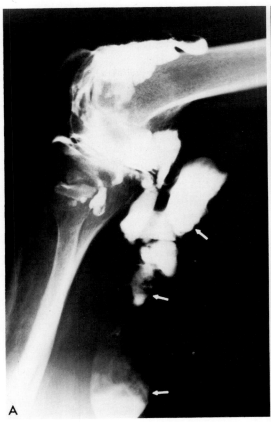
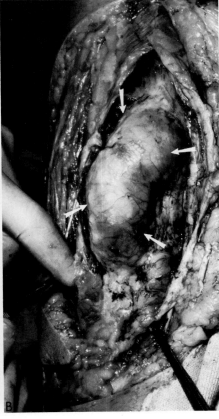

FIGURE 25–30. Rheumatoid arthritis: Synovial cysts.

A A typical popliteal cyst (arrows) is demonstrated during knee arthrography. Its margins are somewhat irregular, indicating synovial inflammation.

B Surgery in a different patient with a popliteal cyst reveals the bulging posterior synovial sac (arrows). (Courtesy of R. Convery, M.D., San Diego, California.)

Illustration continued on opposite page

the specific joint that is involved and the presence or absence of cyst rupture. Each technique has had its proponents, but the data have been inconclusive. Furthermore, scintigraphic arthrography, performed by injecting some type of radiopharmaceutical preparation into the joint, has been used to diagnose synovial cysts,[299] as has CT scanning.[300] The last-mentioned technique appears well suited to the evaluation of synovial cysts of the hip, allowing the full extent of the mass to be delineated. Recently, MR imaging also has been employed in the investigation of synovial cysts.[301, 364, 365] This method is very sensitive to the detection of fluid and, therefore, represents the best available imaging technique in the assessment of synovial cysts as well as ganglia (Fig. 25–31).[366]

The appearance of synovial cysts in rheumatoid arthritis, as in many articular disorders, probably is related to elevation of intra-articular pressure that occurs as a response to the accumulation of joint fluid. The passage of fluid from the joint into the adjacent soft tissue cyst serves to decompress the articulation.[56] As cited previously, an inverse relationship between the degree of articular destruction and the size of synovial cysts is consistent with this protective role for these soft tissue masses.

The wall of the rheumatoid synovial cyst is formed of dense collagen.[19] An inflamed synovium-like lining is present, as is variable lymphocytic and plasma cell infiltration. The sterile contents include synovial fluid and extensive cellular debris. Lymphoid follicles are rarely present.[163]

Although they most frequently are observed in the popliteal region,[164] rheumatoid synovial cysts have been described at other sites, including the calf (related to rheumatoid disease of the knee),[165, 166] the knee (superior,[328] anteromedial,[167] lateral,[293] or retrofemoral aspect[168]), the ankle, the plantar aspect of the foot,[169] the hip,[170–173, 292, 329] the hand and wrist,[174, 175] the elbow,[176–178, 291] and the shoulder.[179–180, 312] Presumably, an extra-articular synovial mass can arise about any involved articulation in this disease.

Sinus Tracts. Cutaneous-joint sinus tracts are recognized as an occasional feature of rheumatoid arthritis. Several mechanisms might contribute to this phenomenon.[58]

Classic "fistulous" rheumatism, described by Bywaters[57] in 1953 and later by Rosin and Toghill,[181] is related to the appearance of chronic skin sinuses near affected joints in rheumatoid arthritis patients (Figs. 25–32 and 25–33). In these patients, erythematous periarticular nodules erupt, forming draining sinuses, often multiple, in the vicinity of the hands and the feet. Initially, the sinus drainage is sterile, although with continued drainage secondary infection with staphylococci or other organisms can be seen. Radiographs reveal marked joint destruction with erosions, subchondral cysts, and osseous fragments. Pathologic features include pannus formation and fragments of necrotic bone and cartilage.

The pathogenesis of classic fistulous rheumatism is not certain. Bywaters[57] suggested that synovial fluid under elevated pressure created by joint motion intruded beneath the cartilage, producing an enlarging bone cyst. With continued physical activity, microfracture and bone necrosis occurred. When large or numerous, the bone fragments were extruded as foreign bodies, which formed abscesses that ruptured to

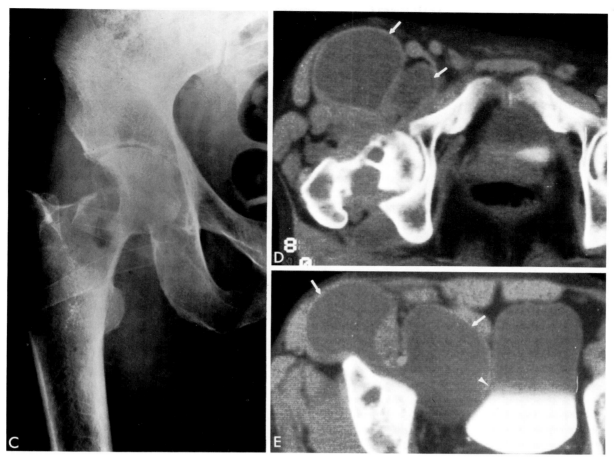

FIGURE 25–30. *Continued*

C–E In a 54 year old man with probable rheumatoid arthritis, plain films and CT scans were used to investigate the nature of a mass in the right groin. The radiograph (**C**) demonstrates a large soft tissue mass, joint space narrowing, and extensive erosion of the femoral neck (a surgical drain is in place). Transaxial CT sections at the levels of the femoral neck (**D**) and acetabular roof (**E**) reveal the size of the synovial cyst (arrows), its lobulated nature, displacement of the bladder (arrowhead), and femoral and acetabular erosions. At surgery, a cystic mass arising from the hip and extending to the iliopsoas bursa was found. Pathologically, hypertrophic synovitis with multinucleated giant cells, palisading histiocytes, and lymphoid follicles was seen. (Courtesy of J. Scavulli, M.D., San Diego, California.)

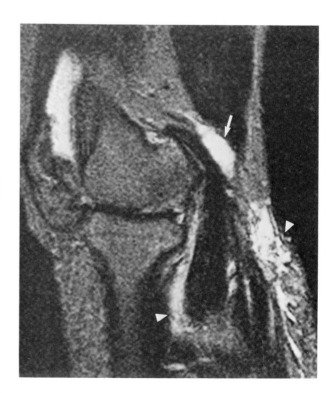

FIGURE 25–31. Rheumatoid arthritis: Synovial cysts. Role of MR imaging. A parasagittal T2-weighted spin echo MR image (TR/TE, 2000/150) of the knee reveals fluid of high signal intensity in the joint and in a synovial cyst (arrow). Note extravasation of fluid, indicating rupture of the cyst contents (arrowheads).

(Courtesy of T. Mattsson, Riyadh, Saudi Arabia.).

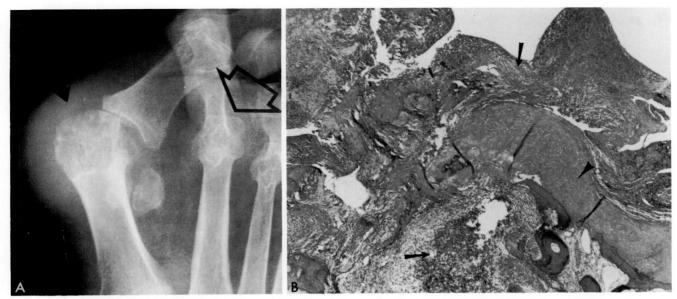

FIGURE 25–32. Rheumatoid arthritis: Sinus tracts in classic "fistulous" rheumatism. A 52 year old woman with rheumatoid arthritis developed sinus tracts spontaneously about the metatarsophalangeal joints. Cultures of the drainage material and of the intra-articular fluid were sterile.

A Radiographic findings include soft tissue swelling, erosions of the first metatarsal head (solid arrow), and subluxation at the second (open arrow) and third metatarsophalangeal joints.

B A photomicrograph (90×) of a metatarsal head demonstrates pannus (arrows) extending across and beneath the articular cartilage (arrowhead). No bone fragments are seen.

(From Shapiro RF, et al: Ann Rheum Dis *34*:489, 1975.)

the skin surface. The common, although not invariable, presence of bone fragments within granulation tissue and sinus tracts in patients with fistulous rheumatism suggests the participation of bone necrosis with subsequent inflammatory response as a major factor in the genesis of this complication. Because a large number of rheumatoid patients reveal bone fragments within joints that never develop sinus tracts and such tracts are relatively unusual in some other arthritides characterized by intra-articular bony and cartilaginous debris, a causal relationship between such fragmentation and sinus tract formation is only speculative.

Prominent subchondral cyst formation in patients with classic fistulous rheumatism suggests the presence of raised intra-articular pressure. As noted previously, synovial cysts may be one defense against the harmful effects of such elevated pressure. It may be possible that in the small joints of the hands and the feet, which are subject to considerable stress or the pressure of weight-bearing, sinus tract formation represents an additional protective mechanism for reducing abnormal intra-articular pressure.

Joint sepsis with subsequent sinus tract formation is a second mechanism of fistulous rheumatism. Septic arthritis is a recognized complication of rheumatoid arthritis, particularly in those patients who reveal high-titer serum rheumatoid factor, extensive joint destruction, systemic rheumatoid disease,[182] and hypocomplementemia[183] and in those who have received intra-articular injections of corticosteroids. Cutaneous sinus tracts may relate directly to septic joints in rheumatoid arthritis[58, 184] or to infectious arthritis occurring after prosthetic joint surgery in this disease.[58] In rheumatoid arthritis patients with septic arthritis and secondary formation of sinus tracts, the clinical course generally is characterized by fever, increasing pain, limitation of motion in one or more joints, and the appearance of sinuses

draining purulent material. Large articulations as well as small ones may be affected, and identical organisms are obtained in cultures of both the sinus drainage and synovial fluid. The implicated agents, although variable, most frequently are staphylococci.

Synovial cyst formation with sinus tract formation is a third, albeit rare, mechanism of fistulous rheumatism (Fig. 25–34). Although there have been reports of spontaneous cutaneous drainage of popliteal cysts in rheumatoid patients,[185] this complication is more frequent after direct aspiration.[58, 165, 313] Sinus tract formation complicating rheumatoid bursitis in which the adjacent articulations are uninvolved is exceedingly rare.[314]

Digital Vessels

Description of the significant visceral vascular lesions that are a common manifestation of rheumatoid arthritis[19, 21, 186] is beyond the scope of this chapter. Necrotizing arteritis in mesenteric, renal, and cerebral locations, subacute arteritis in skeletal muscles, and fibromuscular hyperplasia in peripheral vessels are all recognized in this disease. Changes in synovial capillaries, arteries, and venules also are well known. Vasculitis, complicated by digital gangrene and acro-osteolysis, can be seen in rheumatoid arthritis as well as in other collagen vascular disorders. In rheumatoid arthritis patients, such acro-osteolysis almost invariably is associated with severe erosive arthritis and, usually, with peripheral neuropathy.[187–190] Rarely, lysis of phalanges may be observed in the absence of erosions or neuropathy.[191] Of interest, vasculitis in rheumatoid arthritis has been suggested as a potential cause of ischemic necrosis at numerous skeletal sites, including the phalanges, femoral head, and symphysis pubis.[259]

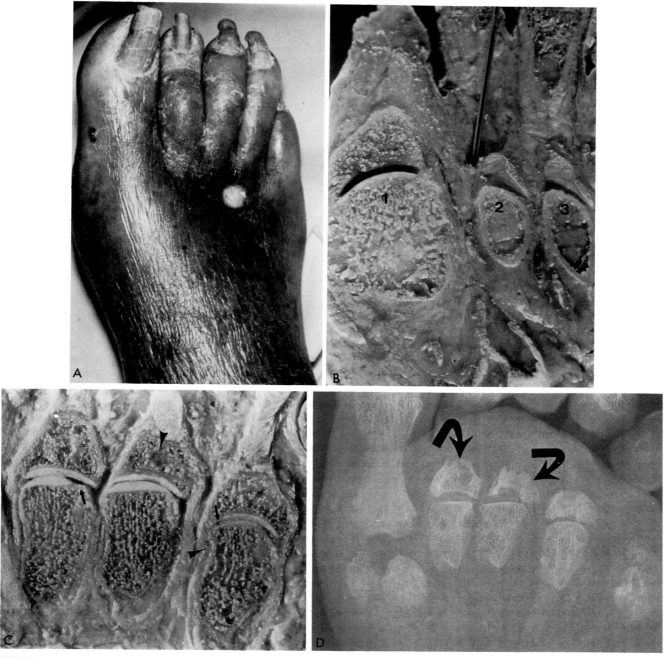

FIGURE 25–33. Rheumatoid arthritis: Sinus tracts in classic "fistulous" rheumatism. A 59 year old man with rheumatoid arthritis developed sterile drainage from the dorsum of the foot.

A A draining sinus tract is evident on the dorsum of the foot between the third and fourth toes.

B A transverse section of the amputated foot outlines a tract (probe) adjacent to the medial aspect of the proximal phalanx of the second toe. The metatarsal heads are numbered.

C A more dorsal section through the second, third, and fourth metatarsophalangeal joints reveals cartilaginous destruction (arrows) and bony erosions (arrowheads).

D The sectional radiograph of the specimen in **C** shows the extent of the erosions of the metatarsal heads and proximal phalanges (curved arrows).

(From Shapiro RF, et al: Ann Rheum Dis *34*:489, 1975.)

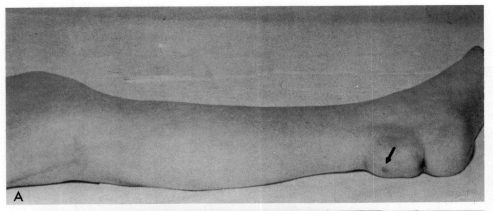

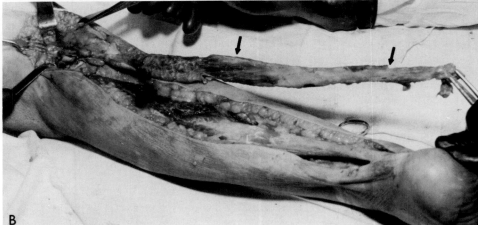

FIGURE 25–34. Rheumatoid arthritis: Synovial cyst formation with sinus tract formation. A 52 year old woman with rheumatoid arthritis developed a giant synovial cyst of the knee, which perforated the skin near the ankle.

A The clinical photograph demonstrates soft tissue swelling, a localized cyst near the Achilles tendon, and an opening (arrow).

B During surgical exploration, the extent of the dissecting popliteal cyst is evident (arrows).

(From Shapiro RF, et al: Ann Rheum Dis *34*:489, 1975.)

Bones

Generalized or periarticular osteoporosis is a common manifestation in patients with rheumatoid arthritis. The pathogenesis of periarticular osteoporosis appears to be related to the adjacent synovial inflammation with hyperemia; however, the cause of generalized osteoporosis in this disease is not entirely clear.[192, 316, 317, 333–336] Reduced physical activity leading to disuse osteoporosis has been implicated in some studies.[367, 368] Corticosteroid[193–196, 248, 315] or salicylate[197] therapy appears to be an additional factor, although low dose corticosteroid treatment in rheumatoid arthritis is not uniformly associated with an increased risk of osteoporosis,[369] and reduced bone formation may be evident in some patients with this disease who have not received corticosteroid therapy.[370] Furthermore, some patients seem to

develop a modified form of the reflex sympathetic dystrophy syndrome superimposed on their rheumatoid process.[198] In these persons, an unusual degree of pain, stiffness, edema, hyperhidrosis, and vasodilatation in the hand and fingers may obscure the underlying articular disease. Diffuse osteoporosis of the spine in rheumatoid arthritis may be most prominent in women over the age of 50 years.[193, 194]

Osteoporosis producing osseous weakening contributes to the fractures that are not uncommonly encountered in patients with rheumatoid arthritis (Table 25–5) (Figs. 25–35 and 25–36). These may occur after minimal trauma or spontaneously in spinal sites (compression fractures of vertebral bodies) or extraspinal locations.[199–201, 330, 371–373] Typical locations include the femur, tibia, fibula, sacrum, and para-acetabular and symphyseal regions. Schneider and Kaye[202] emphasized insufficiency or stress fractures of the

TABLE 25–5. Mechanisms and Sites of Pathologic Fractures in Rheumatoid Arthritis

Mechanism	Typical Sites
Synovial inflammation with erosion of bone	Odontoid process, carpal scaphoid bone, distal portion of ulna
Mechanical erosion of bone	Ribs, articular surfaces of small bones in the hands and feet, medial aspect of the humeral neck
Intraosseous cystic lesions	Proximal portion of ulna, femoral neck, femur and tibia about the knee
Bone deformation	Acetabulum
Generalized osteopenia	Insufficiency fractures of vertebral bodies, pelvis, tubular bones of the lower extremity, small bones of the foot
Ischemic necrosis	Femoral head, vertebral bodies
Osteomyelitis	Variable

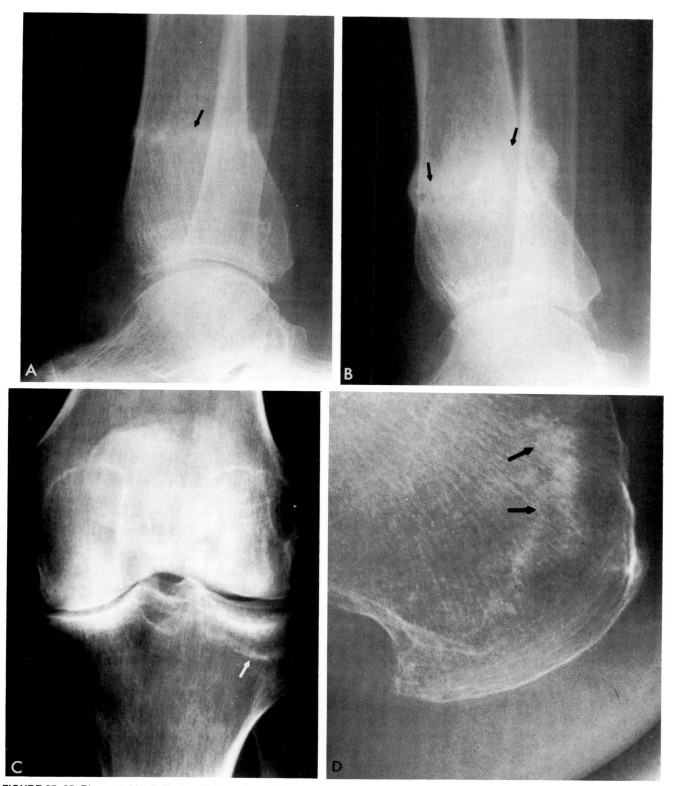

FIGURE 25–35. Rheumatoid arthritis: Insufficiency (stress) fractures.

A, B Radiographs obtained several months apart outline a pathologic fracture of the distal tibia (arrows), which arose from fatigue of the osteoporotic bone.

C An insufficiency fracture of the lateral tibial plateau (arrow) is seen in this patient with rheumatoid knee involvement.

D In another patient with rheumatoid arthritis, a classic insufficiency fracture of the calcaneus (arrows) has produced vertically oriented bony sclerosis.

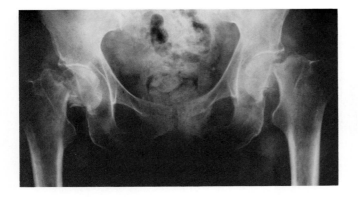

FIGURE 25–36. Rheumatoid arthritis: Insufficiency (stress) fractures. Bilateral displaced fractures of the femoral neck are evident. Note diffuse joint space loss in both hips. An insufficiency fracture of the symphysis pubis (arrowhead) also is evident.

tubular bones of the lower extremity in rheumatoid arthritis. They noted the contribution of osteoporosis, corticosteroid therapy, angular deformity, and flexion contracture in the development of these fractures. Other investigators have made similar observations[253, 254, 287, 319–322] and some have implicated osteomalacia as the cause of such fractures in patients with rheumatoid arthritis.[223] Accurate diagnosis of

insufficiency fractures can be difficult and requires a high index of clinical suspicion, quality radiographs, and even scintigraphy or MR imaging.[374–376]

Erosive abnormality of bone related to the rheumatoid process itself can also lead to fracture and deformity[323] (Figs. 25–37 and 25–38). Thus, pathologic fractures through the odontoid process[203] and olecranon process[204, 324]

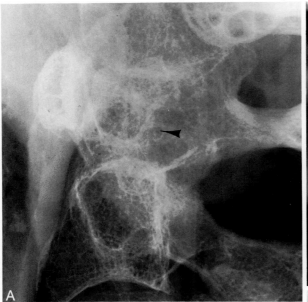

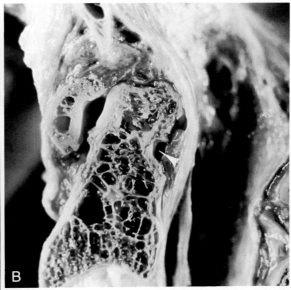

FIGURE 25–37. Rheumatoid arthritis. Fractures through sites of bone erosion—odontoid process.

A, B A lateral radiograph and photograph of a sagittal section through the odontoid process show a typical site of bone erosion in the posterior surface of the dens (arrowheads).

C Lateral tomography in a patient reveals a fracture at the base of the odontoid process (arrowheads).

(**C**, From Resnick, D, Cone R: RadioGraphics 4:549, 1984.)

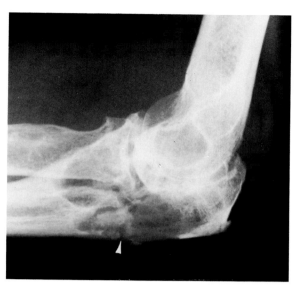

FIGURE 25–38. Rheumatoid arthritis: Fractures through sites of bone erosion—ulnar olecranon. A fracture (arrowhead) through a large cyst is evident.

and acetabular weakening and fracture leading to protrusion deformity[205, 286] are observed. Other sites include the scaphoid and humeral neck (Figs. 25–39 and 25–40) as well as the phalanges of the hand.[325] Similarly, epiphyseal collapse about small and large articulations can be attributed to altered forces acting on osteopenic bones.[326, 327]

Massive osteolysis is a rare finding of unknown pathogenesis that has been observed in rheumatoid arthritis.[255] Patients typically have severe disease, extensive abnormalities of the cervical spine, and neurologic deficit, suggesting that neuropathic osteoarthropathy is one important factor that is responsible for the disappearance of bone. Infection and corticosteroid therapy are additional pathogenetic possibilities. The humeral and femoral heads, elbows, and small bones of the hands and wrists usually are affected (Fig. 25–41).

SERONEGATIVE SPONDYLOARTHROPATHIES

Overview

The three major seronegative spondyloarthropathies—ankylosing spondylitis, psoriasis, and Reiter's syndrome—share with rheumatoid arthritis many radiologic and pathologic features.[377] They, too, involve synovial articulations and are associated with considerable inflammation of the synovial membrane. Fundamental differences exist between the spondyloarthropathies and rheumatoid arthritis, however, especially in the distribution and morphology of osteoarticular lesions.[227, 228]

All three of these spondyloarthropathic processes produce significant abnormalities of cartilaginous joints and entheses as well as synovial articulations. The discovertebral junctions throughout the spine, the symphysis pubis, the manubriosternal joints, and the tendinous and ligamentous attachments in the calcaneus, pelvis, trochanters of the femur, tuberosities of the humerus, and patella are altered to a much greater extent in ankylosing spondylitis, pso-

riasis, and Reiter's syndrome than in rheumatoid arthritis. Involvement of the cartilaginous joints and entheses, when occurring in conjunction with involvement of the synovial joints, shows a characteristic, although not invariable, distribution in each of these seronegative spondyloarthropathies. Ankylosing spondylitis affects primarily the synovial and cartilaginous joints and entheses of the axial skeleton, with less consistent and severe changes in the appendicular skeleton. The distribution of psoriatic arthritis is somewhat variable, although a polyarticular disorder of synovial joints of the appendicular skeleton with prominent involvement of the interphalangeal articulations of the hand and foot, combined with changes at the synovial and cartilaginous joints of the axial skeleton and entheses of the axial and appendicular skeleton, is distinctive. In Reiter's syndrome, asymmetric and "spotty" abnormalities of synovial articulations of the lower extremities frequently are coupled with sacroiliitis, spondylitis, and enthesopathy of the inferior surface of the calcaneus.

In addition to these differences in the distribution of articular abnormalities in the various seronegative spondyloarthropathies and rheumatoid arthritis, differences in the morphology of the lesions also can be evident. In this regard, the radiographic and pathologic characteristics of joint involvement in ankylosing spondylitis, psoriasis, and Reiter's syndrome are fundamentally similar and can be distinguished from those in rheumatoid arthritis. In synovial articulations, the absence of osteoporosis and the presence of bony proliferation and intra-articular bony ankylosis in the seronegative spondyloarthropathies are most helpful in differentiating the changes from those of rheumatoid arthritis. In cartilaginous joints, the extent of osseous erosion and bony proliferation in the former disorders also is helpful in differential diagnosis. At sites of tendon and ligament attachment to bone, an inflammatory enthesopathy leading to

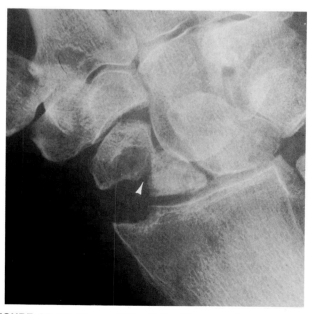

FIGURE 25–39. Rheumatoid arthritis: Fractures through sites of bone erosion—scaphoid. This radiograph documents a fracture of the carpal scaphoid bone through a site of erosion (arrowhead). There is ischemic necrosis of the proximal pole of the bone.
(From Resnick D, Cone R: RadioGraphics 4:549, 1984.)

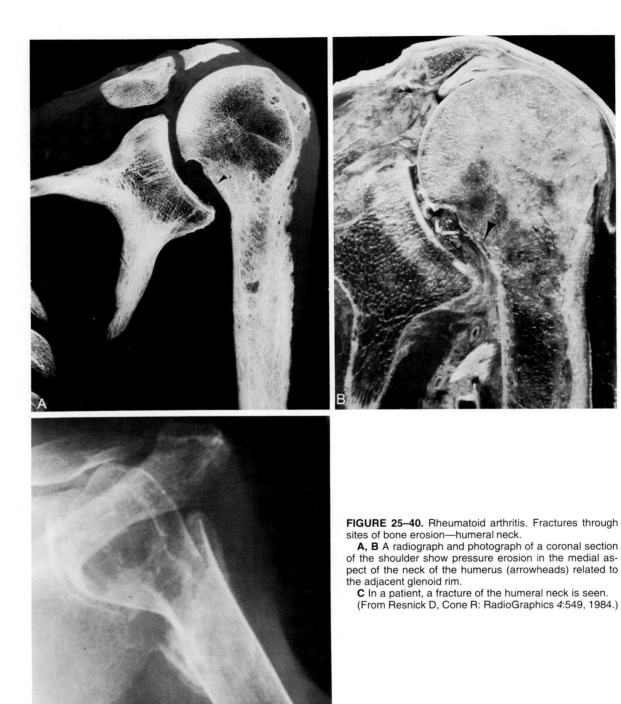

FIGURE 25–40. Rheumatoid arthritis. Fractures through sites of bone erosion—humeral neck.

A, B A radiograph and photograph of a coronal section of the shoulder show pressure erosion in the medial aspect of the neck of the humerus (arrowheads) related to the adjacent glenoid rim.

C In a patient, a fracture of the humeral neck is seen.

(From Resnick D, Cone R: RadioGraphics *4*:549, 1984.)

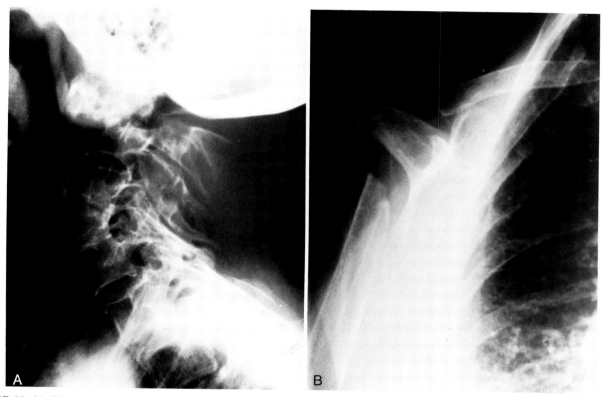

FIGURE 25–41. Rheumatoid arthritis: Massive osteolysis. In association with extensive destruction in the cervical spine with atlantoaxial subluxation and neurologic deficit, osteolysis of the proximal humerus, clavicle, and ribs is evident. (Courtesy of B. J. Manaster, M.D., Salt Lake City, Utah.)

osseous destruction and repair is characteristic of the spondyloarthropathies.

Synovial Joints (Table 25–6)
(Figs. 25–42 to 25–45)

As in rheumatoid arthritis, the predominant target area in the synovial joints in the seronegative spondyloarthropathies appears to be the synovial membrane.[19–22, 89, 225, 229] Furthermore, an inflammatory process of this membrane becomes evident,[278] and, in some instances, massive joint effusions have been recorded.[266] As opposed to the situation in rheumatoid arthritis, however, the inflammatory changes in ankylosing spondylitis, psoriasis, and Reiter's syndrome

are of less intensity,[267] although synovial proliferation and thickening, villous hypertrophy, lymphocytic and plasma cell infiltration, and granulomatous tissue or pannus are observed.[281] Exudation is less marked, and proliferation and reaction of connective tissue ensue. Fibroplasia, which is followed by cartilaginous metaplasia and chondro-ossification, can lead to intra-articular bony ankylosis,[206] a feature that can be apparent in any of the spondyloarthropathies but is most typical of ankylosing spondylitis and psoriasis. The detection of osseous fusion at sites other than the carpal and tarsal areas is relatively unusual in rheumatoid arthritis.

Although cartilaginous destruction can proceed from superficial extension of inflamed synovial tissue in the seronegative spondyloarthropathies (in a manner similar to that

Text continued on page 855

TABLE 25–6. Abnormalities of Synovial Joints in the Seronegative Spondyloarthropathies

Pathologic	Radiologic
Synovial inflammation and production of fluid	Soft tissue swelling and widening of joint space
Mild to moderate hyperemia	Variable osteoporosis
Pannus destruction of cartilage	Narrowing of joint space
Pannus destruction of "unprotected" bone at margin of joint	Marginal bony erosions
Pannus destruction of subchondral bone	Bony erosions and formation of subchondral cysts
Fibroplasia, cartilaginous metaplasia, chondro-ossification and capsular ossification	Bony ankylosis
Bony proliferation in response to damage	Marginal "whiskering," periostitis, subchondral sclerosis
Noninflammatory proliferation of the periosteum	Cortical atrophy, osteolysis

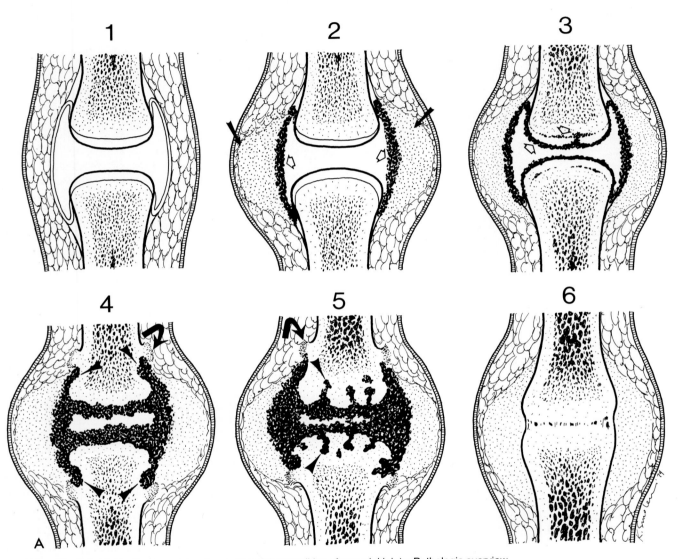

FIGURE 25–42. Seronegative spondyloarthropathies: Abnormalities of synovial joints. Pathologic overview.

A The normal synovial joint is depicted at the upper left (1). Early changes (2) consist of synovial inflammation (open arrows) and soft tissue edema (solid arrows). Osteoporosis may not be evident. Subsequently (3), synovial inflammatory tissue or pannus extends across and beneath the chondral surface (open arrows), leading to cartilaginous erosion or disruption. At later stages (4, 5), marginal and central osseous erosions develop (arrowheads). Associated bony proliferation (curved arrows) becomes evident. Finally (6), intra-articular bony ankylosis may develop.

Illustration continued on opposite page

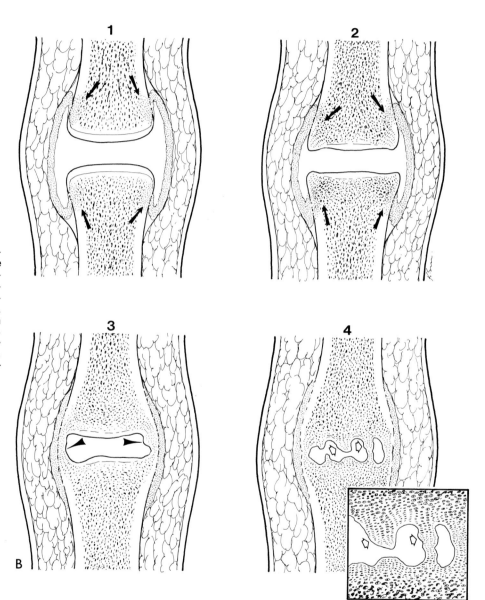

FIGURE 25–42. *Continued*

B Capsular ossification may be an important manifestation of the seronegative spondyloarthropathies. Initially (1, 2), inflammatory changes at the capsular attachment to bone (arrows) can be associated with erosion and bone formation. Subsequently (3), capsular ossification can lead to bridging of the peripheral portions of the joints (arrowheads). Finally (4), endochondral ossification (open arrows) can produce further intra-articular ankylosis.

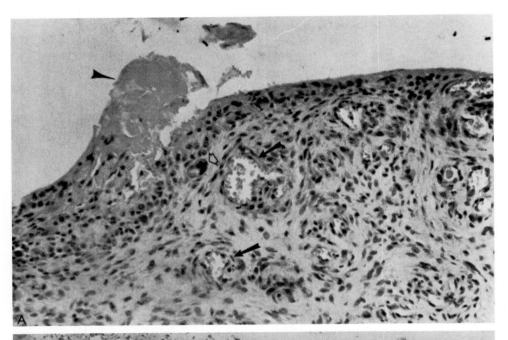

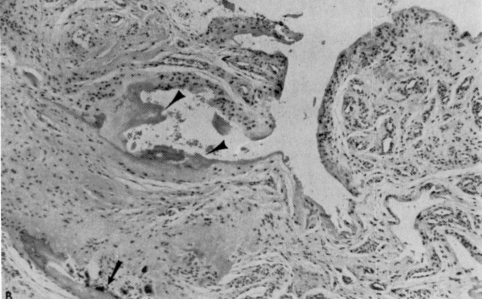

FIGURE 25–43. Seronegative spondyloarthropathies: Abnormalities of synovial joints. Sequential histologic abnormalities in patients with psoriatic arthritis.

A Synovial cell proliferation and fibrosis are associated with vascular invasion (solid arrows) and surface fibrin deposition (arrowhead). A multinucleated giant cell is revealed (open arrow) (230×).

B Fibrin exudate (arrowheads) coats an inflamed and vascular synovial membrane. Osteoclastic resorption of trabeculae is seen (arrow) (92×).

Illustration continued on opposite page

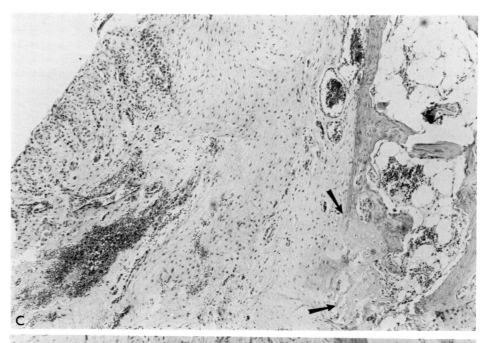

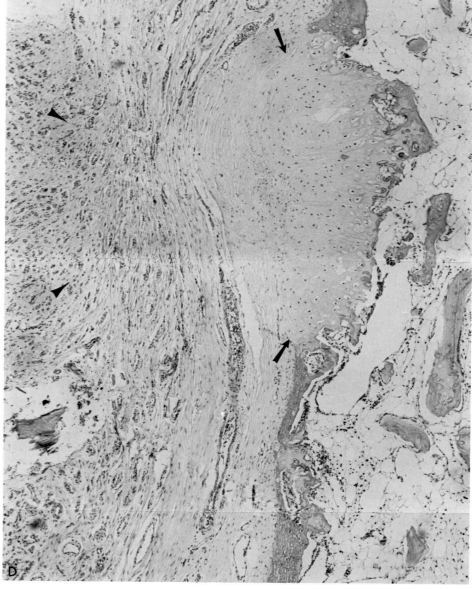

FIGURE 25–43. *Continued*
  C Chondrometaplasia (arrows) beneath a hypervascular synovial membrane is apparent (92×).
  D Observe vascular and fibrous synovial tissue (arrowheads) and prominent chondrometaplasia (arrows) (92×).

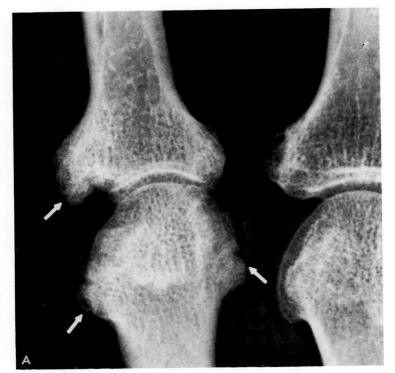

FIGURE 25–44. Seronegative spondyloarthropathies: Abnormalities of synovial joints. Radiographic changes of bony proliferation or "whiskering."

A In a cadaver with ankylosing spondylitis, observe superficial osseous erosion with adjacent bony proliferation (arrows), producing an irregular osseous outline. Osteoporosis is not apparent.

B A radiograph of a coronal section through the second metacarpophalangeal joint demonstrates the exuberant bony proliferation (arrows) about areas of erosion.

C The corresponding gross photograph delineates the nature and extent of the proliferative changes (arrows).

Illustration continued on opposite page

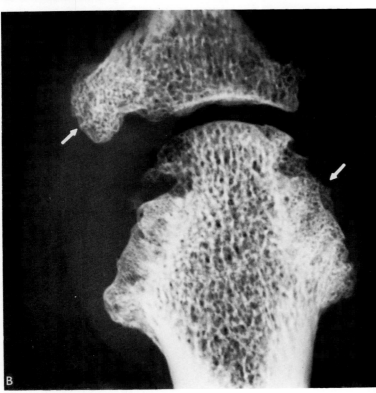

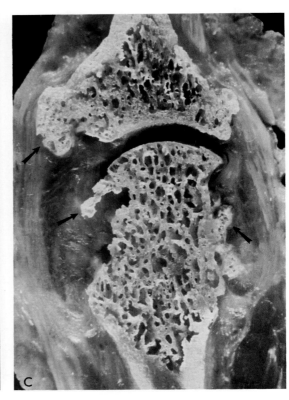

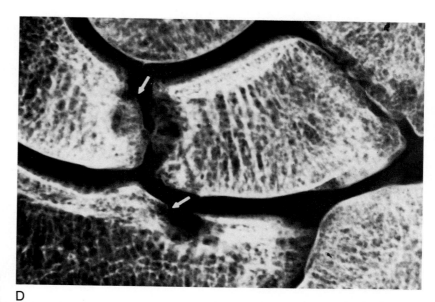

D

FIGURE 25–44. *Continued*

D A radiograph of a coronal section through the wrist delineates superficial erosion of the distal portion of the radius, the scaphoid, and the lunate with adjacent bony excrescences (arrows).

E A corresponding gross photograph demonstrates the irregular proliferative changes (arrows) about sites of erosion.

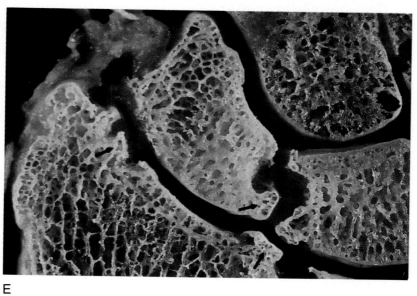

E

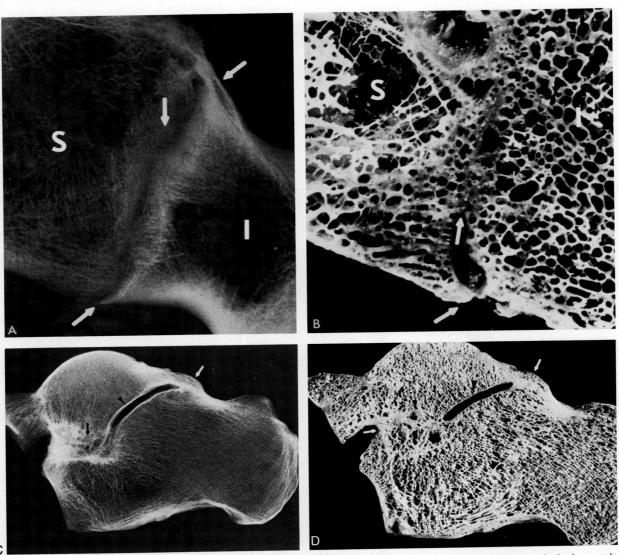

FIGURE 25–45. Seronegative spondyloarthropathies: Abnormalities of synovial joints. Radiographic changes of intra-articular bony ankylosis.
   A In a cadaver with ankylosing spondylitis, a radiograph of a coronal section through the sacroiliac joint demonstrates capsular and ligamentous ossification (arrows) producing osseous fusion of the sacrum (S) and ilium (I).
   B In a different cadaver, a photograph of a similar section through the sacroiliac articulation demonstrates progressive intra-articular ankylosis (arrows) extending from sacrum (S) to ilium (I).
   C, D A radiograph and photograph of a sagittal section of the hindfoot in a cadaver with ankylosing spondylitis reveal ossification with bony bridging at the margins (arrows) of the posterior subtalar joint with a well-preserved central articular space (arrowheads).

which is evident in rheumatoid arthritis), buds of granulation tissue may erode cartilage from beneath, especially in ankylosing spondylitis.[207, 208] Prominent changes in the subchondral bone relate to erosion of the osseous plate and invasion of the calcified zone of cartilage. This process, occurring deep to the cartilaginous layer, can lead to disruption of chondral attachments and shedding or breaking free of the articular surface. The exposure of hyperemic subchondral bone on both sides of the joint might explain the marked tendency to intra-articular osseous fusion in these disorders. Furthermore, the destruction of subchondral bone at a relatively early stage, due to the intimate relationship of the inflammatory tissue that has insinuated itself between the cartilage and bone, can lead to significant erosive changes at a time when the articular space is relatively preserved.

The proclivity to osseous fusion of certain synovial joints, such as the apophyseal and sacroiliac articulations, especially in ankylosing spondylitis, also can be related to abnormalities occurring at the capsuloligamentous attachments, perhaps reflecting another manifestation of a generalized enthesopathy.[90, 206, 209] Capsular ossification apparently can lead to interosseous bridging at the periphery of an involved articulation at a time when synovial inflammation and cartilage destruction are not prominent (Fig. 25–45). In this fashion, a bony shell can be detected that encloses well-preserved articular cartilage.[210, 282] Subsequent removal of the cartilaginous surface may occur by the process of endochondral ossification, in which the subchondral bone plate and the densely calcified cartilage are replaced by porous trabecular bone. The irregular progression of ossification can create radiographically evident, poorly defined ''eroded'' bony surfaces.

The central osseous structures (the sites of erosion by superficial or subchondral pannus and, perhaps, of endochondral ossification), and the peripheral or marginal osseous structures (the sites of destruction by inflamed synovium at the recesses of the articulation), respond in a characteristic fashion in the seronegative spondyloarthropathies.[211] Subchondral eburnation, irregular excrescences at the margins of the joint, and periostitis of adjacent diaphyses, particularly in the phalanges, the metacarpals, and the metatarsals, are distinctive (Fig. 25–44). The exact cause of new bone formation in these disorders is not known, although the fact that the inflammatory abnormalities in involved joints may be intermittent, allowing time during periods of clinical remission in which reactive bone healing can occur, could be significant. Although ankylosing spondylitis, psoriasis, and Reiter's syndrome share one additional feature, the presence of the histocompatibility antigen (HLA) B27,[212] which might suggest that this gene is linked to or functions as a modifying gene that affects bone production,[213] this hypothesis has not been supported by evidence of the lack of this antigen in patients with other bone-forming conditions, such as heterotopic ossification following paralysis.

As the degree of synovial inflammatory changes in the seronegative spondyloarthropathies generally is less than that in rheumatoid arthritis, it might be expected that the extent of osseous erosion in the former disorders will be somewhat limited. In general, this is true. Osseous erosion in ankylosing spondylitis, psoriasis, and Reiter's syndrome may be superficial and quickly obscured by the profound tendency for bone proliferation. Furthermore, collapse of weakened osteoporotic periarticular bone, a prominent finding in some patients with rheumatoid arthritis, also would be expected to be less frequent and extensive in the seronegative spondyloarthropathies, in which osteoporosis is not commonly a significant finding. Despite this general tendency to less severe erosion and collapse of osseous surfaces, however, some patients, particularly those with psoriasis, can reveal striking osteolysis, which may progress to involve large portions of the supporting bone. Cortical atrophy, which may be related to a noninflammatory proliferation of the periosteum, may be an important feature in the production of osteolysis in these patients.[21] Telescoping of one bone into the adjacent one can lead to extensive deformities that can be detected clinically in these circumstances.

Bursae and Tendon Sheaths

Inflammation in synovium-lined bursae and tendon sheaths is recognized in the seronegative spondyloarthropathies. The frequency and severity of this manifestation may be somewhat less than in rheumatoid arthritis, although at certain sites, characteristic clinical and radiologic manifestations occur. Retrocalcaneal bursitis[75–78, 268] in ankylosing spondylitis, psoriasis, or Reiter's syndrome produces preachilles soft tissue swelling and indistinctness as well as osseous erosion of the subjacent calcaneal surface, findings that are virtually indistinguishable from those in rheumatoid arthritis. In some patients, proliferation about the bony erosions can create poorly defined margins, suggesting the presence of ankylosing spondylitis, psoriasis, or Reiter's syndrome rather than rheumatoid arthritis.

Synovial cyst formation and rupture can accompany any inflammatory process associated with increased intra-articular pressure. The available reports on patients with seronegative spondyloarthropathies, however, rarely emphasize these manifestations. This observation, compared with the relatively frequent reported concern for the appearance of synovial cysts in rheumatoid arthritis patients, may indicate only that the clinical manifestations related to cyst formation in ankylosing spondylitis, psoriasis, or Reiter's syndrome are overshadowed by abnormalities at other sites, although the lesser degree of synovial inflammatory changes in the seronegative spondyloarthropathies than in rheumatoid arthritis could result in a decreased prevalence of (clinically bothersome) synovial cysts. Similarly, tenosynovitis, a well-known and frequently encountered manifestation of rheumatoid arthritis, has received less attention in ankylosing spondylitis, psoriasis, and Reiter's syndrome, although occasionally it may be a prominent feature in these latter disorders. In fact, periosteal proliferation in digits in some patients with seronegative spondyloarthropathies can be related to synovitis of adjacent tendon sheaths. Considerable soft tissue swelling in this clinical situation can produce a ''sausage-shaped'' finger or toe.

Erosion of spinous processes of vertebrae, particularly in the cervical spine, can be noted in ankylosing spondylitis, psoriasis, and, to a lesser extent, Reiter's syndrome. Although it is attractive to attribute such abnormality to the enthesopathy that occurs in any of these three disorders, inflammation in interspinous bursae, as noted in rheumatoid arthritis, can contribute to this osseous erosion.[96, 265]

TABLE 25–7. Abnormalities of Cartilaginous Joints and Entheses in the Seronegative Spondyloarthropathies

Pathologic	Radiologic
Inflammation of subchondral bone	Bony erosion and sclerosis
Bony proliferation	Bony ankylosis
Inflammation of capsular, ligamentous, and tendinous attachments	Bony erosion and sclerosis

Cartilaginous Joints and Entheses
(Table 25–7) (Figs. 25–46 to 25–49)

The tendency for ankylosing spondylitis, psoriasis, and Reiter's syndrome to affect cartilaginous articulations and sites of tendon and ligament attachment to bone is well known.[89, 90, 226, 233] At the manubriosternal joint and symphysis pubis, pathologic observations confirm the presence of chronic inflammatory changes in the subchondral bone, characterized initially by cellular infiltration, vascular fibrous tissue, and osteoclastic resorption of trabeculae ("os-

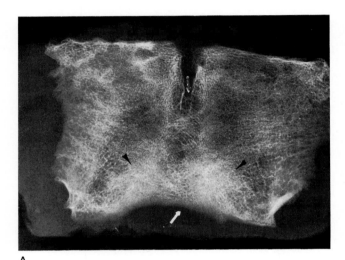

A

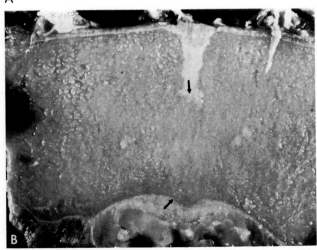

B

FIGURE 25–46. Seronegative spondyloarthropathies: Abnormalities of cartilaginous joints (symphysis pubis). A radiograph and corresponding photograph of a coronal section through the symphysis pubis in a cadaver with ankylosing spondylitis, indicating intra-articular osseous fusion (arrows) with surrounding bony sclerosis (arrowheads).

teitis") and subsequently by the lessening of inflammation and the appearance of progressive fibrosis and bone formation leading to trabecular thickening and intra-articular ossification (Fig. 25–46). Similar abnormalities in the discovertebral joint produce the "osteitis" of the anterior vertebral margin that is accompanied by erosion and sclerosis of bone and the progressive discal ossification that is associated with syndesmophyte formation.[378]

At each of the cartilaginous articulations (the manubriosternal joint, the symphysis pubis, and the discovertebral junction), the changes may relate not only to true chondro-osseous inflammation but also to an enthesopathy at the peripheral capsular attachments,[90] indistinguishable from that present at other sites of ligament and tendon attachment to bone (see later discussion). About the intervertebral discs, osseous erosions can be observed at the anterior or anterolateral attachment and, to a lesser extent, the posterior attachment of the outer fibers of the anulus fibrosus to the corners of the vertebral body. At these sites, lymphocytic and plasma cell infiltration can be associated with adjacent reactive bone production. Initially immature in nature, the newly formed bone frequently is replaced by mature (lamellar) bone (syndesmophytes) (Fig. 25–47). The subsequent growth of the syndesmophytes can be attributed to progressive chondrification of the anulus[214] or recurrence of inflammation with further deposition of bone.[90] Obliteration of the intervening cartilage, be it in the intervertebral disc, symphysis pubis, or manubriosternal articulation, may be attributed to endochondral ossification. Pathologic and radiologic studies of the intervertebral disc in ankylosing spondylitis indicate progressive bony replacement of the cartilage.[279] Calcification of the cartilaginous endplate results in reduplication and migration of the chondro-osseous junction. The process evolves more quickly at the peripheral portions of the disc, resulting in a narrowed structure of lenticular shape.

The pathogenesis of destructive lesions at single or multiple discovertebral junctions during the course of ankylosing spondylitis has stimulated a great debate.[215, 216] Several mechanisms probably contribute to these lesions, including an increasing enthesopathy, pressure destruction of the intervertebral disc related to kyphosis, cartilage node formation, and pseudarthrosis about a fracture site. The last-mentioned mechanism is expected in long-standing disease in which a rigid vertebral column, caused by widespread bony ankylosis, is predisposed to fracture in a manner similar to that of a long tubular bone.[269] Continued motion at the fracture site leads to a pseudarthrosis in which callus formation, hemorrhage, fibrous proliferation, and mild inflammatory changes are seen.[270] Similarly, in disease of long duration, segmental ankylosis, rather than uniform ankylosis, can produce increased stress at unossified discal levels, abnormal spinal motion, and radiologic and pathologic findings similar to those accompanying pseudarthroses.[249, 250] As destructive lesions of intervertebral discs also are observed in early stages of ankylosing spondylitis,[271, 272] other mechanisms must be operational. Inflammation seems a likely cause in these instances. In fact, although erosive disease, termed erosive spondylopathy, at multiple discovertebral junctions generally is followed by more typical spinal and sacroiliac joint abnormalities of ankylosing spondylitis,[273] it also is observed as an isolated or self-limited process.[273–275]

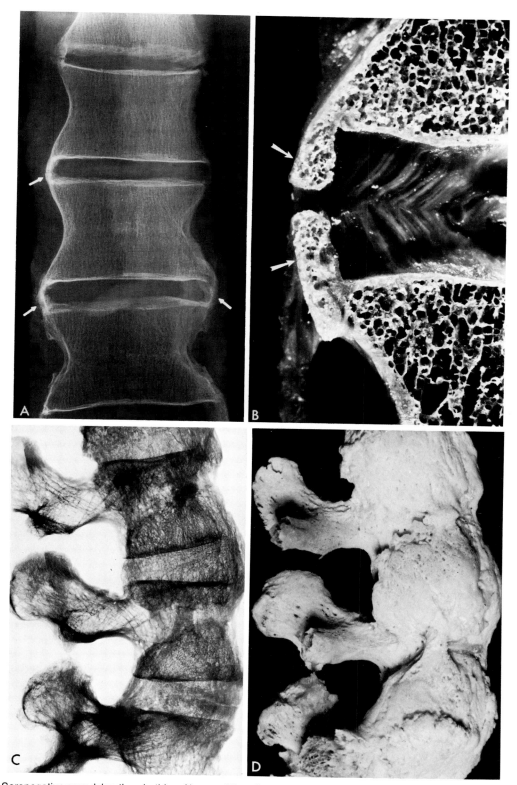

FIGURE 25–47. Seronegative spondyloarthrophathies: Abnormalities of cartilaginous joints (discovertebral junctions).

A A radiograph of a coronal section of the spine in a cadaver with ankylosing spondylitis reveals typical syndesmophytes extending as linear osseous bridges from one vertebral body to the next (arrows).

B On a photograph of a corresponding section from another cadaver with ankylosing spondylitis, the nature of the syndesmophytes is evident (arrows)—they represent chondrification and ossification of the anulus fibrosus.

C, D A radiograph and photograph of a macerated lumbar spine in a cadaver with psoriatic arthritis show extensive discal ossification resulting in spinal ankylosis. Superior articular processes demonstrate irregular new bone formation.

(**C, D**. From Heuck F: Radiologe *22*:572, 1982.)

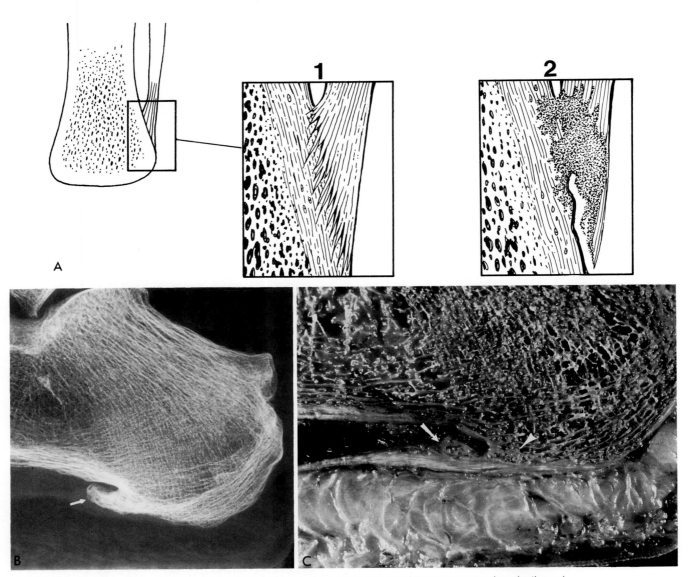

FIGURE 25–48. Seronegative spondyloarthropathies: Abnormalities of attachment of ligaments or tendons (entheses).

A At a normal attachment of tendon to bone (1), interdigitation of the tendinous fibers and bony surface is seen. In the presence of an inflammatory enthesopathy (2), cellular infiltration and granulation tissue erode the tendon and adjacent bone.

B A radiograph of a sagittal section of the calcaneus in a cadaver with ankylosing spondylitis outlines a well-defined osseous excrescence with surrounding proliferation at the ligamentous attachment to the bone (arrow).

C On a photograph of the section, the relationship of the bony enthesophyte to the plantar ligament is evident (arrow). Minor trabecular thickening can be detected (arrowhead).

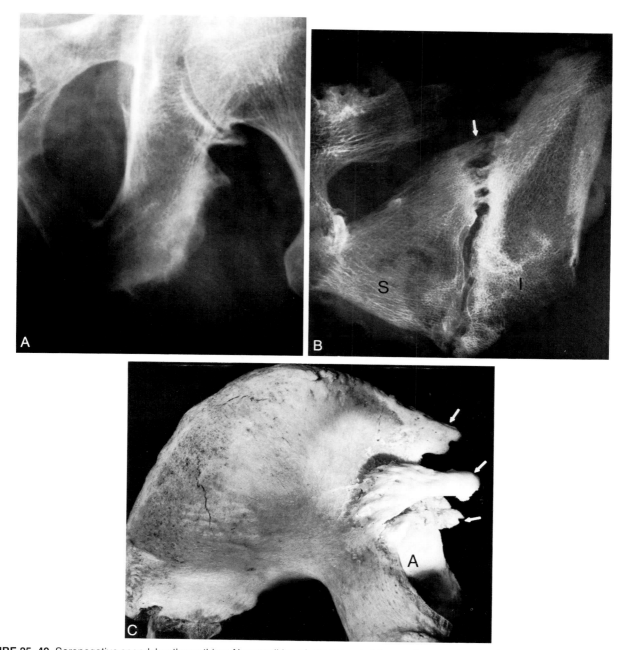

FIGURE 25–49. Seronegative spondyloarthropathies: Abnormalities of attachment of ligaments or tendons (entheses).

A Observe poorly defined erosion and reactive bone formation in the ischial tuberosity in a patient with ankylosing spondylitis. (Courtesy of V. Vint, M.D., San Diego, California.)

B A radiograph of a coronal section of the sacroiliac joint in a cadaver with ankylosing spondylitis demonstrates bone proliferation (arrow) and ossification of the interosseous sacroiliac ligament, producing partial ankylosis. S, Sacrum; I, ilium.

C In a cadaver with psoriatic arthritis, an unusual amount of bone proliferation (arrows) arises above the acetabulum (A) and from the iliac crest. (From Heuck F: Radiologe *22*:572, 1982.)

TABLE 25–8. Rheumatoid Arthritis Versus the Seronegative Spondyloarthropathies

	Rheumatoid Arthritis	Seronegative Spondyloarthropathies
Synovial Joint Involvement	+	+
Soft tissue swelling	+	+
Osteoporosis	+	±
Marginal erosions	+	+
Central erosions and cysts	+	+
Bony ankylosis	±	+
Bony proliferation	−	+
Malalignment and subluxation	+	±
Bursal and Tendon Sheath Involvement	+	+
Soft tissue swelling	+	+
Bony erosions	+	+
Bony proliferation	−	+
Cartilaginous Joint Involvement	±	+
Bony erosions	±	+
Bony proliferation	±	+
Bony ankylosis	±	+
Enthesopathy	±	+
Bony erosions	±	+
Bony proliferation	±	+

+ = Common; ± = less common; − = rare or absent.

An enthesopathy (Figs. 25–48 and 25–49) occurring at other tendinous and ligamentous connections to bone in patients with seronegative spondyloarthropathies is responsible for prominent clinical and radiographic manifestations on the plantar aspect of the calcaneus, the pelvis, the patella, the iliac crest, the ischial and humeral tuberosities, and the femoral trochanters.[19–22, 75–78, 89, 90, 217] At these sites, microscopically evident focal inflammatory lesions consist of varying degrees of cellular infiltration with lymphocytes, plasma cells, and, to a lesser extent, polymorphonuclear leukocytes. Edema, decrease in hematopoietic tissue, and cellular deposits in the adjacent bone marrow are associated with osseous erosion and sclerosis.[276] Bony deposition eventually can obscure the eroded surface, producing a poorly defined or "fluffy" osseous contour. The ligaments themselves are inflamed, with cellular infiltration and vascular invasion. These ligamentous changes are most prominent at their osseous attachments, although changes distant to bone also can be encountered. In rare instances, ligamentous ossification is seen.[277]

SUMMARY

The pathologic and radiographic abnormalities associated with articular involvement in rheumatoid arthritis and the seronegative spondyloarthropathies (ankylosing spondylitis, psoriasis, Reiter's syndrome) are similar in many respects. Involvement of synovial and cartilaginous joints, bursae, tendon sheaths, entheses, tendons, ligaments, soft tissues, and bones can be encountered in any of these disorders. The distribution and extent of abnormalities differ among these diseases, however (Table 25–8). In rheumatoid arthritis, alterations in synovium-lined articulations, bursae, and tendon sheaths frequently overshadow those in cartilaginous joints and sites of tendon and ligament attachment to bone. In ankylosing spondylitis, psoriasis, and Reiter's syndrome, abnormalities at cartilaginous articulations, including the discovertebral and manubriosternal joints and sym-

physis pubis, can be severe. In addition, in these last three conditions, a peculiar enthesopathy produces osseous erosion and proliferation at tendo-osseous junctions.

References

1. Harris ED, DiBona DR, Krane SM: A mechanism for cartilage destruction in rheumatoid arthritis. Trans Assoc Am Physicians *83*:267, 1970.
2. Krane SM: Joint erosion in rheumatoid arthritis. Arthritis Rheum *17*:306, 1974.
3. Janis R, Hamerman D: Articular cartilage changes in early arthritis. Bull Hosp Joint Dis *30*:136, 1969.
4. Evanson JM, Jeffrey JJ, Krane SM: Human collagenase: Identification and characterization of an enzyme from rheumatoid synovium in culture. Science *158*:499, 1967.
5. Lazarus GS, Decker JL, Oliver CH, et al: Collagenolytic activity of synovium in rheumatoid arthritis. N Engl J Med *279*:914, 1968.
6. Harris ED, Evanson JM, DiBona DR, et al: Collagenase and rheumatoid arthritis. Arthritis Rheum *13*:83, 1970.
7. Ziff M, Gribetz HJ, Lospalluto J: Effect of leukocyte and synovial membrane extracts on cartilage mucoprotein. J Clin Invest *39*:405, 1960.
8. Weissmann G, Spilberg I: Breakdown of cartilage protein-polysaccharide by lysosomes. Arthritis Rheum *11*:162, 1968.
9. Oronsky A, Ignarro L, Perper R: Release of cartilage mucopolysaccharide degrading neutral protease from human leukocytes. J Exp Med *138*:461, 1973.
10. Weston PD, Barret AJ, Dingle JT: Specific inhibition of cartilage breakdown. Nature *222*:285, 1969.
11. Luscombe M: Acid phosphatase and catheptic activity in rheumatoid synovial tissue. Nature *197*:1010, 1962.
12. Dingle JT: The immunoinhibition of cathepsin D-mediated cartilage degradation. *In* AJ Barrett, JT Dingle (Eds): Tissue Proteinases. Amsterdam, North Holland Publishing Company, 1971, p 313.
13. Kobayashi I, Ziff M: Electron microscopic studies of the cartilage-pannus junction in rheumatoid arthritis. Arthritis Rheum *18*:475, 1975.
14. Fessel JM, Chrisman OD: Enzymatic degradation of chondromucoprotein by cell-free extract of human cartilage. Arthritis Rheum *7*:398, 1964.
15. Salter RB, McNeil OR, Carbin R: The pathological changes in articular cartilage associated with persistent joint deformity: An experimental investigation. Studies of Rheumatoid Disease, Proceedings of the Third Canadian Conference on Research in the Rheumatoid Diseases, Toronto, University of Toronto Press, 1966, p 33.
16. Krane SM, Emkey RD, Ferzoco L: The enhancement by rheumatoid synovial culture media of ^{45}Ca release from prelabeled fetal bones. Arthritis Rheum *14*:396, 1971.
17. Robinson DR, Smith H, Levine L: Prostaglandin (PG) synthesis by human synovial cultures and its stimulation by colchicine. Arthritis Rheum *16*:129, 1973.
18. Klein DC, Raisz LG: Prostaglandins: Stimulation of bone resorption in tissue culture. Endocrinology *86*:1436, 1970.
19. Gardner DL: Pathology of rheumatoid arthritis. *In* Copeman's Textbook of the Rheumatic Diseases. 5th Ed. Edinburgh, Churchill Livingstone, 1978, p 273.

20. Jaffe HL: Metabolic, Degenerative and Inflammatory Diseases of Bones and Joints. Philadelphia, Lea & Febiger, 1972, p 779.
21. Fassbender HG: Pathology of Rheumatic Diseases. New York, Springer-Verlag, 1975, p 79.
22. Sokoloff L: The pathology of rheumatoid arthritis and allied disorders. *In* JL Hollander, DJ McCarty Jr (Eds): Arthritis and Allied Conditions. 8th Ed. Philadelphia, Lea & Febiger, 1972, p 309.
23. Goldenberg DL, Cohen AS: Synovial membrane histopathology in the differential diagnosis of rheumatoid arthritis, gout, pseudogout, systemic lupus erythematosus, infectious arthritis, and degenerative joint disease. Medicine *57*:239, 1978.
24. Henne W, Pfannenstiel P, Pixberg HU: Knochen- und Gelenkszintigraphie mit 99mTc-markiertem Pyrophosphat bzw. Polyphosphat—ein vorläufiger Erfahrungsbericht. ROFO *119*:187, 1973.
25. Muirden KD, Senator GB: Iron in the synovial membrane in rheumatoid arthritis and other joint diseases. Ann Rheum Dis *27*:38, 1968.
26. Grimley PM, Sokoloff L: Synovial giant cells in rheumatoid arthritis. Am J Pathol *49*:931, 1966.
27. Donald KJ, Kerr JFR: Giant cells in the synovium in rheumatoid arthritis. Med J Aust *1*:761, 1968.
28. Muirden KD, Peace G: Light and electron microscope studies in carrageenin, adjuvant, and tuberculin-induced arthritis. Ann Rheum Dis *28*:392, 1969.
29. Bhan AK, Roy S: Synovial giant cells in rheumatoid arthritis and other joint diseases. Ann Rheum Dis *30*:294, 1971.
30. Muirden KD: Giant cells, cartilage and bone fragments within rheumatoid synovial membrane: Clinico-pathological correlations. Australas Ann Med *19*:105, 1970.
31. Soila P: Roentgen manifestations of adult rheumatoid arthritis. With special regard to the early changes. Acta Rheum Scand (Suppl) *1*:1, 1958.
32. Mall JC, Genant HK, Silcox DC, et al: The efficacy of fine-detail radiography in the evaluation of patients with rheumatoid arthritis. Radiology *112*:37, 1974.
33. Fletcher DE, Rowley KA: The radiological features of rheumatoid arthritis. Br J Radiol *25*:282, 1952.
34. Muirden KD: Peri-articular bone lesions in rheumatoid arthritis (Abstr). Scand J Rheum *4*(Suppl 8):505, 1975.
35. Mills K: Pathology of the knee joint in rheumatoid arthritis. J Bone Joint Surg [Br] *52*:746, 1970.
36. Woods CG, Greenwald AS, Haynes DW: Subchondral vascularity in the human femoral head. Ann Rheum Dis *29*:138, 1970.
37. Duncan H, Mathews CHE, Crouch MM, et al: Bone erosion in rheumatoid arthritis. Henry Ford Hosp Med J *26*:32, 1978.
38. Heersche JNM: Mechanism of osteoclastic bone resorption: A new hypothesis. Calcif Tissue Res *26*:81, 1978.
39. Dorey DK, Bick K: Ultrastructural analysis of glycosaminoglycan hydrolysis in the rat periodontal ligament. I. Evidence for macrophage involvement and bone remodeling. Calcif Tissue Res *24*:135, 1977.
40. Kahn AS, Stewart CC, Teitelbaum SL: Contact-mediated bone resorption by human monocytes in vitro. Science *199*:988, 1978.
41. Mundy GR, Altman AJ, Gondek MD, et al: Direct resorption of bone by human monocytes. Science *196*:1109, 1977.
42. Resnick D: Rheumatoid arthritis of the wrist. The compartmental approach. Med Radiogr Photogr *52*:50, 1976.
43. Brook A, Corbett M: Radiographic changes in early rheumatoid disease. Ann Rheum Dis *36*:71, 1977.
44. Resnick D, Niwayama G, Coutts R: Subchondral cysts (geodes) in arthritic disorders: Pathologic and radiographic appearance of the hip joint. AJR *128*:799, 1977.
45. Cruickshank B, Macleod LG, Shearer WS: Subarticular pseudocysts in rheumatoid arthritis. J Fac Radiologists *5*:218, 1954.
46. Freund E: The pathological significance of intra-articular pressure. Edinburgh Med J *47*:192, 1940.
47. Bywaters EGL: The hand. *In* ME Carter (Ed): Radiological Aspects of Rheumatoid Arthritis. Amsterdam, Excerpta Medica International Congress Series, Vol 61, 1964, p 43.
48. Soila P: The causal relations of rheumatoid disintegration of juxta-articular bone trabeculae. Acta Rheum Scand *9*:231, 1963.
49. Kersley GD, Ross FGM, Fowles SJ, et al: Tomography in arthritis of the small joints. Ann Rheum Dis *23*:280, 1964.
50. Baggenstoss AH, Bickel WH, Ward LE: Rheumatoid granulomatous nodules as destructive lesions of vertebrae. J Bone Joint Surg [Am] *34*:601, 1952.
51. Castillo BA, El Sallab RA, Scott JT: Physical activity, cystic erosions, and osteoporosis in rheumatoid arthritis. Ann Rheum Dis *24*:522, 1965.
52. DeHaas WHD, DeBoer W, Griffioen F, et al: Rheumatoid arthritis of the robust reaction type. Ann Rheum Dis *33*:81, 1974.
53. Jayson MIV, Rubenstein D, Dixon A StJ: Intra-articular pressure and rheumatoid geodes (bone "cysts"). Ann Rheum Dis *29*:496, 1970.
54. Magyar E, Talerman A, Feher M, et al: The pathogenesis of the subchondral pseudocysts in rheumatoid arthritis. Clin Orthop *100*:341, 1974.
55. Jayson MIV, Dixon A StJ: Intra-articular pressure in rheumatoid arthritis of the knee. Part III. Ann Rheum Dis *29*:401, 1970.
56. Genovese GR, Jayson MIV, Dixon A StJ: Protective value of synovial cysts in rheumatoid knees. Ann Rheum Dis *31*:179, 1972.
57. Bywaters EGL: Fistulous rheumatism: A manifestation of rheumatoid arthritis. Ann Rheum Dis *12*:114, 1953.
58. Shapiro RF, Resnick D, Castles JJ, et al: Fistulization of rheumatoid joints: A spectrum of identifiable syndromes. Ann Rheum Dis *34*:489, 1975.
59. Magyar E, Talerman A, Feher M, et al: Giant bone cysts in rheumatoid arthritis. J Bone Joint Surg [Br] *56*:121, 1974.
60. Hunder GG, Ward LE, Ivins JC: Rheumatoid granulomatous lesion simulating malignancy in the head and neck of the femur. Mayo Clin Proc *40*:766, 1965.
61. Jayson MIV, Dixon A StJ, Yeoman P: Unusual geodes ("bone cysts") in rheumatoid arthritis. Ann Rheum Dis *31*:174, 1972.
62. Rennell C, Mainzer F, Multz CV, et al: Subchondral pseudocysts in rheumatoid arthritis. AJR *129*:1069, 1977.
63. Rappoport AS, Sosman JL, Weissman BN: Lesions resembling gout in patients with rheumatoid arthritis. AJR *126*:41, 1976.
64. Resnick D: Gout-like lesions in rheumatoid arthritis. Letter to the Editor. AJR *127*:1062, 1976.
65. Yates DB, Scott JT: Rheumatoid synovitis and joint disease. Relationship between arthroscopic and histological changes. Ann Rheum Dis *34*:1, 1975.
66. Schumacher HR, Kitridou RC: Synovitis of recent onset. Arthritis Rheum *15*:465, 1972.
67. Henderson DRF, Jayson MIV, Tribe CR: Lack of correlation of synovial histology with joint damage in rheumatoid arthritis. Ann Rheum Dis *34*:7, 1975.
68. Pekin TJ, Zvaifler NJ: Hemolytic complement in synovial fluid. J Clin Invest *43*:1372, 1964.
69. Hedberg H: Studies on the depressed haemolytic complement activity of synovial fluid in adult rheumatoid arthritis. Acta Rheum Scand *9*:165, 1963.
70. Resnick D, Gmelich JT: Bone fragmentation in the rheumatoid wrist: Radiographic and pathologic considerations. Radiology *114*:315, 1975.
71. Martel W, Hayes JT, Duff IF: The pattern of bone erosion in the hand and wrist in rheumatoid arthritis. Radiology *84*:204, 1965.
72. Arkless R: Rheumatoid wrists: Cineradiography. Radiology *88*:543, 1967.
73. Hulten O, Gellerstedt N: Über Abnutzungsprodukte in Gelenken und ihre Resorption unter dem Bilde einer Synovitis detritica. Acta Chir Scand *84*:1, 1940.
74. Gamp A, Schilling A: Extraartikuläre Manifestation der chronischen Polyarthritis am Bewegungsapparat: Sehnen-, Sehnenscheiden-, Schleimbeutelenzündung, subkutane Knoten. Z Rheumaforsch *25*:42, 1966.
75. Bywaters EGL: Heel lesions of rheumatoid arthritis. Ann Rheum Dis *13*:42, 1954.
76. Resnick D, Feingold ML, Curd J, et al: Calcaneal abnormalities in articular disorders. Rheumatoid arthritis, ankylosing spondylitis, psoriatic arthritis and Reiter's syndrome. Radiology *125*:355, 1977.
77. Sutro CJ: The os calcis, the tendo Achillis and the local bursae. Bull Hosp Joint Dis *27*:76, 1966.
78. Weston WJ: The bursa deep to tendo Achillis. Australas Radiol *14*:327, 1970.
79. Huston KA, Nelson AM, Hunder GG: Shoulder swelling in rheumatoid arthritis secondary to subacromial bursitis. Arthritis Rheum *21*:145, 1978.
80. Weston WJ: The soft tissue signs of the enlarged ulnar bursa in rheumatoid arthritis. J Can Assoc Radiol *24*:282, 1973.
81. Palmer DG: Tendon sheaths and bursae involved by rheumatoid disease at the foot and ankle. Australas Radiol *14*:419, 1970.
82. Potter TA, Kuhns JG: Rheumatoid tenosynovitis. J Bone Joint Surg [Am] *40*:1230, 1958.
83. Nalebuff EA, Potter TA: Rheumatoid involvement of tendon and tendon sheaths in the hand. Clin Orthop *59*:147, 1968.
84. Marmor L: Rheumatoid flexor tenosynovitis. Clin Orthop *31*:97, 1963.
85. Mackenzie AH: Final diagnosis in 63 patients presenting with multiple palmar flexor tenosynovitis (MPFT) (Abstr). Arthritis Rheum *18*:415, 1975.
86. Gray RG, Gottlieb NL: Hand flexor tenosynovitis in rheumatoid arthritis. Prevalence, distribution, and associated rheumatic features. Arthritis Rheum *20*:1003, 1977.
87. Weston WJ: The intra-synovial fatty masses in chronic rheumatoid arthritis. Br J Radiol *46*:213, 1973.
88. Weston WJ: Erosions of the acromion process of the scapula in rheumatoid arthritis. Australas Radiol *17*:219, 1973.
89. Cruickshank B: Pathology of ankylosing spondylitis. Clin Orthop *74*:43, 1971.
90. Ball J: Enthesopathy of rheumatoid and ankylosing spondylitis. Ann Rheum Dis *30*:213, 1971.
91. Martel W: Cervical spondylitis in rheumatoid disease. A comment on neurologic significance and pathogenesis. Am J Med *44*:441, 1968.
92. Meikle JAK, Wilkinson M: Rheumatoid involvement of the cervical spine. Radiological assessment. Ann Rheum Dis *30*:154, 1971.
93. Martel W, Page JW: Cervical vertebral erosions and subluxations in rheumatoid arthritis and ankylosing spondylitis. Arthritis Rheum *3*:546, 1960.
94. Martel W, Duff IF: Pelvo-spondylitis in rheumatoid arthritis. Radiology *77*:744, 1961.
95. Ball J: Pathology of the rheumatoid cervical spine. Lancet *1*:86, 1958.
96. Bywaters EGL: Origin of cervical disc disease in RA. Arthritis Rheum *21*:737, 1978.
97. Bywaters EGL: Rheumatoid discitis in the thoracic region due to spread from costovertebral joints. Ann Rheum Dis *33*:408, 1974.
98. Martel W: Pathogenesis of cervical discovertebral destruction in rheumatoid arthritis. Arthritis Rheum *20*:1217, 1977.
99. Martel W, Seeger JF, Wicks JD, et al: Traumatic lesions of the discovertebral junction in the lumbar spine. AJR *127*:457, 1976.
100. Seaman WB, Wells J: Destructive lesions of the vertebral bodies in rheumatoid disease. AJR *86*:241, 1961.
101. Gibson HJ: Ankylosing spondylitis. Aetiology and pathology. J Fac Radiologists *8*:193, 1957.
102. Lorber A, Pearson CM, Rene RM: Osteolytic vertebral lesions as a manifestation of rheumatoid arthritis and related disorders. Arthritis Rheum *4*:514, 1961.

103. Shichikawa K, Matsui K, Oze K, et al: Rheumatoid spondylitis. Int Orthop (SICOT) 2:53, 1978.
104. Resnick D, Niwayama G: Intravertebral disc herniations: Cartilaginous nodes. Radiology 126:57, 1978.
105. Kellgren JH, Ball J: Tendon lesions in rheumatoid arthritis. A clinicopathological study. Ann Rheum Dis 9:48, 1950.
106. Backhouse KM, Kay AG, Coomes EN, et al: Tendon involvement in the rheumatoid hand. Ann Rheum Dis 30:236, 1971.
107. Straub LR, Wilson EH Jr: Spontaneous rupture of extensor tendons in the hand associated with rheumatoid arthritis. J Bone Joint Surg [Am] 38:1208, 1956.
108. Ehrlich GE, Peterson LT, Sokoloff L, et al: Pathogenesis of rupture of extensor tendons at the wrist in rheumatoid arthritis. Arthritis Rheum 2:332, 1959.
109. Vaughan-Jackson OJ: Rupture of extensor tendons by attrition at the inferior radio-ulnar joint. Report of two cases. J Bone Joint Surg [Br] 30:528, 1948.
110. Weiss JJ, Thompson GR, Doust V, et al: Rotator cuff tears in rheumatoid arthritis. Arch Intern Med 135:521, 1975.
111. Kersley GD: Spontaneous rupture of muscle as a complication of rheumatoid arthritis. Br Med J 2:942, 1948.
112. Laine VA, Vainio KJ: Spontaneous ruptures of tendons in rheumatoid arthritis. Acta Orthop Scand 24:250, 1955.
113. Razzano CD, Wilde AH, Phalen GS: Bilateral rupture of the infrapatellar tendon in rheumatoid arthritis. Clin Orthop 91:158, 1973.
114. Bedi SS, Ellis W: Spontaneous rupture of the calcaneal tendon in rheumatoid arthritis after local steroid injection. Ann Rheum Dis 29:494, 1970.
115. Rask MR: Achilles tendon rupture owing to rheumatoid disease. Case report with a nine-year follow-up. JAMA 239:435, 1978.
116. Harris ED, Faulkner CS II, Brown FE: Collagenolytic systems in rheumatoid arthritis. Clin Orthop 110:303, 1975.
117. Vaughan-Jackson OJ: Rheumatoid hand deformities considered in the light of tendon imbalance. J Bone Joint Surg[Br] 44:764, 1962.
118. Stack HG, Vaughan-Jackson OJ: The zig-zag deformity in the rheumatoid hand. Hand 3:62, 1971.
119. Smith EM, Juvinall RC, Bender LF, et al: Role of the finger flexors in rheumatoid deformities of the metacarpophalangeal joints. Arthritis Rheum 7:467, 1964.
120. Wise KS: The anatomy of the metacarpophalangeal joints, with observations of the aetiology of ulnar drift. J Bone Joint Surg [Br] 57:485, 1975.
121. Swanson AB, Swanson G de G: Pathogenesis and pathomechanics of rheumatoid deformities in the hand and wrist. Orthop Clin North Am 4:1039, 1973.
122. Hastings DE, Evans JA: Rheumatoid wrist deformities and their relation to ulnar drift. J Bone Joint Surg [Am] 57:930, 1975.
123. Clark IP, James DF, Colwill JC: Intra-articular pressure as a factor in initiating ulnar drift. J Bone Joint Surg [Am] 60:325, 1978.
124. Wilkes LL: Ulnar drift and metacarpophalangeal joint subluxation in the rheumatoid hand: Review of the pathogenesis. South Med J 70:963, 1977.
125. Dorwart BB, Schumacher HR: Hand deformities resembling rheumatoid arthritis. Semin Arthritis Rheum 4:53, 1974.
126. Wells WC: Rheumatism of the heart. Trans Soc Improv Med Surg Knowledge 3:373, 1812.
127. Hillier T: Diseases of Children: Clinical Treatise Based on Lectures Delivered at the Hospital for Sick Children. London, Walton, 1868.
128. Moore CP, Willkens RF: The subcutaneous nodule: Its significance in the diagnosis of rheumatic disease. Semin Arthritis Rheum 7:63, 1977.
129. Meynet P: Rhumatisme articulaire subaigu avec production de tumeurs multiples dans les tissue fibreux periarticulaires et le perioste d'un grand nombre d'os. Lyon Med 20:495, 1875.
130. Garrod AE: A Treatise on Rheumatism and Rheumatoid Arthritis. London, Griffin, 1890.
131. Collins DH: The subcutaneous nodule of rheumatoid arthritis. J Pathol Bacteriol 45:97, 1937.
132. Dawson MH: A comparative study of subcutaneous nodules in rheumatic fever and rheumatoid arthritis. J Exp Med 57:845, 1933.
133. Keil H: The rheumatic subcutaneous nodules and simulating lesions. Medicine 17:261, 1938.
134. Hahn BH, Yardley JH, Stevens MB: "Rheumatoid" nodules in systemic lupus erythematosus. Ann Intern Med 72:49, 1970.
135. Zuckner J, Baldassare A: The nonspecific rheumatoid subcutaneous nodule: Its presence in fibrositis and scleroderma. Am J Med Sci 271:69, 1976.
136. Williams HJ, Biddulph EC, Coleman SS, et al: Isolated subcutaneous nodules (pseudorheumatoid). J Bone Joint Surg [Am] 59:73, 1977.
137. Ellman P, Cudkowicz L, Elwood JS: Widespread serous membrane involvement by rheumatoid nodules. J Clin Pathol 7:239, 1954.
138. Maher JA: Dural nodules in rheumatoid arthritis. Arch Pathol 58:354, 1954.
139. Friedman H: Intraspinal rheumatoid nodule causing nerve root compression. J Neurosurg 32:689, 1970.
140. Steiner JW, Gelbloom AJ: Intracranial manifestations in two cases of systemic rheumatoid disease. Arthritis Rheum 2:537, 1959.
141. Fairburn B: Spinal cord compression by a rheumatoid nodule. J Neurol Neurosurg Psychiatry 38:1056, 1975.
142. Chamberlain MA: Intra-articular rheumatoid nodules of the knee. J Bone Joint Surg [Br] 53:507, 1971.
143. Kampner SL, Kuzell W: Intra-articular rheumatoid nodule of the knee joint. Clin Orthop 114:243, 1976.
144. Raven RW, Weber FP, Price LW: The necrobiotic nodules of rheumatoid arthritis: Case in which the scalp, abdominal wall (involving striped muscle), larynx, pericardium (involving myocardium), pleurae (involving lung), and peritoneum were affected. Ann Rheum Dis 7:63, 1948.
145. Askari A, Moskowitz RW, Goldberg VM: Subcutaneous rheumatoid nodules and serum rheumatoid factor without arthritis. JAMA 229:319, 1974.
146. Sokoloff L, McCluskey RT, Bunim JJ: Vascularity of the early subcutaneous nodule of rheumatoid arthritis. Arch Pathol 55:475, 1953.
147. Nowoslawski A, Brzosko WJ: Immunopathology of rheumatoid arthritis. II. The rheumatoid nodule (the rheumatoid granuloma). Pathol Eur 2:302, 1967.
148. Kreel L, Urquhart W: Two unusual radiological features in rheumatoid arthritis. Br J Radiol 36:715, 1963.
149. Dorfman HD, Norman A, Smith RJ: Bone erosion in relation to subcutaneous rheumatoid nodules. Arthritis Rheum 13:69, 1970.
150. Dalinka MK, Wunder JF: Unusual manifestations of rheumatoid disease. Radiology 97:393, 1970.
151. Ginsberg MH, Genant HK, Yu TF, et al: Rheumatoid nodulosis. An unusual variant of rheumatoid disease. Arthritis Rheum 18:49, 1975.
152. Brower AC, NaPombejara C, Stechschulte DJ, et al: Rheumatoid nodulosis: Another cause of juxta-articular nodules. Radiology 125:669, 1977.
153. Ganda OP, Caplan H: Rheumatoid disease without joint involvement. JAMA 228:338, 1974.
154. Bywaters EGL: A variant of rheumatoid arthritis characterized by recurrent digital pad nodules and palmar fasciitis, closely resembling palindromic rheumatism. Ann Rheum Dis 8:2, 1949.
155. Watt TL, Baumann RR: Pseudoxanthomatous rheumatoid nodules. Arch Dermatol 95:156, 1967.
156. Lowney ED, Simons HM: "Rheumatoid" nodules of the skin. Arch Dermatol 88:853, 1963.
157. Palmer DG: Synovial cysts in rheumatoid disease. Ann Intern Med 70:61, 1969.
158. Gristina AG, Wilson PD: Popliteal cysts in adults and children. Arch Surg 88:357, 1964.
159. Harvey JP, Corcos J: Large cysts in lower leg originating in the knee occurring in patients with rheumatoid arthritis. Arthritis Rheum 3:218, 1960.
160. Perri JA, Rodnan GP, Mankin HJ: Giant synovial cysts of the calf in patients with rheumatoid arthritis. J Bone Joint Surg [Am] 50:709, 1968.
161. Rosewarne MD: Synovial rupture of the knee joint: Confusion with deep vein thrombosis. Clin Radiol 29:417, 1978.
162. Swett HA, Jaffe RB, McIff EB: Popliteal cysts: Presentation as thrombophlebitis. Radiology 115:613, 1975.
163. Wagner T, Abgarowicz T: Microscopic appearance of Baker's cyst in cases of rheumatoid arthritis. Reumatologia 8:21, 1970.
164. Pastershank SP, Mitchell DM: Knee joint bursal abnormalities in rheumatoid arthritis. J Can Assoc Radiol 28:199, 1977.
165. Pavelka K, Susta A, Streda A: Giant cyst of the calf in a patient with rheumatoid arthritis. Scand J Rheumatol 1:145, 1972.
166. Harvey JP, Corcos J: Large cysts in the lower leg originating in the knee occurring in patients with rheumatoid arthritis. Arthritis Rheum 3:218, 1960.
167. Palmer DG: Anteromedial synovial cysts at the knee joint in rheumatoid disease. Australas Radiol 16:79, 1972.
168. Meurman KOA, Luppi A, Turunen MJ: A giant retrofemoral Baker's cyst. Br J Radiol 51:919, 1978.
169. Bienenstock H: Rheumatoid plantar synovial cysts. Ann Rheum Dis 34:98, 1975.
170. Watson JD, Ochsner SF: Compression of the bladder due to "rheumatoid" cysts of the hip joint. AJR 99:695, 1967.
171. Coventry MB, Polley HF, Weiner AD: Rheumatoid synovial cyst of the hip. J Bone Joint Surg [Am] 41:721, 1959.
172. Samuelson C, Ward JR, Albo D: Rheumatoid synovial cyst of the hip. A case report. Arthritis Rheum 14:105, 1971.
173. Gatch WD, Green WT: Cysts of the iliopsoas bursa. Ann Surg 82:277, 1925.
174. Bowerman JW, Muhletaler C: Arthrography of rheumatoid synovial cysts of the knee and wrist. J Can Assoc Radiol 24:24, 1973.
175. Iveson JMI, Hill AGS, Wright V: Wrist cysts and fistulae. An arthrographic study of the rheumatoid wrist. Ann Rheum Dis 34:388, 1975.
176. Leffert RD, Dorfman HD: Antecubital cyst in rheumatoid arthritis—surgical findings. J Bone Joint Surg [Am] 54:1555, 1972.
177. Ehrlich GE, Guttmann GG: Valvular mechanisms in antecubital cysts of rheumatoid arthritis. Arthritis Rheum 16:259, 1973.
178. Ehrlich GE: Antecubital cysts in rheumatoid arthritis—a corollary to popliteal (Baker's) cysts. J Bone Joint Surg [Am] 54:165, 1972.
179. Sharon E, Vieux U, Seckler SG: Giant synovial cyst of the shoulder and perforation of the nasal septum in (a patient with) rheumatoid arthritis. Mt Sinai J Med 45:103, 1978.
180. DeSmit AA, Ting YM, Weiss JJ: Shoulder arthrography in rheumatoid arthritis. Radiology 116:601, 1975.
181. Rosin AJ, Toghill PJ: Fistulous rheumatism—an unusual complication of rheumatoid arthritis. Postgrad Med J 39:96, 1963.
182. Karten I: Septic arthritis complicating rheumatoid arthritis. Ann Intern Med 70:1147, 1969.
183. Hunder GG, McDuffie FC: Hypocomplementemia in rheumatoid arthritis. Am J Med 54:461, 1973.
184. Kellgren JH, Ball J, Fairbrother RW, Barnes KL: Suppurative arthritis complicating rheumatoid arthritis. Br Med J 1:1193, 1958.
185. Gerber NJ, Dixon AS: Synovial cysts and juxta-articular bone cysts (geodes). Semin Arthritis Rheum 3:323, 1974.
186. Kemper JW, Baggenstoss AH, Slocumb CH: The relationship of therapy with

cortisone to the incidence of vascular lesions in rheumatoid arthritis. Ann Intern Med 46:831, 1957.

187. O'Quinn SE, Kennedy CB, Baker DT: Peripheral vascular lesions in rheumatoid arthritis. Arch Dermatol 92:489, 1965.
188. Johnson RL, Smyth CJ, Holt GW, et al: Steroid therapy and vascular lesions in rheumatoid arthritis. Arthritis Rheum 2:224, 1959.
189. Slocumb CH, Mayne JG, Ferguson RH, et al: Some unusual manifestations of rheumatoid arthritis. Postgrad Med 42:309, 1967.
190. Skrifvars B, Laine V, Wegelius O: Sclerosis of the arteries of the extremities in rheumatoid arthritis. Acta Med Scand 186:145, 1969.
191. Rohlfing BM, Basch CM, Genant HK: Acro-osteolysis as the sole skeletal manifestation of rheumatoid vasculitis. Br J Radiol 50:830, 1977.
192. Bjelle AO, Nilsson BE: The relationship between radiologic changes and osteoporosis of the hand in rheumatoid arthritis. Arthritis Rheum 14:646, 1971.
193. Saville PD, Kharmosh O: Osteoporosis of rheumatoid arthritis: Influence of age, sex and corticosteroids. Arthritis Rheum 10:423, 1967.
194. McConkey B, Fraser GM, Bligh AS: Osteoporosis and purpura in rheumatoid disease: Prevalence and relation to treatment with corticosteroids. Q J Med 31:419, 1962.
195. Duncan H: Bone dynamics of rheumatoid arthritis treated with adrenal corticosteroids. Arthritis Rheum 10:216, 1967.
196. Duncan H: Osteoporosis in rheumatoid arthritis and corticosteroid induced osteoporosis. Orthop Clin North Am 3:571, 1972.
197. Jett S, Wu K, Duncan H, et al: Adrenal corticosteroid and salicylate actions on human and canine Haversian bone formation and resorption. Clin Orthop 68:301, 1970.
198. de Takats G: Sympathetic reflex dystrophy. Med Clin North Am 49:117, 1965.
199. Baer GJ: Fractures in chronic arthritis. Ann Rheum Dis 2:269, 1941.
200. Miller B, Markheim HR, Towbin MN: Multiple stress fractures in rheumatoid arthritis. A case report. J Bone Joint Surg [Am] 49:1408, 1967.
201. Taylor RT, Huskisson EC, Whitehouse GH, Hart FD: Spontaneous fractures of pelvis in rheumatoid arthritis. Br Med J 4:663, 1971.
202. Schneider R, Kaye JJ: Insufficiency and stress fractures of the long bones occurring in patients with rheumatoid arthritis. Radiology 116:595, 1975.
203. Martel W, Bole GG: Pathologic fracture of the odontoid process in rheumatoid arthritis. Radiology 90:948, 1968.
204. Rappoport AS, Sosman JL, Weissman BN: Spontaneous fractures of the olecranon process in rheumatoid arthritis. Radiology 119:83, 1976.
205. Hastings DE, Parker SM: Protrusio acetabuli in rheumatoid arthritis. Clin Orthop 108:76, 1975.
206. Aufdermaur M: Die pathologische Anatomie der Spondylitis ankylopoetica. Documenta Rheumatologica. Basel, Geigy, 1953.
207. Bywaters EGL: A case of early ankylosing spondylitis with fatal secondary amyloidosis. Br Med J 2:412, 1968.
208. Pasion EG, Goodfellow JW: Pre-ankylosing spondylitis. Histopathological report. Ann Rheum Dis 34:92, 1975.
209. Geiler G: Die Spondylarthritis ankylopoetica aus pathologischanatomischer Sicht. Dtsch Med Wochenschr 94:1185, 1969.
210. Dihlmann W: Anwendung der Röntgenbildanalyse zur Erkennung der feingeweblichen Veränderungen bei der Spondylitis ankylopoetica. Z Rheumaforsch 1(Suppl):21, 1969.
211. Resnick D, Niwayama G: On the nature and significance of bony proliferation in "rheumatoid variant" disorders. AJR 129:275, 1977.
212. Bluestone R: HL-A antigens in clinical medicine. Disease-A-Month 23:1, 1976.
213. Shapiro RF, Utsinger PD, Wiesner KB, et al: HLA-B27 and modified bone formation. Lancet 1:230, 1976.
214. Francois RJ: Microradiographic study of the intervertebral bridges in ankylosing spondylitis and in the normal sacrum. Ann Rheum Dis 24:481, 1965.
215. Cawley MID, Chalmers TM, Kellgren JH, et al: Destructive lesions of vertebral bodies in ankylosing spondylitis. Ann Rheum Dis 31:345, 1972.
216. Dihlmann W, Delling G: Disco-vertebral destructive lesions (so-called Anderson lesions) associated with ankylosing spondylitis. Skel Radiol 3:10, 1978.
217. Guest CM, Jacobson HG: Pelvic and extrapelvic osteopathy in rheumatoid spondylitis. AJR 65:760, 1951.
218. Brown MM, Hadler NM, Sams WM Jr, et al: Rheumatoid nodulosis. Sporadic and familial diseases. J Rheum 6:286, 1979.
219. Ogilvie-Harris DJ, Fornaiser VL: Synovial iron deposition in osteoarthritis and rheumatoid arthritis. J Rheumatol 7:30, 1980.
220. Cheung HS, Ryan LM, Kozin F, et al: Synovial origins of rice bodies in joint fluid. Arthritis Rheum 23:72, 1980.
221. Moldofsky PJ, Dalinka MK: Multiple loose bodies in rheumatoid arthritis. Skel Radiol 4:219, 1979.
222. Burry HC, Caughey DE, Palmer DG: Benign rheumatoid nodules. Aust NZ J Med 9:697, 1979.
223. O'Driscoll S, O'Driscoll M: Osteomalacia in rheumatoid arthritis. Ann Rheum Dis 39:1, 1980.
224. Rauschning W: Popliteal cysts and their relation to the gastrocnemiosemimembranosus bursa. Studies on the surgical and functional anatomy. Acta Orthop Scand 179(Suppl):9, 1979.
225. Bag J: Articular pathology of ankylosing spondylitis. Clin Orthop 143:30, 1979.
226. Scott DL, Eastmond CJ, Wright V: A comparative radiological study of the pubic symphysis in rheumatic disorders. Ann Rheum Dis 38:529, 1979.
227. Resnick D: Radiology of seronegative spondyloarthropathies. Clin Orthop 143:38, 1979.
228. Loebl DH, Kirby S, Stephenson R, et al: Psoriatic arthritis. JAMA 242:2447, 1979.

229. Fassbender HG: Extra-articular processes in osteoarthropathia psoriatica. Arch Orthop Trauma Surg 95:37, 1979.
230. Snow C, Goldman JA, Casey HL, et al: Rheumatoid nodulosis: A continuum of extra-articular rheumatoid disease. South Med J 72:1572, 1979.
231. de Carvalho A, Graudal H, Jørgensen B: Radiologic evaluation of the progression of rheumatoid arthritis. Acta Radiol 21:115, 1980.
232. Young A, Corbett M, Brook A: The clinical assessment of joint inflammatory activity in rheumatoid arthritis related to radiological progression. Rheumatol Rehabil 19:14, 1980.
233. Niepel GA, Sit'aj Š: Enthesopathy. Clin Rheum Dis 5:857, 1979.
234. Zvaifler NJ: Pathogenesis of the joint disease of rheumatoid arthritis. Am J Med 75:3, 1983.
235. Shiozawa S, Shiozawa K, Fujita T: Morphologic observations in the early phase of the cartilage-pannus junction. Light and electron microscopic studies of active cellular pannus. Arthritis Rheum 26:472, 1983.
236. Mohr W, Westerhellweg H, Wessinghage D: Polymorphonuclear granulocytes in rheumatic tissue destruction. III. An electron microscopic study of PMNs at the pannus-cartilage junction in rheumatoid arthritis. Ann Rheum Dis 40:396, 1981.
237. Mohr W, Menninger H: Polymorphonuclear granulocytes at the pannus-cartilage junction in rheumatoid arthritis. Arthritis Rheum 23:1413, 1980.
238. Ziff M: Factors involved in cartilage injury. J Rheumatol (Suppl II) 10:13, 1983.
239. Bromley M, Fisher WD, Woolley DE: Mast cells at sites of cartilage erosion in the rheumatoid joint. Ann Rheum Dis 43:76, 1984.
240. Hamilton JA: Hypothesis: In vitro evidence for the invasive and tumor-like properties of the rheumatoid pannus. J Rheumatol 10:845, 1983.
241. Mitrovic DR, Gruson M, Ryckewaert A: Local hyperthermia and cartilage breakdown. J Rheumatol 8:193, 1981.
242. Myers DB, Broom ND: Morphological and biomechanical studies of rheumatoid pannus and cartilage. J Rheumatol 9:502, 1982.
243. Duncan H: Cellular mechanisms of bone damage and repair in the arthritic joint. J Rheumatol (Suppl II) 10:29, 1983.
244. Barrie HJ: Histologic changes in rheumatoid disease of the metacarpal and metatarsal heads as seen in surgical material. J Rheumatol 8:246, 1980.
245. Wyllie JC: Histopathology of the subchondral bone lesion in rheumatoid arthritis. J Rheumatol (Suppl II) 10:26, 1983.
246. Levick JR: Joint pressure-volume studies: Their importance, design, and interpretation. J Rheumatol 10:353, 1983.
247. Mohr W, Kohler G, Wessinghage D: Polymorphonuclear granulocytes in rheumatic tissue destruction. Rheumatol Int 1:21, 1981.
248. Hajiroussou VJ, Webley M: Prolonged low-dose corticosteroid therapy and osteoporosis in rheumatoid arthritis. Ann Rheum Dis 43:24, 1984.
249. Wu PC, Fang D, Ho EKW, et al: The pathogenesis of extensive discovertebral destruction in ankylosing spondylitis. Clin Orthop 230:154, 1988.
250. Furst SR, Kindynis P, Gundry C, et al: Pseudo-pseudarthrosis in a patient with ankylosing spondylitis. J Rheumatol 17:258, 1990.
251. Gálvez J, Sola J, Ortuxo G, et al: Microscopic rice bodies in rheumatoid synovial fluid sediments. J Rheumatol 19:1851, 1992.
252. Inoue K, Nishioka J, Hakuda S, et al: Rheumatoid nodules at the cement-bone interface in revision arthroplasty of rheumatoid patients. J Bone Joint Surg [Br] 75:455, 1993.
253. Fam AG, Shuckett R, McGillivray DC, et al: Stress fractures in rheumatoid arthritis. J Rheumatol 10:722, 1983.
254. Casey D, Mirra J, Staple TW: Parasymphyseal insufficiency fractures of the os pubis. AJR 142:581, 1984.
255. Mbuyi-Muamba JM, Dequeker J, Burssens A: Massive osteolysis in a case of rheumatoid arthritis: Clinical, histologic and biochemical findings. Metab Bone Dis Rel Res 5:101, 1983.
256. Popert AJ, Scott DL, Wainwright AC, et al: Frequency of occurrence, mode of development, and significance of rice bodies in rheumatoid joint. Ann Rheum Dis 41:109, 1982.
257. Wisneisky JJ, Askari AD: Rheumatoid nodulosis. A relatively benign rheumatoid variant. Arch Intern Med 141:615, 1981.
258. Herzer P, Scholz S, Fuebl HS, et al: Rheumatoid nodules without rheumatoid arthritis. Rheumatol Int 2:183, 1982.
259. Shupak R, Bernier V, Rabinovich S, et al: Avascular necrosis of bone with rheumatoid vasculitis. J Rheumatol 10:261, 1983.
260. Swinburne K: Oedema of feet and ankles in rheumatoid arthritis. Br Med J 1:1541, 1964.
261. Kalliomaki JL, Vastamaki M: Chronic diffuse oedema of the rheumatoid hand. A sign of lymphatic involvement. Ann Rheum Dis 27:167, 1968.
262. DeSilva RTD, Grennan DM, Palmer DG: Lymphatic obstruction in rheumatoid arthritis: A cause for upper limb oedema. Ann Rheum Dis 39:260, 1980.
263. Andersson I, Marsal L, Nilsson B, et al: Abnormal axillary lymph nodes in rheumatoid arthritis. Acta Radiol 21:645, 1980.
264. Bywaters EGL: Thoracic intervertebral discitis in rheumatoid arthritis due to costovertebral joint involvement. Rheumatol Int 1:83, 1981.
265. Bywaters EGL: Rheumatoid and other diseases of the cervical interspinous bursae and changes in the spinous processes. Ann Rheum Dis 41:360, 1982.
266. Yunus M: Huge knee effusion: A record? Arthritis Rheum 24:109, 1981.
267. Soren A, Waugh TR: The synovial changes in psoriatic arthritis. Rev Rhum Mal Osteoartic 50:390, 1983.
268. Canoso JJ, Wohlgethan JR, Newberg AH, et al: Aspiration of the retrocalcaneal bursa. Ann Rheum Dis 43:308, 1984.

269. Thorngren K-G, Liedberg E, Aspelin P: Fractures of the thoracic and lumbar spine in ankylosing spondylitis. Arch Orthop Trauma Surg *98*:101, 1981.

270. Resnick D, Niwayama G: Discovertebral destruction in a man with chronic back problems. Invest Radiol *16*:89, 1981.

271. Mau G, Helbig B, Mann M: Discitis—a rare early symptom of ankylosing spondylitis. Eur J Pediatr *137*:85, 1981.

272. Wise CM, Irby WR: Spondylodiscitis in ankylosing spondylitis: Variable presentations. J Rheumatol *10*:1004, 1983.

273. Jajic I, Furst Z, Vuksic B: Spondylitis erosiva: Report on 9 patients. Ann Rheum Dis *41*:237, 1982.

274. Fallet GH, Courtois C, Vischer TL, et al: Erosive spondylopathy. Scand J Rheumatol *32*:110, 1980.

275. Courtois C, Fallet GH, Vischer TL, et al: Erosive spondylopathy. Ann Rheum Dis *39*:462, 1980.

276. Albert J, Lagier R: Enthesopathic erosive lesions of patella and tibial tuberosity in juvenile ankylosing spondylitis. ROFO *139*:544, 1983.

277. Pritchett JW: Ossification of the coracoclavicular ligaments in ankylosing spondylitis. A case report. J Bone Joint Surg [Am] *65*:1017, 1983.

278. Revell PA, Mayston V: Histopathology of the synovial membrane of peripheral joints in ankylosing spondylitis. Ann Rheum Dis *41*:579, 1982.

279. Francois RJ: Some pathological features of ankylosing spondylitis as revealed by microradiography and tetracycline labelling. Clin Rheumatol *1*:23, 1982.

280. Ishikawa H, Ohno O, Hirohata K: An electron microscopic study of the synovial-bone junction in rheumatoid arthritis. Rheumatol Int *4*:1, 1984.

281. Soren A: Histodiagnosis and Clinical Correlation of Rheumatoid and Other Synovitis. Philadelphia, JB Lippincott Co, 1978, pp 122, 132, 137.

282. Bywaters EGL: Pathology of the spondyloarthropathies. *In* A Calin (Ed): Spondyloarthropathies. New York, Grune & Stratton, 1984.

283. Guerra J Jr, Newell JD, Resnick D, et al: Gastrocnemio-semimembranosus bursal region of the knee. AJR *136*:593, 1981.

284. Patrone NA, Ramsdell CM: Baker's cyst and venous thrombosis. South Med J *74*:768, 1981.

285. Arnoldi CC, Reimann I, Mortensen S, et al: The effect of joint position on juxta-articular bone marrow pressure. Acta Orthop Scand *51*:893, 1980.

286. Taylor RT, Huskisson EC, Whitehouse GH, et al: Spontaneous fractures of pelvis in rheumatoid arthritis. Br Med J *4*:663, 1971.

287. Haider R, Storey G: Spontaneous fractures in rheumatoid arthritis. Br Med J *1*:1514, 1962.

288. Rauschning W, Lindgren PG: The clinical significance of the valve mechanism in communicating popliteal cysts. Arch Orthop Trauma Surg *95*:251, 1979.

289. Wigley RD: Popliteal cysts: Variations on a theme of Baker. Semin Arthritis Rheum *12*:1, 1982.

290. Rauschning W: Anatomy and function of the communication between knee joint and popliteal bursae. Ann Rheum Dis *39*:354, 1980.

291. Pirani M, Lange-Mechlen I, Cockshott WP: Rupture of a posterior synovial cyst of the elbow. J Rheumatol *9*:94, 1982.

292. Chaiamnuay P, Davis P: An unusual case of inguinal swelling. Arthritis Rheum *27*:239, 1984.

293. Shepherd JR, Helms CA: Atypical popliteal cyst due to lateral synovial herniation. Radiology *140*:66, 1981.

294. Lindgren PG, Rauschning W: Radiographic investigation of popliteal cysts. Acta Radiol *21*:657, 1980.

295. Hermann G, Yeh H-C, Lehr-Janus C, et al: Diagnosis of popliteal cyst: Double contrast arthrography and sonography. AJR *137*:369, 1981.

296. Lukes PJ, Herberts P, Zachrisson BE: Ultrasound in the diagnosis of popliteal cysts. Acta Radiol *21*:663, 1980.

297. Gompels BM, Darlington LG: Evaluation of popliteal cysts and painful calves with ultrasonography: Comparison with arthrography. Ann Rheum Dis *41*:355, 1982.

298. Harper J, Schubert F, Benson MD, et al: Ultrasound and arthrography in detection of ruptured Baker's cysts. Australas Radiol *26*:281, 1982.

299. Abdel-Dayem HM, Barodawala YK, Papademetriou T: Scintigraphic arthrography. Comparison with contrast arthrography and future applications. Clin Nucl Med *7*:516, 1982.

300. Lee KR, Tines SC, Price HI, et al: The computed tomographic findings of popliteal cysts. Skel Radiol *10*:26, 1983.

301. Hull RG, Rennie JAN, Eastmond CJ, et al: Nuclear magnetic resonance (NMR) tomographic imaging for popliteal cysts in rheumatoid arthritis. Ann Rheum Dis *43*:56, 1984.

302. Bromley M, Woolley DE: Histopathology of the rheumatoid lesion. Identification of cell types at sites of cartilage erosion. Arthritis Rheum *27*:857, 1984.

303. Crisp AJ, Chapman CM, Kirkham SE, et al: Articular mastocytosis in rheumatoid arthritis. Arthritis Rheum *27*:845, 1984.

304. Godfrey HP, Ilardi C, Engber W, et al: Quantitation of human synovial mast cells in rheumatoid arthritis and other rheumatic diseases. Arthritis Rheum *27*:852, 1984.

305. Wasserman SI: The mast cell and synovial inflammation. Or, what's a nice cell like you doing in a joint like this? Arthritis Rheum *27*:841, 1984.

306. Mitrovic D: The mechanism of cartilage destruction in rheumatoid arthritis. Arthritis Rheum *28*:1192, 1985.

307. Fassbender HG: Is pannus a residue of inflammation? Arthritis Rheum *27*:956, 1984.

308. Petrie JP, Wigley RD: Proximal dissection of the olecranon bursa in rheumatoid arthritis. Rheumatol Int *4*:139, 1984.

309. Benedek TG: Subcutaneous nodules and the differentiation of rheumatoid arthritis from rheumatic fever. Semin Arthritis Rheum *13*:305, 1984.

310. Kaye BR, Kaye RL, Bobrove A: Rheumatoid nodules. Review of the spectrum of associated conditions and proposal of a new classification, with a report of four seronegative cases. Am J Med *76*:279, 1984.

311. Rush PJ, Bernstein BH, Smith CR, et al: Chronic arthritis following benign rheumatoid nodules of childhood. Arthritis Rheum *28*:1175, 1985.

312. Fedullo LM, Bonakdarpour A, Moyer RA, et al: Giant synovial cysts. Skel Radiol *12*:90, 1984.

313. Ruiz EP, Eguren TT, Palop J, et al: Fistule cutanée d'un kyste poplité chez une patiente atteinte de polyarthrite rhumatoide. Rev Rhum Mal Osteoartic *52*:115, 1985.

314. Bassett LW, Gold RH, Mirra JM: Rheumatoid bursitis extending into the clavicle and to the skin surface. Ann Rheum Dis *44*:336, 1985.

315. Als OS, Gotfredsen A, Christiansen C: The effect of glucocorticoids on bone mass in rheumatoid arthritis patients. Influence of menopausal state. Arthritis Rheum *28*:369, 1985.

316. Als OS, Gotfredsen A, Riis BJ, et al: Are disease duration and degree of functional impairment determinants of bone loss in rheumatoid arthritis? Ann Rheum Dis *44*:406, 1985.

317. Sambrook PN, Ansell BM, Foster S, et al: Bone turnover in early rheumatoid arthritis. I. Biochemical and kinetic indexes. Ann Rheum Dis *44*:575, 1985.

318. Shimizu S, Shiozawa K, Imura S, et al: Quantitative histologic studies on the pathogenesis of periarticular osteoporosis in rheumatoid arthritis. Arthritis Rheum *28*:25, 1985.

319. Wordsworth BP, Vipond S, Woods CG, et al: Metabolic bone disease among inpatients with rheumatoid arthritis. Br J Rheumatol *23*:251, 1984.

320. Fam AG: Stress fractures in RA: An overlooked complication. J Musculoskel Med *1*:27, 1984.

321. Jones G, Jawad A: Another look at stress fractures in rheumatoid arthritis. J Rheumatol *11*:867, 1984.

322. Stromquist B: Hip fracture in rheumatoid arthritis. Acta Orthop Scand *55*:624, 1984.

323. Resnick D, Cone R: Pathological fractures in rheumatoid arthritis: Sites and mechanisms. RadioGraphics *4*:549, 1984.

324. Wordsworth BP, Mowat AG, Watson NA: Fracture through a geode in the proximal ulna. Br J Rheumatol *23*:110, 1984.

325. Lowthian PJ, Calin A: Geode development and multiple fractures in rheumatoid arthritis. Ann Rheum Dis *44*:130, 1985.

326. Monsees B, Destouet JM, Murphy WA, et al: Pressure erosions of bone in rheumatoid arthritis: A subject review. Radiology *155*:53, 1985.

327. Monsees B, Murphy WA: Pressure erosions: A pattern of bone resorption in rheumatoid arthritis. Arthritis Rheum *28*:820, 1985.

328. Coulton BL, Popert A: Massive extension of the suprapatellar pouch into the thigh tissues in rheumatoid disease. Ann Rheum Dis *45*:174, 1986.

329. Pellman E, Kumari S, Greenwald R: Rheumatoid iliopsoas bursitis presenting as unilateral leg edema. J Rheumatol *13*:197, 1986.

330. Godfrey N, Staple TW, Halter D, et al: Insufficiency os pubis fractures in rheumatoid arthritis. J Rheumatol *12*:1176, 1985.

331. Iguchi T, Kurosaka M, Ziff M: Electron microscopic study of HLA-DR and monocyte/macrophage staining cells in the rheumatoid synovial membrane. Arthritis Rheum *29*:600, 1986.

332. Morales-Piga A, Elena-Ibanez A, Zea-Mendoza AC, et al: Rheumatoid nodulosis: Report of a case with evidence of intraosseous rheumatoid granuloma. Arthritis Rheum *29*:1278, 1986.

333. van Soesbergen RM, Lips P, van den Ende, et al: Bone metabolism in rheumatoid arthritis compared with postmenopausal osteoporosis. Ann Rheum Dis *45*:149, 1986.

334. Verstraeten A, Dequeker J: Mineral metabolism in postmenopausal women with active rheumatoid arthritis. J Rheumatol *13*:43, 1986.

335. Verstraeten A, Dequeker J: Vertebral and peripheral bone mineral content and fracture incidence in postmenopausal patients with rheumatoid arthritis: Effect of low dose corticosteroids. Ann Rheum Dis *45*:852, 1986.

336. Ekenstam EA, Ljunghall S, Hallgren R: Serum osteocalcin in rheumatoid arthritis and other inflammatory arthritides. Ann Rheum Dis *45*:484, 1986.

337. Leisen JCC, Duncan H, Riddle JM, et al: The erosive front: A topographic study of the junction between the pannus and the subchondral plate in the macerated rheumatoid metacarpal head. J Rheumatol *15*:17, 1988.

338. Malone DG, Wilder RL, Saavedra-Delgado AM, et al: Mast cell numbers in rheumatoid synovial tissues. Arthritis Rheum *30*:130, 1987.

339. Malone DG, Metcalfe DD: Mast cells and arthritis. Ann Allergy *61*:27, 1988.

340. Cush JJ, Lipsky PE: Cellular basis for rheumatoid inflammation. Clin Orthop *265*:9, 1991.

341. Iguchi T, Matsubara T, Kawai K, et al: Clinical and histologic observations of monoarthritis. Clin Orthop *250*:241, 1990.

342. Allard SA, Muirden KD, Maini RN: Correlation of histopathological features of pannus with patterns of damage in different joints in rheumatoid arthritis. Ann Rheum Dis *50*:278, 1991.

343. Chu CQ, Field M, Feldmann M, et al: Localization of tumor necrosis factor α in synovial tissues and at the cartilage-pannus junction in patients with rheumatoid arthritis. Arthritis Rheum *34*:1125, 1991.

344. Ziff M: Rheumatoid arthritis—its present and future. J Rheumatol *17*:127, 1990.

345. Ziff M: Role of the endothelium in chronic inflammatory synovitis. Arthritis Rheum *34*:1345, 1991.

346. Kursunoglu-Brahme S, Riccio T, Weisman M, et al: Rheumatoid knee: Role of gadopentetate-enhanced MR imaging. Radiology *176*:831, 1990.

347. Björkengren AG, Geborek P, Rydholm U, et al: MR imaging of the knee in

acute rheumatoid arthritis: Synovial uptake of gadolinium-DOTA. AJR *155*:329, 1990.

348. Kaye JJ, Callahan LF, Nance EP Jr, et al: Bony ankylosis in rheumatoid arthritis. Associations with longer duration and greater severity of disease. Invest Radiol *22*:303, 1987.

349. Möttönen TT: Prediction of erosiveness and rate of development of new erosions in early rheumatoid arthritis. Ann Rheum Dis *47*:648, 1988.

350. Maricic M: Giant cystic lesions in rheumatoid arthritis. J Rheumatol *17*:552, 1990.

351. Gubler FM, Maas M, Dijkstra PF, et al: Cystic rheumatoid arthritis. Radiology *177*:829, 1990.

352. Moore EA, Jacoby RK, Ellis RE, et al: Demonstration of a geode by magnetic resonance imaging: A new light on the cause of juxta-articular bone cysts in rheumatoid arthritis. Ann Rheum Dis *49*:785, 1990.

353. Nikpoor N, Aliabadi P, Poss R, et al: Case report 504. Skel Radiol *17*:515, 1988.

354. Schils JP, Resnick D, Haghighi PN, et al: Pathogenesis of discovertebral and manubriosternal joint abnormalities in rheumatoid arthritis: A cadaveric study. J Rheumatol *16*:291, 1989.

355. Pearson ME, Kosco M, Huffer W, et al: Rheumatoid nodules of the spine: Case report and review of the literature. Arthritis Rheum *30*:709, 1987.

356. Grillet B, Dequeker J: Rheumatoid lymphedema. J Rheumatol *14*:1095, 1987.

357. Dacre JE, Scott DL, Huskinsson EC: Lymphoedema of the limbs as an extra-articular feature of rheumatoid arthritis. Ann Rheum Dis *49*:722, 1990.

358. Russell EB, Hunter JB, Pearson L, et al: Remitting seronegative symmetrical synovitis with pitting edema—13 additional cases. J Rheumatol *17*:633, 1990.

359. Ziff M: The rheumatoid nodule. Arthritis Rheum *33*:761, 1990.

360. Segal R, Caspi D, Tishler M, et al: Accelerated nodulosis and vasculitis during methotrexate therapy for rheumatoid arthritis. Arthritis Rheum *31*:1182, 1988.

361. Kerstens PJSM, Boerbooms AMT, Jeurissen MEC, et al: Accelerated nodules during low dose methotrexate therapy for rheumatoid arthritis: An analysis of ten cases. J Rheumatol *19*:867, 1992.

362. Ishikawa H, Ueba Y, Hirohata K: An intra-articular rheumatoid nodule in the hip. A case report. J Bone Joint Surg [Am] *70*:775, 1988.

363. Couret M, Combe B, Chuong VT, et al: Rheumatoid nodulosis: Report of two new cases and discussion of diagnostic criteria. J Rheumatol *15*:1427, 1988.

364. Fielding JR, Franklin PD, Kustan J: Popliteal cysts: A reassessment using magnetic resonance imaging. Skel Radiol *20*:433, 1991.

365. Lieberman JM, Yulish BS, Bryan PJ, et al: Magnetic resonance imaging of ruptured Baker's cyst. J Can Assoc Radiol *39*:295, 1988.

366. Burk DL Jr, Dalinka MK, Kanal E, et al: Meniscal and ganglion cysts of the knee: MR evaluation. AJR *150*:331, 1988.

367. Sambrook PN, Eisman JA, Champion GD, et al: Determinants of axial bone loss in rheumatoid arthritis. Arthritis Rheum *30*:721, 1987.

368. Bijlsma JWJ: Bone metabolism in patients with rheumatoid arthritis. Clin Rheumatol *7*:16, 1988.

369. Sambrook PN, Cohen ML, Eisman JA, et al: Effects of low dose corticosteroids on bone mass in rheumatoid arthritis: A longitudinal study. Ann Rheum Dis *48*:535, 1989.

370. Compston JE, Vedi S, Mellish RWE, et al: Reduced bone formation in nonsteroid treated patients with rheumatoid arthritis. Ann Rheum Dis *48*:483, 1989.

371. Reading JM, Sheehan NJ: Spontaneous fractures of the lower limb in chronic rheumatoid arthritis. J Orthop Rheumatol *4*:173, 1991.

372. Straaton KV, Lopez-Mendez A, Alarcon GS: Insufficiency fractures of the distal tibia misdiagnosed as cellulitis in three patients with rheumatoid arthritis. Arthritis Rheum *34*:912, 1991.

373. Semba CP, Mitchell MJ, Sartoris DJ, et al: Multiple stress fractures in the hindfoot in rheumatoid arthritis. J Rheumatol *16*:671, 1989.

374. Abe H, Nakamura M, Takahashi S, et al: Radiation-induced insufficiency fractures of the pelvis: Evaluation with ^{99m}Tc-methylene diphosphonate scintigraphy. AJR *158*:599, 1992.

375. Deutsch AL, Mink JH, Waxman AD: Occult fractures of the proximal femur: MR imaging. Radiology *170*:113, 1989.

376. Brahme SK, Cervilla V, Vint V, et al: Magnetic resonance appearance of sacral insufficiency fractures. Skel Radiol *19*:489, 1990.

377. Resnick D: Inflammatory disorders of the vertebral column: Seronegative spondyloarthropathies, adult-onset rheumatoid arthritis, and juvenile chronic arthritis. Clin Imaging *13*:253, 1989.

378. Aufdermaur M: Pathogenesis of square bodies in ankylosing spondylitis. Ann Rheum Dis *48*:628, 1989.

26

Rheumatoid Arthritis

Donald Resnick, M.D., and Gen Niwayama, M.D.

Standard textbooks of rheumatology generally contain numerous chapters devoted to rheumatoid arthritis.[1, 2] Furthermore, these chapters appear in the early pages of the book, prior to the consideration of other articular disorders. The extensive discussion provided by these chapters and their early placement emphasize the fundamental role that this disease commands in the practice of rheumatologic medicine. Rheumatoid arthritis is an "everyday" disease whose general clinical, pathologic, and radiologic features are well known to most physicians. An in-depth inspection of the radiographic and pathologic characteristics of rheumatoid arthritis provides a standard by which the other rheumatologic conditions can be measured.

Such an inspection must initially consider the basic pathology and radiology of rheumatoid involvement in synovium-lined articulations, bursae, and tendon sheaths, cartilaginous joints, tendinous and ligamentous attachments to bone, and supporting soft tissue structures. This has been accomplished in Chapter 25. From this reference point, an analysis of the changes produced by rheumatoid arthritis in specific locations of the body is appropriate. Such an analysis is contained within this chapter following a brief summary of the diagnostic criteria and clinical abnormalities of the disease.

DIAGNOSTIC CRITERIA

Rheumatoid arthritis is not a new disease.[466] The first description appears to be that of Landré-Beauvais (1772–1840), who believed the disorder was a variant of gout (goutte asthénique primitive), although evidence contained in paintings of Rubens (1577–1640) suggests that rheumatoid arthritis existed long before its identification by Landré-Beauvais.[466, 467] As indicated in the historical review by Benedek and Rodnan,[466] important contributions regarding this disease included the differentiation of rheumatoid arthritis from other articular disorders by Charcot (1825–1893), the application of the name rheumatoid arthritis by Garrod (1858), the association of the disease with subcutaneous nodules by Adams (1873), the description of a syndrome of rheumatoid arthritis, splenomegaly and leukopenia by Felty (1924), and the discovery of rheumatoid factor on the basis of investigations by Billings (1912), Cecil (1929), and Dawson (1932).

The accurate diagnosis of rheumatoid arthritis is without difficulty in the patient who reveals a generalized symmetric, peripherally located polyarthritis associated with (1) clinically detectable severe morning stiffness, synovial inflammation, and subcutaneous nodules, (2) radiologic evidence of an erosive articular process, (3) laboratory parameters of the disease, including a positive serologic test for rheumatoid factor and an elevated erythrocyte sedimentation rate, and (4) pathologic documentation of typical rheumatoid lesions of the synovium and the soft tissues.[3] More troublesome, however, is establishing the presence of this disease in the person who has atypical clinical and radiologic features. Because of this difficulty, a committee was appointed by the American Rheumatism Association in 1956 to formulate criteria for the diagnosis of rheumatoid arthritis.[4, 5] This committee suggested that four grades of diagnosis be used, which reflected the level of confidence that was provided by examining the patient with suspected rheumatoid disease. The four grades were classic, definite,

probable, and possible. Modifications of these criteria have been proposed subsequently[6] and, in 1987, revised criteria for the classification of rheumatoid arthritis were formulated by an appointed subcommittee of the American Rheumatism Association.[7] The new criteria are as follows:

1. Morning stiffness in and around joints lasting at least 1 hour before maximal improvement.
2. Soft tissue swelling (arthritis) of three or more joint areas observed by a physician.
3. Swelling (arthritis) of the proximal interphalangeal, metacarpophalangeal, or wrist joints.
4. Symmetric swelling (arthritis).
5. Rheumatoid nodules.
6. The presence of rheumatoid factor.
7. Radiographic erosions or periarticular osteopenia, or both, in hand or wrist joints, or in both.

Criteria 1 through 4 must have been present for at least 6 weeks. Rheumatoid arthritis is defined by the presence of four or more criteria, and no further qualifications (classic, definite, or probable) or list of exclusions are required. The subcommittee report, based on a computer analysis of 262 patients with rheumatoid arthritis and 262 control subjects with rheumatic diseases other than rheumatoid arthritis, demonstrated 91 to 94 per cent sensitivity and 89 per cent specificity for rheumatoid arthritis when compared with the control population.[7] However, until the basic causative mechanisms of rheumatoid arthritis are elucidated or an absolutely sensitive and specific test for the disease is found, descriptive criteria will be necessary.[663] Furthermore, it has been suggested that a single radiographic criterion based on a posteroanterior exposure of both hands may not be adequate, and that radiographic evaluation of the feet also should be employed.[664]

CLINICAL ABNORMALITIES
General Features

Although rheumatoid arthritis can be apparent in persons of all ages, it predominates between the ages of 25 and 55 years. Women are affected more commonly than men, the female-to-male ratio of the disease being approximately 2 or 3 to 1.[8, 9] An insidious onset, which is most typical, can be initiated by physical or psychic stress. An acute onset is occasionally apparent, particularly in elderly persons,[10, 631] although some investigators believe that this variety of arthritis in the aged population is not truly rheumatoid arthritis, citing the frequency of seronegativity for rheumatoid factor and peculiar pitting edema in the hands and feet in affected patients.[598] Indeed, a syndrome of remitting, seronegative, symmetric synovitis with pitting edema is believed by some investigators to be a separate clinical entity, which should be distinguished from late-onset rheumatoid arthritis.[665–668]

Various prodromal symptoms have been noted in rheumatoid arthritis, including fatigue, anorexia, weight loss, malaise, and muscular pain and stiffness. These findings can be obscured by prominent articular complaints, which frequently are an early manifestation of the disease. Joint pain and stiffness initially can involve a single joint for a period of weeks or months before more generalized articular findings become manifest. In these instances of monoarthritis, clinical diagnosis can be extremely difficult, as the abnormalities simulate traumatic or infectious synovitis. With the appearance of polyarticular disease, the correct diagnosis becomes more apparent. Spotty joint involvement soon becomes symmetric in distribution. Arthritic attacks generally are sudden in onset, persist for hours to days, and subside without residual disability.[9] The eventual outcome of the joint disease is variable. Some patients demonstrate mild clinical manifestations for a long period of time, whereas in others, rapid, severe, and disabling arthritis soon becomes apparent.

Articular Involvement

Articular involvement becomes manifest as pain that is aggravated on motion, swelling, stiffness, and limitation of movement. Redness, a clinical feature that may be associated with joint inflammation, is extremely rare in rheumatoid arthritis. Any rheumatoid articulation that is associated with prominent redness should be investigated to exclude the possibility of infection.[9] Periarticular soft tissue swelling that is fusiform or spindle-shaped in configuration due to increased intra-articular fluid, synovial hypertrophy, and thickening of adjacent soft tissues is accentuated by atrophy of contiguous muscles.

The most typically affected joints are the proximal interphalangeal and metacarpophalangeal joints of the hand, the wrist, the metatarsophalangeal joints of the foot, the knee, the joints of the shoulder, the ankle, and to a lesser extent, the hip; any joint can be involved, however, including the temporomandibular and cricoarytenoid articulations. Symmetry is the hallmark of joint alteration in this disease; in most patients, a remarkable degree of symmetry is demonstrated in the distribution of the arthritis on both sides of the body. There are some exceptions to this rule, however:

1. Although symmetric abnormalities of groups of joints (e.g., metacarpophalangeal and metatarsophalangeal articulations) can be seen, the identical digits may not be affected on both sides of the body.

2. Initially, monoarticular or pauciarticular abnormalities can be noted that do not obey the rule of symmetry. The reported frequency of monoarthritis in rheumatoid arthritis has varied from approximately 5 to 20 per cent of cases.[11, 12] It may persist for weeks or months; the knee and the wrist are the two articulations that are the most frequent sites of monoarthritis. Monoarticular rheumatism also has been noted after trauma.[13, 652] In general, a monoarticular or pauciarticular distribution in rheumatoid arthritis will soon become symmetric.[14] In some persons, an asymmetric form of the disease persists, which may be less severe than the symmetric form.[15]

3. A markedly asymmetric or unilateral distribution in rheumatoid arthritis can be seen in patients with neurologic deficits.[16–21, 468–470] Unilateral muscular weakening or paralysis protects the ipsilateral side from the effects of the articular disease. This protective appearance can be noted in persons with upper or lower motor neuron lesions and therefore can be encountered in rheumatoid arthritis patients with poliomyelitis, encephalitis, neurovascular syphilis, cerebrovascular accidents, cerebral palsy, meningioma, peripheral nerve injury, and other neurologic conditions. Non-neurologic disorders such as osteoarthritis leading to

decreased use of one or more extremities can reveal a similar protective phenomenon. In fact, overuse of one side of the body compared to the other (e.g., right upper extremity in right-handed people) may produce ipsilateral exaggerated abnormalities of rheumatoid arthritis, leading to an asymmetric appearance.[22, 482] This clinical asymmetry, which can be accompanied by radiographic asymmetry, is more striking in patients with pronounced paralysis[19] and is not evident when a neurologic deficit develops in a patient already suffering from rheumatoid arthritis. In this latter situation, the joints of the paralyzed limbs will remain symptomatic, and, in some cases, actual accentuation of clinical manifestations will develop, predominantly in the paralyzed limbs.[17] Rarely, paralysis occurring after the onset of rheumatoid arthritis may lead to the reduction of synovitis in the paralyzed extremity or extremities.[448]

These observations regarding the importance of physical activity in the development of joint lesions in rheumatoid arthritis have been substantiated by other investigators.[23, 24] More extensive erosive and cystic osseous lesions have been noted in rheumatoid arthritis patients who maintain normal physical activity, perhaps related to fibrin or some immunizing agent that may be forced into the synovium during exercise, increasing the severity of the disease. Increased intra-articular pressure in overused limbs also may accelerate joint destruction.[25] In the hemiplegic person, increased activity of the contralateral limb in compensation for its weakened counterpart coupled with decreased activity of the paralyzed extremity thus would lead to prominent asymmetric articular disease. This manifestation also may relate to vasomotor effects or hemodynamic changes occurring in patients with both rheumatoid arthritis and neurologic disease.[468]

4. Differences in the distribution of rheumatoid arthritis occasionally can be related to the sex of the patient. In women, a symmetric distribution in the small peripheral joints of the extremities is more typical than in men.[26] In male patients, asymmetric abnormalities in small or large joints can be noted. This difference in disease distribution between the two sexes may be influenced by the increased use of altered articulations that can be evident in men with rheumatoid arthritis who are employed in physically demanding occupations. It also should be noted that characteristics other than distribution of articular lesions have reportedly differed between men and women with rheumatoid arthritis. For example, male patients with the disease have been found to have more severe joint destruction, a higher prevalence of rheumatoid nodules, and frequent vasculitis and pulmonary involvement.[471]

5. Atypical cases of ''rheumatoid arthritis'' (those that do not fully meet the necessary criteria for the disease) often are characterized by asymmetric joint alterations. Whether these cases represent true rheumatoid arthritis or a (seronegative) arthritis of the rheumatoid type frequently is not clear.[27]

Despite these exceptions to the rule of symmetry, most patients with rheumatoid arthritis will reveal bilateral and relatively equal articular involvement. The physician must be careful not to apply too stringent an index in the interpretation of symmetry in this disease, however.[28] Application of such an index in many patients with rheumatoid arthritis will lead to an erroneous diagnosis.

Articular manifestations in this disease may initially be episodic.[8, 474] Episodes are generally short-lived, leading to a certain amount of irreparable joint damage. A remission of variable length then can be observed, followed by a second episode of arthritis. Synovial effusions during palindromic episodes show variable leukocyte counts and, in some cases, predominance of mononuclear cells.[474] Ultimately, sustained joint disease becomes manifest.

Soft Tissue, Muscular, and Vascular Involvement

Subcutaneous nodules are evident in approximately one fourth of patients with rheumatoid arthritis.[599, 600, 669] They appear at pressure points, especially the juxta-articular regions of the elbow. Other tendinous and soft tissue locations commonly reveal similar nodules, and these lesions may be demonstrated in distant body sites, including the lungs, pleurae, vocal cords, larynx, scalp, sclerae, peritoneum, and abdominal wall.[29-32] Initially, in certain sites, they appear fixed to the bone and only later become movable structures.[669] Although they may develop rapidly, especially in patients receiving methotrexate therapy,[670] subcutaneous nodules usually have an insidious onset and persist unchanged for months or years. Ulceration, drainage, and sepsis can occur in association with these lesions.

Muscular weakness and atrophy can be prominent in patients with rheumatoid arthritis.[601] These muscular abnormalities can relate to disuse or inflammatory changes. With regard to the inflammatory myopathy, three patterns of cellular infiltration have been defined: arteritis, polymyositis, and focal nodular myositis.[472] None of these patterns is specific for rheumatoid arthritis, and the relationship among them is not clear. A second form of myopathy results from denervation atrophy of muscle fibers.[472] This type of myopathy is a consequence of the peripheral neuropathy seen in the disease. Miscellaneous forms of myopathy result from muscle disuse, dystrophy-like changes, and corticosteroid therapy.

A variety of vascular lesions are noted in this disease. Inflammatory and noninflammatory vascular changes are encountered, leading to many clinical manifestations and complications, including peripheral neuropathy, perforation of the bowel, myocardial infarction, Raynaud's phenomenon, gangrene, and pulmonary hypertension.[33-40, 632]

Systemic Involvement

A discussion of all of the systemic manifestations of rheumatoid arthritis is beyond the scope of this chapter. Note will be made here of only a few such abnormalities.

Neuropathies

In a review of the neuropathology of rheumatoid arthritis, Kim and Collins[472] divided the lesions into categories of encephalopathy, myelopathy, and peripheral neuropathy. With respect to the first category, these authors identified lesions resulting directly from rheumatoid disease (e.g., rheumatoid nodule formation), those secondary to vascular disease (infarction, hemorrhage), and miscellaneous lesions (amyloidosis, infection). Myelopathy can result from direct involvement by rheumatoid disease (vasculitis, rheumatoid

nodules), from vertebral subluxation, which can affect the brain stem or spinal cord, and from miscellaneous causes (hemorrhage, infection).

Peripheral neuropathies in this disease are of several types. A mild or severe sensory and motor neuropathy has been noted.[41-43] Its manifestations include a symmetric distribution, involvement of upper or lower extremities, a "stocking" distribution of sensory impairment, and wrist and foot drop.[9] Vasculitis with or without toxic or metabolic factors may be responsible for this complication. Entrapment or compressive neuropathies also are observed.[44] These neuropathies, which relate to mechanical irritation of a specific peripheral nerve at a vulnerable anatomic site (within fibrous or osseofibrous canals), can affect the median nerve (carpal tunnel syndrome, "double crush" syndrome, and anterior interosseous syndrome), ulnar nerve (cubital canal syndrome, canal of Guyon syndrome, and double crush syndrome), and radial nerve (posterior interosseous syndrome) in the upper extremity; and the sciatic nerve (tibial or common peroneal entrapment by a Baker's cyst), common peroneal nerve (pressure palsy), and posterior tibial nerve (tarsal tunnel syndrome, medial plantar syndrome, lateral plantar syndrome) in the lower extremity (see Chapter 77).

Felty's Syndrome

The association of rheumatoid arthritis, splenomegaly, and leukopenia was first described by Felty in 1924.[9, 45] Additional clinical manifestations of this syndrome include weight loss, anemia, lymphadenopathy, chronic leg ulceration, and abnormal skin pigmentation. Women are affected more frequently than men, and the abnormalities can become severe, with destructive arthritis, systemic complications (including Sjögren's syndrome), and recurrent infections due to the lowered leukocyte count and, perhaps, the reduced chemotactic migration of polymorphonuclear leukocytes in the blood.[473] Leukopenia probably results from hypersplenism, although the demonstration of leukocyte antibodies in patients with this disease may indicate the importance of autoimmune factors in this regard.[46] The anemia appears to be related to hemolysis and can improve with splenectomy[47] or corticosteroid therapy.[48]

Metabolic Bone Disorders

Osteopenia is a well-recognized manifestation of rheumatoid arthritis. In almost all patients, such osteopenia relates to osteoporosis, the severity of which is influenced by the age and sex of the patient, the duration of the disease, the extent of immobilization, and the administration of corticosteroids.[49-51] In addition, osteomalacia related to inadequate intake of vitamin D, malabsorption, and lack of sunshine and hypercalcemia with secondary hyperparathyroidism are two additional mechanisms that may contribute to osteopenia.[452, 634] The subject of osteopenia (and its complications) in rheumatoid arthritis is discussed in Chapter 25.

Sjögren's Syndrome

Sjögren's syndrome is a triad consisting of keratoconjunctivitis sicca, xerostomia, and connective tissue disease (see Chapter 62). The connective tissue disorder, which is evident in 50 to 70 per cent of patients with Sjögren's syndrome, may be identical to rheumatoid arthritis.[7]

LABORATORY ABNORMALITIES

A constellation of laboratory abnormalities exists, which, although not specific, provides significant aid in the accurate diagnosis of rheumatoid arthritis.[52]

A moderate normochromic or hypochromic normocytic anemia is common in this disease. The leukocyte count can be normal, elevated, or, rarely, decreased. The erythrocyte sedimentation rate commonly is markedly elevated and tends to parallel the activity of the disease; exacerbations usually are accompanied by an increase and remissions by a decrease in the sedimentation rate. The C-reactive protein is evident in almost all patients with clinical evidence of disease activity, paralleling the elevation of the erythrocyte sedimentation rate. Alterations in serum proteins also are encountered. Rheumatoid factors, which represent a group of macroglobulins, generally are present in high titer in the serum of patients with this disease. They also are evident in a variety of chronic inflammatory conditions, but are not detected in great concentration in most other articular disorders. An additional serologic reaction is the LE phenomenon, which is positive in 8 to 27 per cent of patients with rheumatoid arthritis. The serum complement level in this disease usually is either normal or slightly elevated.

Additional laboratory abnormalities relate to the dysfunction of various organ systems that can occur in this disease. Alterations in liver and renal function are particularly characteristic.

ABNORMALITIES AT SPECIFIC LOCATIONS

General Distribution

The general radiographic and pathologic features of articular involvement in rheumatoid arthritis are discussed in Chapter 25. A symmetric arthritis showing predilection for the hands, wrists, feet, knees, shoulders, elbows, ankles, and hips is typical (Fig. 26–1). In the axial skeleton, the articulations of the cervical spine are the only sites that are affected consistently or significantly, although changes in the thoracolumbar spine and sacroiliac joints are encountered occasionally. Cartilaginous joints, such as the discovertebral junctions (outside of the cervical region), symphysis pubis, and manubriosternal articulations, and tendinous and ligamentous attachments to bone may be involved, but the frequency and severity of changes at these sites are less pronounced in this disease than in the seronegative spondyloarthropathies (ankylosing spondylitis, psoriasis, and Reiter's syndrome).

Hand

Clinical Abnormalities

The joints of the hand are affected in almost all persons with rheumatoid arthritis. Metacarpophalangeal and proximal interphalangeal joint alterations predominate. On clinical examination, fusiform soft tissue swelling is associated with tenderness elicited by firm pressure at these locations. Clinical (as well as radiologic) evidence of distal interphalangeal joint disease is less frequent and rarely is severe[53]; however, the diagnosis of rheumatoid arthritis cannot be eliminated by the finding of involvement of the distal interphalangeal joints.[635, 636] Swelling on the volar aspect of the

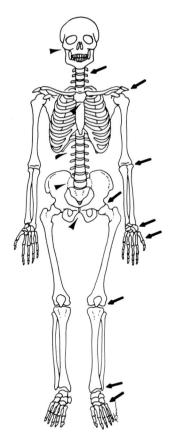

FIGURE 26–1. General distribution of disease in rheumatoid arthritis. Rheumatoid arthritis characteristically is a symmetric arthritis of the small joints of the hands (proximal interphalangeal and metacarpophalangeal joints), feet (metatarsophalangeal joints and interphalangeal joint of the great toe), and wrists (all of its compartments), the knees, the ankles, the elbows, the glenohumeral and acromioclavicular joints, and the hips (arrows). In the axial skeleton, the articulations of the cervical spine typically are affected (arrow). Less constant involvement occurs in the thoracolumbar spine, sacroiliac and temporomandibular joints, symphysis pubis, and manubriosternal joint (arrowheads).

digits reflects the inflammatory changes in the flexor tendon sheaths.[54–56]

In long-standing disease, swan-neck deformities (hyperextension at proximal interphalangeal joints and flexion at distal interphalangeal joints), boutonnière deformities (flexion at proximal interphalangeal joints and hyperextension at distal interphalangeal joints), and hitchhiker's or Z-shaped deformity of the thumb (flexion at the metacarpophalangeal joint and hyperextension at the interphalangeal joint) can be observed (see discussion later in this chapter).[57, 58] The articulations themselves become relatively fixed in position due to fibrous (or less commonly, bony) fusion.

Spontaneous rupture of extensor tendons of the digits is a well-recognized complication of this disease.[59, 60, 671] As at other sites, factors that appear important in the pathogenesis of these tendinous ruptures include abnormal stress, intrinsic tendon abnormality, tenosynovitis, and injury from adjacent osseous structures. Attrition and rupture of flexor tendons in the hand also are observed in rheumatoid arthritis.[480]

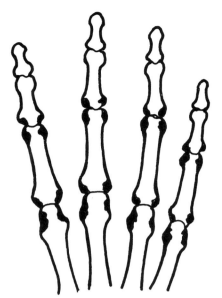

FIGURE 26–2. Metacarpophalangeal and proximal interphalangeal joints: Target areas. In the four ulnar digits, early osseous erosions may appear at the radial and ulnar aspects of the metacarpophalangeal and proximal interphalangeal joints. The initial changes occur on the radial aspect of the phalanges and metacarpal bones at the second and third metacarpophalangeal joints and on the radial and ulnar aspects of the phalanges at the third proximal interphalangeal articulation. Distal interphalangeal joint changes are less constant and severe.

Radiographic-Pathologic Correlation

Early Abnormalities (Figs. 26–2 to 26–5). Radiographic abnormalities of the interphalangeal and metacarpophalangeal joints in rheumatoid arthritis are well de-

scribed.[61–65] Detection of these changes at an early stage may require, in addition to posteroanterior and semipronated oblique views, radiographic examination in semisupinated[66–68] and tangential[69] projections. These changes, which relate to synovial hypertrophy, accumulation of intraarticular fluid, soft tissue edema, and osteochondral destruction in the vicinity of inflammatory pannus,[70–73] are most evident at specific target sites in the hand in rheumatoid arthritis. The second and third metacarpophalangeal joints and the third proximal interphalangeal joint may reveal the earliest abnormalities.[672] Particularly characteristic is indistinctness of osseous outline corresponding to the insertion of the capsule on the dorsoradial aspect of the proximal portion of the proximal phalanges of the four medial digits[74]; this finding differs from a normal pattern of cortical irregularity that has been identified at the base of the proximal phalanges, predominantly on the ulnar aspect of the bone.[483] Soon fusiform soft tissue swelling, periarticular osteoporosis, concentric loss of articular space, and marginal erosions become evident at many or all of the proximal interphalangeal and metacarpophalangeal joints.

The marginal erosions, which occur at the osseous surfaces that do not possess protective cartilage,[62] appear at the radial and ulnar aspects of the articulation. At both proximal interphalangeal and metacarpophalangeal joint locations, the erosions are larger on the proximal bone that constitutes the articulation (the metacarpal head at the metacarpophalangeal joint; the proximal phalanx at the proximal interphalangeal joint) because the unprotected areas are more extensive at these sites. At the metacarpophalangeal joints, the radial aspect of the bone is more significantly affected than the ulnar aspect; the radiovolar portion of the metacarpal head may reveal the most prominent erosion. In the thumb, a characteristic deep erosion may appear at the

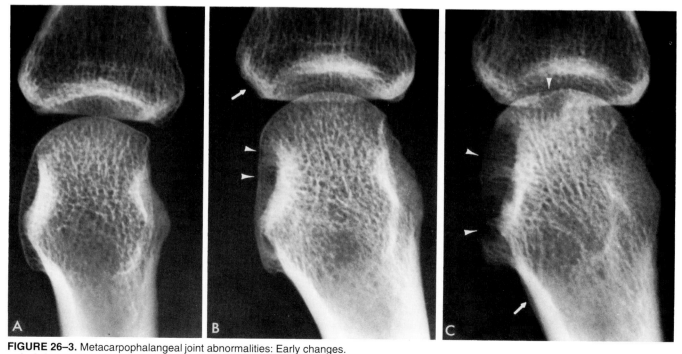

FIGURE 26–3. Metacarpophalangeal joint abnormalities: Early changes.
A–C Sequential articular changes are illustrated. Initially **(A)**, the bones appear normal, with preservation of the subchondral bone plate on the radial aspect of the metacarpal head. Subsequently **(B)**, small radiolucent areas appear beneath the metacarpal head, leading to thinning of the bone plate with focal discontinuity or gaps (arrowheads). Tiny erosions and surface irregularity of the proximal phalanx also are evident (arrow). At a later stage **(C)**, obvious osseous defects are seen (arrowheads). Note mild periosteal proliferation (arrow).

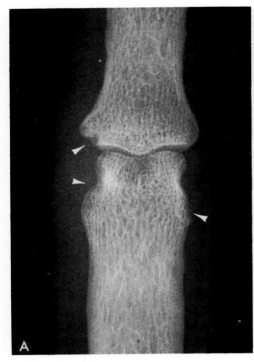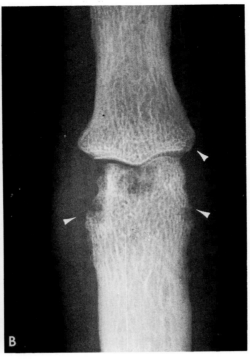

FIGURE 26–4. Proximal interphalangeal joint abnormalities: Early changes. Initial radiographic changes **(A)** include soft tissue swelling, joint space narrowing, and marginal erosions (arrowheads). Subsequently **(B)** (in another digit), further loss of interosseous space and progressive erosions are evident (arrowheads). Note that the erosive changes are more extensive on the proximal phalanx than on the middle phalanx.

ulnar side of the volar aspect of the base of the distal phalanx about the interphalangeal articulation near the insertion of the flexor pollicis longus and at the radial and ulnar sides of the first metacarpophalangeal articulation.[61] Marginal erosions about the distal interphalangeal joints generally are small compared with those of the more proximal digital joints, although any distal interphalangeal joint can reveal focal marginal defects.[635] The erosions at these articulations may be more common if coexisting osteoarthritis is present.[673]

In addition to marginal erosions, two other types of bony erosion have been noted in the hands of patients with rheumatoid arthritis: compressive (pressure) erosions[602, 603] and superficial surface resorption[62] (Table 26–1). Compressive erosions are related to the effect of muscular forces acting on osteoporotic bones and are a prominent feature of many articular disorders, including juvenile chronic arthritis.[75] The muscular forces are considerable, particularly at the metacarpophalangeal joints.[76] In rheumatoid arthritis, destruction of cartilage produces increased forces on the ad-

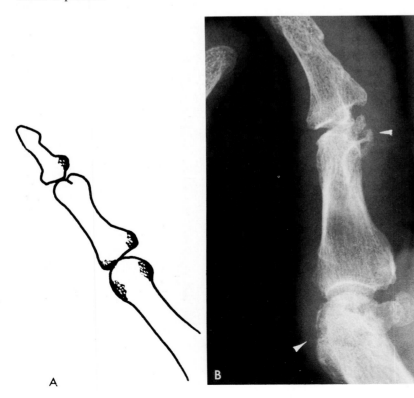

FIGURE 26–5. Abnormalities of the metacarpophalangeal and interphalangeal joints of the thumb: Early changes. Radial and ulnar erosions at the first metacarpophalangeal joint and ulnar erosion on the volar aspect of the bones at the interphalangeal joint are typical (arrowheads and shaded areas).

TABLE 26–1. Types of Bony Erosion in the Hand and Wrist in Rheumatoid Arthritis

Type	Mechanism	Common Sites
Marginal erosion	Pannus destruction of bare areas (without protective cartilage) of bone	Metacarpophalangeal and proximal interphalangeal joints; radial styloid; midportion of scaphoid; triquetrum; capitate; trapezium
Compressive erosion	Collapse of osteoporotic bone by muscular forces	Metacarpophalangeal joints
Surface resorption	Erosion of bone beneath inflamed tendons	Outer aspect of distal end of ulna; dorsal aspect of first metacarpal bone; proximal phalanx of first digit

jacent osteoporotic bone, leading to invagination of the end of one bone into another (the counterpart of this in the hip is protrusio acetabuli). Irregular notching and splaying of the apposing reciprocal bony surfaces are detected.

Superficial surface resorption beneath inflamed tendon sheaths can be evident in the diaphyses and metaphyses of the phalanges without the appearance of abnormalities in the adjacent articulations.[62] This is encountered most typi-

cally on the dorsal aspect of the first metacarpal bone subjacent to the extensor pollicis longus tendon and on the proximal phalanx of the thumb at the insertions of the flexor pollicis brevis and adductor pollicis muscles. The involved cortices appear thin, with fraying of the subperiosteal margin. Associated periosteal proliferation can be seen, although the finding is quite subtle.

Continued Abnormalities (Fig. 26–6). With further destruction of cartilage and bone, the articular space may be obliterated completely. Erosion of central portions of the joint can lead to apparently enclosed radiolucent defects, cysts, or pseudocysts. In most instances, radiographs obtained in multiple projections will reveal that these defects communicate with the articular cavity, corresponding to sites of transchondral extension of pannus.[77] Rarely, true intraosseous rheumatoid nodules can be responsible for these lesions (see Chapter 25). Furthermore, remodeling of bony trabeculae can account for cysts in additional cases. In some patients, particularly those with rheumatoid nodulosis, prominent cystic lesions of the phalanges may be unaccompanied by joint space narrowing or significant synovitis.[78, 79] The cysts usually are distributed symmetrically and most often are located about the proximal interphalangeal and metacarpophalangeal joints (as well as in the wrists and feet).[674]

Although fibrous ankylosis is the characteristic ultimate fate of severe arthritis of metacarpophalangeal and proximal interphalangeal joints, occasional examples of intra-articu-

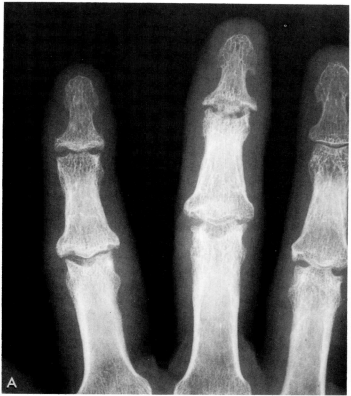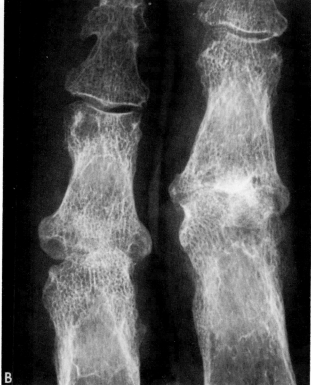

FIGURE 26–6. Abnormalities of the interphalangeal joints: More advanced changes.
A Considerable osseous erosion appears at the proximal interphalangeal and distal interphalangeal joints. Central and marginal defects have produced separation of the bony contours. This degree of separation combined with the extent of changes at the distal interphalangeal joints is unusual in rheumatoid arthritis.
B Secondary proliferative alterations at the proximal interphalangeal joints, consisting of eburnation and osteophytosis, obscure some of the more typical rheumatoid abnormalities. Note, however, marginal erosions and partial intra-articular osseous fusion of the second proximal interphalangeal joint.

lar osseous fusion can be seen in these locations.[675] In almost all such instances, it is the proximal interphalangeal joint that is ankylosed; bony ankylosis of the metacarpophalangeal articulation is exceedingly unusual, with the exception of that in the thumb.[675]

Finger Deviations and Deformities. Deviation and deformity of the fingers are common complications of rheumatoid arthritis affecting the hand and the wrist. Although not diagnostic of the disease,[80] these deformities are well recognized in the rheumatoid arthritis patient and have received a great deal of attention.[57, 58, 71, 76, 81–90, 484]

Mallet Finger. Although extensive synovial inflammation of the distal interphalangeal joints of the four medial digits is relatively uncommon, loosening or disruption of the distal attachment of the extensor tendon to the terminal phalanx may result in the development of a typical mallet or drop finger. With progressive loosening of the collateral ligaments combined with the detrimental effect on cartilage and bone of the intra-articular inflamed synovial tissue, instability of the distal interphalangeal joint can appear.

This relatively uncommon deformity should not be confused with the deviations of the distal interphalangeal articulations that may be secondary to boutonnière and swan-neck collapse deformities.

Boutonnière Deformity (Fig. 26–7A, B). The peculiar anatomy of the three-joint system of the digits (metacarpophalangeal, proximal interphalangeal, and distal interphalangeal articulations) influences the pattern of joint deformity that may accompany rheumatoid arthritis. A collapse deformity (buckling) of this system can lead to hyperextension of one joint and reciprocal flexion of the contiguous articulation.[81] In normal situations, the balanced tendon mechanism and ligamentous restriction prevent collapse deformity of the digits, but in rheumatoid arthritis, the vulnerable balance is compromised by the direct effect of this disease on articulations, tendons, and ligaments. Flexion of the proximal interphalangeal joint combined with hyperextension at the distal interphalangeal joint produces the boutonnière deformity of the digit.

Synovial inflammation and hyperplasia and capsular dis-

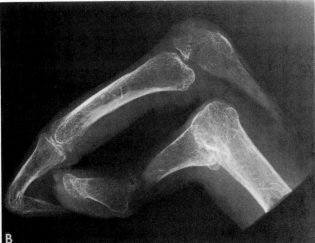

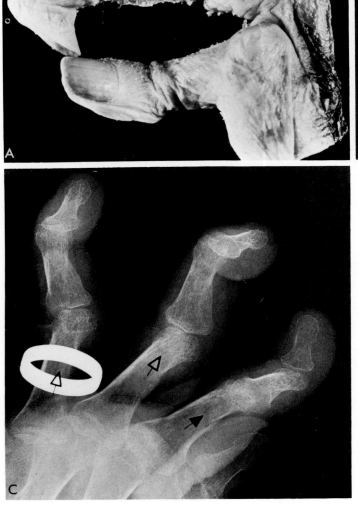

FIGURE 26–7. Boutonnière and swan-neck deformities of digits.
A, B A photograph and radiograph of the first and second digits of a cadaver with rheumatoid arthritis reveal a boutonnière deformity of the thumb (with flexion at the metacarpophalangeal joint and hyperextension at the interphalangeal joint) and a swan-neck deformity of the second finger (extension at the proximal interphalangeal joint and flexion at the distal interphalangeal joint). Observe the destructive articular changes at both metacarpophalangeal articulations.
C Typical swan-neck deformity of the third and fourth digits (open arrows) and a boutonnière deformity of the second digit (closed arrow) are evident in this rheumatoid arthritis patient.

tention are important findings in the initiation of the boutonnière deformity. The insertion of the central slip of the extensor tendon may become lengthened or torn from its attachment to the base of the middle phalanx, thus becoming unable to effect normal extension of the middle phalanx. The proximal interphalangeal joint protrudes upward through the lateral extensions of the extensor tendon like a button through a buttonhole. The abnormal palmar position of the lateral tendons is located beneath the central axis of the joint, and thus these tendons become flexors of the proximal interphalangeal joint. The displacement also results in shortening of these lateral tendons, producing an increased pull in their insertion on the distal phalanx, leading to hyperextension deformity of the distal interphalangeal joint.[81, 91, 92]

Swan-Neck Deformity (Fig. 26–7C). Swan-neck deformity consists of hyperextension of the proximal interphalangeal joint and flexion of the distal interphalangeal joint. Its pathogenesis is complex[81] and not fully agreed on. Although synovitis of the proximal interphalangeal joint, hyperextension of the long extensor tendons, deformity of the metacarpophalangeal articulation, and carpal collapse[485] may be contributory factors, the primary cause of the deformity is a synovitis of the flexor tendon sheath, which restricts interphalangeal joint flexion.[93, 94] This compromises the normal function of the long flexor tendon, which is to flex the distal interphalangeal articulation. The flexor action is then concentrated on the metacarpophalangeal joint. The flexed position at this site leads to tightness of the intrinsic muscles and to exaggerated pull of the intrinsic muscles on the central tendon across the dorsal aspect of the proximal interphalangeal joint. Resulting failure of proximal interphalangeal joint flexion is associated with imbalancing forces on the extensor aspect of the joint, leading to hyperextension at this location.[58] The distal interphalangeal joint becomes flexed as a result of the pull of the extended profundus tendon, which exceeds the pull of the long extensor tendon, which is bowstrung across the proximal interphalangeal joint.[95] Other deforming forces that can accelerate the swan-neck appearance include palmar subluxation of the metacarpophalangeal or wrist joint[81] and contracture of the intrinsic wing-insertions secondary to chronic flexion deformity of the metacarpophalangeal joint.[96] Progressive deterioration of the proximal interphalangeal articulations can be seen with bony ankylosis.[97]

Swan-neck deformity also can occur secondary to a mallet finger deformity itself[91] or as the result of rupture of the flexor digitorum sublimis tendon.[84]

Deformities of the Metacarpophalangeal Joint (Fig. 26–8). A variety of metacarpophalangeal articular deformities and deviations appear in the rheumatoid hand, including ulnar drift, extensor tendon subluxation, and palmar subluxation and flexion of the joint.[81, 98]

The reported frequency of ulnar deviation at the metacarpophalangeal joints in rheumatoid arthritis varies according to the population being studied and the techniques used to investigate the patients. In a typical population, ulnar drift has been recorded in 27 per cent of patients.[58] In patients with more chronic disease, radiographs outline ulnar deviation in 47 per cent of hands in patients with rheumatoid arthritis.[99] Using an angle formed by the intersection of two coordinates, one constructed along the longitudinal axis of each metacarpal at the radial cortex and a second con-

structed along the longitudinal axis of each phalanx at its radial cortex, as a measure of the degree of ulnar deviation, a frequency of ulnar deviation in 384 digits affected by rheumatoid arthritis of 38 per cent[99] was found; palmar subluxation was noted in 20 per cent of digits in rheumatoid arthritis. An earlier investigation of 800 digits in 100 rheumatoid arthritis patients being evaluated for reconstructive hand surgery revealed ulnar deviation in 63 per cent and palmar subluxation in 68 per cent.[100] These reports indicate that the frequency and severity of ulnar deviation and volar subluxation of the metacarpophalangeal joint demonstrable on radiographs are less than those found on clinical examination.[101] The degree of ulnar drift increases with flexion at the metacarpophalangeal joints; the ulnar-deviated fingers pressed tightly against the cassette during radiography appear less deformed. This discrepancy between clinical and radiographic evidence of metacarpophalangeal articular deformity is more striking in patients with reversible ulnar drift; this occurs in systemic lupus erythematosus[102] and Jaccoud's arthropathy.[103]

The pathogenesis of ulnar drift is complex and not fully understood.[97] An inflammatory synovitis of the metacarpophalangeal joint with a rise in intra-articular pressure[86] appears to be the initial factor in the development of this deformity[104]; stabilization at this articulation is sacrificed by destruction of ligamentous, capsular, and muscular tissues.[105–107] Instability and ulnar deviation of extensor tendons may be another primary factor or an aggravating factor in the production of ulnar deviation.[58, 104] An additional contributing factor, metacarpal volar descent, results from ligamentous laxity of the fourth and fifth carpometacarpal joints.[100, 105] Gravity and lateral pressure on the hand produced during everyday maneuvers have been described as causes of ulnar deviation.[9, 108]

A relationship between radial deviation of the wrist and ulnar deviation at the metacarpophalangeal joints, producing the zigzag deformity of the hand in rheumatoid arthritis, has been noted in many patients.[83, 89, 99, 481, 676] Ulnar deviation at the radiocarpal joint allows a more direct alignment of the flexor tendons proximal and distal to the metacarpophalangeal joints, decreasing their ulnar deviating tendencies.[101] With radial deviation of the wrist, a common finding in rheumatoid arthritis, greater volar forces at the mouths of flexor tunnels may result in ulnar deviation at the metacarpophalangeal joints.

Any relationship between radial deviation at the wrist and ulnar deviation at the metacarpophalangeal joints has obvious therapeutic significance. The angle of radiocarpal deviation chosen by the surgeon during wrist arthrodesis may determine the postsurgical outcome.[101] It appears that surgical employment of ulnar deviation at the wrist during arthrodesis can correct ulnar drift at the metacarpophalangeal articulations in some rheumatoid arthritis patients. Similarly, spontaneous radiocarpal compartment fusion in this disease may mechanically block the development of the zigzag malalignment, although the contralateral wrist and hand may have typical deformity.[83]

Thumb Deformities (Fig. 26–9). The malalignments that are most frequently encountered in the thumb in rheumatoid arthritis are collapse deformities (boutonnière deformity) related to disturbance of function at the first metacarpophalangeal joint; swan-neck deformity, related to disturbance of function at the first carpometacarpal joint; and instability,

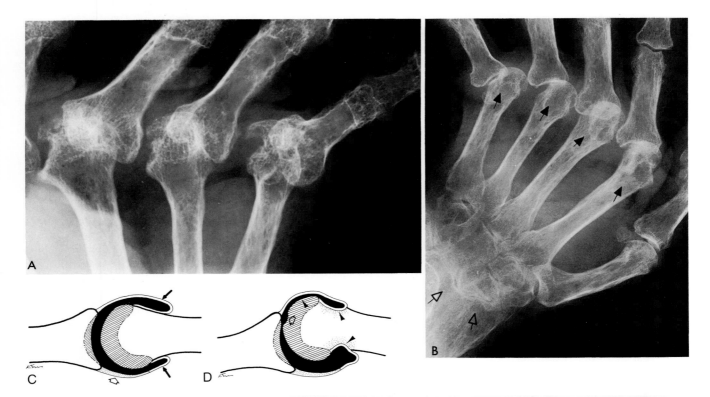

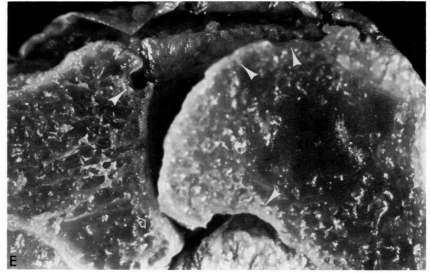

FIGURE 26–8. Metacarpophalangeal joint deformities.

A Ulnar deviation. Severe ulnar deviation at multiple metacarpophalangeal joints is associated with large erosions of the metacarpal heads.

B Ulnar deviation. The simultaneous occurrence of ulnar deviation at the metacarpophalangeal joints (solid arrows) and radial deviation at the radiocarpal joint of the wrist (open arrows) is well shown in this patient. The resulting appearance is termed the zigzag deformity.

C–E Flexion deformity and volar subluxation. On a drawing of a sagittal section of a normal metacarpophalangeal joint **(C)**, note the articular cartilage (hatched areas), prominent synovial pouches (solid arrows), and volar plate (open arrow). In a similar drawing of a flexed rheumatoid metacarpophalangeal joint **(D)**, observe areas in which abnormal synovium is in contact with articular cartilage or bone (arrowheads) and an area of pressure erosion of cartilage (open arrow). On a photograph of an oblique section of a flexed metacarpophalangeal joint in a cadaver with rheumatoid arthritis **(E)**, synovium-derived erosions (arrowheads) and pressure erosion (open arrow) of bone and cartilage are evident.

(C, D. From McMaster M: J Bone Joint Surg [Br] *54*:687, 1972.)

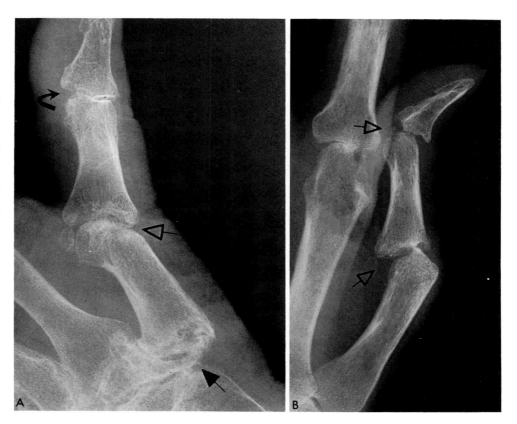

FIGURE 26–9. Deformities of the thumb.

A Swan-neck deformity. Hyperextension at the first metacarpophalangeal joint (open arrow) is seen. Note the severe bony and cartilaginous destruction at the first carpometacarpal (solid arrow) and first metacarpophalangeal joints and less dramatic abnormalities at the interphalangeal joint (curved arrow). At this stage, flexion deformity of the interphalangeal joint has not occurred.

B Boutonnière deformity. Findings include flexion at the first metacarpophalangeal joint and hyperextension at the interphalangeal joint (open arrows). Associated articular destruction in this and the adjacent digit is evident.

stiffness, or pain of the interphalangeal, metacarpophalangeal, and carpometacarpal joints.[81, 109]

The boutonnière deformity (Z-shaped deformity or hitchhiker's thumb) is the most common collapse deformity of the thumb in patients with rheumatoid arthritis.[110] Synovitis of the first metacarpophalangeal joint distends the joint capsule and stretches and displaces ulnarly the extensor pollicis longus tendon and adductor expansion.[111, 112] Radial displacement of the lateral thenar expansions and lengthening of the attachment of the extensor pollicis brevis tendon to the base of the proximal phalanx ensue. The ability to extend the metacarpophalangeal joint is compromised, and a flexion deformity at this location results. Secondary hyperextension of the interphalangeal joint is related to the pull on the distal phalanx of the extensor pollicis longus tendon and the extensor insertions of the intrinsic muscles.[81] Progressive destruction of the metacarpophalangeal joint accompanies and aggravates this deformity.

The swan-neck deformity of the thumb is initiated by destruction and capsular stretching at the first carpometacarpal joint. Radial subluxation of the metacarpal base becomes evident. Altered function at the first carpometacarpal articulation leads to adductor muscle spasm and contracture. With the increasing difficulty that is encountered in abducting the thumb, compensatory changes in the distal joints appear. Hyperextension of the metacarpophalangeal joint and, to a lesser extent, hyperextension of the interphalangeal joint are seen.[113] Secondary flexion at the interphalangeal articulation, occurring in response to hyperextension at the first metacarpophalangeal joint, produces the typical swan-neck deformity. Progressive destruction in the first carpometacarpal articulation can be observed.[114]

In addition to these classic deformities, destruction at either the interphalangeal or carpometacarpal articulation of the thumb can lead to severe instability.

Wrist

Clinical Abnormalities

Wrist involvement is a characteristic feature of rheumatoid arthritis. Although generally accompanied by abnormalities in the fingers, such clinical (and radiologic) involvement can initially appear in the absence of significant digital alterations. Indeed, it has been suggested that wrist involvement may predominate during the first 5 years of disease, although changes in the hand eventually may overtake those in the wrist.[677, 678] Clinical findings can relate to synovitis in any of the compartments of the wrist, adjacent tenosynovitis, and attenuation or injury of several soft tissue, tendinous, and ligamentous structures.[671] Soft tissue swelling is common on both the dorsal (due to synovial hypertrophy in the wrist joint or extensor tendon sheaths) and volar (due to tenosynovitis of the flexor tendon sheaths) aspects of the joint. Extensor carpi ulnaris tenosynovitis creates a painless swelling on the ulnar aspect of the wrist, which may appear early in the course of the disease. Painless bilateral tenosynovitis of the extensor digitorum also creates soft tissue swelling at an early stage of the disease. A characteristic concavity of the dorsum of the hand distal to the wrist is located between the prominent soft tissues of the wrist and the metacarpophalangeal joints. Palmar subluxation and atrophy of the interosseous muscles create hollows between the metacarpals.

Subsequent clinical features of the wrist in rheumatoid arthritis relate to dorsal subluxation of the distal portion of the ulna, the carpal tunnel syndrome attributable to synovitis in the carpal tunnel with dysesthesias along the course of the median nerve, and rupture of one or more extensor tendons.[115, 116] The pathogenesis of extensor tendon rupture of the wrist has been related to rheumatoid involvement of the inferior radioulnar compartment with the production of irregular osseous spikes that injure the adjacent tendon[60] or hypermobility of the ulnar head.[116] Another possible mechanism is tendon necrosis as a result of local granulomatous infiltration.[56] The severity of the clinical findings when the inferior radioulnar joint is involved and the possible association with extensor tendon attrition have caused investigators to advocate various surgical techniques, the most popular of which is excision of the distal end of the ulna (the Darrach procedure).[117–121, 679, 680]

Various wrist deformities can occur during the course of rheumatoid arthritis.[81, 83, 87, 89] Each is associated with typical articular attitudes, which can be detected clinically. Further-more, synovial cysts arising during the disease can create local soft tissue masses.[122]

Radiographic-Pathologic Correlation

Early Abnormalities. The early radiographic and pathologic findings of rheumatoid wrist disease have been well delineated.[61, 62, 123] A complete understanding of these abnormalities requires an in-depth knowledge of normal wrist anatomy (see Chapter 22) and the arthrographic changes in the wrist in rheumatoid arthritis (see Chapter 13).

Distal End and Styloid Process of the Ulna. Erosion and swelling around the distal end of the ulna and the ulnar styloid process are early manifestations of rheumatoid arthritis and are related to abnormality of the prestyloid recess of the radiocarpal compartment, the inferior radioulnar compartment, and the extensor carpi ulnaris tendon and sheath[124] (Figs. 26–10 and 26–11).

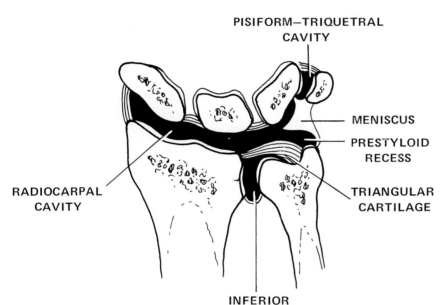
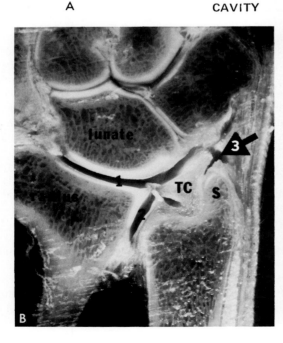
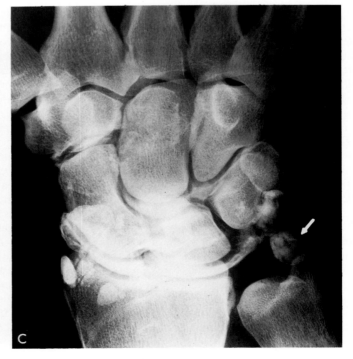

FIGURE 26–10. Distal end and styloid process of ulna: Normal relationships.

A A drawing of a coronal section through the radiocarpal compartment of a normal wrist. The triangular fibrocartilage separates the inferior radioulnar compartment, or cavity, from the radiocarpal compartment. The meniscus homologue, which is firmly attached to the triquetrum, separates the pisiform-triquetral compartment from the radiocarpal compartment. Note the prestyloid recess, which is a constant diverticulum, or limb, of the radiocarpal compartment. The recess is intimate with the ulnar styloid process.

B Corresponding coronal section showing radiocarpal (1) and inferior radioulnar (2) compartments. The prestyloid recess (3) is seen to good advantage as it approaches the styloid process (S) of the ulna. TC, Triangular fibrocartilage.

C Posteroanterior arthrogram of normal wrist of cadaver showing radiocarpal and midcarpal compartments filled with contrast material. Note the large prestyloid recess (arrow), which approximates the ulnar styloid process.

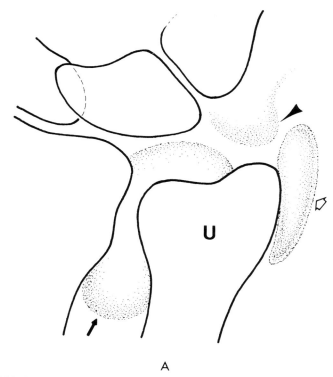
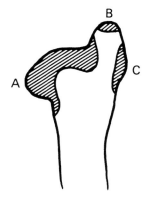

A. EROSIONS RELATED TO
    INFERIOR RADIOULNAR
    COMPARTMENT

B. EROSIONS RELATED TO
    PRESTYLOID RECESS

C. EROSIONS RELATED TO
    EXTENSOR CARPI ULNARIS
    TENDON SHEATH

A   B

FIGURE 26–11. Abnormalities of the distal end and styloid process of the ulna: Sites of early soft tissue swelling and osseous erosion.
  A Soft tissue swelling about the distal end of the ulna (U) may appear as distention of the prestyloid recess of the radiocarpal compartment (arrowhead), of the inferior radioulnar compartment (solid arrow), or of the extensor carpi ulnaris tendon sheath (open arrow).
  B Early osseous erosions appear at three distinct areas in the distal portion of the ulna.

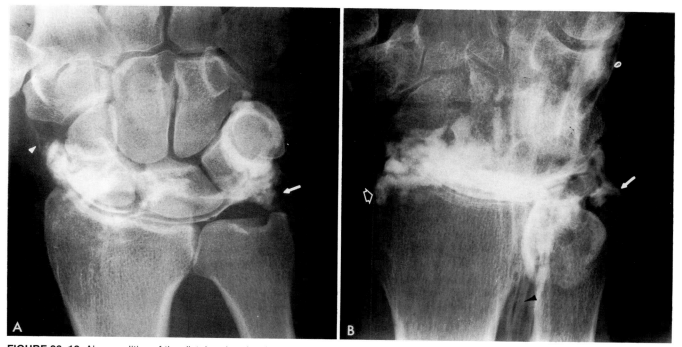

FIGURE 26–12. Abnormalities of the distal end and styloid process of the ulna: Prestyloid recess.
  A In early rheumatoid arthritis, contrast arthrography of the radiocarpal compartment can outline a corrugated synovial pattern that is most severe in the prestyloid recess (arrow). Observe also lymphatic filling (arrowhead) and visualization of the pisiform-triquetral compartment.
  B In another rheumatoid arthritis patient, contrast medium–filled radiocarpal and inferior radioulnar compartments are seen. Note the corrugated pattern within the prestyloid recess (solid arrow) and elsewhere (open arrow). Communication (arrowhead) with sheaths of extensor tendons is evident.

The prestyloid recess of the radiocarpal compartment is intimate with the ulnar styloid process and may extend circumferentially around the process or contact only its undersurface (Fig. 26–12). A corrugated synovial pattern frequently is visualized in arthrograms of the rheumatoid wrist, most prominently in the prestyloid recess of the radiocarpal compartment, where the pattern may be associated with filling of the adjacent lymphatic structures.[464] The latter phenomenon probably reflects locally increased permeability of the inflamed synovial membrane in conjunction with lymphatic hyperplasia.[125, 126] Prominent congested synovial folds can obliterate the small opening into the prestyloid recess of the radiocarpal compartment, with the result that radiocarpal arthrography may fail to make this diverticulum visible. The inflamed synovial tissue within the prestyloid recess is in contact with, and may produce erosions of, the tip of the ulnar styloid process. These erosions begin as focal radiolucent areas within the subchondral bone. As erosion progresses, however, the ulnar styloid tip becomes increasingly irregular.

Proliferative synovitis within the inferior radioulnar compartment frequently is coincident with rheumatoid arthritis and results in localized prominence of the soft tissue[127, 128] (Fig. 26–13). Contrast filling of this compartment through defects in the triangular fibrocartilage has been noted in radiocarpal arthrograms of 70 per cent[129] and 58 per cent[130] of patients with rheumatoid arthritis. The diseased synovium extends over the radial and the palmar surfaces of the distal portion of the ulna and the adjacent ulnar aspect of the distal end of the radius. Radiographic findings include shallow surface defects, which progress to become extensive scalloped erosions, and sharply angular surfaces on the distal portions of the radius and ulna. The intimate relationship of the radius and the ulna often leads to secondary compression erosions.[61, 62]

Tendinitis and tenosynovitis of the extensor carpi ulnaris tendon and its sheath represent the third factor that contributes to abnormality of the distal ulna and the ulnar styloid process (Fig. 26–14). Proliferative synovitis within the sheath is visualized easily in arthrograms of the wrist because of the frequent communication of the sheath with the radiocarpal compartment.[129, 130] This synovitis results in swelling of the soft tissue along the outer aspect of the ulnar head. Subjacent resorption of bone and periostitis occur along the medial margin of the distal ulna beneath the inflamed tendon and sheath.[61, 62, 124]

Radial Styloid Process and Scaphoid. Synovial inflammation within the radiocarpal compartment leads to rheumatoid erosion of the distal end of the radius and the adjacent scaphoid bone[131] (Fig. 26–15). Although not so frequent as erosive abnormality of the ulnar styloid process, erosion of the radial styloid process has been noted in 11 per cent of rheumatoid wrists.[62] At this site, there is an unprotected or ''bare'' area on the surface of the bone adjacent to the radial collateral ligament. Alterations on the lateral midportion of the scaphoid bone likewise are characteristic and have been noted in 36 per cent of rheumatoid wrists.[62] This site also is devoid of cartilage and vulnerable to erosion. Irregular defects of variable size and eventual fragmentation of the bone are not unusual.[132] Erosion and surface irregularity at this site must be distinguished from a normal degree of notching of the scaphoid, which is not uncommon.[133]

Palmar Aspect of the Distal Radius. Radiocarpal arthrograms of the normal wrist show multiple finger-like projections that extend for a short distance beneath the distal end of the radius (Fig. 26–16). These projections are the palmar radial recesses. In arthrograms of the rheumatoid wrist, the outline of a corrugated synovial lining within these recesses is visible.[130] Radiographs of the rheumatoid wrist frequently reveal erosion of the neighboring bone. These erosions appear as irregular radiolucent shadows overlying the midportion of the distal radius in posteroanterior radiographs. Their palmar location is recognized more readily on steep oblique and lateral radiographs.

Triquetral and Pisiform Bones. Erosions of the triquetrum and the pisiform bones are common in early rheumatoid arthritis and occur at three sites: the proximal medial portion of the triquetrum, the distal medial portion of the triquetrum, and the adjacent surfaces of the triquetrum and the pisiform[134] (Fig. 26–17). Abnormalities at these three sites have been noted in 38 per cent, 23 per cent, and 41 per cent, respectively, of 100 rheumatoid arthritis patients.

Initially, a shallow marginal erosion can be seen on the proximal portion of the triquetrum at the medial limit of the radiocarpal compartment (Fig. 26–18). Repeated contact with an irregular ulnar styloid process that projects through the opening of the prestyloid recess exacerbates enlargement of the osseous defect.[135] These well-recognized compressive forces on the triquetrum[62] may lead to flattening, sclerosis, and fragmentation of the ulnar styloid process and the triquetrum.[132, 136]

The medial limit of the midcarpal compartment is another site at which marginal erosion of the triquetral bone occurs (Fig. 26–18). Abnormal pooling of contrast material may be seen at this site in an arthrogram of a wrist in a patient with rheumatoid arthritis. An associated marginal erosion of the adjacent hamate bone is frequent.

The pisiform-triquetral compartment is seen tangentially in ''reverse'' oblique radiographs made with the wrist in a semisupinated position (Fig. 26–19). Arthrography of the wrist in rheumatoid arthritis frequently reveals a corrugated synovial pattern and lymphatic filling in this area. Plain radiographs may disclose superficial or deep erosion on the palmar surface of the triquetral bone and the dorsal surface of the pisiform bone. Because these abnormalities are not visible on posteroanterior radiographs and because they may be present even in the absence of narrowing of the radiocarpal and the midcarpal compartments and in the absence of erosion of the radial and the ulnar styloid processes, radiography in the reverse oblique projection is suggested for evaluation of the wrist in rheumatoid arthritis.

Midcarpal, Carpometacarpal, and Intermetacarpal Compartments. Although early erosive changes most frequently occur at the sites already described, abnormalities are not uncommon in several other areas of the wrist (Fig. 26–20). Marginal erosion of the trapezium adjacent to the attachment of the radial collateral ligament and on the radial aspect of the capitate bone has been noted.[62, 137] Marginal erosion of the radial aspect of the base of the first metacarpal bone indicates rheumatoid involvement of the first carpometacarpal compartment; scalloped erosion of the base of one or more of the other four metacarpal bones reflects synovial proliferation within the intermetacarpal compartments.

Continued Abnormalities. Continued synovial inflam-

Text continued on page 890

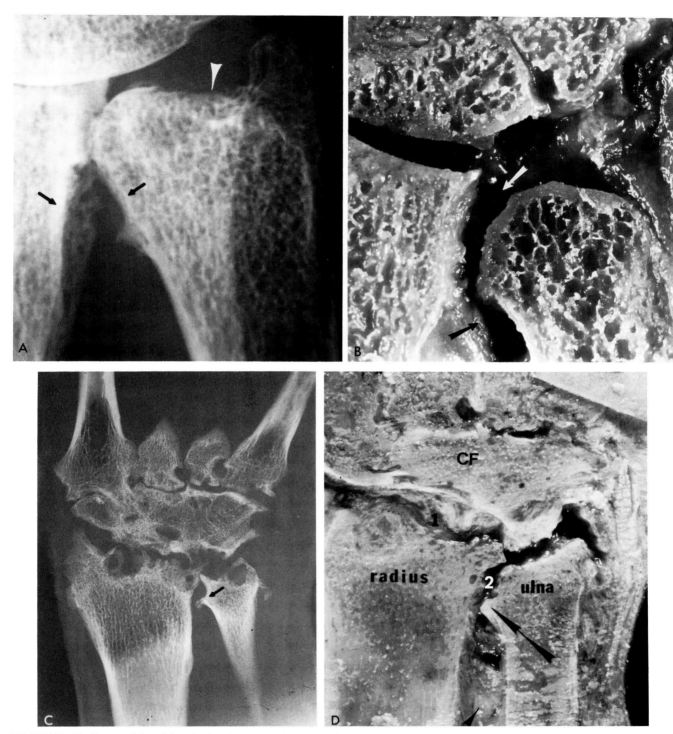

FIGURE 26–13. Abnormalities of the distal end and styloid process of the ulna: Inferior radioulnar compartment.

A Magnification radiograph outlines osseous erosion (arrows) of apposing surfaces of distal portion of the radius and distal end of the ulna due to rheumatoid synovitis of the inferior radioulnar compartment. Observe notchlike irregularity of the ulnar end (arrowhead).

B A photograph of a coronal section of the wrist in a cadaver with rheumatoid arthritis demonstrates synovial inflammation in the inferior radioulnar compartment (arrows) with osseous erosion of the distal part of the radius and the distal portion of the ulna. Changes in other areas of the wrist also are evident.

C Radiograph of coronal section of wrist of cadaver with advanced rheumatoid arthritis. Extensive erosive abnormalities and carpal fusion are evident. Note the irregular bony spicules (arrow) of the ulna.

D Photograph of same coronal section as in **C**. Considerable synovial alterations can be seen at the radiocarpal (1) and the inferior radioulnar (2) compartments. Carpal fusion (CF) and bony spicules (arrow) of the ulna also are seen to good advantage. Note the saclike distal contour of the inferior radioulnar compartment (arrowhead).

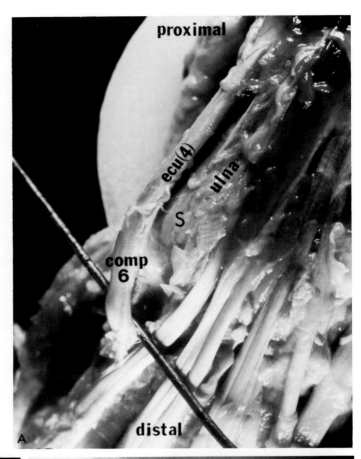

FIGURE 26–14. Abnormalities of the distal end and styloid process of the ulna: Extensor carpi ulnaris tendon and tendon sheath.

A Gross specimen showing compartments on dorsum of wrist enclosing extensor tendons and sheaths. The sixth compartment (comp 6) has been dissected to reveal the extensor carpi ulnaris tendon (ecu 4). Note the intimate relationship of this tendon with the posterior and outer aspects of the distal ulna and the ulnar styloid process (S).

B Wrist of rheumatoid patient showing swelling of soft tissue (arrow) and subjacent resorption of bone with periosteal proliferation (arrowhead). Additional alterations include changes on apposing surfaces of the distal radius and distal ulna.

C An additional radiograph (magnification) delineates surface resorption of the outer aspect of the ulna (arrows) on the basis of extensor carpi ulnaris tendinitis and tenosynovitis.

Illustration continued on opposite page

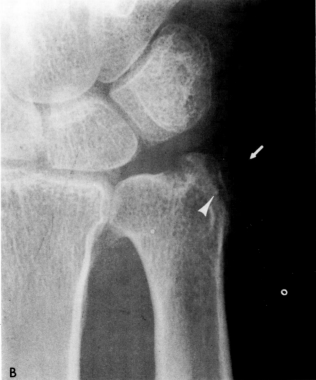

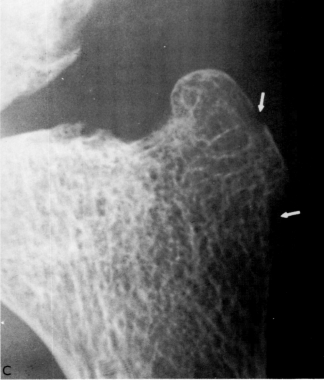

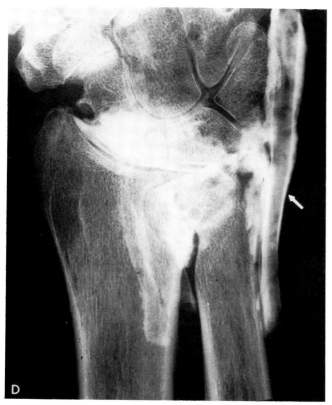

FIGURE 26–14. *Continued*

D Arthrogram of rheumatoid wrist showing radiocarpal, inferior radioulnar, and midcarpal compartments filled with contrast material. Note the communication of the radiocarpal compartment with the sheath (arrow) of the extensor carpi ulnaris tendon. The tendon is identifiable within the sheath.

E Coronal section of rheumatoid wrist showing close relation of irregular extensor carpi ulnaris tendon (4) and sheath (arrows) to distal end and styloid process (S) of ulna.

F Sagittal section of rheumatoid wrist demonstrating irregular extensor carpi ulnaris tendon and sheath (arrows) passing along outer aspect of ulnar styloid process (S). All but this portion of the distal end of the ulna was removed before the specimen was photographed.

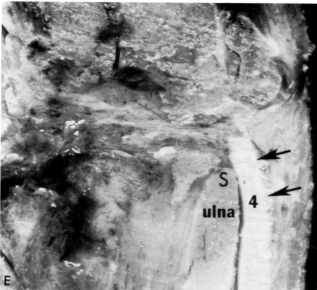

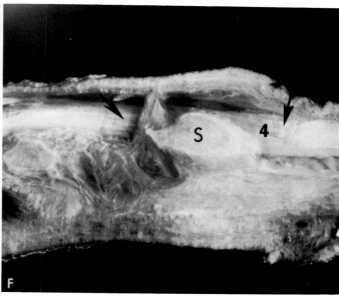

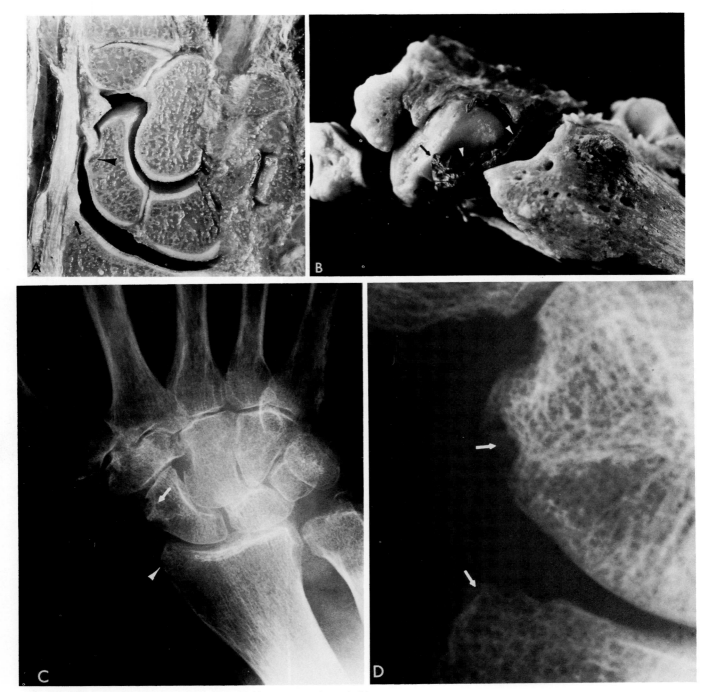

FIGURE 26–15. Abnormalities of the radial styloid process and scaphoid.

A Coronal section demonstrating normal anatomy along the radial aspect of radiocarpal and midcarpal compartments. Marginal areas on the radial styloid process (arrow) and the scaphoid bone (arrowhead) are vulnerable to erosion.

B Photograph of gross specimen made after injection of latex (arrowheads) into the radiocarpal compartment. The radial aspect of the compartment (arrow), which is adjacent to the midportion of the scaphoid bone, is seen clearly.

C Radiograph of rheumatoid wrist showing erosion on radial styloid process (arrowhead) and lateral midportion of scaphoid bone (arrow), characteristic of rheumatoid arthritis. Widespread abnormalities are present throughout the wrist.

D A magnification radiograph of the scaphoid and distal end of the radius outlines marginal erosions of both bones (arrows). Soft tissue swelling also is evident.

Illustration continued on opposite page

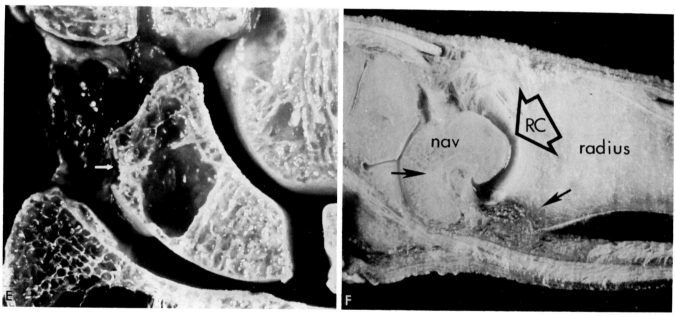

FIGURE 26–15. *Continued*

   E On a photograph of a coronal section of a rheumatoid cadaveric wrist, observe marginal erosions of the scaphoid bone (arrow) with associated cysts.

   F Sagittal section of rheumatoid wrist of cadaver demonstrates synovial proliferation and osseous erosion (arrows) of radius and scaphoid bone (nav) at limits of radiocarpal compartment (RC).

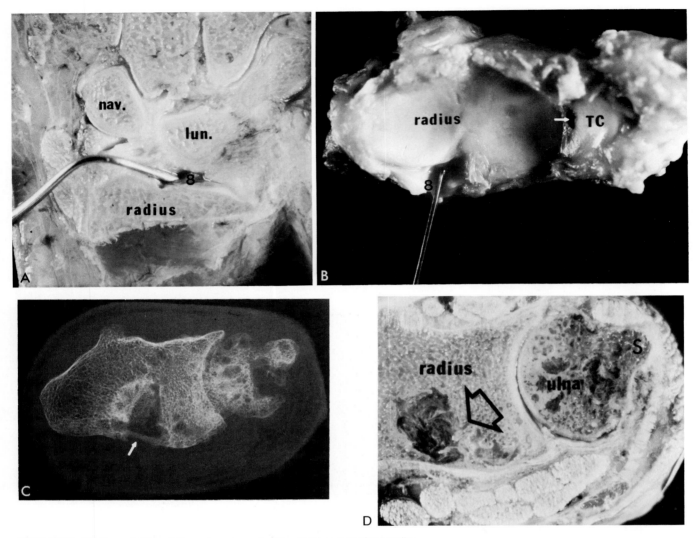

FIGURE 26–16. Abnormalities of the palmar aspect of the distal portion of the radius.

   A Coronal section of normal cadaveric wrist showing probe in the palmar radial recesses (8) as they pass beneath the distal end of the radius. nav, scaphoid; lun, lunate.

   B Gross specimen from different cadaveric wrist showing probe in palmar radial recesses (8) beneath the distal end of the radius. Note the defect (arrow) in the triangular fibrocartilage (TC).

   C Radiograph of transverse section of the distal end of the radius in a cadaver with advanced rheumatoid arthritis. Osseous erosion (arrow) on the palmar aspect of the radius and abnormalities of the ulna can be seen.

   D Photograph of same section as in **C** showing synovial proliferation with invasion of bone (arrow). S, Styloid process of ulna.

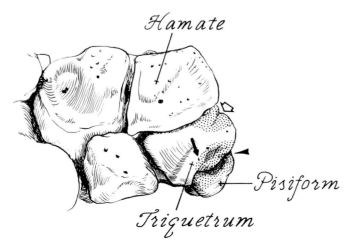

FIGURE 26–17. Distribution of abnormalities of the triquetrum and the pisiform. Osseous changes occur predominantly at three sites: on the triquetrum at the ulnar limit of the radiocarpal compartment (solid arrow), on the triquetrum at the ulnar limit of the midcarpal compartment (open arrow), and on the triquetrum and pisiform related to the pisiform-triquetral compartment (arrowhead).

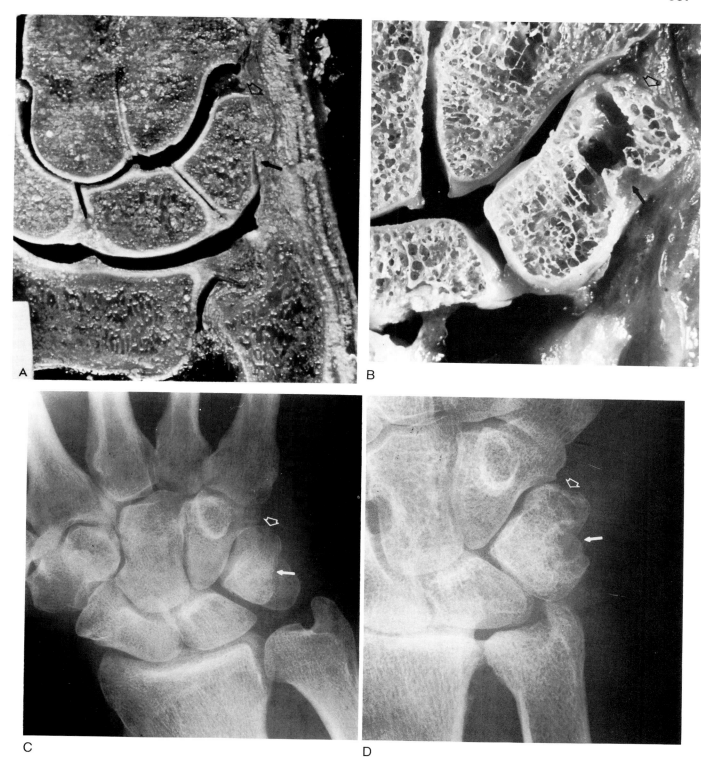

FIGURE 26–18. Abnormalities of the triquetrum and the pisiform: Radiocarpal and midcarpal compartments.

A Coronal section of normal wrist showing relation of ulnar or medial limit of midcarpal and radiocarpal compartments to triquetrum. The triquetrum has two marginal areas that are vulnerable to erosion—one at the medial limit of the radiocarpal compartment (solid arrow), the other at the medial limit of the midcarpal compartment (open arrow).

B A photograph of a coronal section of a rheumatoid wrist reveals marginal erosion of the triquetrum related to synovial proliferation of the radiocarpal (solid arrow) and the midcarpal (open arrow) compartments.

C Radiograph of the wrist in a patient with rheumatoid arthritis showing marginal erosions (open and solid arrows) on the triquetrum. The erosions are related to abnormality at the ulnar or medial limit of the midcarpal compartment and, to a lesser extent, the ulnar limit of the radiocarpal compartment.

D Radiograph of wrist of another patient, who had more advanced rheumatoid arthritis. The marginal erosions (open and solid arrows) and associated abnormalities throughout the wrist can be identified more easily.

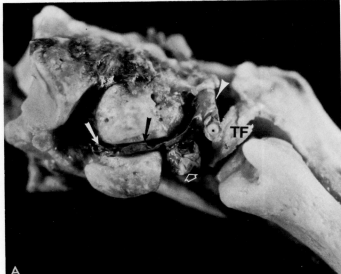

FIGURE 26–19. Abnormalities of the triquetrum and the pisiform: Pisiform-triquetral compartment.

A Specimen from wrist of normal cadaver photographed after latex has been introduced into the radiocarpal compartment. Note that this compartment (arrowhead) is continuous with the pisiform-triquetral compartment (solid arrows), which extends between the triquetrum and the pisiform. Note also the large proximal recess (open arrow) of the pisiform-triquetral compartment, the triangular fibrocartilage (TF) and the prestyloid recess (dot) of the radiocarpal compartment.

B "Reverse" oblique radiograph of rheumatoid wrist in semisupinated position showing erosion (arrows) on apposing surfaces of triquetrum and pisiform.

C Reverse oblique arthrogram of rheumatoid wrist in semisupinated position. The contrast material has passed from the radiocarpal compartment to the pisiform-triquetral compartment, which has a large proximal recess (open arrow). Note the corrugated irregularity (solid arrows).

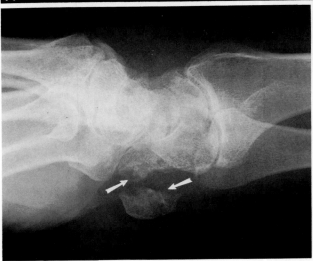

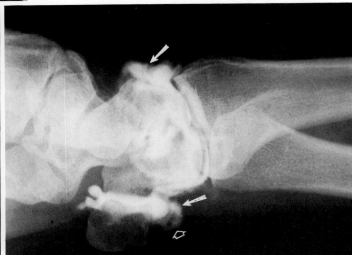

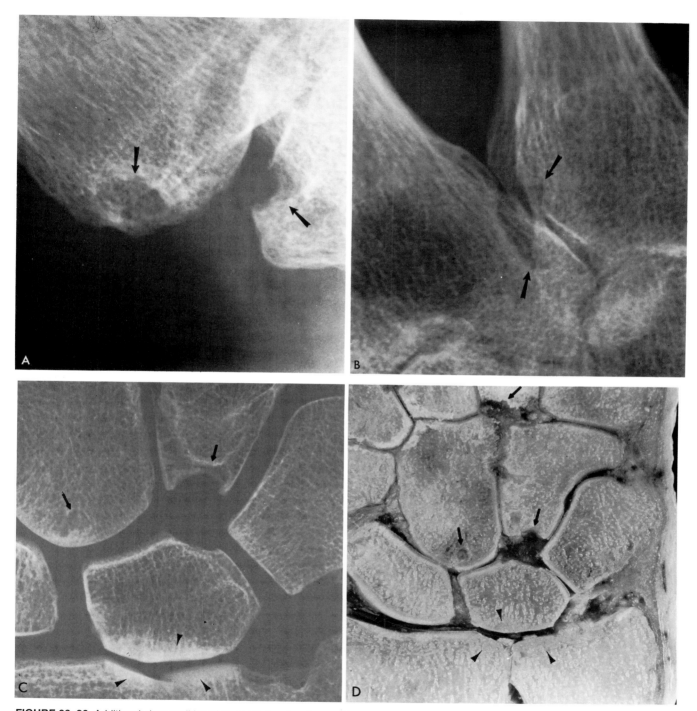

FIGURE 26–20. Additional abnormalities of the carpal and metacarpal bones.
  A Marginal erosions are frequent at the base of the first metacarpal bone and adjacent trapezium (arrows).
  B Scalloped osseous erosions (arrows) may appear about the intermetacarpal compartments.
  C, D A radiograph and corresponding photograph of a coronal section of a wrist in rheumatoid arthritis show bone erosions in multiple areas, including the proximal portion of the hamate, capitate, and metacarpal bases (arrows). Observe sclerosis of apposing portions of lunate, radius, and ulna (arrowheads). In this region, the cartilaginous surfaces have disappeared. The triangular cartilage is destroyed.

mation within the wrist soon results in significant alteration in all the compartments, characterized by progressive loss and obliteration of the articular space, further osseous erosion, and bony ankylosis (Fig. 26–21). This pancompartmental distribution is characteristic of rheumatoid arthritis and allows differentiation from selective compartmental changes that are encountered in a variety of other disease processes affecting the wrist.[123]

Although qualitative analysis of rheumatoid alterations in the wrist is not difficult, application of quantitative techniques in this analysis for the purpose of assessing the progress of the disease can be tedious. Trentham and Masi[138] have introduced the carpometacarpal ratio as a sensitive quantitative index of progression of carpal involvement in rheumatoid arthritis (Fig. 26–22). This index, which also has been used (and modified) by other investigators,[139, 637, 681, 796] is calculated by dividing the length of the carpus (the distance from the dense volar-ulnar margin of the distal radius to the base of the third metacarpal bone at its cortical midpoint) by that of the third metacarpal (the

greatest length of the metacarpal bone). It is a measure of cartilaginous loss and bony compression at the radiolunate, lunate-capitate, and capitate–third metacarpal spaces, frequent sites of joint space narrowing in rheumatoid arthritis.[137] Although useful, this technique encounters certain difficulties such as obscuration of the reference points by the rheumatoid process and distortion of the measurement by the various wrist deformities that characterize this disease. Similar difficulties appear when other quantitative measurements (such as the carpal-ulnar distance) are used to evaluate progression of rheumatoid disease of the wrist.[139]

Intra-articular osseous fusion can lead to carpal masses of variable size. Most frequently, such ankylosis affects the midcarpal compartment and, to a lesser extent, the common carpometacarpal compartment of the wrist.[675] Radiocarpal compartmental bony ankylosis is less common; at this site, as elsewhere in the skeleton, fibrous ankylosis is more typical.

Wrist Malalignment and Deformity. Incongruity in

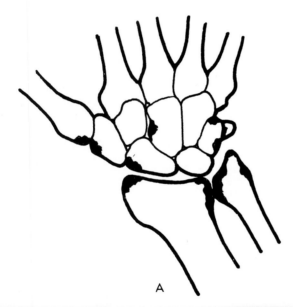

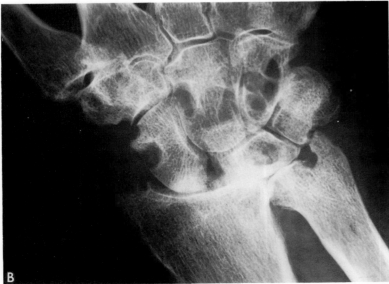

FIGURE 26–21. Pancompartmental abnormalities of the rheumatoid wrist.

A Some of the typical sites of osseous erosion in rheumatoid arthritis are indicated. Note that all of the compartments in the wrist soon are involved.

B A radiograph demonstrates typical pancompartmental osseous erosions of rheumatoid arthritis.

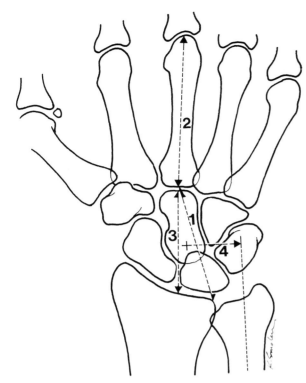

FIGURE 26–22. Indices used to measure quantitatively the progression of carpal involvement in rheumatoid arthritis. The carpometacarpal ratio (see Trentham DE, Masi AT: Arthritis Rheum 19:939, 1976) is calculated by dividing carpal length (1) by length of the third metacarpal bone (2) (mean normal in men, 0.61; mean normal in women, 0.58). A similar ratio (McMurtry RY, et al: J Bone Joint Surg [Am] 60:955, 1978) can be determined by a modification of this technique, dividing carpal length (3) by that of the third metacarpal bone (mean normal, 0.54 ± 0.03). With either of these measurements, a decreased value in rheumatoid arthritis indicates carpal collapse. A carpal ulnar distance is a measurement of the perpendicular distance (4) from the center of rotation for radial and ulnar deviation to the distal projection of the longitudinal axis of the ulna.[139] This distance, when divided by the length of the third metacarpal bone, results in a value of 0.30 ± 0.03 in normal wrists. With an ulnar shift of the carpus in rheumatoid arthritis, the ratio decreases.

cartilaginous and osseous surfaces, laxity of the articular capsule and the ligaments, and muscular and tendinous imbalance can cause malalignment of a wrist in rheumatoid arthritis.[123] Radiographic interpretation of these malalignments requires knowledge of normal wrist alignment (see Chapter 22).

Radiocarpal Malalignment (Fig. 26–23). Destruction of the triangular fibrocartilage and dorsal subluxation of the distal end of the ulna disrupt the normal concavity of the radiocarpal compartment. The proximal row of carpal bones migrates in a medial (ulnar) and a palmar direction along the inclined articular surface of the distal radius.[140] When the scaphoid and the lunate migrate medially, both bones flex toward the palm. In a posteroanterior radiograph, the scaphoid bone looks foreshortened.[141] The radial deviation at the radiocarpal compartment that results from medial migration of the scaphoid and the lunate may be apparent in as many as 70 per cent of wrists in rheumatoid arthritis patients.[141] The obtuse angle created by this type of deformity may measure as much as 145 degrees.[99]

Imbalance of the muscles and the tendons contributes to radial deviation at the wrist, and imbalance of the tendons also may be associated with ulnar deviation at the metacarpophalangeal joints, producing the zigzag deformity of the hand.[99]

Intercarpal Malalignment (Fig. 26–24). Although both palmar flexion instability (palmar or volar intercalated segment instability, or VISI) and dorsiflexion instability (dorsal intercalated segment instability, or DISI) occur in the wrist in rheumatoid arthritis, the authors' experience shows the latter to be more frequent. Palmar flexion instability is manifested by medial migration of the proximal row of carpal bones with resulting palmar flexion of the lunate and the scaphoid bones. Dorsiflexion instability is sometimes related to abnormality of the distal attachment of the palmar radiocarpal ligaments and disruption of the scapholunate ligament.[142] The scapholunate angle increases, and scapholunate dissociation becomes apparent. We have noted such dissociation in approximately 25 per cent of patients with long-standing rheumatoid involvement of the wrist. Other authors have reported a slightly lower frequency.[143] Arkless[144] investigated 110 wrists of 55 patients with rheumatoid arthritis and noted 58 wrists in which the lunate failed to return to its supraradial position in ulnar deviation. In 50 per cent of the wrists in which abnormal lunate dynamics were demonstrated, excessive separation was seen between the scaphoid and the lunate bones. Rough movement of a wrist may produce sclerosis[144] and osseous debris[132] in this portion of the radiocarpal compartment. Other investigators[143] have noted additional sites of intercarpal dissociation.

Inferior Radioulnar and Distal Ulnar Malalignment (Fig. 26–25). Rheumatoid arthritis deformities on the ulnar aspect of the wrist include distal and dorsal subluxation of the ulna and diastasis of the inferior radioulnar compartment. Martel and coworkers[62] reported the latter finding in 41 of 100 consecutive rheumatoid arthritis patients; other investigators[143] have reported this finding less frequently. The association of radiographically apparent diastasis of the distal radius and the distal ulna with dorsal subluxation of the ulna is not constant because posterior displacement of the ulnar head does not always produce detectable widening at the inferior radioulnar compartment on posteroanterior radiographs.[143]

Synovial proliferation in the wrist in rheumatoid arthritis destroys the triangular fibrocartilage, the ulnar collateral ligament, and the articular capsule—the supporting structures of the distal portion of the ulna.[145] In addition, the extensor carpi ulnaris tendon undergoes both palmar and medial subluxation, which impairs its function as a dorsal stabilizer of the distal part of the ulna.[116] Palmar flexion and palmar displacement of the radius and the hand with respect to the ulna also are seen. Palmar displacement of the ulna is rare.[653]

The caput ulnae syndrome,[116] which consists of pain, limited motion, and dorsal prominence of the distal end of the ulna, may be noted in the rheumatoid arthritis patient. The abnormally located, eroded head of the ulna projects into the compartments of the extensor tendons on the dorsum of the wrist and produces fraying of the surfaces of the tendons. Mechanical attrition in association with tenosynovitis may lead to weakening of these tendons. Subsequent

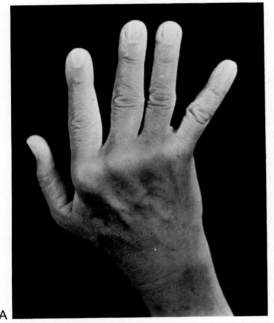

FIGURE 26–23. Wrist malalignment and deformity: Radiocarpal malalignment.

A Hand and wrist of patient with rheumatoid arthritis showing zigzag deformity caused by radial deviation at radiocarpal compartment and ulnar deviation at metacarpophalangeal joints.

B Posteroanterior radiograph of rheumatoid wrist showing medial displacement of proximal row of carpal bones (arrow) in relation to distal end of the radius and distal end of the ulna. The obtuse angle created by the intersection of lines A and B is evidence of considerable radial deviation at the radiocarpal compartment.

C Radiograph showing typical zigzag deformity caused by radial deviation at wrist (angle created by intersection of lines A and B) and ulnar deviation at metacarpophalangeal joints (angle created by intersection of lines C and D).

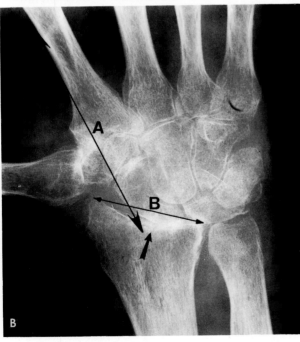

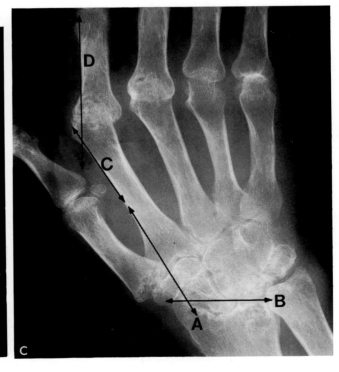

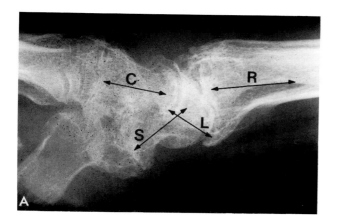

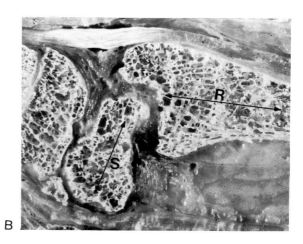

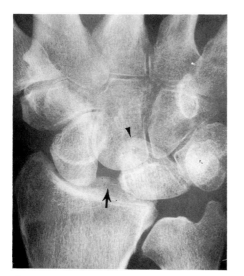

FIGURE 26–24. Wrist malalignment and deformity: Intercarpal malalignment.

A Lateral radiograph showing dorsiflexion instability of rheumatoid wrist. The longitudinal axis of the lunate (L) is dorsiflexed in relation to that of the radius (R). Note that the angle between the longitudinal axis of the lunate and that of the scaphoid (S) is larger than normal (30 to 60 degrees). Note also the longitudinal axis of the capitate (C).

B Macerated sagittal section of wrist of cadaver with rheumatoid arthritis showing dorsiflexion instability. Note the vertical position of the scaphoid (S) in relation to the longitudinal axis of the radius (R).

C Posteroanterior radiograph of rheumatoid wrist showing scapholunate dissociation. The interosseous space (arrow) between the scaphoid and the lunate is wider than normal. The scaphoid appears to be foreshortened. Because the lunate is dorsiflexed, it is superimposed on the capitate (arrowhead).

D Macerated coronal section of wrist of cadaver with rheumatoid arthritis. Disruption of the interosseous ligament between the scaphoid and the lunate has allowed separation of the two bones (arrow). Note the osseous erosions of the distal end of the radius (arrowheads). The capitate bone and the radiocarpal (RC) and midcarpal compartments also are well shown.

E A radiograph of the same section as in **D** reveals the scapholunate dissociation (arrow) and the severity of the other rheumatoid changes.

Illustration continued on following page

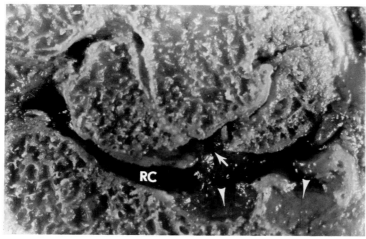

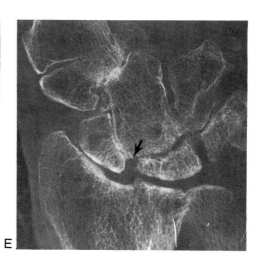

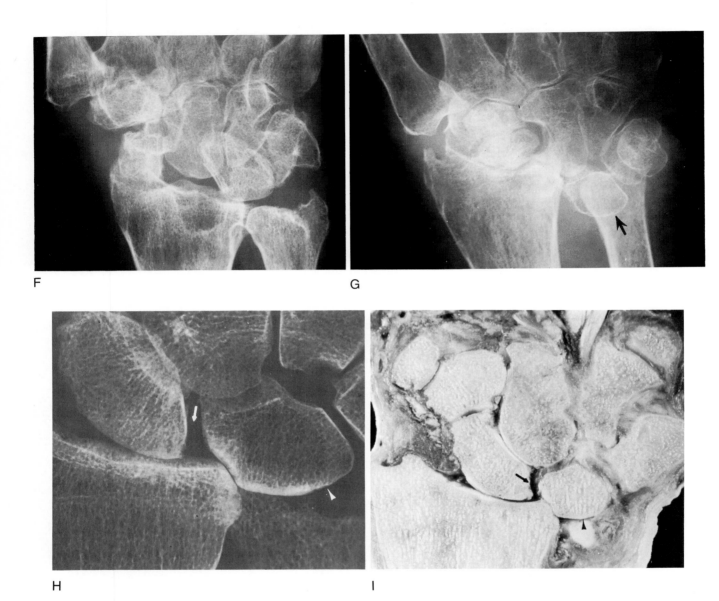

F

G

H

I

FIGURE 26–24. *Continued*

  F, G Radiographs from two additional patients with rheumatoid arthritis, in which the extent of carpal deformity is striking. In one **(F)**, a large gap appears between an eroded scaphoid and lunate, and the capitate is moving proximally. In the other **(G)**, the lunate (arrow) is located between the radius and ulna.

  H, I A radiograph and photograph of a coronal section of a cadaveric rheumatoid wrist reveal disruption of the interosseous ligament between scaphoid and lunate, with separation of the two bones (arrows), and proximal and ulnar migration of the lunate (arrowheads), with sclerosis and mechanical erosion of the lunate and radius. Additional osseous erosions also are apparent.

Illustration continued on opposite page

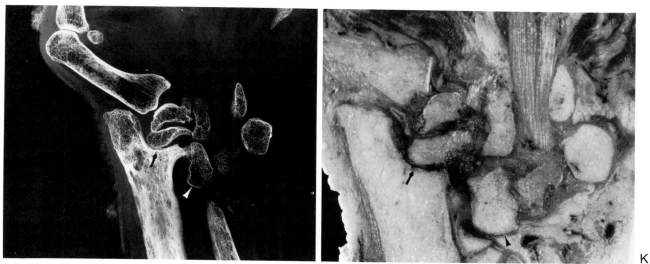

FIGURE 26–24. *Continued*

J, K In a different cadaver with rheumatoid arthritis, a radiograph and photograph of a coronal section of the wrist reveal more severe deformity. Findings include proximal migration of the lunate (arrowheads) and mechanical erosion of bone at the radioscaphoid space (arrows).

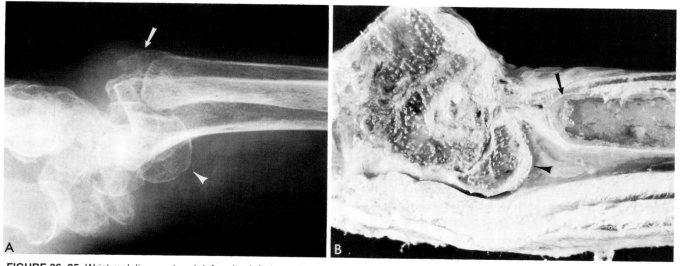

FIGURE 26–25. Wrist malalignment and deformity: Inferior radioulnar and distal ulnar malalignment.

A A lateral radiograph reveals severe dorsal subluxation of the distal part of the ulna (arrow) in addition to significant and widespread osseous and articular changes. Note the abnormal position of the lunate (arrowhead) overlying the distal end of the radius.

B A photograph of a sagittal section of a deformed rheumatoid cadaveric wrist demonstrates mild dorsal subluxation of the distal end of the ulna (arrow) and dorsal tilting of the lunate (arrowhead).

rupture of the extensor tendons commencing on the ulnar aspect of the wrist can occur, necessitating surgical intervention.

Elbow

Clinical Abnormalities

The elbow frequently is involved in rheumatoid arthritis. In a study of over 50 patients with a 5 to 25 year history of the disease, Freyberg[146] noted clinical or radiologic evidence of elbow disease in 34 per cent of persons. Lower (10 to 20 per cent) and higher (60 to 70 per cent) frequencies of elbow abnormalities in patients with rheumatoid arthritis also have been recorded.[147-149] Involvement of this joint, which commonly is bilateral but may be more marked in the dominant extremity, usually is associated with polyarthritis, although rarely a monoarticular onset of rheumatoid disease in the elbow can be encountered.[150] Clinical symptoms and signs are variable but can lead to considerable disability due to limitation of both flexion and extension of the joint.[148] Additional clinical manifestations include local pain and tenderness, swelling over the lateral aspect of the joint between the radial head and the olecranon,[151] antecubital soft tissue masses related to synovial cysts with compression of adjacent nerves,[152, 153, 604, 682] and paraolecranon nodules, synovial cysts, or bursitis (Fig. 26–26). Control of clinical problems may require synovectomy with or without radial head resection[147, 148, 154–157] or excisional arthroplasty.[158, 159] After the former procedure, transfer of forces to the medial aspect of the joint can lead to progressive collapse of the lateral edge of the coronoid process of the ulna.[486]

Although a variety of subcutaneous bursae are affected in rheumatoid arthritis, it is involvement of the olecranon bursa that has received the greatest attention. Olecranon bursitis is seen not only in rheumatoid arthritis but also in gout and in association with trauma or infection. With rheumatoid (or gouty) involvement, palpable nodules within the bursa are noted. Aspiration of the bursal fluid in rheumatoid arthritis allows analysis of cell counts; the mean value of the white blood cell count of this fluid in one series of patients[487] was approximately 3000 cells/cu mm, differing from the lower values expected in traumatic bursitis and the higher values seen in septic bursitis. Chyliform synovial effusions in the olecranon bursa are seen in rheumatoid arthritis, and histologic evaluation may reveal cholesterol-rich rheumatoid nodules in the bursal wall.[488] Such nodules can be demonstrated during bursography[487] as soft tissue radiodense shadows within the air-filled bursa. Furthermore, bursography can directly document bursal rupture, a rare complication associated with swelling of the forearm.[489] MR imaging also can be applied to the analysis of olecranon bursitis in patients with rheumatoid arthritis.

Radiographic-Pathologic Correlation

Synovial inflammation in the elbow with progressive destruction of cartilage and bone produces the familiar radiographic findings of rheumatoid arthritis, including soft tissue swelling with a positive "fat pad" sign,[160, 161] regional or periarticular osteoporosis, joint space narrowing, and bony erosions (Fig. 26–27). Although joint space diminu-

tion commonly affects the entire joint, the humeroradial aspect may be involved more prominently than the humeroulnar aspect. Erosion and deformity of the radial head, the coronoid process of the ulna,[462] and the distal portion of the humerus are most typical. More severe changes are characterized by extensive osteolysis of large portions of the humerus, radius, and ulna, prominent cystic lesions of the olecranon process that can fracture spontaneously or after minor trauma,[162] osteophytosis,[149] and, rarely, bony ankylosis[149, 163] (Fig. 26–28).

Glenohumeral Joint

Clinical Abnormalities

Clinical symptoms of disability related to glenohumeral joint involvement in rheumatoid arthritis are not infrequent.[164-170] Pain, tenderness, and restricted motion can be evident. Associated subacromial bursitis can result in prominent soft tissue swelling.[171, 172, 683] Synovial rupture of the joint can lead to an acute exacerbation of clinical manifestations.[173, 490, 605]

Radiographic-Pathologic Correlation

Progressive destruction of the chondral surface of the glenoid cavity and humeral head leads to diffuse loss of joint space. The diminution of articular space can be accompanied by marginal erosions, especially in the lateral portion of the humeral head,[786] and by subchondral cystic lesions and sclerosis of apposing surfaces of the glenoid and humerus (Fig. 26–29). In this joint, osteophytes can be a prominent radiographic finding.[131, 167, 174, 606, 654]

Although osseous erosions occur on the glenoid cavity or rim and the humerus, they are more prominent at the latter site. Particularly characteristic are superficial irregularities, deep erosive changes, and cystic changes on the superolateral aspect of the humeral head adjacent to the greater tuberosity (Fig. 26–29). These osseous abnormalities resemble the Hill-Sachs compression fracture occurring after anterior glenohumeral joint dislocation (although the Hill-Sachs lesion is localized to the posterolateral aspect of the humeral head) and the marginal erosions of other synovial processes, such as ankylosing spondylitis. Continued destruction leads to extension of the bony erosions so that the entire anatomic neck and greater tuberosity as well as the glenoid cavity become altered. Deformity with flattening of the articular surfaces can appear. Furthermore, a deep bone erosion may develop on the medial aspect of the surgical neck of the humerus, related to abnormal pressure exerted by the adjacent glenoid margin; it usually is accompanied by elevation of the humerus with respect to the glenoid cavity, due to rotator cuff atrophy or tear (see subsequent discussion) and eventually may lead to a pathologic fracture of the humeral neck.[607, 608]

Rotator cuff atrophy or tear is common in long-standing rheumatoid arthritis owing to the damaging effect of the inflamed synovial tissue on the undersurface of the tendons adjacent to the greater tuberosity (Fig. 26–30). This complication can be visualized radiographically as progressive elevation of the humeral head with respect to the glenoid cavity, narrowing of the space between the top of the humerus and the inferior surface of the acromion, sclerosis

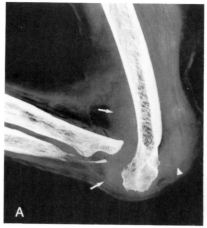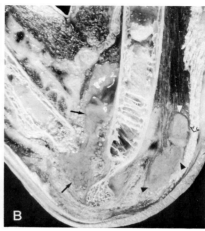

FIGURE 26–26. Abnormalities of the elbow: Paraolecranon nodules, cysts, and bursitis. A sagittal sectional radiograph **(A)** and photograph **(B)** of the elbow in a rheumatoid cadaver show extensive destruction of the humerus and radius. Note synovial inflammatory tissue in the joint (solid arrows) with posterior extension (arrowheads), leading to distortion of the triceps tendon (open arrow). A posterior soft tissue mass is evident.

and cyst formation on adjacent portions of humeral head and acromion, reversal (or concavity) of the normal convex shape of the inferior acromion, and accentuation of cystic and sclerotic changes on the superolateral aspect of the head of the humerus owing to abutment of this surface against the acromion on abduction of the shoulder; it is visualized arthrographically as abnormal communication between the glenohumeral joint and subacromial (subdeltoid) bursa in association with intra-articular findings, including nodular filling defects, irregular capsular attachments, and lymphatic filling.[175] Although these radiographic abnormalities are difficult to distinguish from those associated with rotator cuff tears in patients without rheumatoid arthritis, the combination of superior subluxation of the humeral head in relation to the glenoid cavity and diffuse joint space narrowing of the glenohumeral articulation is suggestive of rotator cuff tear in association with rheumatoid arthritis or another synovial disorder.

In some instances, rheumatoid arthritis can lead to the appearance of one or more synovial cysts in the neighboring soft tissues (Fig. 26–30). Their demonstration is provided by glenohumeral joint arthrography, during which the synovial cysts may be filled and their irregular synovial lining may be outlined, or by MR imaging, in which the precise location and size of the cyst can be defined.

Acromioclavicular Joint

Pain, tenderness to direct palpation, and local soft tissue swelling can indicate rheumatoid involvement of the acromioclavicular joint.[684] Clinical and radiographic abnormalities in this location may be more common than those of the glenohumeral joint,[176] although alterations at both these sites combined with abnormalities of the coracoclavicular ligament attachment and osteolysis of the superior ribs can be evident in a single patient.[131, 177–181]

Bilateral or unilateral abnormalities are observed on radiographs (Fig. 26–31). Soft tissue swelling superior to the joint and subchondral osteoporosis and erosions, predominating on the clavicle, are early findings. Subsequently, larger erosive changes on the clavicle and, to a lesser extent, the acromion are detected that may progress to extensive osteolysis of the outer one third of the clavicle, disruption of adjacent ligamentous and capsular structures,

and subluxation. The joint then appears widened. The eroded clavicular end can be irregular in outline or smoothly tapered. Reconstitution of bone can lead to eventual narrowing of the interosseous space.

In most patients, these radiographic changes relate pathologically to the presence of inflamed synovial tissue within the acromioclavicular joint. An additional site of acromion and clavicular erosion, adjacent to the joint, also may be evident. At this latter site, periostitis and bony irregularity result from abnormal synovial tissue in the subacromial (subdeltoid) bursa.[182] In fact, continuity of pannus among the glenohumeral joint, subacromial bursa, and acromioclavicular joint can be documented on arthrographic and pathologic examinations in some patients with rheumatoid arthritis.[183]

Coracoclavicular Joint

An elongated, shallow erosion can be seen along the undersurface of the distal end of the clavicle in rheumatoid arthritis[184, 185] (Figs. 26–32 and 26–33). It usually commences 2 to 4 cm from the distal end of the bone and may be associated with irregularity in the osseous outline of the adjacent coracoid process. This erosion eventually can deepen and extend further, giving the bone a tapered appearance. Usually, but not invariably, additional abnormalities in the glenohumeral and acromioclavicular joints are evident.

The pathogenesis of this erosive change is not clear. It may be related to rheumatoid involvement of the coracoclavicular ligament; the occurrence of the clavicular erosion within the distribution of inflamed ligamentous fibers lends support to this concept. A second potential mechanism of inferior clavicular erosion is the presence of synovial inflammation in the neighboring bursae or articulations that occasionally are evident in this area. Finally, as the distance between the coracoid process and clavicle appears to be diminished in many patients with this finding, it is possible that in long-standing rheumatoid arthritis with significant disturbance at the acromioclavicular and glenohumeral joints, abnormal motion in the shoulder may produce mechanical factors that contribute to erosive changes in the inferior aspect of the clavicle. In this respect, the findings may be similar to those observed in the ribs in rheumatoid arthritis.[179, 186]

Text continued on page 905

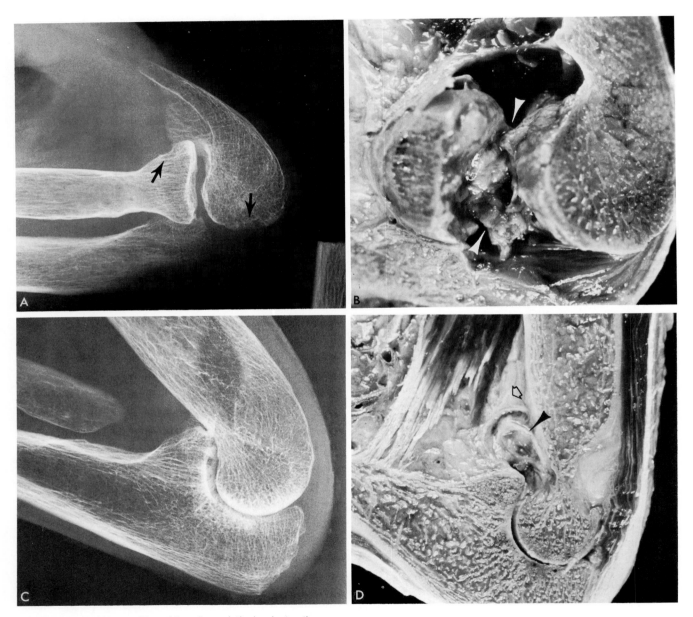

FIGURE 26–27. Abnormalities of the elbow: Articular destruction.

A, B Humeroradial space. On a radiograph and photograph of a sagittal section of a rheumatoid elbow joint, observe erosions of the distal end of the humerus and proximal part of the radius (arrows) with considerable inflammatory pannus within the joint (arrowheads).

C, D Humeroulnar space. This radiograph and photograph of a sagittal section of a rheumatoid elbow joint indicate considerable narrowing and bony eburnation of the humeroulnar space. Note the synovial proliferation (arrowhead) with displacement of the anterior fat pad (open arrow).

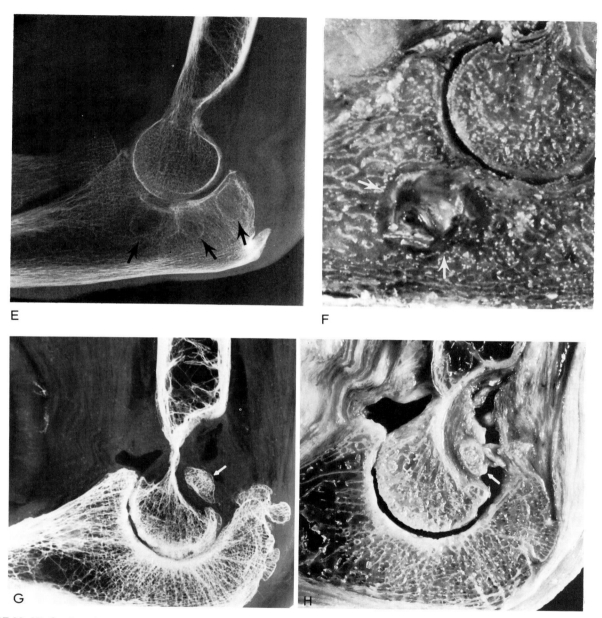

FIGURE 26–27. *Continued*

E, F Humeroulnar space. In a similar sagittal sectional radiograph and photograph, observe cysts (arrows) within the proximal portion of the ulna corresponding to sites of synovial inflammatory tissue.

G, H Humeroulnar space. In a sagittal sectional radiograph and photograph, note narrowing of the articular space due to destruction of cartilage and the presence of an osteochondral fragment (arrows) within the olecranon fossa. Osteophytes also are apparent, arising from the olecranon process.

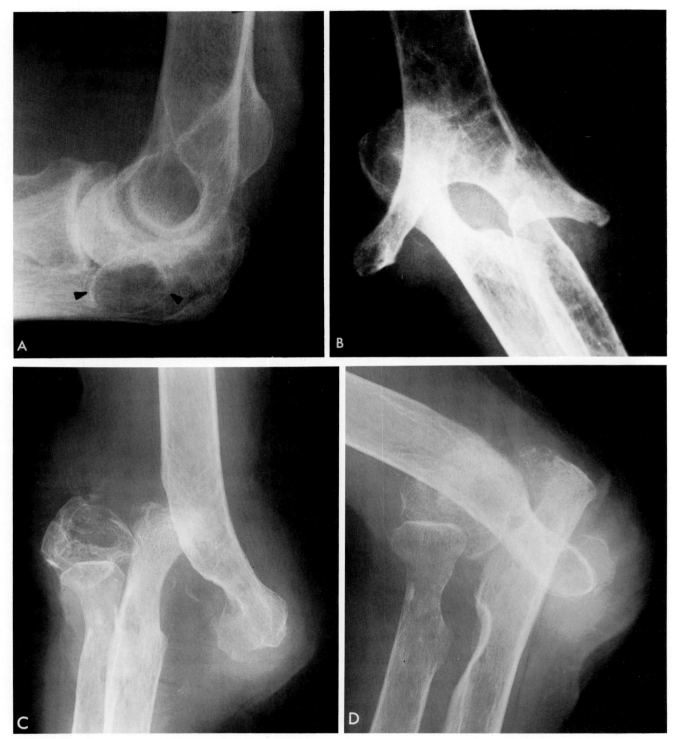

FIGURE 26–28. Abnormalities of the elbow: Articular destruction.

A Prominent cysts (arrowheads) in the ulnar olecranon occasionally may fracture spontaneously.

B The severity of the rheumatoid process is illustrated in this elbow radiograph. The appearance simulates that of neuropathic osteoarthropathy.

C, D A frontal and lateral radiograph of the elbow in a different patient with rheumatoid arthritis demonstrate a fracture of the distal portion of the humerus, which occurred after minor trauma. The fragment and the radius and ulna are displaced, predominantly in a proximal, radial, and posterior direction.

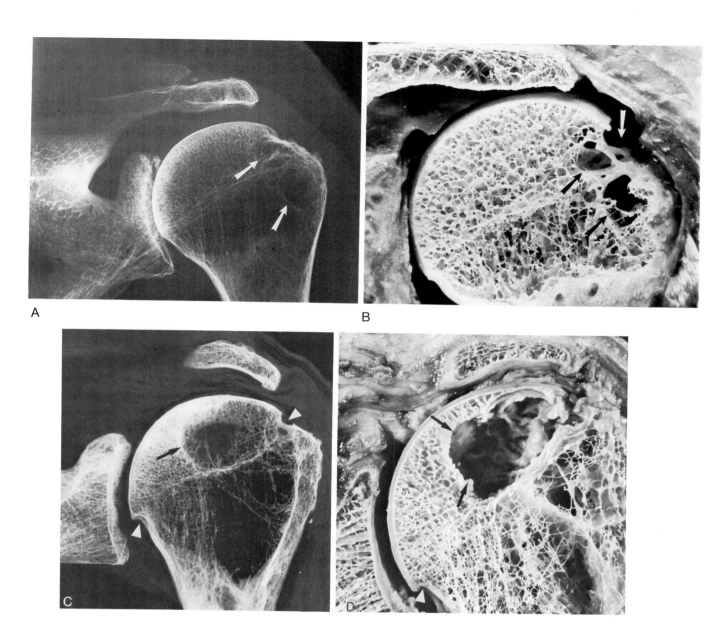

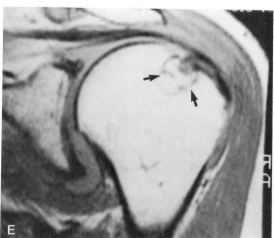

FIGURE 26–29. Abnormalities of the glenohumeral joint: Articular destruction.

A, B A radiograph and photograph of a coronal section of the articulation illustrate joint space narrowing, bony eburnation, and erosive and cystic changes predominantly on the lateral aspect of the humeral head (arrows).

C, D In a different cadaver, a radiograph and photograph reveal marginal erosions (arrowheads) and a large intraosseous cystic lesion (arrows), which communicates with the surface of the bone.

E A coronal proton density weighted spin echo MR image (TR/TE, 1000/20) in a 50 year old woman with rheumatoid arthritis shows intra-articular fluid of intermediate signal intensity and erosion of the superolateral portion of the humeral head (arrows).

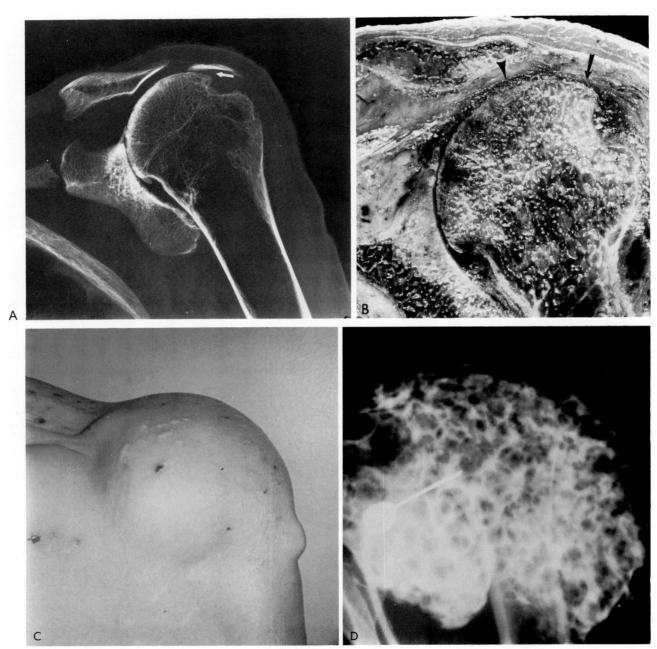

FIGURE 26–30. Abnormalities of the glenohumeral joint: Periarticular abnormalities.

   A, B Rotator cuff tear and atrophy. Radiograph and photograph of a coronal section of a rheumatoid glenohumeral joint indicate the presence of severe articular changes and rotator cuff atrophy. Note joint space narrowing and sclerosis, erosion of the superolateral aspect of the humeral head, elevation of the humeral head with respect to the glenoid, and narrowing of the acromiohumeral head distance (arrows). The rotator cuff is atrophic (arrowhead).

   C, D Bursal distention. A clinically apparent soft tissue mass in this patient with rheumatoid arthritis represents a massively distended subacromial (subdeltoid) bursa. Contrast opacification of the bursa reveals irregular filling defects.

Illustration continued on opposite page

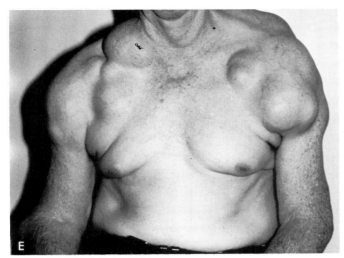

FIGURE 26–30. *Continued*
E–G Cyst formation. The clinical photograph **(E)** from this patient with rheumatoid arthritis demonstrates multiple bilateral synovial cysts about the shoulders. The soft tissue swelling also is evident on a radiograph of the left shoulder **(F)** in association with osteoporosis and bony erosion, destruction, and fragmentation of the humerus, scapula, and clavicle. Contrast opacification of the cysts **(G)** reveals their widespread distribution, irregular outline, and enclosed nodules. (**E–G**, Courtesy of G. Williams, M.D., S. Carstens, M.D., and V. Vint, M.D., La Jolla, California.)

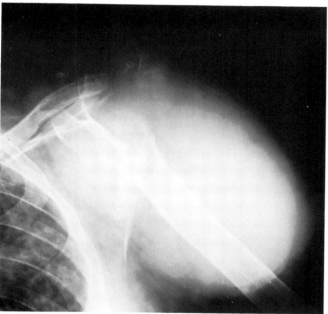

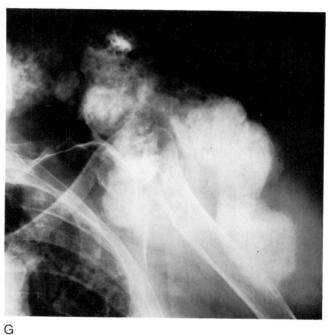

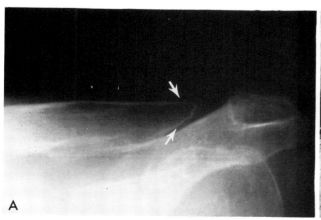

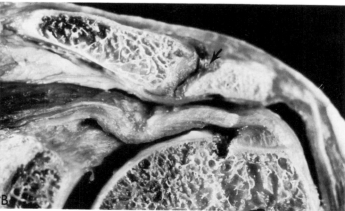

FIGURE 26–31. Abnormalities of the acromioclavicular joint.
A On this radiograph observe tapering of the distal end of the clavicle (arrows) with widening of the acromioclavicular joint.
B A photograph of a coronal section of the acromioclavicular joint of a cadaver with rheumatoid arthritis demonstrates synovial proliferation (arrow) with destruction of articular cartilage, fibrocartilaginous disc, and adjacent bone.

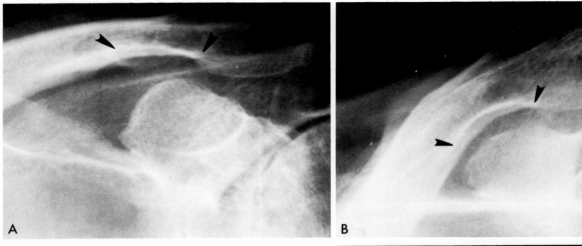

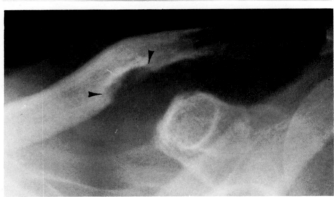

FIGURE 26–32. Abnormalities of the coracoclavicular joint. Three examples of scalloped erosions (arrowheads) of the undersurface of the distal end of the clavicle in rheumatoid arthritis. A somewhat similar appearance may be seen in ankylosing spondylitis and hyperparathyroidism. (From Resnick D, Niwayama G: Radiology *120*:75, 1976.)

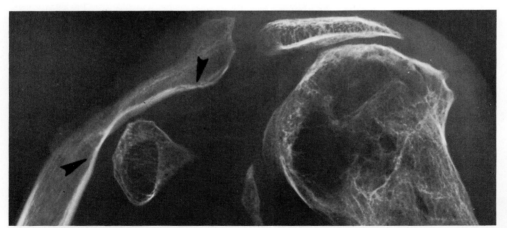

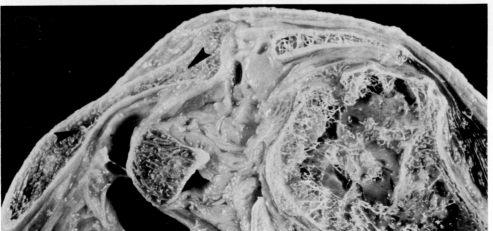

FIGURE 26–33. Abnormalities of the coracoclavicular joint. Radiograph and photograph of a macerated coronal section of a rheumatoid shoulder joint show an elongated clavicular erosion (arrowheads), undulating clavicular outline, and adjacent coracoid process. The rotator cuff is torn, with the irregular humeral head assuming a high position close to the acromion. (From Resnick D, Niwayama G: Radiology *120*:75, 1976.)

Sternoclavicular and Manubriosternal Joints

Although clinical evidence of abnormalities in one or both sternoclavicular joints is not uncommonly elicited by careful history and physical examination, particularly in long-standing disease, radiologic evidence of sternoclavicular changes is more difficult to detect because of the inadequacies of routine sternoclavicular joint radiography.[454] Tomograms may be required to demonstrate significant articular disease in this location. Using conventional tomographic technique, subchondral and marginal erosions have been detected in approximately 30 per cent of patients suffering from rheumatoid arthritis.[187] Rarely, extensive osteolysis of the medial end of the clavicle with or without associated osteolysis of the distal end of the clavicle can be seen (Fig. 26–34).

Using conventional tomography to study the manubriosternal joint, investigators have noted abnormalities in 30 to 70 per cent of patients with rheumatoid arthritis.[188–191, 491, 685] The changes, which can include osteoporosis, slight irregularity of the osseous surfaces, eburnation, decreased height of the intervening fibrocartilage, and bony ankylosis (Fig. 26–35), are less frequent and less severe than in ankylosing spondylitis[188, 190, 192, 492] and must be distinguished from minor bony changes and osseous fusion, which can be encountered in degenerative joint disease and "normal" persons.[193, 491] The manubriosternal joint changes in rheumatoid arthritis usually occur after abnormalities become evident in other articulations, although, uncommonly, they may appear early in the course of the disease.[189] The pathogenesis of manubriosternal joint abnormalities is not certain; they may relate to extension of synovial disease from neighboring costochondral joints, traumatic or degenerative processes, primary involvement of cartilaginous joints in the rheumatoid disease process, or transformation of the joint into one with a synovial cavity, with subsequent inflammation. Histologic and microradiographic analysis has indicated active inflammation of the articulation in some

patients and the absence of inflammation and the presence of fibrous replacement in others.[194] Occasionally, inflammatory synovial tissue within a cavity of the manubriosternal joint has been detected.[194, 686]

In the many rheumatoid arthritis patients with minor or moderate articular disease of the manubriosternal joint and in the few with more severe sternal destruction[195, 638] or articular subluxation,[196, 638] a decrease in sternal mobility by fibrosis, ankylosis, or malalignment can lead to impaired respiration and pulmonary infection.[197, 198, 461] Although subluxation and dislocation of this joint in rheumatoid arthritis are regarded as rare complications of the disease by most investigators,[493] other authors suggest that such deformity is not uncommon, is easily overlooked, and is associated with severe thoracic kyphosis[638] or cervicothoracic spinal erosion.[494] This latter hypothesis—the association of sternal and spinal abnormalities—has gained support from pathologic observations confirming the coexistence of severe deformities in both anatomic sites in cadavers with rheumatoid arthritis[494] and from reports of spontaneous fractures of the sternum in older patients with osteoporosis who have exaggerated kyphosis of the thoracic spine.[495, 687]

Forefoot

Clinical Abnormalities

Clinical abnormalities of the forefoot are especially common in rheumatoid arthritis (80 to 90 per cent of patients) and may be the initial manifestation of the disease (10 to 20 per cent of patients).[9, 199–206] The metatarsophalangeal joints of the lateral digits are affected most frequently. Intermittent or constant pain, tenderness, and soft tissue swelling can be prominent findings, even in the early stage of the disease. With more long-standing arthritis, a shuffling gait and characteristic deformities appear. These deformities include forefoot spread (spreading of the metatarsal bones due to changes in the deep transverse ligaments),

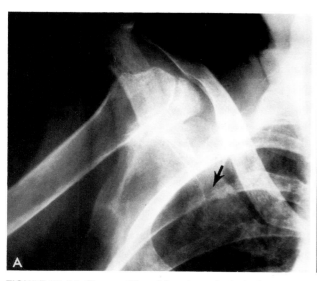
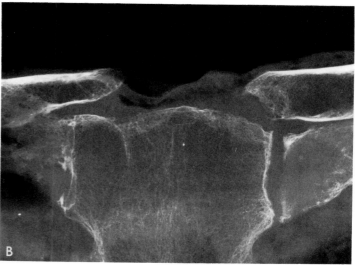

FIGURE 26–34. Abnormalities of the sternoclavicular joint.
A This radiograph reveals striking abnormalities of the glenohumeral, acromioclavicular, coracoclavicular, and sternoclavicular joints. Note the resorption of the humeral head, medial and lateral ends of the clavicle, and undersurface of the distal part of the clavicle. In addition, resorption of the superior surface of several ribs can be seen (arrow).
B A radiograph of a coronal section of the sternoclavicular joint in this cadaver outlines the extent of erosion and osteolysis that may occur in the medial end of the clavicle in rheumatoid arthritis. Subluxation also is evident.

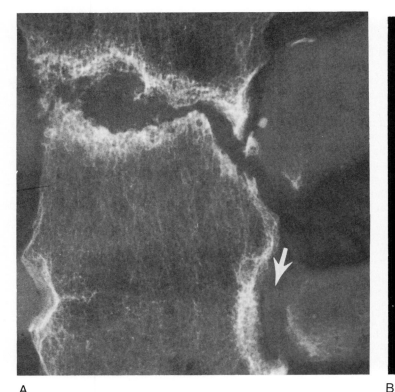

A

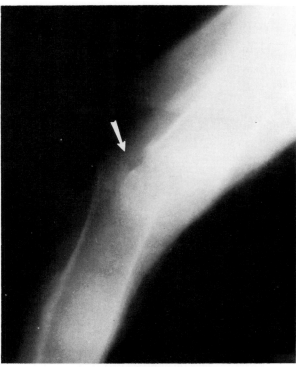

B

FIGURE 26–35. Abnormalities of the manubriosternal joint.
A Radiographic abnormalities of the manubriosternal joint are illustrated in this coronal section of the sternum. They include osseous erosions and sclerosis. Note irregularity of the costosternal joints (arrow).
B A lateral radiograph in this rheumatoid patient reveals spontaneous subluxation of the manubriosternal joint (arrow).

hallux valgus, fibular deviation of the first to fourth digits (lateral deviation of the toes at the metatarsophalangeal joints), hammer toe (acute flexion of the distal or proximal interphalangeal joints, or both, with the distal phalanx pointing directly downward), and "cock-up" toe (hyperextension of the toe at the metatarsophalangeal joint with subluxation of the phalanx above the metatarsal head). Painful callosities are evident beneath the metatarsal heads (especially the second and third) and distal phalanges. In these locations, bursitis and spontaneous sinus tracts can be seen.[207–210] Involvement of the bursae between the metatarsal heads can lead to swelling and Morton's metatarsalgia.[497, 500] Additional findings in rheumatoid arthritis include insufficiency (stress) fractures, peripheral neuropathy, tendon injury and rupture, widespread edema, and hallux rigidus.[9, 200, 204, 205, 211, 496–498] A variety of surgical procedures may be required to control the clinical manifestations.[212–215]

Radiographic-Pathologic Correlation

Radiologic abnormalities of the forefoot also are frequent in rheumatoid arthritis.[216, 217, 688] Furthermore, these abnormalities commonly are the initial manifestation of the disease, antedating changes in the hand and the wrist. Earliest alterations appear at the metatarsophalangeal joints, particularly the fifth. With progression, one or more metatarsophalangeal joints are affected in a relatively symmetric fashion in both feet. At these sites, changes predominate on the medial aspect of the metatarsal head with the exception of that in the fifth digit, at which site soft tissue swelling

and subjacent osseous erosion on the lateral aspect of the bone can be a very early and important finding of the disease (Fig. 26–36). Although significant cartilaginous and osseous lesions are infrequent in the interphalangeal articulations of the second to fifth digits, the interphalangeal joint of the great toe is commonly and characteristically affected.[218]

Early radiographic alterations at the metatarsophalangeal joints consist of soft tissue swelling, periarticular osteoporosis, concentric joint space narrowing, and marginal and central osseous defects, corresponding to pathologic evidence of synovial inflammation, with resultant cartilaginous and bony destruction (Fig. 26–37). Small subchondral radiolucent areas and surface irregularities are especially common on the medial aspect of the first to fourth metatarsal heads and on the medial and lateral aspects of the fifth metatarsal head. Although they are soon accompanied by osseous lesions of the adjacent portions of the proximal phalanges, the changes at the latter site are less prominent than those of the metatarsal bones. Progressive diminution and obliteration of the articular spaces are associated with enlarging bony defects and destruction. Some proliferative changes with sclerosis, osteophytosis, and periostitis of adjacent phalangeal shafts can appear, although they are overshadowed by the presence and degree of osteolysis. Intraarticular bony ankylosis is distinctly unusual at metatarsophalangeal (as well as interphalangeal) articulations.

In the great toe, the changes in the metatarsal head and the proximal phalanx about the metatarsophalangeal joint are accompanied by osteoporosis, joint space loss, and erosions of the adjacent sesamoids[219] (Fig. 26–38). To visualize the sesamoid abnormalities adequately, tangential radiographs frequently are required.[220, 221] With the development of deformities of the first digit such as hallux valgus and medial rotation of the toe, sesamoid displacement becomes apparent. The frequency of hallux valgus deformity rises with increasing duration of the disease, with the rise much more distinct in female patients.[200] Rheumatoid hallux valgus results primarily from pathologic changes in the supporting ligamentous structures and less so from intra-articular involvement and poor footwear.[222] Extensive joint space narrowing, sclerosis, and osteophytosis in some patients with rheumatoid arthritis lead to the appearance of hallux rigidus identical to that occurring in osteoarthritis or gout. Hallux varus is a relatively uncommon finding in this disease.

The interphalangeal joint of the great toe participates in the rheumatoid process, and radiographic changes at this site can be detected in as many as 50 per cent of foot radiographs[218] (Fig. 26–39). Especially characteristic is an elongated surface irregularity that appears on the medial margin of the proximal phalanx adjacent to the interphalangeal joint, and that may be associated with smaller erosions on the medial aspect of the adjacent distal phalanx. Abnormalities on the lateral aspect of the joint and articular space loss may not accompany this medial erosion. Although moderate-sized erosions about the central portion of the joint and articular subluxation occasionally are noted, severe destructive arthritis, as may be evident in psoriasis and

Reiter's syndrome, is unusual at this site in rheumatoid arthritis.

Mild joint space loss, superficial marginal and central osseous erosions, and subchondral sclerosis can be seen at other interphalangeal joints in the foot in rheumatoid arthritis.

The radiographic characteristics of the deformed forefoot in rheumatoid arthritis include fibular deviation of the toes (with the exception of the fifth digit) and dorsiflexion and lateral subluxation or dislocation of the proximal phalanges at the metatarsophalangeal articulations (Fig. 26–40). These and other phalangeal displacements and deformities can obscure significant articular abnormalities and complicate the evaluation of joint space loss at metatarsophalangeal and interphalangeal joints.

The radiographic evaluation of forefoot lesions in rheumatoid arthritis also is made difficult when information regarding previous surgical procedures is fragmentary or unavailable. Surgical resection of the metatarsal and phalangeal heads can simulate the findings of severe osseous destruction related to the disease itself.

Midfoot

Clinical Abnormalities

In the midfoot in rheumatoid arthritis, weakness of the muscles and stretching of the inflamed ligaments may be followed by postural deformities.[200] The most frequent midtarsal deformity in this disease is pes planovalgus,[499] which

Text continued on page 913

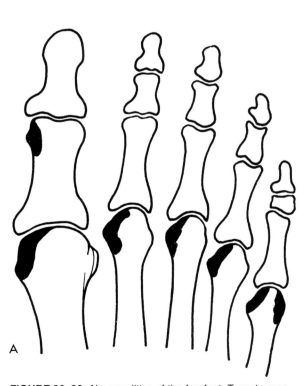
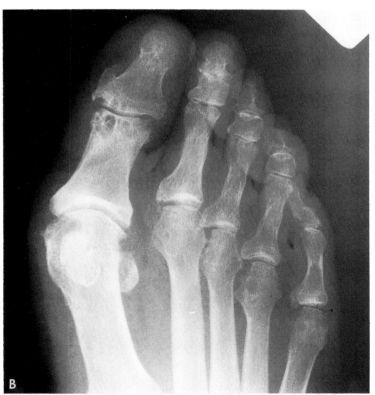

FIGURE 26–36. Abnormalities of the forefoot: Target areas.
  A The early osseous erosions of rheumatoid arthritis appear on the medial aspect of the first to fourth metatarsal bones, the medial and lateral aspects of the fifth metatarsal bone, and the medial aspect of the distal portion of the proximal phalanx of the great toe.
  B A radiograph reveals the early erosions. All the metatarsal heads are involved, particularly the medial aspects. Note the prominent changes at the interphalangeal joint of the great toe and the relative absence of findings in other interphalangeal articulations.

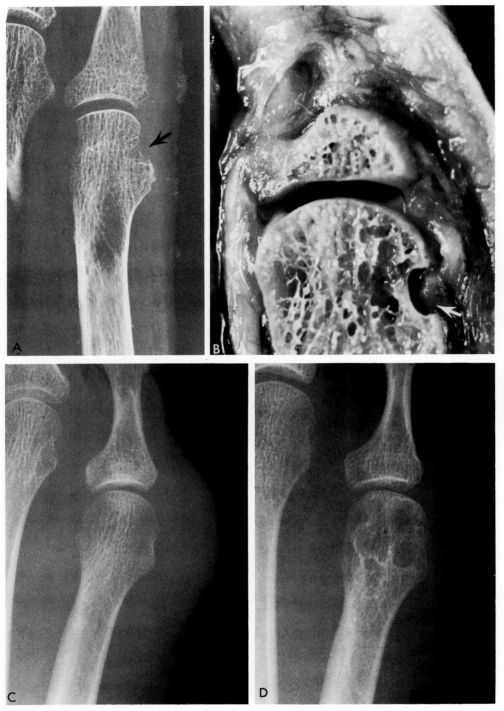

FIGURE 26–37. Abnormalities of the metatarsophalangeal joints (second through fifth toes).

A, B A radiograph and photograph of two different transverse sections through the fifth metatarsophalangeal joint reveal an early and characteristic erosion (arrows) on the outer aspect of the metatarsal head. This may be the initial radiographic manifestation of the disease.

C, D Early changes may consist of soft tissue swelling due to bursal inflammation **(C)** or cystic erosions **(D)** about the fifth metatarsophalangeal joint.

Illustration continued on opposite page

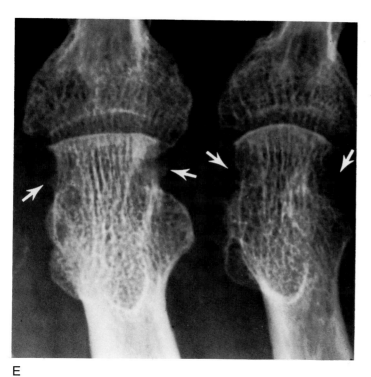

E

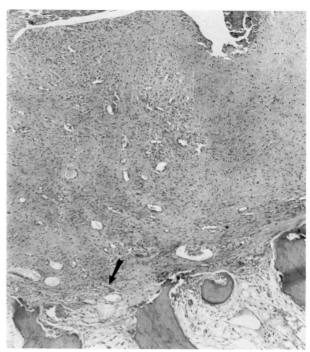

F

FIGURE 26–37. *Continued*

 E A magnification radiograph outlines the typical osseous erosions (arrows) that appear on the metatarsal heads.

 F In this photomicrograph (86×), the cartilaginous layer is totally replaced by rheumatoid pannus. Fibrin deposits are seen on the surface, and the original chondro-osseous junction is well vascularized with fibroblastic cellular proliferation (arrow).

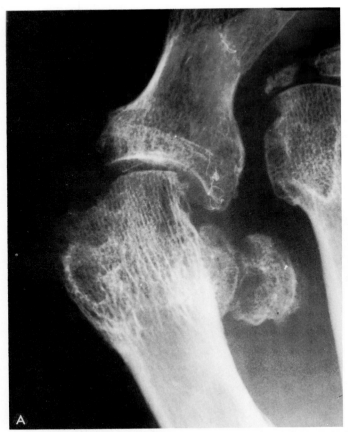

FIGURE 26–38. Abnormalities of the metatarsophalangeal joint of the great toe and adjacent sesamoids.

A Note the extensive erosions of the medial and lateral aspects of the metatarsal head and adjacent sesamoids, with hallux valgus deformity.

B, C Routine radiograph **(B)** and transverse T1-weighted spin echo MR image (TR/TE, 600/20) **(C)** from a 69 year old man with rheumatoid arthritis. In the radiograph, extensive erosions are seen about several metatarsophalangeal joints, especially the first and fifth. Fibular deviation of the toes and dislocation of the second and third metatarsophalangeal joints are apparent. In the MR image, pannus and fluid of low signal intensity within the metatarsophalangeal joints, particularly the first, are evident (open arrows). Note erosions of multiple metatarsal heads (arrowheads).

Illustration continued on opposite page

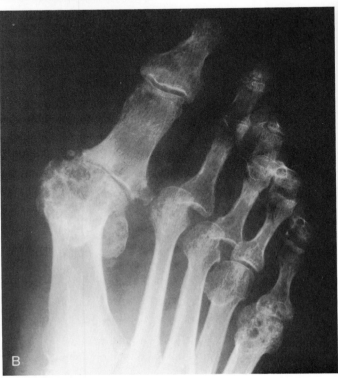

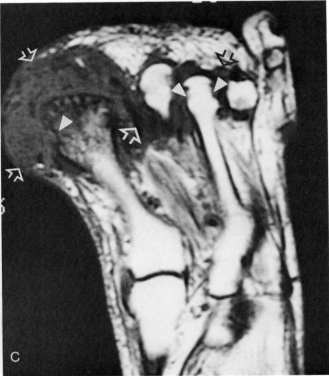

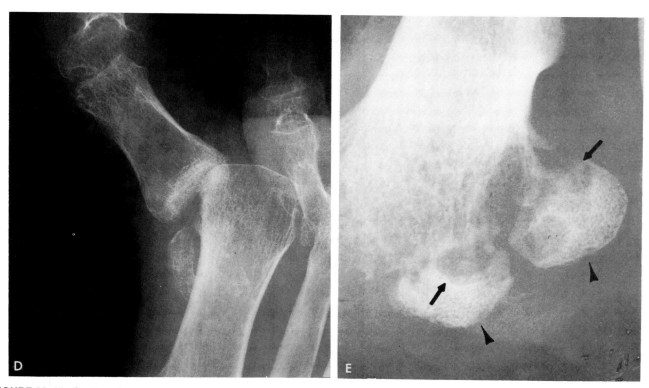

FIGURE 26–38. *Continued*

D Hallux varus deformity, an unusual manifestation of this disease, with medial sesamoid displacement is dramatically illustrated in this radiograph.

E On a radiograph of a coronal section of the first metatarsal head in a cadaver with rheumatoid arthritis, subluxation and osseous erosion of the sesamoids and adjacent first metatarsal bone are readily apparent (arrows). The sesamoid changes predominate in the subchondral regions, although surface resorption also is seen (arrowheads).

(**E**, from Resnick D, et al: Radiology *123*:57, 1977.)

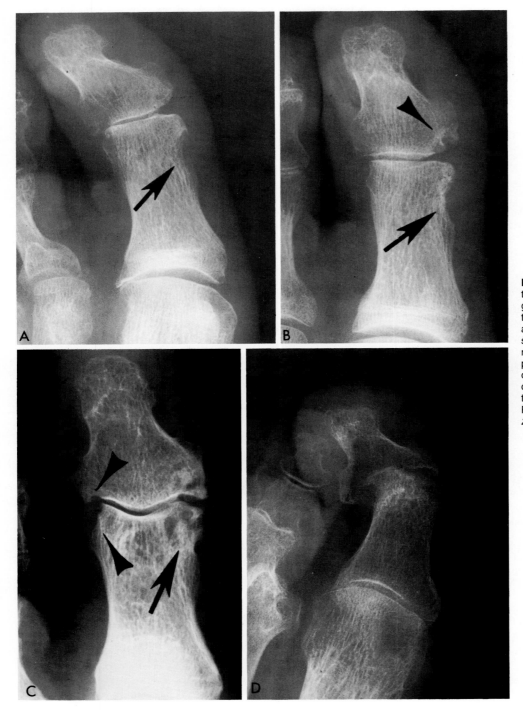

FIGURE 26–39. Abnormalities of the interphalangeal joint of the great toe. The spectrum of alterations is indicated in these four examples. Note the prominent erosion that occurs on the distal medial aspect of the proximal phalanx (arrows), additional osseous erosions (arrowheads) and, in one example **(D)**, lateral subluxation of the distal phalanx. (From Resnick D: J Can Assoc Radiol *26*:255, 1975.)

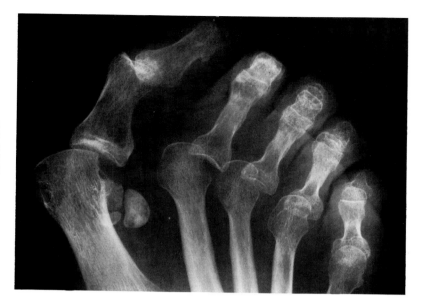

FIGURE 26–40. Forefoot deformities. Fibular deviation and subluxation of the phalanges typically occur at the first to fourth digits. The relatively mild nature of the osseous erosions in comparison with the degree of deformity that is evident in this patient is somewhat unusual.

was noted in 50 per cent of the women and 40 per cent of the men in one series of patients with rheumatoid arthritis.[223] This deformity may relate to rupture of an inflamed tibialis posterior tendon.[689] Tarsal block may contribute to midfoot deformity.[216]

Radiographic-Pathologic Correlation

Proper radiographic evaluation of the early stages of rheumatoid involvement in the midfoot, as elsewhere, occasionally requires soft tissue techniques to be able to discern synovial abnormalities,[224] and evaluation of the late stages of such involvement requires standing films to discern the presence and the extent of deformity. Even without these techniques, radiographic changes in the midfoot in rheumatoid arthritis are common. In a radiographic study of 75 feet in 39 patients with rheumatoid arthritis, alterations were encountered in the talocalcaneonavicular joint (39 per cent), the tarsometatarsal joints (36 per cent), the posterior subtalar joint (29 per cent), the cuneonavicular, intercuneiform, or cuneocuboid joint (28 per cent), and the calcaneocuboid joint (25 per cent)[225] (Figs. 26–41 to 26–43). Other authors also have indicated rheumatoid predilection for the talocalcaneonavicular joint[200]; changes are particularly frequent in the talonavicular portion of this articular cavity. The radiographs may reveal symmetric joint space loss, focal sclerosis, and osteophytosis. Erosions are infrequent and small, and osseous fusion occasionally is seen. Adjacent sesamoid bones can be affected.[504] Although a dorsal synovial effusion may displace the extrasynovial fat planes on the talar head and neck,[224] this is not a common finding on routine radiographs.[225] Posterior subtalar joint involvement, which is less characteristic than that of the talocalcaneonavicular joint, can lead to enlargement of its posterior recess[226] and development of a subtalar mass proximal to the calcaneal tuberosity.[224]

Abnormality in the calcaneocuboid joint includes articular space narrowing or osseous fusion and shallow subchondral irregularities. A synovial mass lateral to the articulation occasionally is evident.

The cuneonavicular, intercuneiform, cuneocuboid, and cuboideonavicular joints frequently are altered concomitantly (Fig. 26–44); this is not surprising in view of the

communication among these joints, which can be observed on anatomic[227] and arthrographic[225] studies. Joint space narrowing and osseous fusion can be seen in these locations.

Tarsometatarsal changes in the lateral, intermediate, and medial compartments frequently occur together, although isolated involvement of the medial cavity can be noted (Fig. 26–44). As elsewhere in the midfoot, the radiographic abnormalities include joint space narrowing, bony ankylosis, and superficial erosions.

In many patients with rheumatoid arthritis, the entire midfoot on both sides is altered. Occasionally, with complete obliteration and osseous fusion of all of the articular spaces, large tarsal bony masses are created. Osteophytes on the dorsum of the foot may accompany these extensive changes. In almost all patients with such changes, the metatarsophalangeal joints and other articulations also participate in the rheumatoid process. Rarely, in rheumatoid arthritis, subluxation[501] or dislocation[502, 503] of the midfoot is seen. Typically, one of the subtalar joints is the primary site of the deformity.

Heel

Clinical Abnormalities

Clinical lesions of the heel that are encountered in rheumatoid arthritis and the seronegative spondyloarthropathies (ankylosing spondylitis, psoriasis, and Reiter's syndrome) are retrocalcaneal bursitis, Achilles tendinitis, and plantar fasciitis.[200, 228–230] Retrocalcaneal bursitis is characterized by a fluctuating mass that falls to the sides of the Achilles tendon; Achilles tendinitis is associated with pain, local tenderness to palpation, and a thickened or swollen tendinous structure; and plantar fasciitis can lead to redness, swelling, and tenderness of the plantar surface of the calcaneus. In rheumatoid arthritis, retrocalcaneal bursitis is more frequent than Achilles tendinitis or plantar fasciitis; all three conditions may be observed in the seronegative spondyloarthropathies. Moderate to severe heel pain (talalgia) is more characteristic of these latter disorders than of rheumatoid arthritis,[230, 231, 690] although retrocalcaneal bursitis in the rheumatoid arthritis patient occasionally can be a

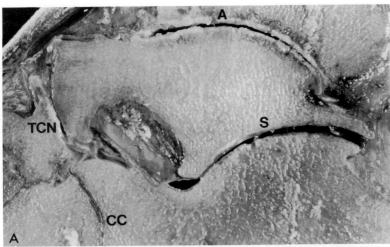

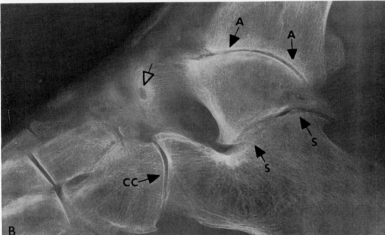

FIGURE 26–41. Abnormalities of the talocalcaneal joints. A photograph and corresponding radiograph of a sagittal section of a foot in rheumatoid arthritis reveal cartilage loss, joint space narrowing, and irregular subchondral bone in the subtalar joint (S). Associated ankle (A) alterations are evident. The superior portion of the calcaneocuboid joint (CC) is relatively spared. Note the involvement of the talonavicular portion of the talocalcaneonavicular articulation (TCN), with cartilage loss and a well-defined subchondral talar cyst (open arrow). (From Resnick D: J Can Assoc Radiol 27:99, 1976.)

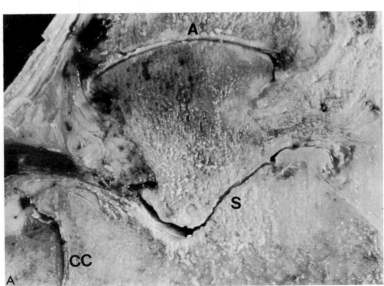

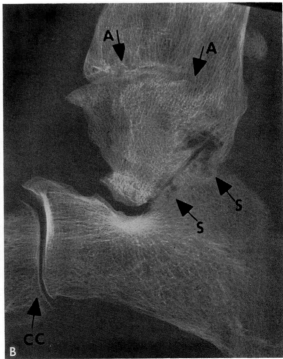

FIGURE 26–42. Abnormalities of the talocalcaneal joints. A photograph and radiograph of a lateral sagittal section through the subtalar joint (S) reveal extensive involvement, with cartilage loss, joint space narrowing, and erosions, particularly about the posterior aspect of the cavity. Reactive sclerosis is evident. Ankle (A) alterations were present but are not well shown on the radiograph. The calcaneocuboid joint (CC) is relatively spared.

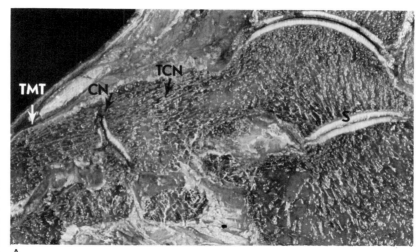

A

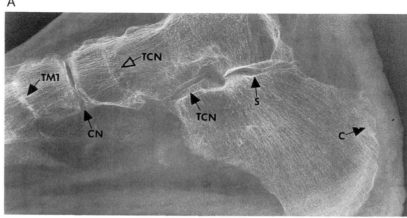

B

FIGURE 26–43. Abnormalities of the talocalcaneal joint. In a medial section of this cadaveric foot, osseous fusion of the talonavicular portion of the talocalcaneonavicular joint (TCN) has completely obliterated the articular cavity. Similarly, the intermediate tarsometatarsal joint (TMT) is almost completely fused. Minor abnormalities of the cuneonavicular joint (CN) and posterior calcaneus (C) are noted. The subtalar joint (S) is relatively spared. (From Resnick D: J Can Assoc Radiol 27:99, 1976.)

FIGURE 26–44. Abnormalities of the tarsometatarsal joints.

A Joint space loss in the lateral and intermediate tarsometatarsal cavities (TMT) is associated with diffuse alterations of the talonavicular portion of the talocalcaneonavicular (TCN) joint and cuneonavicular (CN) and calcaneocuboid (CC) joints.

B Bony fusion between the bases of the first and second metatarsal bones and the medial and intermediate cuneiforms at the tarsometatarsal joints (TMT) is noted. Similar bridging of the calcaneocuboid cavity (CC) is apparent. Changes of the cuneonavicular joint (CN) consist of articular space obliteration and reactive sclerosis.

(From Resnick D: J Can Assoc Radiol 27:99, 1976.)

presenting or major feature of the disease. Bywaters[228] noted heel pain in 2.5 per cent of 250 rheumatoid arthritis patients, whereas Vainio[223] elicited this complaint in 9 per cent of 955 adults with rheumatoid arthritis.

Radiographic-Pathologic Correlation

Synovitis, accumulation of bursal fluid, and surrounding soft tissue edema in association with retrocalcaneal bursitis can produce a soft tissue mass on the posterosuperior aspect of the calcaneus, which obliterates the normal radiolucent region that extends between the top of the bone and the Achilles tendon, and which projects into the inferior portion of the preachilles fat pad[228, 229, 231, 232] (Fig. 26–45). Subjacent erosion of the calcaneus on both its posterior and superior aspects is characteristic. The resulting erosion may be well or poorly defined, the latter appearance related to a minimal amount of new bone formation.

Achilles tendinitis leads to enlargement and blurring of

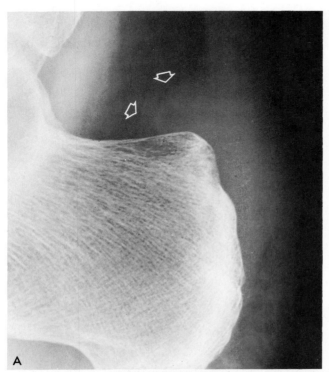

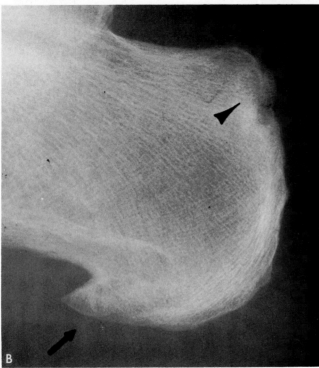

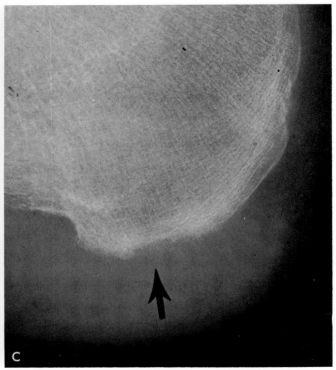

FIGURE 26–45. Abnormalities of the calcaneus: Posterosuperior and inferior aspects.

A A low kV soft tissue radiograph defines a thickened Achilles tendon and a fluid-filled retrocalcaneal bursa (open arrows), which projects into the preachilles fat pad. Focal osteoporosis of the neighboring calcaneus is evident. (Courtesy of J. Weston, M.D., Lower Hutt, New Zealand.)

B Observe erosion of the posterosuperior aspect of the calcaneus (arrowhead) and a well-defined plantar calcaneal enthesophyte (arrow).

C Superficial erosion (arrow) on the plantar aspect of the calcaneus is evident.

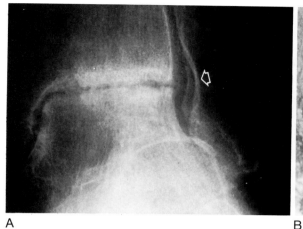
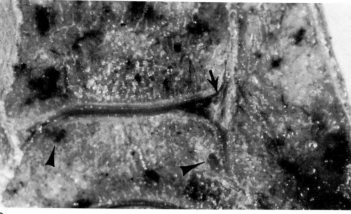

A   B

FIGURE 26–46. Abnormalities of the ankle.
A An anteroposterior radiograph delineates diffuse loss of articular space, significant erosions of the tibia and talus with surrounding sclerosis, and scalloping of the medial aspect of the distal fibula (arrow).
B A photograph of a coronal section of the ankle in a cadaver with rheumatoid arthritis indicates synovial proliferation (arrow) and mild cartilaginous and osseous destruction (arrowheads).

the tendon, with accompanying soft tissue swelling. The osseous attachments of the Achilles tendon can appear irregular, with enthesophyte formation.

Well-defined calcaneal excrescences also are observed on the plantar aspect of the bone in patients with rheumatoid arthritis (Fig. 26–45). They are identical to those seen in ''normal'' persons, which presumably result from a degenerative process. Poorly marginated plantar outgrowths with adjacent sclerosis, as seen in the seronegative spondyloarthropathies, are rare in rheumatoid arthritis. Although erosions on the undersurface of the calcaneus are seen in rheumatoid arthritis, they are infrequent and of small size.

Spontaneous Achilles tendon rupture has been described in patients with rheumatoid arthritis,[233] some of whom have received local corticosteroid injections.[234] These ruptures may have resulted from collagenolysis of the tendon as a result of its proximity to an inflamed retrocalcaneal bursa. Tendon inflammation itself or enthesitis[691] may be a contributing factor in other patients with this complication. Such tendon rupture appears to be more frequent in the hands and the wrists, although tenosynovitis, especially of the peroneal and posterior tibial tendons, is a well-known feature of the disease, and rupture of the last of these tendons may lead to flatfoot deformity.[689]

Ankle

The frequency of clinical and radiologic abnormalities in the ankle in rheumatoid arthritis is lower than that in the knee and the articulations of the hand, wrist, and foot.[235–238] In the presence of synovitis of the ankle, soft tissue swelling, limitation of motion, and pain can be evident. Pain also may be associated with synovial inflammation in the neighboring posterior tibial and peroneal tendons.

Synovial hypertrophy in the tibiotalar articulation can lead to radiographically evident masses that are anterior, posterior, or lateral to the joint margin.[235–236] Instillation of contrast material into the tibiotalar space more directly delineates the degree of synovial irregularity and capsular distention and demonstrates the communication of the abnormal joint with adjacent tendon sheaths or the posterior

subtalar joint.[239] These tendinous and articular communications, however, can be a normal finding on ankle arthrography,[226, 240] although their rate of occurrence may be greater in rheumatoid arthritis patients. Visualization of lymphatics and synovial cysts is an additional finding on arthrography in these patients.

Continued disease activity leads to cartilaginous and osseous destruction manifested radiographically as joint space loss and marginal and central bony erosions (Fig. 26–46).

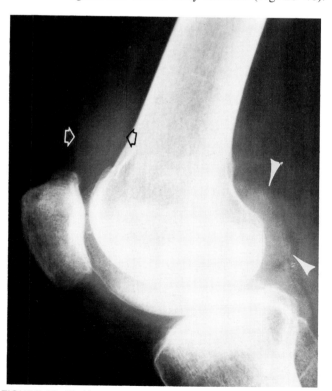

FIGURE 26–47. Abnormalities of the knee: Synovial effusion. On a lateral radiograph, an effusion is indicated by an enlarged suprapatellar pouch (greater than 10 mm in thickness) (arrows) between two radiolucent fat collections, one above the patella and one anterior to the distal end of the femur, and by increased radiodensity in the posterior recesses (arrowheads).

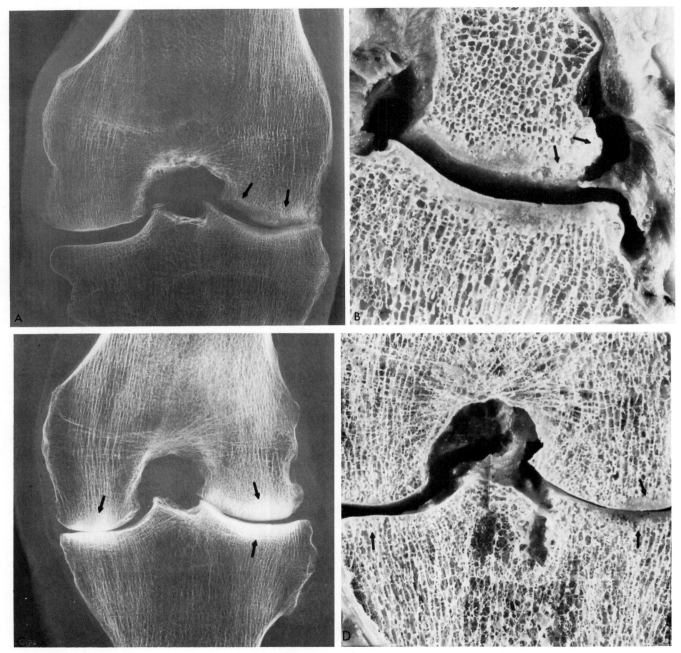

FIGURE 26–48. Abnormalities of the knee: Femorotibial compartments.

   A, B A radiograph and photograph of a macerated coronal section of the knee demonstrate superficial erosion, especially of the lateral femoral condyle (arrows) and intercondylar notch. Adjacent eburnation of femur and tibia is evident.

   C, D In a different cadaver, diffuse loss of articular space in both the medial and lateral femorotibial compartments is associated with subchondral sclerosis (arrows).

Illustration continued on opposite page

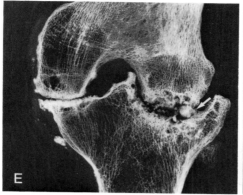 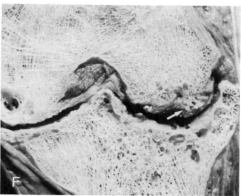

FIGURE 26–48. *Continued*
  E, F A radiograph and a photograph of a macerated coronal section of the knee in a third cadaver illustrate severe femorotibial involvement. The lateral compartment is affected more severely with depression of the tibial plateau, and intra-articular bone fragments are evident (arrows).

Subluxation and progressive osteoporosis may be complicated by the appearance of insufficiency (stress) fractures.

Knee

Clinical Abnormalities

The knee frequently is affected in rheumatoid arthritis. The extensive synovial lining at this site reveals inflammation, often at an early stage of the disease. Pain and swelling appear. The presence of a joint effusion is documented by careful physical examination[9, 241] and can be further substantiated by radiography accomplished in the lateral projection (Fig. 26–47) (see Chapter 22). Additional early clinical manifestations in the rheumatoid knee are loss of full extension of the joint and atrophy of the quadriceps musculature, the latter related to reflex inhibition of the muscle caused by the presence of intra-articular fluid.[505] Increased fluid accumulation in the joint can be accompanied by small or large synovial cysts, especially on the posterior aspect of the knee.[242] Their presence, extent, and degree of synovial irregularity can be outlined during knee arthrography (as a result of opacification of these structures, which communicate with the neighboring articulation)[506] or by ultrasonography or MR imaging (see later discussion). Acute rupture of synovial cysts can lead to clinical findings that simulate those of thrombophlebitis.

With increasing knee abnormalities, rheumatoid arthritis patients may have difficulty in walking and demonstrate loss of normal joint motion. Progressive articular involvement coupled with alterations in the menisci[507] and surrounding ligamentous and soft tissue structures leads to instability and contracture.[463]

Radiographic-Pathologic Correlation

The inflamed synovial tissue has a detrimental effect on cartilage and bone.[243, 252] Characteristically, symmetric abnormalities occur in both the medial and the lateral femorotibial compartments (Fig. 26–48) and may be combined with similar changes in the patellofemoral compartment. This bicompartmental or tricompartmental distribution, which can be depicted on radiography, is an important clue to the correct diagnosis, although it may be simulated by the distribution of disease in other synovial processes. Occasionally, the lateral femorotibial compartment is involved more severely than the medial, leading to a valgus deformity of the knee. As in other rheumatoid joints, the initial and more severe cartilaginous and osseous abnormalities

occur at the margins of the articulation. Thus, small erosions on the medial and lateral margins of the tibia and the femur may be the first radiographic finding. These lesions occasionally are preceded by or soon accompanied by diffuse loss of the interosseous distance between femur and tibia in both the medial and lateral compartments and by the development of subchondral erosions and cysts. The cysts are of variable size and occasionally become large enough to simulate neoplasm and to produce collapse of the subarticular bone.[244] Pathologically, communication between the cyst and articular cavity is demonstrated commonly, but not invariably, associated with transchondral extension of inflamed synovium.

Although accurate radiographic evaluation of the patellofemoral compartment is made difficult by the grooved contour of the anterior femoral surface and the dependence of patellar position on the presence and size of any joint effusion and the precise attitude of the knee during radiography, lateral and axial radiographs frequently demonstrate joint space loss and subchondral erosions and cysts of the patella (Fig. 26–49).

Subchondral eburnation and, to a lesser extent, osteophytes are not infrequently observed in the knee in rheumatoid arthritis, particularly in the distal femur and proximal tibia. These changes usually are evident in longstanding disease and may be accompanied by complete obliteration of the interosseous space. Furthermore, flexion deformity may complicate the later stages of rheumatoid arthritis, obscuring many of the intra-articular abnormalities.[463]

Varus or valgus deformity with or without subluxation also can be evident. In these attitudes, the femorotibial compartment on the convex side of the deformed knee can appear widened, suggesting asymmetric compartmental destruction. Pathologically, however, both femorotibial compartments are affected. Bony ankylosis of the knee joint indeed is rare in rheumatoid arthritis.

The authors have not found radiographs obtained with the patient standing as useful in the evaluation of the knee in rheumatoid arthritis as they are in the appraisal of the knee in degenerative disease. This may relate to the symmetric or diffuse nature of cartilaginous destruction that accompanies the rheumatoid process. Occasionally, however, "standing" radiographs will reveal complete obliteration of the articular space when initial films outline only mild to moderate joint space loss.

The aggressive nature of the diseased synovium in the

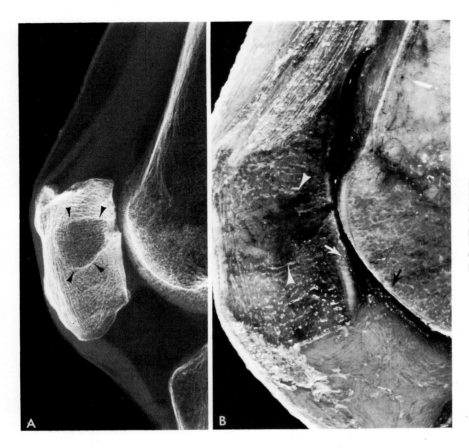

FIGURE 26–49. Abnormalities of the knee: Patellofemoral compartment. On a radiograph and photograph of a sagittal section of a rheumatoid knee, note cartilaginous loss on the patellar and femoral surfaces (arrows) and a large patellar cyst (arrowheads), which is communicating with the patellofemoral compartment.[509]

knee in rheumatoid arthritis has led many authors to advocate synovectomy during the early or more advanced stages of the disease.[245–248] The regeneration of abnormal synovium, sometimes within a period of months to a few years after surgical intervention, limits the usefulness of this procedure in many persons.[249, 250] This regenerated synovial tissue frequently is histologically and enzymatically identical to that in the nonoperated knee joint.[251] It can lead to further destruction of cartilage and bone, and the only available recourse to the surgeon may be total joint replacement.[253–255] After such replacement, regeneration of rheumatoid synovial tissue is infrequent,[508] although it has been observed.[692]

Rare manifestations of rheumatoid involvement in or about the knee include intra-articular rheumatoid nodules, which can lead to mechanical derangement,[256, 257] and spontaneous rupture of the infrapatellar tendon.[258]

Proximal Tibiofibular Joint

Approximately one third of rheumatoid arthritis patients with knee joint involvement will reveal additional changes in the proximal tibiofibular articulation consisting of joint space loss and osseous erosion[259] (Fig. 26–50). This is not surprising, as the synovial joint between the proximal tibia and fibula may communicate with the knee joint in 10 per cent of adults. Furthermore, aggressive synovial tissue in one joint could readily destroy the intervening connective tissue in those patients in whom the knee and proximal tibiofibular joint do not normally communicate. Subluxation of the fibular head has been described in rheumatoid

arthritis, perhaps related to synovial hypertrophy with secondary capsular and ligamentous injury.[509]

Hip

Clinical Abnormalities

The frequency of abnormalities of the hip is far less than that of the knee. The prevalence of hip alterations increases with the duration and the severity of rheumatoid arthritis, especially in those patients receiving corticosteroids.[9, 260] Pain, tenderness, shortening of the limb, gait abnormalities, and decreased range of motion, particularly internal rotation, extension, and abduction, are the observed clinical manifestations. Soft tissue swelling on the anterior aspect of the joint and over the greater trochanter (due to bursitis) can be evident in as many as 15 per cent of patients with rheumatoid arthritis.[512] With more chronic and severe involvement, muscle atrophy, adjacent rheumatoid nodules over the sacrum and ischial tuberosities, and a mass in the groin or leg edema related to synovial cyst formation may be encountered.[9, 261–263, 510, 511, 639]

Radiographic-Pathologic Correlation

Radiographic abnormalities of the hip generally are bilateral and symmetric in distribution,[264, 265] although, rarely, asymmetric or unilateral alterations are seen. The most typical early abnormality is loss of joint space[266] (Fig. 26–51). In almost all patients, diminution of articular space is concentric, reflecting thinning and loss of the cartilaginous coat over much of the femoral and acetabular surfaces. The femoral head moves inward along the axis of the femoral

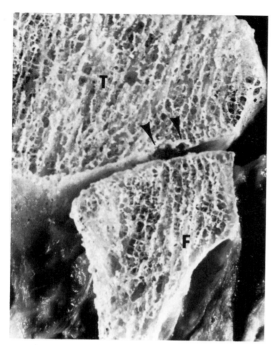

FIGURE 26–50. Abnormalities of the proximal tibiofibular joint. A photograph of a macerated sagittal section through the proximal tibiofibular joint in a cadaver with rheumatoid arthritis demonstrates joint space narrowing and osseous erosions (arrowheads). T, Tibia; F, fibula.

neck (axial migration).[264, 265, 267] Much less frequently, greater loss of joint space appears on the superior aspect of the joint, producing upward or superior migration of the femoral head with respect to the acetabulum, similar to that which accompanies osteoarthritis.[265]

The degree of articular space loss may increase with progression of the disease. Eventually, this space can be completely obliterated, and the femoral head and acetabulum protrude into the pelvis[265, 268] (Fig. 26–52). Acetabular protrusion, which is defined as inward movement of the acetabular line so that the distance between this line and the laterally located ilioischial line is 3 mm or more in men and 6 mm or more in women,[269] is particularly characteristic of rheumatoid arthritis, although it can be observed in seronegative spondyloarthropathies, infection, osteoarthritis (with medial migration of the femoral head), osteomalacia, Paget's disease, idiopathic protrusion (Otto pelvis), and additional disorders.[693] Protrusio acetabuli has been noted in 14 per cent of rheumatoid arthritis patients with hip disease, especially elderly women with long-standing arthritis.[268] The deformity commonly is bilateral and associated with subchondral cystic lesions, osseous collapse of the acetabular roof and femoral head, and osteoporosis. It progresses more rapidly in patients who bear their weight on these joints and are physically active and in those who are receiving corticosteroid medication.[694] The precise role played by steroids in the pathogenesis of protrusio acetabuli is not clear; a high frequency of steroid intake in patients with this deformity may reflect only the severity of the entire disease process, although it also may indicate that a direct steroid-related effect on para-acetabular bone can promote acetabular protrusion.[268, 270] In long-standing rheumatoid arthritis, the radiographic appearance of bilaterally protruded acetabula containing small, eroded femoral heads is especially distinctive.

Osseous erosions and cysts also are well-known radiographic and pathologic manifestations of rheumatoid hip disease.[271–273] Radiographically, the earliest lucent zones appear at the chondro-osseous margin of the femoral head

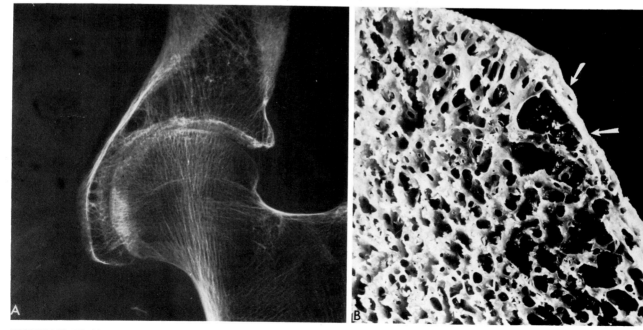

FIGURE 26–51. Abnormalities of the hip: Early changes.
A A radiograph of a coronal section of a rheumatoid cadaveric hip indicates diffuse loss of articular space with migration of the femoral head inward or axially along the axis of the femoral neck.
B A photograph of the superolateral aspect of a macerated femoral head demonstrates a pseudocystic lesion (arrows) with trabecular destruction and compression. These early defects usually are located at the chondro-osseous margin of the head of the femur.

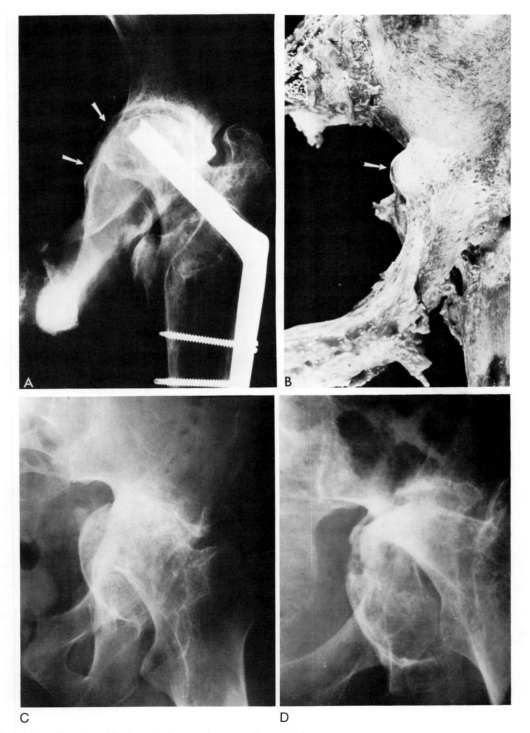

FIGURE 26–52. Abnormalities of the hip: Late changes with acetabular protrusion.

A, B A radiograph and photograph of a macerated hemipelvis and femur in a cadaver with rheumatoid arthritis reveal acetabular protrusion (arrows) and a smooth, small femoral head. Obviously, prior surgical treatment of an intertrochanteric fracture was accomplished.

C, D Two additional examples of protrusion deformity with acetabular fragmentation are shown. Observe the small size of the femoral head, which, in one case, is grossly deformed.

FIGURE 26–53. Abnormalities of the hip: Large cystic lesions.

A Occasionally radiographs reveal large lucent lesions of the femoral head and neck in rheumatoid arthritis. In this example, the osteolytic focus resembles a solitary bone cyst, and its relationship to rheumatoid arthritis cannot be defined. Although this patient had severe rheumatoid disease, the hip is relatively spared. However, similar lesions are noted in patients with rheumatoid arthritis as a result of pannus invasion of bone or, perhaps, intraosseous rheumatoid nodule formation.

B A photograph of a macerated coronal section of the proximal femur in a cadaver with rheumatoid arthritis indicates a large destructive lesion of the lateral aspect near the junction of the femoral head and neck. Sclerosis in the neighboring bone is minimal. Pannus could be traced from the articular surface into the lesion.

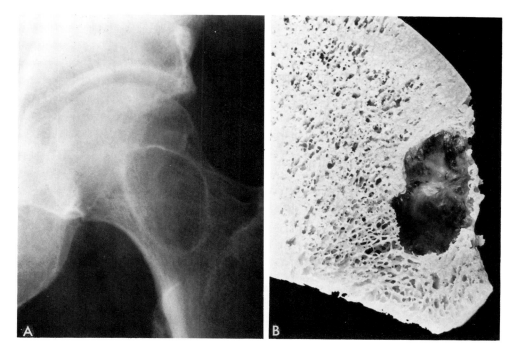

near the femoral neck (Fig. 26–51*B*). Additional lesions are observed as surface irregularities throughout the femoral head and, to a lesser degree, the acetabulum. They are usually multiple and without sclerotic margins. Both the marginal and central osseous defects are commonly associated with joint space loss. The lesions reflect pannus invasion of bone at the chondro-osseous junction and of cartilage and bone in the central articular areas. Rarely, large pseudoneoplastic foci of bone destruction can be seen in either the femoral head or the femoral neck[274–276, 513] (Fig. 26–53), perhaps reflecting true intraosseous rheumatoid

nodule formation, or, more likely, extension of aggressive synovial tissue from the joint.[277]

Some degree of sclerosis can appear about the hip after a considerable period of time.[278, 279] This sclerosis, which frequently is combined with mild osteophytosis of the femur and acetabulum, may be related to a reparative response of the diseased bone and cartilage or secondary degenerative joint disease (Fig. 26–54). In these instances, differentiation of rheumatoid arthritis with superimposed osteoarthritis from primary osteoarthritis can be difficult. The presence of symmetric loss of joint space and the

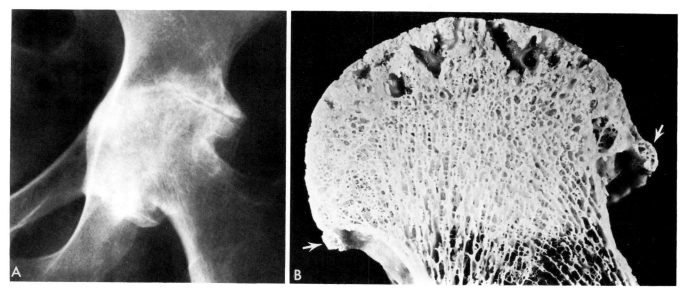

FIGURE 26–54. Abnormalities of the hip: Sclerosis and osteophytosis.

A In this rheumatoid arthritis patient, osteophytes on the femoral and acetabular margins are combined with diffuse loss of joint space and subchondral eburnation. Although the resulting radiographic picture resembles that of osteoarthritis alone, the presence of widespread articular space loss suggests that the degenerative abnormalities have been superimposed on an inflammatory arthritis.

B A photograph of a macerated coronal section of a femoral head in a rheumatoid arthritis patient demonstrates the presence of medial and lateral femoral osteophytes (arrows), in addition to widespread erosive and cystic changes. This represents the superimposition of degenerative joint disease on rheumatoid arthritis.

absence of prominent osteophytes and significant thickening along the femoral neck (buttressing) in rheumatoid arthritis are helpful clues.

The eventual outcome of rheumatoid hip disease often is complete obliteration of the articular space and fibrous ankylosis. Bony ankylosis is exceedingly rare. Very uncommonly, spontaneous recovery of the joint space has been noted in rheumatoid arthritis (as in osteoarthritis), which in some instances is associated with arthroplasty of the contralateral hip.[280] The exact mechanism for this unusual phenomenon is not known, although presumably it is related to the accumulation of fibrocartilaginous plugs as a healing response to the hyaline cartilaginous erosion that has occurred during the active phase of the disease.

Osteonecrosis of the femoral head is not uncommon in those rheumatoid arthritis patients who are being treated with corticosteroids. Its pathogenesis is not entirely clear, although vascular occlusion, abnormalities of lipid metabolism, and osseous collapse due to osteoporosis are potential causes. The radiographic appearance of osteonecrosis of the femoral head in this clinical setting will depend on the presence and severity of cartilaginous and osseous destruction that has been produced by the synovial inflammation of rheumatoid arthritis. If this destruction is severe, collapse of the femoral head is associated with significant loss of articular space, and the combination of findings is difficult to differentiate from that in uncomplicated rheumatoid hip disease; if osteonecrosis occurs in a relatively normal joint, the combination of osseous collapse, cyst formation, and sclerosis without joint space loss is identical to that of osteonecrosis occurring in patients without rheumatoid disease.

In those patients with rheumatoid arthritis who develop disabling hip disease, arthroplasty or other surgical procedures may be required.[281–286] In most instances, the clinical and radiologic appearance of the hip in the postoperative period is identical to that which is noted after similar surgery in nonrheumatoid persons, although a higher frequency of infection[287] has been recorded in rheumatoid arthritis patients, which may be related to the previous surgical attempts that commonly have taken place in these persons.[288] Other factors, such as the debilitating nature of the disease, the sedentary life that is common in these frequently bedridden patients, the high frequency of pulmonary disease and decubitus ulcers, the need for corticosteroid medication, and a peculiar susceptibility to septic arthritis, also may be important (see discussion later in this chapter). It also has been noted that a high frequency of problems related to trochanteric osteotomy occurs in patients with rheumatoid arthritis, perhaps related to the presence of abnormal bone or lateral displacement of the femoral head.[514]

Sacroiliac Joint

As opposed to the frequent and severe clinical and radiologic abnormalities that characterize sacroiliac joint disease in ankylosing spondylitis, changes in this location in rheumatoid arthritis are relatively infrequent and mild. An association of such changes with an age of disease onset greater than 40 years, elevation of the erythrocyte sedimentation rate, and widespread involvement of the appendicular joints and cervical spine has been observed.[515] Furthermore, the frequency of radiographic signs of sacroiliac joint disease in rheumatoid arthritis is reported to be higher in those patients who possess the HLA-B27 antigen.[516, 517] As both rheumatoid arthritis and ankylosing spondylitis can coexist in the same patient, the latter disease must be considered in any patient with rheumatoid arthritis who has significant abnormality of the sacroiliac joint and is positive for the HLA-B27 antigen.

Asymptomatic radiographic abnormalities of the sacroiliac joint can be present in as many as 25 to 35 per cent of patients with severe, long-standing disease.[289–294, 655] Abnormalities, which may be more frequent in women than in men,[291] can be bilateral or unilateral in distribution, but symmetric alterations, which are the rule in ankylosing spondylitis, are not frequent in rheumatoid arthritis. Joint space narrowing varies in severity; it frequently is mild, but occasionally complete obliteration of the articulation with segmental osseous fusion is encountered (Fig. 26–55). Osseous erosions have predilection for the iliac aspect of the joint; they are superficial and well marginated and are associated with absent or only mild sclerosis. Ossification of the sacroiliac ligament located above the synovial part of the sacroiliac joint is uncommon in rheumatoid arthritis. Pathologic examination frequently demonstrates cartilaginous degeneration and fibrous ankylosis not unlike that occurring in osteoarthritis.[295] Inflammatory pannus rarely is observed.

It has been reported that conventional tomographic evaluation of the sacroiliac joints in rheumatoid arthritis patients may reveal a higher frequency of sacroiliitis than is evident on routine radiography, and that with conventional tomograms, subchondral erosions and bony ankylosis may be noted.[453] CT and MR imaging also have been used effectively to study the sacroiliac joint.

Symphysis Pubis

The symphysis pubis, which frequently is affected in ankylosing spondylitis and other seronegative spondyloarthropathies, is not commonly altered in rheumatoid arthritis. Occasionally, in patients with chronic disease, radiographic abnormalities are detected, which generally are silent clinically.[294, 296, 297] These include subchondral erosion, mild eburnation, and narrowing of the interosseous space. Associated abnormalities of the pelvis may consist of superficial erosive changes in the ischial tuberosities and the iliac crests. If severe alterations are detected in the symphysis pubis, sites of ligamentous attachment to the pelvis, and sacroiliac articulations in patients with documented rheumatoid arthritis, the possibility of superimposed ankylosing spondylitis must be considered (see Chapter 28).

Parasymphyseal insufficiency fractures of the os pubis have been described in patients with rheumatoid arthritis as well as in those with postmenopausal osteoporosis.[518] The resulting radiographic abnormalities, consisting of lysis, sclerosis, and fragmentation of bone, can resemble those of malignant neoplasm.

Costovertebral Joints and Ribs

Abnormalities of the thoracic cage in patients with rheumatoid arthritis can include erosions on the superior margin of the posterior aspect of the upper (third, fourth, fifth)

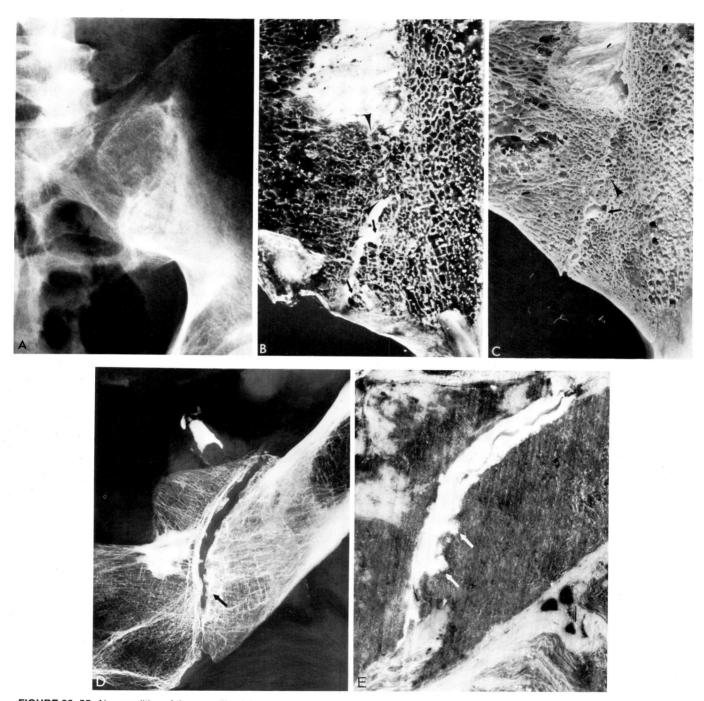

FIGURE 26–55. Abnormalities of the sacroiliac joint.

A A radiograph of a rheumatoid arthritis patient reveals focal erosions and reactive sclerosis, particularly on the iliac aspect of the sacroiliac joint. The articular space is diminished. These changes can be distributed in a unilateral or bilateral fashion. The degree of bony eburnation that is present in this case is unusual in rheumatoid arthritis.

B, C Coronal sections of the sacroiliac joint of two cadavers with rheumatoid arthritis demonstrate osseous erosions, especially in the ilium (arrows), and segmental intra-articular osseous fusion (arrowheads).

D, E In a third cadaver with rheumatoid arthritis, a radiograph and photograph of a transverse section through the lower portion of the sacroiliac joint demonstrate superficial erosion of bone, especially in the ilium (arrows). A bone island in the sacrum is seen incidentally.

ribs.[178, 186] The erosions are visible approximately 5 to 10 cm from the midline of the body and exist more laterally in the lower ribs.[519] They are identical to those that are encountered in other collagen vascular disorders, neurologic processes, and chronic obstructive lung disease.[298] It is probable that rib erosions in rheumatoid arthritis, as well as some other processes, are due to pressure effect from the scapula. Their appearance in those persons who reveal osteoporosis, kyphosis, and restricted shoulder motion supports this concept.[186] Furthermore, such rib erosions increase in frequency in rheumatoid arthritis patients with long-standing disease; they have been observed in 15 per cent of such patients.[519] Radionuclide examination with bone-seeking radiopharmaceutical agents has revealed no accentuated activity at the sites of rib erosion.[520]

Costovertebral joint (between the head of the rib and facets on the vertebral bodies) and costotransverse joint (between the tubercle of the rib and the transverse process of the vertebra) involvement occasionally is seen in rheumatoid arthritis patients,[299] although changes are difficult to demonstrate on radiographic examination. An inflammatory synovitis at these locations can produce osseous erosion, joint space narrowing, ankylosis, and enlargement of the posterior aspects of the ribs. Spread of such disease to the neighboring intervertebral discs has been emphasized as a mechanism of thoracic discitis in rheumatoid arthritis patients.[300, 525]

Thoracic and Lumbar Spine

In comparison to the distinctive alterations of the cervical spine, which represent a common and well-known manifestation of rheumatoid arthritis, abnormalities of the thoracic and lumbar spine are relatively infrequent in this disease. Occasionally a report notes the presence of destructive lesions of vertebral bodies in the thoracic and lumbar segments,[277, 301–303, 640, 695] which histologically may resemble rheumatoid nodules. These granulomatous white nodular foci involve the vertebral body and may extend to the vertebral endplates, allowing collapse of the subchondral bone and intervertebral discal abnormality. Similarly, rare examples of rheumatoid nodules within the extradural space producing compression of the spinal cord have been described.[304–308] These latter nodules can be located in any portion of the vertebral column, from the cranial region to the cauda equina, and may extend outside the spinal canal to involve adjacent osseous structures and musculature. Synovial cysts arising from the apophyseal joints may have a similar appearance.[450]

Rheumatoid arthritic changes in the apophyseal joints of the thoracic and lumbar spine only rarely are reported. In 1964, Lawrence and coworkers[309] detected an increased frequency of apophyseal joint destruction and subluxation and of intervertebral disc space narrowing of the lumbar spine in rheumatoid arthritis patients compared with controls, although these investigators noted the difficulty in delineating apophyseal joint changes accurately on routine radiography. Bywaters,[300] in a discussion of his investigation on rheumatoid involvement of the costovertebral joints, indicated that the changes in the adjacent apophyseal joints were less frequent, an observation that was confirmed by Ball.[310] Martel and Duff[294] found no examples of apophyseal joint

ankylosis in the dorsolumbar spine of patients with rheumatoid arthritis, although such changes were not uncommon in the cervical region. On the other hand, Sims-Williams and collaborators,[311] using stereoscopic views of the apophyseal joints of the lumbar spine in six patients with rheumatoid arthritis, distinguished superficial erosions that resembled typical rheumatoid defects in all cases. Similar apophyseal joint lesions of both the thoracic and lumbar spine were described by Shichikawa and associates[312]; these investigators detected evidence of fibrin deposition, proliferative vascular tissue, and cartilage destruction on histologic evaluation of a lower lumbar apophyseal joint.

Alterations at the discovertebral junction of the thoracic and lumbar spine also have been noted.[300, 311–313, 525, 640, 696, 787] Intervertebral disc space narrowing, irregularity of the subchondral margins of the vertebral bodies, "erosion," and sclerosis can be evident on radiography of these sites (Fig. 26–56A,B). The cause of the radiographic changes and their relationship to the more commonly observed discovertebral lesions of the cervical spine have been the subjects of much debate. Such discovertebral changes could relate to (1) apophyseal joint instability with abnormal motion at the corresponding discovertebral junction, leading to cartilaginous node formation; (2) apophyseal joint synovitis with extension into the vertebral body–intervertebral disc junction; (3) costovertebral joint synovitis (in the thoracic spine) with extension into the vertebral body–intervertebral disc junction; (4) synovial infiltration into fissures within the degenerating nucleus pulposus of the intervertebral disc and subsequent inflammation; (5) neuropathic alterations secondary to analgesic or steroid therapy; and (6) enthesopathy (similar to that occurring in ankylosing spondylitis), resulting in inflammation of ligaments and adjacent areolar tissue, with extension into the vertebral body–intervertebral disc junction. Histologic evidence has been gathered for the first,[313] third,[300, 525] and sixth[312] of these mechanisms, although the interpretation of the findings is not uniform, even among experienced pathologists. In the authors' experience,[313, 686] discovertebral trauma related to apophyseal joint instability appears to have a prominent role in the production of alterations of the discovertebral junction in the cervical, thoracic, and lumbar spine. Although this certainly need not be the only important mechanism in this regard, the similarity of the radiographic appearance of spines of patients with rheumatoid arthritis to that in other disorders associated with cartilaginous node formation cannot be disregarded.[314] Such a mechanism also could explain the association of discovertebral junction destruction in the rare rheumatoid arthritis patient with intravertebral nodules (which could lead to osseous weakening, allowing discal displacement).

Patients with rheumatoid arthritis who are receiving corticosteroid medication are predisposed to develop ischemic necrosis of bone. Although the femoral head is the typical target site of this complication, vertebral bodies in the thoracic and lumbar segments of the spine can be affected. Radiographic abnormalities include vertebral collapse and fragmentation. Radiolucent fracture lines, which may accumulate gas from surrounding tissues (vacuum vertebral body), are an important clue, allowing correct diagnosis (Fig. 26–56C,D). The finding is not unlike that accompanying ischemic necrosis of the femoral head (crescent sign).

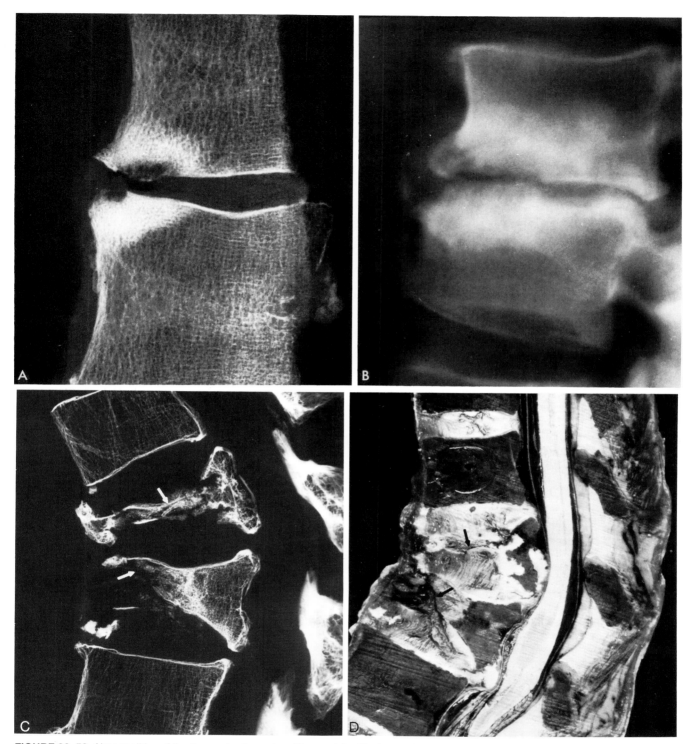

FIGURE 26–56. Abnormalities of the thoracolumbar spine: Discovertebral lesions and ischemic necrosis.

A In a sagittal section of the upper lumbar spine in a cadaver with rheumatoid arthritis, intervertebral disc space narrowing, vacuum phenomena, intraosseous lucent area, sclerosis, and osteophytosis are observed along the anterior aspect of the discovertebral junction. The findings commonly are related to cartilaginous node formation, perhaps due to recurrent discovertebral trauma in association with apophyseal joint instability.

B On a lateral conventional tomogram of the lumbar spine in a rheumatoid arthritis patient, a similar appearance is evident. The findings of disc space narrowing, poorly defined osseous erosion, and sclerosis, which resemble those in infection and intervertebral osteochondrosis, are encountered in rheumatoid arthritis. Their pathogenesis is debated.

C, D A radiograph and photograph of a sagittal section of the thoracolumbar segment of the spine in a rheumatoid cadaver demonstrate findings of corticosteroid-induced ischemic necrosis of bone. Observe collapse of two vertebral bodies with fractures (arrows) and cartilaginous node formation. Exaggerated kyphosis and compression of the spinal cord are apparent.

Cervical Spine

Clinical Abnormalities

Although considerable controversy exists regarding the occurrence of thoracolumbar spinal abnormalities in rheumatoid arthritis, there is little disagreement regarding the prevalence of cervical spinal changes in this disease. Furthermore, the clinical significance of these abnormalities rarely is challenged. Cervical spine involvement can lead to severe pain and disability as well as to a variety of neurologic manifestations,[698] although some patients with significant radiographic evidence of disease may be entirely asymptomatic. In rheumatoid arthritis, the cervical spine commonly is affected along with peripheral articular sites, although initial or predominant involvement of the cervical spine can occur without obvious clinical (or radiographic) abnormalities at other locations.[315, 316]

Approximately 60 to 80 per cent of rheumatoid arthritis patients develop symptoms and signs related to cervical spine abnormalities at some time during their illness. Pain is the most common clinical manifestation of cervical spine involvement.[315-320] It may be brief or sustained in duration. In patients with atlantoaxial subluxation, pain may be expressed in the temporal and retro-orbital region; occipital pain is considered to arise from level C2-C3 or below.[9] Weakness and abnormal mobility also can be evident. Neurologic manifestations include paresthesias, paresis, and muscle wasting; in some instances, quadriplegia and death occur.[321-326] Vertebrobasilar vascular insufficiency can lead to transient blindness, nystagmus, vertigo, and loss of consciousness; the anterior spinal arteries may be occluded, producing anterior horn cell lesions.[9] Pulsatile masses related to pseudoaneurysms have been described.[641]

Radiographic-Pathologic Correlation

General Features. The entire cervical spine partakes in the rheumatoid process; changes may be evident as far cephalad as the base of the occiput and as far caudad as the C7-T1 junction.[609] Furthermore, synovial and cartilaginous articulations, the joints of Luschka, tendinous and ligamentous attachments, and soft tissues of the cervical region can reveal significant abnormalities in this disease. Recognition of changes in all these sites requires optimal radiography, which, in addition to standard radiographs, must include an open-mouth frontal projection (for the odontoid process) and a lateral view of the flexed neck (for the C1-C2 articulations); it often requires a swimmer's view (for the lower cervical and upper thoracic region) and conventional tomography, CT, or MR imaging as well. Because a rheumatoid arthritis patient may have spinal instability with neurologic compromise, care often is required in positioning the patient for these imaging studies and, in many instances, the entire examination is not feasible. In those patients who can undergo complete radiographic evaluation, the frequency of radiographic changes of the cervical spine is consistently high (and may reach 85 per cent).[358] Radiographic abnormalities in the cervical spine have been reported to correlate with those in the peripheral joints and with the presence of serum rheumatoid factor and subcutaneous nodules.[537, 697] Reports that indicate a relatively low frequency of cervical spine alterations in this disease may not have included all the necessary radiographic projections; for example, an apparently normal cervical spine can reveal considerable subluxation at the C1-C2 junction merely with the addition of a lateral view of the flexed neck. Similarly, subtle discovertebral or odontoid erosions may be entirely hidden without the aid of conventional tomography. When all radiographic parameters are used, demonstration of abnormalities throughout the cervical spine is frequent, although they usually predominate in the upper cervical region.

Occipitoatlantoaxial Articulations

Atlantoaxial Subluxation (Fig. 26–57). Various types of malalignment at the atlantoaxial region have been described in rheumatoid arthritis. The major types, each of which is discussed in the following pages, include anterior atlantoaxial subluxation, vertical subluxation (also known as cranial settling and atlantoaxial impaction), lateral subluxation, and posterior subluxation. Subluxations of all types in this region have been noted in 40 to 85 per cent of patients with rheumatoid arthritis.[699]

Abnormal separation between the anterior arch of the atlas and the odontoid process (dens) of the axis, designated anterior atlantoaxial subluxation, is a characteristic finding in rheumatoid arthritis, which may be evident in an early stage of the disease, at a time at which other cervical spine abnormalities, including odontoid erosion, are not apparent.[327-331, 533, 538, 700] Its recorded rate of occurrence varies with the precise methods of patient selection and radiographic examination and the criteria used to indicate subluxation. Generally, the interosseous distance between the posterior aspect of the anterior arch of the atlas and the anterior aspect of the odontoid process does not exceed 2.5 mm in adults,[332] although slight variation in the normal measurement exists in men and women.[333] The points of measurement have been a subject of debate. Some investi-

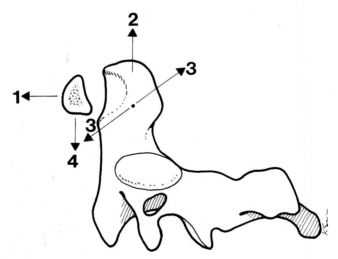

FIGURE 26–57. Abnormalities of the cervical spine: Directions of atlantoaxial subluxation. There are varying types of subluxation that may occur at the atlantoaxial articulations in a rheumatoid arthritis patient. Most typically anterior movement of the atlas with respect to the axis (1) is seen. Vertical translocation of the odontoid process (cranial settling) (2) also can occur. Lateral subluxation (3) can be recorded on frontal radiographs as asymmetry becomes apparent between the odontoid process and the lateral masses of the atlas. In addition, the anterior arch of the atlas can move inferiorly (4) with respect to the odontoid process, a finding associated with cranial settling. Finally, in the presence of severe erosion of the odontoid process, the anterior arch can move posteriorly against the eroded bone or, rarely, behind the eroded odontoid process.

gators use the minimum perpendicular measurement between the two bones, although others use the superior, middle, or inferior aspects of the space. The inferior aspect is most popular.[526] It also should be obvious that slight variation in reported distances can be related to differences in focal spot-target-film distances. As a minimal degree of flexion and extension motion occurs normally at the atlanto-odontoid articulation, a cranial shift of the atlas relative to the dens can be seen in extension and a small gap in the superior aspect of the atlantoaxial space can be noted in flexion[330]; in addition, the angle of inclination of C1 and C2 normally increases slightly in flexion.[334] An interosseous interval between atlas and odontoid process less than 2.5 mm that changes considerably on flexion and extension also can be abnormal.

The consensus of prior reports on anterior atlantoaxial subluxation in rheumatoid patients indicates a frequency of 20 to 25 per cent[318, 331, 335] (Fig. 26–58). This frequency rises with increasing severity of the disease, although in patients with significant odontoid erosions, an abnormally wide gap between the atlas and odontoid process may indicate not a lax or disrupted transverse ligament but rather an increased incongruity of apposing osseous surfaces. In postmortem studies, anterior subluxation has been noted in 11 to 46 per cent of cases of rheumatoid arthritis.[699]

The pathogenesis of anterior atlantoaxial subluxation relates to the presence of transverse ligament laxity due to synovial inflammation and hyperemia of the adjacent articulations, especially that between the posterior surface of the odontoid process and the anterior surface of the ligament (see Chapter 22). Of interest, analysis of biopsy specimens obtained from ligamentous structures between the posterior arch of the atlas and the spinous process of the axis in patients with rheumatoid arthritis and atlantoaxial subluxation has revealed focal inflammation.[701] Although the more

pertinent anterior ligaments were not evaluated, the presence of such inflammation provides a possible explanation for ligamentous laxity in cases of anterior atlantoaxial subluxation.[702] The mechanism of this C1-C2 derangement has been studied by cineradiography.[329] During flexion, the atlas slowly separates anteriorly from the axis. With increasing displacement, the cervical canal is progressively compressed by the posterior arch of the atlas. During extension, atlantoaxial subluxation persists as long as the plane of the atlas is angled below the horizontal. When the horizontal plane is reached, the atlas slides backward until it rests against the odontoid process. In some instances, a rapid movement is associated with a "clicking" sensation.

In addition to anterior movement of the atlas with respect to the odontoid process, vertical subluxation at C1-C2 also can be observed in patients with rheumatoid arthritis,[336–339, 343, 610] which, when extensive, can be fatal (Fig. 26–59). This complication, which also is referred to as atlantoaxial impaction[527] or cranial settling,[528] is diagnosed by applying one or more of a number of radiographic measurements that assess the relationship of the tip of the odontoid process to landmarks at the base of the skull[340, 703, 704, 707] (see Chapter 22). In one series of patients with rheumatoid arthritis, a diagnosis of cranial settling has been made on the basis of the location of the tip of the odontoid process at a level that is 8 mm or more above McGregor's line in men or 9.7 mm above this line in women.[527] The coexistence of odontoid erosions, however, can make such measurements very difficult to obtain. An alternative method, employed by Redlund-Johnell and others, relies on the minimum distance between McGregor's line and the midpoint of the inferior margin of the body of the axis as determined in a lateral radiograph of the neck in neutral position.[705] As settling progresses, the anterior arch of the atlas gradually assumes a position near the lower portion of the axis. When severe,

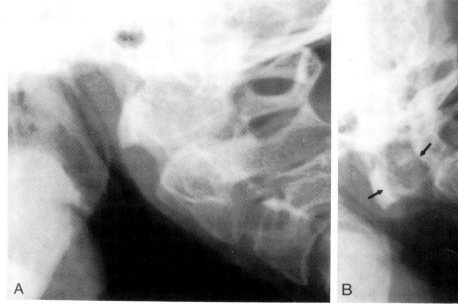
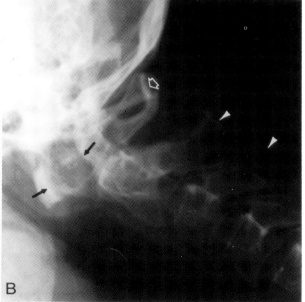

FIGURE 26–58. Abnormalities of the cervical spine: Anterior atlantoaxial subluxation. Lateral radiographs of the cervical spine obtained during extension **(A)** and flexion **(B)** of the neck reveal severe atlantoaxial subluxation evident in the flexed position. Note the abnormal distance (solid arrows) between the posterior surface of the anterior arch of the atlas and the anterior surface of the odontoid process. The spinolaminar line of the atlas (open arrow) does not align with that of the other cervical vertebrae (arrowheads), confirming the presence of anterior subluxation. (Courtesy of V. Vint, M.D., San Diego, California.)

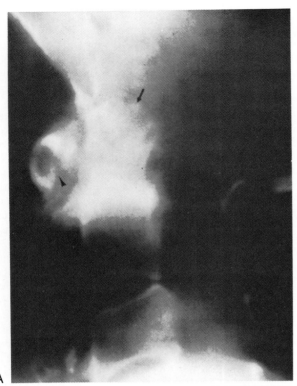

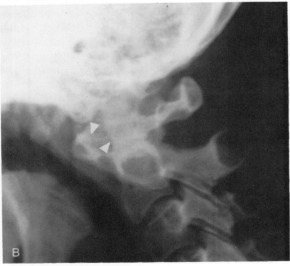

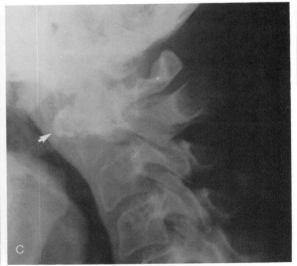

FIGURE 26–59. Abnormalities of the cervical spine: Vertical translocation of the odontoid process (cranial settling).

A Conventional tomography of the cervical spine in the lateral projection confirms the existence of vertical translocation of the odontoid process. Its tip (arrow) is located in the foramen magnum, and the anterior arch of the atlas (arrowhead) is opposite the lower portion of the odontoid process. (Courtesy of V. Vint, M.D., San Diego, California.)

B, C In a different patient with rheumatoid arthritis, lateral radiographs of the cervical spine were obtained 9 years apart. In the earlier study **(B)**, anterior atlantoaxial subluxation (arrowheads) is evident. In the later study **(C)**, cranial settling has occurred with the anterior arch of the atlas (arrow) having moved inferiorly with respect to the axis. Note the apparent absence of anterior atlantoaxial subluxation in **C**, suggesting improvement in the radiographic findings, which definitely is not the case.

such settling is easily diagnosed on radiographs obtained in a lateral projection or on conventional tomograms or CT scans. It should be recognized, however, that changes in the position of the cervical spine may have a significant influence on the radiographic values used to diagnose vertical subluxation; indeed, even in healthy persons, flexion of the neck may result in a more superior position of the dens.[710]

Cranial settling has been observed in 5 to 22 per cent of patients with rheumatoid arthritis.[527, 528] In general, vertical translocation of the dens results from disruption and collapse of osseous and articular structures that exist between the occiput and the atlas, and between the atlas and the axis.[339, 341, 708, 709] Although neurologic dysfunction associated with vertical migration of the odontoid process, a movement that results in its more intimate relationship with the base of the brain, might be expected to be more severe

than that seen in association with forward subluxation, this is not always the case.[339] Associated erosion of the tip of the odontoid process may serve as a protective mechanism in many of the persons who reveal vertical translocation of the dens; however, because of the proximity to the dens of such important structures as the medulla oblongata, the proximal portion of the spinal cord, and the vertebral arteries, it is mandatory to recognize vertical subluxation at C1-C2 when it is present. MR imaging represents a very effective method in the further evaluation of such subluxation as well as its effects on the spinal cord (see later discussion).[706]

Lateral subluxation of the atlantoaxial joints also has been observed in rheumatoid arthritis patients.[342, 451, 711] In these patients, asymmetry is recorded between the odontoid process (and body of the axis) and the atlas. This complication has been diagnosed when the lateral masses of the atlas were displaced more than 2 mm with respect to those of the axis,[527, 529] and it has been observed in 10 to 20 per cent of rheumatoid arthritis patients. Because of the anatomy of the region, lateral subluxation and anterior subluxation generally coexist.[526] The sequence of events that leads to lateral subluxation of the atlantoaxial joints includes articular space narrowing, bony erosion, disruption of the articular capsules, and, in severe cases, collapse of the lateral masses of the axis, allowing the atlas to shift and tilt laterally. Bone erosion may be the most important factor in the development of this deformity.[530] These changes are optimally visualized on anteroposterior radiographs and conventional tomograms or CT scans (Fig. 26–60). Clinically, patients with lateral subluxation reveal a fixed head tilt toward the side of osseous collapse and rotation of the face toward the opposite side.[529] Associated clinical findings

are limited neck motion, headache, and severe peripheral arthritis.

In the presence of an eroded odontoid process, the atlas may assume a more posterior position in relation to the axis (Fig. 26–61). Rarely, the anterior arch of the atlas may move up and then over the odontoid process, resulting in posterior atlantoaxial subluxation.[531, 532, 611] Other pathologic aberrations allowing posterior atlantoaxial subluxation are incompetence of the anterior arch of the atlas and fractures of the odontoid process.[612, 613]

The clinical course of patients with atlantoaxial subluxation is variable. In some persons, only mild symptoms and signs appear, which do not progress. In others, clinical and radiographic deterioration becomes evident (the distance between the anterior arch of the atlas and the odontoid process can reach 12 to 15 mm), and the patient may de-

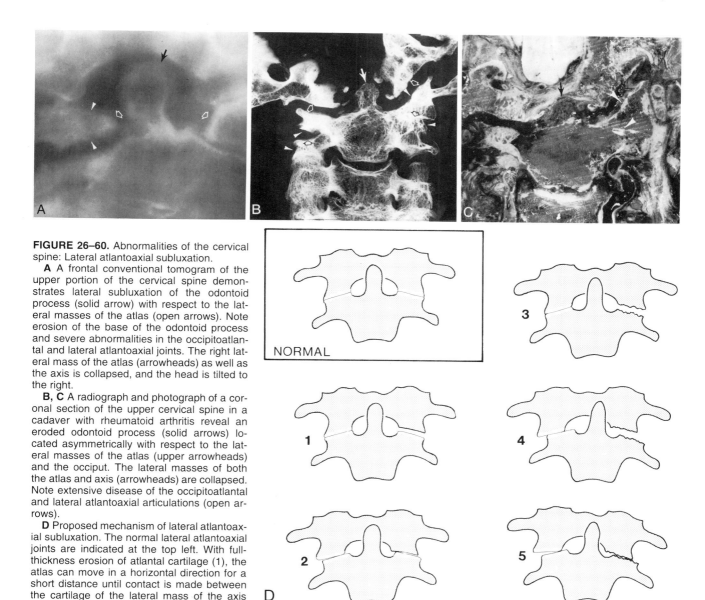

FIGURE 26–60. Abnormalities of the cervical spine: Lateral atlantoaxial subluxation.

A A frontal conventional tomogram of the upper portion of the cervical spine demonstrates lateral subluxation of the odontoid process (solid arrow) with respect to the lateral masses of the atlas (open arrows). Note erosion of the base of the odontoid process and severe abnormalities in the occipitoatlantal and lateral atlantoaxial joints. The right lateral mass of the atlas (arrowheads) as well as the axis is collapsed, and the head is tilted to the right.

B, C A radiograph and photograph of a coronal section of the upper cervical spine in a cadaver with rheumatoid arthritis reveal an eroded odontoid process (solid arrows) located asymmetrically with respect to the lateral masses of the atlas (upper arrowheads) and the occiput. The lateral masses of both the atlas and axis (arrowheads) are collapsed. Note extensive disease of the occipitoatlantal and lateral atlantoaxial articulations (open arrows).

D Proposed mechanism of lateral atlantoaxial subluxation. The normal lateral atlantoaxial joints are indicated at the top left. With full-thickness erosion of atlantal cartilage (1), the atlas can move in a horizontal direction for a short distance until contact is made between the cartilage of the lateral mass of the axis and the denuded osseous surface of the lateral mass of the atlas (2). Alternatively, cartilaginous and osseous erosion of apposing surfaces of atlas and axis (3) allows greater offset between the two bones. Movement continues until the medial margin of the lateral mass of the atlas contacts the odontoid process (4). The head now can tilt toward the side of involvement (5).

(**D**, Modified from N Bogduk, GAC Major, J Carter: Ann Rheum Dis *43*:341, 1984).

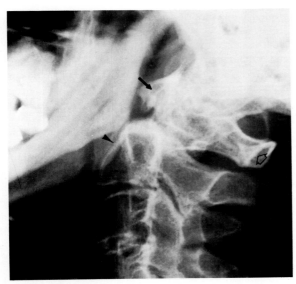

FIGURE 26–61. Abnormalities of the cervical spine: Posterior atlantoaxial subluxation. A lateral radiograph reveals posterior displacement of the anterior arch of the atlas (solid arrow) with respect to the axis (arrowhead) owing to erosion of the odontoid process. Note the malalignment of the spinolaminar line of the atlas (open arrow) with respect to that of the other vertebrae.

velop disabling neurologic abnormalities that require operative intervention to ensure stability.[327, 344–346, 797] In a study of the clinical significance of atlantoaxial subluxation in patients with rheumatoid arthritis, Weissman and collaborators[527] made the following observations: The critical distance of anterior subluxation was 9 mm, as patients with lesser degrees of subluxation did not develop cord compression if atlantoaxial impaction were absent; there was no correlation between the radiographic progression of subluxation and the development of spinal cord compression; and cord compression was more likely to occur in men, in the presence of atlantoaxial impaction, and possibly in the presence of lateral atlantoaxial subluxation. Boden and coworkers[797] emphasized the correlations of the posterior atlantoodontoid interval (and the diameter of the subaxial sagittal canal) with the presence and severity of paralysis. Occasional reports of spontaneous improvement in radiographic abnormalities[347] may indicate an illusion due to vertical deterioration in a spine that already is the site of anteroposterior C1-C2 displacement (Fig. 26–59B, C).[328, 539]

Odontoid Process Erosion. Odontoid process erosions have been detected in 14 to 35 per cent of patients with rheumatoid arthritis, varying with the severity of the disease.[330] They occur as the natural consequence of synovial inflammation in adjacent articulations (Fig. 26–62). Thus, they predominate in the osseous portions that are intimate with the synovium-lined spaces between the anterior arch of C1 and the anterior aspect of the odontoid process, and between the posterior surface of the odontoid process and the transverse ligament. At both of these sites, early superficial erosions can be difficult to detect on routine radiography and may require conventional tomography for adequate evaluation. On radiographs and conventional tomograms, the lateral projection is best. With progression, larger scalloped defects appear that can surround the base of the dens circumferentially. Furthermore, defects of the

odontoid tip at sites of ligamentous attachment and of the base of the odontoid process related to the nearby lateral atlantoaxial joints also can be seen.

Further erosion of the odontoid process, which usually is associated with atlantoaxial subluxation, can lead to considerable osteolysis.[348] The dens may be reduced to a small osseous spicule that resembles the hypoplastic odontoid process seen in a variety of congenital disorders. With severe dissolution of the odontoid process, it rarely may slip beneath the transverse ligament, leading to anterior atlantoaxial subluxation with an intact ligamentous structure.[315] In addition, pathologic fracture of the weakened dens can be seen in patients after minimal trauma.[349, 457] The fracture line commonly is irregular, passing through erosions of the anterior and posterior surfaces of the bone. In these cases, the anterior arch of the atlas and the superior odontoid fragment move forward as a unit during flexion of the neck, documenting the intactness of the transverse ligament. Progressive resorption and disappearance of the superior fragment also can be detected, a situation similar to that noted after odontoid process fractures in patients without rheumatoid arthritis.[350]

Local sclerosis can accompany odontoid process erosions. Rarely, bony proliferation becomes more marked, with periostitis along the anterior aspect of the dens.[330] An identical finding is detected more frequently in ankylosing spondylitis. Bony production with eburnation and osteophytosis can be apparent in any of the atlantoaxial joints in long-standing rheumatoid arthritis.

Other Manifestations. Loss of interosseous space and superficial and deep subchondral erosions can be seen in all the synovial articulations between the occiput, the atlas, and the axis in patients with rheumatoid arthritis. Reactive sclerosis about eroded areas is unusual. Atlantoaxial rotatory subluxation has been observed in rheumatoid arthritis but has not been fully described.[700] Bony ankylosis between occiput and atlas or atlas and axis and atlanto-occipital subluxations or dislocations[614] occasionally are apparent.

Subaxial Articulations

Subaxial Subluxation and Dislocation (Fig. 26–63). Subluxation of varying severity is observed at one or more subaxial levels in patients with rheumatoid arthritis.[329–331, 351–353, 615, 616, 700] The frequency of these abnormalities, which have been noted in 9 per cent of unselected clinic patients,[330] increases with the chronicity and severity of the articular disorder. Associated myelopathy occurs,[536] is uncommon, and may be related in some cases to cervical cord compression by extradural granulation tissue.[541] Frequently the subluxations are of slight or moderate degree, although cases of subaxial dislocation also are encountered.[615] When localized to one area, changes are particularly characteristic at the C3-C4 and C4-C5 levels[331]; however, multilevel subluxations are more typical, producing a "doorstep" or "stepladder" appearance on lateral radiographs. The degree of subluxation is not uniform at all areas in multilevel disease. Anterior subluxation is far more frequent than posterior subluxation.

In most cases, subluxations are not fixed in the abnormal position. Rather, changes in alignment can be demonstrated on lateral radiographs taken during flexion and extension of the neck. In fact, a normally aligned cervical spine in a neutral position can reveal considerable subluxation at multiple levels during flexion of the neck.

Patients have been described with significant subluxation at multiple levels of the cervical spine who developed quadriplegia and massive osteolysis about joints of the upper extremity, perhaps related to their neurologic deficit[354, 535] (see Chapter 25).

Apophyseal Joint Abnormalities (Fig. 26–63). In the apophyseal joints of the subaxial region, joint space narrowing and superficial erosions are common. Sclerosis is not characteristic. In extreme cases, articular disorganization is evident. During flexion of the neck, instability produces tilting of the lateral masses of one vertebra on the next, with abnormal widening of the articular spaces. Generally, fibrous ankylosis is the terminal event; however, bony ankylosis of one or more articulations can be seen,[539] and, in rare instances, ankylosis of these joints throughout the cervical spine can produce an appearance that simulates that of ankylosing spondylitis.[617]

Discovertebral Joint Abnormalities (Fig. 26–64). At the discovertebral junction of the cervical spine in rheumatoid arthritis, intervertebral disc space narrowing, subchondral osseous irregularity, and adjacent eburnation are the typical findings. The pathogenesis of these discovertebral lesions is a subject of great debate (see Chapter 25); trauma due to apophyseal joint instability with intraosseous displacement of discal material (cartilaginous nodes[355]) and extension of abnormal synovium-like tissue from the adjacent joints of Luschka[356] are the two suggested mechanisms that currently are most popular. Erosions can be confined to one aspect of the junction, usually the posterior, or diffusely involve the entire joint. Surrounding eburnation also can be localized or generalized in distribution. Multiple levels of the cervical spine typically are affected.

A characteristic manifestation of rheumatoid discitis is the absence of osteophytosis. Thus, considerable subchondral irregularity and erosion, intervertebral disc space narrowing, and sclerosis can be seen without osteophyte formation. The absence of osteophytes serves to distinguish the cervical spinal abnormalities of rheumatoid arthritis from those of degenerative disc disease (intervertebral osteochondrosis and spondylosis deformans).

Spinous Process Erosions (Fig. 26–65). Erosions and destruction of one or more spinous processes can be detected, particularly in the lower cervical (and upper thoracic) region. Martel observed such abnormalities in 11 per cent of 100 rheumatoid arthritis patients.[330] Tapered and sharpened spinous elements can be related to inflammation of the adjacent supraspinous ligaments or neighboring bursae.[534] In the presence of severe disc space loss at any level in the cervical spine, close approximation and contact of neighboring spinous processes can lead to pressure resorption with interdigitation of adjacent osseous surfaces.[329]

Osteoporosis. Generalized osteoporosis of cervical vertebrae is common in this disease and, in some cases, is aggravated by the administration of corticosteroids. The exaggerated radiolucency of the vertebral bodies can accentuate radiographically evident eburnation that is encountered about the discovertebral junctions.

Diffuse Locations. Although the foregoing discussion has used a regional approach to cervical spine changes, diffuse involvement of the entire cervical spine is common, particularly in long-standing rheumatoid arthritis (Table 26–2).[447, 540] The resulting radiographic picture, consisting of atlantoaxial subluxation, odontoid and apophyseal joint

TABLE 26–2. Cervical Spine Abnormalities in Rheumatoid Arthritis

Occipitoatlantoaxial Articulations
Atlantoaxial subluxation
Odontoid erosion and fracture
Apophyseal joint erosion, sclerosis, and fusion

Subaxial Articulations
Subaxial subluxation
Apophyseal joint erosion, sclerosis, and fusion
Intervertebral disc space narrowing
Erosion and sclerosis of vertebral body margins
Spinous process erosion
Osteoporosis

erosions, subaxial subluxations, intervertebral disc space narrowing, marginal sclerosis of vertebrae, and spinous process destruction, is virtually pathognomonic of this disease. The degree of atlantoaxial subluxation may correlate well with the severity of other rheumatoid changes in the cervical spine, especially vertebral endplate and spinous process erosions and intervertebral subluxations.[329, 357] It also may correlate with seropositivity for rheumatoid factor and is more prevalent in men than in women if an equal number of patients of both sexes are examined. Certain features, such as subluxation, have been correlated with the administration of corticosteroids, perhaps owing to exaggerated osseous and tendinous weakening.[359] Furthermore, an association between cervical and peripheral arthritis has been recorded.[359, 360, 537]

Some investigators have suggested that specific radiographic findings in the cervical spine occur in 30 per cent or more of patients with rheumatoid arthritis with a disease duration of less than 10 years.[697] These findings are odontoid erosions, subaxial subluxations, superficial apophyseal joint erosions, and both apophyseal joint sclerosis and discovertebral joint narrowing with osteophytosis at the fourth through seventh cervical levels. Some of these abnormalities, such as subaxial subluxations and superficial apophyseal joint erosions, may not increase in frequency in subsequent decades of disease, whereas others, such as erosions of the odontoid process, eventually may become more common.[697]

Other Joints

Rheumatoid arthritis affects other articulations. These include the temporomandibular joint,[401–405, 618, 712–714, 788, 789] the cricoarytenoid joint,[406–409, 449, 619, 642] and perhaps even the articulations of the inner ear.[410] At the temporomandibular joint, radiographic changes include erosions, osteoporosis, joint space narrowing, decreased range of motion, and flattening of the glenoid fossa of the temporal bone (Fig. 26–66). These abnormalities, which may be evident in as many as 80 per cent of patients (compared to 34 per cent of "normal" controls)[411] are more apparent on conventional tomograms or CT scans than on routine radiographs, may be detected with MR imaging, and are similar to changes of ankylosing spondylitis and psoriasis.[405] In rheumatoid arthritis, asymmetric abnormalities and increased destruction of the temporomandibular joint have been associated with an edentulous state.[524]

Text continued on page 938

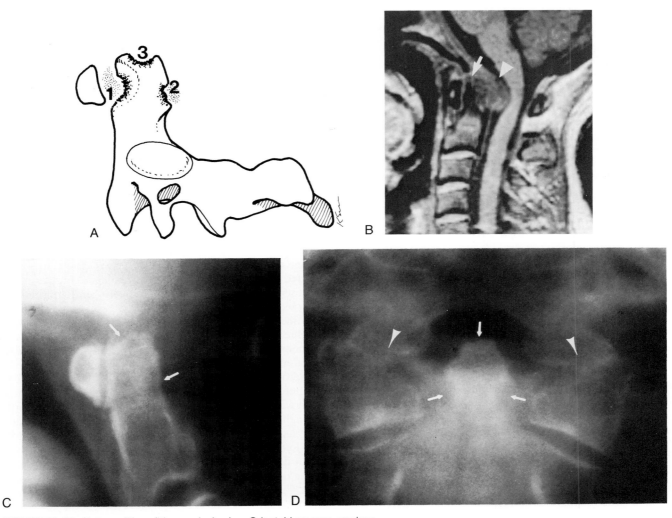

FIGURE 26–62. Abnormalities of the cervical spine: Odontoid process erosions.

  A Odontoid process erosions occur in areas that are intimate with the synovial articulations between the anterior arch of the atlas and the dens (1) and between the dens and the transverse ligament of the atlas (2) and in areas that are intimate with the ligamentous attachments (3) at the tip of the odontoid process.

  B A sagittal multiplanar gradient echo (MPGR) MR image (TR/TE, 300/9; flip angle, 15 degrees) reveals prominent synovial inflammation in the posterior median atlantoaxial joint (arrowhead) with erosion of the odontoid process (arrow) and compression of the spinal cord.

  (**B**, Courtesy of S. Moreland, M.D., San Diego, California.)

  C A lateral conventional tomogram illustrates osseous erosion at the tip and posterior surface of the dens (arrows) in this rheumatoid arthritis patient.

  D A frontal conventional tomogram reveals erosion on the lateral aspect and tip of the dens (arrows). Note joint space narrowing between the occiput and atlas (arrowheads).

Illustration continued on opposite page

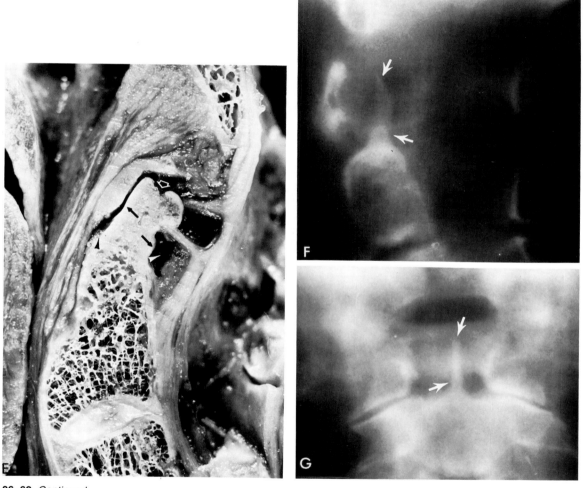

FIGURE 26–62. *Continued*

E In a photograph of a macerated sagittal section of the axis, observe the erosion of the odontoid process (solid arrows) related to synovial proliferation in the posterior and anterior median atlantoaxial joints (arrowheads). The tip of the odontoid process also is eroded (open arrow).

F, G Lateral and frontal conventional tomograms reveal severe destruction of the odontoid process (arrows), which has been reduced to an irregular, pointed protuberance.

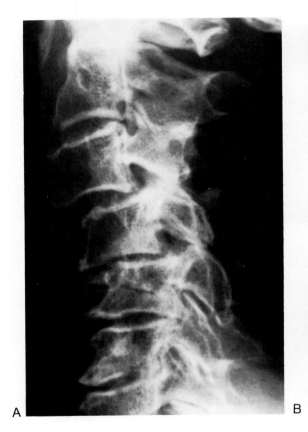

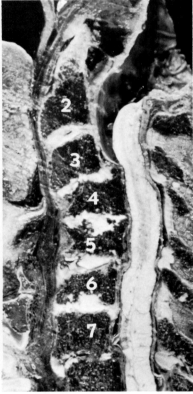

FIGURE 26–63. Abnormalities of the cervical spine: Subaxial subluxation and apophyseal joint changes.

A Note the "stepladder" appearance due to subluxation at multiple cervical levels associated with narrowing of the intervertebral disc spaces and narrowing, sclerosis, and subluxation of the apophyseal joints.

B In a photograph of a sagittal section of a rheumatoid spine, subaxial subluxation is most evident in the middle cervical region (vertebral bodies are numbered). Observe compression of the anterior aspect of the spinal cord by the fourth and fifth vertebral bodies and extensive discovertebral irregularity.

FIGURE 26–64. Abnormalities of the cervical spine: Discovertebral joint changes.

A On this lateral radiograph observe narrowing of multiple intervertebral discs and irregularity and sclerosis of adjacent vertebral surfaces (arrows). These findings in the absence of osteophytes strongly suggest the diagnosis of rheumatoid arthritis.

B On a radiograph of a sagittal section of a cervical spine in a cadaver with rheumatoid arthritis, note the loss of intervertebral disc height at the C6-C7 level with "erosion" and sclerosis of the vertebral bodies. The findings are reminiscent of those in infective spondylitis.

C A coronal section of the cervical spine in a cadaver with rheumatoid arthritis delineates inflammatory changes in the joints of Luschka (arrows), discal fissuring, and narrowing of the intervertebral disc spaces (arrowheads).

(**C** Courtesy of E. G. L. Bywaters, M.D., London, England.)

D In another cadaver with rheumatoid arthritis, a photograph of a coronal section of the lower cervical spine demonstrates, at multiple levels, considerable destruction in the joints of Luschka (arrows) and adjacent intervertebral discs.

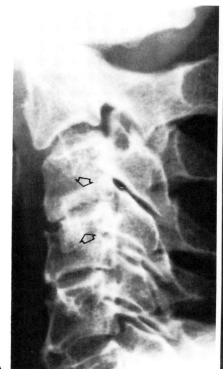

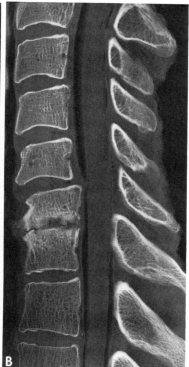

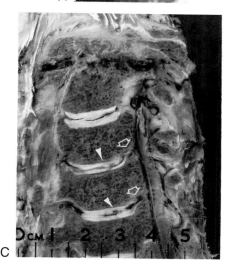

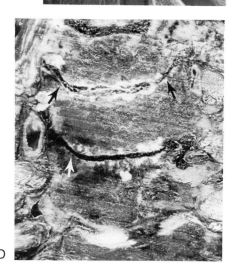

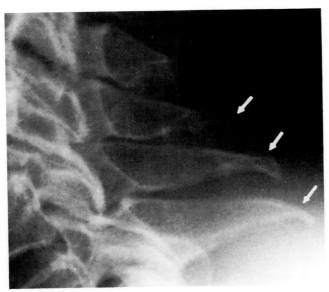

FIGURE 26–65. Abnormalities of the cervical spine: Spinous process erosions. The spinous processes in the lower cervical spine are sharpened or tapered (arrows). Apophyseal joint alterations also are seen.

Cricoarytenoid and cricothyroid joint alterations lead to hoarseness, pain radiating to the ears, and dyspnea.[9] Dyspnea is related, in part, to the presence of a narrow rima glottidis due to ankylosis of the cricoarytenoid articulation, which can result in respiratory obstruction. Laryngoscopy outlines inflammatory swelling of the arytenoid cartilage, thyroid cartilage, and vocal cords, which may become paralyzed. Radiologic detection of cartilaginous destruction is difficult[521] and may require low voltage technique[522] or CT.[642] Histologic evaluation reveals an acute phase charac-

terized by synovitis, joint effusion, and synovial proliferation, and a chronic phase associated with pannus formation, joint destruction, and fibrous ankylosis or, rarely, bony ankylosis.[523] Rheumatoid nodules have been identified in the larynx.[523]

Arthritis of the articulations of the inner ear is reported in patients with rheumatoid arthritis, although the pathogenesis of the abnormalities in this site is debated. Indeed, the precise anatomic characteristics of the ossicular joints is not agreed upon.[715]

COEXISTENT OSSEOUS AND ARTICULAR DISEASE

Septic Arthritis

Infections are frequent in rheumatoid arthritis patients, especially after the introduction of steroids and immunosuppressive agents.[361] Pulmonary infections (including bronchitis, bronchiectasis, pneumonia, abscess, and empyema),[362–364] skin infections, osteomyelitis,[546] and septic arthritis[365–367] all have been noted. Commonly, these infections are silent clinically, unaccompanied by fever or leukocytosis.[363]

The cause of the increased susceptibility to infection in rheumatoid arthritis patients is not known.[368, 656] Investigators have indicated that the response of polymorphonuclear leukocytes to chemotaxis is impaired in adult and juvenile patients with rheumatoid arthritis,[369] although results of studies have not been uniform in this regard.[620] Leukocytes in the joint fluid in rheumatoid arthritis may demonstrate decreased phagocytosis of bacteria.[370] Decreased antigenic stimulation of IgM in rheumatoid arthritis patients also has been noted.[371] Bacteriolytic activity of sera and synovial fluid from patients with rheumatoid arthritis is low compared with that from normal persons or patients with os-

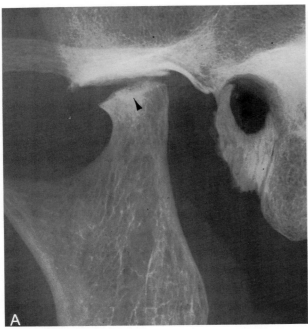
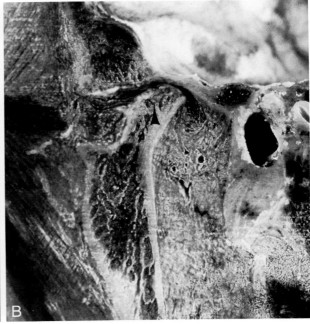

FIGURE 26–66. Abnormalities of the temporomandibular joint. In a sagittal section of the temporomandibular joint in a cadaver with rheumatoid arthritis, a radiograph **(A)** and photograph **(B)** document flattening and sclerosis of the mandibular condyle (arrowheads) and glenoid fossa, joint space narrowing, and partial destruction of the intra-articular disc.

teoarthritis.[372] It also is possible that any chronically arthritic joint is predisposed to infection.[717] The marked neovascularity of the subsynovium in the arthritic joint may become plugged by microorganisms, leading to focal ischemia of the subsynovial tissue and subchondral bone.[718] All of these observations may have relevance to the higher frequency of infection that occurs in rheumatoid arthritis.

The reported frequency of suppurative arthritis in patients with rheumatoid disease has varied from less than 1 per cent[365, 366, 373] to 12 per cent.[374] Two to 50 per cent of patients with suppurative arthritis may have underlying rheumatoid arthritis.[375–378] Indeed, rheumatoid arthritis appears to be the most common predisposing factor to septic arthritis. Many series of patients with both suppurative and rheumatoid arthritis have been reported in the literature.[376, 379–387, 621] Pyarthrosis is more frequent in elderly rheumatoid arthritis patients with severe disability.[379] In most patients, nodular erosive disease has been present for 10 to 20 years.[379, 381] Systemic steroid medication had been administered in most reported cases,[379, 388] although septic arthritis may appear in rheumatoid arthritis patients treated with other medications.[380] In the majority of persons, the source of the joint infection is obvious; it may be an ulcerating nodule, an infected prosthesis, a skin infection, or an intraarticular injection.[366, 380, 381] Additional sources of sepsis have included urinary tract infection, pneumonia, and sinusitis.[379] The most frequently reported infecting organism has been *Staphyloccocus aureus*[376, 380–385, 790]; other agents have included coliform bacteria,[376, 382, 383] Pasteurella,[389] Streptococcus,[379, 381, 385, 455] Haemophilus,[390] pneumococcus,[378, 391] *Pseudomonas aeruginosa*,[383] Salmonella,[385] *Bacteroides fragilis*,[387, 544] and *B. melaninogenicus*,[543] fungi,[545, 716] and mycobacteria.[456] Tuberculous articular infection has been described as a complication of rheumatoid arthritis.[542, 790]

Septic arthritis complicating rheumatoid disease frequently affects multiple joints[376]; it is more unusual to find polyarticular involvement in uncomplicated septic arthritis in the adult patient. Although any joint can be infected in rheumatoid arthritis patients, the knee is the most common site of pyarthrosis; other sites include the wrist, the elbow, the glenohumeral joint, the ankle, the hip, the sacroiliac joint, and the metacarpophalangeal and metatarsophalangeal joints. Sternoclavicular joint localization is not unusual[365, 366, 376, 392] and may have diagnostic significance.[379] The onset of pyarthrosis in the person with rheumatoid arthritis may produce only subtle clinical changes; a source of infection, onset of chills, or any deterioration in the clinical state should arouse suspicion of a superimposed articular infection.[548] An enlarging synovial cyst[558] and a soft tissue mass[559] are additionally reported signs of septic arthritis in patients with rheumatoid arthritis, although none of these findings is specific for infection.[622] Local pain and swelling of an involved joint may simulate exacerbation of the rheumatoid process. Furthermore, a syndrome of sterile arthritis that mimics septic arthritis occurs in persons with rheumatoid arthritis, increasing the difficulty of distinguishing between patients with rheumatoid arthritis alone and those with both rheumatoid arthritis and septic arthritis.[719] Joint aspiration to demonstrate a specific organism and to determine its response to antibiotics is essential for correct diagnosis and treatment. The importance of early diagnosis

TABLE 26–3. Radiographic Features of Septic Arthritis Complicating Rheumatoid Arthritis

Monoarticular or polyarticular distribution
Predilection for knee involvement
Asymmetric changes
Progressive soft tissue swelling and joint effusion
Rapid and poorly defined bony erosion

is underscored by the fact that infection constitutes the most common cause of death in rheumatoid arthritis patients.[361] The literature cites a mortality rate as high as 35 per cent in patients with suppurative arthritis complicating rheumatoid arthritis.[379, 382]

In most reported radiographic investigations,[376, 379, 380] cortical destruction and erosive abnormalities were noted but were difficult to distinguish from the underlying rheumatoid alterations (Table 26–3). It would appear, however, that certain radiographic observations are of diagnostic aid.[383, 385] Radiographic evidence of any rapid deterioration of a joint should be suspect. In particular, an enlarging soft tissue mass and a progressive effusion within a joint affected by rheumatoid arthritis in the absence of recent trauma must be viewed with caution, especially when the articular space becomes widened (Figs. 26–67 and 26–68). Asymmetric joint disease and poorly defined and rapid destruction of bone are other useful signs of infection in the patient with rheumatoid arthritis. Rarely, spontaneous dislocation is the presenting clinical and radiologic finding.[547] Imaging with bone-seeking radiopharmaceutical agents or gallium generally is not helpful in identifying those patients with rheumatoid arthritis who have septic arthritis as well,[549, 576] although exceptions to this rule occur (Fig. 26–69).

Amyloidosis

Disorders characterized by paraproteinemia, such as multiple myeloma, macroglobulinemia, and amyloidosis, may develop in rheumatoid arthritis[393, 557] (see Chapter 60). Perhaps prolonged antigenic stimulation of the reticuloendothelial system in patients with chronic rheumatoid arthritis terminates in neoplastic proliferation. Amyloid deposits commonly are noted within joints in rheumatoid arthritis.[394] Alternatively, articular manifestations of amyloid disease with or without multiple myeloma can simulate rheumatoid arthritis.[395, 396]

Gout

The coexistence of rheumatoid arthritis and gout is not common, although it is being reported with increasing frequency[458, 459, 550, 551, 657, 720] (see Chapter 43). Typically, men are affected, gout is the initial disease, and rheumatoid arthritis develops years later. The confirmation of the presence of both disorders in the same person is complicated by false positive serologic test results for rheumatoid factor in patients with chronic tophaceous and nontophaceous gout[397–399] and by overlap of clinical and radiologic features of one disease with the other.[400] Furthermore, persistent hyperuricemia may decrease the subsequent clinical expression of rheumatoid arthritis.[552]

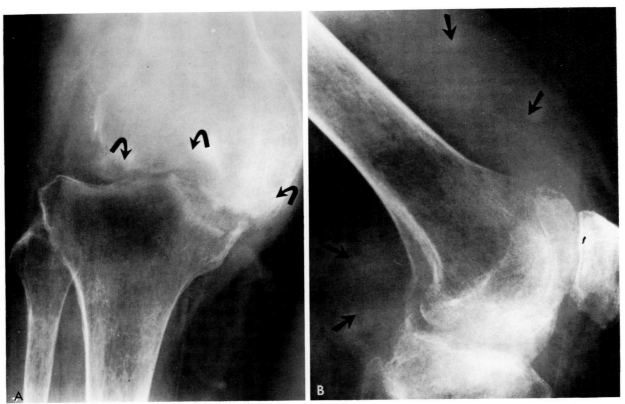

FIGURE 26–67. Rheumatoid arthritis (Still's disease) and septic arthritis. This 29 year old woman with Still's disease developed pain and swelling of the right knee of 2 weeks' duration. Aspiration of the knee yielded cultures of *Escherichia coli.* A large effusion (straight arrows) is evident. The bones are osteoporotic and the distal femoral surface is grossly irregular (curved arrows). Subluxation is seen. (From Resnick D: Radiology *114*:581, 1975.)

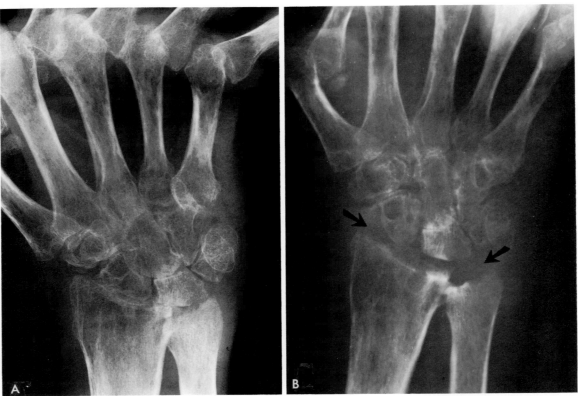

FIGURE 26–68. Rheumatoid arthritis and septic arthritis. A 47 year old man with advanced rheumatoid arthritis and vasculitis, being treated with steroids, underwent a right amputation below the knee for gangrene of the foot. Wrist swelling and pain subsequently were apparent, and cultures were positive for *Staphylococcus aureus.*

  A Initial radiographic examination demonstrates severe rheumatoid alterations, including osteoporosis, joint space narrowing, erosions, and subluxation.

  B Five months later, the radiocarpal joint is markedly widened (arrows). No change in the bony abnormalities is seen.

  (From Resnick D: Radiology *114*:581, 1975.)

940

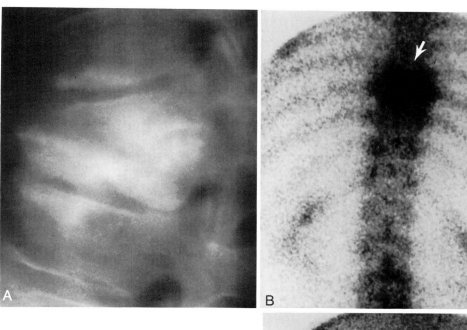

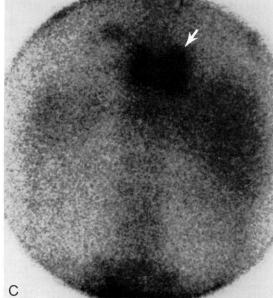

FIGURE 26–69. Rheumatoid arthritis and infection of the intervertebral disc. In this patient with long-standing rheumatoid arthritis, a subacute onset of back pain was associated with staphylococcal septicemia and documented infection of the intervertebral disc.

A The lateral radiograph of the lower thoracic spine shows collapse of adjacent vertebral bodies, destruction of the intervertebral disc, and bone eburnation. The appearance is that of infection, although similar abnormalities occasionally are encountered in rheumatoid arthritis patients who do not have superimposed infection.

B, C Technetium phosphate **(B)** and gallium **(C)** scans delineate accentuated radionuclide activity (arrows).

(Courtesy of V. Vint, M.D., San Diego, California.)

Calcium Pyrophosphate Dihydrate (CPPD) Crystal Deposition Disease

The coexistence of rheumatoid arthritis and calcium pyrophosphate dihydrate (CPPD) crystal deposition disease is encountered occasionally. This situation should be distinguished from that in which patients with CPPD crystal deposition disease alone demonstrate clinical manifestations resembling rheumatoid arthritis, the pseudo-rheumatoid arthritis pattern (see following discussion). It appears likely that the coexistence of true rheumatoid arthritis and CPPD crystal deposition disease is but a chance occurrence; however, accurate diagnosis of both disorders requires evaluation of the radiographs.[553] Radiographic examination outlines changes compatible with crystal deposition disease (intra- and periarticular calcification and pyrophosphate arthropathy) and others indicative of an erosive articular process (osteoporosis, marginal and central osseous erosions). Accurate interpretation of the radiograph is not difficult (Fig. 26–70). Bony erosion is not a manifestation of CPPD crystal deposition disease (see Chapter 44) and, when present, should arouse suspicion of a superimposed articular process. Similarly, calcification and an arthropathy resembling degenerative disease are not features of rheumatoid arthritis alone, so that the recognition of these atypical features, as well as others, including asymmetry and the absence of osteoporosis,[623] should suggest that a superimposed articular process may be present. Proper radiographic analysis is important, as clinical differentiation of rheumatoid arthritis and CPPD crystal deposition disease can be difficult. Some patients with CPPD crystal deposition disease show a pseudo–rheumatoid arthritis pattern of joint involvement, which is characterized by intermittent acute attacks of arthritis. In these latter persons, soft tissue swelling, intra- and periarticular calcification, joint space narrowing, osseous sclerosis, and fragmentation indicate severe manifestations of CPPD crystal deposition disease and should not be mistaken for rheumatoid arthritis.

Ankylosing Spondylitis

Rheumatoid arthritis and ankylosing spondylitis may coexist in the same patient (see Chapter 28). In these persons,

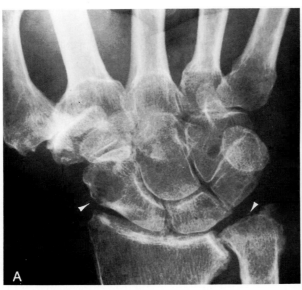
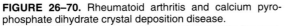
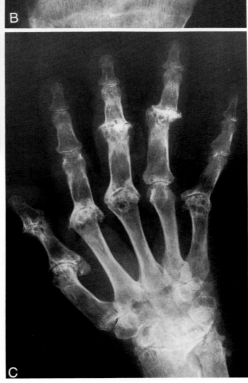

FIGURE 26–70. Rheumatoid arthritis and calcium pyrophosphate dihydrate crystal deposition disease.

A, B A 79 year old man had significant articular complaints in the hands, wrists, elbows, knees, and feet. Serum rheumatoid factor was positive in a titer of 1 to 512. In **A**, marginal erosions of rheumatoid arthritis in the radial styloid, midbody of the scaphoid, distal end of the ulna, and apposing portions of the radius and ulna (arrowheads) can be observed. No chondrocalcinosis is seen. In **B**, chondrocalcinosis within the cartilage of the knee is evident.

C In this 82 year old man with well-documented rheumatoid arthritis and a positive serologic test for rheumatoid factor (titer, 1 to 1024), calcium pyrophosphate dihydrate crystals were recovered from the knee. Observe severe abnormalities of the wrist and hand, representing a combination of rheumatoid arthritis and crystal deposition disease. Rheumatoid arthritis–like alterations include involvement of all wrist compartments, erosions of the distal portions of the radius and ulna, and marginal erosions and cysts within metacarpal heads and phalanges. The degree of bony sclerosis and the extent of osteophytosis are unusual features for uncomplicated rheumatoid arthritis and may be related to the superimposition of the crystalline disorder.

(From Resnick D, et al: Radiology *140*:615, 1980.)

clinical (symmetric peripheral joint disease, synovial thickening, subcutaneous nodules, and positive serologic test results for rheumatoid factor) and radiologic (osteoporosis, soft tissue swelling, joint space narrowing, marginal erosions, and deformities of peripheral articulations) manifestations of rheumatoid arthritis are combined with those of ankylosing spondylitis (axial skeletal disease with pain, tenderness, restricted motion, sacroiliitis and spondylitis, and the presence of the HLA-B27 antigen).[460, 554, 555, 721–724]

Diffuse Idiopathic Skeletal Hyperostosis

Not surprisingly, rheumatoid arthritis and diffuse idiopathic skeletal hyperostosis, both common disorders in middle-aged and elderly patients, may occur together.[412] In patients with both disorders, atypical clinical features include a high frequency of flexion contractures of the elbows, the ankles, the wrists, or the knees; atypical radiologic features include the absence of osteoporosis and the presence of bony sclerosis and proliferation about erosions, osteophytes, and intra-articular bony ankylosis (see Chapter 41).

Psoriasis and Pemphigoid

Persons with psoriatic skin disease can develop true rheumatoid arthritis with all of its clinical and radiologic manifestations. These patients must be distinguished from those with psoriatic arthritis, who reveal a symmetric rheumatoid arthritis–like distribution of articular disease and have negative serologic test results for rheumatoid factor (see Chapter 29).

Another skin disease, pemphigoid, has been noted in association with rheumatoid arthritis.[413, 414] In pemphigoid, which is a bullous cutaneous disorder occurring mainly in older persons, immunoglobulins and complement are bound in the dermoepidermal junction. In this regard, coexistence of pemphigoid with rheumatoid arthritis and other collagen vascular disorders may be more than a chance occurrence.[415, 416]

Collagen Vascular Disorders

Rheumatoid arthritis can be combined with other collagen vascular disorders (scleroderma, polyarteritis nodosa, systemic lupus erythematosus, and dermatomyositis) in various overlap syndromes and in mixed connective tissue disease (see Chapter 37). In some of these disorders (e.g., mixed connective tissue disease), specific laboratory parameters allow accurate diagnosis. In others, the exact nature of the disease is more perplexing and diagnosis is complicated by the occurrence of rheumatoid arthritis–like clinical and radiographic features in patients with ''pure'' collagen vascular disorders (e.g., scleroderma and systemic lupus erythematosus).

Pigmented Villonodular Synovitis and Giant Cell Tumor of Tendon Sheath

Pigmented villonodular synovitis is a diffuse proliferative synovial disorder of unknown cause usually confined to a single joint; giant cell tumor of a tendon sheath is a histologically similar process localized to the lining of a tendon

(see Chapters 84 and 95). Rarely, pigmented villonodular synovitis[417] or giant cell tumor[418, 419] can be evident in a joint or a tendon sheath of a patient with rheumatoid arthritis.[465] Although this combination of diseases may represent no more than a coincidence, it is possible that rheumatoid arthritis predisposes a person to develop pigmented villonodular synovitis or giant cell tumor of a tendon sheath. The observation that repeated hemorrhage can induce histologic changes similar to those of pigmented villonodular synovitis in an experimental situation[420] may indicate that bleeding in a joint affected by rheumatoid arthritis also could provoke such a reaction. It likewise is possible that under certain unknown circumstances, the characteristics of the proliferating synovium in rheumatoid arthritis change, leading to the histologic appearance of pigmented villonodular synovitis or a giant cell tumor of a tendon sheath.[513] As hyperplasia of the synovial lining in a pattern resembling pigmented villonodular synovitis has been identified also in osteoarthritis and ischemic necrosis of bone,[556] the stimulus for such synovial change may be the presence of intra-articular fragments of cartilage or bone. The diagnosis of pigmented villonodular synovitis or a giant cell tumor of a tendon sheath in patients with rheumatoid arthritis is difficult. An increasing effusion and progressive erosion in any joint affected by rheumatoid arthritis or the appearance of an asymmetric mass about an interphalangeal joint of a hand in a patient with rheumatoid arthritis in association with subjacent osseous destruction should arouse suspicion that one of these complicating conditions is present.

RADIOLOGIC ASSESSMENT OF DISEASE EXTENT AND PROGRESSION

Although the previous discussion would indicate that characteristic radiographic abnormalities occur during the course of rheumatoid arthritis and many such changes occur within the first few years of disease,[739, 740] certain limitations exist in the application of this technique to the assessment of disease extent and progression. The occurrence of normal irregular bony surfaces at such sites as the metacarpal and metatarsal heads and the phalanges of the hand creates difficulty in the accurate delineation of early osseous erosion in rheumatoid arthritis. Knowledge of the specific target areas of the disease and experience gained from analysis of a large number of rheumatoid arthritis patients are indispensable in correct radiologic interpretation; however, intraobserver and interobserver differences even among experts with regard to the presence of definite radiographic abnormality have been documented.[560, 644] Such differences by themselves, however, do not negate the value of any grading system if there is high correlation with regard to the manner in which two or more readers interpret the radiographs. That is, if two observers are consistent in their degree of differing opinion, the data conceivably still could be used in any scoring system that is devised (see subsequent discussion).[727]

The identification of an ideal series of radiographs in the evaluation of a patient with suspected rheumatoid arthritis is recognized as important by radiologists and rheumatologists alike but has led to a great deal of controversy and disagreement. Some investigators recommend a complete joint survey, others a limited survey, and a few are satisfied with one or two radiographs. Most authors agree that the key to the early and accurate radiographic diagnosis of rheumatoid arthritis lies in the analysis of the hands, wrists, and feet[643, 726, 731]; however, what constitutes the proper projections in each of these anatomic regions is debated. For example, with respect to the hands, proponents of a single posteroanterior radiograph can be found,[561] whereas other diagnosticians favor a more complete radiographic series that includes specialized projections of the digits.[562] Differences of opinion exist regarding the best radiographic views in other articular sites as well. Furthermore, the necessity of additional diagnostic techniques (see subsequent discussion) and specific radiographic screen-film systems[563] is not clear.

The limitation of radiography in the evaluation of the patient with rheumatoid arthritis is evident also by the difficulty encountered in establishing a grading system that can measure improvement or progression of disease. As osteoporosis, joint space narrowing, and bone erosion are considered characteristic radiographic features of rheumatoid arthritis, most attempts at grading the severity of articular involvement have emphasized one or more of these features.[726–728, 730, 735] Problems arise as a result of an independence in some cases of one radiographic feature with respect to another (e.g., progression of bony erosion with lack of progression of joint space loss) or of one joint with respect to another (e.g., progression of disease in the second metacarpophalangeal joint and absence of progression in the third metacarpophalangeal joint) and as a result of the difficulty in defining the changing size of an osseous erosion or the extent of joint space loss, especially in the presence of effusion, subluxation, or deformity.[733] Furthermore, how is the significance of a new radiographic finding weighed against the extension of an old one (e.g., bone erosion)?[564] How is the importance of intra-articular bony ankylosis in the wrist judged or how are the features of osteoarthritis in the hand separated from those of rheumatoid arthritis?[564]

Even if a standard radiographic examination with regard to projection and technique were established and an acceptable grading system based on specific site(s) and morphologic characteristics were developed, the precise relationship of clinical, laboratory, and radiologic findings in rheumatoid arthritis would be unclear. Although some studies indicate an association between radiologic progression and limitation of joint motion[566, 725] and between such progression and high values of the erythrocyte sedimentation rate as well as the presence of rheumatoid factor in the blood,[565] less correlation is reported between radiologic deterioration and joint swelling, joint tenderness, and rheumatoid nodules on clinical examination[566, 725] or between radiologic deterioration and the presence of antinuclear antibodies and the level of the Rose-Waaler titer on laboratory examination.[565] Although some investigators have found good correlation between specific radiographic abnormalities and particular clinical manifestations,[732] other researchers confirm the inconstant correlation of disease activity derived from clinical, laboratory, and radiologic parameters.[567] These data are consistent with the observation that radiographic abnormalities in rheumatoid arthritis, reflecting bone and cartilage destruction, may progress or become stationary but are largely irreversible.[566] In general, radiographically evident bone erosions show little change in patients with significant clinical improvement[568]; in these

persons, the lack of progression of such erosions on radiographs may be a more reliable indicator of therapeutic success. Although radiographic evidence of healing of bone erosions, characterized by a decreased size and a sclerotic margin, has been recorded,[569, 736–738] it is infrequent and requires a period of observation that is quite long, usually a matter of years. Therefore, in planning a radiologic protocol that is appropriate in the patient receiving treatment for rheumatoid arthritis, physicians should use longer intervals between examinations and yet standardize radiographic technique. Such longer intervals generally are not successful in any study of rheumatoid arthritis in which a control population, consisting of rheumatoid arthritis patients receiving only placebo "medication," is included, as such persons may reveal clinical deterioration during the study period, necessitating a change in therapy.

The somewhat gloomy picture regarding radiographic assessment of patients with rheumatoid arthritis that has just been painted should not be considered evidence that the authors believe the situation is hopeless, without remedy. Rather, it should serve as a reminder that despite the presence of radiographic abnormalities in rheumatoid arthritis that can be predicted on the basis of an understanding of the pathology of the disease, further investigation is required to delineate the ideal manner in which to apply this technique and to place plain film radiography in its proper place alongside other available diagnostic methods, particularly scintigraphy and MR imaging.[729, 734] Such investigation currently is taking place (see subsequent discussion).[624, 645]

OTHER DIAGNOSTIC TECHNIQUES

Fine-Detail Radiography with Magnification

Fine-detail radiography with magnification, which is discussed in detail elsewhere in the book (Chapter 4), allows identification of subtle abnormalities, especially about the small joints of the hand and the foot and about the calcaneus, at a time when conventional radiographs are negative or equivocal.[421, 570–572, 625] Small erosions can be delineated at an early stage by disruption of the subchondral bone plate of the metacarpal and metatarsal heads and phalanges. In addition, this technique allows detection of soft tissue swelling and patterns of bone resorption (intracortical tunneling, trabecular thinning).

Low KV Radiography and Xeroradiography

Application of low KV radiography allows analysis of soft tissues by maximizing the low radiographic contrast between soft tissue structures[422] (see Chapter 5). In rheumatoid arthritis, this technique delineates capsular distention and periarticular edema at an early stage, before cartilaginous and osseous destruction become evident.[128, 423–425] It may be especially applicable to the joints of the hand, the wrist, and the foot, and it correlates better with clinical and scintigraphic findings than does routine radiography.

Xeroradiography represents an additional technique that is useful in the evaluation of soft tissue as well as cartilaginous and osseous structures[426–429, 573] (see Chapter 6). Bony erosions and joint space diminution are well evaluated by this technique. Abnormalities of the retrocalcaneal bursa and Achilles tendon also are identified.

Arthrography

Arthrography has a limited role in the routine evaluation of rheumatoid arthritis patients. In those persons in whom the diagnosis is unclear or in whom the differentiation of soft tissue swelling and synovial thickening is difficult, contrast opacification of joints will allow direct assessment of the presence and extent of synovial hypertrophy and inflammation (see Chapter 13). An irregular or corrugated appearance of the contrast material and lymphatic filling are two arthrographic signs of synovitis, although they are not specific for rheumatoid synovitis. In the wrist, arthrography delineates the integrity of ligamentous structures; intercompartmental communication in the wrist in rheumatoid arthritis documents defects in the intercarpal ligaments or the triangular fibrocartilage, although similar defects can be seen in other articular disorders, as well as in older patients without arthritis.

In certain situations, arthrography has a definite advantage over routine radiography in patients with rheumatoid arthritis. Rotator cuff disruption, synovial cysts (Fig. 26–71), and sinus tracts are definitively delineated during arthrographic examination. It may be used to delineate the synovial changes that occur during treatment of the disease.[574]

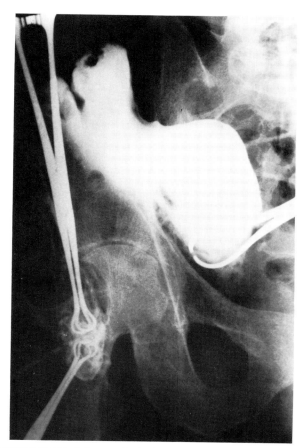

FIGURE 26–71. Arthrography in rheumatoid arthritis. Intraoperative arthrogram in a 50 year old man with rheumatoid arthritis, who had a mass in the groin, confirms the existence of a large synovial cyst arising from an abnormal hip and extending into the pelvis. (Courtesy of J. Scavulli, M.D., San Diego, California.)

Scintigraphy

As in other articular disorders, radionuclide examination using bone- or joint-seeking pharmaceutical agents represents a sensitive method for evaluating disease activity in rheumatoid arthritis[430–440, 646, 741, 742] (see Chapter 15). Technetium pertechnetate and technetium phosphate scans outline joint inflammation, which may antedate clinical activity, and these studies may be used to monitor response to therapy.[658] A typical abnormal radionuclide pattern in rheumatoid arthritis consists of a symmetrically distributed peripheral joint process that can be distinguished from that which is seen in the seronegative spondyloarthropathies.[439] In rheumatoid arthritis, activity usually is prominent in the wrist, the metacarpophalangeal and proximal interphalangeal (and occasionally the distal interphalangeal) joints of the hand, the metatarsophalangeal and interphalangeal joints of the foot, the knee, and the elbow (Fig. 26–72). Enhanced uptake of the radiopharmaceutical agent in the cervical spine, atlantoaxial region, and temporomandibular joint has been observed.[575] Accumulation in areas of bursitis and soft tissue nodules also can be seen. Gallium-67 and indium-111 have been used to investigate joint inflammation in patients with rheumatoid arthritis. As in the case of the technetium compounds mentioned earlier, increased accumulation indicates activity of the synovial disease.[576, 659, 798] Another technetium compound, technetium human immunoglobulin G, also has shown promise in the detection of synovial inflammation in rheumatoid arthritis.[791]

The total body retention of technetium phosphate compounds is elevated in persons with rheumatoid arthritis, a finding compatible with altered bone metabolism in the disease (see Chapter 25).

Computed Tomography

Although the application of CT scanning to the evaluation of disorders of the musculoskeletal system is discussed in detail in Chapter 8, a few comments related to the use of this technique in rheumatoid arthritis patients are appropriate here. CT generally is not required in assessing the distribution and the extent of joint involvement in this disease; plain film radiography, arthrography, and scintigraphy are superior in this respect. In certain locations, such as the foot[626, 627] and hip, the complexity of articular anatomy creates difficulty in accurate plain film diagnosis, especially in a patient with rheumatoid arthritis who manifests considerable bone destruction and deformity. Acetabular protrusion (Fig. 26–73) and ischemic necrosis of the femoral head are two examples of problems seen in patients with rheumatoid arthritis that can be evaluated with CT. In the former situation, the degree of displacement and the thickness of the acetabular floor can be determined, information that can be vital to an orthopedic surgeon planning total joint replacement. In the latter situation, distortion of the trabecular pattern within the femoral head, specifically alteration of the normal ''asterisk'' sign,[577] can be diagnostic of ischemic necrosis at a stage when plain films are normal or equivocally abnormal. It is clear, however, that CT does not allow the diagnosis of ischemic necrosis of the femoral head at an earlier stage than it can be identified by scintigraphy or MR imaging.

CT is well suited to the evaluation of para-articular

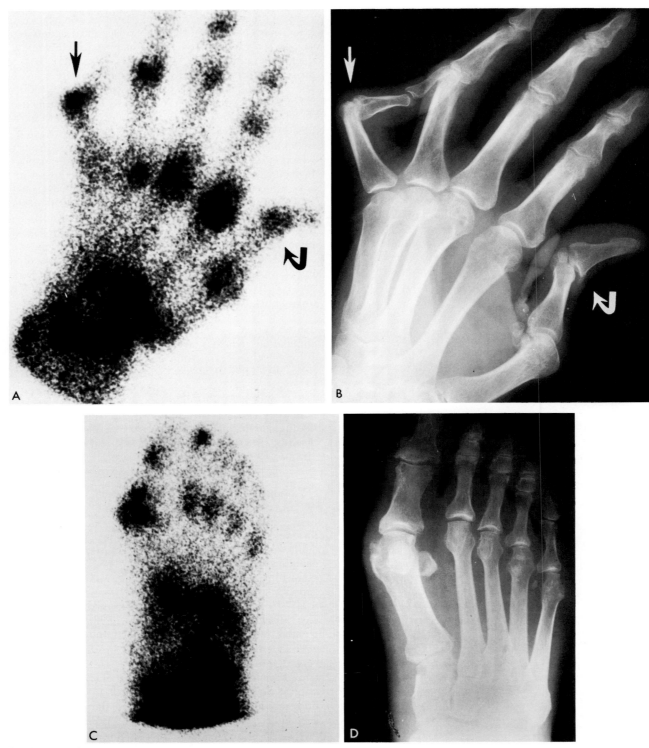

FIGURE 26–72. Scintigraphy in rheumatoid arthritis.
   A Radionuclide scan of right hand demonstrates uniform wrist activity and greater proximal than distal joint involvement. Note deformities of first (curved arrow) and fifth (arrow) digits.
   B Radiograph of same hand as in **A** shows typical deformities. Areas of greatest radionuclide activity correlate well with radiographic changes.
   C Radionuclide scan of left foot shows typical distribution of activity greatest in proximal joints. Corresponding symmetric abnormalities were seen in this patient's right foot.
   D Radiograph of same foot as in **C** reveals extensive erosive disease corresponding to sites of abnormality on the radionuclide scan. Again, marked radionuclide uptake is seen in areas of greatest radiographic change.
   (From Weissberg D, et al: AJR *131*:665, 1978. Copyright 1978, American Roentgen Ray Society.)

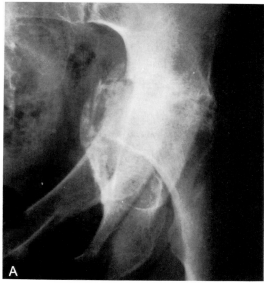

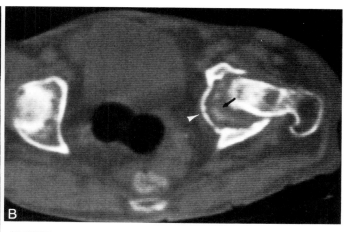

FIGURE 26–73. Computed tomography in rheumatoid arthritis. This 61 year old woman had a long history of rheumatoid arthritis. Four months prior to admission to the hospital, she fell at home and subsequently developed increasing pain in the hip. After evaluation, which included these imaging studies, a total hip arthroplasty was performed. At the time of surgery, a proliferative synovitis and fibrous tissue covering the acetabulum were evident. There was no evidence of infection.

A The routine radiograph reveals fragmentation of the femoral head and acetabulum, acetabular protrusion, and bone eburnation.

B On a transaxial section at the level of the hip, CT confirms the presence of a deformed femoral head. Intra-articular bone fragments are seen (arrow). Observe the thin acetabular shell (arrowhead) protruding into the pelvis. The opposite hip, not well shown at this level, was minimally abnormal.

masses, which, in rheumatoid arthritis, commonly are related to synovial cyst formation. Although in the knee, arthrography alone represents a direct way to outline such cysts, the combination of arthrography and CT is ideally applied to outlining synovial cysts in other locations, particularly the hip and shoulder. The exact extent and location of the mass and its relationship to regional blood vessels and nerves can be ascertained (Fig. 26–74).

CT has been advocated as a useful, noninvasive method in the diagnosis and management of cervical spine abnormalities in the rheumatoid arthritis patient. The craniocervical junction and atlantoaxial region are well displayed in the transaxial images obtainable with CT,[578–582, 647, 648] although multiplanar reconstruction of images occasionally is

required.[579, 580, 628] With regard to the atlantoaxial junction, CT has been reported to be a method by which the synovial tissue between the odontoid process and the transverse ligament can be evaluated and signs of impending rupture of the latter ligament can be delineated.[581] Similarly, at this level, additional manifestations of rheumatoid arthritis that can be assessed with CT have included spinal cord compression, erosions of the odontoid process, subluxation, and calcification,[581] although some of these latter abnormalities are equally well determined with other methods, including plain film radiography. In a comparison of CT and conventional radiography in the assessment of the upper cervical spine in patients with rheumatoid arthritis, Braunstein and collaborators[582] emphasized the importance of the latter

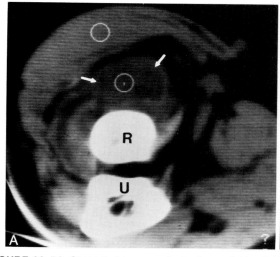

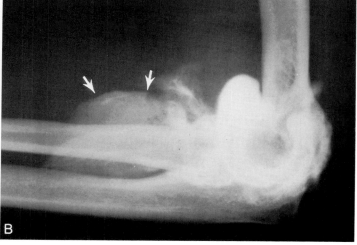

FIGURE 26–74. Computed tomography in rheumatoid arthritis. A 60 year old man with a long history of rheumatoid arthritis developed a mass about the elbow.

A A transaxial CT scan through the forearm identifies a cystic area (10 Hounsfield units) (arrows) adjacent to the radius (R) and ulna (U).

B Elbow arthrography with positive contrast agent results in opacification of the synovial cyst (arrows).

technique as the initial examination of choice. These investigators found that CT, with its unique capacity to allow transaxial imaging, was well suited to the visualization of the transverse ligament of the atlas and spinal cord, but it rarely provided additional *significant* information. Conversely, Raskin and associates[578] found that cord compression, as seen with CT, correlated well with clinically apparent neurologic status, and that CT was a useful and noninvasive technique in the assessment of atlantoaxial subluxation. These sentiments were echoed by other investigators,[579] who have reported that CT ideally allowed identification of alterations of the spinal canal, cord, and foramina and that the information that was generated by this technique could influence the surgeon's choice of an appropriate operative procedure.

One further application of CT is related to the diagnosis and the monitoring of osteopenia, specifically osteoporosis, in the axial skeleton of patients with rheumatoid arthritis and other disorders. This method of assessing bone mineral content is discussed in Chapter 52.

Ultrasonography

The many uses of ultrasonography as applied to the musculoskeletal system are discussed in Chapter 11. With regard to rheumatoid arthritis, ultrasonography has proved capable in the analysis of para-articular masses, such as synovial cysts and tendon sheath involvement (especially in the hands and wrists).[743–745]

Magnetic Resonance Imaging

The role of MR imaging in the assessment of musculoskeletal disorders has expanded dramatically during the last 10 years (see Chapters 9, 10, and 70). Although disagreement exists with regard to the precise scanning protocols that should be used, this imaging method can be applied effectively to the evaluation of the patient with rheumatoid arthritis. General applications of MR imaging in this evaluation include detection of articular disease, assessment of activity of such disease, determination of the nature of some of the complications of rheumatoid arthritis, and analysis of the extent of articular and para-articular changes in specific locations, such as the spine and temporomandibular joint.[746]

Preliminary data suggested that this technique was sensitive to changes in water composition and, therefore, allowed detection and localization of sites of inflammation. In rheumatoid arthritis, this sensitivity allowed the delineation of inflammatory articular effusions and their response to treatment.[583, 629, 649] Although such information could be obtained by joint examination and aspiration, MR imaging could be applied to the assessment of changes in those articulations (such as the hip and sacroiliac joint) that were deep and difficult to palpate with the hand or puncture with a needle. Early on, also, it became apparent that the technique allowed evaluation of intra-articular structures, such as hyaline cartilage and fibrocartilage, and of adjacent tendons and ligaments.[650, 651] Furthermore, MR imaging represented a safe and effective means to outline the extent of synovial cyst formation and the spinal cord.[583, 660]

It is now recognized that MR imaging is a very sensitive imaging method in the detection of articular diseases and that, in some instances, the imaging abnormalities depicted are almost specific for rheumatoid arthritis.[747–750] Descriptions have been published of the MR imaging appearance of rheumatoid arthritis changes in virtually all appendicular joints, although especially in those of the hand and foot, wrist, knee, and glenohumeral joint. Effusions, joint space narrowing, marginal erosions, and subchondral cystic lesions are among the described alterations, and some of these findings have been detected prior to their appearance on routine radiographs.[751, 752, 799] The specificity of the abnormalities, in part, is based on their distribution, with the application of the same diagnostic rules that are used in the interpretation of the routine radiographs. Accompanying changes in periarticular tendons and tendon sheaths can assist in this diagnosis.[753, 792] It should be noted, however, that the differentiation of synovial fluid and inflammatory synovial tissue, or pannus, in the rheumatoid joint on standard spin echo and gradient echo sequences may be difficult (although possible[793]), and modification of the MR imaging technique may be required in this situation (see subsequent discussion). Furthermore, although joint space loss can be inferred on the basis of the positions of the apposing bones about the involved joint, direct and accurate assessment of articular cartilage by MR imaging remains a problem, despite the multiple techniques that have been employed.[754, 794] Problems in this regard relate to the difficulties encountered in differentiating superficial portions of cartilage from joint fluid and deep portions of cartilage from subchondral bone and in detecting intrachondral signal alterations in a consistent fashion (see Chapter 70).

MR imaging has been used to assess the activity of rheumatoid arthritis and also its response to a variety of therapeutic regimens. A number of investigators have employed gadolinium-containing contrast agents injected intravenously, prior to the MR imaging examination, to better assess the extent of synovial proliferation in the rheumatoid joint.[662, 755–760, 795, 800, 803] If employed correctly, with the acquisition of MR images before and immediately after the injection of the gadolinium agent, differentiation of synovial inflammatory tissue and fluid is possible. On routine spin echo studies, without such injection, low intensity signal derives both from fluid and from pannus on T1-weighted images and high intensity signal characterizes both fluid and pannus on T2-weighted images. Immediately after intravenous injection of a gadolinium-containing agent, the effusion remains of low signal intensity on T1-weighted spin echo images, and the synovium demonstrates enhancement with increased signal intensity on these images (Figs. 26–75 to 26–78). Delayed imaging after intravenous injection of the contrast medium is characterized by seepage of contrast agent across the inflammatory pannus with an increase in the signal intensity of joint fluid on T1-weighted spin echo images. The changing pattern of distribution of gadolinium-containing agent in the joint has led some investigators to employ rapid gradient echo sequences to allow quantitative assessment of the rate of gadolinium accumulation in the synovial tissue.[757] Despite the nonspecific nature of the findings,[761] the use of intravenous injection of gadolinium contrast agent as an adjunct in MR imaging of joints involved in the rheumatoid process (or in other synovial inflammatory disorders) shows promise as a means to determine the extent of the process and its response to therapy.[758] It should be recognized, however, that the gadolinium compound is costly and that the examina-

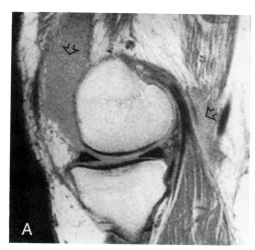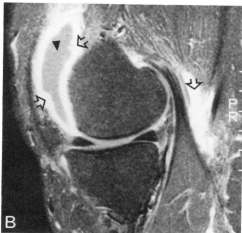

FIGURE 26–75. MR imaging in rheumatoid arthritis. Differentiation of effusion and pannus using intravenous gadolinium contrast agent.
A Initial proton density weighted parasagittal spin echo MR image (TR/TE, 1200/30) prior to intravenous injection of gadolinium compound reveals relatively low signal intensity of fluid or pannus, or both, in the knee joint and within a synovial cyst (open arrows).
B Immediately after the intravenous injection of the gadolinium agent, a proton density weighted parasagittal spin echo MR image (TR/TE, 1600/30), obtained with fat saturation technique (chemical shift saturation, or ChemSat), reveals enhancement of the inflamed synovial membrane in the joint and bursa (open arrows). The fluid (arrowhead) remains of low signal intensity.

FIGURE 26–76. MR imaging in rheumatoid arthritis. Differentiation of effusion and pannus using intravenous gadolinium contrast agent. This patient had an acutely swollen knee.

A A coronal T1-weighted spin echo MR image (TR/TE, 800/20) demonstrates collections of low signal intensity distributed throughout the knee (arrows).

B A coronal T2-weighted spin echo MR image (TR/TE, 2000/60) shows diffuse, nearly uniform brightening of these collections (arrows).

C A coronal T1-weighted spin echo MR image (TR/TE, 800/20) after the intravenous administration of gadolinium contrast agent allows clear distinction between joint fluid, which is of low signal intensity (arrows), and inflammatory pannus, which demonstrates enhancement with an increase in signal intensity (arrowheads).

(From Kursunoglu-Brahme S, et al: Radiology *176*:831, 1990.)

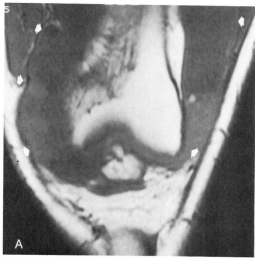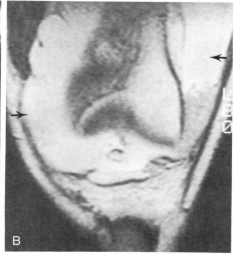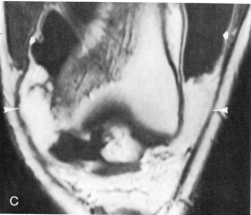

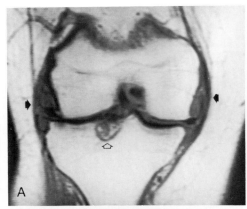
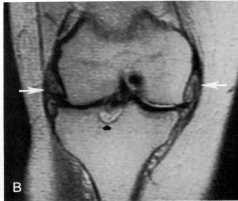
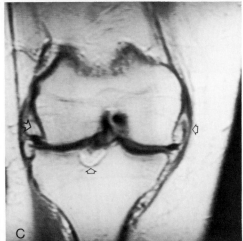

FIGURE 26–77. MR imaging in rheumatoid arthritis. Differentiation of effusion and pannus using intravenous gadolinium contrast agent.

A A coronal T1-weighted spin echo MR image (TR/TE, 800/20) shows small collections of low signal intensity on either side of the joint (solid arrows). An erosion is evident in the proximal portion of the tibia (open arrow).

B A coronal T2-weighted spin echo MR image (TR/TE, 2000/60) reveals slight to moderate enhancement of these collections (large arrows). The osseous erosion in the tibia also appears brighter (small arrow).

C A coronal T1-weighted spin echo MR image (TR/TE, 800/20) obtained immediately after the intravenous administration of gadolinium contrast agent shows diffuse, fairly uniform enhancement of the collections (open arrows). These collections represent pannus; no evidence of a joint effusion is present.

(From Kursunoglu-Brahme S, et al: Radiology *176*:831, 1990.)

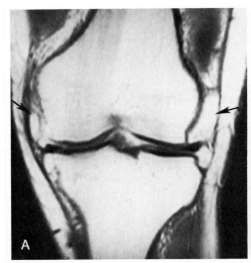
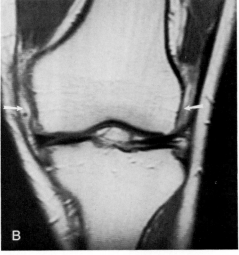

FIGURE 26–78. MR imaging in rheumatoid arthritis: Monitoring of response to treatment using intravenous gadolinium contrast agent.

A Prior to treatment, a coronal T1-weighted spin echo MR image (TR/TE, 800/20) obtained immediately after the intravenous injection of gadolinium contrast agent reveals collections of enhanced signal intensity (arrows), representing inflammatory pannus.

B One month after arthrocentesis and treatment with intra-articular steroids, a repeat coronal T1-weighted spin echo MR image (TR/TE, 800/20) obtained immediately after the intravenous injection of gadolinium agent shows a decrease in the amount of pannus (arrows) and a loss of signal intensity, presumably reflecting healing and fibrosis of the synovial inflammatory process.

(From Kursunoglu-Brahme S, et al: Radiology *176*:831, 1990.)

tion time is increased when images are required both before and after its injection. Furthermore, it appears that some of the newer MR imaging sequences, such as three-dimensional or volumetric acquisition using gradient recalled echo techniques, such as gradient recalled acquisition in the steady state (GRASS) with spoiling (SPGR) or fast low-angle shot (FLASH), when combined with fat suppression, or newer methods, such as magnetization transfer contrast sequences, may allow differentiation of inflamed synovium and fluid without the requirement for the intravenous injection of gadolinium agent.[804]

A variety of musculoskeletal complications of rheumatoid arthritis are well evaluated with MR imaging. These include, but are not limited to, ischemic necrosis of bone (see Chapters 70 and 80), bursitis, synovial cyst formation, tendon injury and disruption, and insufficiency fractures. Fluid collections and abnormal synovium within the iliopsoas, subdeltoid-subacromial, retrocalcaneal, olecranon, and prepatellar bursae (as well as other bursal cavities) are easily demonstrated with this technique (Fig. 26–79).[762, 764] Similarly, synovial cysts about any involved joint are delineated with MR imaging.[763, 765] In superficial articulations, such as the knee, ultrasonography is equally effective in the assessment of such synovial cysts, although in deeper locations, including the hip and spine, MR imaging has distinct advantages. Tendon injury and rupture, which may affect the hand, foot, knee, and shoulder in patients with rheuma-

toid arthritis, are best assessed with MR imaging. Disruption of the tendons of the rotator cuff, the quadriceps mechanism, and the tibialis posterior tendon are a few specific examples in which this imaging method can be very useful. Insufficiency fractures, an important complication of rheumatoid arthritis, occurring in the sacrum, femoral neck, parasymphyseal bone, tubular bones of the lower extremity, and elsewhere, reveal characteristic signal intensity abnormalities with MR imaging. For example, with standard spin echo techniques, such fractures demonstrate serpentine linear shadows of low signal intensity surrounded by larger regions of intermediate signal intensity on T1-weighted images, with the areas of intermediate signal, presumably representing surrounding edematous foci, becoming brighter on T2-weighted images. Indeed, MR imaging is at least equivalent and probably superior to bone scintigraphy with regard to its sensitivity in the detection of these fractures (see Chapters 67 and 70).

The evaluation of the rheumatoid spine with MR imaging deserves special emphasis (Figs. 26–80 and 26–81). Although this technique can be used to assess any spinal segment, most reports have emphasized its value when applied to the analysis of rheumatoid arthritis changes in the cervical region.[766–778, 801, 802] Abnormalities about the craniocervical junction are particularly well shown with MR imaging. In common with routine radiography, conventional tomography, and CT scanning, MR imaging allows assess-

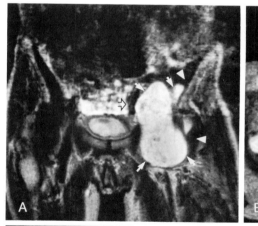

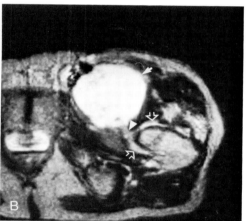

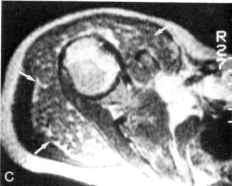

FIGURE 26–79. MR imaging in rheumatoid arthritis: Identification of bursitis.

A, B Iliopsoas bursitis. A 64 year old man with long-standing rheumatoid arthritis developed a progressively enlarging, painful mass in the left inguinal region. A coronal T2-weighted spin echo MR image (TR/TE, 2000/90) **(A)** shows the cyst (solid arrows) medial to the psoas muscle (arrowheads) and lateral to the external iliac vessels (open arrow). A transaxial T2-weighted spin echo MR image (TR/TE, 2000/90) **(B)** again reveals the cyst (solid arrow) with an opening (arrowhead) to a fluid-filled hip joint (open arrows). At surgery, a grossly dilated fluid-filled iliopsoas bursa, with chronically inflamed synovium, was identified.

(**A, B,** From Lupetin AR, Daffner RH: J Comput Assist Tomogr *14*:1035, 1990.)

C Subacromial bursitis. In this 34 year old woman, a transaxial T2-weighted spin echo MR image (TR/TE, 1800/70) shows the distended bursa (arrows) containing fluid of high signal intensity and areas of low signal intensity, perhaps representing fibrous synovial nodules.

(**C,** Courtesy of J. Milsap, Jr., M.D., Atlanta, Georgia.)

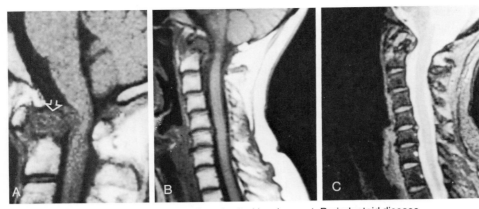

FIGURE 26–80. MR imaging in rheumatoid arthritis: Evaluation of spinal involvement. Periodontoid disease.
  A A sagittal T1-weighted spin echo MR image (TR/TE, 450/30) of the upper cervical spine reveals a mass of intermediate signal intensity (arrow) that is eroding the odontoid process and causing cord compression. (From Neuhold A, et al: Medicamundi *32*:38, 1987.)
  B, C Sagittal T1-weighted spin echo (TR/TE, 600/11) **(B)** and multiplanar gradient recalled (MPGR) **(C)** MR images show similar involvement in a different patient. Note the high signal intensity about the odontoid process in **C**. (Courtesy of C. Gundry, M.D., Minneapolis, Minnesota.)

ment of the relationship of the occiput, atlas, and axis and, therefore, is useful in delineating the extent of subluxation in this spinal segment. Also, in common with routine radiography, positions of flexion and extension of the patient's neck can be employed during MR imaging to accentuate the abnormal findings.[774, 802] In a departure from standard radiography, MR imaging allows direct visualization of the spinal cord so that sites of physical distortion of the cord by displaced vertebrae or inflammatory masses, or both, can be detected.[769] As indicated previously, several types of subluxation develop at the occipitoatlantoaxial

junction, and each, including anterior, vertical (cranial settling), lateral, and posterior displacement, is equally apparent on the MR images.[774] The severity of myelopathy correlates better with the MR imaging findings than those noted with conventional radiography,[766] a result that is not unexpected owing to the ability of the former method to allow direct assessment of altered soft tissues, especially retrodental pannus.[767, 770, 771, 775, 777] Medullary compression by the tip of the odontoid process in instances of cranial settling is far better appreciated on MR images than on standard radiographs.[775] In instances of cord compression,

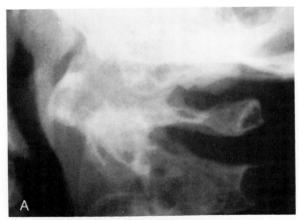

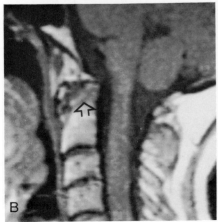

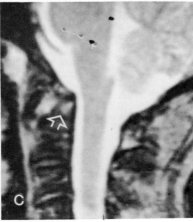

FIGURE 26–81. MR imaging in rheumatitis: Evaluation of spinal involvement. Periodontoid disease.
  A A routine radiograph reveals severe erosion of the odontoid process.
  B A sagittal T1-weighted spin echo MR image (TR/TE, 550/20) demonstrates the odontoid erosion (open arrow).
  C This erosion is seen to better advantage (open arrow) on a sagittal gradient echo (MPGR) image (TR/TE, 450/15; flip angle, 15 degrees). Note the bright signal between the anterior arch of the atlas and the eroded dens, reflecting abnormality in the median anterior atlantoaxial joint.

areas of abnormal signal intensity within the spinal cord itself, perhaps reflecting edema, have been detected in rheumatoid arthritis patients using MR imaging.[776] After stabilizing procedures, such as posterior occipitocervical fusion, the regions of inflammatory tissue may decrease in size when examined with MR imaging, suggesting that this method may be useful in the analysis of rheumatoid arthritis patients who reveal residual symptoms or develop new symptoms and signs in the postoperative period.[778] Although the advantages of MR imaging as an imaging method for the analysis of the cervical spine in patients with rheumatoid arthritis are obvious, the technique appears to be less effective in the evaluation of changes in the apophyseal joints and spinous processes.[772]

MR imaging has been used effectively to assess the temporomandibular joint in patients with rheumatoid arthritis and other rheumatic diseases.[662, 714] Alterations of the mandibular condyle, articular portions of the temporal bone, intra-articular disc, and adjacent soft tissues may be delineated, although some investigators favor arthrotomography in the early diagnosis of arthritic alterations at this site.[713]

ETIOLOGY

Only a few pertinent observations are recorded here; the interested reader should consult standard textbooks, which contain excellent discussions of potential causes of rheumatoid arthritis.[3, 441, 479]

The cause of rheumatoid arthritis is not known. Hypotheses suggesting that the disorder is due to a metabolic or nutritional factor, an endocrine disturbance, or a neurologic imbalance are unproved. No solid evidence is available currently to indicate an inherited genetic predisposition to rheumatoid arthritis, although the recently reported increased frequencies of the C and D locus histocompatibility antigens, HLA-Cw 3 and HLA-DRw 4, are interesting in this regard,[3, 442, 475, 476, 633, 779] and, in some instances, the presence of particular antigens has been correlated with the severity of radiographic abnormalities.[476, 661, 780] The specificity of these antigens as well as others[477] for rheumatoid arthritis is not so strong as the HLA-B27 locus for ankylosing spondylitis and associated diseases. Although many of the clinical and laboratory features of rheumatoid arthritis are consistent with infection, meticulous bacteriologic studies have failed to recover an infectious agent consistently from the blood, the synovial fluid, the synovial tissues, or the subcutaneous nodules.[441] Investigators have failed to transmit the disease from one person to another by injecting joint fluid.

Adequate evidence has now been accumulated to show that intra-articular immune complexes (antigen-antibody) that activate the complement system, stimulating inflammatory cellular infiltrates, exist in the abnormal synovium in rheumatoid arthritis.[3] Polymorphonuclear leukocytes phagocytose the immune complexes and release lysosomal enzymes, initiating or propagating the inflammatory synovitis.[443] A similar mechanism may be operational in the production of extra-articular lesions.[444] The elevated rate of immunoglobulin turnover and the abnormal immunocyte accumulation in the diseased synovium support the role of immunologic processes in rheumatoid arthritis. The specific antigen responsible for these processes has not been identified, however.

In recent years, the importance of the Epstein-Barr virus in the causation and the pathogenesis of rheumatoid arthritis has been considered. According to Depper and Zvaifler,[478] there are three basic ways in which this virus and rheumatoid arthritis might be related: (1) the virus could initiate the primary event in the disease through a direct infection of the articular cavity or through the formation of immune complexes; (2) the virus could enhance the production of rheumatoid factor and potentiate or perpetuate the intra-articular inflammation; and (3) the virus may not be handled well by patients with rheumatoid arthritis, resulting in an increased production of antibodies directed toward virus-related antigens. Of these possibilities, the second appears most attractive.

DIFFERENTIAL DIAGNOSIS

General Abnormalities

When a radiographic examination reveals a symmetrically distributed articular disorder affecting the proximal interphalangeal and metacarpophalangeal joints of the hands, the wrists, the metatarsophalangeal joints of the feet, the calcanei, the knees, and the elbows, characterized by osteoporosis, fusiform soft tissue swelling, concentric joint space loss, and marginal and central erosions, the diagnosis of rheumatoid arthritis is obvious. When the radiographs of rheumatoid arthritis patients disclose some degree of asymmetry, mild or absent osteoporosis, or preservation of joint space, an accurate appraisal is much more difficult. Fortunately, these latter features are not common in the disease, although they are observed occasionally.

Seronegative "Rheumatoid" Arthritis

Many patients with polyarticular inflammatory disease are serologically negative (seronegative) for rheumatoid factor, and the precise nature of their joint abnormality is variable and often not clear. As some of these persons fulfill other criteria for the disease, they indeed may have rheumatoid arthritis, although, in the absence of rheumatoid factor in the serum and the commonly associated absence of rheumatoid nodules, the remaining criteria for the disease are less specific and could be fulfilled by patients with other articular processes.[584, 805, 806] There is additional evidence to suggest that seronegative ''rheumatoid'' arthritis is not rheumatoid arthritis at all: (1) a disparity is seen in the prognosis of the disease in patients with and without rheumatoid factor; (2) certain clinical features, in addition to rheumatoid nodules, such as keratoconjunctivitis sicca, vasculitis, interstitial lung disease, and Felty's syndrome, are associated with seropositivity; and (3) a family history of disease is more frequent in those patients who are seropositive for rheumatoid factor.[584] Of course, these data could be interpreted in an alternative way: seronegative ''rheumatoid'' arthritis is a mild but definite variant of true rheumatoid arthritis. Previous studies, however, have indicated that some patients with seronegative joint disease can clearly be separated from those with rheumatoid arthritis. The seronegative spondyloarthropathies (ankylosing spondylitis, psoriasis, and Reiter's syndrome) and forms of juvenile chronic arthritis are examples of diseases that are now known to differ from rheumatoid arthritis.[585, 586] It is to be expected that further investigation will allow identification of other well-defined rheumatic syndromes in patients with seronegative arthritis.

Currently, it appears certain that patients who have seronegative ''rheumatoid'' arthritis can be divided into two major groups of persons: those with otherwise typical rheumatoid arthritis who are serologically negative for rheumatoid factor and those with some other form of arthritis. In the former group, some of these patients will become seropositive or became seronegative as a result of therapy.[27, 782] With regard to the latter group, certain members share clinical and radiologic features that eventually will allow their separation into a more homogeneous disease category. For example, a clinical entity consisting of seronegativity, oligoarthritis or polyarthritis, asymmetric joint involvement in the lower extremity, low back pain, sacroiliitis, painless mucosal ulcerations, a family history of a known spondyloarthropathy, and serologic positivity for HLA-B27 antigen has been identified in young men.[587]

With this overview of the clinical dilemma, it is apparent that previous studies comparing seropositive rheumatoid arthritis and seronegative ''rheumatoid'' arthritis must be viewed with a degree of caution. Because we really are comparing apples and oranges, it becomes difficult to delineate meaningful data reflecting real differences between patients with true rheumatoid arthritis who are seropositive and those with true rheumatoid arthritis who are seronegative. Certainly, with respect to radiologic abnormalities, many of the persons with seronegative ''rheumatoid'' arthritis have atypical features and, in fact, the observer often can predict such seronegativity when reviewing the radiographs. One such feature is the asymmetry of the articular involvement. According to Bland and Brown,[588] less frequent involvement of the metacarpophalangeal and metatarsophalangeal joints is seen in seronegative disease, whereas Burns and Calin[589] have reported the presence of osteosclerosis, new bone formation, intra-articular bony ankylosis, predominant carpal involvement, and the relative absence of classic subchondral erosions in a seronegative group of patients. Edelman and Russell[590] observed less deformity and fewer bone erosions in patients with seronegative disease. El-Khoury and coworkers[781] found osteosclerosis, carpal predominance, intra-articular bone fusion, and new bone formation in seronegative patients, although greater asymmetry of disease was not apparent.

These results and others indicate that the presence of one or more radiographic features that are otherwise atypical for rheumatoid arthritis should alert the observer that the patient probably is seronegative for rheumatoid factor. The greater the number of such features, the greater is the likelihood of seronegativity. The authors of this chapter believe that the disease in such patients is best regarded as ''rheumatoid-like'' arthritis, indicating that the radiographic abnormalities are explained by a pathologic process (synovial inflammation) that resembles that of true rheumatoid arthritis. The specific nature of the process generally is not clear. Some of the patients have rheumatoid arthritis. Indeed, in certain situations, even classic seropositive rheumatoid arthritis can have unusual radiologic features; for example, men with rheumatoid arthritis and patients with both rheumatoid arthritis and diffuse idiopathic skeletal hyperostosis may exhibit atypical radiographic abnormalities. Other persons with rheumatoid-like arthritis will later develop clinical evidence of a recognizable seronegative spondyloarthropathy. Many will continue to display clinical and radiologic features that resist any further classification.[783]

Spondyloarthropathies

Rheumatoid arthritis characteristically has articular lesions that differ in distribution and morphology from those of the seronegative spondyloarthropathies (ankylosing spondylitis, psoriasis, Reiter's syndrome). Ankylosing spondylitis (which shows predilection for the axial skeleton, although it also may produce appendicular articular disease), psoriasis (which may affect axial and appendicular skeleton as well as distal interphalangeal articulations), and Reiter's syndrome (which leads to asymmetric arthritis of the lower extremity with or without sacroiliac and spinal alterations) each may be associated with prominent findings in synovial and cartilaginous joints and entheses (sites of ligament and tendon attachment to bone). In the synovial joints, the absence of osteoporosis and the presence of bony proliferation and intra-articular osseous fusion commonly are encountered in the seronegative spondyloarthropathies, differing from the features of rheumatoid arthritis. Similarly, ankylosing spondylitis, psoriasis, and Reiter's syndrome can produce significant and extensive abnormalities of cartilaginous joints and entheses; these sites are much less frequently and severely affected in rheumatoid arthritis. Thus, prominent erosion and sclerosis of the symphysis pubis, manubriosternal joint, and ligamentous attachments of the pelvis, femur, and calcaneus are typical of seronegative spondyloarthropathies. Widespread spondylitis and sacroiliitis also are characteristic of these latter disorders; sacroiliac changes in rheumatoid arthritis are uncommon and mild, whereas spinal alterations in this disease usually are confined to the cervical region.

Gout

Gouty arthritis is associated with asymmetric articular disease of the appendicular skeleton, characterized by soft tissue masses, eccentric osseous erosions, bony proliferation, preservation of joint space, and absence of osteoporosis. Generally, the features are easily differentiated from those of rheumatoid arthritis, although occasional rheumatoid arthritis patients, especially men, do reveal goutlike abnormalities. Furthermore, the radiographic changes in long-standing rheumatoid arthritis and gout can be remarkably similar, particularly in the joints of the hand, the foot, and the wrist. Differentiation of the two disorders is not difficult on the basis of clinical and laboratory features.[445]

Collagen Vascular Disorders

Joint involvement in systemic lupus erythematosus and scleroderma can resemble that in rheumatoid arthritis.[446] Classically, however, the arthropathy of systemic lupus erythematosus is a deforming, nonerosive process, which initially is reversible. Cartilaginous destruction due to pressure erosion at areas of contact between malpositioned osseous structures and periarticular bony ''hook'' erosions caused by capsular and ligamentous changes can be observed in systemic lupus erythematosus, but marginal and central osseous defects and diffuse joint space narrowing are unusual in this disease, unless coexistent rheumatoid arthritis is present. Alternatively, the deformities in rheumatoid arthritis almost universally are associated with joint space narrowing and bony erosion.

In scleroderma, articular changes may be especially prominent in the distal interphalangeal joints of the fingers and the first carpometacarpal and inferior radioulnar compartments of the wrist, and they generally are associated with tuftal resorption and soft tissue and capsular calcification.

Mixed connective tissue disease and overlap syndromes can lead to radiographic abnormalities of more than one collagen vascular disorder. Thus, rheumatoid arthritis–like alterations are combined with those of scleroderma or systemic lupus erythematosus, providing clues to the mixed nature of the collagen disease.

Calcium Pyrophosphate Dihydrate (CPPD) Crystal Deposition Disease

This articular disorder is manifested radiographically as articular and periarticular calcification and pyrophosphate arthropathy. The calcification involves various structures, including cartilage (chondrocalcinosis), and is most prominent in the knees, the wrists, the metacarpophalangeal joints, and the symphysis pubis. Pyrophosphate arthropathy leads to joint space narrowing, eburnation, cyst formation, collapse, and fragmentation. The resulting radiographic picture does not realistically resemble that of rheumatoid arthritis.

The arthropathy of hemochromatosis is very similar to that of idiopathic CPPD crystal deposition disease.

Abnormalities at Specific Sites

Hand and Wrist

Symmetric changes at metacarpophalangeal and proximal interphalangeal joints (including the interphalangeal joint of the thumb) are common in rheumatoid arthritis; abnormalities of distal interphalangeal articulations are less frequent and rarely are severe. This pattern of distribution differs from that in other disorders.[630] Psoriatic arthritis leads to significant abnormalities of distal interphalangeal

joints as well as of more proximal articulations. Osteoarthritis (inflammatory or noninflammatory) most typically affects distal interphalangeal, proximal interphalangeal, and metacarpophalangeal joints. Gouty arthritis can involve any joint of the hand, including the distal interphalangeal joints. CPPD crystal deposition disease has predilection for the metacarpophalangeal articulations.

Rheumatoid arthritis initially can be manifested as soft tissue swelling, joint space narrowing, and osseous erosions in one or two locations of the wrist; radiocarpal, inferior radioulnar, and pisiform-triquetral compartmental changes are especially common. Soon, however, pancompartmental alterations become manifest. The diffuse nature of wrist involvement in rheumatoid arthritis is an important characteristic of this disease (Table 26–4). In patients without a significant history of accidental or occupational trauma, osteoarthritis leads to articular abnormalities that invariably are confined to the first carpometacarpal compartment or the trapezioscaphoid space of the midcarpal compartment, or it involves both. CPPD crystal deposition disease favors the radiocarpal compartment; scleroderma may selectively involve the first carpometacarpal and inferior radioulnar compartments; and gout produces pancompartmental disease with predominant involvement of the common carpometacarpal compartment.

Elbow

Radiographic abnormalities of the elbow in rheumatoid arthritis are sufficiently characteristic in most instances to allow accurate diagnosis. Joint space narrowing, osseous erosions, and cysts frequently are accompanied by soft tissue prominence related to rheumatoid nodules and olecranon bursitis. The elbow is involved in other polyarticular disorders, including gout, CPPD crystal deposition disease, and seronegative spondyloarthropathies, but obvious differences in radiographic findings between these diseases and rheumatoid arthritis usually are apparent. Olecranon bursitis can be secondary to gout, infection, and trauma.

TABLE 26–4. Compartmental Analysis of Hand and Wrist Disease[1]

	DIP[2] Joints	PIP[2] Joints	MCP[2] Joints	Radio-carpal Joint	Inferior Radioulnar Joint	Midcarpal Joint	Pisiform-Triquetral Joint	Common Carpo-metacarpal Joint	First Carpo-metacarpal Joint
Rheumatoid arthritis		+	+	+	+	+	+	+	+
Osteoarthritis	+	+	+			+[3]			+
Inflammatory osteoarthritis	+	+	±			+[3]			+
Calcium pyrophosphate dihydrate crystal deposition disease			+	+		+[3]			+
Gouty arthritis	+	+	+	+	+	+		+[4]	+
Scleroderma[5]	+	+			+				+

[1]Only the typical locations for each disease are indicated.
[2]DIP, Distal interphalangeal; PIP, proximal interphalangeal; MCP, metacarpophalangeal.
[3]Has predilection for trapezioscaphoid area of midcarpal joint.
[4]Very severe abnormalities may be present in this compartment.
[5]Some patients have coexistent rheumatoid arthritis.

Glenohumeral Joint

Marginal erosions of the humeral head are seen in rheumatoid arthritis, ankylosing spondylitis, and infection, as well as in other disorders. In ankylosing spondylitis, the size of the defect may be considerably larger than in rheumatoid arthritis. Septic arthritis of the glenohumeral joint usually is monoarticular, differing from the polyarticular nature of rheumatoid arthritis.

Rotator cuff tears may complicate rheumatoid arthritis as well as other synovial processes of the glenohumeral joint, including ankylosing spondylitis and infection. Such tears also can result from trauma and are very common in elderly persons. In those instances in which disruption of the rotator cuff is unassociated with a primary articular process, radiographs document the elevated position of the humeral head with respect to the glenoid cavity, although joint space loss between the humeral head and glenoid cavity is absent or mild.

Acromioclavicular Joint

Resorption of the distal clavicle and widening of the acromioclavicular joint are observed in rheumatoid arthritis, ankylosing spondylitis, infection, other collagen vascular disorders, and hyperparathyroidism, and after trauma. When the changes are secondary to an articular process, prominent acromial abnormalities may accompany the clavicular alterations. In hyperparathyroidism, subchondral resorption of bone is evident on both the acromial and the clavicular aspects of the articulation, but the acromial alterations are relatively mild. Posttraumatic osteolysis of the distal end of the clavicle is accompanied by a pertinent clinical history of acute or chronic injury and frequently by radiographic evidence of fracture and dislocation. Osteolysis predominates in the clavicle, although mild acromial abnormalities also may be seen.

Coracoclavicular Joint

Resorption of the undersurface of the distal clavicle is seen in rheumatoid arthritis, hyperparathyroidism, and ankylosing spondylitis. In ankylosing spondylitis, bone proliferation is an associated radiographic manifestation.

Sternoclavicular and Manubriosternal Joints

Changes in the sternoclavicular and manubriosternal joints are not specific for rheumatoid arthritis. Similar abnormalities accompany the seronegative spondyloarthropathies. At the manubriosternal articulation, alterations in the seronegative spondyloarthropathies are more marked than in rheumatoid arthritis.

Forefoot

The most common sites of articular disease of the forefoot in rheumatoid arthritis are the metatarsophalangeal joints and the interphalangeal joint of the great toe. Although these same articulations are involved in psoriasis, Reiter's syndrome, and gout, extensive abnormality of other interphalangeal joints in one or more digits can be evident in any of these three latter disorders (Table 26–5). Furthermore, forefoot abnormalities usually are symmetric in distribution in rheumatoid arthritis and asymmetric in psoriasis, Reiter's syndrome, and gouty arthritis.

At the interphalangeal joint of the great toe, the changes

TABLE 26–5. Compartmental Analysis of Forefoot Disease[1]

	Metatarsophalangeal Joints	Interphalangeal Joint of Great Toe	Other Interphalangeal Joints
Rheumatoid arthritis	+	+	
Gouty arthritis	+	+	+
Psoriatic arthritis	+	+[2]	+
Reiter's syndrome	+	+[2]	+
Osteoarthritis	+[3]		

[1]Only the typical locations of each disease are indicated.
[2]Severe destructive changes may be observed.
[3]Has predilection for the metatarsophalangeal joint of the first digit.

of rheumatoid arthritis predominate on the medial aspect of the joint, especially along the distal portion of the proximal phalanx. Although joint space narrowing and mild subchondral erosions and cysts are encountered in the interphalangeal joint in rheumatoid arthritis, severe destruction usually is not apparent. This latter finding is evident in gout, psoriasis, and Reiter's syndrome.

Midfoot

Diffuse changes with predilection for the talonavicular portion of the talocalcaneonavicular joint characterize midfoot involvement in rheumatoid arthritis. The talonavicular space also is affected in CPPD crystal deposition disease and in neuropathic osteoarthropathy (especially in diabetic patients), but both of these disorders are associated with bony sclerosis and fragmentation, findings that are not common in rheumatoid arthritis. Midfoot changes also are evident in seronegative spondyloarthropathies and gouty arthritis. In gout, abnormalities may predominate at the tarsometatarsal joints.

Heel

Retrocalcaneal bursitis producing soft tissue swelling and subjacent osseous erosion occurs not only in rheumatoid arthritis but also in ankylosing spondylitis, psoriasis, and Reiter's syndrome (Table 26–6). The changes are virtually indistinguishable in these four disorders, although poorly defined erosions and bony sclerosis are more typical of the seronegative spondyloarthropathies.

Tendon thickening can be seen in any of these four diseases. Nodular prominence of the Achilles tendon also can be encountered in gout (due to tophi) and hyperlipoproteinemia (due to xanthoma). Abnormalities on the plantar aspect of the calcaneus in rheumatoid arthritis consist of superficial erosions and well-defined enthesophytes. In the seronegative spondyloarthropathies, prominent erosions, considerable sclerosis, and exuberant, poorly defined excrescences are seen.

Knee

In rheumatoid arthritis, symmetric involvement of the medial femorotibial and lateral femorotibial compartments with or without patellofemoral compartmental changes is seen. In osteoarthritis, asymmetric alterations of the medial and lateral femorotibial compartments (the medial side is more frequently the predominant side of involvement) can

TABLE 26–6. Abnormalities of the Heel

	Retrocalcaneal Bursitis with Posterosuperior Calcaneal Erosion	Achilles Tendinitis	Enthesophyte at Posterior Attachment of Achilles Tendon	Well-defined Plantar Calcaneal Enthesophyte	Poorly Defined Plantar Calcaneal Enthesophyte
Rheumatoid arthritis	+	+	+	+	
Ankylosing spondylitis	+	+	+		+[1]
Psoriatic arthritis	+	+	+		+[1]
Reiter's syndrome	+	+			+[1]
Gouty arthritis	+[2]	+[3]			
Xanthoma	+[2]	+[3]			

[1]Poorly defined enthesophytes may become better defined with healing.
[2]Erosion of calcaneus can occur beneath tophus or xanthoma.
[3]Nodular thickening of the tendon may be seen.

be combined with patellofemoral compartmental disease. In CPPD crystal deposition disease, patellofemoral abnormalities occurring alone or in combination with asymmetric medial and lateral femorotibial alterations are typical. Although any of these three disorders can be associated with varus or valgus angulation of the knee, a varus deformity is especially characteristic of osteoarthritis, whereas valgus deformity is not uncommon in rheumatoid arthritis and CPPD crystal deposition disease.

Marginal erosions of femur and tibia are evident in rheumatoid arthritis, seronegative spondyloarthropathies, gout, and infection, especially tuberculosis. In the seronegative spondyloarthropathies, the erosive changes commonly are poorly marginated and associated with bony proliferation. In gout and tuberculosis, such erosions may be unaccompanied by joint space narrowing.

Popliteal cysts can occur in association with any articular process leading to the accumulation of joint fluid and elevation of intra-articular pressure. Examples of such processes are rheumatoid arthritis, ankylosing spondylitis, psoriasis, gout, infection, juvenile chronic arthritis, and the peripheral arthritis of inflammatory bowel disease. Popliteal cysts also can follow trauma and frequently are associated with meniscal tears or other internal derangements of the knee.

Hip

Symmetric loss of articular space with axial migration of the femoral head with respect to the acetabulum is typical of rheumatoid involvement of the hip. In osteoarthritis, superior or medial migration is more frequent than axial migration, reflecting the asymmetric nature of the cartilaginous destruction. Axial migration of the femoral head can accompany the hip disease of CPPD crystal deposition disease and ankylosing spondylitis, although both of these disorders are associated with osteophytes and sclerosis. In long-standing rheumatoid arthritis, however, osteophytes may appear as a manifestation of secondary degenerative joint disease. Furthermore, occasionally a patient with rheumatoid arthritis reveals superior loss of articular space simulating the pattern of osteoarthritis.

Acetabular protrusion is a common manifestation of severe rheumatoid hip disease. It is associated with diffuse loss of interosseous space and an eroded and often diminutive femoral head. Protrusio acetabuli also can be encountered in patients with osteoarthritis, familial or idiopathic

protrusion deformities (Otto pelvis), ankylosing spondylitis, infection, osteomalacia, and Paget's disease (Table 26–7).

An idiopathic variety of chronic inflammatory hip disease (coxitis) has been described, mainly in the French literature, that is characterized by radiographic features resembling those of rheumatoid arthritis.[591–594] It occurs at any age but is most frequent in young adults. Men or women may be affected. Rapid onset of pain and an intermittent and inflammatory pattern of symptoms are typical. The process will remain localized to one or both hips. Less commonly, pauciarticular or, rarely, polyarticular disease is seen. Radiographic features confirm the inflammatory nature of the process in the hip and include diffuse loss of interosseous space, subchondral osteolysis, the later development of blunt and triangular osteophytes, especially in the lateral aspect of the femoral head, and, infrequently, periarticular osteoporosis (Figs. 26–82 and 26–83). As other disease processes, such as rheumatoid arthritis, the seronegative spondyloarthropathies, infection, and osteoarthritis, can begin as monoarticular inflammatory hip disease,[595–597] the accurate diagnosis of idiopathic coxitis is difficult and is made primarily on the basis of a long period of observation and the application of a number of clinical, radiographic, laboratory, and histologic criteria.

Sacroiliac Joint

Sacroiliac joint abnormalities are not common or prominent in rheumatoid arthritis. When evident, they generally are asymmetric in distribution and consist of minor subchondral erosions, minimal eburnation, and absent or focal intra-articular bony ankylosis (Table 26–8). These characteristics differ from those of ankylosing spondylitis (bilateral symmetric disease with extensive erosions, sclerosis, and bony fusion), psoriasis and Reiter's syndrome (bilateral symmetric, bilateral asymmetric, or unilateral disease with

TABLE 26–7. Some Causes of Protrusio Acetabuli

Rheumatoid arthritis
Ankylosing spondylitis
Osteoarthritis (medial migration pattern)
Infection
Paget's disease
Osteomalacia
Irradiation
Acetabular trauma

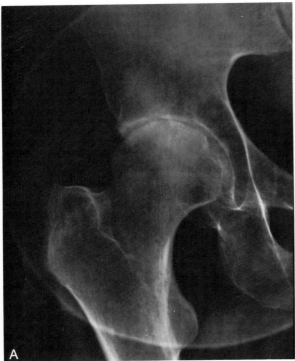

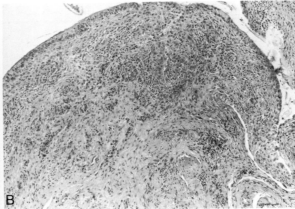

FIGURE 26–82. Idiopathic chronic monoarticular inflammatory hip disease (coxitis). A 42 year old woman developed constant pain in the right groin. Serologic tests for rheumatoid factor and LE preparations consistently were negative. Monoarticular disease of the hip was the only finding on clinical examination. Thirteen years after the radiographic and pathologic studies were accomplished, only one other joint (a metatarsophalangeal articulation) was involved.

A The radiograph of the right hip reveals diffuse loss of joint space, sclerosis, and indistinctness of the subchondral bone in the central and lateral portions of the femoral head.

B Biopsy of the synovial membrane shows hypervascularity and cellular infiltration (20×).

(Courtesy of M. Lequesne, M.D., Paris, France.)

changes identical to those of ankylosing spondylitis), gout (bilateral or unilateral abnormalities with large erosions), degenerative joint disease (bilateral or unilateral disease with prominent subchondral sclerosis), osteitis condensans ilii (bilateral symmetric alterations of the lower ilium with significant bony eburnation), hyperparathyroidism (bilateral symmetric abnormalities with widening of the interosseous space, erosions, and sclerosis), and infection (unilateral disease with poorly defined osseous defects and reactive sclerosis).

Symphysis Pubis

Although not a common site of involvement in rheumatoid arthritis, erosions and sclerosis of bone at this location can simulate the findings in seronegative spondyloarthropathies and posttraumatic or postoperative osteitis pubis.

Costovertebral Joints and Ribs

The rib erosions in rheumatoid arthritis are identical to those that accompany neurologic disorders and other collagen vascular diseases. Occasionally in a patient with rheumatoid arthritis, costovertebral joint erosion, eburnation, and ankylosis simulate the changes in ankylosing spondylitis.

Spine

Unlike ankylosing spondylitis, psoriatic arthritis, and Reiter's syndrome, rheumatoid arthritis produces infrequent abnormalities of the thoracic and lumbar spine. Rheumatoid changes in the cervical spine consisting of apophyseal joint erosion and malalignment, intervertebral disc space narrowing with adjacent eburnation and without osteophytes, and multiple subluxations, including that at the atlantoaxial junction, are virtually diagnostic when they occur as a group. They differ from the cervical alterations of ankylosing spondylitis (widespread apophyseal joint ankylosis and syndesmophytes), psoriatic arthritis (apophyseal joint narrowing and eburnation, and prominent anterior vertebral bone formation), diffuse idiopathic skeletal hyperostosis (flowing ossification and excrescences along the anterior aspect of the spine with preservation of intervertebral disc height), and juvenile chronic arthritis (apophyseal joint ankylosis with hypoplasia of vertebral bodies and intervertebral discs). Atlantoaxial subluxation alone is not a pathognomonic sign of rheumatoid arthritis, however. It also is observed in ankylosing spondylitis, psoriatic arthritis, Reiter's syndrome, and juvenile chronic arthritis, as well as after trauma or local infection. Such subluxation occurring after an infectious condition in the head or neck is designated Grisel's syndrome; it is more common in children than in adults and may be explained by the existence of a periodontoidal vascular plexus that drains the posterior su-

TABLE 26–8. Comparison of Sacroiliac Joint Abnormalities in Rheumatoid Arthritis and Ankylosing Spondylitis

	Rheumatoid Arthritis	Ankylosing Spondylitis
Distribution	Asymmetric or unilateral	Bilateral and symmetric
Erosions	Superficial	Deep
Sclerosis	Mild or absent	Moderate or severe[1]
Bony ankylosis	Rare, segmental	Common, diffuse

[1]Sclerosis may disappear in long-standing disease.

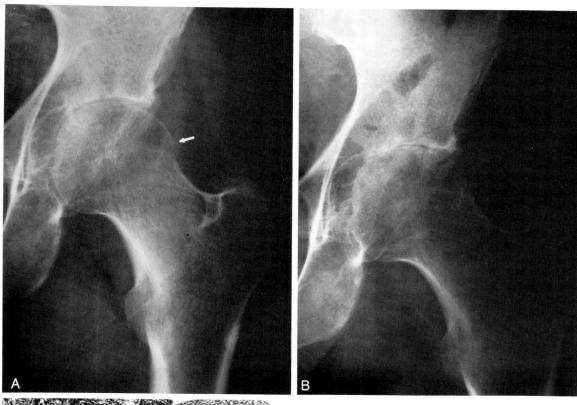

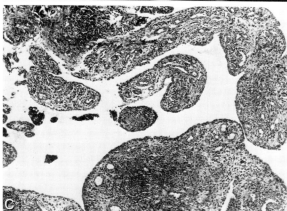

FIGURE 26–83. Idiopathic chronic monoarticular inflammatory hip disease (coxitis). A 41 year old man had a 2 year history of pain in the left hip. No other joints were involved. Serologic testing for rheumatoid factor was persistently negative. Two years after these radiographic and pathologic studies, the disease remained monoarticular in distribution.

A An initial radiograph shows moderate concentric joint space narrowing, periarticular osteoporosis, and a small triangular osteophyte (arrow) in the lateral aspect of the femoral head.

B One year later, joint space narrowing has progressed. Subchondral indistinctness, especially laterally, is seen.

C Histologic evaluation demonstrates hypertrophic synovial villi, proliferation of synoviocytes, hypervascularity, and nodular infiltrates of lymphocytes and plasma cells (20×).

(Courtesy of M. Lequesne, M.D., Paris, France.)

perior pharyngeal region.[784, 785] Odontoid erosions can be evident in a variety of synovial disorders, and intervertebral disc space narrowing with adjacent osseous irregularity can be apparent after trauma or infection.

SUMMARY

Rheumatoid arthritis is a common articular disorder with a characteristic radiographic picture. A symmetric polyarticular disease of the synovial joints of the appendicular skeleton is apparent, with prominent abnormalities of the proximal interphalangeal and metacarpophalangeal joints of the hand, the wrist, the metatarsophalangeal joints of the foot, the posterior and plantar aspects of the calcaneus, the knee, the elbow, the glenohumeral and acromioclavicular joints, the ankle, and the hip; these abnormalities commonly are combined with changes in the cervical spine. This distribution of synovial joint involvement, although not invariable, is sufficiently common to allow accurate diagnosis in most patients with this disorder, especially when the involvement is characterized by fusiform soft tissue swelling, regional or periarticular osteoporosis, marginal and central osseous erosions and cysts, and diffuse loss of interosseous space.

Occasionally a rheumatoid arthritis patient will have a coexistent articular disorder that complicates the radiologic (and clinical) picture. Such diseases can include septic arthritis, ankylosing spondylitis, CPPD crystal deposition disease, gout, diffuse idiopathic skeletal hyperostosis, psoriasis, and other collagen vascular disorders. In these cases, careful analysis of the radiographic changes usually provides some clue indicating the presence of a second disease.

References

1. Scott JT (Ed): Copeman's Textbook of the Rheumatic Diseases. 5th Ed. Edinburgh, Churchill Livingstone, 1978.
2. Hollander JL, McCarty DJ Jr (Eds): Arthritis and Allied Conditions. 8th Ed. Philadelphia, Lea & Febiger, 1972.
3. Currey HLF: Aetiology and pathogenesis of rheumatoid arthritis. In JT Scott (Ed): Copeman's Textbook of the Rheumatic Diseases. 5th Ed. Edinburgh, Churchill Livingstone, 1978, p 261.
4. Ropes MW, Bennett GA, Cobb S, et al: Proposed diagnostic criteria for rheumatoid arthritis. Ann Rheum Dis 16:118, 1957.
5. Ropes MW, Bennett GA, Cobb S, et al: Diagnostic criteria for rheumatoid arthritis, 1958 revision. Ann Rheum Dis 18:49, 1959.
6. Lawrence JS: Report from the subcommittee on diagnostic criteria in rheumatoid arthritis. In PH Bennett, PHN Wood (Eds): Population Studies of the Rheumatic Diseases. International Congress Series No. 148. Amsterdam, Excerpta Medica Foundation, 1968, pp 175, 454.
7. Arnett FC, Edworthy SM, Bloch DA, et al: The American Rheumatism Association 1987 revised criteria for the classification of rheumatoid arthritis. Arthritis Rheum 31:315, 1988.
8. Ragan C: The clinical picture of rheumatoid arthritis. In JL Hollander, DJ McCarty Jr (Eds): Arthritis and Allied Conditions. 8th Ed. Philadelphia, Lea & Febiger, 1972, p 318.
9. Buchanan WW: Clinical features of rheumatoid arthritis. In JT Scott (Ed): Copeman's Textbook of the Rheumatic Diseases. 5th Ed. Edinburgh, Churchill Livingstone, 1978, p 333.
10. Corrigan AB, Robinson RG, Terenty TR, et al: Benign rheumatoid arthritis of the aged. Br Med J 1:444, 1974.
11. Villiaumey J, Strauss J, DiMenza C, et al: Les monoarthrites rhumatoides. Rev Rhum Mal Osteoartic 40:627, 1973.
12. David-Chaussé J, Ricard A-M, Dehais J: 22 cas de monoarthrites rhumatismales de l'adulte (hanches exclues). Rev Rhum Mal Osteoartic 39:775, 1972.
13. Bloch-Michel H, Benoist M, Degott C, et al: Monoarthrites rhumatoïdes post-traumatiques. Nouv Presse Med 2:695, 1973.
14. Fleming A, Crown JM, Corbett M: Early rheumatoid disease. I. Onset. Ann Rheum Dis 35:357, 1976.
15. Short CL, Bauer W: The course of rheumatoid arthritis in patients receiving simple medical and orthopaedic measures. N Engl J Med 238:142, 1948.
16. Bywaters EGL, Dressner E: Hemiplegia and rheumatoid arthritis. Arthritis Rheum 11:79, 1968.
17. Thompson M, Bywaters EGL: Unilateral rheumatoid arthritis following hemiplegia. Ann Rheum Dis 21:370, 1962.
18. Kamermann JS: Protective effect of traumatic lesions on rheumatoid arthritis. Ann Rheum Dis 25:361, 1966.
19. Glick EN: Asymmetrical rheumatoid arthritis after poliomyelitis. Br Med J 3:26, 1967.
20. Bland J, Eddy W: Hemiplegia and rheumatoid hemiarthritis. Arthritis Rheum 11:72, 1968.
21. Yaghmai I, Rooholamini SM, Faunce HF: Unilateral rheumatoid arthritis: Protective effect of neurologic deficits. AJR 128:299, 1977.
22. Soila P: A roentgenological study of asymmetry in rheumatoid arthritis. A preliminary communication. Acta Rheumatol Scand 9:264, 1963.
23. Castillo BA, El Sallab RA, Scott JT: Physical activity, cystic erosions, and osteoporosis in rheumatoid arthritis. Ann Rheum Dis 24:522, 1965.
24. Norton WL, Ziff M: Electron microscopic observations on the rheumatoid synovial membrane. Arthritis Rheum 9:589, 1966.
25. Dixon AS, Grant C: Acute synovial rupture in rheumatoid arthritis. Clinical and experimental observations. Lancet 1:742, 1964.
26. Resnick D: Gout-like lesions in rheumatoid arthritis. Letter to the Editor. AJR 127:1062, 1976.
27. Dixon AS: "Rheumatoid arthritis" with negative serological reaction. Ann Rheum Dis 19:209, 1960.
28. Bywaters EGL: Symmetrical joint involvement. Ann Rheum Dis 34:376, 1975.
29. McFarland GBJ, Hoffer MM: Rheumatoid nodules in synovial membrane and tendons. Clin Orthop 58:165, 1968.
30. Kellgren JH, Ball J: Tendon lesions in rheumatoid arthritis: A clinicopathological study. Ann Rheum Dis 9:48, 1950.
31. Webb J, Payne WH: Rheumatoid nodules of the vocal cords. Ann Rheum Dis 31:122, 1972.
32. Baker RJ, Johnson WC, Burgoon CF: Unusual skin lesions of rheumatoid arthritis. Dermatologica 143:305, 1971.
33. Epstein WV, Engleman EP: The relation of the rheumatoid factor content of serum to clinical neurovascular manifestations of rheumatoid arthritis. Arthritis Rheum 2:250, 1959.
34. Schmid FR, Cooper NS, Ziff M, et al: Arteritis in rheumatoid arthritis. Am J Med 30:56, 1961.
35. Karten I: Arteritis, myocardial infarction and rheumatoid arthritis. JAMA 210:1717, 1969.
36. Mongan E, Cass R, Jacox R, et al: A study of the relation of seronegative and seropositive rheumatoid arthritis to each other and to necrotizing vasculitis. Am J Med 47:23, 1969.
37. Aronoff A, Bywaters EGL, Fearnley GR: Lung lesions in rheumatoid arthritis. Br Med J 2:228, 1955.
38. Cummings JK, Taleisnik J: Peripheral gangrene as a complication of rheumatoid arthritis. Report of a case and a review of the literature. J Bone Joint Surg [Am] 53:1001, 1971.
39. Wilkinson M, Torrance WN: Clinical background of rheumatoid vascular disease. Ann Rheum Dis 26:475, 1967.
40. Lindsay MK, Tavadia HB, Whyte AS, et al: Acute abdomen in rheumatoid arthritis due to necrotizing arteritis. Br Med J 2:592, 1973.
41. Ferguson RH, Slocumb CH: Peripheral neuropathy in rheumatoid arthritis. Bull Rheum Dis 11:251, 1961.
42. Hart FD, Golding JR: Rheumatoid neuropathy. Br Med J 1:1594, 1960.
43. Chamberlain MA, Bruckner FE: Rheumatoid neuropathy. Ann Rheum Dis 29:609, 1970.
44. Nakano KK: The entrapment neuropathies of rheumatoid arthritis. Orthop Clin North Am 6:837, 1975.
45. Felty AR: Chronic arthritis in the adult associated with splenomegaly and leukopenia. A report of 5 cases of an unusual clinical syndrome. Johns Hopkins Hosp Bull 35:16, 1924.
46. Rosenthal FD, Beeley JM, Gelsthorpe K, et al: White-cell antibodies and the aetiology of Felty's syndrome. Q J Med 43:187, 1974.
47. Moore RA, Brunner CM, Sandusky WR, et al: Felty's syndrome: Long term follow-up after splenectomy. Ann Intern Med 75:381, 1971.
48. Pengelly CDR: Felty's syndrome. Good response to adrenocorticosteroids: Possible mechanism of the anaemia. Br Med J 2:986, 1966.
49. Kennedy AC, Smith DA, Anderson JA, et al: Osteoporosis in rheumatoid arthritis: Its natural history and statistical predilection. Rheumatology 4:441, 1974.
50. Mueller MN, Jurist JM: Skeletal status in rheumatoid arthritis. Arthritis Rheum 16:66, 1973.
51. Duncan H: Osteoporosis in rheumatoid arthritis and corticosteroid induced osteoporosis. Orthop Clin North Am 3:571, 1972.
52. Ziff M, Baum J: Laboratory findings in rheumatoid arthritis. In JL Hollander, DJ McCarty Jr (Eds): Arthritis and Allied Conditions. 8th Ed. Philadelphia, Lea & Febiger, 1972, p 367.
53. McCarty DJ, Gattner RA: A study of distal interphalangeal joint tenderness in rheumatoid arthritis. Arthritis Rheum 9:325, 1966.
54. Gray RG, Gottlieb NL: Hand flexor tenosynovitis in rheumatoid arthritis. Prevalence, distribution, and associated rheumatic features. Arthritis Rheum 20:1003, 1977.
55. Millender LH, Nalebuff EA, Albin R, et al: Dorsal tenosynovectomy and tendon transfer in the rheumatoid hand. J Bone Joint Surg [Am] 56:601, 1974.
56. Backhouse KM, Kay AGL, Coomes EN, et al: Tendon involvement in the rheumatoid hand. Ann Rheum Dis 30:236, 1971.

57. Inglis AE: Rheumatoid arthritis in the hand. Am J Surg 109:368, 1965.
58. Brewerton DA: Hand deformities in rheumatoid disease. Ann Rheum Dis 16:183, 1957.
59. Straub LR, Wilson EH Jr: Spontaneous rupture of extensor tendons in the hand associated with rheumatoid arthritis. J Bone Joint Surg [Am] 38:1208, 1956.
60. Vaughan-Jackson OJ: Rupture of extensor tendons by attrition at the inferior radio-ulnar joint. Report of two cases. J Bone Joint Surg [Br] 30:528, 1948.
61. Martel W: The pattern of rheumatoid arthritis in the hand and wrist. Radiol Clin North Am 2:221, 1964.
62. Martel W, Hayes JT, Duff IF: The pattern of bone erosion in the hand and wrist in rheumatoid arthritis. Radiology 84:204, 1965.
63. Berens DL, Lockie LM, Lin RK, et al: Roentgen changes in early rheumatoid arthritis. Wrists-hands-feet. Radiology 82:645, 1964.
64. Soila P: Roentgen manifestations of adult rheumatoid arthritis with special regard to the early changes. Acta Rheum Scand Suppl 1:1, 1958.
65. Fletcher DE, Rowley KA: The radiological features of rheumatoid arthritis. Br J Radiol 25:282, 1952.
66. Norgaard F: Earliest roentgenological changes in polyarthritis of the rheumatoid type: Rheumatoid arthritis. Radiology 85:325, 1965.
67. Clemmesen S: A critical evaluation of Norgaard's technique for early roentgenological diagnosis of rheumatoid arthritis. Acta Rheumatol Scand 12:241, 1966.
68. Norgaard F: Earliest roentgen changes in polyarthritis of the rheumatoid type. Continued investigations. Radiology 92:299, 1969.
69. Brewerton DA: A tangential radiographic projection for demonstrating involvement of metacarpal heads in rheumatoid arthritis. Br J Radiol 40:233, 1967.
70. Kuczynski K: The synovial structures of the normal and rheumatoid digital joint. Hand 3:41, 1971.
71. Brewerton DA: Pathological anatomy of rheumatoid finger joints. Hand 3:121, 1971.
72. Bywaters EGL: Pathogenesis of finger joint lesions in rheumatoid arthritis. Ann Rheum Dis 28(Suppl):5, 1969.
73. Landsmeer JMF: Observations on the joints of the human finger. Ann Rheum Dis 28(Suppl):11, 1969.
74. Norgaard F: Tidligste rontgenologiske forandringer ved polyarthritis. Ugeskr Laeger 125:1312, 1963.
75. Martel W, Holt JF, Cassidy JT: Roentgenologic manifestations of juvenile rheumatoid arthritis. AJR 88:400, 1962.
76. Smith EM, Juvinall RC, Bender LF, et al: Role of the finger flexors in rheumatoid deformities of the metacarpophalangeal joints. Arthritis Rheum 7:467, 1964.
77. Cruickshank B, MacLeod JG, Shearer WS: Subarticular pseudocysts in rheumatoid arthritis. J Fac Radiologists 5:218, 1954.
78. Ginsberg MH, Genant HK, Yu TF, et al: Rheumatoid nodulosis. An unusual variant of rheumatoid disease. Arthritis Rheum 18:49, 1975.
79. Brower AC, NaPombejara C, Stechschulte DJ, et al: Rheumatoid nodulosis: Another cause of juxta-articular nodules. Radiology 125:669, 1977.
80. Dorwart BB, Schumacher HR: Hand deformities resembling rheumatoid arthritis. Semin Arthritis Rheum 4:53, 1974.
81. Swanson AB, Swanson GG: Pathogenesis and pathomechanics of rheumatoid deformities in the hand and wrist. Orthop Clin North Am 4:1039, 1973.
82. McMaster M: The natural history of the rheumatoid metacarpophalangeal joint. J Bone Joint Surg [Br] 54:687, 1972.
83. Stack HG, Vaughan-Jackson OJ: The zig-zag deformity in the rheumatoid hand. Hand 3:62, 1971.
84. Vaughan-Jackson OJ: Rheumatoid hand deformities considered in the light of tendon imbalance. J Bone Joint Surg [Am] 44:764, 1962.
85. Wise KS: The anatomy of the metacarpophalangeal joints with observations of the aetiology of ulnar drift. J Bone Joint Surg [Br] 57:485, 1975.
86. Clark IP, James DF, Colwill JC: Intra-articular pressure as a factor in initiating ulnar drift. J Bone Joint Surg [Am] 60:325, 1978.
87. Hastings DE, Evans JA: Rheumatoid wrist deformities and their relation to ulnar drift. J Bone Joint Surg [Am] 57:930, 1975.
88. Wilkes LL: Ulnar drift and metacarpophalangeal joint subluxation in the rheumatoid hand: Review of the pathogenesis. South Med J 70:963, 1977.
89. Shapiro JS: A new factor in the etiology of ulnar drift. Clin Orthop 68:32, 1970.
90. Heywood AWB: Correction of the rheumatoid boutonnière deformity. J Bone Joint Surg [Am] 51:1309, 1969.
91. Littler JW, Eaton RG: Redistribution of forces in the correction of the boutonnière deformity. J Bone Joint Surg [Am] 49:1267, 1967.
92. Flatt AE: Surgical rehabilitation of the arthritic hand. Arthritis Rheum 2:278, 1959.
93. Kay A: Development of deformities in the rheumatoid hand: A preliminary report. Ann Rheum Dis 28(Suppl):95, 1969.
94. Harrison SH: Rheumatoid deformities of the proximal interphalangeal joints of the hand. Ann Rheum Dis 28(Suppl):20, 1969.
95. Straub LR: The etiology of finger deformities in the hand affected by rheumatoid arthritis. Bull Hosp Joint Dis 21:322, 1960.
96. Stack HG: Muscle function in the fingers. J Bone Joint Surg [Br] 44:899, 1962.
97. Swezey RL: Dynamic factors in deformity of the rheumatoid arthritic hand. Bull Rheum Dis 22:649, 1971–1972.
98. Smith RJ, Kaplan EB: Rheumatoid deformities at the metacarpophalangeal joints of the fingers. J Bone Joint Surg [Am] 49:31, 1967.
99. Resnick D: Inter-relationships between radiocarpal and metacarpophalangeal joint deformities in rheumatoid arthritis. J Can Assoc Radiol 27:29, 1976.
100. Swanson AB, DeGroot GA, Hehl RW, et al: Pathogenesis of rheumatoid deformities in the hand. In RL Cruess, NS Mitchell (Eds): Surgery of Rheumatoid Arthritis. Philadelphia, JB Lippincott, 1971, p 143.
101. Pahle JA, Raunio P: The influence of wrist position on finger deviation in the rheumatoid hand. A clinical and radiological study. J Bone Joint Surg [Br] 51:664, 1969.
102. Aptekar RG, Lawless OJ, Decker JL: Deforming non-erosive arthritis of the hand in systemic lupus erythematosus. Clin Orthop 100:120, 1974.
103. Murphy WA, Staple TW: Jaccoud's arthropathy reviewed. AJR 118:300, 1973.
104. Fearnley GR: Ulnar deviation of the fingers. Ann Rheum Dis 10:126, 1951.
105. Zancolli E: Structural and Dynamic Basis of Hand Surgery. Philadelphia, JB Lippincott, 1968.
106. Backhouse KM: The mechanics of normal digital control in the hand and an analysis of ulnar drift of rheumatoid arthritis. Ann R Coll Surg Engl 43:154, 1968.
107. Hakstian RW, Tubiana R: Ulnar deviation of the fingers. J Bone Joint Surg [Am] 49:299, 1967.
108. Lush B: Ulnar deviation of the fingers. Ann Rheum Dis 11:219, 1952.
109. Ratliff AHC: Deformities of the thumb in rheumatoid arthritis. J Bone Joint Surg [Br] 54:557, 1972.
110. Clayton ML: Surgery of the thumb in rheumatoid arthritis. J Bone Joint Surg [Am] 44:1376, 1962.
111. Nalebuff EA: Diagnosis, classification, and management of rheumatoid thumb deformities. Bull Hosp Joint Dis 29:119, 1968.
112. McFarlane RM: Observations on the functional anatomy of the intrinsic muscles of the thumb. J Bone Joint Surg [Am] 44:1073, 1962.
113. Swanson AB: Disabling arthritis at the base of the thumb—treatment by resection of the trapezium and flexible (silicone) implant arthroplasty. J Bone Joint Surg [Am] 54:456, 1972.
114. Burton RI: Basal joint arthrosis of the thumb. Orthop Clin North Am 4:331, 1973.
115. Ehrlich GE, Peterson LT, Sokoloff L, et al: Pathogenesis of rupture of extensor tendons at the wrist in rheumatoid arthritis. Arthritis Rheum 2:332, 1959.
116. Backdahl M: The caput ulnae syndrome in rheumatoid arthritis. A study of the morphology, abnormal anatomy and clinical picture. Acta Rheumatol Scand 5(Suppl):5, 1963.
117. Darrach W: Anterior dislocation of the head of the ulna. Ann Surg 56:802, 1912.
118. Cracchiolo A, Marmor L: Resection of the distal ulna in rheumatoid arthritis. Arthritis Rheum 12:415, 1969.
119. Rana NA, Taylor AR: Excision of the distal end of the ulna in rheumatoid arthritis. J Bone Joint Surg [Br] 55:96, 1973.
120. Kessler I, Hect O: Present application of the Darrach procedure. Clin Orthop 72:254, 1970.
121. Black RM, Boswick JA Jr, Wiedel J: Dislocation of the wrist in rheumatoid arthritis. The relationship to distal ulna resection. Clin Orthop 124:184, 1977.
122. Iveson JMI, Hill AGS, Wright V: Wrist cysts and fistulae. An arthrographic study of the rheumatoid wrist. Ann Rheum Dis 34:388, 1975.
123. Resnick D: Rheumatoid arthritis of the wrist. The compartmental approach. Med Radiogr Photogr 52:50, 1976.
124. Resnick D: Rheumatoid arthritis of the wrist: Why the ulnar styloid? Radiology 112:29, 1974.
125. Stenstrom R, Wegelius O: Clearance of 125I-labeled urographin from knee joints in rheumatoid arthritis. Acta Rheumatoid Scand 16:151, 1970.
126. Wiljasalo M, Julkunen H, Salven I: Lymphography in rheumatic diseases. Ann Med Intern Fenn 55:125, 1966.
127. Weston WJ: The soft tissue signs of the enlarged ulnar bursa in rheumatoid arthritis. J Can Assoc Radiol 24:282, 1973.
128. Fischer E: Weichstrahldiagnostik des vergrösserten recessus sacciformis des distalen Radio-ulnargelenks. Radiologe 15:157, 1975.
129. Harrison MO, Freiberger RH, Ranawat CS: Arthrography of the rheumatoid wrist joint. AJR 112:480, 1971.
130. Resnick D: Arthrography in the evaluation of arthritic disorders of the wrist. Radiology 113:331, 1974.
131. Berens DL, Lin RK: Roentgen Diagnosis of Rheumatoid Arthritis. Springfield, Ill, Charles C Thomas, 1969.
132. Resnick D, Gmelich J: Bone fragmentation in the rheumatoid wrist: Radiographic and pathologic considerations. Radiology 114:315, 1975.
133. Swezey RL, Alexander SJ: Notching of the carpal navicular. Ann Rheum Dis 28:45, 1969.
134. Resnick D: Early abnormalities of the pisiform and triquetrum in rheumatoid arthritis. Ann Rheum Dis 35:46, 1976.
135. Lewis OJ, Hamshere RJ, Bucknill TM: The anatomy of the wrist joint. J Anat 106:539, 1970.
136. Arkless R: Rheumatoid wrists: Cineradiography. Radiology 88:543, 1967.
137. VanDam G: The hand. In ME Carter (Ed): Radiological Aspects of Rheumatoid Disease. Proceedings of an International Symposium, Amsterdam, 1963. Amsterdam, Excerpta Medica, 1964, p 63.
138. Trentham DE, Masi AT: Carpo:metacarpal ratio. A new quantitative measure of radiologic progression of wrist involvement in rheumatoid arthritis. Arthritis Rheum 19:939, 1976.
139. McMurtry RY, Youm Y, Flatt AE, et al: Kinematics of the wrist. II. Clinical applications. J Bone Joint Surg [Am] 60:955, 1978.
140. Linscheid RL: The mechanical factors affecting deformity at the wrist in rheumatoid arthritis. In Proceedings of the Twenty-fourth Annual Meeting of the

American Society for Surgery of the Hand, New York, January 17–18, 1969. J Bone Joint Surg [Am] *51*:790, 1969.

141. Pekin TJ Jr, Zvaifler NJ: Navicular displacement in rheumatoid arthritis: Its recognition and significance (Abstr). Arthritis Rheum 6:292, 1963.

142. Linscheid RL, Dobyns JH, Beabout JW, et al: Traumatic instability of the wrist. Diagnosis, classification, and pathomechanics. J Bone Joint Surg [Am] *54*:1612, 1972.

143. Collins LC, Lidsky MD, Sharp JT, et al: Malposition of carpal bones in rheumatoid arthritis. Radiology *103*:95, 1972.

144. Arkless R: Rheumatoid wrists: Cineradiography. Radiology 88:543, 1967.

145. Straub LR, Ranawat CS: The wrist in rheumatoid arthritis. Surgical treatment and results. J Bone Joint Surg [Am] *51*:1, 1969.

146. Freyberg RH: A study of the time of onset of structural joint damage in rheumatoid arthritis (Abstr). Arthritis Rheum *11*:481, 1968.

147. Stein H, Dickson RA, Bentley G: Rheumatoid arthritis of the elbow. Pattern of joint involvement and results of synovectomy with excision of the radial head. Ann Rheum Dis *34*:403, 1975.

148. Porter BB, Richardson C, Vainio K: Rheumatoid arthritis of the elbow: The results of synovectomy. J Bone Joint Surg [Br] 56:427, 1974.

149. deSeze S, Debeyre N, Djian A, et al: The elbow joint. *In* ME Carter (Ed): Radiological Aspects of Rheumatoid Disease. Proceedings of an International Symposium, Amsterdam, 1963. Amsterdam, Excerpta Medica, 1964, p 115.

150. May V, Aristoff H, Glowinski J: La monoarthrite rhumatoïde du coude. Rev Rhum Mal Osteoartic *39*:801, 1972.

151. Bilka PJ: Physical examination of the arthritic patient. Bull Rheum Dis 20:596, 1970.

152. Ehrlich GE, Guttmann GG: Valvular mechanisms in antecubital cysts of rheumatoid arthritis. Arthritis Rheum *16*:259, 1973.

153. Leffert RD, Dorfman HD: Antecubital cyst in rheumatoid arthritis—surgical findings. J Bone Joint Surg [Am] *54*:1555, 1972.

154. Inglis AE, Ranawat CS, Straub LR: Synovectomy and debridement of the elbow in rheumatoid arthritis. J Bone Joint Surg [Am] 53:652, 1971.

155. Torgerson WR, Leach RE: Synovectomy of the elbow in rheumatoid arthritis. J Bone Joint Surg [Am] 52:371, 1970.

156. Wilson DW: Synovectomy of the elbow for rheumatoid arthritis. Proc R Soc Med *64*:264, 1971.

157. Wilson DW, Arden GP, Ansell BM: Synovectomy of the elbow in rheumatoid arthritis. J Bone Joint Surg [Br] 55:106, 1973.

158. Hurri L, Pulkki T, Vainio K: Arthroplasty of the elbow in rheumatoid arthritis. Acta Chir Scand *127*:459, 1964.

159. Dickson RA, Stein H, Bentley G: Excision arthroplasty of the elbow in rheumatoid disease. J Bone Joint Surg [Br] *58*:227, 1976.

160. Jackman RJ, Pugh DG: The positive elbow fat pad sign in rheumatoid arthritis. AJR *108*:812, 1970.

161. Weston WJ: The synovial changes at the elbow in rheumatoid arthritis. Australas Radiol *15*:170, 1971.

162. Rappoport AS, Sosman JL, Weissman BN: Spontaneous fractures of the olecranon process in rheumatoid arthritis. Radiology *119*:83, 1976.

163. Bouman WRJJ: The elbow joint. *In* ME Carter (Ed): Radiological Aspects of Rheumatoid Disease. Proceedings of an International Symposium, Amsterdam, 1963. Amsterdam, Excerpta Medica, 1964, p 125.

164. Weissenbach RJ, Francon F, Perles L: L'articulation scapulo-humerale dans le rhumatisme chronique infectieux. Arch Rheumatol 4:25, 1941.

165. Weil MP, Perroy A, Sichere RM, et al: L'articulation de l'epaule dans le rhumatisme evolutif. Rev Rhum Mal Osteoartic *18*:613, 1951.

166. Laine VAI, Vainio KJ, Pekanmaki K: Shoulder affections in rheumatoid arthritis. Ann Rheum Dis *13*:157, 1954.

167. deSeze S, Debeyre N, Manuel R: The shoulder. *In* ME Carter (Ed): Radiological Aspects of Rheumatoid Disease. Proceedings of an International Symposium, Amsterdam, 1963. Amsterdam, Excerpta Medica, 1964, p 147.

168. McNair MM, Boyle JA, Buchanan WW, et al: A clinical and radiological study of rheumatoid arthritis with a note on the findings in osteoarthrosis. I. The shoulder joint. Clin Radiol 20:269, 1969.

169. Booth RE, Marvel JP: Differential diagnosis of shoulder pain. Orthop Clin North Am 6:353, 1975.

170. Sbarbaro JL: The rheumatoid shoulder. Orthop Clin North Am 6:593, 1975.

171. Huston KA, Nelson AM, Hunder GG: Shoulder swelling in rheumatoid arthritis secondary to subacromial bursitis. Arthritis Rheum *21*:145, 1978.

172. Weston WJ: The enlarged subdeltoid bursa in rheumatoid arthritis. Br J Radiol *42*:481, 1969.

173. Lane PWF, Dyer NH, Hawkins CF: Synovial rupture of the shoulder joint. Br Med J *1*:356, 1972.

174. Meijers KAE: Shoulder joint. *In* ME Carter (Ed): Radiological Aspects of Rheumatoid Disease. Proceedings of an International Symposium, Amsterdam, 1963. Amsterdam, Excerpta Medica, 1964, p 137.

175. DeSmet AA, Ting YM, Weiss JJ: Shoulder arthrography in rheumatoid arthritis. Radiology *116*:601, 1975.

176. Nakata H, Russell WJ: Chest roentgenograms in rheumatoid arthritis: Hiroshima-Nagasaki. AJR *108*:819, 1970.

177. Alpert M, Meyers M: Osteolysis of the acromial end of clavicles in rheumatoid arthritis. AJR 86:251, 1961.

178. Ennevaara K: Painful shoulder joint in rheumatoid arthritis: Clinical and radiological study of 200 cases with special reference to arthrography of the glenohumeral joint. Acta Rheumatol Scand *11*(Suppl):1, 1967.

179. Alpert M, Feldman F: Rib lesions in rheumatoid arthritis. Radiology 82:872, 1964.

180. Beranbaum SL, Ozoktay S: Roentgen study of advanced rheumatoid arthritis of the shoulder joint. St Barnabas Hosp Med Bull *1*:39, 1963.

181. Zuckner J, Martin JM: The acromioclavicular joint in rheumatoid arthritis (Abstr). Arthritis Rheum *13*:360, 1970.

182. Weston WJ: Erosions of the acromion process of the scapula in rheumatoid arthritis. Australas Radiol *17*:219, 1973.

183. Sharon E, Vieux U, Seckler SG: Giant synovial cyst of the shoulder and perforation of the nasal septum in (a patient with) rheumatoid arthritis. Mt Sinai J Med *45*:103, 1978.

184. Martel W: The shoulder: discussion. *In* ME Carter (Ed): Radiological Aspects of Rheumatoid Disease. Proceedings of an International Symposium, Amsterdam, 1963. Amsterdam, Excerpta Medica, 1964, p 165.

185. Resnick D, Niwayama G: Resorption of the undersurface of the distal clavicle in rheumatoid arthritis. Radiology *120*:75, 1976.

186. Park WM, Ward D, Ball J, et al: Rheumatoid disease and rib defects. Ann Rheum Dis 30:466, 1971.

187. Kalliomaki JL, Viitanen S-M, Virtama P: Radiological findings of sternoclavicular joints in rheumatoid arthritis. Acta Rheumatol Scand *14*:233, 1968.

188. Dihlmann W: Röntgendiagnostik der Iliosakralgelenke und ihrer nahen Umgebung. Stuttgart, G Thieme, 1967.

189. Laitenen H, Saksanen S, Suoranta H: Involvement of the manubriosternal articulation in rheumatoid arthritis. Acta Rheumatol Scand *16*:40, 1970.

190. Dilsen N, McEwen C, Poppel M, et al: A comparative roentgenologic study of rheumatoid arthritis and rheumatoid (ankylosing) spondylitis. Arthritis Rheum 5:341, 1962.

191. Hart FD, Robinson KC, Allchin FM, et al: Ankylosing spondylitis. Q J Med *18*:217, 1949.

192. Savill DL: The manubriosternal joint in ankylosing spondylitis. J Bone Joint Surg [Br] 33:56, 1951.

193. Passler HW: Zur normalen und pathologischen Anatomie und Zur Pathologie des Brustbeins. Beitr Pathol Anat 87:659, 1931.

194. Kormano M: A microradiographic and histological study of the manubriosternal joint in rheumatoid arthritis. Acta Rheumatol Scand *16*:47, 1970.

195. Perrin RL, Roller WR, Perkins DG: Sternal destruction in rheumatoid arthritis. Skel Radiol 2:95, 1977.

196. Rapoport RJ, Carrera GF, Kozin F: Manubriosternal joint subluxation in rheumatoid arthritis. J Rheumatol 6:174, 1979.

197. Ashley GT: The morphological and pathological significance of synostosis at the manubriosternal joint. Thorax 9:159, 1954.

198. Solovay J, Gardner C: Involvement of the manubriosternal joint in Marie-Strumpell disease. AJR 65:749, 1951.

199. Short CL, Bauer W, Reynolds WE: Rheumatoid Arthritis. Cambridge, Mass, Harvard University Press, 1957.

200. Calabro JJ: A critical evaluation of the diagnostic features of the feet in rheumatoid arthritis. Arthritis Rheum 5:19, 1962.

201. Thould AK, Simon G: Assessment of radiological changes in hands and feet in rheumatoid arthritis. Ann Rheum Dis 25:220, 1966.

202. Minaker K, Little H: Painful feet in rheumatoid arthritis. Can Med Assoc J *109*:724, 1973.

203. Calabro JJ: The feet in rheumatoid arthritis (Abstr). AIR—Arch Int Rheumatol 2:249, 1959.

204. Calabro JJ: The feet as an aid in the differential diagnosis of arthritis (Abstr). Arthritis Rheum 3:435, 1960.

205. Dixon AS: The rheumatoid foot. *In* AGS Hill (Ed): Modern Trends in Rheumatology. Vol II. London, Butterworths, 1971, p 158.

206. Dixon AS: Medical aspects of the rheumatoid foot. Proc R Soc Med 63:677, 1970.

207. Bienenstock H: Rheumatoid plantar synovial cysts. Ann Rheum Dis *34*:98, 1975.

208. Bywaters EGL: Fistulous rheumatism. A manifestation of rheumatoid arthritis. Ann Rheum Dis *12*:114, 1953.

209. Rosin AJ, Toghill PJ: Fistulous rheumatism. An unusual complication of rheumatoid arthritis. Postgrad Med J 39:96, 1963.

210. Shapiro RF, Resnick D, Castles JJ, et al: Fistulization of rheumatoid joints: A spectrum of identifiable syndromes. Ann Rheum Dis *34*:489, 1975.

211. Jayson MIV, Barks JS: Oedema in rheumatoid arthritis: Changes in the coefficient of capillary filtration. Br Med J 2:555, 1971.

212. Schwartzmann JR: The surgical management of foot deformities in rheumatoid arthritis. Clin Orthop 36:86, 1964.

213. Clayton ML: Surgical treatment of the rheumatoid foot. *In* NJ Giannestras (Ed): Foot Disorders. Philadelphia, Lea & Febiger, 1967, p 319.

214. Faithful DK, Savill DL: Review of the results of excision of the metatarsal heads in patients with rheumatoid arthritis. Ann Rheum Dis 30:201, 1971.

215. Barton NJ: Arthroplasty of the forefoot in rheumatoid arthritis. J Bone Joint Surg [Br] 55:126, 1973.

216. Isemein L, Fournier AM: The foot. *In* ME Carter (Ed): Radiological Aspects of Rheumatoid Disease. Proceedings of an International Symposium, Amsterdam, 1963. Amsterdam, Excerpta Medica, 1964, p 83.

217. Martel W: Acute and chronic arthritis of the foot. Semin Roentgenol 5:391, 1970.

218. Resnick D: The interphalangeal joint of the great toe in rheumatoid arthritis. J Can Assoc Radiol 26:255, 1975.

219. Resnick D, Niwayama G, Feingold ML: The sesamoid bones of the hands and feet: Participators in arthritis. Radiology *123*:57, 1977.

220. Gheith SL, Dixon AS: Tangential x-ray of the forefoot in rheumatoid arthritis. Ann Rheum Dis *31*:92, 1973.

221. Kirkup JR, Vidigal E, Jacoby RK: The hallux and rheumatoid arthritis. Acta Orthop Scand 48:527, 1977.
222. Haines RW, McDougall A: The anatomy of hallux valgus. J Bone Joint Surg [Br] 36:272, 1954.
223. Vainio S: The rheumatoid foot: A clinical study with pathological and roentgenological comments. Ann Chir Gynaecol Fenn 45:Suppl 1, 1956.
224. Weston WJ, Anttila P: Synovial lesions of the midtarsal and posterior subtaloid joints in rheumatoid arthritis. Australas Radiol 16:84, 1972.
225. Resnick D: Roentgen features of the rheumatoid mid and hindfoot. J Can Assoc Radiol 27:99, 1976.
226. Resnick D: Radiology of the talocalcaneal articulations. Anatomic considerations and arthrography. Radiology 111:581, 1974.
227. Romanes GJ: Cunningham's Textbook of Anatomy. 11th Ed. London, Oxford University Press, 1972.
228. Bywaters EGL: Heel lesions of rheumatoid arthritis. Ann Rheum Dis 13:42, 1954.
229. Sutro CJ: The os calcis; the tendo Achillis and the local bursae. Bull Hosp Joint Dis 27:76, 1966.
230. Gerster JC, Vischer TL, Bennani A, et al: The painful heel. Comparative study in rheumatoid arthritis, ankylosing spondylitis, Reiter's syndrome, and generalized osteoarthrosis. Ann Rheum Dis 36:343, 1977.
231. Resnick D, Feingold ML, Curd J, et al: Calcaneal abnormalities in articular disorders. Rheumatoid arthritis, ankylosing spondylitis, psoriatic arthritis and Reiter's syndrome. Radiology 125:355, 1977.
232. Weston WJ: The bursa deep to tendo Achillis. Australas Radiol 14:327, 1970.
233. Rask MR: Achilles tendon rupture owing to rheumatoid disease. Case report with a nine-year follow-up. JAMA 239:435, 1978.
234. Bedi SS, Ellis W: Spontaneous rupture of the calcaneal tendon in rheumatoid arthritis after local steroid injection. Ann Rheum Dis 29:494, 1970.
235. Palmer DG: Tendon sheaths and bursae involved by rheumatoid disease at the foot and ankle. Australas Radiol 14:419, 1970.
236. Saunders CG, Weston WJ: Synovial mass lesions in the anteroposterior projection of the ankle joint. J Can Assoc Radiol 22:275, 1971.
237. Kirkup JR: Ankle and tarsal joints in rheumatoid arthritis. Scand J Rheumatol 3:50, 1974.
238. Vidigal E, Jacoby RJ, Dixon AS, et al: The foot in rheumatoid arthritis. Ann Rheum Dis 34:292, 1975.
239. Hug G, Dixon AS: Ankle joint synoviography in rheumatoid arthritis. Ann Rheum Dis 36:532, 1977.
240. Fulp MJ: Arthrography of the ankle. J Am Podiatry Assoc 63:502, 1973.
241. Cary GR: Methods for determining the presence of subtle knee joint effusion. J La State Med Soc 118:147, 1966.
242. Genovese GR, Jayson MIV, Dixon AS: Protective value of synovial cysts in rheumatoid knees. Ann Rheum Dis 31:179, 1972.
243. Mills K: Pathology of the knee joint in rheumatoid arthritis. A contribution to the understanding of synovectomy. J Bone Joint Surg [Br] 52:746, 1970.
244. Magyar E, Talerman A, Fehér M, et al: Giant bone cysts in rheumatoid arthritis. J Bone Joint Surg [Br] 56:121, 1974.
245. Ranawat CS, Desai K: Role of early synovectomy of the knee joint in rheumatoid arthritis. Arthritis Rheum 18:117, 1975.
246. Aidem HP, Baker LD: Synovectomy of the knee joint in rheumatoid arthritis. JAMA 187:4, 1964.
247. Paradies LH: Synovectomy for rheumatoid arthritis of the knee. J Bone Joint Surg [Am] 57:95, 1975.
248. Marmor L: Surgery of the rheumatoid knee. Synovectomy and debridement. J Bone Joint Surg [Am] 55:535, 1973.
249. Goldie I: Pathomorphologic features in original and regenerated synovial tissue after synovectomy in rheumatoid arthritis. Clin Orthop 77:295, 1971.
250. Ranawat CS, Straub LR, Freyberg R, et al: A study of regenerated synovium after synovectomy of the knee in rheumatoid arthritis. Arthritis Rheum 14:117, 1971.
251. Patzakis MJ, Mills DM, Bartholomew BA, et al: A visual, histological, and enzymatic study of regenerating rheumatoid synovium in the synovectomized knee. J Bone Joint Surg [Am] 55:287, 1973.
252. Kulka JP, Bocking D, Ropes MW, et al: Early joint lesions of rheumatoid arthritis. Report of eight cases with knee biopsies of lesions less than one year's duration. Arch Pathol 59:129, 1955.
253. Turner RA, Brown EM, Sbarbaro JL, et al: Arthroplasty of the knee with tibial and/or femoral metallic implants in rheumatoid arthritis. Rheumatologic evaluation. Arthritis Rheum 15:1, 1972.
254. Wilson FC: Total replacement of the knee in rheumatoid arthritis. A prospective study of the results of treatment with the Walldius prosthesis. J Bone Joint Surg [Am] 54:1429, 1972.
255. Potter TA, Weinfeld MS, Thomas WH: Arthroplasty of the knee in rheumatoid arthritis and osteoarthritis. A follow-up study after implantation of the McKeever and MacIntosh prostheses. J Bone Joint Surg [Am] 54:1, 1972.
256. Kampner SL, Kuzell W: Intra-articular rheumatoid nodule of the knee joint. Clin Orthop 114:243, 1976.
257. Huang TL, Fossier C, Ray RD, et al: Intra-articular rheumatoid nodule of the knee joint associated with recurrent subluxation of the patella. A case report. J Bone Joint Surg [Am] 61:438, 1979.
258. Razzano CD, Wilde AH, Phalen GS: Bilateral rupture of the infrapatellar tendon in rheumatoid arthritis. Clin Orthop 91:158, 1973.
259. Resnick D, Newell J, Guerra J, et al: The proximal tibiofibular joint. Anatomic-pathologic-radiographic correlation. AJR 131:133, 1978.

260. Bossingham DH, Schorn D, Morgan G: Patterns of hip involvement in rheumatoid arthritis (RA) (Abstr). Ann Rheum Dis 37:293, 1978.
261. Samuelson C, Ward JR, Albo D: Rheumatoid synovial cyst of the hip. A case report. Arthritis Rheum 14:105, 1971.
262. Watson JD, Ochsner SF: Compression of bladder due to "rheumatoid" cysts of hip joint. AJR 99:695, 1967.
263. Torisu T, Chosa H, Kitano M: Rheumatoid synovial cyst of the hip joint. A case report. Clin Orthop 137:191, 1978.
264. Hermodsson I: Roentgen appearances of arthritis of the hip. Acta Radiol Diagn 12:865, 1972.
265. Resnick D: Patterns of migration of the femoral head in osteoarthritis of the hip: Roentgenographic-pathologic correlation and comparison with rheumatoid arthritis. AJR 124:62, 1975.
266. Duthie JJR, Brown PE, Truelove LH, et al: Course and prognosis in rheumatoid arthritis. A further report. Ann Rheum Dis 23:193, 1964.
267. Arlet J: Monoarthrites "rhumatismales" chroniques de la hanche (20 observations anatomo-cliniques). Rev Rhum Mal Osteoartic 39:789, 1972.
268. Hastings DE, Parker SM: Protrusio acetabuli in rheumatoid arthritis. Clin Orthop 108:76, 1975.
269. Armbuster T, Guerra J, Resnick D, et al: The adult hip: An anatomic study. Part I. The bony landmarks. Radiology 128:1, 1978.
270. Duncan H: Bone dynamics of rheumatoid arthritis in patients treated with adrenal cortico-steroids. Arthritis Rheum 10:216, 1967.
271. Resnick D, Niwayama G, Coutts R: Subchondral cysts (geodes) in arthritic disorders: Pathologic and radiographic appearance of the hip joint. AJR 128:799, 1977.
272. Cruickshank B, Macleod IG, Shearer WS: Subarticular pseudocysts in rheumatoid arthritis. J Fac Radiologists 5:218, 1954.
273. Soila P: The causal relations of rheumatoid disintegration of juxtaarticular bone trabeculae. Acta Rheum Scand 9:231, 1963.
274. Hunder GG, Ward LE, Ivins JC: Rheumatoid granulomatous lesion simulating malignancy in the head and neck of the femur. Mayo Clin Proc 40:766, 1965.
275. Colton CL, Darby AJ: Giant granulomatous lesions of the femoral head and neck in rheumatoid arthritis. Ann Rheum Dis 29:626, 1970.
276. Doury P, Mine J, Delahaye R-P, et al: La coxite rhumatoïde à forme pseudotumorale. Ann Med Interne 130:31, 1979.
277. Baggenstoss AH, Bickel WH, Ward LE: Rheumatoid granulomatous nodules as destructive lesions of vertebrae. J Bone Joint Surg [Am] 34:601, 1952.
278. Steven GS: Analysis of radiographic appearances in chronic arthritis. Proc R Soc Med 42:354, 1949.
279. Hermodsson I: Roentgen picture of osteo-arthritis in the hip joint in cases of polyarthritis rheumatica chronica. Acta Radiol 29:139, 1948.
280. Pascual E, Steinberg ME, Schumacher HR: Restoration of the hip joint space in long standing rheumatoid arthritis following contralateral cup arthroplasty. Clin Orthop 111:121, 1975.
281. Schwartzmann JR: Arthroplasty of the hip in rheumatoid arthritis. A follow-up study of sixty-eight hips. J Bone Joint Surg [Am] 41:705, 1959.
282. Peterson LFA: Surgery for rheumatoid arthritis—timing and techniques: The lower extremity. J Bone Joint Surg [Am] 50:587, 1968.
283. Clayton ML: Care of the rheumatoid hip. Clin Orthop 90:70, 1973.
284. Conaty JP: Surgery of the hip and knee in patients with rheumatoid arthritis. J Bone Joint Surg [Am] 55:301, 1973.
285. Brattstrom H, Cedell C-A, Hagstam A, et al: Cup arthroplasty in patients with rheumatoid arthritis. Acta Orthop Scand 45:89, 1974.
286. Johnson KA: Arthroplasty of both hips and both knees in rheumatoid arthritis. J Bone Joint Surg [Am] 57:901, 1975.
287. Harris J, Lightowler CDR, Todd RC: Total hip replacement in inflammatory hip disease using the Charnley prosthesis. Br Med J 2:750, 1972.
288. Poss R, Ewald FC, Thomas WH, et al: Complications of total hip replacement arthroplasty in patients with rheumatoid arthritis. J Bone Joint Surg [Am] 58:1130, 1976.
289. Sharp J: The differential diagnosis of ankylosing spondylitis. Br Med J 1:975, 1957.
290. Dixon AS, Lience E: Sacro-iliac joint in adult rheumatoid arthritis and psoriatic arthropathy. Ann Rheum Dis 20:247, 1961.
291. Sievers K, Laine V: The sacro-iliac joint in rheumatoid arthritis in adult females. Acta Rheumatol Scand 9:222, 1963.
292. Dixon AS: The sacroiliac joint in adult rheumatoid arthritis. In ME Carter (Ed): Radiological Aspects of Rheumatoid Disease. Proceedings of an International Symposium, Amsterdam, 1963. Amsterdam, Excerpta Medica, 1964, p 267.
293. Wilkinson M, Meikle JAK: Tomography of the sacroiliac joints. Ann Rheum Dis 25:433, 1966.
294. Martel W, Duff IF: Pelvo-spondylitis in rheumatoid arthritis. Radiology 77:744, 1961.
295. Resnick D, Niwayama G, Goergen TG: Degenerative disease of the sacro-iliac joint. Invest Radiol 10:608, 1975.
296. Kormano M: Symphysial changes in rheumatoid arthritis. Scand J Rheumatol 4:17, 1975.
297. Kormano M: Radiographic appearance of the pubic symphysis in old age and in rheumatoid arthritis. Acta Rheumatol Scand 17:286, 1971.
298. Sargent EN, Turner AF, Jacobson G: Superior marginal rib defects—an etiologic classification. AJR 106:491, 1969.
299. Cohen MJ, Ezekiel J, Persellin RH: Costovertebral and costotransverse joint involvement in rheumatoid arthritis. Ann Rheum Dis 37:473, 1978.

300. Bywaters EGL: Rheumatoid discitis in the thoracic region due to spread from costovertebral joints. Ann Rheum Dis 33:408, 1974.
301. Glay A, Rona G: Nodular rheumatoid vertebral lesions versus ankylosing spondylitis. AJR 94:631, 1965.
302. Lorber A, Pearson CM, Rene RM: Osteolytic vertebral lesions as manifestation of rheumatoid arthritis and related disorders. Arthritis Rheum 4:514, 1961.
303. Seaman WB, Wells J: Destructive lesions of vertebral bodies in rheumatoid disease. AJR 86:241, 1961.
304. Linquist PR, McDonnell DE: Rheumatoid cyst causing extradural compression. J Bone Joint Surg [Am] 52:1235, 1970.
305. Maher JA: Dural nodules in rheumatoid arthritis. Arch Pathol 58:354, 1954.
306. Ellman P, Cudkowicz L, Elwood JS: Widespread serous membrane involvement by rheumatoid nodules. J Clin Pathol 7:239, 1954.
307. Friedman H: Intraspinal rheumatoid nodule causing nerve root compression. J Neurosurg 32:689, 1970.
308. Fairburn B: Spinal cord compression by a rheumatoid nodule. J Neurol Neurosurg Psychiatry 38:1056, 1975.
309. Lawrence JS, Sharp J, Ball J, Bier F: Rheumatoid arthritis of the lumbar spine. Ann Rheum Dis 23:205, 1964.
310. Ball J: Discussion of rheumatoid discitis in the thoracic region. Ann Rheum Dis 33:408, 1974.
311. Sims-Williams H, Jayson MIV, Baddeley H: Rheumatoid involvement of the lumbar spine. Ann Rheum Dis 36:524, 1977.
312. Shichikawa K, Matsui K, Oze K, Ota H: Rheumatoid spondylitis. Int Orthop (SICOT) 2:53, 1978.
313. Resnick D: Thoracolumbar spine abnormalities in rheumatoid arthritis. Ann Rheum Dis 37:389, 1978.
314. Resnick D, Niwayama G: Intravertebral disc herniations: Cartilaginous (Schmorl's) nodes. Radiology 126:57, 1978.
315. Bland JH: Rheumatoid arthritis of the cervical spine. Bull Rheum Dis 18:471, 1967.
316. Bland JH: Rheumatoid arthritis of the cervical spine. J Rheumatol 1:319, 1974.
317. Sharp J, Purser DW, Lawrence JS: Rheumatoid arthritis of the cervical spine in the adult. Ann Rheum Dis 17:303, 1958.
318. Conlon PW, Isdale IC, Rose BS: Rheumatoid arthritis of the cervical spine. An analysis of 333 cases. Ann Rheum Dis 25:120, 1966.
319. Robinson HS: Rheumatoid arthritis—atlanto-axial subluxation and its clinical presentation. Can Med Assoc J 94:470, 1966.
320. Ornilla E, Ansell BM, Swannell AJ: Cervical spine involvement in patients with chronic arthritis undergoing orthopaedic surgery. Ann Rheum Dis 31:364, 1972.
321. Hopkins JS: Lower cervical rheumatoid subluxation with tetraplegia. J Bone Joint Surg [Br] 49:46, 1967.
322. Ahlgren P, Fog J: Atlanto-epistrophical subluxation in rheumatoid arthritis. Acta Rheumatol Scand 14:210, 1968.
323. Webb FWS, Hickman JA, Brew DS: Death from vertebral artery thrombosis in rheumatoid arthritis. Br Med J 2:537, 1968.
324. Whaley K, Dick WC: Fatal subaxial dislocation of the cervical spine in rheumatoid arthritis. Br Med J 2:31, 1968.
325. Sukoff MH, Kadin MM, Moran T: Transoral decompression for myelopathy caused by rheumatoid arthritis of the cervical spine. Case report. J Neurosurg 37:493, 1972.
326. Martel W, Abell MR: Fatal atlanto-axial luxation in rheumatoid arthritis. Arthritis Rheum 6:224, 1963.
327. Rana NA, Hancock DO, Taylor AR, et al: Atlanto-axial subluxation in rheumatoid arthritis. J Bone Joint Surg [Br] 55:458, 1973.
328. Mathews JA: Atlanto-axial subluxation in rheumatoid arthritis. A 5-year follow-up study. Ann Rheum Dis 33:526, 1974.
329. Park WM, O'Neill M, McCall IW: The radiology of rheumatoid involvement of the cervical spine. Skel Radiol 4:1, 1979.
330. Martel W: The occipito-atlanto-axial joints in rheumatoid arthritis. In ME Carter (Ed): Radiological Aspects of Rheumatoid Disease. Proceedings of an International Symposium, Amsterdam, 1963. Amsterdam, Excerpta Medica, 1964, p 189.
331. Sharp J: Atlanto-axial joints. In Proceedings of the International Symposium on Rheumatoid Arthritis, Amsterdam, 1963. Amsterdam, Excerpta Medica, 1964, p 211.
332. Jackson H: Diagnosis of minimal atlanto-axial subluxation. Br J Radiol 23:672, 1950.
333. Hinck VC, Hopkins CE: Measurement of the atlanto-dental interval in the adult. AJR 84:945, 1960.
334. Coutts MB: Atlanto-epistropheal subluxations. Arch Surg 29:297, 1934.
335. Mathews JA: Atlanto-axial subluxation in rheumatoid arthritis. Ann Rheum Dis 28:260, 1969.
336. Swinson DR, Hamilton EBD, Mathews JA, et al: Vertical subluxation of the axis in rheumatoid arthritis. Ann Rheum Dis 31:359, 1972.
337. Davis FW Jr, Markley HE: Rheumatoid arthritis with death from medullary compression. Ann Intern Med 35:451, 1951.
338. Martel W: The occipito-atlanto-axial joints in rheumatoid arthritis and ankylosing spondylitis. AJR 86:223, 1961.
339. Rana NA, Hancock DO, Taylor AR, Hill AGS: Upward translocation of the dens in rheumatoid arthritis. J Bone Joint Surg [Br] 55:471, 1973.
340. McGregor M: The significance of certain measurements of the skull in the diagnosis of basilar impression. Br J Radiol 21:171, 1948.
341. Martel W, Page JW: Cervical vertebral erosions and subluxations in rheumatoid arthritis and ankylosing spondylitis. Arthritis Rheum 3:546, 1960.
342. Burry HC, Tweed JM, Robinson RG, et al: Lateral subluxation of the atlanto-axial joint in rheumatoid arthritis. Ann Rheum Dis 37:525, 1978.
343. Kornblum D, Clayton ML, Nash HH: Nontraumatic cervical dislocations in rheumatoid spondylitis. JAMA 149:431, 1952.
344. Hamblen DL: Occipito-cervical fusion. Indications, techniques, and results. J Bone Joint Surg [Br] 49:33, 1967.
345. Ferlic DC, Clayton ML, Leidholt JD, et al: Surgical treatment of the symptomatic unstable cervical spine in rheumatoid arthritis. J Bone Joint Surg [Am] 57:349, 1975.
346. Wilson PD Jr, Dangelmajer RC: The problem of atlanto-axial dislocation in rheumatoid arthritis (Abstr). J Bone Joint Surg [Am] 45:1780, 1963.
347. Isdale IC, Conlon PW: Atlanto-axial subluxation: A six year follow-up report. Ann Rheum Dis 30:387, 1971.
348. Rosenberg F, Bataille R, Sany J, et al: Lyse de l'odontoïde au cours de la polyarthrite rhumatoïde. Rev Rhum Mal Osteoartic 45:249, 1978.
349. Martel W, Bole GG: Pathologic fracture of the odontoid process in rheumatoid arthritis. Radiology 90:948, 1968.
350. Freiberger RH, Wilson PD Jr, Nicholas JA: Acquired absence of the odontoid process. A case report. J Bone Joint Surg [Am] 47:1231, 1965.
351. Cabot A, Becker A: The cervical spine in rheumatoid arthritis. Clin Orthop 131:130, 1978.
352. Seignon B, Tellart-Chaudeur MO, Gougeon J: Les lésions destructices du rachis cervical moyen et inférieur au cours de la polyarthrite rhumatoïde. Etude des complications neurologiques. Un cas avec quadriplégie. Revue générale. Sem Hôp Paris 51:1157, 1975.
353. Crellin RQ, Maccabe JJ, Hamilton EBD: Severe subluxation of the cervical spine in rheumatoid arthritis. J Bone Joint Surg [Br] 52:244, 1970.
354. Williams LE, Bland JH, Lipson RL: Cervical spine subluxations and massive osteolysis in the upper extremities in rheumatoid arthritis. Arthritis Rheum 9:348, 1966.
355. Martel W: Pathogenesis of cervical discovertebral destruction in rheumatoid arthritis. Arthritis Rheum 20:1217, 1977.
356. Bywaters EGL: Origin of cervical disc disease in RA. Arthritis Rheum 21:737, 1978.
357. Park WM, O'Brien W: Computer-assisted analysis of radiographic neck lesions in chronic rheumatoid arthritis. Acta Radiol (Diagn) 8:529, 1969.
358. Bland JH, Buskirk FW, Davis PH, et al: Rheumatoid arthritis of the cervical spine. Arthritis Rheum 5:637, 1962.
359. Rasker JJ, Cosh JA: Radiological study of cervical spine and hand in patients with rheumatoid arthritis of 15 years' duration: An assessment of the effects of corticosteroid treatment. Ann Rheum Dis 37:529, 1978.
360. Lawrence JS: Radiological cervical arthritis in populations. Ann Rheum Dis 35:365, 1976.
361. Baum J: Infection in rheumatoid arthritis. Arthritis Rheum 14:135, 1971.
362. Aronoff A, Bywaters EGL, Fearnley GR: Lung lesions in rheumatoid arthritis. Br Med J 2:228, 1955.
363. Huskisson EC, Hart FD: Severe, unusual, and recurrent infections in rheumatoid arthritis. Ann Rheum Dis 31:118, 1972.
364. Walker WC, Wright V: Pulmonary lesions and rheumatoid arthritis. Medicine 47:501, 1968.
365. DeAndrade JR, Tribe CR: Staphylococcal septicaemia with pyoarthrosis in rheumatoid arthritis. Report of three fatal cases. Br Med J 1:1516, 1962.
366. Gaulhofer-de Klerck EH, VanDam G: Septic complications in rheumatoid arthritis. Acta Rheumatol Scand 9:254, 1963.
367. Rimoin DL, Wennberg JE: Acute septic arthritis complicating chronic rheumatoid arthritis. JAMA 196:617, 1966.
368. Johnson JS, Vaughan JH, Hench PK, et al: Rheumatoid arthritis, 1970–1972. Ann Intern Med 78:937, 1973.
369. Mowat AG, Baum J: Chemotaxis of polymorphonuclear leukocytes from patients with rheumatoid arthritis. J Clin Invest 50:2541, 1971.
370. Bodel PT, Hollingsworth JW: Comparative morphology, respiration, and phagocytic function of leukocytes from blood and joint fluid in rheumatoid arthritis. J Clin Invest 45:580, 1966.
371. Bandilla KK, Pitts NC, McDuffie FC: Immunoglobulin M deficiency in the immune response of patients with rheumatoid arthritis. Arthritis Rheum 13:214, 1970.
372. Pruzanski W, Leers WD, Wardlaw AC: Bacteriolytic and bactericidal activity of sera and synovial fluids in rheumatoid arthritis (Abstr). Arthritis Rheum 14:409, 1971.
373. Gibberd FB: A survey of four hundred and six cases of rheumatoid arthritis. Acta Rheumatol Scand 11:62, 1965.
374. Ball J: Post-mortem findings and articular pathology in rheumatoid arthritis. In JJR Duthie, WRM Alexander (Eds): Rheumatic Diseases. Pfizer Medical Monograph 3. Baltimore, Williams & Wilkins, 1968.
375. Argen RJ, Wilson CH Jr, Wood P: Suppurative arthritis. Clinical features of 42 cases. Arch Intern Med 117:661, 1966.
376. Kellgren JH, Ball J, Fairbrother RW, et al: Suppurative arthritis complicating rheumatoid arthritis. Br Med J 1:1193, 1958.
377. Ward J, Cohen AS, Bauer W: The diagnosis and therapy of acute suppurative arthritis. Arthritis Rheum 3:522, 1960.
378. Wilkens RF, Healey LA, Decker JL: Acute infectious arthritis in the aged and chronically ill. Arch Intern Med 106:354, 1960.
379. Karten I: Septic arthritis complicating rheumatoid arthritis. Ann Intern Med 70:1147, 1969.
380. Myers AR, Muller LM, Pinals RS: Pyarthrosis complicating rheumatoid arthritis. Lancet 2:714, 1969.

381. Russell AS, Ansell BM: Septic arthritis. Ann Rheum Dis *31*:40, 1972.
382. Gristina AG, Rovere GD, Shoji H: Spontaneous septic arthritis complicating rheumatoid arthritis. J Bone Joint Surg [Am] *56*:1180, 1974.
383. Resnick D: Pyarthrosis complicating rheumatoid arthritis. Roentgenographic evaluation of 5 patients and a review of the literature. Radiology *114*:581, 1975.
384. Mitchell WS, Brooks PM, Stevenson RD, et al: Septic arthritis in patients with rheumatoid disease: A still underdiagnosed complication. J Rheumatol *3*:124, 1976.
385. Gelman MI, Ward JR: Septic arthritis: A complication of rheumatoid arthritis. Radiology *122*:17, 1977.
386. Kuntz JL, Mansilla D, Pasquali JL, et al: Arthrites septiques spontanées au cours de la polyarthrite rhumatoïde. Sem Hôp Paris *53*:241, 1977.
387. Ryden A-C, Schwan A, Agell B-O: A case of septic arthritis in multiple joints due to *Bacteroides fragilis* in a patient with rheumatoid arthritis. Acta Orthop Scand *49*:98, 1978.
388. Tondreau RL, Hodes PJ, Schmidt ER Jr: Joint infections following steroid therapy: Roentgen manifestations. AJR *82*:258, 1959.
389. Barth WF, Healy LA, Decker JL: Septic arthritis due to *Pasteurella multocida* complicating rheumatoid arthritis. Arthritis Rheum *11*:394, 1968.
390. Norden CW, Sellers TF Jr: *Hemophilus influenzae* pyarthrosis in an adult. JAMA *189*:694, 1964.
391. Dyer HR, Gum OB: Pneumococcal arthritis complicating rheumatoid arthritis. South Med J *59*:537, 1966.
392. Allum TGL: Suppuration in rheumatoid arthritis. Letter to the Editor. Br Med J *1*:1479, 1958.
393. Zawadzki ZA, Benedek TG: Rheumatoid arthritis, dysproteinemic arthropathy, and paraproteinemia. Arthritis Rheum *12*:555, 1969.
394. Hajzok O, Tomik F, Hajzokova M: Amyloidosis in rheumatoid arthritis. A study of 48 histologically confirmed cases. Z Rheumatol *35*:356, 1976.
395. Goldberg A, Brodsky I, McCarty D: Multiple myeloma with paramyloidosis presenting as rheumatoid disease. Am J Med *37*:653, 1964.
396. Gordon DA, Pruzanski W, Ogryzlo MA, et al: Amyloid arthritis simulating rheumatoid disease in five patients with multiple myeloma. Am J Med *55*:142, 1973.
397. Eisman J, Fan PT: Rheumatoid factor in patients with gout. Arthritis Rheum *20*:1147, 1977.
398. McCarty DJ: Diagnostic mimicry in arthritis—patterns of joint involvement associated with calcium pyrophosphate dihydrate crystal deposits. Bull Rheum Dis *25*:804, 1974–1975.
399. Wallace S, Robinson H, Masi AT, et al: Preliminary criteria for the classification of the acute arthritis of primary gout. Arthritis Rheum *20*:895, 1977.
400. Talbott JH, Altman RD, Yu T-F: Gouty arthritis masquerading as rheumatoid arthritis or vice versa. Semin Arthritis Rheum *8*:77, 1978.
401. Russell LA, Bayles TB: The temporomandibular joint in rheumatoid arthritis. J Am Dent Assoc *28*:533, 1941.
402. Uotila E: The temporomandibular joint in adult rheumatoid arthritis. A clinical and roentgenologic study. Acta Odont Scand *22*(Suppl 39):1, 1964.
403. Goodwill CJ, Steggles BG: Destruction of the temporo-mandibular joints in rheumatoid arthritis. Ann Rheum Dis *25*:133, 1966.
404. Ericson S, Lundberg M: Alterations in the temporomandibular joint at various stages of rheumatoid arthritis. Acta Rheumatol Scand *13*:257, 1967.
405. Resnick D: Temporomandibular joint involvement in ankylosing spondylitis. Comparative study with rheumatoid arthritis and psoriasis. Radiology *112*:587, 1974.
406. Montgomery WW, Perone PM, Schall LA: Arthritis of the cricoarytenoid joint. Ann Otol Rhinol Laryngol *64*:1025, 1955.
407. Baker OA, Bywaters EGL: Laryngeal stridor in rheumatoid arthritis due to cricoarytenoid joint involvement. Br Med J *1*:1400, 1957.
408. Bienenstock H, Ehrlich GE, Freyberg RH: Rheumatoid arthritis of the cricoarytenoid joint: A clinicopathologic study. Arthritis Rheum *6*:48, 1963.
409. Copeman WSC: Rheumatoid arthritis of the crico-arytenoid joints. Br Med J *2*:1398, 1957.
410. Goodwell CJ, Lord IJ, Jones RPK: Hearing in rheumatoid arthritis. A clinical and audiometric survey. Ann Rheum Dis *31*:170, 1972.
411. Chalmers IM, Blair GS: Rheumatoid arthritis of the temporomandibular joint. A clinical and radiological study using circular tomography. Q J Med *42*:369, 1973.
412. Resnick D, Curd J, Shapiro RF, et al: Radiographic abnormalities of rheumatoid arthritis in patients with diffuse idiopathic skeletal hyperostosis. Arthritis Rheum *21*:1, 1978.
413. Lillicrap DA: Rheumatoid arthritis and pemphigoid. Proc R Soc Med *56*:921, 1963.
414. Salo OP, Rasanen JA: Pemphigoid and rheumatoid arthritis. A clinical and immunological study. Ann Clin Res *4*:173, 1972.
415. Peck SM, Lefkovits AM: Bullous pemphigoid with polymyositis and coexisting contact dermatitis. Arch Dermatol *94*:672, 1966.
416. Jordon RE, Muller SA, Hale WL, et al: Bullous pemphigoid associated with systemic lupus erythematosus. Arch Dermatol *99*:17, 1969.
417. Torisu T, Watanabe H: Pigmented villonodular synovitis occurring in a rheumatoid patient. A case report. Clin Orthop *91*:134, 1973.
418. Jimenez-Diaz C, Fernandez-Criado M, Navarro V, et al: Sur une forme polyarticulaire de synovite villonodulaire pigmentaire. Rev Rhum Mal Osteoartic *34*:11, 1967.
419. Reginato A, Martinez V, Schumacher HR, et al: Giant cell tumor associated with rheumatoid arthritis. Ann Rheum Dis *33*:333, 1974.
420. Young JM, Hudacek AG: Experimental production of pigmented villonodular synovitis in dogs. Am J Pathol *30*:799, 1954.
421. Mall JC, Genant HK, Silcox DC, et al: The efficacy of fine-detail radiography in the evaluation of patients with rheumatoid arthritis. Radiology *112*:37, 1974.
422. Melson GL, Staple TW, Evens RG: Soft tissue radiographic technique. Semin Roentgenol *8*:19, 1973.
423. Makela P: Studies on soft tissue radiography of the hands in rheumatoid arthritis. Academic dissertation. Turku, Finland, University of Turku, 1978.
424. Makela P, Haataja M: Soft tissue radiography for evaluating clinical activity of rheumatoid arthritis. Acta Radiol (Diagn) *19*:389, 1978.
425. Makela P, Haataja M: Soft tissue radiography of the hands in the rheumatoid arthritis. Scand J Rheumatol *5*:113, 1976.
426. Lovell CR, Brock M, Jayson MIV, et al: Xeroradiography in assessment of the rheumatoid hand. Ann Rheum Dis *36*:464, 1977.
427. Gerster JC, Hauser H, Fallet GH: Xeroradiographic techniques applied to assessment of Achilles tendon in inflammatory or metabolic disease. Ann Rheum Dis *34*:479, 1975.
428. Verow PW, Dippy J: Soft tissue changes in early rheumatoid arthritis as seen on xeroradiography and non-screen radiographs. Clin Radiol *29*:585, 1978.
429. Reichmann S, Astrand K, Deichgraber E, et al: Soft tissue xeroradiography of the shoulder joint. Acta Radiol (Diagn) *16*:572, 1975.
430. Dick WC, Neufeld RR, Prentice AG, et al: Measurement of joint inflammation. A radioisotopic method. Ann Rheum Dis *29*:135, 1970.
431. Weiss TE, Schuler SE: Joint imaging as a clinical aid in diagnosis and therapy of arthritic and related diseases. Bull Rheum Dis *25*:791, 1974.
432. Green FA, Hays MT: The pertechnetate joint scan. II. Clinical correlations. Ann Rheum Dis *31*:278, 1972.
433. Remans J, Berghs H, Drieskens L, et al: Scintiscan evaluation of rheumatoid hands for monitoring the anti-inflammatory effects of drugs. J Belge Rhumatol Med Phys *31*:211, 1976.
434. Sturrock RD, Nicholson R, Wojtulewski JA: Technetium counting in rheumatoid arthritis. Evaluation in the small joints of the hands. Arthritis Rheum *17*:417, 1974.
435. Remans J, Berghs H, Drieskens L, et al: Proximal interphalangeal arthroscintigraphy in rheumatoid arthritis. Ann Rheum Dis *37*:440, 1974.
436. Berry H, Huskisson EC: Isotopic indices as a measure of inflammation in rheumatoid arthritis. Ann Rheum Dis *33*:523, 1974.
437. Oka M, Rekonen A, Ruotsi A: Tc-99m in the study of systemic inflammatory activity in rheumatoid arthritis. Acta Rheumatol Scand *17*:27, 1971.
438. Huskisson EC, Scott J, Balme HW: Objective measurement of rheumatoid arthritis using technetium index. Ann Rheum Dis *35*:81, 1976.
439. Weissberg D, Resnick D, Taylor A, et al: Rheumatoid arthritis and its variants: Analysis of scintiphotographic, radiographic, and clinical examinations. AJR *131*:665, 1978.
440. Hoffer PB, Genant HK: Radionuclide joint imaging. Semin Nucl Med *6*:121, 1976.
441. Robinson WD: The etiology of rheumatoid arthritis. *In* JL Hollander, DJ McCarty Jr (Eds): Arthritis and Allied Conditions. 8th Ed. Philadelphia, Lea & Febiger, 1972, p 297.
442. McMichael AJ, Sasazuki T, McDevitt HO, et al: Increased frequency of HLA-Cw3 and HLA-Dw4 in rheumatoid arthritis. Arthritis Rheum *20*:1037, 1977.
443. Zvaifler NJ: Rheumatoid synovitis. An extravascular immune complex disease. Arthritis Rheum *17*:297, 1974.
444. Conn DL, McDuffie FC, Dyck PJ: Immunopathological study of sural nerves in rheumatoid arthritis. Arthritis Rheum *15*:135, 1972.
445. Hoffman GS: Polyarthritis: The differential diagnosis of rheumatoid arthritis. Semin Arthritis Rheum *8*:115, 1978.
446. Rabinowitz TG, Twersky J, Guttadauria M: Similar bone manifestations of scleroderma and rheumatoid arthritis. AJR *121*:35, 1974.
447. Chevrot A, Correas G, Pallardy G: Atteinte cervicale de la polyarthrite rhumatoïde. Etude de 577 dossiers. J Radiol Electrol Med Nucl *59*:545, 1978.
448. Smith RD: Effect of hemiparesis on rheumatoid arthritis. Arthritis Rheum *22*:1419, 1979.
449. Chalmers A, Traynor JA: Cricoarytenoid arthritis as a cause of acute upper airway obstruction. J Rheumatol *6*:541, 1979.
450. Brushan C, Hodges FJ III, Wityk JJ: Synovial cyst (ganglion) of the lumbar spine simulating extradural mass. Neuroradiology *18*:263, 1979.
451. Seignon B, Tellart MO, Etienne JC, et al: L'arthrite atloïdoaxoïdienne laterale au cours de la polyarthrite rhumatoïde. A propos de dix observations. Sem Hôp Paris *55*:979, 1979.
452. O'Driscoll S, O'Driscoll M: Osteomalacia in rheumatoid arthritis. Ann Rheum Dis *39*:1, 1980.
453. Elhabali M, Scherak O, Seidl G, et al: Tomographic examinations of sacroiliac joints in adult patients with rheumatoid arthritis. J Rheumatol *6*:417, 1979.
454. Yood RA, Goldenberg DL: Sternoclavicular joint arthritis. Arthritis Rheum *23*:232, 1980.
455. Houston BD, Crouch ME, Finch RG: Streptococcus MG-Intermedius (*Streptococcus milleri*) septic arthritis in a patient with rheumatoid arthritis. J Rheumatol *7*:89, 1980.
456. DeMerieux P, Keystone EC, Hutcheon M, et al: Polyarthritis due to *Mycobacterium kansasii* in a patient with rheumatoid arthritis. Ann Rheum Dis *39*:90, 1980.
457. Storms GEMG, Kruijsen MWM, Van Beusekom HJ, et al: Pathological fracture of the odontoid process in rheumatoid arthritis. Neth J Med *23*:120, 1980.
458. Jessee EF, Toone E, Owen DS, et al: Coexistent rheumatoid arthritis and chronic tophaceous gout. Arthritis Rheum *23*:244, 1980.

459. Rizzoli AJ, Trujeque L, Bankhurst AD: The coexistence of gout and rheumatoid arthritis. J Rheumatol 7:316, 1980.

460. Major P, Resnick D, Dalinka M, et al: Coexisting rheumatoid arthritis and ankylosing spondylitis. Am J Rheum 134:1076, 1980.

461. Holt ME, Rooney PJ: Manubrio-sternal joint subluxation in rheumatoid arthritis. J Rheumatol 7:260, 1980.

462. Foster DR, Park WM, McCall IW, et al: The supinator notch sign in rheumatoid arthritis. Clin Radiol 131:195, 1980.

463. Waugh W, Newton G, Tew M: Articular changes associated with a flexion deformity in rheumatoid and osteoarthritic knees. J Bone Joint Surg [Br] 62:180, 1980.

464. DeSilva RTD, Grennan DM, Palmer DG: Lymphatic obstruction in rheumatoid arthritis: A cause for upper limb oedema. Ann Rheum Dis 39:260, 1980.

465. Myers BW, Masi AT, Feiginbaum SL: Pigmented villonodular synovitis and tenosynovitis: A clinical epidemiologic study of 166 cases and literature review. Medicine 59:223, 1980.

466. Benedek TG, Rodnan GP: A brief history of the rheumatic diseases. Bull Rheum Dis 32:59, 1982.

467. Appelboom T, deBoelpaepe C, Ehrlich GE, et al: Rubens and the question of antiquity of rheumatoid arthritis. JAMA 245:483, 1981.

468. Ueno Y, Sawada K, Imura H: Protective effect of neural lesion on rheumatoid arthritis. Arthritis Rheum 26:118, 1983.

469. Hamilton S: Unilateral rheumatoid arthritis in hemiplegia. J Can Assoc Radiol 34:49, 1983.

470. Hammoudeh M, Kahn MA, Kuscher I: Unilateral rheumatoid arthritis. Arthritis Rheum 24:1218, 1981.

471. Lewis RB, Sanders LL, Lipsmeyer E: Characteristics of rheumatoid arthritis in a male population. J Rheumatol 7:559, 1980.

472. Kim RC, Collins GH: The neuropathology of rheumatoid disease. Hum Pathol 12:5, 1981.

473. Howe GB, Fordham JN, Brown KA, et al: Polymorphonuclear cell function in rheumatoid arthritis and in Felty's syndrome. Ann Rheum Dis 40:370, 1981.

474. Schumacher HR: Palindromic onset of rheumatoid arthritis. Clinical, synovial fluid, and biopsy studies. Arthritis Rheum 25:361, 1982.

475. Karr RW, Rodey GE, Lee T, et al: Association of HLA-DRw4 with rheumatoid arthritis in black and white patients. Arthritis Rheum 23:1241, 1980.

476. Young A, Jaraquemada D, Awad J, et al: Association of HLA-DR4/Dw4 and DR2/Dw2 with radiologic changes in a prospective study of patients with rheumatoid arthritis. Arthritis Rheum 27:20, 1984.

477. Schiff B, Mizrachi Y, Orgad S, et al: Association of HLA-Aw31 and HLA-DR1 with adult rheumatoid arthritis. Ann Rheum Dis 41:403, 1982.

478. Depper JM, Zvaifler NJ: Epstein-Barr virus. Its relationship to the pathogenesis of rheumatoid arthritis. Arthritis Rheum 24:755, 1981.

479. Bennett JC: The etiology of rheumatoid arthritis. In WN Kelley, ED Harris, Jr, S Ruddy, CB Sledge (eds): Textbook of Rheumatology. Philadelphia, WB Saunders Co, p. 887.

480. Mannerfelt L, Norman O: Attrition ruptures of flexor tendons in rheumatoid arthritis caused by bony spurs in the carpal tunnel. J Bone Joint Surg [Br] 51:270, 1969.

481. Read GO, Solomon L, Biddulph S: Relationship between finger and wrist deformities in rheumatoid arthritis. Ann Rheum Dis 42:619, 1983.

482. Owsianik WDJ, Kundi A, Whitehead JN, et al: Radiological articular involvement in the dominant hand in rheumatoid arthritis. Ann Rheum Dis 39:508, 1980.

483. Stelling CB, Keats MM, Keats TE: Irregularities at the base of the proximal phalanges: false indicator of early rheumatoid arthritis. AJR 138:695, 1982.

484. Rombouts JJ, Rombouts-Lindemans C: L'atteinte de la main au cours de la polyarthrite rhumatoide. Louvain Med 99:693, 1980.

485. Shapiro JS: Wrist involvement in rheumatoid swan-neck deformity. J Hand Surg 7:484, 1982.

486. Rymaszewski LA, Mackay I, Amis AA, et al: Long-term effects of excision of the radial head in rheumatoid arthritis. J Bone Joint Surg [Br] 66:109, 1984.

487. Goldin DS, Stangler DA, Canoso JJ: Rheumatoid subcutaneous bursitis. J Rheumatol 8:974, 1981.

488. Taccari E, Teodori S: Rheumatoid chyliform bursitis: pathogenetic role of rheumatoid nodules. Arthritis Rheum 27:221, 1984.

489. Macfarlane JD, Van DerLinden SJ: Leaking rheumatoid olecranon bursitis as a cause of forearm swelling. Ann Rheum Dis 40:309, 1981.

490. Delcambre B, Siame JL, Leroux JL: Rupture capsulaire de l'épaule dans un cas de polyarthrite rhumatoïde responsable d'un oedème pseudophlébitique du membre supérieur. Rev Rheum Mal Osteoartic 48:455, 1981.

491. Sebes JI, Salazar JE: The manubriosternal joint in rheumatoid disease. AJR 140:117, 1983.

492. Grosbois B, Pawlotsky Y, Chales G, et al: Etude clinique et radiologique de l'articulation manubrio-sternale. Rev Rhum Mal Osteoartic 48:495, 1981.

493. Wiseman MJ: Dislocation of the manubriosternal joint in rheumatoid arthritis. Ann Rheum Dis 40:307, 1981.

494. Khong TK, Rooney PJ: Manubriosternal joint subluxation in rheumatoid arthritis. J Rheumatol 9:712, 1982.

495. Itani M, Evans GA, Park WM: Spontaneous sternal collapse. J Bone Joint Surg [Br] 64:432, 1982.

496. McGuigan L, Burke D, Fleming A: Tarsal tunnel syndrome and peripheral neuropathy in rheumatoid disease. Ann Rheum Dis 42:128, 1983.

497. Awerbuch MS, Shephard E, Vernon-Roberts B: Morton's metatarsalgia due to intermetatarsophalangeal bursitis as an early manifestation of rheumatoid arthritis. Clin Orthop 167:214, 1982.

498. Bouysset M, Bouvier M, Bonvoisin B, et al: Fractures spontanées sur pied rhumatoide. Lyon Med 250:95, 1983.

499. Mann RA: Acquired flatfoot in adults. Clin Orthop 181:46, 1983.

500. Claustre J, Bonnel F, Constans JP, et al: L'espace intercapitometatarsien. Rev Rhum Mal Osteoartic 50:435, 1980.

501. Pastershank SP: Mid-foot dissociation in rheumatoid arthritis. J Can Assoc Radiol 32:166, 1981.

502. Ang JC, Rubenstein J, English E: Subtalar dislocation in rheumatoid arthritis. J Rheumatol 9:671, 1982.

503. Gonzalez-Lanza M, Elena A, Vadillo JAG: Subtalar dislocation in rheumatoid arthritis. J Rheumatol 11:113, 1984.

504. Moilanen A, Vilppula A: A rare condition of rheumatoid arthritis. ROFO 139:706, 1983.

505. Spencer JD, Hayes KC, Alexander IJ: Knee joint effusion and quadriceps reflex inhibition in man. Arch Phys Med Rehabil 65:171, 1984.

506. Fujikawa K: Arthrographic studies of the rheumatoid knee. Part I. Synovial proliferation. Ann Rheum Dis 40:332, 1981.

507. Fujikawa K, Tanaka Y, Matsubayashi T, et al: Arthrographic study of the rheumatoid knee. Part 2. Articular cartilage and menisci. Ann Rheum Dis 40:344, 1981.

508. Boerbooms AMT, Vanderbroek WJM, VanRens TJG, et al: 99mTc-pertechnetate uptake after total knee replacement in rheumatoid arthritis. Acta Orthop Scand 53:125, 1982.

509. Jager M, Schmidt JM: Subluxation in proximalen Tibiofibulargelenk auf dem Boden einer Synovialitis bei chronischer Polyarthritis. Akt Rheumatol 6:103, 1981.

510. Levy R, Hermann G, Haimov M, et al: Rheumatoid synovial cyst of the hip. Arthritis Rheum 25:1382, 1982.

511. Jacobs P, The HSG, Bijlsma A, et al: Rheumatoid synovial cyst of the hip. Arthritis Rheum 26:814, 1983.

512. Raman D, Haslock I: Trochanteric bursitis—a frequent cause of hip pain in rheumatoid arthritis. Ann Rheum Dis 41:602, 1982.

513. Gerster JC, Anani P, deGoumoens P, et al: Lytic lesions of the femoral neck in rheumatoid arthritis simulating pigmented villonodular synovitis or malignancy. Clin Rheumatol 1:30, 1982.

514. Ranawat CS, Dorr LD, Inglis AE: Total hip arthroplasty in protrusio acetabuli of rheumatoid arthritis. J Bone Joint Surg [Am] 62:1059, 1980.

515. DeCarvalho A, Graudal H: Sacroiliac joint involvement in classical or definite rheumatoid arthritis. Acta Radiol (Diagn) 21:417, 1980.

516. Dahlquist SR, Nordmark LG, Bjelle A: HLA-B27 and involvement of sacroiliac joints in rheumatoid arthritis. J Rheumatol 11:27, 1984.

517. Graudal H, deCarvalho A, Lissen L: The course of sacroiliac involvement in rheumatoid arthritis. Scand J Rheumatol 32:(Suppl)34, 1979.

518. Casey D, Mirra J, Staple TW: Parasymphyseal insufficiency fractures of the os pubis. AJR 142:581, 1984.

519. McKendry RJR, Hogan DB: Superior margin rib defects in rheumatoid arthritis. J Rheumatol 8:673, 1981.

520. Hogan DB, McKendry RJR: Radionuclide appearance of rheumatoid rib erosions. Clin Nucl Med 6:366, 1981.

521. Jurik AG, Pedersen U: Rheumatoid arthritis of the crico-arytenoid and crico-thyroid joints: A radiological and clinical study. Clin Radiol 35:233, 1984.

522. Jurik AG: Visualization of the intralaryngeal joints. A low voltage radiological study. Clin Radiol 33:687, 1982.

523. Bridger MWM, Jahn AF, Van Nostrand AWP: Laryngeal rheumatoid arthritis. Laryngoscope 90:296, 1980.

524. Larheim TA, Storhaug K, Tveito L: Temporomandibular joint involvement and dental occlusion in a group of adults with rheumatoid arthritis. Acta Odontol Scand 41:301, 1983.

525. Bywaters EGL: Thoracic intervertebral discitis in rheumatoid arthritis due to costovertebral joint involvement. Rheumatol Int 1:83, 1981.

526. Jackson H: Atlanto-axial subluxation. Radiology 148:864, 1983.

527. Weissman BNW, Alibadi P, Weinfeld MS, et al: Prognostic features of atlanto-axial subluxation in rheumatoid arthritis. Radiology 144:745, 1982.

528. El-Khoury GY, Wener MH, Menezes AH, et al: Cranial settling in rheumatoid arthritis. Radiology 137:637, 1980.

529. Halla JT, Fallahi S, Hardin JG: Non-reducible rotational head tilt and lateral mass collapse. Arthritis Rheum 25:1316, 1982.

530. Bogduk N, Major GAC, Carter J: Lateral subluxation of the atlas in rheumatoid arthritis: A case report and post-mortem study. Ann Rheum Dis 43:341, 1984.

531. Teigland J, Magnaes B: Rheumatoid backward dislocation of the atlas with compression of the spinal cord. Scand J Rheumatol 9:253, 1980.

532. Weiner S, Bassett L, Spiegel T: Superior, posterior, and lateral displacement of C1 in rheumatoid arthritis. Arthritis Rheum 25:1378, 1982.

533. deCarvalho A, Graudal H: The course of atlanto-axial involvement and disc narrowing of the cervical spine in rheumatoid arthritis. ROFO 135:32, 1981.

534. Bywaters EGL: Rheumatoid and other diseases of the cervical interspinous bursae, and changes in the spinous processes. Ann Rheum Dis 41:360, 1982.

535. Mbuyi-Muamba JM, Dequeker J, Burssens A: Massive osteolysis in a case of rheumatoid arthritis: Clinical, histologic, and biochemical findings. Metab Bone Dis Rel Res 5:101, 1983.

536. Halla JT, Fallahi S: Cervical discovertebral destruction, subaxial subluxation, and myelopathy in a patient with rheumatoid arthritis. Arthritis Rheum 24:944, 1981.

537. Winfield J, Young A, Williams P, et al: Prospective study of the radiological changes in hands, feet, and cervical spine in adult rheumatoid disease. Ann Rheum Dis 42:613, 1983.

538. Winfield J, Cooke D, Brook AS, et al: A prospective study of the radiological changes in the cervical spine in early rheumatoid disease. Ann Rheum Dis 40:109, 1981.

539. Pellicci PM, Ranawat CS, Tsairis P, et al: A prospective study of the progression of rheumatoid arthritis of the cervical spine. J Bone Joint Surg [Am] 63:342, 1981.

540. Lipson SJ: Rheumatoid arthritis of the cervical spine. Clin Orthop 182:143, 1984.

541. Kudo H, Iwano K, Yoshizawa H: Cervical cord compression due to extradural granulation tissue in rheumatoid arthritis. J Bone Joint Surg [Br] 66:426, 1984.

542. Bryan WJ, Doherty JH Jr, Sculco TP: Tuberculosis in a rheumatoid patient. Clin Orthop 171:206, 1982.

543. Dodd MJ, Griffiths ID, Freeman R: Pyogenic arthritis due to bacteroides complicating rheumatoid arthritis. Ann Rheum Dis 41:248, 1982.

544. Hart CA, Godfrey VM, Woodrow JC, et al: Septic arthritis due to *Bacteroides fragilis* in a wrist affected by rheumatoid arthritis. Ann Rheum Dis 41:623, 1982.

545. Feld R, Fornasier VL, Bombardier C, et al: Septic arthritis due to Saccharomyces species in a patient with chronic rheumatoid arthritis. J Rheumatol 9:637, 1982.

546. Crook PR, Gray J: Bacteroides causing osteomyelitis in rheumatoid arthritis. Ann Rheum Dis 41:645, 1982.

547. Gompels BM, Darlington LG: Septic arthritis in rheumatoid disease causing bilateral shoulder dislocation: Diagnosis and treatment assisted by grey scale ultrasonography. Ann Rheum Dis 40:609, 1981.

548. Harvey AR, Buchanan WW: Clinical clues to the recognition of septic arthritis in the patient with rheumatoid arthritis. IM 3:91, 1982.

549. Coleman RE, Samuelson CO Jr, Baim S, et al: Imaging with Tc-99m MDP and Ga-67 citrate in patients with rheumatoid arthritis and suspected septic arthritis: Concise communication. J Nucl Med 23:479, 1982.

550. Atdjian M, Fernandez-Madrid F: Coexistence of chronic tophaceous gout and rheumatoid arthritis. J Rheumatol 8:989, 1981.

551. Moser CD: Koinzidenz von akuter Gicht und rheumatoider Arthritis im Fruhstadium der Erkrankung. Akt Rheumatol 6:73, 1981.

552. Agudelo CA, Turner RA, Panetti M, et al: Does hyperuricemia protect from rheumatoid inflammation? A clinical study. Arthritis Rheum 27:443, 1984.

553. Resnick D, Williams G, Weisman M: Rheumatoid arthritis and pseudorheumatoid arthritis in calcium pyrophosphate dihydrate crystal deposition disease. Radiology 140:615, 1981.

554. Lemmer JP, Irby WR: Co-existence of HLA-B27 ankylosing spondylitis and DR4 seropositive nodular rheumatoid arthritis in a patient with membranous nephropathy. J Rheumatol 8:661, 1981.

555. Alexander EL, Bias WB, Arnett FC: The co-existence of rheumatoid arthritis with Reiter's syndrome and/or ankylosing spondylitis: A model of dual HLA-associated disease susceptibility and expression. J Rheumatol 8:398, 1981.

556. Vigorita VJ: Pigmented villonodular synovitis-like lesions in association with rare cases of rheumatoid arthritis, osteonecrosis, and advanced degenerative joint disease. Report of five cases. Clin Orthop 183:115, 1984.

557. Fam AG, Lewis AJ, Cowan DH: Multiple myeloma and amyloid bone lesions complicating rheumatoid arthritis. J Rheumatol 8:845, 1981.

558. Rubin BR, Gupta VP, Levy RS, et al: Anaerobic abscess of a popliteal cyst in a patient with rheumatoid arthritis. J Rheumatol 9:733, 1982.

559. Keller C, Leden I, Lidgren L, et al: Anaerobic bacterial coxitis and pseudocystic tumour in rheumatoid arthritis. Scand J Rheumatol 9:216, 1980.

560. Mewa AAM, Pui M, Cockshott WP, et al: Observer differences in detecting erosions in radiographs of rheumatoid arthritis. J Rheumatol 10:216, 1983.

561. Edwards CW, Edwards SE, Huskisson EC: The value of radiography in the management of rheumatoid arthritis. Clin Radiol 34:413, 1983.

562. Norgaard F: A follow-up study of the earliest radiological changes in rheumatoid polyarthritis. Br J Radiol 53:63, 1980.

563. DeSmet AA, Goin JE, Arnett GR, et al: Comparison of two detail screen-film systems using a rheumatoid erosion model. Invest Radiol 18:359, 1983.

564. Gofton JP: Problems associated with the measurement of radiologic progression of disease in rheumatoid arthritis. J Rheumatol 10:177, 1983.

565. DeCarvalho A, Graudal H: Radiographic progression of rheumatoid arthritis related to some clinical and laboratory parameters. Acta Radiol (Diagn) 21:551, 1980.

566. DeCarvalho A, Graudal H: Relationship between radiological and clinical findings in rheumatoid arthritis. Acta Radiol (Diagn) 21:797, 1980.

567. Scott DL, Grindulis KA, Struthers GR, et al: Progression of radiological changes in rheumatoid arthritis. Ann Rheum Dis 43:8, 1984.

568. Pullar T, Hunter JA, Capell HA: Does second-line therapy affect the radiological progression of rheumatoid arthritis? Ann Rheum Dis 43:18, 1984.

569. Jalava S, Reunanen K: Healing of erosions in rheumatoid arthritis. Scand J Rheumatol 11:97, 1982.

570. Buckland-Wright JC: Advances in the radiological assessment of rheumatoid arthritis. Br J Rheumatol (Suppl)22:34, 1983.

571. Buckland-Wright JC: Microfocal radiographic examination of erosions in the wrist and hand of patients with rheumatoid arthritis. Ann Rheum Dis 43:160, 1984.

572. DeSmet AA, Goin JE, Martin R: A radiographic model for simulating rheumatoid erosions. Invest Radiol 18:352, 1983.

573. Kessler M, Lissner J, Schattenkirchner M, et al: Xeroradiographie und konventionelles Röntgenverfahren bei chronischer Polyarthritis. ROFO 134:162, 1981.

574. Omnetti CM, Gutierrez E, Hliba E, et al: Synoviorthesis with ³²P-colloidal chromic phosphate in rheumatoid arthritis—clinical, histopathologic and arthrographic changes. J Rheumatol 9:229, 1982.

575. Pocock DG, Agnew JE, Wood EJ, et al: Radionuclide imaging of the neck in rheumatoid arthritis. Rheumatol Rehabil 21:131, 1982.

576. McCall IW, Sheppard H, Haddaway M, et al: Gallium-67 scanning in rheumatoid arthritis. Br J Radiol 56:241, 1983.

577. Dihlmann W: Computed tomography of the hip joint. Medicamundi 28:29, 1983.

578. Raskin RJ, Schnapf DJ, Wolf CR, et al: Computerized tomography in evaluation of atlanto-axial subluxation in rheumatoid arthritis. J Rheumatol 10:33, 1983.

579. Kaufman RL, Glenn WV Jr: Rheumatoid cervical myelopathy: Evaluation by computerized tomography with multiplanar reconstruction. J Rheumatol 10:42, 1983.

580. Kaiser MC, Veiga-Pires JA, Capesius P: Atlanto-axial impaction and compression of the medulla oblongata and proximal spinal cord in rheumatoid arthritis evaluated by CT scanning. Br J Radiol 56:764, 1983.

581. Castor WR, Miller JDR, Russell AS, et al: Computed tomography of the craniocervical junction in rheumatoid arthritis. J Comput Assist Tomogr 7:31, 1983.

582. Braunstein EM, Weissman BN, Seltzer SE, et al: Computed tomography and conventional radiographs of the craniocervical region in rheumatoid arthritis. A comparison. Arthritis Rheum 27:26, 1984.

583. Hull RG, Rennie AN, Eastmond CJ, et al: Nuclear magnetic resonance (NMR) tomographic imaging for popliteal cysts in rheumatoid arthritis. Ann Rheum Dis 43:56, 1984.

584. Calin A, Marks SH: The case against seronegative rheumatoid arthritis. Am J Med 70:992, 1981.

585. Masi AT, Feigenbaum SL: Is seronegative rheumatoid arthritis a valid clinical diagnosis? IM 5:56, 1984.

586. Masi AT, Feigenbaum SL: Seronegative rheumatoid arthritis. Fact or fiction? Arch Intern Med 143:2167, 1983.

587. Prakash S, Mehra NK, Bhargava S, et al: HLA B27 related ''unclassifiable'' seronegative spondyloarthropathies. Ann Rheum Dis 42:640, 1983.

588. Bland JH, Brown EW: Seronegative and seropositive rheumatoid arthritis. Ann Intern Med 60:88, 1964.

589. Burns TM, Calin A: The hand radiograph as a diagnostic discriminant between seropositive and seronegative ''rheumatoid arthritis'': A controlled study. Ann Rheum Dis 42:605, 1983.

590. Edelman J, Russell AS: A comparison of patients with seropositive and seronegative rheumatoid arthritis. Rheumatol Int 3:47, 1983.

591. Lequesne M, deSèze S: Les coxites rhumatismales isolées (monarthrites de la hanche). Diagnostic par la méthode des critères et des exclusions. Rev Rhum Mal Osteoartic 37:53, 1970.

592. Lequesne M, Azema B: La coxite inflammatoire isolée. Critères. Rev Rhum Mal Osteoartic 39:809, 1972.

593. Villiaumey J, Strauss J, DiMenza C, et al: Les monarthrities rhumatoïdes. Rev Rhum Mal Osteoartic 40:627, 1973.

594. Arlet J: Monoarthrites ''rhumatismales'' chroniques de la hanche. Rev Rhum Mal Osteoartic 39:789, 1972.

595. Fletcher MR, Scott JT: Chronic monarticular synovitis. Diagnostic and prognostic features. Ann Rheum Dis 34:171, 1975.

596. Pitkeathey D, Griffiths H, Catto M: Monarthritis: A study of forty-five cases. J Bone Joint Surg [Br] 46:685, 1964.

597. Goldenberg D, Egan M, Cohen A: Inflammatory synovitis in degenerative joint disease. J Rheumatol 9:204, 1982.

598. McCarty DJ, O'Duffy JD, Pearson L, et al: Remitting seronegative symmetrical synovitis with pitting edema. RS₃PE syndrome. JAMA 254:2763, 1985.

599. Benedek TG: Subcutaneous nodules and the differentiation of rheumatoid arthritis from rheumatic fever. Semin Arthritis Rheum 13:305, 1984.

600. Kaye BR, Kaye RL, Bobrove A: Rheumatoid nodules. Review of the spectrum of associated conditions and proposal of a new classification, with a report of four seronegative cases. Am J Med 76:279, 1984.

601. Halla JT, Koopman WJ, Fallahi S, et al: Rheumatoid myositis. Clinical and histologic features and possible pathogenesis. Arthritis Rheum 27:737, 1984.

602. Monsees B, Murphy WA: Pressure erosions: A pattern of bone resorption in rheumatoid arthritis. Arthritis Rheum 28:820, 1985.

603. Monsees B, Destouet JM, Murphy WA, et al: Pressure erosions of bone in rheumatoid arthritis: A subject review. Radiology 155:53, 1985.

604. Keret D, Porter KM: Synovial cyst and ulnar nerve entrapment. A case report. Clin Orthop 188:213, 1984.

605. DeJager JP, Fleming A: Shoulder joint rupture and pseudothrombosis in rheumatoid arthritis. Ann Rheum Dis 43:503, 1984.

606. Dijkstra J, Dijkstra PF, Klundert W: Rheumatoid arthritis of the shoulder. Description and standard radiographs. ROFO 142:179, 1985.

607. Levine RB, Sullivan KL: Rheumatoid arthritis: Skeletal manifestations observed on portable chest roentgenograms. Skel Radiol 13:295, 1985.

608. Resnick D, Cone R: Pathological fractures in rheumatoid arthritis: Sites and mechanisms. RadioGraphics 4:549, 1984.

609. Komusi T, Munro T, Harth M: Radiologic review: The rheumatoid cervical spine. Semin Arthritis Rheum 14:187, 1985.

610. Redlund-Johnell I, Pettersson H: Vertical dislocation of the C1 and C2 vertebrae in rheumatoid arthritis. Acta Radiol (Diagn) 25:133, 1984.

611. Lipson SJ: Cervical myelopathy and posterior atlanto-axial subluxation in patients with rheumatoid arthritis. J Bone Joint Surg [Am] 67:593, 1985.

612. Redlund-Johnell I: Posterior atlanto-axial dislocation in rheumatoid arthritis. Scand J Rheumatol *13*:337, 1984.

613. Santavirta S, Sandelin J, Slatis P: Posterior atlanto-axial subluxation in rheumatoid arthritis. Acta Orthop Scand *56*:298, 1985.

614. Redlund-Johnell I: Atlanto-occipital dislocation in rheumatoid arthritis. Acta Radiol (Diagn) *25*:165, 1984.

615. Redlund-Johnell I: Subaxial caudal dislocation of the cervical spine in rheumatoid arthritis. Neuroradiology *26*:407, 1984.

616. King TT: Editorial: Rheumatoid subluxations of the cervical spine. Ann Rheum Dis *44*:807, 1985.

617. Wong RL, Wilson AJ, Ingenito FS, et al: Apophyseal joint ankylosis of the cervical spine in adult-onset rheumatoid arthritis. Arthritis Rheum *28*:958, 1985.

618. Syrjanen SM: The temporomandibular joint in rheumatoid arthritis. Acta Radiol (Diagn) *26*:235, 1985.

619. Lawry GV, Finerman ML, Hanafee WN, et al: Laryngeal involvement in rheumatoid arthritis. A clinical, laryngoscopic, and computerized tomographic study. Arthritis Rheum *27*:873, 1984.

620. Wandall JH: Leucocyte function in patients with rheumatoid arthritis: quantitative in-vivo leucocyte mobilisation and in-vitro function of blood and exudate leucocytes. Ann Rheum Dis *44*:694, 1985.

621. Kraft SM, Panush RS, Longley S: Unrecognized staphylococcal pyarthrosis with rheumatoid arthritis. Semin Arthritis Rheum *14*:196, 1985.

622. Call RS, Ward JR, Samuelson CO Jr: ''Pseudoseptic'' arthritis in patients with rheumatoid arthritis. West J Med *143*:471, 1985.

623. Doherty M, Dieppe P, Watt I: Low incidence of calcium pyrophosphate dihydrate crystal deposition in rheumatoid arthritis, with modification of radiographic features in coexistent disease. Arthritis Rheum *27*:1002, 1984.

624. Sharp JT, Bluhm GR, Brook A, et al: Reproducibility of multiple-observer scoring of radiologic abnormalities in the hands and wrists of patients with rheumatoid arthritis. Arthritis Rheum *28*:16, 1985.

625. Hartley RM, Liang MH, Weissman BN, et al: The value of conventional views and radiographic magnification in evaluating early rheumatoid arthritis. Arthritis Rheum *27*:744, 1984.

626. Seltzer SE, Weissman BN, Braunstein EM, et al: Computed tomography of the hindfoot with rheumatoid arthritis. Arthritis Rheum *28*:1234, 1985.

627. Seltzer SE, Weissman BN, Braunstein EM, et al: Computed tomography of the hindfoot. J Comput Assist Tomogr *8*:488, 1984.

628. Rafii M, Zwanger-Mendelson S, Firooznia H, et al: Fusion of the lateral joints in fixed atlantoaxial dislocation: A computed tomography demonstration. CT *8*:203, 1984.

629. Hammer M, Schwarzrock R, Hundeshagen H, et al: NMR-tomographie der kniegelenke bei Patienten mit rheumatischen Gelenkerkrankugen. Z Rheumatol *44*:152, 1985.

630. Sartoris DJ, Resnick D: Target area approach to arthritis of the small articulations. Contemp Diagn Radiol *8*:1, 1985.

631. Deal CL, Meenan RF, Goldenberg DL, et al: The clinical features of elderly-onset rheumatoid arthritis. A comparison with younger-onset disease of similar duration. Arthritis Rheum *28*:987, 1985.

632. Schneider HA, Yonker RA, Katz P, et al: Rheumatoid vasculitis: Experience with 13 patients and review of the literature. Semin Arthritis Rheum *14*:280, 1985.

633. Walton K, Dyer PA, Grennan DM, et al: Clinical features, autoantibodies and HLA-DR antigens in rheumatoid arthritis. J Rheumatol *12*:223, 1985.

634. van Soesbergen RM, Lips P, van den Ende A, et al: Bone metabolism in rheumatoid arthritis compared with postmenopausal osteoporosis. Ann Rheum Dis *45*:149, 1986.

635. Jacob J, Sartoris D, Kursungolu S, et al: Distal interphalangeal joint involvement in rheumatoid arthritis. Arthritis Rheum *29*:10, 1986.

636. Halla JT, Fallahi S, Hardin JG: Small joint involvement: A systematic roentgenographic study in rheumatoid arthritis. Ann Rheum Dis *45*:327, 1986.

637. Alarcón GS, Koopman WJ: The carpometacarpal ratio: A useful method for assessing disease progression in rheumatoid arthritis. J. Rheumatol *12*:846, 1985.

638. Kelly MC, Hopkinson ND, Zaphiropoulos GC: Manubriosternal dislocation in rheumatoid arthritis: The role of thoracic kyphosis. Ann Rheum Dis. *45*:345, 1986.

639. Pellman E, Kumari S, Greenwald R: Rheumatoid iliopsoas bursitis presenting as unilateral leg edema. J Rheumatol *13*:197, 1986.

640. Heywood AWB, Meyers OL: Rheumatoid arthritis of the thoracic and lumbar spine. J Bone Joint Surg [Br] *68*:362, 1986.

641. Fedele FA, Ho G Jr, Dorman BA: Pseudoaneurysm of the vertebral artery: A complication of rheumatoid cervical spine disease. Arthritis Rheum *29*:136, 1986.

642. Brazeau-Lamontagne L, Charlin B, Levesque R-Y, et al: Cricoarytenoiditis: CT assessment in rheumatoid arthritis. Radiology *158*:463, 1986.

643. Scott DL, Coulton BL, Popert AJ: Long term progression of joint damage in rheumatoid arthritis. Ann Rheum Dis *45*:373, 1986.

644. Fries JF, Bloch DA, Sharp JT, et al: Assessment of radiologic progression in rheumatoid arthritis. A randomized controlled trial. Arthritis Rheum *29*:1, 1986.

645. Sharp JT, Young DY, Bluhm GR, et al: How many joints in the hands and wrists should be included in a score of radiologic abnormalities used to assess rheumatoid arthritis? Arthritis Rheum *28*:1326, 1985.

646. de Silva M, Kyle V, Hazleman B, et al: Assessment of inflammation in the rheumatoid knee joint: Correlation between clinical, radioisotopic, and thermographic methods. Ann Rheum Dis *45*:277, 1986.

647. Toolanen G, Larsson S-E, Fagerlund M: Medullary compression in rheumatoid atlanto-axial subluxation evaluated by computed tomography. Spine *11*:191, 1986.

648. Mendelsohn DB, Hertzanu Y: Atlantoaxial impaction simulating a posterior fossa mass on computed tomography. A case report. Spine *11*:66, 1986.

649. Beltran J, Noto AM, Herman LJ, et al: Joint effusions; MR imaging. Radiology *158*:133, 1986.

650. Adams ME, Li DKB: Magnetic resonance imaging in rheumatology. J Rheumatol *12*:1038, 1985.

651. Baker DG, Schumacher HR Jr, Wolf GL: Nuclear magnetic resonance evaluation of synovial fluid and articular tissues. J Rheumatol *12*:1062, 1985.

652. Currey J, Therkildsen LHK, Bywaters EGL: Monoarticular rheumatoid-like arthritis of seven years' duration following fracture of the radial head. Ann Rheum Dis *45*:783, 1986.

653. Schultz RJ, Siegler G, Diwan L: Palmar displacement of the distal end of the ulna in rheumatoid arthritis. A case report. J Bone Joint Surg [Am] *68*:1280, 1986.

654. Dijkstra J, Dijkstra PF, Klundert W: Rheumatoid arthritis of the shoulder. Description and standard radiographs. RÖFO *142*:179, 1985.

655. Gersoff WK, Burkus JK: Dislocation of the sacroiliac joint associated with rheumatoid arthritis. A case report. Clin Orthop *209*:219, 1986.

656. McCarthy DA, Holburn CM, Pell BK, et al: Scanning electron microscopy of rheumatoid arthritis peripheral blood polymorphonuclear leucocytes. Ann Rheum Dis *45*:899, 1986.

657. Strader KW, Agudelo CA: Coexistence of rheumatoid nodulosis and gout. J Rheumatol *13*:818, 1986.

658. Möttönen T, Hannonen P, Rekonen A, et al: Joint scintigraphy and erosions. Ann Rheum Dis *45*:966, 1986.

659. Uno K, Matusi N, Nohira K, et al: Indium-III leukocyte imaging in patients with rheumatoid arthritis. J Nucl Med *27*:339, 1986.

660. McAfee PC, Bohlman HH, Han JS, et al: Comparison of nuclear magnetic resonance imaging and computed tomography in the diagnosis of upper cervical spinal cord compression. Spine *11*:295, 1986.

661. Jaraquemada D, Ollier W, Awad J, et al: HLA and rheumatoid arthritis: A combined analysis of 440 British patients. Ann Rheum Dis *45*:627, 1986.

662. Smith H-J, Larheim TA, Aspestrand F: Rheumatic and nonrheumatic disease in the temporomandibular joint: Gadolinium-enhanced MR imaging. Radiology *185*:229, 1992.

663. Arnett FC: Revised criteria for the classification of rheumatoid arthritis. Bull Rheum Dis *38*:1, 1989.

664. Paimela L: The radiographic criterion in the 1987 revised criteria for rheumatoid arthritis. Reassessment in a prospective study of early disease. Arthritis Rheum *35*:255, 1992.

665. Chaouat D, Le Parc J-M: The syndrome of seronegative symmetrical synovitis with pitting edema (RS3 PE syndrome): A unique form of arthritis in the elderly? Report of 4 additional cases. J Rheumatol *16*:1211, 1989.

666. Chaouat D, Perier JY, LeParc JM, et al: Polyarthrite subaiguë oedémateuse bénigne du sujet âge. Neuf observations. Presse Med *19*:1705, 1990.

667. Russell EB, Hunter JB, Pearson L, et al: Remitting, seronegative, symmetric synovitis with pitting edema—13 additional cases. J Rheumatol *17*:633, 1990.

668. Pariser KM, Canoso JJ: Remitting, seronegative (A) symmetrical synovitis with pitting edema—two cases of RS₃PE syndrome. J Rheumatol *18*:1260, 1991.

669. Ziff M: The rheumatoid nodule. Arthritis Rheum *33*:761, 1990.

670. Segal R, Caspi D, Tishler M, et al: Accelerated nodulosis and vasculitis during methotrexate therapy for rheumatoid arthritis. Arthritis Rheum *31*:1182, 1988.

671. Taleisnik J: Rheumatoid arthritis of the wrist. Hand Clinics *5*:257, 1989.

672. Buckland-Wright JC, Walker SR: Incidence and size of erosions in the wrist and hand of rheumatoid patients: A quantitative microfocal radiographic study. Ann Rheum Dis *46*:463, 1987.

673. Abbott GT, Bucknall RC, Whitehouse GH: Osteoarthritis association with distal interphalangeal joint involvement in rheumatoid arthritis. Skel Radiol *20*:495, 1991.

674. Gubler FM, Maas M, Dijkstra PF, et al: Cystic rheumatoid arthritis: Description of a nonerosive form. Radiology *177*:829, 1990.

675. Kaye JJ, Callahan LF, Nance EP Jr, et al: Bony ankylosis in rheumatoid arthritis. Associations with longer duration and greater severity of disease. Invest Radiol *22*:303, 1987.

676. DiBenedetto MR, Lubbers LM, Coleman CR: Relationship between radial inclination angle and ulnar deviation of the fingers. J Hand Surg [Am] *16*:36, 1991.

677. Hendrix RW, Urban MA, Schroeder JL, et al: Carpal predominance in rheumatoid arthritis. Radiology *164*:219, 1987.

678. Hindley CJ, Stanley JK: The rheumatoid wrist: Patterns of disease progression. A review of 50 wrists. J Hand Surg [Br] *16*:275, 1991.

679. Newman RJ: Excision of the distal ulna in patients with rheumatoid arthritis. J Bone Joint Surg [Br] *69*:203, 1987.

680. Cope R: The surgery of the rheumatoid wrist: Postoperative appearances and complications of the more common procedures. Skel Radiol *17*:576, 1989.

681. Mann FA, Wilson AJ, Gilula LA: Radiographic evaluation of the wrist: What does the hand surgeon want to know? Radiology *184*:15, 1992.

682. White SH, Goodfellow JW, Mowat A: Posterior interosseous nerve palsy in rheumatoid arthritis. J Bone Joint Surg [Br] *70*:468, 1988.

683. Thevenon A, Cocheteux P, Duquesnoy B, et al: Subacromial bursitis with rice bodies as a presenting feature of seronegative rheumatoid arthritis. Arthritis Rheum *30*:715, 1987.

684. Petersson CJ: The acromioclavicular joint in rheumatoid arthritis. Clin Orthop *223*:86, 1987.

685. Doube A, Clarke AK: Symptomatic manubriosternal joint involvement in rheumatoid arthritis. Ann Rheum Dis *48*:516, 1989.

686. Schils JP, Resnick D, Haghighi PN, et al: Pathogenesis of discovertebral and manubriosternal joint abnormalities in rheumatoid arthritis: A cadaveric study. J Rheumatol *16*:291, 1989.

687. Chen C, Chandnani V, Kang HS, et al: Insufficiency fracture of the sternum caused by osteopenia: Plain film findings in seven patients. AJR *154*:1025, 1990.

688. Möttönen TT: Prediction of erosiveness and rate of development of new erosions in early rheumatoid arthritis. Ann Rheum Dis *47*:648, 1988.

689. Downey DJ, Simkin PA, Mack LA, et al: Tibialis posterior tendon rupture: A cause of rheumatoid flat foot. Arthritis Rheum *31*:441, 1988.

690. Bouysset M, Tebib J, Weil G, et al: The rheumatoid heel: Its relationship to other disorders in the rheumatoid foot. Clin Rheumatol *8*:208, 1989.

691. Matsumoto K, Hukuda S, Nishioka J, et al: Rupture of the Achilles tendon in rheumatoid arthritis with histologic evidence of enthesitis. A case report. Clin Orthop *280*:235, 1992.

692. Goldring SR, Wojno WC, Schiller AL, et al: In patients with rheumatoid arthritis, the tissue reaction associated with loosened total knee replacements exhibits features of a rheumatoid synovium. J Orthop Rheumatol *1*:9, 1988.

693. Kindynis Ph, Garcia J: Protrusion acétabulaire. J Radiol *71*:415, 1990.

694. Barrie HJ: Pathology of femoral heads in patients with rheumatoid disease. J Rheumatol *17*:448, 1990.

695. Pearson ME, Kosco M, Huffer W, et al: Rheumatoid nodules of the spine: Case report and review of the literature. Arthritis Rheum *30*:709, 1987.

696. Matsumine A, Shichikawa K, Yamashita K, et al: Rheumatoid arthritis causing paraplegia. A case report. J Bone Joint Surg [Am] *70*:1410, 1988.

697. Wolfe BK, O'Keeffe D, Mitchell DM, et al: Rheumatoid arthritis of the cervical spine: Early and progressive radiographic features. Radiology *165*:145, 1987.

698. Agarwal AK, Kraus DR, Eisenbeis CH Jr, et al: Anatomical and neurological characteristics of cervical spine involvement in rheumatoid arthritis. J Orthop Rheumatol *2*:77, 1989.

699. Bland JH: Rheumatoid subluxation of the cervical spine. J Rheumatol *17*:134, 1990.

700. Halla JT, Hardin JG, Vitek J, et al: Involvement of the cervical spine in rheumatoid arthritis. Arthritis Rheum *32*:652, 1989.

701. Konttinen YT, Bergroth V, Santavirta S, et al: Inflammatory involvement of cervical spine ligaments in patients with rheumatoid arthritis and atlantoaxial subluxation. J Rheumatol *14*:531, 1987.

702. Konttinen YT, Santavirta S, Kauppi M, et al: Atlantoaxial laxity in rheumatoid arthritis. Acta Orthop Scand *60*:379, 1989.

703. Kawaida H, Sakou T, Morizono Y: Vertical settling in rheumatoid arthritis. Diagnostic value of the Ranawat and Redlund-Johnell methods. Clin Orthop *239*:128, 1989.

704. Kauppi M, Sakaguchi M, Konttinen YT, et al: A new method of screening for vertical atlantoaxial dislocation. J Rheumatol *17*:167, 1990.

705. Redlund-Johnell I, Pettersson H: Radiographic measurement of the craniovertebral region, designed for evaluation of abnormalities in rheumatoid arthritis. Acta Radiol (Diag) *25*:33, 1984.

706. Tumiati B, Casoli P: Syringomyelia in a patient with rheumatoid subluxation of the cervical spine. J Rheumatol *18*:1403, 1991.

707. Morizono Y, Sakou T, Kawaida H: Upper cervical involvement in rheumatoid arthritis. Spine *12*:721, 1987.

708. Slatis P, Santavirta S, Sandelin J, et al: Cranial subluxation of the odontoid process in rheumatoid arthritis. J Bone Joint Surg [Am] *71*:189, 1989.

709. Santavirta S, Hopfner-Hall, Kainen D, Paukku P, et al: Atlantoaxial facet joint arthritis in the rheumatoid cervical spine. A panoramic zonography study. J Rheumatol *15*:217, 1988.

710. Kauppi M: The effect of flexion-extension movement on vertical atlantoaxial subluxation measurements. J Rheumatol *18*:1804, 1991.

711. Halla JT, Hardin JG Jr: The spectrum of atlantoaxial facet joint involvement in rheumatoid arthritis. Arthritis Rheum *33*:325, 1990.

712. Goupille P, Fouquet B, Cotty P, et al: The temporomandibular joint in rheumatoid arthritis: Correlations between clinical and computed tomography features. J Rheumatol *17*:1285, 1990.

713. Larheim TA, Smith H-J, Aspestrand F: Temporomandibular joint abnormalities associated with rheumatic disease: Comparison between MR imaging and arthrotomography. Radiology *183*:221, 1992.

714. Larheim TA, Smith H-J, Aspestrand F: Rheumatic disease of the temporomandibular joint: MR imaging and tomographic manifestations. Radiology *175*:527, 1990.

715. Camilleri AE: Nature of the ossicular joints and their involvement in rheumatoid arthritis. Ann Rheum Dis *50*:271, 1991.

716. Campen DH, Kaufman RL, Beardmore TD: Candida septic arthritis in rheumatoid arthritis. J Rheumatol *17*:86, 1990.

717. Goldenberg DL: Infectious arthritis complicating rheumatoid arthritis and other chronic rheumatic disorders. Arthritis Rheum *32*:496, 1989.

718. Mahowald ML: Animal models of infectious arthritis. Clin Rheum Dis *12*:403, 1986.

719. Singleton JD, West SG, Nordstrom DM: ''Pseudoseptic'' arthritis complicating rheumatoid arthritis: A report of six cases. J Rheumatol *18*:1319, 1991.

720. Martinez-Cordero E, Bessudo-Babani A, Perez SCT, et al: Concomitant gout and rheumatoid arthritis. J Rheumatol *15*:1307, 1988.

721. Hoos R, Sprekeler S, Botzenhardt U: Spondylitis ankylosans und chronische Polyarthritis stellen keine sich ausschließenden Krankheits-einheiten dar. Akt Rheumatol *16*:135, 1991.

722. Fallet GH, Barnes CG, Berry H, et al: Coexisting rheumatoid arthritis and ankylosing spondylitis. J Rheumatol *14*:1135, 1987.

723. Helfgott SM, Lazarides G, Sandberg-Cook J: Cooccurrence of rheumatoid arthritis and ankylosing spondylitis. J Rheumatol *15*:1451, 1988.

724. Hart FD, Lipner AE: Co-existent ankylosing spondylitis and seropositive rheumatoid arthritis. J Orthop Rheumatol *4*:56, 1991.

725. Fuchs HA, Callahan LF, Kaye JJ, et al: Radiographic and joint count findings of the hand in rheumatoid arthritis. Related and unrelated findings. Arthritis Rheum *31*:44, 1988.

726. van der Heijde DMFM, van Leeuwen MH, van Riel PLCM, et al: Biannual radiographic assessments of hands and feet in a three-year prospective followup of patients with early rheumatoid arthritis. Arthritis Rheum *35*:26, 1992.

727. Sharp JT: Radiologic assessment as an outcome measure in rheumatoid arthritis. Arthritis Rheum *32*:221, 1989.

728. Hindley CJ, Stanley JK: Radiographic assessment of the rheumatoid wrist and hand. J Orthop Rheumatol *5*:15, 1992.

729. Brower AC: Use of the radiograph to measure the course of rheumatoid arthritis. The gold standard versus fool's gold. Arthritis Rheum *33*:316, 1990.

730. Kaye JJ, Nance EP, Callahan LF, et al: Observer variation in quantitative assessment of rheumatoid arthritis. Part II. A simplified scoring system. Invest Radiol *22*:41, 1987.

731. Isomäki H, Kaarela K, Martio J: Are hand radiographs the most suitable for the diagnosis of rheumatoid arthritis? Arthritis Rheum *31*:1452, 1988.

732. Kaye JJ, Callahan LF, Nance EP Jr, et al: Rheumatoid arthritis: Explanatory power of specific radiographic findings for patient clinical status. Radiology *165*:753, 1987.

733. Kaye JJ, Fuchs HA, Moseley JW, et al: Problems with the Steinbroker staging system for radiographic assessment of the rheumatoid hand and wrist. Invest Radiol *25*:536, 1990.

734. Brower AC: Radiographic assessment of disease progression in rheumatoid arthritis. Rheum Dis Clin North Am *17*:471, 1991.

735. Kaye JJ: Radiographic methods of assessment (scoring of rheumatic disease). Rheum Dis Clin North Am *17*:457, 1991.

736. Kremer JM, Lee JK: A long-term prospective study of the use of methotrexate in rheumatoid arthritis. Update after a mean of fifty-three months. Arthritis Rheum *31*:577, 1988.

737. Buckland-Wright JC, Clarke GS, Walker SR: Erosion number and area progression in the wrists and hands of rheumatoid patients: A quantitative microfocal radiographic study. Ann Rheum Dis *48*:25, 1989.

738. Rau R, Herborn G, Karger T, et al: Retardation of radiologic progression in rheumatoid arthritis with methotrexate therapy. A controlled study. Arthritis Rheum *34*:1236, 1991.

739. Fuchs HA, Kaye JJ, Calahan LF, et al: Evidence of significant radiographic damage in rheumatoid arthritis within the first 2 years of disease. J Rheumatol *16*:585, 1989.

740. Sharp JT: Scoring radiographic abnormalities in rheumatoid arthritis. J Rheumatol *16*:568, 1989.

741. Möttönen TT, Hannonen P, Toivanen J, et al: Value of joint scintigraphy in the prediction of erosiveness in early rheumatoid arthritis. Ann Rheum Dis *47*:183, 1988.

742. Olsen N, Halberg P, Halskov O, et al: Scintimetric assessment of synovitis activity during treatment with disease modifying antirheumatic drugs. Ann Rheum Dis *47*:995, 1988.

743. Flaviis LD, Scaglione P, Nessi R, et al: Ultrasonography of the hand in rheumatoid arthritis. Acta Radiol (Diag) *29*:457, 1988.

744. Fornage BD: Soft-tissue changes in the hand in rheumatoid arthritis: Evaluation with US. Radiology *173*:735, 1989.

745. Murakami DM, Bassett LW, Seeger LL: Advances in imaging in rheumatoid arthritis. Clin Orthop *265*:83, 1991.

746. Kaye JJ: Arthritis: Roles of radiography and other imaging techniques in evaluation. Radiology *177*:601, 1990.

747. Foley-Nolan D, Stack JP, Ryan M, et al: Magnetic resonance imaging in the assessment of rheumatoid arthritis—a comparison with plain film radiographs. Br J Rheumatol *30*:101, 1991.

748. Beltran J, Caudill JL, Herman LA, et al: Rheumatoid arthritis: MR imaging manifestations. Radiology *165*:153, 1987.

749. Gilkeson G, Polisson R, Sinclair H, et al: Early detection of carpal erosions in patients with rheumatoid arthritis: A pilot study of magnetic resonance imaging. J Rheumatol *15*:1361, 1988.

750. Krahe VT, Landwehr P, Stolzenburg T, et al: Magnetische Resonanz tomographie (MRT) der Hand bei chronischer polyarthritis. ROFO *152*:206, 1990.

751. Kieft GJ, Dijkmans BAC, Bloem JL, et al: Magnetic resonance imaging of the shoulder in patients with rheumatoid arthritis. Ann Rheum Dis *49*:7, 1990.

752. Moore EA, Jacoby RK, Ellis RE, et al: Demonstration of a geode by magnetic resonance imaging: A new light on the cause of juxta-articular bone cysts in rheumatoid arthritis. Ann Rheum Dis *49*:785, 1990.

753. Sanchez RB, Quinn SF: MRI of inflammatory synovial processes. Magn Res Imaging *7*:529, 1989.

754. Yao L, Sinha S, Seeger LL: MR imaging of joints: Analytic optimization of GRE techniques at 1.5T. AJR *158*:339, 1992.

755. Reiser MF, Bongartz GP, Erlemann R, et al: Gadolinium-DTPA in rheumatoid arthritis and related diseases: First results with dynamic magnetic resonance imaging. Skel Radiol *18*:591, 1989.

756. Bjorkengren AG, Geborek P, Rydholm U, Holtäs S, Petterson H: MR imaging of the knee in acute rheumatoid arthritis: Synovial uptake of gadolinium-DOTA. AJR 155:329, 1990.

757. König H, Sieper J, Wolf K-J: Rheumatoid arthritis: Evaluation of hypervascular and fibrous pannus with dynamic MR imaging enhanced with Gd-DTPA. Radiology 176:473, 1990.

758. Kursunoglu-Brahme S, Riccio T, Weisman MH, et al: Rheumatoid knee: Role of gadopentetate-enhanced MR imaging. Radiology 176:831, 1990.

759. Adam G, Dammer M, Bohndorf K, et al: Rheumatoid arthritis of the knee: Value of gadopentetate dimeglumine–enhanced MR imaging. AJR 156:125, 1991.

760. Whitten CG, Moore TE, Yuh WTC, et al: The use of gadopentetate dimeglumine in magnetic resonance imaging of synovial lesions. Skel Radiol 21:215, 1992.

761. Pages M, Poey C, Lassoued S, et al: MR imaging of the knee in rheumatoid arthritis and other rheumatic diseases. AJR 157:1128, 1991.

762. Varma DGK, Richli WR, Charnsangavej C, et al: MR appearance of the distended iliopsoas bursa. AJR 156:1025, 1991.

763. Fielding JR, Franklin PD, Kustan J: Popliteal cysts: A reassessment using magnetic resonance imaging. Skel Radiol 20:433, 1991.

764. Toohey AK, LaSalle TL, Martinez S, et al: Iliopsoas bursitis: Clinical features, radiographic findings, and disease associations. Semin Arthritis Rheum 20:41, 1990.

765. Dungan DH, Seeger LL, Grant EG: Case report 707. Skel Radiol 21:52, 1992.

766. Yamashita Y, Takahashi M, Sakamoto Y, et al: Atlantoaxial subluxation. Radiography and magnetic resonance imaging correlated to myelopathy. Acta Radiol (Diag) 30:135, 1989.

767. Pettersson H, Larsson EM, Holtäs S, et al: MR imaging of the cervical spine in rheumatoid arthritis. AJNR 9:573, 1988.

768. Einig M, Higer HP, Meairs S, et al: Magnetic resonance imaging of the craniocervical junction in rheumatoid arthritis: Value, limitations, indications. Skel Radiol 19:341, 1990.

769. Breedveld FC, Algra PR, Vielvoye CJ, et al: Magnetic resonance imaging in the evaluation of patients with rheumatoid arthritis and subluxations of the cervical spine. Arthritis Rheum 30:624, 1987.

770. Semble EL, Elster AD, Loeser RF, et al: Magnetic resonance imaging of the cranioevertebral junction in rheumatoid arthritis. J Rheumatol 15:1367, 1988.

771. Neuhold A, Seidl G, Wicke L: MRI in atlanto-odontoid arthritis. Medicamundi 32:39, 1987.

772. Bundschuh C, Modic MT, Kearney F, et al: Rheumatoid arthritis of the cervical spine: Surface-coil MR imaging. AJR 151:181, 1988.

773. Chérié-Lignière G, Montagnani G, Panarace G, et al: Magnetic resonance imaging for the study of cervical myelopathy in rheumatoid arthritis. Clin Exp Rheumatol 6:343, 1988.

774. Reynolds H, Carter SW, Murtagh FR, et al: Cervical rheumatoid arthritis: Value of flexion and extension views in imaging. Radiology 164:215, 1987.

775. Kawaida H, Sakou T, Morizono Y, et al: Magnetic resonance imaging of upper cervical disorders in rheumatoid arthritis. Spine 14:1144, 1989.

776. Aisen AM, Martel W, Ellis JH, et al: Cervical spine involvement in rheumatoid arthritis: MR imaging. Radiology 165:159, 1987.

777. Dvorak J, Grob D, Baumgartner H, et al: Functional evaluation of the spinal cord by magnetic resonance imaging in patients with rheumatoid arthritis and instability of upper cervical spine. Spine 14:1057, 1989.

778. Larsson E-M, Holtäs S, Zygmunt S: Pre- and postoperative MR imaging of the craniocervical junction in rheumatoid arthritis. AJR 152:561, 1989.

779. Silman A, Ollier B, McDermott M: HLA: Linkage with rheumatoid arthritis or seropositivity. J Rheumatol 15:1189, 1988.

780. Van Zebren D, Hazes JMW, Zwinderman AH, et al: Association of HLA-DR4 with a more progressive disease course in patients with rheumatoid arthritis. Results of a followup study. Arthritis Rheum 34:822, 1991.

781. El-Khoury GY, Larson RK, Kathol MH, et al: Seronegative and seropositive rheumatoid arthritis: Radiographic differences. Radiology 168:517, 1988.

782. Husby G, Gran JT: The differentiation between seronegative rheumatoid arthritis and other forms of seronegative polyarthritis. A review with suggested criteria. Clin Exp Rheumatol 5:97, 1987.

783. Gran JT, Husby G: Seronegative rheumatoid arthritis and HLA-DR4: Proposal for criteria. J Rheumatol 14:1079, 1987.

784. Wetzel FT, La Rocca H: Grisel's syndrome. A review. Clin Orthop 240:141, 1989.

785. Mathern GW, Batzdorf U: Grisel's syndrome. Cervical spine clinical, pathologic, and neurologic manifestations. Clin Orthop 244:131, 1989.

786. Babini JC, Gusis SE, Babini SM, et al: Superolateral erosions of the humeral head in chronic inflammatory arthropathies. Skel Radiol 21:515, 1992.

787. Redlund-Johnell I, Larsson E-M: Subluxation of the upper thoracic spine in rheumatoid arthritis. Skel Radiol 22:105, 1993.

788. Goupille P, Fouquet B, Valat J-P: Computed tomography of the temporomandibular joint in rheumatoid arthritis. J Rheumatol 19:1315, 1992.

789. Goupille P, Fouquet B, Cotty P, et al: Articulation temporo-mandibulaire et polyarthrite rhumatoide. Rev Rhum Mal Osteoartic 59:213, 1992.

790. Soria LM, Solé JMN, Sacanell AR, et al: Infectious arthritis in patients with rheumatoid arthritis. Ann Rheum Dis 51:402, 1992.

791. de Bois MHW, Arndt J-W, van der Velde EA, et al: ^{99m}Tc human immunoglobulin scintigraphy—a reliable method to detect joint activity in rheumatoid arthritis. J Rheumatol 19:1371, 1992.

792. Rubens DJ, Blebea JS, Totterman SMS, et al: Rheumatoid arthritis: Evaluation of wrist extensor tendons with clinical examination versus MR imaging—a preliminary report. Radiology 187:831, 1993.

793. Singson RD, Zalduondo FM: Value of unenhanced spin-echo MR imaging in distinguishing between synovitis and effusion of the knee. AJR 159:569, 1992.

794. Rominger MB, Bernreuter WK, Kenney PJ, et al: MR imaging of the hands in early rheumatoid arthritis: Preliminary results. RadioGraphics 13:37, 1993.

795. Yanagawa A, Takano K, Nishioka K, et al: Clinical staging and gadolinium-DTPA enhanced images of the wrist in rheumatoid arthritis. J Rheumatol 20:781, 1993.

796. Nattrass GR, King GJW, McMurtry RY, et al: An alternative method for determination of the carpal height ratio. J Bone Joint Surg (Am) 76:88, 1994.

797. Boden SD, Dodge LD, Bohlman HH, et al: Rheumatoid arthritis of the cervical spine. A long-term analysis with predictors of paralysis and recovery. J Bone Joint Surg [Am] 75:1282, 1993.

798. Sewell KL, Ruthazer R, Parker JA: The correlation of indium-111 joint scans with clinical synovitis in rheumatoid arthritis. J Rheumatol 20:2015, 1993.

799. Poleksic L, Zdravkovic D, Jablanovic D, et al: Magnetic resonance imaging of bone destruction in rheumatoid arthritis: comparison with radiography. Skeletal Radiol 22:577, 1993.

800. Waterton JC, Rajanayagam V, Ross BD, et al: Magnetic resonance methods for measurement of disease progression in rheumatoid arthritis. Magn Res Imag 11:1033, 1993.

801. Glew D, Watt I: MRI in rheumatoid disease of the cervical spine. Clinical MRI 3:83, 1993.

802. Roca A, Bernreuter WK, Alarcón GS: Functional magnetic resonance imaging should be included in the evaluation of the cervical spine in patients with rheumatoid arthritis. J Rheumatol 20:1485, 1993.

803. Gubler FM, Algra PR, Dijkstra PF, et al: Gadolinium-DTPA enhanced magnetic resonance imaging of bone cysts in patients with rheumatoid arthritis. Ann Rheum Dis 52:716, 1993.

804. Peterfy CG, Majumdar S, Lang P, et al: MR imaging of the arthritic knee: Improved discrimination of cartilage, synovium, and effusion with pulsed saturation transfer and fat-suppressed T1-weighted sequences. Radiology 191:413, 1994.

805. Aho K, Kurki P: Seropositive versus seronegative rheumatoid arthritis—time for a new definition. J Rheumatol 21:388, 1994.

806. Buchanan WW, Singal DP: Seronegative rheumatoid arthritis: Tell it as it is. J Rheumatol 21:391, 1994.

27

Juvenile Chronic Arthritis

Donald Resnick, M.D., and Gen Niwayama, M.D.

Juvenile rheumatoid arthritis first was described in 1864 by Cornil,[1] although a 1483 painting by Botticelli, ''Portrait of a Youth,'' in which some features of the disease possibly are displayed, would suggest that juvenile rheumatoid arthritis is older than Cornil's description would indicate.[134] Thirty-three years after Cornil's description, Still,[2] an English pediatrician, detailed an articular condition in 22 children that appeared to be distinct from the adult type of rheumatoid arthritis because of its predilection for large joints rather than small ones, its propensity for producing joint contractures and muscle wasting, and its association with significant extra-articular manifestations, such as splenomegaly, lymphadenopathy, anemia, fever, pleuritis, and pericarditis. Since this report, the designation of Still's disease frequently has been used to describe rheumatoid arthritis in children.[3-7]

Through the years, there has been a natural tendency to label many articular disorders of children as juvenile rheumatoid arthritis despite variable clinical and radiologic manifestations and an unpredictable disease course. Largely through the work of Ansell and Bywaters[8, 9] and Schaller and Wedgwood,[10, 135] it now is recognized that a number of separate disorders can lead to chronic arthritis in children, and that, in many patients, scrutiny of clinical and radiographic features will allow a more precise diagnosis. Currently, no uniformly accepted classification system for juvenile chronic arthritis exists, however.[187]

CLASSIFICATION

In arriving at a workable classification of articular disease in children, the physician must first exclude certain groups of disorders with characteristic features.[8, 198] Infectious diseases, bleeding diatheses, neoplasms such as leukemia and neuroblastoma, collagen vascular disorders including scleroderma, systemic lupus erythematosus, and dermatomyositis, Sjögren's syndrome, rheumatic fever, and post-dysenteric arthritis as well as some rarer conditions all are eliminated in this fashion. The remaining group of diseases is designated as juvenile chronic arthritis (or polyarthritis). Within this group are certain disorders, such as ankylosing spondylitis, psoriatic arthritis, and the arthritis associated with inflammatory bowel disease, whose true nature may be revealed only after a follow-up period of variable length. At the time of their initial presentation, however, it frequently was impossible to classify these children with arthritis into one specific subgroup of juvenile chronic arthritis. In view of this difficulty, reviews of clinical and radiologic manifestations in large numbers of children with chronic arthritis must be interpreted cautiously as they commonly include patients with heterogeneous types of arthritis. In some reports, serologic histocompatibility antigen (HLA) typing[176] has allowed subtypes of juvenile chronic arthritis to be better defined. For example, the frequency of DR4 antigen is increased in those children who are serologically positive for rheumatoid factor or who have polyarticular disease; similarly, DR5 antigen is present more frequently in children with systemic symptoms and signs, DR5 and DR8 antigens in children with involvement

TABLE 27–1. Juvenile Chronic Arthritis Classification

Juvenile-onset adult type (seropositive) rheumatoid arthritis
Seronegative chronic arthritis (Still's disease)
 Classic systemic disease
 Polyarticular disease
 Pauciarticular or monoarticular disease
Juvenile-onset ankylosing spondylitis
Psoriatic arthritis
Arthritis of inflammatory bowel disease
Other seronegative spondyloarthropathies
Miscellaneous arthritis

of a few joints, and B27 antigen in children with abnormalities of the axial skeleton.[141, 177, 199]

The following subgroups of juvenile chronic arthritis now are recognized (Tables 27–1 and 27–2) (Fig. 27–1).

Juvenile-Onset Adult Type (Seropositive) Rheumatoid Arthritis

An articular disease that resembles and behaves like the adult counterpart has been noted in 10 per cent of 954 children with juvenile chronic arthritis[11] (Fig. 27–1A). A frequency of approximately 5 per cent is suggested by some investigators.[135] This subgroup is more frequent in girls than in boys.[183] Although this pattern of disease has been detected in children as young as 5 years of age, it is more common after the age of 10 years.[8, 11–14] The clinical onset usually is polyarticular, with early involvement of the interphalangeal and metacarpophalangeal joints of the hand, the wrist, the knee, and the metatarsophalangeal and interphalangeal joints of the foot. Severe destructive arthritis is common, occurring in more than 50 per cent of patients. Subcutaneous nodules, particularly about the elbow, which histologically are identical to those in adult-onset rheumatoid arthritis, can be detected in approximately 10 to 20 per cent of children.[8] Manifestations of vasculitis, which are rare at the onset of disease, increase in frequency thereafter. Iridocyclitis is not present.

Radiologic changes in juvenile-onset adult type rheumatoid arthritis commonly are apparent when the child first is evaluated. Soft tissue swelling, periarticular osteoporosis, and periostitis in the hands and the feet can be prominent. Periosteal bone formation can involve large segments of the metaphyses of phalanges, metacarpals, and metatarsals. It is the frequency and the severity of periostitis that consti-

TABLE 27–2. Juvenile Chronic Arthritis: Clinical and Radiographic Features

Disorder	Clinical Features	Sites of Articular Involvement	Radiographic Features
Juvenile-onset adult type (seropositive) rheumatoid arthritis	Female predominance >10 years old Polyarticular involvement ± Subcutaneous nodules ± Vasculitis Seropositive for rheumatoid factor	MCP and IP joints of hand Wrist Knee MTP and IP joints of foot Cervical spine	Soft tissue swelling Osteoporosis Periostitis Erosions ± Joint space loss Atlantoaxial subluxation
Still's disease Systemic disease	Affects males and females equally <5 years old Systemic manifestations Mild articular manifestations	Unusual and mild joint involvement*	
Polyarticular disease	Affects males and females equally Variable age Polyarticular involvement Symmetric	MCP and IP joints of hand Wrist Knee Ankle Intertarsal, MTP, and IP joints of foot Cervical spine	Soft tissue swelling Osteoporosis Periostitis Growth disturbances ± Erosions ± Joint space loss Intra-articular bony ankylosis Apophyseal joint ankylosis with hypoplasia of cervical vertebrae and discs Scoliosis
Pauciarticular or monoarticular disease	Female predominance Young age Iridocyclitis ± Systemic manifestations Asymmetric	Knee Ankle Elbow Wrist	Soft tissue swelling Osteoporosis Growth disturbances ± Joint space loss ± Erosions
Juvenile-onset ankylosing spondylitis	Male predominance 10–12 years old Polyarticular or pauciarticular involvement Predilection for the lower extremity Asymmetric ± Back pain ± Iridocyclitis ± Family history HLA-B27 positive	Ankle Knee Intertarsal joints Calcaneus Hip ± Sacroiliac joint ± Spine	± Sacroiliitis ± Spondylitis Joint space loss Intra-articular bony ankylosis Erosions Bony proliferation

*When present, findings are similar to polyarticular or pauciarticular disease.
˜ MCP, metacarpophalangeal; IP, interphalangeal; MTP, metatarsophalangeal.

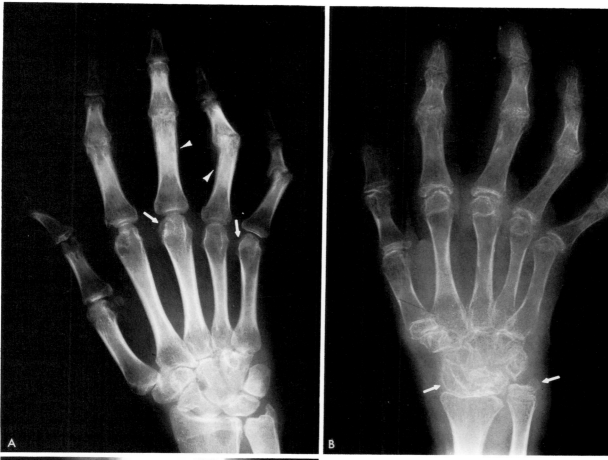

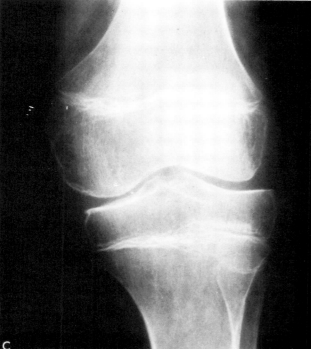

FIGURE 27–1. Juvenile chronic arthritis: Subgroups of disease.

A Juvenile-onset adult type (seropositive) rheumatoid arthritis. An 18 year old girl with seropositive rheumatoid arthritis for approximately 6 years. Observe that the radiographic abnormalities are similar to those seen in adult-onset disease. Involvement occurs in all the compartments of the wrist and in the metacarpophalangeal and proximal interphalangeal joints, with less striking changes in the distal interphalangeal joints. Radiographic changes include soft tissue swelling, periarticular osteoporosis, joint space narrowing, and marginal erosions. At some metacarpophalangeal joints, considerable erosive alterations are not accompanied by severe loss of joint space (arrows). Also note intra-articular osseous fusion at several proximal interphalangeal joints and periostitis of phalangeal shafts (arrowheads).

B Seronegative chronic arthritis (Still's disease): Polyarticular disease. An 11 year old girl, seronegative for rheumatoid factor, had symmetric articular disease of the hands, wrists, knees, feet, and cervical spine. The radiograph outlines considerable generalized osteoporosis, periarticular soft tissue swelling, superficial erosions of carpal bones and metacarpal heads with irregularity of shape, joint space narrowing, epiphyseal collapse, and enlargement of epiphyses, particularly those of the distal radius and distal ulna (arrows). The crenated or "crinkled" appearance of the carpus and metacarpal heads is distinctive. Flexion contractures of several digits are evident.

C Seronegative chronic arthritis (Still's disease): Pauciarticular disease. A 9 year old girl initially had monoarticular disease of the knee and subsequently developed involvement of several other joints. The radiograph reveals soft tissue swelling, osteoporosis, and enlargement of the epiphyses of the distal portion of the femur and proximal portion of the tibia. Mild joint space narrowing can be seen.

Illustration continued on following page

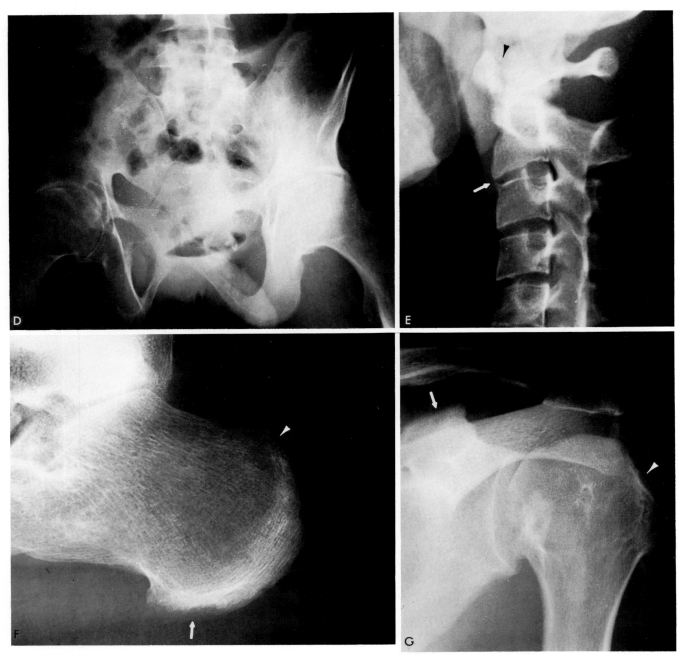

FIGURE 27–1. *Continued*

D–G Juvenile-onset ankylosing spondylitis. A 20 year old man had a 4 year history of arthritis involving the low back, hips, feet, heels, and shoulders. The radiograph of the pelvis **(D)** demonstrates bilateral complete intra-articular osseous fusion of the synovial and ligamentous portions of the sacroiliac joints and concentric joint space narrowing of the hips with femoral and acetabular osteophytes. In the cervical spine **(E),** apophyseal joint bony ankylosis and syndesmophytosis (arrow) are associated with a minor degree of atlantoaxial subluxation (arrowhead). Observe that significant hypoplasia of vertebral bodies and intervertebral discs is not evident. The plantar aspect of the calcaneus **(F)** is eroded and sclerotic, with an irregular contour (arrow). Osseous erosion of the posterosuperior aspect of the bone also is seen (arrowhead). A radiograph of the shoulder **(G)** demonstrates extensive and poorly defined erosion on the lateral aspect of the humeral head (arrowhead), called the hatchet deformity, and bony proliferation of the coracoid process (arrow).

Illustration continued on opposite page

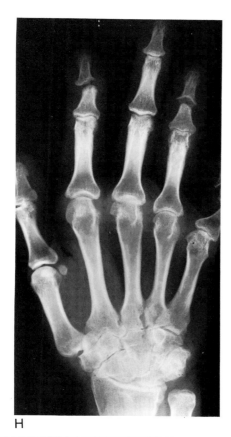

H

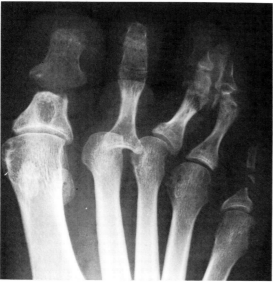

FIGURE 27–1. *Continued*

H, I Juvenile-onset psoriatic arthritis. A 25 year old woman had a 10 year history of psoriatic skin disease and arthritis. Radiographs revealed polyarticular involvement of the joints of the hand, wrist, and foot. Observe extensive destruction of multiple distal interphalangeal joints in both the hand and the foot and subluxations.

tute a fundamental difference between juvenile-onset and adult-onset disease.

Significant osseous erosions also are encountered in children in this subgroup of disease.[8, 10, 15, 183] These erosions can have a marginal distribution and may be unaccompa-

nied by loss of the interosseous space; the appearance of significant erosive abnormality in the absence of joint space loss should be emphasized as a diagnostic sign of juvenile-onset rheumatoid arthritis. When joint space loss is evident, it commonly is diffuse, producing symmetric diminution of the articular space, particularly in the hip (at which site it may be combined with acetabular protrusion) and the knee. Atlantoaxial subluxation is not uncommon.

The prognosis of polyarthritis in children who become seropositive for rheumatoid factor generally is poor. It should be emphasized, however, that a significant percentage of patients with this subgroup of juvenile chronic arthritis do not reveal such seropositivity at the onset of their disease.[198]

Seronegative Chronic Arthritis (Still's Disease)

In this largest subgroup (approximately 70 per cent) of juvenile chronic arthritis, children develop systemic or articular (or both) symptoms and signs in the absence of positive serologic test results for rheumatoid factor. Within this subgroup are certain clinical varieties, such as classic systemic disease, polyarticular disease, and pauciarticular or monoarticular disease.

Classic Systemic Disease. This pattern, which usually is seen in boys and girls below the age of 5 years and represents approximately 20 per cent of cases of juvenile chronic arthritis, is associated with severe extra-articular clinical manifestations. An acute febrile onset (with high and remittent fever) may or may not be accompanied by arthritis. The affected child has toxic symptoms, with irritability, listlessness, anorexia, and weight loss. A rash accompanies the fever in approximately 80 to 90 per cent of children. Discrete or confluent macular or maculopapular lesions are detected on the trunk and the extremities, and occasionally on the neck and the face[10, 16]; these lesions generally are fleeting or evanescent. Generalized lymphadenopathy and hepatosplenomegaly can simulate the findings in leukemia or lymphoma. The enlarged lymph nodes are related topographically to inflamed articulations and are characterized pathologically by nonspecific follicular hyperplasia.[9] Lymphedema in the upper or lower extremities, or in both locations, may be evident.[200]

Pericarditis and myocarditis represent serious manifestations of Still's disease.[10, 16–20] Endocarditis is not observed. Pleuritis and interstitial pulmonary disease have been recorded. Amyloidosis also can complicate Still's disease, leading to renal enlargement, uremia, and even death.[21]

Although joint manifestations are common, they generally are mild in nature. Myalgia and arthralgia may precede actual arthritis. Radiologic findings are unusual, although occasionally chronic and disabling articular changes can become evident.

Laboratory features include moderate anemia, elevated erythrocyte sedimentation rate, and leukocytosis.

There are reports of neonatal-onset articular disease with systemic manifestations whose clinical findings do not precisely coincide with the classic form of systemic disease described earlier.[142, 195] Abnormalities include rash, diffuse multisystem involvement, chronic arthritis, short, bowed bones with wide metaphyses, and alterations in the central nervous system. Investigators who believe it is a distinct disorder have proposed the name neonatal-onset multisystem inflammatory disease (NOMID).[201] Among its most characteristic features are initial presentation in the newborn and bizarre enlargement of the ossified portions of the epiphyses about the involved joints. The epiphyses ossify eratically, possess coarsened trabeculation, and contain peripheral portions that appear spiculated.[201] Additional findings include prominent periostitis about the diaphyses and metaphyses of affected tubular bones, persistence of the anterior fontanelle and the formation of wormian bones in the skull, and a gibbus deformity of the thoracolumbar spine.[195, 201] The pathogenesis of NOMID appears to be a chronic unremitting inflammatory process that begins at birth and affects many organs.[201]

Polyarticular Disease (Fig. 27–1*B*). Polyarticular arthritis may occur at the onset of Still's disease or as a later complication in a child with systemic manifestations. This pattern is evident in approximately 20 per cent of patients with juvenile chronic arthritis. Some reports indicate boys and girls are affected in equal numbers; others suggest a strong female preponderance.[135] Symmetric involvement of the metacarpophalangeal and proximal interphalangeal joints of the hands, the wrists, the knees, the ankles, and the intertarsal, metatarsophalangeal, and interphalangeal joints of the feet is typical. The cervical spine frequently is a site of early abnormality and characteristically is the only region of the vertebral column that is affected. Clinically apparent loss of extension of the neck is common. Accompanying systemic manifestations, which may be less severe than in the classic systemic variety of disease, include rash, splenomegaly, lymphadenopathy, and carditis. Fever and leukocytosis also can be apparent. The entire clinical spectrum may resemble that in rheumatic fever.

In the initial stages of polyarthritis, radiographic findings are soft tissue swelling, osteoporosis, and advanced skeletal maturation. In the hands and the feet, abnormalities of shape (squaring) of the carpal and tarsal bones frequently are combined with initial loss of joint space and subsequent intra-articular bony ankylosis. Synovitis of flexor tendon sheaths may produce periostitis of the diaphyses and metaphyses of phalanges, metacarpals, and metatarsals. Premature fusion of the epiphyses of the bones is not uncommon, accounting for characteristic defects of growth. The epiphyses may appear enlarged or ballooned in relation to the diaphyses, and decrease in bone length is characteristic. Osseous erosion is unusual, and when present it rarely is severe.

In the larger articulations, such as the knee, osteoporosis and epiphyseal overgrowth are more typical than articular space loss and erosive change. In the hip, radiographic abnormalities may be detected in as many as 40 per cent of patients who are followed for 10 years or more.[22] This involvement, which may produce major clinical disability, is associated with enlargement and osteoporosis of the femoral capital epiphysis, failure of growth and premature fusion of the femoral neck, coxa valga deformity, hypoplasia of the iliac bones, and protrusio acetabuli. Joint space diminution and erosions are late findings. Similar alterations can appear in the glenohumeral joint and the elbow.

Cervical spine abnormalities may be a presenting feature in 2 per cent of patients.[11] Apophyseal joint erosions, narrowing, and bony ankylosis predominate in the upper cervical region, particularly at the C2-C3 level. Associated hypoplasia of the vertebral bodies and intervertebral discs is characteristic. Thoracolumbar spinal abnormalities of Still's disease are relatively infrequent, although osteoporosis with or without compression fractures (perhaps related to steroid administration) and scoliosis are encountered.

Children with polyarthritis and systemic onset generally have a poor prognosis, similar to that of children with polyarthritis from disease onset and of children with polyarthritis who are seropositive for rheumatoid factor.[198]

Pauciarticular or Monoarticular Disease (Fig. 27–1*C*). This pattern, which is observed in young children and may represent 30 to 70 per cent of all cases of juvenile chronic arthritis, generally is confined to large joints, most frequently the knees, the ankles, the elbows, and the wrists.[10, 23, 24] The small joints of the hands and the hips may be spared. This clinical pattern of arthritis carries with it a serious threat of blindness from iridocyclitis.[16] Additional systemic manifestations are infrequent, although occasionally lymphadenopathy, splenomegaly, fever, and rash are observed. Laboratory findings may be entirely unremarkable. In recent years, two distinct subgroups of this pattern of disease have been identified on the basis of clinical and immunogenetic evidence.[135] Pauciarticular disease, type I, is composed of children, predominantly girls, who are young in age (5 years or younger).[202] Chronic iridocyclitis is frequent, as are positive tests for antinuclear antibodies. Sacroiliitis and spondylitis are absent, and the prognosis for ultimate joint function is good. Pauciarticular disease, type II, is composed of children who are older at the time of onset of disease. Boys principally are affected, and the peripheral joints in the lower extremities characteristically are involved. Iridocyclitis may be observed, and sacroiliitis may become apparent at the time of follow-up evaluation. It is obvious that some patients who initially manifest this subgroup of disease will later show evidence of a seronegative spondyloarthropathy. Because of this and other factors that complicate the division of pauciarticular and monoarticular disease into specific categories, it appears easier to divide such diseases on the basis of the number of joints that are affected. This is done in the following paragraphs, although this division, too, is not without difficulty.

A monoarticular type of juvenile chronic arthritis has been reported in 5 to 35 per cent of patients,[23, 25–27] the frequency being affected by the method of patient selection, the time of clinical evaluation, and the length of follow-up examination. Children who initially exhibited monoarticular disease subsequently may develop pauciarticular disease or rarely polyarthritis. In general, there is no way of predicting which children with monoarthritis will later develop more widespread articular abnormality.[128]

Pauciarticular arthritis has been reported in 35 to 60 per cent of patients,[25, 28, 29] although there are differing opinions regarding the number of joints that can be involved and still represent a pauciarticular presentation. Estimates have included the following: more than one but fewer than four joints,[30, 31] more than one but fewer than five joints,[11, 32] and more than one but fewer than six joints.[24, 33] One or two major articulations may be affected in combination with two or three joints of the fingers and the toes.[25] The disease may be self-limited, arresting within several years without residual deformity.

In monoarticular or pauciarticular Still's disease, radiographically demonstrable abnormalities of bone growth may appear at an early stage. Increased size and accelerated maturation of epiphyseal ossification centers, longitudinal overgrowth of bones adjacent to an affected articulation, and regional atrophy and remodeling of bone are observed.[11, 23, 160] Soft tissue swelling and osteoporosis are seen, but bony erosion is a late manifestation.

Juvenile-Onset Ankylosing Spondylitis
(Fig. 27–1D–G)

Children with this disease, particularly boys, develop sacroiliitis and spondylitis in the presence of the histocompatibility antigen HLA-B27.[34–38] Although the mean age of onset of disease is 10 to 12 years, the variation is wide, ranging from 3 to 15 years of age.[8] An asymmetric arthritis generally is observed, and the articulations of the lower limbs are affected, particularly the ankle, the knee, and the intertarsal joints. Occasionally, presenting symptoms and signs may involve the hip or an interphalangeal joint of the toe,[11] and prominent findings related to retrocalcaneal bursitis may be seen. The joints of the upper extremity are relatively spared. Clinical manifestations may be encountered in the sacroiliac joints, but radiographic changes in these articulations and those of the spine are difficult to interpret in young children and frequently are delayed until the latter part of the second decade of life. Acute iridocyclitis is not a common presenting feature of the disease but subsequently is apparent in as many as 25 per cent of patients.[8] A family history of ankylosing spondylitis is not infrequent. HLA-B27 may be detected in approximately 90 per cent of affected children.

Radiographic abnormalities in juvenile-onset ankylosing spondylitis have been well described.[39] Sacroiliac joint alterations appear as the disease progresses. Although they initially may be unilateral or asymmetric in distribution, they soon become bilateral and symmetric. Articular space widening, indistinct joint margins, erosions, and sclerosis can be noted. Eventually, joint space diminution and osseous ankylosis can be evident. The spinal changes also progress with increasing duration of the disease, and these may be seen in the thoracic, the lumbar, and less frequently the cervical regions of the vertebral column. They include osteitis or sclerosis of vertebral corners, squaring of the anterior vertebral surface, syndesmophytosis, and apophyseal joint bony ankylosis. Atlantoaxial subluxation is unusual.[40]

Radiographic findings in the appendicular skeleton are most common in the hips, the knees, and the shoulders, and they are less common in the small joints of the hands and the feet. Joint space narrowing, erosions, bony proliferation, and even intra-articular osseous fusion are typical of the changes that accompany any of the seronegative spondyloarthropathies. The inferior and posterior aspects of the calcaneus, the ischial tuberosities, and the trochanters of the proximal portion of the femur may be affected.

The radiographic abnormalities of juvenile-onset ankylosing spondylitis are virtually indistinguishable from those of adult-onset disease.[40] A high frequency of peripheral joint abnormalities, especially early in the disease course, may be more characteristic of the juvenile variety of the disease. The differentiation of radiographic features of juvenile-onset ankylosing spondylitis from other varieties of juvenile chronic arthritis (juvenile-onset adult type rheumatoid arthritis; Still's disease) can be difficult. In the latter

conditions, sacroiliac joint abnormalities may be encountered, consisting of erosions, sclerosis, and decreased articular space, although the prevalence of these findings generally is lower than in juvenile-onset ankylosing spondylitis.[41] Furthermore, in children with ankylosing spondylitis, the appearance of spondylitis in the thoracic and lumbar segments, the lower rate of occurrence of cervical spinal alterations, the sparing of the articulations of the hands and the wrists, and the absence of severe osteoporosis and growth disturbances are additional features that differ from those in other varieties of juvenile chronic arthritis.

Psoriatic Arthritis (Fig. 27–1H, I)

In a small subgroup of children with juvenile chronic arthritis, articular involvement may antedate psoriatic skin disease and can be characterized by severe and progressive joint destruction. A family history of psoriasis in these children is common. The age of onset is variable (usually 9 or 10 years of age),[8, 42, 43] and abnormalities of the nails may be the initial clinical manifestation. Asymmetric articular involvement with periods of remission and exacerbation is most characteristic.[178] Radiographic abnormalities can simulate those in adults with psoriatic arthritis, including distal interphalangeal joint destruction, phalangeal tuftal resorption, and sacroiliitis.

Juvenile-onset psoriatic arthritis usually has an oligoarticular onset, although progression to polyarthritis is reported to be common.[203, 249] Diffuse swelling of a finger or toe owing to tenosynovitis, occasional chronic iridocyclitis, and, perhaps, a slight female predominance are other characteristics of the disease. An increased prevalence of the antigens HLA-B17 and HLA-A2 has been noted in some reports.[203]

Arthritis of Inflammatory Bowel Disease

In this type, spinal, sacroiliac, and peripheral articular findings accompany enteritis and colitis, although such findings also may develop in a child prior to recognition of inflammatory bowel disease.[254] Furthermore, diarrhea and serologic evidence of previous Shigella or Salmonella infection may be evident in cases of childhood Reiter's syndrome, although this syndrome may appear in children without bowel symptoms and signs.[123–125, 250]

Other Seronegative Spondyloarthropathies

In addition to ankylosing spondylitis, psoriatic arthritis, and the arthritis of inflammatory bowel disease, other varieties of seronegative spondyloarthropathy affect children. These include Reiter's syndrome[136, 137] and reactive arthritis. Furthermore, it is expected that additional syndromes will be identified.[180] In this regard, a disorder characterized by involvement of the axial skeleton, enthesopathy, and the presence of the HLA-B27 antigen has been described.[138, 139, 179, 196] Findings include a male predominance, late age of disease onset, positive family history of arthritis, oligoarthropathy, and involvement of the sacroiliac joint. New bone formation is observed at sites of ligament and tendon attachment, including those in the pelvis and the calcaneus. Osteopenia may be prominent. Many of these characteristics are identical to those seen in all of the seronegative

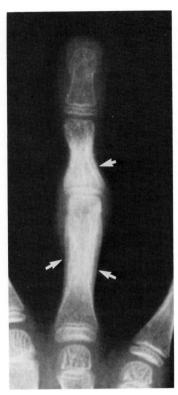

FIGURE 27–2. Seronegative enthesopathy and arthropathy (SEA) syndrome. This young child developed enthesopathy and dactylitis, was seropositive for HLA-B27 antigen, and did not reveal clinical or radiographic evidence of sacroiliitis. The radiograph shows soft tissue swelling and contracture about the proximal interphalangeal joint of the fourth finger and periosteal reaction in the diaphyses and metaphyses of the proximal and middle phalanges (arrows). (Courtesy of C. Pineda, M.D., Mexico City, Mexico.)

spondyloarthropathies and, indeed, some patients who exhibit this syndrome initially will eventually develop ankylosing spondylitis, psoriatic arthritis, Reiter's syndrome, or inflammatory bowel disease.

In recent years, increased emphasis has been given to the clinical features and eventual outcome in children with HLA-B27 antigen–associated seronegative (for rheumatoid factor) enthesopathy and arthropathy, a constellation of findings that has been designated the SEA syndrome.[204, 205] Although a significant proportion of patients with this syndrome develop back complaints and radiographic evidence of sacroiliitis, thereby fulfilling diagnostic criteria for ankylosing spondylitis, during the first 5 years of disease or thereafter,[199, 206] this is not a constant association.[204, 205, 207, 208] Enthesitis in peripheral locations, as well as dactylitis (Fig. 27–2), may be the sole manifestation of seronegative "spondyloarthropathy" in children.[205] The proportion of Caucasian children with the SEA syndrome who develop ankylosing spondylitis appears to be lower than that in other ethnic groups,[204] although long-term follow-up studies of patients with this syndrome are not available at the present time.

Arnett and collaborators[166] have reported another possibly distinct subset of seronegative spondyloarthropathy that occurs in children and young adults, especially women, characterized by the presence of the antigen HLA-B27 and the absence of rheumatoid factor and antinuclear antibodies

in the blood. Findings include cervical spine involvement and polyarticular disease in the appendicular skeleton that is symmetric and destructive, simulating rheumatoid arthritis.

Polyarthropathy Associated with Other Disorders

Included in this miscellaneous group are articular findings related to such conditions as systemic lupus erythematosus[126] and familial Mediterranean fever.

RADIOGRAPHIC ABNORMALITIES

The radiographic abnormalities associated with juvenile chronic arthritis depend on the specific subgroup that is being investigated. In the following discussion, emphasis is placed on those features that can be encountered in juvenile-onset adult type (seropositive) rheumatoid arthritis and the polyarticular and pauciarticular types of seronegative chronic arthritis (Still's disease). As was outlined previously, certain differences in radiographic characteristics and distribution exist between these two groups; however, many similarities also are evident, facilitating inclusion of both groups in the following analysis.[4, 11, 44, 45, 188, 209]

General Features (Table 27–3) (Fig. 27–3)

Soft Tissue Swelling. Periarticular fusiform soft tissue swelling is a common early manifestation of arthritis. It is variable in extent, although large joint effusions sometimes are apparent. Asymmetric or eccentric soft tissue prominence can relate to tenosynovitis.

Osteopenia. Juxta-articular or diffuse osteoporosis may be encountered. In addition, band-like metaphyseal lucent zones may be seen, particularly in the distal femur, proximal tibia, distal radius, distal tibia, and distal fibula (although rarely in other locations, including the cervical spine). They are identical to those seen in childhood

TABLE 27–3. Juvenile Chronic Arthritis Versus Adult-Onset Rheumatoid Arthritis: General Radiographic Characteristics*

Finding	Juvenile Chronic Arthritis	Adult-Onset Rheumatoid Arthritis
Soft tissue swelling	Common	Common
Osteoporosis	Common	Common
Joint space loss	Late manifestation	Early manifestation
Bony erosions	Late manifestation	Early manifestation
Intra-articular bony ankylosis	Common	Rare
Periostitis	Common	Rare
Growth disturbances	Common	Absent
Epiphyseal compression fractures	Common	Less common
Joint subluxation	Common	Common
Synovial cysts	Uncommon	Common

*Characteristics will vary depending on the specific subgroups of juvenile chronic arthritis.

leukemia.[45, 46] The pathogenesis of this type of lucent finding in juvenile chronic arthritis, although not fully understood, may be related to a depression in endochondral bone formation in response to a severe systemic illness[47] or trabecular atrophy due to persistent hyperemia in the vascular metaphyseal regions,[45] or both. Subsequent development of transverse radiodense "growth recovery" lines has been noted.

Osteoporosis in children with juvenile chronic arthritis may lead to fractures. Several types have been identified, including compression fractures of the epiphyses (see later discussion), diaphyseal and metaphyseal fractures of tubular bones, and compression fractures of vertebral bodies. The frequency of such fractures is increased in patients with severe disease and in those who are immobilized or receiving corticosteroid therapy.

Joint Space Abnormalities. Diminution of the interosseous space in juvenile chronic arthritis is less frequent than in adult-onset rheumatoid arthritis and, when present, usually is a late manifestation of the disease.[4, 11, 45, 48] The combination of osteoporosis and soft tissue swelling without cartilaginous (or osseous) destruction is an important radiographic characteristic of this disease. Preservation of joint space is especially characteristic of monoarticular disease.[45] In some patients, however, particularly those with juvenile-onset adult type (seropositive) rheumatoid arthritis, loss of articular space may be more rapid. In later stages of juvenile chronic arthritis, intra-articular bony ankylosis is frequent, especially in the small joints of the hands and the wrists (and in the apophyseal articulations of the cervical spine as well). Martel and coworkers[45] observed such ankylosis in 15 of 80 patients (19 per cent) with juvenile chronic arthritis, and they attributed the finding to periosteal new bone formation or immobilization.

Bony Erosion. Destruction of bone also is a relatively late manifestation of juvenile chronic arthritis, although patients with juvenile-onset adult type (seropositive) rheumatoid arthritis may reveal osseous erosion at an earlier stage of their disease, especially in the hands and feet. The erosive abnormalities may be distributed at the margins of the articulation (in a fashion identical to that in adult-onset rheumatoid arthritis) or along the entire articular surface of the bone. In the latter situation, pocketed or etched osseous defects create irregular surfaces, an appearance that is especially frequent in the carpal and tarsal areas.

Periostitis. As in many conditions that affect the immature skeleton, periosteal bone formation is a frequent and prominent manifestation of juvenile chronic arthritis. Martel and collaborators[45] noted periostitis in 18 of 80 patients (23 per cent) with this disease. It is most common in periarticular regions of phalanges, metacarpals, and metatarsals, although periosteal proliferation of metaphyses and diaphyses of long bones also may be observed. Periostitis can appear early in the course of the disease in combination with osteoporosis and soft tissue swelling, simulating the appearance of osteomyelitis. Its pathogenesis may include inflammation of the joint capsule and adjacent periosteum, tenosynovitis, and chronic hyperemia,[45] and it is facilitated by the relative ease with which the periosteum of a child is lifted from the underlying bone and stimulated to form new bone. The extent of bony proliferation may become extreme, and the eventual appearance of enlarged, rectangular tubular bones of the hands and the feet is not uncommon.

Growth Disturbances. Growth disturbances are a remarkable feature of juvenile chronic arthritis.[11, 45, 49] They may become profound, particularly when the onset of the disorder occurs in early life. The absence of these abnormalities in adult-onset rheumatoid arthritis is noteworthy.

Epiphyseal enlargement due to accelerated growth stimulated by hyperemia is frequent about small and large articulations. Commonly affected locations include the distal portion of the femur, the proximal portion of the tibia, and the radial head.[209] This overgrowth is further accentuated by the adjacent constricted appearance of the metaphysis and diaphysis. In addition, relative sparing of the subchondral region of the epiphysis leads to characteristic epiphyseal ballooning, an appearance that suggests that the hyperemic joint capsule attaching to the epiphysis or metaphysis at some distance from the joint is the predominant factor influencing epiphyseal overgrowth.[45] Long-standing elevation of intra-articular pressure, by provoking epiphyseal hypertension and intraosseous engorgement, may be an additional factor in the occurrence of growth disturbances of the epiphyses.[148] Soft tissue swelling and osteoporosis frequently are associated with enlargement of the epiphysis, although joint space narrowing and osseous erosion may not be apparent. Accelerated osseous growth and maturation in the wrist and the midfoot lead to an increase in the number and the size of the carpal and the tarsal bones.

Disturbance of normal growth of the diaphysis leads to a variety of appearances of the bones in juvenile chronic arthritis. Bony atrophy with osteoporosis and reduction in diameter, overgrowth, or undergrowth may be seen. In the hands and the feet, short, broad phalanges, metacarpals, and metatarsals simulate the changes in various bone dysplasias, and an accurate diagnosis of an articular disorder on the basis of radiographic features can be difficult.[50] In the lower extremities, leg-length discrepancies are seen, the specific pattern and severity being influenced by a variety of factors. For example, monoarticular or pauciarticular involvement that includes the knee in a child below the age of 9 years results in mild to moderate lengthening of the affected side.[160] In other instances and locations, the outcome is characterized by shortening of the involved region. Such shortening is more common in children whose disease began after the age of 9 years.

Typical growth abnormalities in juvenile chronic arthritis also are observed in the mandible and the cervical spine (see discussion later in this chapter).

The pathogenesis of the growth disturbances in this disease may be multifactorial. Growth accentuation due to hyperemia and growth inhibition due to chronic illness, prolonged steroid therapy, immobilization, and neurogenic factors may be important.[45] Premature epiphyseal fusion in patients with brachydactyly may be either the cause or the result of cessation of bone growth. Additional factors promoting growth abnormalities in juvenile chronic arthritis include inflammation of periarticular connective tissues, epiphyseal destruction, subluxation, muscle spasm and fibrosis, and contracture, all of which may lead to altered mechanical stresses, influencing patterns of osseous development.[45]

Epiphyseal Compression Fractures. Epiphyseal compression fractures accompanying juvenile chronic arthritis were emphasized by Martel and collaborators.[45] These fractures are evident in the weight-bearing epiphyses of the

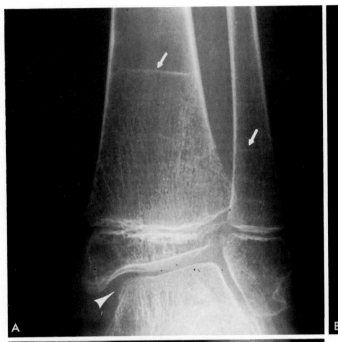

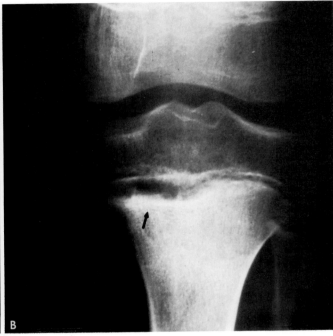

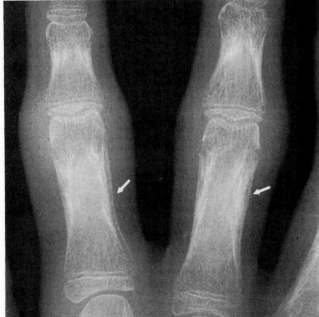

FIGURE 27–3. Juvenile chronic arthritis: General radiographic abnormalities.

A Osteoporosis and growth recovery lines. Observe diffuse osteopenia of the tibia, fibula, and talus and radiodense bands or growth recovery lines (arrows). The tilting of the articular surface of the tibial epiphysis and talus is a typical but nondiagnostic sign of the disease (arrowhead).

B Disturbance of endochondral bone formation. The considerable alterations of the proximal tibial metaphysis consisting of widening and consolidation of bone (arrow) presumably are related to disturbance of endochondral bone formation. The tibia on the opposite side was less severely involved. (Courtesy of S. Houston, M.D., Saskatoon, Saskatchewan, Canada.)

C Periostitis. Prominent periosteal proliferation of numerous phalanges (arrows) is associated with osteoporosis and periarticular soft tissue swelling. Joint space diminution and erosions are not significant features in this child.

Illustration continued on opposite page

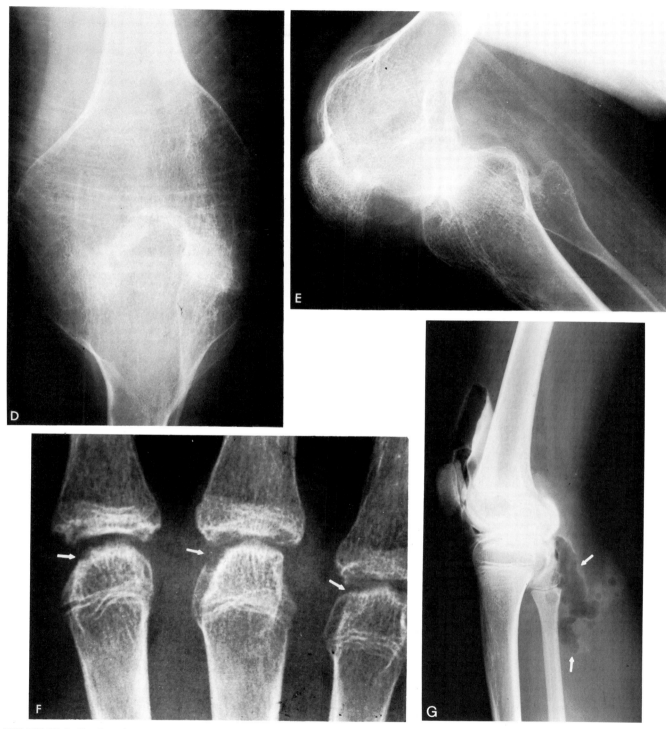

FIGURE 27–3. *Continued*

D, E Growth disturbances. Striking enlargement or ballooning of the epiphyses of the distal femur and proximal tibia are observed. Note the tapered diminutive diaphyses, particularly in the fibula. Osteoporosis and a flexion contracture of the joint are seen.

F Epiphyseal compression fractures. The irregular outline of the metacarpal heads (arrows) is produced by compression of weakened osteoporotic bones.

G Synovial cyst. Knee arthrography in a 10 year old boy outlines communication between the articular cavity and a popliteal cyst (arrows). (**G,** Courtesy of M. Ozonoff, M.D., Newington, Connecticut.)

lower extremity as well as in the epiphyses of the hands and the feet. They are produced by abnormal stress (resulting from muscle spasm and subluxation) acting on weakened osteoporotic bone. Flattening and deformity of the epiphyseal ossification centers and formation of dense intraosseous foci due to trabecular compression are evident. Cupping of the ossification centers of the proximal phalanges owing to compression by the metacarpals and the metatarsals is frequent.

Joint Subluxation. In juvenile chronic arthritis, subluxation and dislocation can be observed in any articulation but are most common in the hip.[51, 52] These complications result from large intra-articular effusions or, more importantly, from ligamentous destruction and muscle foreshortening due to fibrosis.[45] Soft tissue swelling and osteoporosis may be the only accompanying radiographic features.

Soft Tissue Calcification. Periarticular soft tissue calcific deposits may be recorded in this disease.[45] They appear to be located in the joint capsule, the ligaments, or the muscles. Ossification in the synovial membrane[11] and vascular calcification,[11, 45, 53] particularly of the digital arteries, also have been noted.

The exact cause of periarticular calcification in juvenile chronic arthritis is not known, although an association of this finding with intra-articular corticosteroid therapy, or other forms of intra-articular treatment, has been recorded.[143, 210] After such therapy, calcifications have appeared at variable times, generally between 2 and 12 months after the corticosteroid injections. Capsular and periarticular collections have predominated, although an intra-articular location of the calcific deposits has been seen.[143]

Synovial Cysts. Although synovial cysts are a well-recognized manifestation of adult-onset rheumatoid arthritis, they are not observed commonly in juvenile chronic arthritis.[54–57] Theoretically, such cysts could develop about any involved articulation, although they are noted most frequently in the popliteal region of the knee.[144] The cysts typically occur during an exacerbation of the joint disease. The nature of the clinically detectable soft tissue mass is revealed during arthrography with contrast opacification of the juxta-articular synovium-lined sac. Ultrasonography or MR imaging also can be used to demonstrate this lesion.[145, 211, 255]

Abnormalities in Specific Locations

Hand (Fig. 27–4). Any articulation of the hand may be affected in juvenile chronic arthritis; the frequency of such involvement is less than that in the wrist, and it increases with progression of the disease. Asymmetric abnormalities of both hands are most typical. Swelling and regional osteoporosis can develop about distal interphalangeal, proximal interphalangeal, and metacarpophalangeal joints.[212] Periostitis of metacarpal and phalangeal shafts, preservation of joint space, and absence of significant erosions are most common. Epiphyseal collapse and deformity also are characteristic.

A variety of finger deformities eventually may appear during the course of the disease.[58] Boutonnière deformity (characterized by flexion of the proximal interphalangeal joint and hyperextension at the distal interphalangeal joint)

and flexion deformity (characterized by flexion at both the proximal interphalangeal and distal interphalangeal joints) appear more frequently than swan-neck deformity (characterized by hyperextension at the proximal interphalangeal joint and flexion at the distal interphalangeal joint).

Deviation of the fingers in a horizontal plane also is frequent in juvenile chronic arthritis. In contrast to the situation in adult-onset rheumatoid arthritis, in which ulnar deviation of the metacarpophalangeal joints frequently is associated with radial deviation of the wrist,[59] radial deviation of the metacarpophalangeal articulations in association with ulnar deviation of the wrist is more typical in juvenile-onset disease.[129] In those children who have radial deviation of the wrist, flexion deformity rather than ulnar deviation of the metacarpophalangeal joints usually is observed.

Wrist (Fig. 27–5). Abnormalities of the wrist are extremely common in juvenile chronic arthritis.[45, 58, 60, 213] Soft tissue prominence, osteoporosis, and irregular carpal ossification centers are seen. Marginal erosions may be evident in older children with adult type (seropositive) rheumatoid arthritis; in fact, in these persons, the radiographic findings in the wrist resemble changes in adult-onset rheumatoid arthritis, including a pancompartmental distribution, ulnar styloid erosions, and tenosynovitis.

Intra-articular bony ankylosis of the compartments of the wrist may be prominent. Generally, although not invariably, at least one of the three major articulations of the wrist (radiocarpal, midcarpal, common carpometacarpal) remains unankylosed, allowing some motion. Investigators have observed a high frequency of bony ankylosis in the common carpometacarpal joint. In a review of 100 consecutive patients with juvenile chronic arthritis, Maldonado-Cocco and collaborators[146] reported bone ankylosis in the wrist in 47 per cent of cases. The common carpometacarpal joint was affected most frequently, usually in association with ankylosis of the intercarpal articulation. The specific site of fusion was between the base of the second or third metacarpal (or both) and the adjacent trapezoid and capitate. Exclusive ankylosis of the intercarpal or radiocarpal joint was infrequent, and the first carpometacarpal joint was never fused. Ankylosis of the carpus was unrelated to the type of disease onset and was more common in persons with disease of longer duration. In the authors' experience, diffuse narrowing and ankylosis of the midcarpal and common carpometacarpal articulations commonly appear with or without joint space narrowing of the radiocarpal articulation.[214] The resulting radiographic picture is characterized in some patients by grouping of the carpal bones and metacarpal bases into an ossific mass that is separated from the distal part of the radius. A similar pattern with more prominent sparing of the radiocarpal compartment has been noted in adult-onset Still's disease (see later discussion).

Narrowing and ankylosis of various compartments of the wrist in juvenile chronic arthritis can lead to shortening of the carpus. The degree of shortening can be measured as an expression of the distance between the distal radial physeal growth plate and the proximal end of the third metacarpal bone,[61] although growth disturbances of the third metacarpal bone may introduce some diagnostic errors when this technique of measurement is used.[215] Similar shortening of the carpal bones can be seen in multiple epiphyseal dysplasia, Turner's syndrome, arthrogryposis, and the otopalatodigital syndrome.

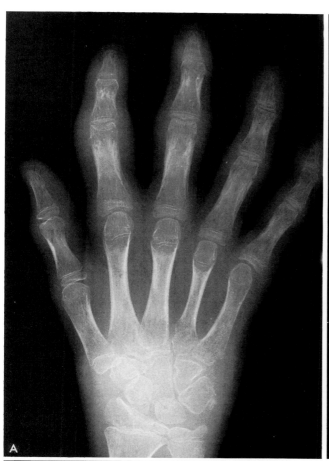

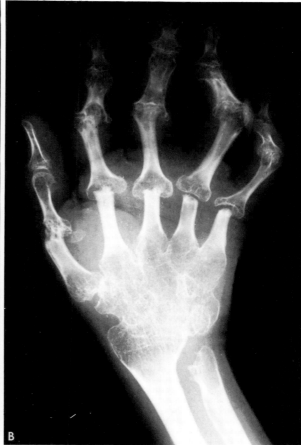

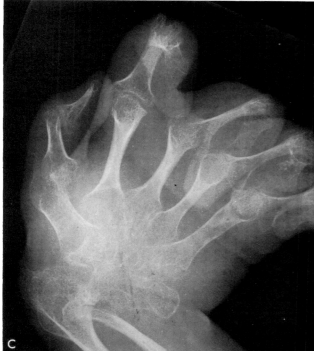

FIGURE 27–4. Abnormalities of the hand.

A The typical changes in this child with polyarticular Still's disease include periarticular soft tissue swelling and osteoporosis about metacarpophalangeal and proximal interphalangeal joints as well as the wrist, mild joint space narrowing and erosive abnormalities, and periosteal bone formation in the phalanges.

B Severe abnormalities in another child with Still's disease consist of bony ankylosis of the carpal bones, metacarpal bases, and distal radius; growth disturbances of the distal ulna; and erosion, compression, and flexion deformities of the proximal interphalangeal joints. Interpretation of the changes about the metacarpophalangeal joints is complicated by the fact that previous surgical procedures had been performed.

C Severe flexion deformities of the proximal interphalangeal and distal interphalangeal joints are combined with osteoporosis, erosion, collapse, and subluxation at the metacarpophalangeal joints and carpal ankylosis. Observe the typical "ulnar bayonet" deformity associated with ulnar migration of the carpal bones at the radiocarpal joint. Bony ankylosis at the first metacarpophalangeal joint also is evident.

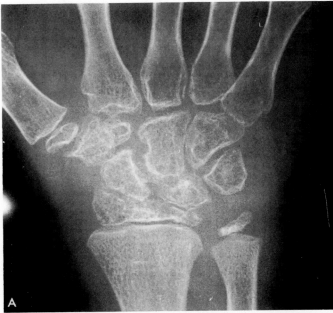

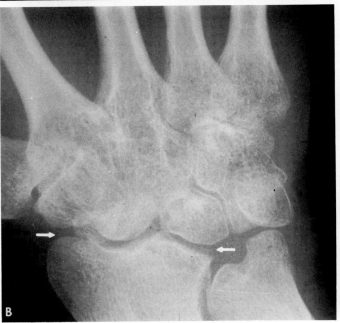

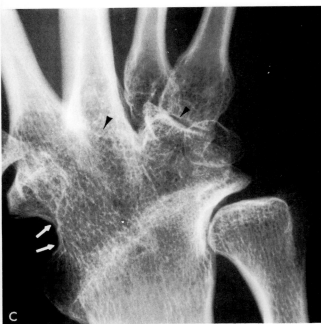

FIGURE 27–5. Abnormalities of the wrist.

A In a young child, erosions of multiple carpal bones have led to crenated osseous contours. There is evidence of joint space narrowing and acceleration of bone maturation in this patient.

B Observe extensive joint space narrowing and intra-articular bony ankylosis of portions of the midcarpal and common carpometacarpal joints with relative sparing of the radiocarpal articulation (arrows). At the last-mentioned site, deformity of the articular surface of the distal radius is evident. Overgrowth of the ulna and ulnar styloid also can be seen.

C In this patient, bony ankylosis of the radiocarpal and midcarpal compartments is prominent (arrows). Joint space narrowing and partial ankylosis at the common carpometacarpal joint also are apparent (arrowheads).

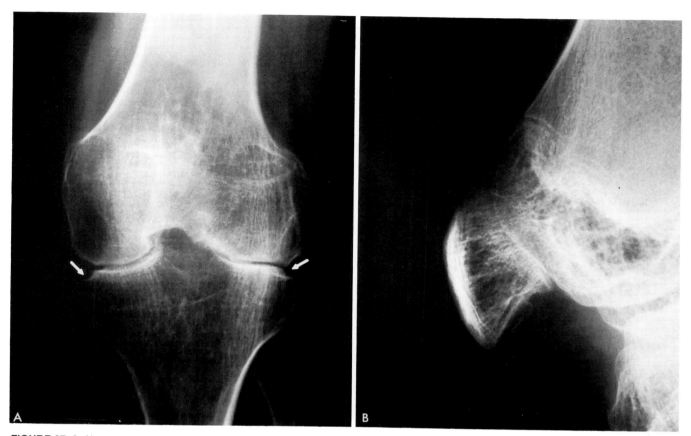

FIGURE 27–6. Abnormalities of the knee.

A The major radiographic abnormalities in this 23 year old woman who had had arthritis for approximately 10 years consist of diffuse joint space narrowing and marginal erosions (arrows), which simulate the findings in adult-onset rheumatoid arthritis, although slight overgrowth of the femoral epiphysis indicates that the disease began at a relatively young age.

B On a lateral radiograph of a knee, note the flattening of the inferior portion of the patella, resulting in a square configuration of the bone.

Growth disturbances and articular destruction can lead to significant wrist deformities in juvenile chronic arthritis.[58] The ulna may be relatively short compared to the radius, producing ulnar deviation at the wrist.[213] An associated "ulnar bayonet" deformity is initiated as the carpal bones migrate in an ulnar direction, sliding off the distal end of the radius. The degree of deformity may become extreme.

The carpal tunnel syndrome related to tenosynovitis can complicate cases of juvenile chronic arthritis.[62]

Knee (Fig. 27–6). Radiographic abnormalities of the knee in juvenile chronic arthritis include osteoporosis, soft tissue swelling, enlargement with ballooning of the distal femoral and proximal tibial epiphyses, flattening of the femoral condyles, widening of the intercondylar notch, joint space narrowing, and marginal or central osseous erosions.[147, 181] These findings are virtually identical to those in hemophilia. Alterations in patellar shape also have been observed in both juvenile chronic arthritis and hemophilia. These alterations consist of flattening of the inferior pole of the patella, resulting in squaring of the bone. It has been suggested that a square patella is more characteristic of juvenile chronic arthritis than of hemophilia,[63] although the value of this sign in differentiating these two disorders probably is limited.

Hip (Fig. 27–7). Involvement of the hip is common[11, 51, 64] and eventually may necessitate synovectomy[150] or total joint replacement.[65, 121, 218, 257] The frequency of radiograph-

ically evident hip abnormalities in patients with juvenile chronic arthritis is approximately 35 to 45 per cent,[22, 45] although this frequency is related intimately to the duration of the disease process.[66] In younger patients, impairment of iliac bone development and coxa valga deformity are not uncommon. The femoral capital epiphysis may be enlarged and irregular in outline, and premature fusion of the growth plate can be evident. Articular space narrowing (diffuse) and osseous erosion also may develop as a joint deteriorates, and osteophytosis can appear.[130] Restoration of the joint space has been reported in association with vigorous physical therapy and continued ambulation.[67, 182] Such restoration is associated with clinical improvement, although subsequent radiologic and clinical deterioration has been observed.[149] Protrusio acetabuli is more frequent in older children and is probably aggravated by chronic inflammation and continued weight-bearing.[45] It has been suggested that the direction of the acetabular protrusion is more cephalad, or superior, in juvenile chronic arthritis than in adult-onset rheumatoid arthritis.[216] Osteonecrosis of the femoral head has been described in patients with juvenile chronic arthritis. Generally, it is regarded as a complication of corticosteroid therapy, although synovitis with resultant elevation of intracapsular pressure theoretically could contribute to femoral head ischemia.[217]

Intra-articular bone ankylosis of the hip occasionally is evident in patients with juvenile chronic arthritis; however,

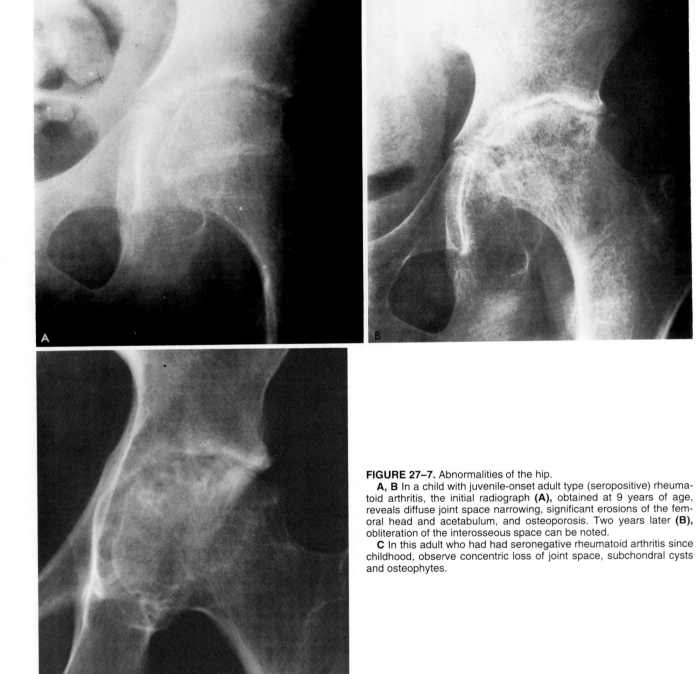

FIGURE 27–7. Abnormalities of the hip.

A, B In a child with juvenile-onset adult type (seropositive) rheumatoid arthritis, the initial radiograph **(A),** obtained at 9 years of age, reveals diffuse joint space narrowing, significant erosions of the femoral head and acetabulum, and osteoporosis. Two years later **(B),** obliteration of the interosseous space can be noted.

C In this adult who had had seronegative rheumatoid arthritis since childhood, observe concentric loss of joint space, subchondral cysts and osteophytes.

in some instances, the change may indicate that a diagnosis of juvenile-onset ankylosing spondylitis is more appropriate. Of interest, a patient with ankylosis of the hip secondary to severe juvenile chronic arthritis, who maintained motion by developing a pseudarthrosis through the proximal femoral growth plate, has been reported.[68]

Foot and Ankle (Fig. 27–8). The radiographic abnormalities of the tarsus in this disease are similar to those in the carpus. Enlargement and irregularity of the tarsal bones, joint space narrowing, and intra-articular bony ankylosis can be seen. Such ankylosis is most frequent in the intertarsal joints, but it may be observed in the tarsometatarsal and

ankle articulations as well.[219, 220] Metatarsophalangeal and interphalangeal joint alterations consist of osteoporosis, epiphyseal enlargement, brachydactyly, and periostitis. Articular space diminution and erosions also are observed. At the ankle, tilting or angulation of the distal tibial epiphysis may be encountered. Late deformities include clawing of the toes, hammer toes, hindfoot varus or valgus, pes cavus, and hallux valgus.[152]

Other Articulations of the Appendicular Skeleton (Fig. 27–9). Alterations of the humeral head parallel those of the femoral head, with osteoporosis, bone enlargement, joint space narrowing, erosions,[251] and subluxation. The

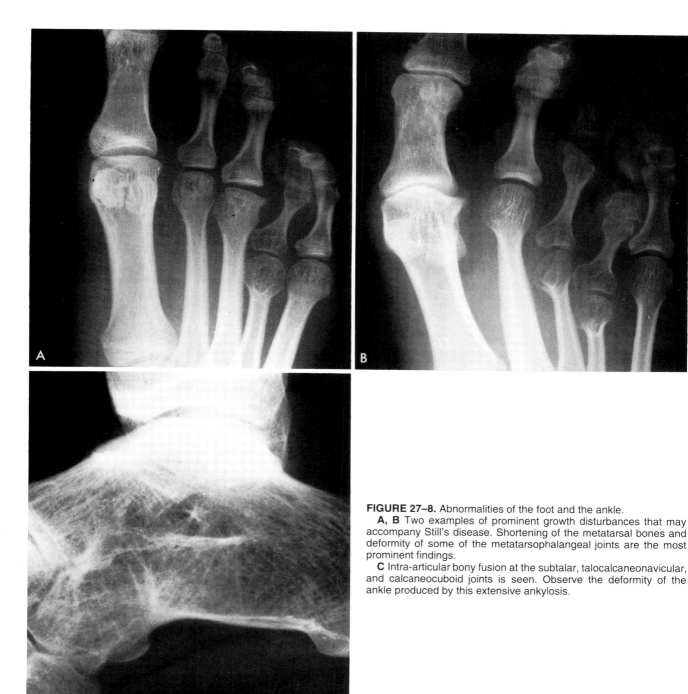

FIGURE 27–8. Abnormalities of the foot and the ankle.

A, B Two examples of prominent growth disturbances that may accompany Still's disease. Shortening of the metatarsal bones and deformity of some of the metatarsophalangeal joints are the most prominent findings.

C Intra-articular bony fusion at the subtalar, talocalcaneonavicular, and calcaneocuboid joints is seen. Observe the deformity of the ankle produced by this extensive ankylosis.

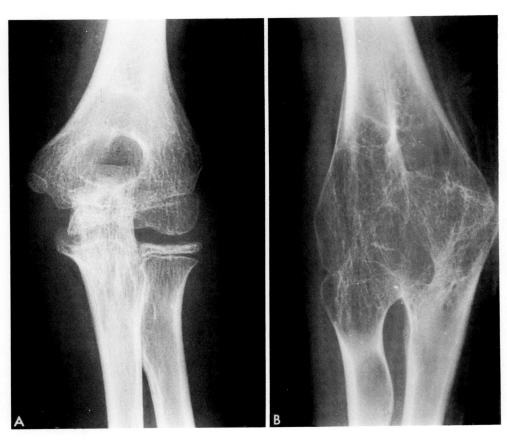

FIGURE 27–9. Abnormalities of the elbow.
A The radiographic findings include soft tissue swelling, osteoporosis, and irregularity with increased density of the radial head.
B In another child, bony ankylosis of the humeroradial and humeroulnar spaces is seen.

glenoid fossa may demonstrate an abnormal shape. In the elbow, the radial head may become significantly enlarged, a finding that also is seen in hemophilia. Shortening of the ulna can be associated with bowing of the radius.[11]

Sacroiliac Joint (Table 27–4). Although children with juvenile-onset ankylosing spondylitis, psoriatic arthritis, and inflammatory bowel disease can reveal significant sacroiliac joint abnormalities, changes in this articulation in other varieties of juvenile chronic arthritis are relatively

infrequent. Furthermore, documenting the presence of an abnormal sacroiliac joint can be difficult because of the widened articular space and indistinct subchondral bone that characterize the normal sacroiliac joint in the pediatric age group. Martel and coworkers[45] observed sacroiliac joint alterations in 5 per cent of 80 patients with juvenile chronic arthritis, although they did not indicate whether the changes were related to juvenile-onset ankylosing spondylitis. In reports that exclude patients with the latter subgroup of

TABLE 27–4. Comparison of Radiographic Abnormalities

	Juvenile Chronic Arthritis*	Adult-Onset Rheumatoid Arthritis	Juvenile-Onset Ankylosing Spondylitis	Adult-Onset Ankylosing Spondylitis
Cervical spine				
C1-C2 subluxation	+	+ +	+	+
Apophyseal joint ankylosis	+ +	±	+ +	+ +
Hypoplasia of vertebral bodies and intervertebral discs	+ +	−	±	−
Thoracolumbar spine				
Apophyseal joint ankylosis	±	−	+ +	+ +
Syndesmophytes	−	−	+ +	+ +
Sacroiliac joints				
Erosions	+	+	+ +	+ +
Ankylosis	±	±	+ +	+ +
Peripheral joints				
Early involvement	+ +	+ +	+ +	±
Erosions	±	+ +	+	+
Joint space narrowing	±	+ +	+	+
Bony proliferation and periostitis	+ +	±	+ +	+ +

+ + = very common; + = common; ± = uncommon; − = rare or absent.
*Characteristics of juvenile-onset adult type rheumatoid arthritis and Still's disease.

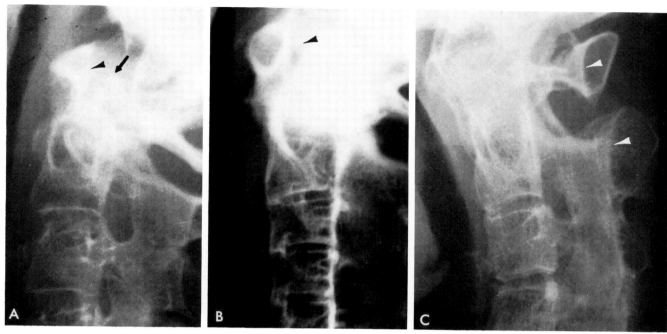

FIGURE 27–10. Abnormalities of the cervical spine: Atlantoaxial subluxation.
A In a patient who developed juvenile-onset adult type (seropositive) rheumatoid arthritis, the odontoid process is eroded (arrow) and the anterior arch of the atlas is subluxed slightly posteriorly (arrowhead) in this lateral radiograph, obtained during extension of the neck. Apophyseal joint space narrowing and bony ankylosis at some levels can be noted.
B In a patient with Still's disease, the space between the anterior arch of the atlas and the odontoid process is widened (arrowhead), indicating anterior subluxation of the atlas. Observe apophyseal joint ankylosis and hypoplastic vertebral bodies and intervertebral discs.
C In this person with juvenile-onset ankylosing spondylitis, atlantoaxial subluxation is indicated by the forward position of the spinolaminar line of the atlas (upper arrowhead) compared with that of the axis (lower arrowhead). Observe widespread bony ankylosis of apophyseal joints with a minor degree of hypoplasia of vertebral bodies and intervertebral discs.

disease, the estimated frequency of sacroiliitis in juvenile chronic arthritis has varied from approximately 8 to 20 per cent.[41] In these cases, erosions without adjacent sclerosis and osseous fusion after prolonged periods of immobilization have been noted. Pathologic examination of sacroiliac joints has revealed loss of articular space and cartilaginous fusion without inflammation (perhaps related to disuse) or chronic inflammatory changes similar to those of adult-onset rheumatoid arthritis.[69]

Cervical Spine (Table 27–4) (Figs. 27–10 to 27–12). Radiographic abnormalities of the cervical spine are a significant feature of juvenile chronic arthritis,[127] although neurologic alterations resulting from such cervical spine abnormalities are less frequent than in adult-onset rheumatoid arthritis.[153] Subluxation may develop in any vertebral segment but is most characteristic at the atlantoaxial level. Atlantoaxial subluxation (greater than 4 or 5 mm between the posterior surface of the anterior arch of the first cervical vertebra and the anterior surface of the odontoid process)[122] can be observed in juvenile-onset ankylosing spondylitis and Still's disease but is most characteristic of juvenile-onset adult type (seropositive) rheumatoid arthritis.[11, 70] It should be remembered that atlantoaxial instability in the child is not diagnostic of juvenile chronic arthritis, being observed in trauma and a variety of conditions including those, such as Down's syndrome, with hypoplasia of the odontoid process and congenital weakening of the surrounding ligaments, and those associated with inflammation in the neck. The last-mentioned situation frequently is called Grisel's syndrome; in this disorder nontraumatic at-

lantoaxial subluxation accompanies peripharyngeal inflammatory disease.[154] The cause of this syndrome is unknown, but the recent demonstration of vascular continuity between the pharyngovertebral veins and the periodontoidal venous plexus and suboccipital epidural sinuses suggests that hematogenous spread of infection is a pathogenetic factor.[154]

Erosions of the anterior, posterior, and superior surfaces of the odontoid process also may be seen in juvenile chronic arthritis.[221] Apophyseal joint space narrowing and bony ankylosis in association with subchondral erosions predominate in the upper cervical spine, especially at the C2-C3 and C3-C4 levels; it is distinctly unusual to see significant ankylosis of the lower cervical spine without more proximal involvement. Exceptionally, the apophyseal joints throughout the cervical spine are ankylosed.

Growth disturbances consist of decreased vertical and anteroposterior diameters of the vertebral bodies at levels of apophyseal joint ankylosis. The adjacent intervertebral discs also are diminished in height (or completely obliterated) and may contain calcification. The changes apparently are related to growth disturbances, disuse atrophy, and remodeling and also are described in the dorsolumbar spine, suggesting involvement of the adjacent apophyseal joints.[45]

The resulting radiographic appearance in juvenile chronic arthritis, with dwarf-like alterations of both the vertebral bodies and intervertebral discs and apophyseal joint ankylosis, is indeed distinctive. Although apophyseal joint ankylosis can be seen in ankylosing spondylitis, the vertebral bodies are not significantly diminished in size, nor are the intervertebral discs diminutive because the disease onset

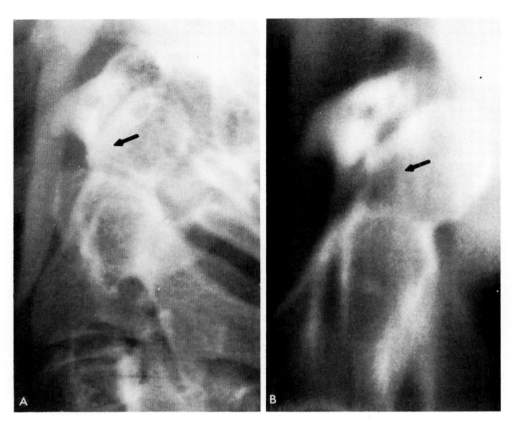

FIGURE 27–11. Abnormalities of the cervical spine: Odontoid erosion. A young adult with juvenile-onset adult type (seropositive) rheumatoid arthritis reveals odontoid erosions (arrows) **(A)**, better demonstrated on conventional tomography **(B).**

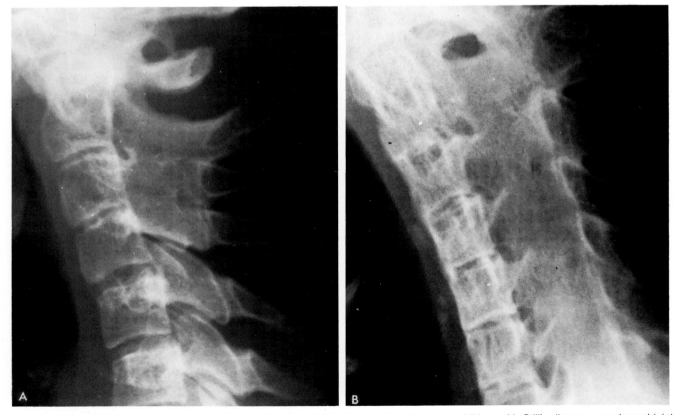

FIGURE 27–12. Abnormalities of the cervical spine: Apophyseal joint bony ankylosis. In two children with Still's disease, apophyseal joint ankylosis is evident. The process usually is first evident in the upper cervical region and progresses to the lower vertebrae. Hypoplasia of vertebral bodies and intervertebral discs is prominent in both **A** and **B.** Atlantoaxial subluxation also is evident in **A.**

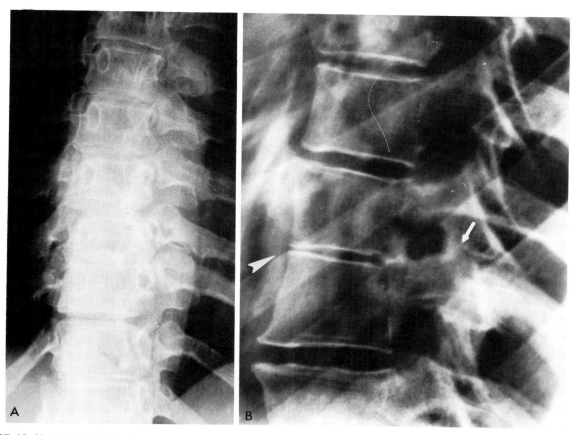

FIGURE 27–13. Abnormalities of the thoracic spine.
 A A mild scoliosis of the lower thoracic spine, convex to the right, is evident.
 B Observe apophyseal joint ankylosis (arrow) and hypoplasia of the intervertebral disc and adjacent portions of the vertebral bodies (arrowhead).

generally occurs at a more advanced age. Furthermore, in ankylosing spondylitis, syndesmophytes are characteristic. Congenital fusion of vertebral bodies (Klippel-Feil deformity) may simulate the changes in juvenile chronic arthritis, although in the former disorder, the spinous processes of several vertebrae also may be incorporated into a single ossific mass and elevation of the scapula with an omovertebral bone can be seen. Fibrodysplasia ossificans progressiva can be accompanied by vertebral alterations that resemble those of juvenile chronic arthritis, but additional abnormalities, such as soft tissue ossification, ensure accurate diagnosis of the former condition.

Thoracic and Lumbar Spine (Table 27–4) (Fig. 27–13). The thoracolumbar spine is not commonly affected in juvenile chronic arthritis. Compression fractures of vertebral bodies can be observed,[11, 45] particularly in those patients who have received steroid medication. Compression fractures usually are evident in the thoracic region in association with osteoporosis. Healing may occur slowly after withdrawal of the corticosteroids.

Scoliosis, which may appear rapidly, also has been noted in children with long-standing juvenile chronic arthritis.[11, 71, 151] Its pathogenesis is not clear, although abnormal spinal curvature may be related to muscle imbalance or asymmetric involvement of the apophyseal articulations. Additional potential factors in the development of scoliosis include torticollis, contracture of the hip, and pelvic tilt.[151] The degree of abnormal spinal curvature is variable but has been reported to be mild to moderate in the majority of cases.[222]

Mandible, Temporomandibular Joint, and Other Facial Structures (Fig. 27–14). Underdevelopment of the jaw (micrognathia) with limitation of bite is not uncommon in patients with juvenile chronic arthritis (approximately 10 to 20 per cent), frequently occurring in association with temporomandibular joint abnormalities.[223, 224] Micrognathia also may be encountered without restricted motion at the temporomandibular articulations, however, and may be associated with significant abnormalities of the cervical spine.[72, 73] In fact, symptoms and signs of arthritis of the temporomandibular joint are relatively infrequent in patients who have undergrowth of the mandible, although radiography and tomography may indicate characteristic abnormalities of periarticular bone.[45, 156] Micrognathia is more typical in those children whose disease begins early in life and in those with systemic or polyarticular disease than in those with pauciarticular or monoarticular arthritis. With regard to the relationship of micrognathia and early onset disease, Larheim[159] has reported that the dystrophic appearance of the temporomandibular joint in patients with juvenile chronic arthritis resembles the normal appearance seen in the first months of life.

Radiographic abnormalities have been observed in as many as 40 per cent of patients with juvenile chronic arthritis,[157, 158] although the frequency of detectable lesions

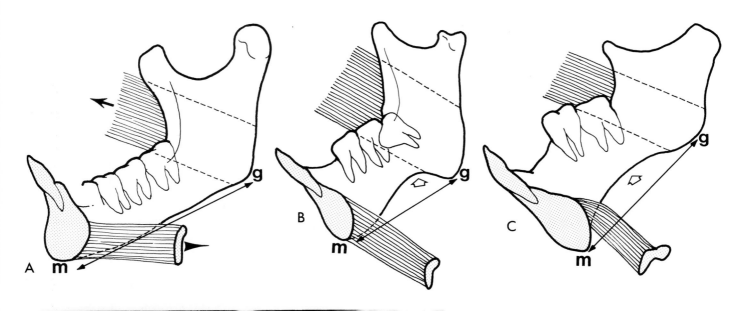

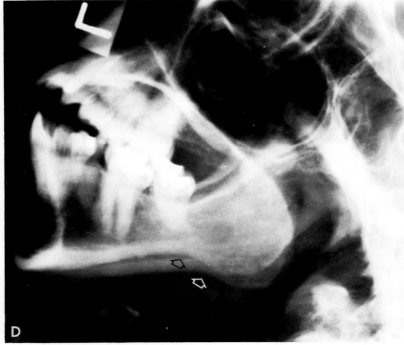

FIGURE 27–14. Abnormalities of the mandible and temporomandibular joint.

A–C Antegonial notching. In the normal situation **(A),** a relatively straight line can be drawn along the inferior surface of the mandible from the gonion (g) to the menton (m). Note the sites of attachment and pull of the masseter muscle (arrow) and genio-hyoid muscle (arrowhead). In acquired conditions, including juvenile chronic arthritis **(B),** a short ante-gonial notch is seen (open arrow) in association with abnormality of the mandibular condyle. In a variety of congenital disorders **(C),** a long curve can be seen (open arrow) rather than an acute arch. Furthermore, the angle formed between the horizontal portion of the mandibular body and the ascending ramus may be more obtuse.

D In this child with juvenile chronic arthritis, note the short antegonial notches (arrows). Additional findings are articular changes in the temporomandibular joints (not well shown here) and bird-face.

(A–C, Modified after Becker MH, et al: Radiology *121*:149, 1976.)

is influenced by the type of patient population that is being studied and the methods of examination. Initially, unilateral or asymmetric lesions predominate; however, symmetric involvement is seen later.[157] The abnormalities have been reported to be more frequent in patients with early onset disease, polyarticular involvement, splenomegaly and kidney involvement, and anemia.[158] Radiographic changes include shortening of the body and vertical rami of the mandible with widening of the mandibular notches. Both mandibular condyles frequently are flattened and poorly differentiated, although the temporomandibular joints themselves may appear normal. Articular space narrowing, bony erosion, and abnormal joint motion may be encountered in some persons. Intra-articular osseous fusion also has been noted.[74]

Martel and collaborators[45] have reviewed the possible mechanisms by which micrognathia might develop in patients with juvenile chronic arthritis. The vertical height of the ramus and the length of the mandible are determined primarily by the condylar growth center. Bone arises from the condylar cartilage, which itself is derived by apposition from a layer of precartilaginous connective tissue, which lies beneath the fibrous articular surface.[75] As the precartilaginous zone is not protected by a suprajacent cartilaginous barrier, it may be vulnerable to injury, especially in early life, in the presence of synovial inflammatory tissue. Although this relationship between articular inflammation and mandibular growth gains further support from the appearance of micrognathia as a sequel to chronic middle ear infection,[76] the absence of clinical and radiologic abnormalities of the temporomandibular joint in some children with mandibular hypoplasia should be noted. Other systemic factors indeed may be important in ensuring normal growth of this bone.

Antegonial notching of the mandible has been emphasized as an additional radiographic manifestation of juvenile chronic arthritis.[77] This notching represents a concavity on the undersurface of the mandibular body just anterior to the angular process (gonion). It may appear in a variety of congenital (Treacher Collins syndrome, camptomelic dwarfism, neurofibromatosis) and acquired (temporomandibular joint arthritis or infection, trauma) disorders. In acquired conditions, including juvenile chronic arthritis, the antegonial notch is shorter than in the congenital diseases. In juvenile chronic arthritis, mandibular hypoplasia is associated with muscular imbalance. The masseter and medial pterygoid muscles cause the bone in the region of the angle to grow inferiorly, producing antegonial notching.[78]

Additional abnormalities of the facial skeleton have been reported in juvenile chronic arthritis.[79] Bird-face, observed in 10 to 30 per cent of patients,[80, 81] has been related to arrested mandibular growth in combination with normal growth of other facial structures, leading to convexity of the facial profile. In some cases, the abrupt appearance of bird-face in this disease may be attributed to acute collapse of osseous structures about the temporomandibular joint,[79] a process that also has been identified in adult-onset rheumatoid arthritis.[82, 83]

Arthritis of the cricoarytenoid joints has been observed in juvenile chronic arthritis.[84] The synovium-lined space between the cricoid and arytenoid cartilages can participate in articular inflammation in both adult-onset and juvenile-onset disease.[85, 225] Cricoarytenoid arthritis can lead to airway obstruction. Radiographic changes generally are lacking.

OTHER DIAGNOSTIC TECHNIQUES

Scintigraphy

The value of bone scintigraphy and related radionuclide techniques in the assessment of musculoskeletal disorders is discussed in detail in Chapter 15. Although specific indications for the use of such techniques in the evaluation of children with juvenile chronic arthritis have not received a great deal of emphasis, general guidelines can be suggested. Bone scanning remains an effective method with high sensitivity and low specificity. Bone scintigraphy may be combined with single photon emission computed tomography (SPECT) to increase sensitivity in the detection of one or more foci of abnormal radiopharmaceutical accumulation.[226] As has been described in patients with adult-onset rheumatoid arthritis (see Chapter 26), the major application of bone scintigraphy in those persons with juvenile chronic arthritis relates to the determination of disease distribution. The method allows simultaneous assessment of all major articulations of the human body, and monoarticular, oligoarticular, or polyarticular patterns of disease can be identified. The localization of increased activity of the bone-seeking radiopharmaceutical agent to a single joint is associated with an increased probability of a nonrheumatic disorder, such as neoplasm or infection, or a posttraumatic abnormality,[227] although this scintigraphic pattern does not eliminate the possibility of some form of juvenile chronic arthritis. When scintigraphic patterns show involvement of multiple articulations, the diagnosis of noninfectious inflammatory disease becomes far more likely.

Computed Tomography

As indicated in Chapter 8, CT scanning is best applied to the analysis of regions of complex anatomy, such as the hip, shoulder, spine, and temporomandibular joint. With regard to arthritis, CT is most useful for assessing the extent of bone involvement and the nature of para-articular masses, and for monitoring joint aspiration. In general, however, the value of CT in the evaluation of children with juvenile chronic arthritis is limited.[209]

Magnetic Resonance Imaging

An ever-increasing role is anticipated for MR technique as an imaging method for pediatric joint disease, related primarily to its ability to allow direct visualization of non-ossified portions of epiphyseal cartilage. This benefit already has been used to advantage in the assessment of such disorders as developmental dysplasia of the hip (see Chapter 86) and Legg-Calvé-Perthes disease (see Chapter 81). In children with juvenile chronic arthritis, MR imaging has allowed detection of alterations in the articular cartilage of the knee,[228–230] hip,[228–230] elbow,[228] and other joints, although difficulties arise owing to deficiencies of many of the standard imaging sequences that have been used in the analysis of minor or localized chondral defects (see Chapter 70) (Fig. 27–15). The differentiation of joint fluid and synovial inflammatory tissue in juvenile chronic arthritis remains a

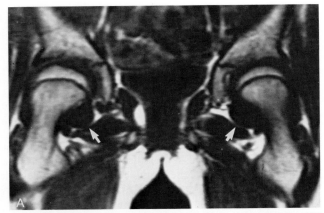

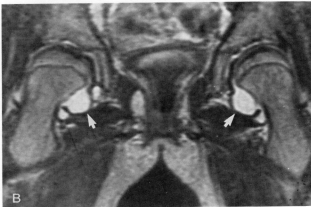

FIGURE 27–15. Juvenile chronic arthritis: MR imaging. Hip involvement in a 10 year old girl.

A Coronal T1-weighted (TR/TE, 400/20) spin echo MR image reveals mild flattening of both femoral heads and acetabula and bilateral joint effusions (arrows).

B Coronal T2-weighted (TR/TE, 2000/70) spin echo MR image again demonstrates large effusions (arrows). Despite this arthrographic effect, visualization of articular cartilage is poor.

(Courtesy of D. Bong, M.D., Vancouver, British Columbia, Canada.)

difficult task when standard spin echo imaging sequences are used,[228] although the addition of intravenously administered gadolinium compounds improves such differentiation in a manner similar to that in adult-onset rheumatoid arthritis (Fig. 27–16).[231] Images obtained after contrast enhancement also may allow improved assessment of cartilage integrity and detection of loculated collections of joint fluid.[231] The success of this injection technique requires that

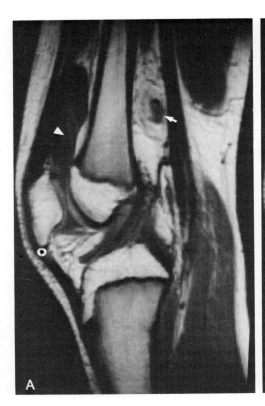

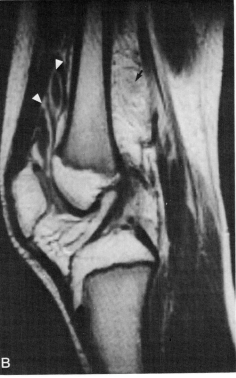

FIGURE 27–16. Juvenile chronic arthritis: MR imaging using intravenous gadolinium contrast agent. Severe pauciarthritis in a 13 year old girl.

A Initial unenhanced T1-weighted sagittal spin echo MR image (TR/TE, 560/26) shows a large effusion (arrowhead) and lymph node (arrow). The joint fluid is of low signal intensity.

B After intravenous administration of gadolinium tetraazacyclododecanetetraacetic acid (DOTA), a repeat T1-weighted spin echo sagittal MR image (TR/TE, 560/26) reveals enhancement of portions of the suprapatellar and cruciate regions (arrowheads), consistent with synovial inflammatory tissue, and of the lymph node (arrow). Note that some unenhanced joint fluid remains, especially in the suprapatellar recess.

(Reproduced with permission from Hervé-Somma CMP, et al: Radiology *182*:93, 1992.)

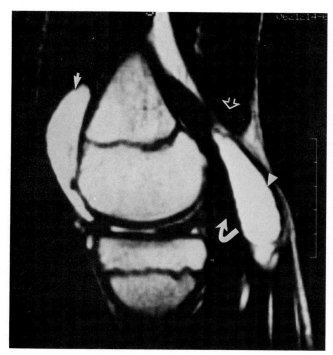

FIGURE 27–17. Juvenile chronic arthritis: Synovial cyst demonstrated by MR imaging. In a 14 year old girl, a parasagittal T2-weighted spin echo MR image (TR/TE, 3000/80) shows fluid of high signal intensity both in the suprapatellar recess (closed arrow) and in a synovial cyst (arrowhead). The latter is located between the semimembranosus muscle (open arrow) and medial head of the gastrocnemius muscle (curved arrow). (Courtesy of C. Kusnick, M.D., Irvine, California.)

nonenhanced images in the same plane and with the same imaging factors be obtained and that enhanced images be acquired without delay.

The identification of atrophic or hypoplastic menisci in the knees of patients with juvenile chronic arthritis with MR imaging is of interest.[230, 231] The cause of this finding is not clear, although enzymatic degradation of these fibrocartilaginous structures or interference with their nutrition owing to adjacent pannus may be contributory. Similarly, the cruciate ligaments may appear mildly or severely hypotrophic.[231]

The identification of the sites and extent of intra- or periarticular bone destruction in juvenile chronic arthritis is possible using MR imaging.[229] Marginal or central osseous defects are apparent, and the signal characteristics of the cyst-like intraosseous lesions are compatible with the presence of fluid or pannus, or both, within them.

That synovial cysts in this disease can be detected with MR imaging (Fig. 27–17) is not surprising,[211, 228] although, as indicated earlier, such cysts are not a frequently reported complication of juvenile chronic arthritis.

Additional applications of MR imaging in children with juvenile chronic arthritis include analysis of the temporomandibular joint and the assessment of such complications as ischemic necrosis of bone and growth disturbances.[230] The technique also is useful in the evaluation of the spine and spinal cord (Fig. 27–18).

It should be emphasized, however, that successful MR imaging examinations in young children may require careful sedation with its inherent medical risks.

PATHOLOGIC ABNORMALITIES

Synovial inflammation in juvenile chronic arthritis resembles that in adult-onset rheumatoid arthritis, although the inflammatory process may be less florid in children, with less extensive fibrinous exudate and less proliferation of lining and synovial stroma cells[9, 86] (Figs. 27–19 and 27–20). Macroscopically evident villous hypertrophy of the synovial membrane can be associated with varying degrees of fibrin accumulation in the lining and subintimal layers, cellular hyperplasia, and inflammatory cellular response.[87] Plasma cells and lymphocytes can infiltrate the synovium, particularly in perivascular locations. Macrophages can be identified in the subintimal layer. Increased vascularity of the synovial membrane can be associated with endothelial cell hypertrophy or hyperplasia of capillaries and venules as well as of large vessels. Rarely, cartilaginous debris is observed.[155]

Granulation tissue may extend over the cartilage or between cartilage and subchondral bone and may contain enclosed osseous fragments.

Subcutaneous nodules are identified in 10 to 20 per cent of patients with juvenile chronic arthritis.[8, 88] In children with seropositive disease, the histologic characteristics of the nodule resemble those in the adult variety of disease; in some children, particularly those with seronegative arthritis, the histologic appearance of the nodular lesions may be distinctive.[89] Instead of central necrosis, bands of fibrin are observed, which are surrounded by connective tissue cells and polymorphonuclear leukocytes. Palisading of cells, typical of the adult type of rheumatoid nodule, is not evident. Rather, the juvenile type of nodule resembles that which is seen in rheumatic fever.

SPECIAL TYPES OF JUVENILE CHRONIC ARTHRITIS

Adult-Onset Still's Disease

In the earlier discussion of the classification of juvenile chronic arthritis, note was made of a subgroup of children who develop an adult variety of rheumatoid arthritis. These children are designated as having juvenile-onset adult type (seropositive) rheumatoid arthritis. It is not surprising, therefore, that some adults may develop a disorder that is indistinguishable from Still's disease. In 1956 and 1971, Bywaters and Isdale[90, 91] described 14 women (age of disease onset, 17 to 35 years) who developed an illness characterized by a Still's disease type of rash, fever, and involvement of the cervical spine and peripheral and sacroiliac joints. Pauciarticular abnormalities predominated, with predilection for the knees, the fingers, and the wrists. The course of the joint disease was mild, and only a few of the patients developed radiographic alterations. The reported changes included a peculiar limited variety of carpal ankylosis, apophyseal joint fusion in the cervical spine, and patchy sclerosis about the sacroiliac joint. Serologic tests for rheumatoid factor almost uniformly were negative. Synovial biopsies indicated edema and mild inflammatory changes.

Subsequent reports have described other patients (both men and women) with adult-onset Still's disease,[92–96, 232, 252, 253] emphasizing that the age of 16 years cannot be regarded as a strict cut-off point dividing juvenile-onset and

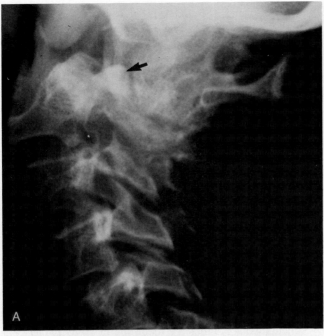

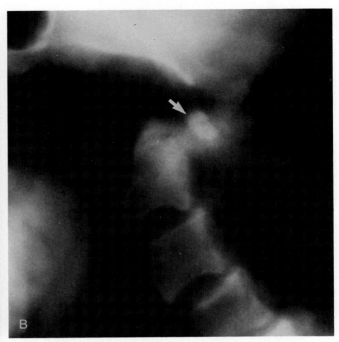

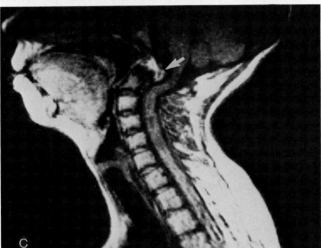

FIGURE 27–18. Juvenile chronic arthritis: Atlantoaxial subluxation demonstrated by routine techniques and MR imaging. A 27 year old woman with juvenile chronic arthritis.

A, B Routine radiography and conventional tomography reveal posterior displacement of the anterior arch of the atlas (arrows), which is located behind an eroded odontoid process.

C A T1-weighted sagittal spin echo MR image (TR/TE, 700/28) shows the effect of the displaced arch of the atlas (arrow) on the spinal cord, which is flattened and angulated at this level.

(Courtesy of M. Murphey, M.D., Washington, D.C.)

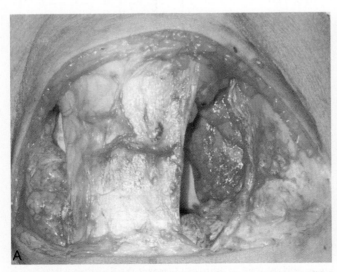

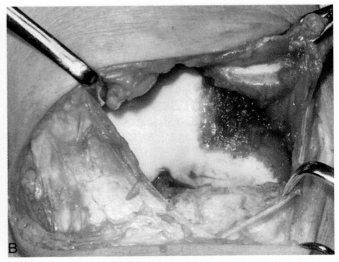

FIGURE 27–19. Juvenile chronic arthritis: Pathologic abnormalities. Two photographs of the knee during surgical intervention document hyperemic synovial inflammatory tissue extending across the anterior surface of the distal femur. (Courtesy of M. Ozonoff, M.D., Newington, Connecticut.)

adult-onset diseases. Furthermore, a distinctive radiographic pattern of articular disease of the wrist has been noted in affected patients[97]: narrowing of portions of the common carpometacarpal and midcarpal compartments without osseous erosions, which may culminate in bony ankylosis (Figs. 27–21 and 27–22). Selective involvement of the spaces between the second and third metacarpal bones and the adjacent trapezoid and capitate, between the trapezoid and capitate, between the capitate and hamate, and between the capitate and lunate can be identified. More diffuse wrist abnormalities also may be encountered, although the absence of erosive disease is remarkable. The metacarpophalangeal joints characteristically are spared. Intertarsal and tarsometatarsal alterations, including intra-articular bone ankylosis,[161] also can occur (Fig. 27–23). These changes can become evident as early as 4 to 6 months or as late as 20 to 30 months after the onset of disease. Additional abnormalities have included periarticular calcification,[162] especially about distal interphalangeal joints of the hand.[163] The calcification at the latter site has been reported to be transient, to involve the capsule, and to be associated with destruction of cartilage and bone.[163]

Similar patterns of ankylosis of the carpal (and tarsal) bones can be observed in children with juvenile chronic arthritis, although such ankylosis appears to be more frequent in children who are 10 years of age or older and in those who have had their disease for at least 2 or 3 years.[31] Predilection for the common carpometacarpal joint (particularly the space about the bases of the second and third metacarpal bones) has been cited. The finding of ankylosis of the carpus without evidence of articular disease of the fingers is much more frequent in children than in adults, although it may be observed in men with rheumatoid arthritis. It thus appears that pericapitate bony ankylosis is characteristic of juvenile chronic arthritis no matter what the age of disease onset. Furthermore, this finding is more frequent in the systemic variety (Still's disease) of the disease, particularly in adults.[131] When seen in juvenile chronic arthritis, pericapitate involvement is more likely to be associated with severe pancompartmental disease of the wrist; in adult-onset Still's disease, pericapitate alterations may occur without radiocarpal involvement.[214]

It is to be expected that, with further investigation, the syndrome of adult-onset Still's disease has become better defined.[191] Although earlier reports emphasized the occurrence of this syndrome in young adults, similar cases in middle-aged and elderly patients have been identified.[164, 184, 256] Such initial reports also stressed the nonprogressive nature of the process; however, it now appears that the prognosis of the disease is variable,[190] and in some patients, severe joint destruction, particularly in the hip (Fig. 27–24), eventually may occur.[233] In fact, two types of disease evolution have been seen: a self-remitting process with or without cyclic exacerbations, and a persistent disease with continuous activity for more than a year and progressive joint involvement.[165] The association of the antigen HLA-Bw35 with the less aggressive pattern of disease has been reported,[165] as has hypercalcemia and the antigen HLA-DRw6 with the more aggressive pattern of disease.[185, 190] Some investigations have failed to verify the prognostic implications of specific antigens; rather, an unfavorable outcome of the disease has been associated with root joint arthritis, polyarthritis, and a ''juvenile rheumatoid arthritis–like'' rash.[234] Most recent studies, however, have emphasized a poor prognosis in 30 to 75 per cent of patients.[234–237] The higher percentages, in part, may reflect selection bias.[234]

The cause of adult-onset Still's disease is not known. Many of its features, including lymphadenopathy, splenomegaly, sore throat, and remittent nature, suggest that an infectious agent could trigger the disease in genetically predisposed persons.[234, 238]

ETIOLOGY AND PATHOGENESIS

A specific cause for juvenile chronic arthritis has not been discovered. Trauma and infection (perhaps related to rubella virus[189]) may be precipitating or provocative factors, but documentation that either of these factors is responsible for the disease has not been obtained.[9, 239]

The frequency of the histocompatibility antigen HLA-B27 in this disease has been assessed in several investigations, with variable results. It is apparent that reports suggesting an increased frequency of specific histocompatibility antigens in juvenile chronic arthritis must be interpreted cautiously because of the heterogeneous nature of the disorder. Edmonds and coworkers[98] noted a higher frequency of this antigen in those children who ultimately developed either sacroiliitis or ankylosing spondylitis, although the overall occurrence of HLA-B27 antigen in patients with seronegative juvenile chronic arthritis was 25 per cent, compared with 8 per cent in controls.[99] The clinical and radiologic manifestations of those patients carrying HLA-B27 antigen (an older age of onset, a predominance of boys over girls, and the predilection for lower limb arthropathy) probably indicate that many suffer from juvenile-onset ankylosing spondylitis and will ultimately develop sacroiliitis and spondylitis.[9, 100–102] Heredity also may be important in the psoriatic subgroup, as well as in other varieties of the disease.[9, 103, 132, 165]

An immunologic basis for juvenile chronic arthritis also has been implicated by some authors.[9, 104–107, 133] The immunologic abnormalities detected in this disorder, however, may well represent secondary events rather than being of pathogenetic significance.[239]

DIFFERENTIAL DIAGNOSIS

As juvenile chronic arthritis does not affect a homogeneous group of patients, its radiographic characteristics are not uniform. Differentiation among the various subgroups of the disease may be possible on the basis of the distribution of abnormalities and their morphologic characteristics (discussed previously). Furthermore, differentiation of juvenile chronic arthritis from other articular disorders usually is accomplished by careful analysis of radiologic alterations.

Hemophilia

The differential diagnosis of juvenile chronic arthritis and hemophilia can be difficult, particularly when observations are confined to a single articulation. Soft tissue swelling, osteoporosis, subchondral osseous irregularity, interosseous space diminution, and growth disturbances can be evident in both disorders. In the knee, the ankle, or the

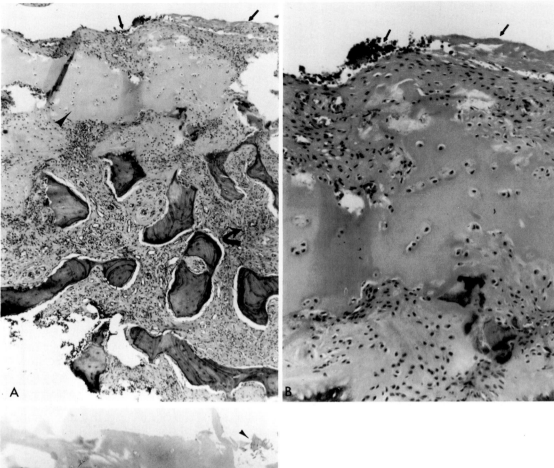

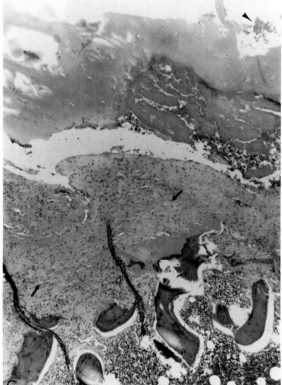

FIGURE 27–20. Juvenile chronic arthritis: Pathologic abnormalities.

A Synovial inflammation has resulted in pannus (straight arrows) on the surface of the hyaline cartilage (arrowhead). Fibrous stroma and numerous vascular channels are seen between trabeculae (curved arrow). The articular lumen is at the top of the picture (100×).

B At higher magnification (250×), fibrin deposits are identified (arrows) on the surface of the pannus.

C Observe subchondral pannus (arrows) and superficial fibrin deposits (arrowhead) (100×).

Illustration continued on opposite page

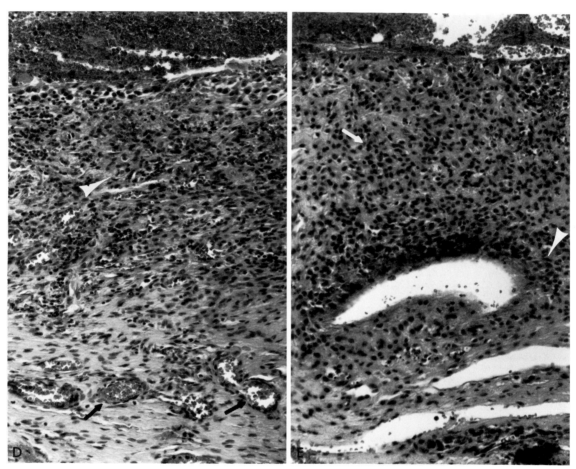

FIGURE 27–20. *Continued*
  D At the top of this photomicrograph (200×) is the articular lumen containing erythrocytes. The synovial tissue reveals numerous vessels (arrows) and proliferating cells (arrowhead), including plasma cells and lymphocytes.
  E An adjacent area reveals the erythrocytes within the articular lumen (at the top of the picture), proliferating synovial cells (arrow), and perivascular collections of plasma and lymphoid cells (arrowhead) (200×).

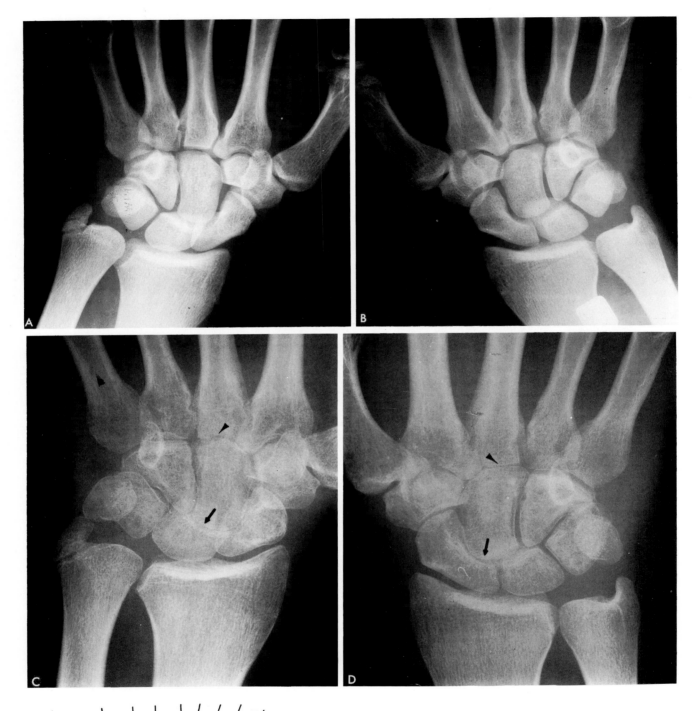

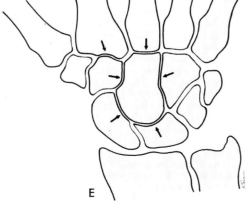

FIGURE 27–21. Adult-onset Still's disease. Wrist involvement. This 21 year old man developed classic systemic manifestations of Still's disease and bilateral wrist pain.

A, B Frontal radiographs of both wrists essentially are unremarkable except for a fragment adjacent to the right ulnar styloid process.

C, D Approximately 2 months later, narrowing of the midcarpal (arrows) and common carpometacarpal (arrowheads) compartments of both wrists is seen. The radiocarpal compartments are relatively spared. Soft tissue swelling and osteoporosis are evident.

E A drawing indicates the pericapitate location (arrows) that characterizes the joint space loss in adult-onset Still's disease.

(**A–D,** courtesy of M. Palayew, M.D., Montreal, Quebec, Canada.)

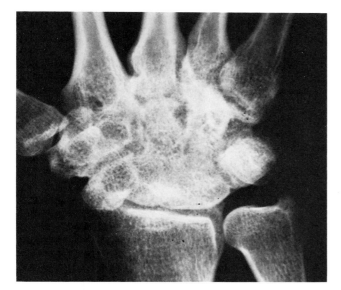

FIGURE 27–22. Adult-onset Still's disease. Wrist involvement. This 44 year old woman had had Still's disease since the age of 25 years. A frontal radiograph shows bone ankylosis of the midcarpal, common carpometacarpal, and intermetacarpal compartments of the wrist. The radiocarpal compartment is moderately narrowed. (Courtesy of J. Esdaile, M.D., Montreal, Quebec, Canada.)

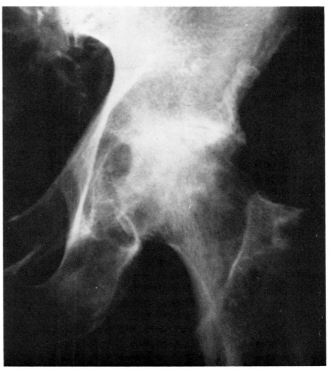

FIGURE 27–24. Adult-onset Still's disease. Hip involvement. The findings include diffuse loss of joint space, axial migration of the femoral head, and bone sclerosis.

elbow, the resulting radiographic picture may be identical in the two conditions. Polyarticular disease and significant involvement of the small joints of the hand and the wrist are less frequent in hemophilia than in juvenile chronic arthritis, whereas radiodense joint effusions and multiple subchondral cystic lesions are somewhat more common in

hemophilic arthropathy. Squaring or flattening of the inferior pole of the patella may be more characteristic of juvenile chronic arthritis.[63]

Idiopathic Multicentric Osteolysis

Idiopathic multicentric osteolysis (IMO) is a disorder characterized by multifocal articular destruction beginning in infancy or childhood[108–110] (see Chapter 94). IMO can be further classified into two types: multicentric osteolysis with nephropathy (no family history of disease, poor prognosis, with proteinuria and renal failure) and hereditary multicentric osteolysis (family history of disease). Although the clinical and radiographic features of IMO are somewhat variable, pain and swelling of the hands, the wrists, the feet, the ankles, and the elbows are typical. These findings may persist during childhood and then remit during adolescence, resulting in deformities of the hands and the feet. Because of a remarkable predilection for the carpal and tarsal bones, the disorder also is referred to as carpal and tarsal osteolysis[111, 112] or disappearing carpal bones.[113] Radiographic characteristics include osteoporosis, progressive osteolysis, and deformity, findings that may simulate the changes in juvenile chronic arthritis. Clinical features of IMO that are helpful in differentiating it from juvenile chronic arthritis are an association of episodes of trauma with articular symptoms and signs and the absence of both clinical signs of systemic disease and inflammatory changes in biopsy specimens. Histologically, in IMO, the synovium, the articular cartilage, and the bone appear to be normal, and proliferation of fibrous tissue is seen.[110] Hydroxyproline levels in the urine occasionally are elevated.[110]

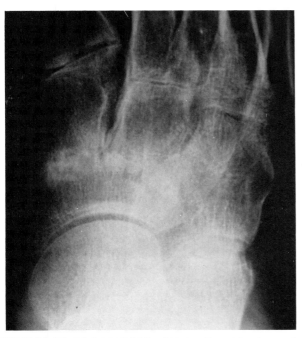

FIGURE 27–23. Adult-onset Still's disease. Tarsal involvement. A 26 year old woman had had Still's disease since the age of 20 years. Observe joint space narrowing, particularly in the naviculocuneiform, calcaneocuboid, intercuneiform, and intermediate and lateral tarsometatarsal articulations. (Courtesy of J. Esdaile, M.D., Montreal, Quebec, Canada.)

Mucopolysaccharidoses and Related Disorders

Articular abnormalities accompanying mucopolysaccharidoses may simulate those in juvenile chronic arthritis, although characteristic findings are noted on skeletal surveys in patients with mucopolysaccharidoses (Morquio, Hurler, Hunter, Sanfilippo, Scheie, and Maroteaux-Lamy syndromes)[114] (see Chapter 88). In many of these syndromes, periarticular involvement is apparent, leading to alterations in ligamentous and tendinous structures. Joint abnormalities may become particularly prominent in Scheie's syndrome and Farber's syndrome.[115] In addition, Winchester's syndrome can lead to articular changes that may simulate those of juvenile chronic arthritis.[116] An onset in infancy, a pattern of autosomal recessive inheritance, arthralgias, joint stiffening and deformity, coarsened facial features, peripheral corneal opacification, and dwarfism are typical features of this syndrome. Destruction and osteolysis of carpal and tarsal bones, as well as of bones in other sites, are accompanied by profound osteoporosis.

Kniest's syndrome (Swiss cheese cartilage) consists of disproportionate dwarfism, kyphoscoliosis, a peculiar flat and rounded facies, hearing loss, enlarged articular structures, and deformed extremities.[117-119] The small and large articulations of the upper and the lower extremities are enlarged symmetrically, with fixed flexion contractures.[119] The fingers are elongated and knobby, an appearance that resembles the Heberden's and Bouchard's nodes of degenerative joint disease. On radiographs of involved joints, osteoporosis, delay in appearance and fragmentation of epiphyseal ossification centers, joint space narrowing, and osseous enlargement are encountered. These findings may be most prominent in the hands, where flattening of multiple metacarpal heads is distinctive. Platyspondyly with irregular and elongated vertebral bodies and narrowing of the interpediculate distances may be evident in the spine. Odontoid hypoplasia can be apparent. Histologic evaluation indicates friable cartilage with irregularity in both cellular size and matrix staining; the combination of hypertrophied chondrocytes surrounded by loose matrix containing large holes resembles Swiss cheese.[120]

Familial Arthropathy and Congenital Camptodactyly (Fig. 27–25)

One or more familial syndromes with flexion deformities of the fingers have been described. In 1965, Jacobs and Downey observed two families in which members, soon after birth, developed arthropathy and flexion contractures.[167] The syndrome was called familial hypertrophic synovitis, as synovial biopsies were characterized by hypertrophic, avascular villi and giant cells. In 1978, Athreya and Schumacher studied three siblings with the same disorder[168]; light and electron microscopy of the synovial mem-

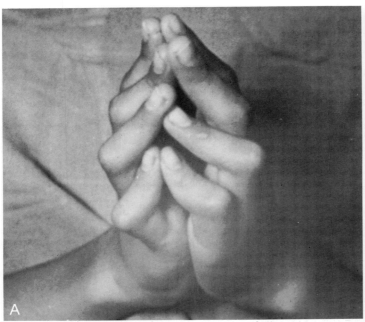
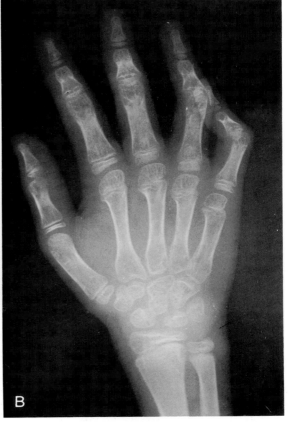

FIGURE 27–25. Familial arthropathy and congenital camptodactyly. This 12 year old boy developed flexion contractures of the fingers at the age of 5 years. Several family members had a similar abnormality. Swelling of the wrists, elbows, and knees was apparent. Arthroscopy of the knee revealed that the synovial membrane had prominent villi. Synovial biopsy documented considerable fibrosis with mild chronic inflammation.

A Clinical photograph reveals the flexion deformities, especially affecting the fourth and fifth fingers of each hand.

B A radiograph shows osteopenia and flexion contractures at the proximal interphalangeal joints.

(Courtesy of M. Martinez-Lavin, M.D., Mexico City, Mexico.)

brane allowed identification of synovial hyperplasia, necrotic villi, deposition of eosinophilic and periodic acid–Schiff (PAS)-positive material, and multinucleated giant cells. Similar observations were recorded by Ochi and associates[169] in 1983, in an investigation of two sisters with congenital camptodactyly and joint effusions. Pathologic abnormalities in involved tendons were those of an advanced tenosynovitis. Further reports of an identical or similar syndrome have appeared.[170, 171, 192–194, 240, 241] The distribution of involved fingers has varied among these reports, and changes in other articulations, such as the knees, have been a characteristic but not uniform feature. Pericardial involvement has occurred in some patients[171, 192, 194] but not in others. Chondrocalcinosis was identified in one case.[241]

From these data, it appears that several inherited disorders can lead to flexion deformities of the fingers and arthropathy, the patterns of inheritance are not uniform or clear, and the radiographic abnormalities, consisting mainly of osteoporosis and deformity (flattening of the metacarpal and metatarsal heads, coxa vara, and contractures of the fingers, wrists, and elbows), are easily distinguishable from those of juvenile chronic arthritis.

Other Disorders

Multiple epiphyseal dysplasia (and spondyloepiphyseal dysplasia) can lead to irregularity of many epiphyses with secondary degenerative joint abnormalities,[197] which can be confused with the changes of juvenile chronic arthritis (see Chapter 87).

Progressive pseudorheumatoid arthritis of childhood is a term applied to a hereditary arthropathy affecting major and minor joints in which findings include restricted articular motion, swelling about interphalangeal articulations, platyspondyly, and irregularities of vertebral bodies that simulate those in Scheuermann's disease.[172–175] Symptoms usually appear between the ages of 3 and 8 years, and the disease appears to have an autosomal recessive pattern of inheritance.

Infection or synovial hemangiomas can produce abnormalities of single articulations, which also simulate the findings of juvenile chronic arthritis. Similarly, neuromuscular disorders may lead to skeletal abnormalities of certain articulations that are indistinguishable from those of juvenile chronic arthritis.[186]

Although rheumatoid nodules that develop in childhood usually are accompanied by manifestations of juvenile chronic arthritis, rheumatic fever, or other systemic disorders such as systemic lupus erythematosus or granuloma annulare,[242, 243] such nodules also can be identified in children without rheumatic diseases. The term "benign rheumatoid nodules of childhood" has been offered as an appropriate designation in this latter situation.[244] Clinically and histologically, benign rheumatoid nodules are identical to nodules seen in juvenile chronic arthritis. Initial reports emphasized that even when patients were monitored clinically for periods as long as 10 years, no evidence of rheumatic disease appeared.[245] Rare cases have since been described, however, in which rheumatoid arthritis has appeared within months or as long as 50 years after the initial diagnosis of benign rheumatoid nodules had been made.[246, 247]

Other entities to be considered in the differential diagnosis of juvenile chronic arthritis include multicentric reticulohistiocytosis (see Chapter 61) and fibroblastic rheumatism. The latter is characterized by cutaneous nodules, sclerodactyly, Raynaud's phenomena, and rapidly progressive and symmetric polyarthritis.[248]

SUMMARY

Juvenile chronic arthritis is composed of a variety of conditions that affect articular structures in children. Several distinct subgroups of patients can be recognized. Juvenile-onset adult type (seropositive) rheumatoid arthritis is characterized by articular disease that resembles and behaves like its adult counterpart. Radiographic abnormalities of the joints of the hand, the wrist, the knee, and the foot consist of soft tissue swelling, osteoporosis, joint space narrowing, and osseous erosions. Periostitis may be prominent.

A second subgroup is composed of patients with seronegative chronic arthritis (Still's disease). Children with Still's disease may have classic systemic disease with severe extra-articular manifestations (fever, rash, lymphadenopathy, hepatosplenomegaly, pericarditis, and myocarditis). Other children with Still's disease have polyarticular, pauciarticular, or monoarticular involvement. The joints of the hand, the wrist, the foot, the knee, and the cervical spine may be affected. In addition to soft tissue swelling and osteoporosis, abnormal skeletal maturation can lead to significant growth disturbances. Periostitis and intra-articular bony ankylosis frequently are evident.

A third subgroup consists of patients with juvenile-onset ankylosing spondylitis. Characteristically, asymmetric involvement of the articulations of the lower extremity later is associated with sacroiliitis and spondylitis. Radiographic changes in the hip, the glenohumeral joint, the knee, and the calcaneus are similar to those noted in adult-onset ankylosing spondylitis. Patients frequently possess the histocompatibility antigen HLA-B27.

Additional varieties of juvenile chronic arthritis include psoriatic arthritis, arthritis of inflammatory bowel disease, Reiter's syndrome, and polyarthropathy associated with other disorders.

Although specific radiographic features of juvenile chronic arthritis depend on the subgroup of patients that is being evaluated, certain characteristics are sufficiently common in most patients to allow differentiation of juvenile chronic arthritis from various adult diseases. Loss of articular space and osseous erosions are relatively late manifestations of juvenile disease. Metaphyseal radiolucency, periostitis, intra-articular bony ankylosis, epiphyseal compression fractures, subluxation or dislocation, and growth disturbances are common. Although changes may be observed in many different skeletal sites, abnormalities of the hand, the wrist, the foot, the knee, the hip, the cervical spine, the mandible, and the temporomandibular joint are especially characteristic.

Differential diagnosis of juvenile chronic arthritis includes hemophilia, idiopathic multicentric osteolysis, mucopolysaccharidoses, epiphyseal dysplasias, multicentric reticulohistiocytosis, and infection.

References

1. Calabro JJ: Juvenile rheumatoid arthritis. *In* JL Hollander, DJ McCarty Jr (Eds): Arthritis and Allied Conditions. 8th Ed. Philadelphia, Lea & Febiger, 1972, p 387.
2. Still GF: On a form of chronic joint disease in children. Med Chir Trans *80:*47, 1897.
3. Barkin RE: The clinical course of juvenile rheumatoid arthritis. Bull Rheum Dis *3:*19, 1952.
4. Sairanen E: On rheumatoid arthritis in children: Clinico-roentgenological study. Acta Rheum Scand Suppl *2:*1, 1958.
5. Schlesinger BE, Forsyth CC, White RHR, et al: Observations on the clinical course and treatment of 100 cases of Still's disease. Arch Dis Child *36:*65, 1961.
6. Bywaters EGL: Categorization in medicine: A survey of Still's disease. Ann Rheum Dis *26:*185, 1967.
7. Calabro JJ, Marchesano JM: The early natural history of juvenile rheumatoid arthritis. Med Clin North Am *52:*567, 1968.
8. Ansell BM: Chronic arthritis in childhood. Ann Rheum Dis *37:*107, 1978.
9. Ansell BM, Bywaters EGL: Juvenile chronic polyarthritis, *In* JT Scott (Ed): Copeman's Textbook of the Rheumatic Diseases. 5th Ed. Edinburgh, Churchill Livingstone, 1978, p 365.
10. Schaller J, Wedgwood RJ: Juvenile rheumatoid arthritis: A review. Pediatrics *50:*940, 1972.
11. Ansell BM, Kent PA: Radiological changes in juvenile chronic polyarthritis. Skel Radiol *1:*129, 1977.
12. Goel KM, Shanks RA: Follow-up study of 100 cases of juvenile rheumatoid arthritis. Ann Rheum Dis *33:*25, 1974.
13. Sievers K, Ahvonen P, Aho K, et al: Serological patterns in juvenile rheumatoid arthritis. Rheumatism *19:*88, 1963.
14. Cassidy JT, Valkenburg HA: A five-year prospective study of rheumatoid factor tests in juvenile rheumatoid arthritis. Arthritis Rheum *10:*83, 1967.
15. Bianco NE, Panush RS, Stillman JS, et al: Immunologic studies of juvenile rheumatoid arthritis. Arthritis Rheum *14:*685, 1971.
16. Calabro JJ: The three faces of juvenile rheumatoid arthritis. Hosp Pract *9:*61, 1974.
17. Sokoloff C: The heart in rheumatoid arthritis. Am Heart J *45:*635, 1953.
18. Lebowitz WB: The heart in rheumatoid arthritis (rheumatoid disease). A clinical and pathological study of sixty-two cases. Ann Intern Med *58:*102, 1963.
19. Franco AE, Levine HD, Hall AP: Rheumatoid pericarditis; report of 17 cases diagnosed clinically. Ann Intern Med *77:*837, 1972.
20. Scharf J, Levy J, Benderly A, et al: Pericardial tamponade in juvenile rheumatoid arthritis. Arthritis Rheum *19:*760, 1976.
21. Schnitzer TJ, Ansell BM: Amyloidosis in juvenile chronic polyarthritis. Arthritis Rheum *20*(Suppl 2):245, 1977.
22. Ansell BM, Unlu M: Hip involvement in juvenile chronic polyarthritis. Ann Rheum Dis *29:*687, 1970.
23. Cassidy JT, Brody GL, Martel W: Monoarticular juvenile rheumatoid arthritis. J Pediatr *70:*867, 1967.
24. Gristina AG, Kelsey WM, Green DL, et al: Pauciarticular juvenile arthritis. South Med J *69:*440, 1976.
25. Boone JE, Baldwin J, Levine C: Juvenile rheumatoid arthritis. Pediatr Clin North Am *21:*885, 1974.
26. Edström G: Rheumatoid arthritis and Still's disease in children. Arthritis Rheum *1:*497, 1958.
27. Bywaters EGL, Ansell BM: Monoarticular arthritis in children. Ann Rheum Dis *24:*116, 1965.
28. Green WT: Monoarticular and pauciarticular arthritis in children. JAMA *115:*2023, 1940.
29. Griffin PP, Tachdjian MO, Green WT: Pauciarticular arthritis in children. JAMA *184:*145, 1963.
30. Calabro JJ, Parrino GR, Atchoo PD, et al: Chronic iridocyclitis in juvenile rheumatoid arthritis. Arthritis Rheum *13:*406, 1970.
31. Laaksonen AL: A prognostic study of juvenile rheumatoid arthritis. Acta Paediatr Scand *166*(Suppl):1, 1966.
32. Calabro JJ, Marchesano JM: Juvenile rheumatoid arthritis. N Engl J Med *277:*696, 1967.
33. Schaller J, Kupfer C, Wedgwood RI: Iridocyclitis in juvenile rheumatoid arthritis. Pediatrics *44:*92, 1969.
34. Ladd JR, Cassidy JT, Martel W: Juvenile ankylosing spondylitis. Arthritis Rheum *14:*579, 1971.
35. Edström G, Thune S, Wittbom-Cigén G: Juvenile ankylosing spondylitis. Acta Rheum Scand *6:*161, 1960.
36. Jacobs P: Ankylosing spondylitis in children and adolescents. Arch Dis Child *38:*492, 1963.
37. Schaller J, Bitnum S, Wedgwood RJ: Ankylosing spondylitis with childhood onset. J Pediatr *74:*505, 1969.
38. Ellefsen F: Juvenile ankylosing spondylitis. Acta Rheum Scand *13:*14, 1967.
39. Kleinman P, Rivelis M, Schneider R, et al: Juvenile ankylosing spondylitis. Radiology *125:*775, 1977.
40. Resnick D: Patterns of peripheral joint disease in ankylosing spondylitis. Radiology *110:*523, 1974.
41. Bywaters EGL, Ansell BM: Sacroiliitis in juvenile chronic polyarthritis. Z Rheumaforsch *24:*122, 1965.
42. Angevine CD, Pless IB, Baum J, et al: Psoriatic arthritis in a child. Arthritis Rheum *16:*278, 1973.
43. Lambert JR, Ansell BM, Stephenson E, et al: Psoriatic arthritis in childhood. Clin Rheum Dis *2:*339, 1976.
44. Middlemiss JH: Juvenile rheumatoid arthritis (Still's disease). Proc R Soc Med *44:*805, 1951.
45. Martel W, Holt JF, Cassidy JT: Roentgenologic manifestations of juvenile rheumatoid arthritis. AJR *88:*400, 1962.
46. LoPresti JM: Juvenile rheumatoid arthritis, with report of case in 15 month old child. Clin Proc Child Hosp *5:*74, 1949.
47. Thomas LB, Forkner CE Jr, Frei E III, et al: Skeletal lesions of acute leukemia. Cancer *14:*608, 1961.
48. Portis RB: Pathology of chronic arthritis of children (Still's disease). Am J Dis Child *55:*1000, 1938.
49. Ansell BM, Bywaters EGL: Growth in Still's disease. Ann Rheum Dis *15:*295, 1956.
50. Bruland H: Pseudo-chondrodystrophia rheumatica (rheumatic dwarfism): Review and discussion of 2 cases. Acta Rheum Scand *6:*209, 1960.
51. Jacqueline F, Boujot A, Canet L: Involvement of hips in juvenile rheumatoid arthritis. Arthritis Rheum *4:*500, 1961.
52. Vainio K, Sairenen E: Uber huftgelenk-luxation bei rheumatoider arthritis. Z Orthop *86:*217, 1955.
53. Forsyth CC: Calcification of digital vessels in a child with rheumatoid arthritis. Arch Dis Child *35:*296, 1960.
54. Schmidt MC, Workman JB, Barth WF: Dissection or rupture of a popliteal cyst. Arch Intern Med *134:*694, 1974.
55. Barbaric ZL, Young LW: Synovial cysts in juvenile rheumatoid arthritis. AJR *116:*655, 1972.
56. Baldassare AR, Auclair RJ, Carls GL, et al: Dissecting popliteal cyst in a child with juvenile rheumatoid arthritis. J Rheumatol *4:*186, 1977.
57. Bamzai A, Krieger M, Kretschmer RR: Synovial cysts in juvenile rheumatoid arthritis. Ann Rheum Dis *37:*101, 1978.
58. Chaplin D, Pulkki T, Saarimaa A, et al: Wrist and finger deformities in juvenile rheumatoid arthritis. Acta Rheum Scand *15:*206, 1969.
59. Resnick D: Inter-relationships between radiocarpal and metacarpophalangeal joint deformities in rheumatoid arthritis. J Can Assoc Radiol *27:*29, 1976.
60. Granberry WM: The hand of the child with juvenile rheumatoid arthritis (Abstr). Arthritis Rheum *21:*561, 1978.
61. Poznanski AK, Hernandez RJ, Guire KE, et al: Carpal length in children—a useful measurement in the diagnosis of rheumatoid arthritis and some congenital malformation syndromes. Radiology *129:*661, 1978.
62. Ishikawa K, Patiala H, Raunio P, et al: Carpal tunnel syndrome in juvenile rheumatoid arthritis. Arch Orthop Unfallchir *82:*85, 1975.
63. Chlosta EM, Kuhns LR, Holt JF: The "patellar ratio" in hemophilia and juvenile rheumatoid arthritis. Radiology *116:*137, 1975.
64. Albright JA, Albright JP, Ogden JA: Synovectomy of the hip in juvenile rheumatoid arthritis. Clin Orthop *106:*48, 1975.
65. Arden GP, Ansell BM, Hunter MJ: Total hip replacement in juvenile chronic polyarthritis and ankylosing spondylitis. Clin Orthop *84:*130, 1972.
66. Isdale IC: Hip disease in juvenile rheumatoid arthritis. Ann Rheum Dis *29:*603, 1970.
67. Bernstein B, Forrester D, Singsen B, et al: Hip joint restoration in juvenile rheumatoid arthritis. Arthritis Rheum *20:*1099, 1977.
68. Stovell PB, Ahuja SC, Inglis AE: Pseudarthrosis of the proximal femoral epiphysis in juvenile rheumatoid arthritis. J Bone Joint Surg [Am] *57:*860, 1975.
69. Carter ME, Loewi G: Anatomical changes in normal sacro-iliac joints during childhood and comparison with the changes in Still's disease. Ann Rheum Dis *21:*121, 1962.
70. Nathan FF, Bickel WH: Spontaneous axial subluxation in a child as the first sign of juvenile rheumatoid arthritis. J Bone Joint Surg [Am] *50:*1675, 1968.
71. Rombouts JJ, Rombouts-Lindemans C: Scoliosis in juvenile rheumatoid arthritis. J Bone Joint Surg [Br] *56:*478, 1974.
72. Rönning O, Väliaho ML, Laaksonen AL: The involvement of the temporomandibular joint in juvenile rheumatoid arthritis. Scand J Rheumatol *3:*89, 1974.
73. Engel MB, Richmond JB, Brodie AG: Mandibular growth disturbance in rheumatoid arthritis of childhood. Am J Dis Child *78:*728, 1949.
74. Martis CS, Karakasis DT: Ankylosis of the temporomandibular joint caused by Still's disease. Oral Surg *35:*462, 1973.
75. Rushton MA: Growth at mandibular condyle in relation to some deformities. Br Dent J *76:*57, 1944.
76. Brodie AG: *In* The Temporomandibular Joint. Springfield, Ill, Charles C Thomas, 1951, p 61.
77. Becker MH, Coccaro PJ, Converse JM: Antegonial notching of the mandible: An often overlooked mandibular deformity in congenital and acquired disorders. Radiology *121:*149, 1976.
78. Hovell JH: Variations in mandibular form. Ann R Coll Surg *37:*1, 1965.
79. Rönning O, Väliaho ML: Involvement of the facial skeleton in juvenile rheumatoid arthritis. Ann Radiol *18:*347, 1975.
80. Forestier J, Jacqueline F, Canet L: Le rhumatisme inflammatoire chronique de l'enfant (étude clinique et radiologique). Rhumatologie *11:*51, 1959.
81. Bache C: Mandibular growth and dental occlusion in juvenile rheumatoid arthritis. Acta Rheum Scand *10:*142, 1964.
82. Marbach JJ, Spiera H: Rheumatoid arthritis of the temporomandibular joints. Ann Rheum Dis *26:*538, 1967.
83. Goodwill CJ, Steggles BG: Destruction of the temporo-mandibular joints in rheumatoid arthritis. Ann Rheum Dis *25:*133, 1966.

84. Jacobs JC, Hui RM: Cricoarytenoid arthritis and airway obstruction in juvenile rheumatoid arthritis. Pediatrics 59:292, 1977.
85. Bienenstock H, Ehrlich GE, Freyberg RH: Rheumatoid arthritis of the cricoarytenoid joint: A clinicopathologic study. Arthritis Rheum 6:48, 1963.
86. Fassbender HG: Pathology of Rheumatic Diseases. New York, Springer-Verlag, 1975, p 211.
87. Wynne-Roberts CR, Anderson CH, Turano AM, et al: Light- and electron-microscopic findings of juvenile rheumatoid arthritis synovium: Comparison with normal juvenile synovium. Semin Arthritis Rheum 7:287, 1978.
88. Kölle G: Klinisches Bild und Verlauf der juvenilen rheumatoiden Arthritis und des Still-Syndroms. Monatsschr Kinderheilkd 118:488, 1970.
89. Bywaters EGL, Glynn LE, Zeldis A: Subcutaneous nodules of Still's disease. Ann Rheum Dis 17:278, 1958.
90. Bywaters EGL: Still's disease in the adult. Ann Rheum Dis 30:121, 1971.
91. Isdale IC, Bywaters EGL: The rash of rheumatoid arthritis and Still's disease. Q J Med 25:377, 1956.
92. Aptekar RG, Decker JL, Bujak JS, et al: Adult onset juvenile rheumatoid arthritis. Arthritis Rheum 16:715, 1973.
93. Fabricant MS, Chandor SB, Friou GJ: Still's disease in adults: A cause of prolonged undiagnosed fever. JAMA 225:273, 1973.
94. Gupta RC, Mills DM: Still's disease in an adult: A link between juvenile and adult rheumatoid arthritis. Am J Med Sci 269:137, 1975.
95. Caroit M, Mathieu M, Kahn MF: Maladie de Still de l'adulte et syndrome de Wissler-Fanconi. Rev Rhum Mal Osteoartic 49:1, 1973.
96. Bujak JS, Aptekar RG, Decker JL, et al: Juvenile rheumatoid arthritis presenting in the adult as fever of unknown origin. Medicine 52:431, 1973.
97. Medsger TA Jr, Christy WC: Carpal arthritis with ankylosis in late onset Still's disease. Arthritis Rheum 19:232, 1976.
98. Edmonds J, Morris RI, Metzger AL, et al: Follow-up study of juvenile chronic polyarthritis with particular reference to histocompatibility antigen W 27. Ann Rheum Dis 33:289, 1974.
99. Hall A, Ansell BM, James DCO, et al: HL-A antigens in juvenile chronic polyarthritis (Still's disease). Ann Rheum Dis 34(Suppl):36, 1975.
100. Sturrock RD, Dick HM, Henderson N, et al: Association of HL-A27 and AJ in juvenile rheumatoid arthritis and ankylosing spondylitis. J Rheumatol 1:269, 1974.
101. Rachelefsky GS, Terasaki PI, Katz R, et al: Increased prevalence of W 27 in juvenile rheumatoid arthritis. N Engl J Med 290:892, 1974.
102. Mitsui H, Juji T, Sonozaki H, et al: Distribution of HLA-B27 in patients with juvenile rheumatoid arthritis. Ann Rheum Dis 36:86, 1977.
103. Gibson DJ, Carpenter CB, Stillman JS, et al: Re-examination of histocompatibility antigens found in patients with juvenile rheumatoid arthritis. N Engl J Med 293:636, 1975.
104. Hoyeraal HM, Mellbye OJ: Humoral immunity in juvenile rheumatoid arthritis. Ann Rheum Dis 33:248, 1974.
105. Hoyeraal HM, Mellbye OJ: High levels in serum complement factors in juvenile rheumatoid arthritis. Ann Rheum Dis 33:243, 1974.
106. Munthe E: Complexes of IgG and IgG rheumatoid factor in synovial tissues of juvenile rheumatoid arthritis. Scand J Rheumatol 1:153, 1972.
107. Hedberg H: The total complement activity of synovial fluid in juvenile forms of arthritis. Acta Rheumatol Scand 17:279, 1971.
108. Tyler T, Rosenbaum HD: Idiopathic multicentric osteolysis. AJR 126:23, 1976.
109. Kohler E, Babbitt D, Huizenga B, et al: Hereditary osteolysis. A clinical, radiological and chemical study. Radiology 108:99, 1973.
110. Whyte MP, Murphy WA, Kleerekoper M, et al: Idiopathic multicentric osteolysis. Report of an affected father and son. Arthritis Rheum 21:367, 1978.
111. Beals RK, Bird CB: Carpal and tarsal osteolysis: A case report and review of the literature. J Bone Joint Surg [Am] 57:681, 1975.
112. Erickson CM, Hirschberger M, Stickler GB: Carpal-tarsal osteolysis. J Pediatr 93:779, 1978.
113. Normand ICS, Dent CE, Smellie JM: Disappearing carpal bones. Proc R Soc Med 55:978, 1962.
114. McKusick VA: The mucopolysaccharidoses. In Heritable Disorders of Connective Tissue. 3rd Ed. St Louis, CV Mosby, 1966.
115. Bierman SM, Edgington T, Newcomer VD, et al: Farber's disease: Disorder of mucopolysaccharide metabolism with articular, respiratory, and neurologic manifestations. Arthritis Rheum 9:620, 1966.
116. Winchester P, Grossman H, Lim WN, et al: A new acid mucopolysaccharidosis with skeletal deformities simulating rheumatoid arthritis. AJR 106:121, 1969.
117. Kniest W: Zur Abgrenzung der Dysostosis enchondralis von der Chondrodystrophie. Z Kinderheilkd 70:633, 1952.
118. Brill PW, Kim HJ, Beratis NG, et al: Skeletal abnormalities in the Kniest syndrome with mucopolysacchariduria. AJR 125:731, 1975.
119. Frayha R, Melhem R, Idriss H: The Kniest (Swiss cheese cartilage) syndrome. Description of a distinct arthropathy. Arthritis Rheum 22:286, 1979.
120. Rimoin DL, Hollister DW, Silberberg R, et al: Kniest (Swiss cheese cartilage) syndrome: Clinical, radiographic, histologic and ultrastructural studies. Clin Res 21:296, 1973.
121. Colville J, Raunio P: Total hip replacement in juvenile rheumatoid arthritis. Analysis of 59 hips. Acta Orthop Scand 50:197, 1979.
122. Locke GR, Gardner JI, Van Epps EF: Atlas-dens interval (ADI) in children. A survey based on 200 normal cervical spines. AJR 97:135, 1966.
123. Iveson JMI, Nanda BS, Hancock JAH, et al: Reiter's disease in three boys. Ann Rheum Dis 34:364, 1975.
124. Lockie GN, Hunger GG: Reiter's syndrome in children. A case report and review. Arthritis Rheum 64:767, 1971.
125. Conaglen J, Grennan DM, Signal T, et al: Juvenile Reiter's syndrome. Aust NZ J Med 9:193, 1979.
126. Ragsdale CG, Petty RE, Cassidy JT, et al: The clinical progression of apparent juvenile rheumatoid arthritis to systemic lupus erythematosus. J Rheumatol 7:50, 1980.
127. Mäkelä AL, Mäkinen E, Lorenz K, et al: Veränderungen an der Halswirbelsäule bei juveniler rheumatoider Arthritis. ROFO 131:420, 1979.
128. Blockey NJ, Gibson AAM, Goel KM: Monarticular juvenile rheumatoid arthritis. J Bone Joint Surg [Br] 62:368, 1980.
129. Granberry WM, Mangum GL: The hand in the child with juvenile rheumatoid arthritis. J Hand Surg 5:105, 1980.
130. Mitnick JS, Mitnick HJ, Genieser NB: Proliferative changes of the hip in juvenile rheumatoid arthritis. Radiology 136:369, 1980.
131. Esdaile JM, Tannenbaum H, Hawkins D: Adult Still's disease. Am J Med 68:825, 1980.
132. Rosenberg AM, Petty RE: Similar patterns of juvenile rheumatoid arthritis within families. Arthritis Rheum 23:951, 1980.
133. Balogh Z, Merétey K, Falus A, et al: Serological abnormalities in juvenile chronic arthritis: A review of 46 cases. Ann Rheum Dis 39:129, 1980.
134. Alarcón-Segovia D, Laffon A, Alcocer-Varela J: Probable depiction of juvenile arthritis by Sandro Botticelli. Arthritis Rheum 26:1266, 1983.
135. Schaller JG: Chronic arthritis in children. Juvenile rheumatoid arthritis. Clin Orthop 182:79, 1984.
136. Rosenberg AM, Petty RE: Reiter's disease in children. Am J Dis Child 133:394, 1979.
137. Singsen BH, Bernstein HB, Koster-King KG, et al: Reiter's syndrome in childhood. Arthritis Rheum 20:402, 1977.
138. Rosenberg AM, Petty RE: A syndrome of seronegative enthesopathy and arthropathy in children. Arthritis Rheum 25:1041, 1982.
139. Jacobs JC, Berdon WE, Johnston AD: HLA-B27-associated spondyloarthritis and enthesopathy in childhood: Clinical, pathologic, and radiographic observations in 58 patients. J Pediatr 100:521, 1982.
140. Thompson GH, Khan MA, Bilenker RM: Spontaneous atlanto-axial subluxation as a presenting manifestation of juvenile ankylosing spondylitis. Spine 7:78, 1982.
141. Forre O, Doblong JH, Hoyeraal HM, et al: HLA antigens in juvenile arthritis. Genetic basis for the different subtypes. Arthritis Rheum 26:35, 1983.
142. Hassink SG, Goldsmith DP: Neonatal onset multisystem inflammatory disease. Arthritis Rheum 26:668, 1983.
143. Gilsanz V, Bernstein BH: Joint calcification following intra-articular corticosteroid therapy. Radiology 151:647, 1984.
144. Rennebohm RM, Towbin RB, Crowe WE, et al: Popliteal cysts in juvenile rheumatoid arthritis. AJR 40:123, 1983.
145. Costello PB, Kennedy AC, Green FA: Shoulder joint rupture in juvenile rheumatoid arthritis producing bicipital masses and a hemorrhagic sign. J Rheumatol 7:563, 1980.
146. Maldonado-Cocco JA, Garcia-Morteo O, Spindler AJ, et al: Carpal ankylosis in juvenile rheumatoid arthritis. Arthritis Rheum 23:1251, 1980.
147. Fiszman P, Ansell BM, Renton P: Radiological assessment of knees in juvenile chronic arthritis (juvenile rheumatoid arthritis). Scand J Rheumatol 10:145, 1981.
148. Bunger C, Harving S, Bunger EH: Intraosseous pressure in the patella in relation to simulated joint effusion and knee position. Acta Orthop Scand 53:745, 1982.
149. Garcia-Morteo O, Babini JC, Maldonado-Cocco JA, et al: Remodeling of the hip joint in juvenile rheumatoid arthritis. Arthritis Rheum 24:1570, 1981.
150. Mogensen B, Brattstrom H, Ekelund L, et al: Synovectomy of the hip in juvenile chronic arthritis. J Bone Joint Surg [Br] 64:295, 1982.
151. Svantesson H, Marhaug G, Haeffner F: Scoliosis in children with juvenile rheumatoid arthritis. Scand J Rheumatol 10:65, 1981.
152. Rana NA: Juvenile rheumatoid arthritis of the foot. Foot Ankle 3:2, 1982.
153. Fried JA, Athreya B, Gregg JR, et al: The cervical spine in juvenile rheumatoid arthritis. Clin Orthop 179:102, 1983.
154. Parke WW, Rothman RH, Brown MD: The pharyngovertebral veins: An anatomical rationale for Grisel's syndrome. J Bone Joint Surg [Am] 66:568, 1984.
155. Rothschild BM, Hanissian AS: Severe generalized (charcot-like) joint destruction in juvenile rheumatoid arthritis. Clin Orthop 155:75, 1981.
156. Larheim TA: Comparison between three radiographic techniques for examination of the temporomandibular joints in juvenile rheumatoid arthritis. Acta Radiol (Diagn) 22:195, 1981.
157. Larheim TA, Dale K, Tveito L: Radiographic abnormalities of the temporomandibular joint in children with juvenile rheumatoid arthritis. Acta Radiol (Diagn) 22:277, 1981.
158. Larheim TA, Hoyeraal HM, Stabrun AE, Hannaes HR: The temporomandibular joint in juvenile rheumatoid arthritis. Scand J Rheumatol 11:5, 1982.
159. Larheim TA: Radiographic appearance of the normal temporomandibular joint in newborns and small children. Acta Radiol (Diagn) 22:593, 1981.
160. Simon S, Whiffen J, Shapiro F: Leg-length discrepancies in monoarticular and pauciarticular juvenile rheumatoid arthritis. J Bone Joint Surg [Am] 63:209, 1981.
161. Healey LA, Willkens RF: Tarsal arthritis with ankylosis in late onset Still's disease. Arthritis Rheum 25:1254, 1982.

162. Laroche M, Fauchier C, Franck JL, et al: Maladie de still de l'adulte (2 observations). Rev Med Toulouse *18:*547, 1982.

163. DeMulder PHM, Van de Putte LBA: Adult-onset Still's disease: Destructive distal interphalangeal arthritis associated with transient capsular calcification. Ann Rheum Dis *41:*544, 1982.

164. Del Paine DW, Leek JC: Still's arthritis in adults: Disease or syndrome? J Rheumatol *10:*758, 1983.

165. Terkeltaub R, Esdaile JM, Decary F, et al: HLA-Bw35 and prognosis in adult Still's disease. Arthritis Rheum *24:*1469, 1981.

166. Arnett FC, Bias WB, Stevens MB: Juvenile-onset chronic arthritis. Clinical and roentgenographic features of a unique HLA-B27 subset. Am J Med *69:*369, 1980.

167. Jacobs JC, Downey JA: Juvenile rheumatoid arthritis. *In* Downey JA, Low NL (eds): The Child with Disabling Illness. Philadelphia, WB Saunders, 1974, p 5.

168. Athreya BH, Schumacher HR: Pathologic features of a familial arthropathy associated with congenital flexion contractures of fingers. Arthritis Rheum *21:*429, 1978.

169. Ochi T, Iwase R, Okabe N, et al: The pathology of the involved tendons in patients with familial arthropathy and congenital camptodactyly. Arthritis Rheum *26:*896, 1983.

170. Malleson P, Schaller JG, Dega F, et al: Familial arthritis and camptodactyly. Arthritis Rheum *24:*1199, 1981.

171. Martinez-Lavin M, Buendia A, Delgado E, et al: A familial syndrome of pericarditis, arthritis, and camptodactyly. N Engl J Med *309:*224, 1983.

172. Spranger J, Albert C, Schilling F: A progressive connective tissue disease with features of juvenile rheumatoid arthritis and osteochondrodysplasia. Eur J Pediatr *133:*186, 1980.

173. Wynne-Davies R, Hall C, Ansell BM: Spondylo-epiphyseal dysplasia tarda with progressive arthropathy. J Bone Joint Surg [Br] *64:*442, 1982.

174. Spranger J, Albert C, Schilling F, et al: Progressive pseudorheumatoid arthropathy of childhood (PPAC): A hereditary disorder simulating juvenile rheumatoid arthritis. Am J Med Genet *14:*399, 1983.

175. Spranger J, Albert C, Schilling F, et al: Progressive pseudorheumatoid arthritis of childhood (PPAC). A hereditary disorder simulating rheumatoid arthritis. Eur J Pediatr *140:*34, 1983.

176. Howard JF, Sigsbee A, Glass DN: HLA genetics and inherited predisposition to JRA. J Rheumatol *12:*7, 1985.

177. Friis J, Morling N, Pedersen FK, et al: HLA-B27 in juvenile chronic arthritis. J Rheumatol *12:*119, 1985.

178. Shore A, Ansell BM: Juvenile psoriatic arthritis—an analysis of 60 cases. J Pediatr *100:*529, 1982.

179. Gerster J-C, Piccinin P: Enthesopathy of the heels in juvenile onset seronegative B-27 spondyloarthropathy. J Rheumatol *12:*310, 1985.

180. Jabs DA, Houk JL, Bias WB, et al: Familial granulomatous synovitis, uveitis, and cranial neuropathies. Am J Med *78:*801, 1985.

181. Pettersson H, Rydholm U: Radiologic classification of knee joint destruction in juvenile chronic arthritis. Pediatr Radiol *14:*419, 1984.

182. Patriquin HB, Camerlain M, Trias A: Late sequelae of juvenile rheumatoid arthritis of the hip: A follow-up study into adulthood. Pediatr Radiol *14:*151, 1984.

183. Williams RA, Ansell BM: Radiological findings in seropositive juvenile chronic arthritis (juvenile rheumatoid arthritis) with particular reference to progression. Ann Rheum Dis *44:*685, 1985.

184. Wouters JMGW, van Rijswijk MH, van de Putte LBA: Adult onset Still's disease in the elderly: A report of two cases. J Rheumatol *12:*791, 1985.

185. Wouters JMGW, Froeling PGA, van de Putte LBA: Adult-onset Still's disease complicated by hypercalcaemia: Possible relationship with rapidly destructive polyarthritis. Ann Rheum Dis *44:*345, 1985.

186. Richardson ML, Helms CA, Vogler JB III, et al: Skeletal changes in neuromuscular disorders mimicking juvenile rheumatoid arthritis and hemophilia. AJR *143:*893, 1984.

187. Cassidy JT, Levinson JE, Bass JC, et al: A study of classification criteria for a diagnosis of juvenile rheumatoid arthritis. Arthritis Rheum *29:*274, 1986.

188. Pettersson H, Rydholm U: Radiologic classification of joint destruction in juvenile chronic arthritis. Acta Radiol (Diagn) *26:*719, 1985.

189. Chantler JK, Tingle AJ, Petty RE: Persistent rubella virus infection associated with chronic arthritis in children. N Engl J Med *313:*1117, 1985.

190. Wouters JMGW, Reekers P, van de Putte LBA: Adult-onset Still's disease. Disease course and HLA associations. Arthritis Rheum *29:*415, 1986.

191. Mann BA, Williams RC Jr: Adult Still's disease—implications of a new syndrome. West J Med *142:*686, 1985.

192. Laxer RM, Cameron BJ, Chaisson D, et al: The camptodactyly-arthropathy-pericarditis syndrome. Case report and literature review. Arthritis Rheum *29:*439, 1986.

193. Martin JR, Huang S-N, Lacson A, et al: Congenital contractural deformities of the fingers and arthropathy. Ann Rheum Dis *44:*826, 1985.

194. Bulutlar G, Yazici H, Özdoğan H, et al: A familial syndrome of pericarditis, arthritis, camptodactyly, and coxa vara. Arthritis Rheum *29:*436, 1986.

195. Kaufman RA, Lovell DJ: Infantile-onset multisystem inflammatory disease: Radiologic findings. Radiology *160:*741, 1986.

196. Mielants H, Veys E: Enthesopathy of the heels in juvenile onset seronegative B27 positive spondyloarthropathy. J Rheumatol *13:*657, 1986.

197. Stanescu V, Stanescu R, Maroteaux P: Articular degeneration as a sequela of osteochondrodysplasia. Clin Rheum Dis *11:*239, 1985.

198. Cassidy JT, Levinson JE, Brewer EJ Jr: The development of classification criteria for children with juvenile rheumatoid arthritis. Bull Rheum Dis *38:*1, 1989.

199. Burgos-Vargas R, Clark P: Axial involvement in the seronegative enthesopathy and arthropathy syndrome and its progression to ankylosing spondylitis. J Rheumatol *16:*192, 1989.

200. Athreya BH, Ostrov BE, Eichenfield AH, et al: Lymphedema associated with juvenile rheumatoid arthritis. J Rheumatol *16:*1338, 1989.

201. Torbiak RP, Dent PB, Cockshott WP: NOMID—a neonatal syndrome of multisystem inflammation. Skel Radiol *18:*359, 1989.

202. Cook DJ, Benson WG, Shore A, et al: Pauciarticular juvenile rheumatoid arthritis presenting in an adult. J Rheumatol *15:*1865, 1988.

203. Hamilton ML, Gladman DD, Shore A, et al: Juvenile psoriatic arthritis and HLA antigens. Ann Rheum Dis *49:*694, 1990.

204. Olivieri I, Foto M, Ruju GP, et al: Low frequency of axial involvement in Caucasian pediatric patients with seronegative enthesopathy and arthropathy syndrome after 5 years of disease. J Rheumatol *19:*469, 1992.

205. Olivieri I, Pasero G: Longstanding isolated juvenile onset HLA-B27 associated peripheral enthesitis. J Rheumatol *19:*164, 1992.

206. Petty RE: HLA-B27 and rheumatic diseases of childhood. J Rheumatol *17:*7, 1990.

207. Sheerin KA, Giannini EH, Brewer EJ Jr, et al: HLA-B27–associated arthropathy in childhood: Long term clinical and diagnostic outcome. Arthritis Rheum *31:*1165, 1988.

208. Siegel DM, Baum J: HLA-B27 associated dactylitis in children. J Rheumatol *15:*976, 1988.

209. Reed MH, Wilmot DM: The radiology of juvenile rheumatoid arthritis. A review of the English language literature. J Rheumatol *18:*2, 1991.

210. Sparling M, Malleson P, Wood B, et al: Radiographic followup of joints injected with triamcinolone hexacetonide for the management of childhood arthritis. Arthritis Rheum *33:*821, 1990.

211. Stannard MW, Fink CW: Diagnosis of synovial cysts in children by magnetic resonance imaging. J Rheumatol *16:*540, 1989.

212. Zerin JM, Sullivan DB, Martel W: Distal interphalangeal joint abnormalities in children with polyarticular juvenile rheumatoid arthritis. J Rheumatol *18:*889, 1991.

213. Evans DM, Ansell BM, Hall MA: The wrist in juvenile arthritis. J Hand Surg [Br] *16:*293, 1991.

214. Bjorkengren AG, Pathria MN, Sartoris DJ, et al: Carpal alterations in adult-onset Still disease, juvenile chronic arthritis, and adult-onset rheumatoid arthritis: Comparative study. Radiology *165:*545, 1987.

215. Zerin JM, Rockwell DT, Garn SM, et al: Carpo-metacarpal growth disturbance and the assessment of carpal narrowing in children with juvenile rheumatoid arthritis. Invest Radiol *26:*727, 1991.

216. Harris CM, Baum J: Involvement of the hip in juvenile rheumatoid arthritis. A longitudinal study. J Bone Joint Surg [Am] *70:*821, 1988.

217. Kobayakawa M, Rydholm U, Wingstrand H, et al: Femoral head necrosis in juvenile chronic arthritis. Acta Orthop Scand *60:*164, 1989.

218. Learmonth ID, Heywood AWB, Kaye J, et al: Radiological loosening after cemented hip replacement for juvenile chronic arthritis. J Bone Joint Surg [Br] *71:*209, 1989.

219. Morgante D, Pathria M, Sartoris D, et al: Subtalar and intertarsal joint involvement in hemophilia and juvenile chronic arthritis: Frequency and diagnostic significance of radiographic abnormalities. Foot Ankle *9:*45, 1988.

220. Garcia-Morteo O, Gusis SE, Somma LF, et al: Tarsal ankylosis in juvenile and adult onset rheumatoid arthritis. J Rheumatol *15:*298, 1988.

221. Espada G, Babini JC, Maldonado-Cocca JA, et al: Radiologic review: The cervical spine in juvenile rheumatoid arthritis. Semin Arthritis Rheum *17:*185, 1988.

222. Ross AC, Edgar MA, Swann M, et al: Scoliosis in juvenile chronic arthritis. J Bone Joint Surg [Br] *69:*175, 1987.

223. Stabrun AE, Larheim TA, Höyeraal HM, et al: Reduced mandibular dimensions and asymmetry in juvenile rheumatoid arthritis. Pathogenetic factors. Arthritis Rheum *31:*602, 1988.

224. Myall RWT, West RA, Horwitz H, et al: Jaw deformity caused by juvenile rheumatoid arthritis and its correction. Arthritis Rheum *31:*1305, 1988.

225. Malleson P, Riding K, Petty R: Stridor due to cricoarytenoid arthritis in pauciarticular onset juvenile rheumatoid arthritis. J Rheumatol *13:*952, 1986.

226. Murray IPC, Dixon J: The role of single photon emission computed tomography in bone scintigraphy. Skel Radiol *18:*493, 1989.

227. Jones MM, Moore WH, Brewer EJ, et al: Radionuclide bone/joint imaging in children with rheumatic complaints Skel Radiol *17:*1, 1988.

228. Yulish BS, Lieberman JM, Newman AJ, et al: Juvenile rheumatoid arthritis: Assessment with MR imaging. Radiology *165:*149, 1987.

229. Verbruggen LA, Shahabpour M, Van Roy P, et al: Magnetic resonance imaging of articular destruction in juvenile rheumatoid arthritis. Arthritis Rheum *33:*1426, 1990.

230. Senac MO Jr, Deutsch D, Bernstein BH, et al: MR imaging in juvenile rheumatoid arthritis. AJR *150:*873, 1988.

231. Hervé-Somma CMP, Sebag GH, Prieur A-M, et al: Juvenile rheumatoid arthritis of the knee: MR evaluation with Gd-DOTA. Radiology *182:*93, 1992.

232. Brandwein SR, Salusinsky-Sternbach M: Adult Still's disease in only one of identical twins. J Rheumatol *16:*1599, 1989.

233. Cabane J, Michon A, Ziza J-M, et al: Comparison of long term evolution of adult onset and juvenile onset Still's disease, both followed up for more than 10 years. Ann Rheum Dis *49:*283, 1990.

234. Pouchot J, Sampalis JS, Beaudet F, et al: Adult Still's disease: Manifestations, disease course, and outcome in 62 patients. Medicine 70:118, 1991.
235. Cush JJ, Medsger TA Jr, Christy WC, et al: Adult-onset Still's disease. Clinical course and outcome. Arthritis Rheum 30:186, 1987.
236. Wouters JMGW, van de Putte LBA: Adult-onset Still's disease: Clinical and laboratory features, treatment and prognosis of 45 cases. Q J Med 61:1055, 1986.
237. Ohta A, Yamaguchi M, Kaneoka H, et al: Adult Still's disease: Review of 228 cases from the literature. J Rheumatol 14:1139, 1987.
238. Wouters JMGW, Van der Veen J, Van de Putte LBA, et al: Adult onset Still's disease and viral infections. Ann Rheum Dis 47:764, 1988.
239. Lang BA, Shore A: A review of current concepts on the pathogenesis of juvenile rheumatoid arthritis. J Rheumatol 17(Suppl 21):1, 1990.
240. Hamza M, Elleuch M, Ferchiou A, et al: Report of a patient with camptodactyly, arthropathy, and epiphyseal dysplasia. Arthritis Rheum 31:935, 1988.
241. Hamza M, Bardin T: Camptodactyly, polyepiphyseal dysplasia and mixed crystal deposition disease. J Rheumatol 16:1153, 1989.
242. Brantley SD, Schlesinger AE, Orzel JA, et al: Intraosseous rheumatoid nodule. Pediatr Radiol 17:432, 1987.
243. Truhan AP, Pachman LM, Esterly NB: Granuloma annulare. Arthritis Rheum 30:117, 1987.
244. Kaye BR, Kaye RL, Bobrove A: Rheumatoid nodules. Am J Med 76:279, 1984.
245. Draheim JH, Johnson LC, Helwig EB: A clinicopathologic analysis of rheumatoid nodules occurring in 54 children. Am J Pathol 35:678, 1959.
246. Mastboom WJB, van der Staak FHJM, Festen C, et al: Subcutaneous rheumatoid nodules. Arch Dis Child 63:662, 1988.
247. Olive A, Maymo J, Lloreta J, et al: Evolution of benign rheumatoid nodules into rheumatoid arthritis after 50 years. Ann Rheum Dis 46:624, 1987.
248. Hernandez RJ, Headington JT, Kaufman RA, et al: Case report 511. Skel Radiol 8:43, 1989.
249. Southwood TR, Petty RE, Malleson PN, et al: Psoriatic arthritis in children. Arthritis Rheum 32:1007, 1989.
250. Cuttica RJ, Scheines EJ, Garay SM, et al: Juvenile onset Reiter's syndrome. A retrospective study of 26 patients. Clin Exp Rheumatol 10:285, 1992.
251. Babini JC, Gusis SE, Babini SM, et al: Superolateral erosions of the humeral head in chronic inflammatory arthropathies. Skel Radiol 21:515, 1992.
252. Bambery P, Thomas RJ, Malhotra HS, et al: Adult onset Still's disease: Clinical experience with 18 patients over 15 years in Northern India. Ann Rheum Dis 51:529, 1992.
253. Coffernils M, Soupart A, Pradier O, et al: Hyperferritinemia in adult onset Still's disease and the hemophagocytic syndrome. J Rheumatol 19:1425, 1992.
254. Van Gundy ET, Kaufman SS, Danford DA, et al: Chronic monoarticular arthritis and acute pericardial tamponade in a child with Crohn's disease. J Rheumatol 20:2140, 1993.
255. Sureda D, Quiroga S, Arnal C, et al: Juvenile rheumatoid arthritis of the knee: Evaluation with US. Radiology 190:403, 1994.
256. Uson J, Pena JM, del Arco A, et al: Still's disease in a 72-year-old man. J Rheumatol 20:1608, 1993.
257. Hastings DE, Orsini E, Myers P, et al: An unusual pattern of growth disturbance of the hip in juvenile rheumatoid arthritis. J Rheumatol 21:744, 1994.

28

Ankylosing Spondylitis

Donald Resnick, M.D., and Gen Niwayama, M.D.

Ankylosing spondylitis is a chronic inflammatory disorder of unknown cause that affects principally the axial skeleton, although the appendicular skeleton also may be involved significantly. Alterations occur in synovial and cartilaginous joints and in sites of tendon and ligament attachment to bone. This chapter summarizes the important clinical, radiologic, and pathologic aspects of this disorder.

HISTORICAL ASPECTS

There is little doubt that ankylosing spondylitis has existed for thousands of years. Descriptions of this disease supplemented with skeletal remains found in museum collections document the existence of ankylosing spondylitis long before the modern era.[1, 2] The first detailed analysis appears to be that of an Irish physician and traveler, Bernard Connor (or O'Connor),[3, 216] who, in 1691, published a volume describing a skeleton with spondylitis[4] which he had obtained "in some church yard or charnel house." Connor observed bones that "were here so straightly and intimately joyned, their ligaments perfectly Bony, and their Articulations so effaced, that they really made but one uniform continuous Bone." Although in the succeeding years further descriptions of ankylosing spondylitis were published,[3, 5] it was not until the later years of the nineteenth century that, in reports by von Bechterew,[6] Strumpell,[7] and Marie,[8] accurate clinical descriptions were recorded.[1] The accuracy of von Bechterew's description of the disease has been questioned, however, leading some physicians to believe he was an excellent neurologist but a poor rheumatologist.[217] Even after these classic publications, the concept of ankylosing spondylitis as a distinct disease was clouded by its similarities to degenerative disorders of the spine. Finally, in 1904, Fraenkel[9] and Simmonds[10] emphasized in patients with ankylosing spondylitis the peculiar abnormalities of the posterior joints of the vertebral column that were unassociated with alterations of the intervertebral disc spaces. With the discovery and perfection of radiographic techniques in the late nineteenth and early twentieth centuries, a more complete understanding of the disease process emerged.[2]

NOMENCLATURE

Although ankylosing spondylitis is now the accepted name for this disease, many synonyms and eponyms have been used in the past. Such designations as rhizomelic spondylitis,[8] Marie-Strumpell's disease, von Bechterew's syndrome, pelvospondylitis ossificans, and spondylitis ossificans ligamentosa have appeared. In the United States, the name rheumatoid spondylitis was popular and was used even by the American Rheumatism Association until 1963. The incontrovertible evidence that this disease does not represent rheumatoid arthritis of the spine, however, cannot be ignored. Prominent sacroiliac joint abnormalities and spinal ligamentous calcification and ossification are not features of rheumatoid arthritis. Furthermore, rheumatoid arthritis predominates in women (whereas ankylosing spondylitis is more frequent in men) and is associated with rheumatoid nodules and a high frequency of positive serologic tests for rheumatoid factor (whereas this frequency is very low in ankylosing spondylitis). Profound clinical and radiologic dissimilarities exist in the two disorders, and although some pathologic aspects are similar, many differences can be found during the gross and microscopic examination of involved tissues in rheumatoid arthritis and ankylosing spondylitis.

Ankylosing spondylitis is an appropriate term for this articular disorder. Spondylitis, derived from the Greek word *spondylos,* meaning vertebra, implies inflammation of one or more vertebrae. Ankylosis is derived from the Greek word *ankylos,* meaning stiffening of a joint. On considering that this distinctive disease is associated with chronic inflammation of multiple articular structures, which frequently results in osseous ankylosis, the designation ankylosing spondylitis indeed does appear appropriate, and this term was adopted by the American Rheumatism Association in 1963.

DIAGNOSTIC CRITERIA

In conferences held in Rome and New York, two sets of specific criteria for the diagnosis of ankylosing spondylitis were developed[11, 12] (Table 28–1). Decrease in spinal mobility and limitation of chest expansion are fundamental in both sets of criteria. Although Moll and Wright[13] and others[218] have outlined certain limitations in the close application of these criteria, their usefulness or value cannot be denied. It must be recognized, however, that ankylosing spondylitis is but one of the seronegative spondyloarthropathies, and overlap among the clinical and radiologic features exists in the various disorders that comprise the seronegative spondyloarthropathies. With this in mind, classification criteria for the entire group of spondyloarthropathic conditions also have been developed.[318] These criteria are as follows: inflammatory spinal pain or synovitis, together with at least one of the following—positive family history, psoriasis, inflammatory bowel disease, urethritis, acute diarrhea, alternating buttock pain, enthesopathy, or radiographically evident sacroiliitis.[318]

PREVALENCE

Even though the frequency of ankylosing spondylitis has been described in previous reports, it is difficult to deter-

TABLE 28–1. Clinical Criteria for Ankylosing Spondylitis*

Rome Criteria (Kellgren, Jeffrey, Ball, 1963[11])
1. Low back pain and stiffness for more than 3 months
2. Pain and stiffness in the thoracic region
3. Limited motion in the lumbar spine
4. Limited chest expansion
5. History of evidence of iritis or its sequelae

Ankylosing spondylitis is present if bilateral sacroiliitis is associated with any one of these criteria

New York Criteria (Bennett and Wood, 1968[12])
1. Limitation of motion of the lumbar spine in anterior flexion, lateral flexion, and extension
2. A history of pain or the presence of pain at the dorsolumbar junction or in the lumbar spine
3. Limitation of chest expansion to one inch or less

   Definite ankylosing spondylitis is present if:
   a. Grade 3–4 bilateral sacroiliitis is associated with at least one clinical criterion
   b. Grade 3–4 unilateral or Grade 2 bilateral sacroiliitis is associated with clinical criterion 1 or with both clinical criteria 2 and 3
   or
   Probable ankylosing spondylitis is present if Grade 3–4 bilateral sacroiliitis is associated with none of these criteria

*After Moll JMH: *In* JT Scott (Ed): Copeman's Textbook of Rheumatic Diseases. 5th Ed. Edinburgh, Churchill Livingstone, 1978.

mine the true incidence of this disease because of the techniques of patient selection that were employed in many of these studies. Certainly ankylosing spondylitis is a common cause of back pain and disability, especially in young men. It has been estimated that 5 to 10 per cent of military patients with rheumatic symptoms and signs have ankylosing spondylitis.[14, 15] The prevalence of this disease in a general population is more difficult to determine, although a figure of approximately 0.1 per cent commonly is quoted.[16–18] This prevalence is lower in blacks[19] and in certain Indian tribes.[20] The precise ratio of the disease in men compared to women is not known, with reports varying from 4 to 1 to 10 to 1.[21–24] The true prevalence of ankylosing spondylitis in women may be much higher than these reports have indicated,[319] as some investigators,[25–27, 385] although not all,[294, 295, 320] have suggested that the disease may be more subtle and difficult to diagnose in female patients. In fact, community-based surveys have suggested that the ratio of men to women who have bilateral sacroiliitis is approximately 1 to 1 in those persons who possess the histocompatibility antigen HLA-B27.[219]

Radiographic and pathologic evaluation of spines has provided another method for determining the frequency of ankylosing spondylitis. Schmorl has recorded a frequency of 0.1 per cent in necropsy studies of approximately 10,000 vertebral columns, whereas Bochman, examining antemortem spinal radiographs obtained for a variety of reasons, noted the disease in 1.5 per cent of cases.[3]

The reported ratio of ankylosing spondylitis to rheumatoid arthritis has varied from 1 to 5 to 1 to 15.[3, 23, 28]

CLINICAL ABNORMALITIES

General Features

The onset of ankylosing spondylitis generally occurs between the ages of 15 and 35 years (average age of onset, 26 to 27 years)[23] in both men and women, although an earlier onset has been noted in some female patients.[29] In approximately 15 to 20 per cent of patients, the disorder begins in the second decade of life, and in 10 per cent of patients, it appears after the age of 39 years.[21] Indeed, in recent years, an increasing age of onset of the disease, with a better ultimate prognosis, has been emphasized.[321, 322] Ankylosing spondylitis occurring in children (juvenile-onset ankylosing spondylitis) also is well recognized (see Chapter 27). Clinical and radiologic manifestations may be influenced by the age of onset of the disease; in younger patients, neck and peripheral joint abnormalities[220, 221] may be more frequent, whereas in older patients, laterally displaced syndesmophytes (or osteophytes) are more common.[30] In juvenile-onset disease, hip involvement and persistence of peripheral arthritis also have been emphasized.[220] Less severe hip disease appears to be a feature of late-onset disease.[321]

An insidious onset of disease, which occurs in 75 to 80 per cent of patients, can lead to considerable delay in accurate diagnosis.[31, 32] Early clinical manifestations generally are noted in the back (70 to 80 per cent of patients), although they may appear in the peripheral joints (10 to 20 per cent of patients)[33] or in the chest.[34] Sciatic pain may be the initial symptom in 5 to 10 per cent of patients.[1, 2] Constitutional findings include anorexia, weight loss, and low grade fever. With respect to the natural history of the disease, most investigators regard it as remarkably benign. Many believe that there exists a large population with relatively asymptomatic and unrecognized abnormalities. A consensus is that in fewer than 20 per cent of patients with adult-onset ankylosing spondylitis does the disease progress to a condition of significant disability.[224] Furthermore, a predictable pattern of disease generally emerges in the first 10 years, and peripheral joint involvement, particularly that of the hip, represents a sign of poor prognosis.[224]

Axial Skeletal Symptoms and Signs

Clinical manifestations related to the spine and the sacroiliac joints are characteristic of ankylosing spondylitis.[1–3, 23, 35–37] Initially, transient aching pain and stiffness of variable intensity in the low back are observed, which subsequently may become persistent. With evolution of the disease, spread to the higher levels of the vertebral column is frequent. Although the progression may be segmental, beginning in the sacroiliac region and extending first to the lumbar spine and then to the thoracic and cervical regions, symptoms and signs may bypass any level of the spine.

Local pain and tenderness over the sacroiliac joints can be prominent in the early phases of the disease. With ankylosis of these joints, the clinical manifestations may become mild or disappear completely. Pain radiating into the lower extremities, resembling sciatica, can be observed in approximately 50 per cent of patients at some stage of the disorder and generally is unassociated with neurologic findings.[2] Yet myelography may be performed to investigate this finding; the appearance of residual contrast material within the spinal canal from a previous myelographic examination is extremely common on radiographic evaluation of the spine in patients with ankylosing spondylitis. CT[323] or MR imaging also can be used effectively to investigate sciatica in the patient with ankylosing spondylitis.

In the lumbar spine, paravertebral muscle spasm,

straightening of the vertebral column, tenderness to percussion, and muscle atrophy are observed; in the thoracic spine, similar abnormalities may be accompanied by diminished chest expansion and exaggeration of the normal kyphotic curvature.[38] Slight, moderate, or marked limitation of movement can be evident in the cervical spine. The head and neck protrude forward and the patient eventually may be forced to gaze constantly at the floor. Muscle spasm and radicular pain are additional manifestations of cervical spinal alterations.

The cauda equina syndrome can be observed in patients with ankylosing spondylitis.[39–40] Although its pathogenesis in this disease is not clear, the occurrence of loss of cutaneous sensation in the sacral and lower lumbar dermatomes, muscle weakness, and disturbed sphincter function may be related to arachnoiditis with subsequent loss of meningeal elasticity.[41] Myelography reveals a voluminous dural sac with arachnoid diverticula.[41, 42] These diverticula also produce characteristic osseous erosions of the laminae that can be detected with CT scanning or MR imaging (see later discussion).

Peripheral Skeletal Symptoms and Signs

Peripheral articular manifestations are apparent initially in approximately 10 to 20 per cent of patients[33] and eventually in as many as 50 per cent of patients.[23, 43] Involvement of peripheral joints in ankylosing spondylitis usually is seen simultaneously with or shortly after that of central articulations. Less commonly, peripheral joint abnormalities or enthesitis antedates spinal and sacroiliac findings and, rarely, appears as a very late manifestation of the disease.[263, 264] In most persons, the manifestations are mild and transient in nature[21] and are overshadowed by more prominent manifestations in the central skeleton. Asymmetric involvement of a few joints is typical. The hips, shoulders, knees, ankles, wrists, elbows, and small joints of the hands and feet can be affected.[44, 45] The sternoclavicular, manubriosternal, and temporomandibular joints also may be involved. Pain and swelling can simulate the findings of rheumatoid arthritis, although asymmetry is more frequent and residual destruction and deformity are less frequent in ankylosing spondylitis than in rheumatoid arthritis.

Involvement of the proximal or "root" joints (the hips and the shoulders) is particularly characteristic and may lead to severe clinical disability. In fact, bilateral hip abnormalities can produce significant limitation of motion and contracture; ambulation may subsequently become impossible.[46, 47] In a study of 87 patients with ankylosing spondylitis, many of whom had long-standing and severe disease, Dwosh and collaborators[46] noted clinical hip disease in 33 patients (38 per cent), which tended to begin early in the disease course. Typical findings included regional pain, limitation of motion, muscle atrophy, and flexion contractures. Hip abnormalities accounted for 50 per cent of the severe disability that was apparent in the entire study group.

Pain and tenderness over bony protuberances are elicited in many persons with ankylosing spondylitis. These manifestations may appear on the undersurface of the calcaneus, the symphysis pubis, the iliac crest, the trochanters of the femur, the ischial tuberosities, and the costal cartilages. The response to firm palpation of centrally and peripherally located entheses has been used as one method of clinical assessment in this disease.[324]

Extraskeletal Symptoms and Signs

Iritis occurs in 20 per cent of patients with ankylosing spondylitis[2] and may be the presenting feature of the disease.[48] Wilkinson and Bywaters[21] observed that this complication was more frequent in patients with peripheral arthropathy.

Spondylitic heart disease can lead to cardiac enlargement, conduction defects, and pericarditis, particularly in patients with chronic disease, peripheral arthritis, and prominent constitutional symptoms and signs.[49–51] Typically, aortic insufficiency due to inflammation of the aortic valve and aorta resembles the finding in syphilitic aortitis. Aortic aneurysms can be seen.

Pulmonary involvement in ankylosing spondylitis can become manifest as peculiar fibrosis and cavitation in the upper lobes, which simulate the findings in tuberculosis.[52, 53] Pleuritis also can be apparent.[54] Although a higher frequency of pulmonary tuberculosis had been recorded previously in patients with ankylosing spondylitis, recent studies have failed to document this association.

Additional systemic manifestations of ankylosing spondylitis include an association with inflammatory bowel disease (see Chapter 31) and with amyloidosis.[55–59] Cruickshank[55] observed that 6 per cent of patients with spondylitis die from renal failure due to amyloid involvement of the kidneys.

Radiation therapy during the course of ankylosing spondylitis can lead to certain complications. Aplastic anemia, leukemia, and transverse myelitis have been encountered in spondylitic patients treated with this method.[60, 61] Radiation-induced carcinomas of the skin and viscera and sarcomas of bone and soft tissue have been recorded in this clinical setting.[62, 63]

Laboratory Findings

In general, laboratory parameters are not useful in diagnosing or following patients with ankylosing spondylitis. The erythrocyte sedimentation rate frequently is elevated during the active phase and may become normal in later phases of the disease.[23] Results of serologic tests for rheumatoid and LE factors characteristically are negative, although 1 to 2 per cent of patients with ankylosing spondylitis may be positive for rheumatoid factor. Complement levels in articular fluid may be increased.[1, 2] Mild leukocytosis and anemia can be observed.

Many patients with ankylosing spondylitis possess the histocompatibility antigen HLA-B27. This finding may have profound implications (see discussion later in this chapter).

RADIOGRAPHIC-PATHOLOGIC CORRELATION

The general radiologic[3, 23, 30, 35, 36, 64–68, 203, 205] and pathologic[55, 69–71, 204] features of ankylosing spondylitis, particularly in the axial skeleton, have been well described.

General Distribution

Ankylosing spondylitis affects synovial and cartilaginous joints as well as sites of tendon and ligament attachment to bone (entheses). An overwhelming predilection exists for involvement of the axial skeleton, especially the sacroiliac, apophyseal, discovertebral, and costovertebral articulations (Fig. 28–1).

Classically, changes initially are noted in the sacroiliac joints and next appear at the thoracolumbar and lumbosacral junctions[35]; with disease chronicity, the midlumbar, the upper thoracic, and the cervical vertebrae may become involved.[21, 36] This characteristic pattern of spinal ascent by no means is invariable, however; it may occur slowly or rapidly[3, 36] and is less frequent in spondylitis accompanying psoriasis and Reiter's disease.[65] Spinal ascent in ankylosing spondylitis may become arrested at any stage, although radiographic abnormalities of the sacroiliac joint without vertebral changes are unusual except in the early phase of the disorder,[21] having been noted in 3 per cent[3] and 4 per cent[36] of patients followed for 1 to 5 years and for 10 years, respectively. Rarely, a higher prevalence of isolated sacroiliac joint abnormalities is reported.[229] Isolated sacroiliac joint abnormalities may be more frequent in women with the disease.[68, 229] Furthermore, in female patients, the combination of sacroiliac joint and cervical spinal abnormalities

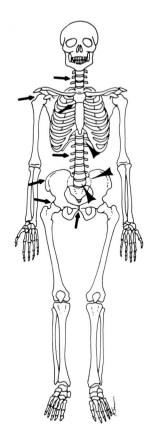

FIGURE 28–1. Ankylosing spondylitis: Distribution of articular disease. Initial abnormalities are most frequent in the sacroiliac joint and the thoracolumbar and lumbosacral junctions (arrowheads). Subsequent abnormalities are common in the entire vertebral column, the tendinous insertions in the pelvis and proximal femur, sternal joints, symphysis pubis, hips, and glenohumeral joints (arrows).

without significant thoracic or lumbar spinal changes appears more common than in male patients. Resnick and coworkers[68] noted this combination in 5 of 16 women (31 per cent) and in only 2 of 55 men (4 per cent); radiographic changes in the various segments of the spine, when present, did not differ significantly in these male and female patients, although the women revealed more frequent and severe osteitis pubis. Although other investigators have observed a higher prevalence of cervical spine abnormalities in women with the disease,[222, 296, 297] the finding has not been uniform[223, 325] nor always statistically significant.[219] A greater frequency of osteitis pubis and a lesser frequency of hip involvement in women have been noted in additional reports.[298, 320] Spinal alterations without sacroiliac joint changes in either men or women are unusual in classic ankylosing spondylitis,[23, 299] occurring in 0 to 3 per cent of patients, whereas this distribution is more frequent in psoriatic spondylitis.

Peripheral joint involvement in ankylosing spondylitis is not rare, especially in women.[68, 219, 223, 312] This involvement becomes more frequent with disease chronicity. The frequency of radiographically evident abnormalities in peripheral locations in cases of long-standing ankylosing spondylitis is greater than 50 per cent if all articulations are included, approaches 50 per cent if only the hips are excluded, and is approximately 30 per cent if both the hips and the glenohumeral joints are excluded.[72] Although initially only one or two peripheral areas may be involved, the eventual pattern is one of more diffuse articular disease. Radiographic changes predominate in the hips and the glenohumeral joints, followed in descending order of frequency by the knees, the hands, the wrists, and the feet, including the calcaneus. Bilateral abnormalities are common, although the degree of symmetry is less striking than in cases of rheumatoid arthritis.

Radiographic abnormalities also can be encountered in the symphysis pubis (frequently in combination with sacroiliac joint abnormalities), the manubriosternal, acromioclavicular, and sternoclavicular joints, and the temporomandibular joints (frequently in combination with cervical spine abnormalities). Changes also are evident at tendinous and ligamentous attachments to bone, such as the iliac crests, ischial tuberosities, greater and lesser trochanters, spinous processes, and inferior surface of the calcanei.

General Radiographic and Pathologic Abnormalities

Synovial Articulations (Fig. 28–2)

The classic histologic descriptions of synovial joint alterations in ankylosing spondylitis stress that the synovitis is similar or identical to that in rheumatoid arthritis.[70, 73, 225] Cellular infiltration with lymphocytes and plasma cells and fibrin deposition are expressions of nonspecific synovitis. In general, however, the inflammatory process in ankylosing spondylitis is more discrete and of lower intensity than in rheumatoid arthritis.[71] The density of the inflammatory cell infiltration and the extent of necrosis are less dramatic. Connective tissue reaction and proliferation with little exudation are apparent. Hyperplastic villi are noted, but severe pannus formation is less frequent. Marked fibroplasia may be followed by cartilaginous metaplasia with chondral os-

sification. In this manner, intra-articular bony ankylosis can be evident.[71, 74, 75] This ankylotic process in the small articulations of the axial skeleton also can result from ossification of the joint capsule.[69] The induction of bone formation at the peripheral capsular attachments is not unlike the enthesopathy that occurs at tendinous and ligamentous osseous attachments in this disease (see later discussion). After peripheral ankylosis, the remainder of the joint may be replaced partially or completely by endochondral ossification.

Additional pathologic features occurring in and around the synovial joints in ankylosing spondylitis relate to subchondral bone sclerosis and periosteal elevation.[76] Although the exact stimulus for such bone formation is not clear, it represents an important radiographic and pathologic characteristic of ankylosing spondylitis (and other seronegative spondyloarthropathies, such as psoriasis and Reiter's syndrome) and is not prominent in rheumatoid arthritis.

The basic similarity of pathologic alterations in synovial joints in ankylosing spondylitis and rheumatoid arthritis accounts for the overlap in their radiographic features. Both cause some degree of osteoporosis, joint space narrowing, and osseous erosion. Certain findings are more characteristic of ankylosing spondylitis than of rheumatoid arthritis, however. Prominent periarticular osteoporosis is not common in ankylosing spondylitis. In fact, subchondral eburnation is typical. Periostitis also is observed, resulting in irregular or shaggy periarticular osseous surfaces. Periosteal proliferation can extend into the metaphyses and the diaphyses of the neighboring bones.

Extensive and diffuse joint space diminution is more frequent in rheumatoid arthritis than in ankylosing spondylitis. It may be noted in the latter disease, particularly in the wrist, the metacarpophalangeal joints, the hip, and the knee. In ankylosing spondylitis, intra-articular bony ankylosis is common in the synovial joints of both the axial (the sacroiliac, the costovertebral, and the apophyseal joints) and the extra-axial (the hip, the wrist, and the articulations of the midfoot) skeleton. Such ankylosis can involve the entire joint surface or only the peripheral and capsular segments. In adult-onset rheumatoid arthritis, fibrous ankylosis is more characteristic except in the carpal and tarsal areas, at which sites massive osseous fusion may be evident.

The osseous erosions in ankylosing spondylitis typically are smaller and more localized than those of rheumatoid arthritis, although large erosions of metacarpal, metatarsal, and humeral heads can be encountered. Subchondral cyst formation and significant subluxations are two additional features that are more frequent in rheumatoid arthritis than in ankylosing spondylitis.

Cartilaginous Articulations (Fig. 28–3)

In the cartilaginous joints of the axial skeleton (the discovertebral junction, the symphysis pubis, and the manubriosternal articulation), profound pathologic changes occur in ankylosing spondylitis.[69–71, 77, 226, 227, 300] The fundamental process, as judged mainly by observations at the discovertebral junction, appears to be inflammatory in nature, as shown by mild to moderate cellular infiltration (plasma cells and lymphocytes) and fibrin accumulation. Swelling of the nuclei of fibrocytes in the outer layer of the anulus fibrosus is followed by chondroid transformation of the connective tissue. Columns of chondrocytes appear at the junction of the intervertebral disc with the vertebral edge, and these subsequently undergo calcification and become vascularized from the subjacent bone. Ossification produces syndesmophytes that extend from one vertebral body to another. The adjacent bony surface is eroded, with surrounding eburnation. Elsewhere at the discovertebral junction, endochondral ossification and excessive discal calcification and ossification are evident.[226]

On radiographic examination, findings include erosion and sclerosis of adjacent bony surfaces and osseous bridging. Eventually, extensive bony ankylosis of the entire articulation may be evident. These alterations in cartilaginous joints are typical of seronegative spondyloarthropathies and are not characteristic of skeletal involvement in rheumatoid arthritis.

Entheses (Fig. 28–4)

Abnormalities in ligamentous attachments (enthesopathy[310]) are a prominent feature of ankylosing spondylitis and other seronegative spondyloarthropathies. Inflammation with cellular infiltration by lymphocytes, plasma cells, and polymorphonuclear leukocytes is associated with erosion and eburnation of the subligamentous bone.[69] Similar changes are evident in surrounding connective tissue.[228] On radiographs, poorly defined erosive abnormalities with surrounding sclerosis are observed. As the lesions heal, the sclerosis decreases, the osseous surface becomes less irregular, and well-defined bony excrescences appear.

Radiographic and Pathologic Abnormalities at Specific Sites

Sacroiliac Joint (Figs. 28–5 and 28–6)

Sacroiliitis is the hallmark of ankylosing spondylitis.[21–23, 36, 64–66, 70, 78–81, 326, 327] It occurs early in the course of the disease. Although an asymmetric or unilateral distribution can be evident on initial radiographic examination, radiographic changes at later stages of the disease almost invariably are bilateral and symmetric in distribution. This symmetric pattern is an important diagnostic clue in this disease and may permit its differentiation from other disorders that affect the sacroiliac joint, such as rheumatoid arthritis, psoriasis, Reiter's syndrome, and infection.

Changes in the sacroiliac joint occur in both the synovial and ligamentous (superior and posterior) portions. They predominate in the ilium, a predilection that is shared by many other processes that involve this joint. Although the exact reason for the predominant involvement of the ilium is obscure, mechanical or anatomic features may be important. The iliac cartilage is thinner than that of the sacrum[82] and possesses normal right-angle "splits"[83] as well as degenerative clefts.[82] Inflammatory synovial tissue might easily gain access to the subchondral bone of the ilium through these anatomic and pathologic gaps in the chondral surface, whereas the sacral surface, possessing a thicker layer of protective cartilage, might be less vulnerable. Initial changes consist of patchy periarticular osteoporosis, particularly about the middle and lower thirds of the joint cavity, and loss of definition, superficial erosion, and focal sclerosis of subchondral bone. A poorly defined subchondral bone plate is an important radiographic sign of sacroiliitis that is not observed in degenerative sacroiliac joint disease.

Further erosive changes lead to considerable fraying of the osseous surface and widening of the interosseous space. This progression of bone destruction is paralleled by increasing eburnation of surrounding osseous tissue. The entire subchondral bony surface eventually may become sclerotic, especially in the ilium.[328, 329] The wide and poorly defined band of sclerosis in this disease differs from the thin and well-defined sclerotic margin typical of degenerative disease and from the localized sclerotic areas characteristic of rheumatoid arthritis. In some cases, the pattern of sclerosis in ankylosing spondylitis simulates that of osteitis condensans ilii.

As proliferative bony changes in the sacroiliac joint become more prominent, irregular bony bridges traverse the articular cavity. This process of osseous fusion initially is incomplete, isolating one or more cartilaginous islands. Later, complete ankylosis can be observed, obliterating the entire joint cavity. Periarticular eburnation subsequently can become diminished and the radiodensity of the bone may return to normal, although a star-shaped area of bony condensation may remain in the upper one third of the joint cavity.

Blurring and irregularity of the ligamentous portion of the sacroiliac space are frequent in ankylosing spondylitis. Calcification and ossification of the ligament can be observed. When extensive and combined with intra-articular ankylosis, bony fusion of the entire sacroiliac space (synovial and ligamentous) is seen. Rarely, such ankylosis may be combined with significant subluxation of the joint.[189]

This description of radiographic abnormalities of the sacroiliac joint in ankylosing spondylitis indicates that characteristic, if not diagnostic, changes in this location do occur, and that the radiographic evaluation is fundamental to the early and correct diagnosis of the disease. In fact, establishing the diagnosis in the absence of radiographic alterations in the sacroiliac joints is difficult. It must be emphasized, however, that meticulous radiographic technique is required[230] and even with such technique, diagnostic difficulties are encountered.[231] The complex anatomy and undulating articular surfaces of the sacroiliac joint resist ideal demonstration on routine plain film examination, requiring angulation of the x-ray beam. A series of films may be required.[232] Intra- and interobserver variation in the interpretation of the sacroiliac joint radiographs is well documented,[233] and further difficulty is encountered as a result of the presence of sacroiliac joint changes on radiographs of a "normal" or "control" population[234] and of degenerative-like alterations in some patients, especially women, with sacroiliitis.[235] Even the application of a grading system to the radiographic analysis of sacroiliitis does little to overcome the diagnostic difficulties. As a result, in recent years, emphasis has been directed to additional techniques, such as scintigraphy, MR imaging, and CT scanning, that may be used to image the sacroiliac joints (see discussion later in this chapter) (Fig. 28–7).

Spine (Table 28–2)

Abnormalities of the spine can be seen in the discovertebral junction, apophyseal joint, costovertebral joints, posterior ligamentous attachments, and atlantoaxial joints.[21, 23, 36, 64–66, 84] Although initially apparent at the thoracolumbar and lumbosacral junctions, changes eventually can be noted throughout the vertebral column. Early findings may be

Text continued on page 1019

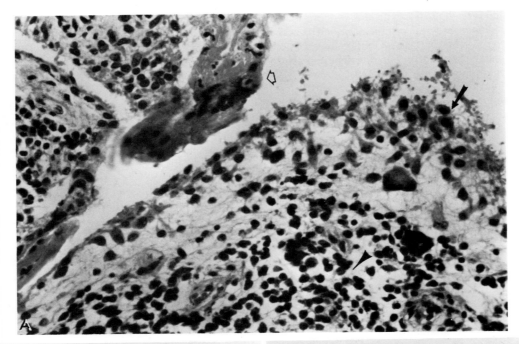

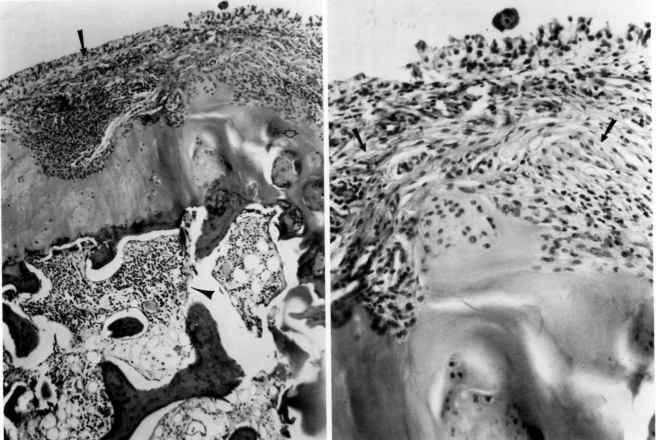

FIGURE 28–2. Synovial joints. General radiologic and pathologic abnormalities.
   A Synovial changes. Abnormalities resemble those of rheumatoid arthritis. Proliferation of the surface lining cells of the synovium (solid arrow), dense infiltration with lymphoid and plasmacytoid cells (arrowhead), and fibrinous cellular exudate (fibrin and inflammatory cells) (open arrow) are evident (200×).
   B Articular cartilage changes. Inflammatory pannus (solid arrow) covers the cartilaginous surface. Observe focal chondrocyte proliferation (open arrow) and subchondral lymphoid cell aggregates (arrowhead) (80×).
   C Articular cartilage changes. Pannus with fibroblastic and lymphoid cells and small capillaries (arrows) covers the cartilaginous surface (200×).

Illustration continued on opposite page

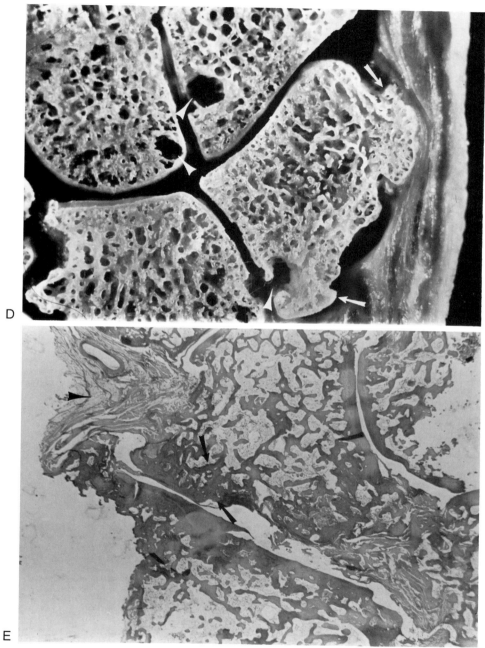

FIGURE 28–2 *Continued*
D Subchondral bone changes. A photograph of a macerated coronal section of the wrist in a cadaver with ankylosing spondylitis reveals osseous proliferation of the triquetrum (arrows), creating an irregular bony outline. Note multiple subchondral cysts and erosions (arrowheads).
E Subchondral bone changes. A photomicrograph (3×) of the radial aspect of the wrist in this same cadaver indicates hyperplastic cartilage, subchondral osteosclerosis (arrows), particularly of the scaphoid, and synovial fibrosis (arrowhead).

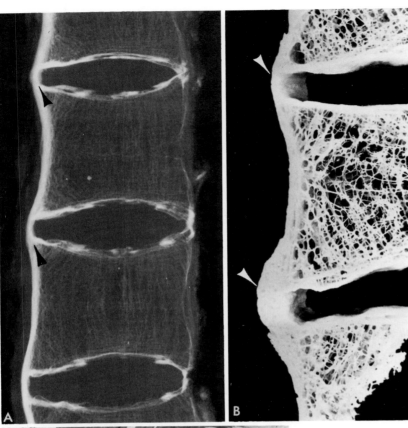

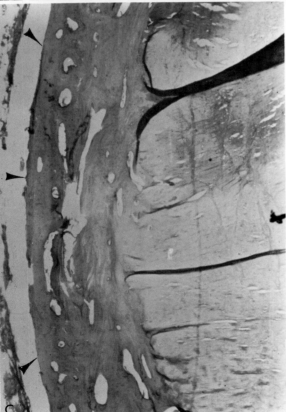

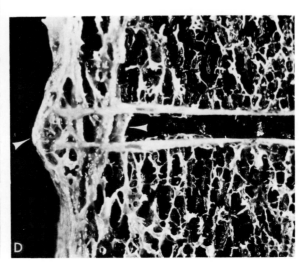

FIGURE 28–3. Cartilaginous articulations: General radiologic and pathologic abnormalities. Discovertebral junction.

A, B A radiograph and photograph of a sagittal section of the spine (the left side of each picture is anterior) reveal typical syndesmophytes (arrowheads) extending from one vertebral body to another. Note their vertical direction and slender configuration.

C On a photomicrograph (10×) of the discovertebral region, the nature of the syndesmophyte (arrowheads) is clear. It represents ossification of the outer fibers of the anulus fibrosus.

D On a macerated sagittal section of the spine, progressive ossification (arrowheads) of the intervertebral disc can be seen. Eventually, the entire disc may be obliterated.

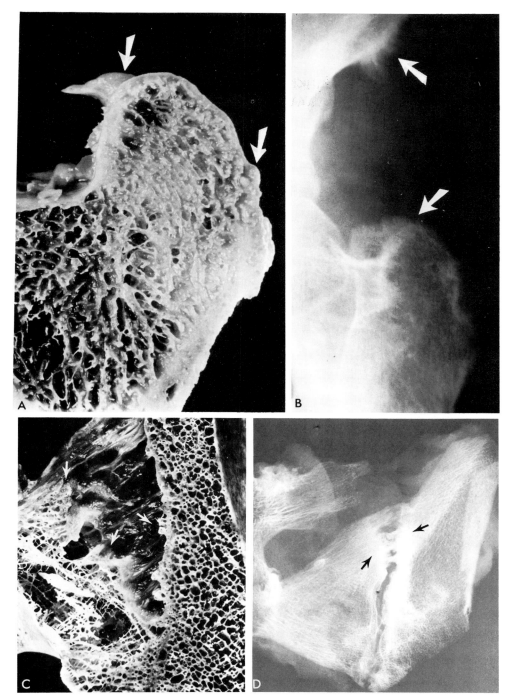

FIGURE 28–4. Entheses: General radiologic and pathologic abnormalities. Femoral trochanter and sacroiliac joint.
  A A photograph of a coronal section through the greater trochanter reveals mild osseous excrescences (arrows) related to enthesopathy.
  B Radiographic findings include irregular hyperostosis of the trochanter and the iliac crest (arrows).
  C, D A photograph and radiograph of two coronal sections of the sacroiliac joint show inflammatory enthesopathy at the sacral and ilial attachments of the interosseous ligament (arrows) above the true synovium lined portion of the joint (which itself demonstrates bony ankylosis in **C**). Osseous proliferation predominates.

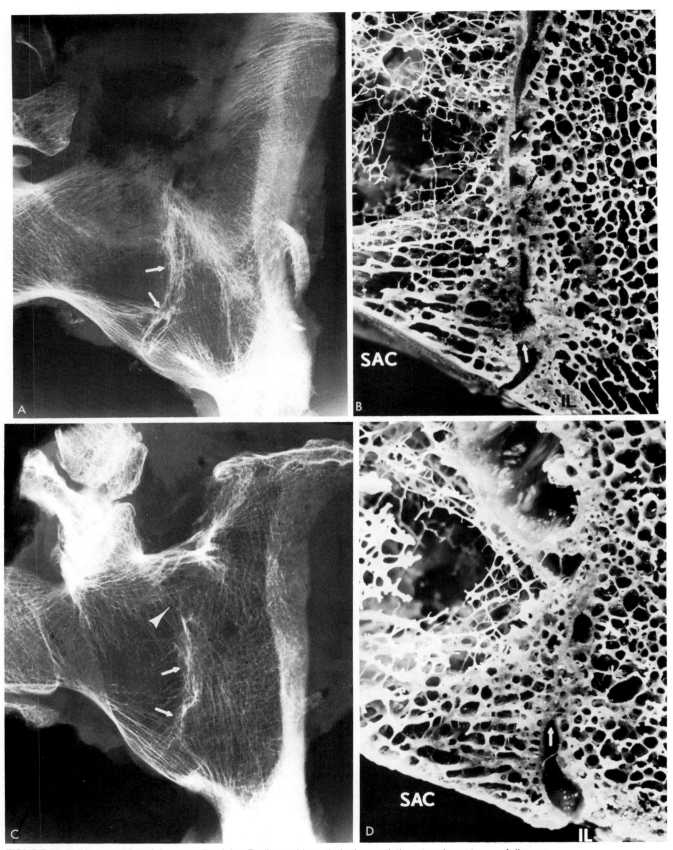

FIGURE 28–5. Abnormalities of the sacroiliac joint. Radiographic-pathologic correlation at various stages of disease.

A, B A coronal sectional radiograph and photograph reveal superficial erosions (arrowhead) and partial ossification (arrows) of the articular cavity. SAC, Sacrum; IL, ilium.

C, D In another coronal sectional radiograph and photograph, more complete bony ankylosis (arrows) of the joint is observed. In addition, the ligamentous space above the synovial joint is ossified (arrowhead) on the radiograph.

Illustration continued on opposite page

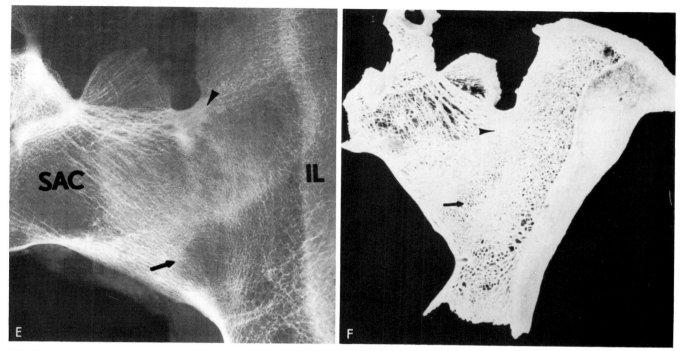

FIGURE 28–5 *Continued*
E, F This coronal sectional radiograph and corresponding photograph reveal complete ossification of the entire synovial (arrows) and ligamentous (arrowheads) space.

more difficult to detect than concomitant abnormalities in the sacroiliac joints, and it is unusual to find significant spinal alterations without sacroiliac joint changes.[85] Occasionally, coned-down views of the lower thoracic and upper lumbar vertebrae delineate abnormalities at an early stage

TABLE 28–2. Terminology Commonly Applied to Spinal Abnormalities in Ankylosing Spondylitis

Term	Definition
Osteitis	Enthesopathy occurring at discovertebral junction associated with erosion, sclerosis, and syndesmophytosis
"Shiny corner" sign	Increased radiodensity of the corners of the vertebral body related to "osteitis"
Squaring	Straightened or convex anterior margin of the vertebral body related to erosion
Syndesmophyte	Ossification within the anulus fibrosus leading to thin, vertical radiodense areas
Bamboo spine	Undulating vertebral contour due to extensive syndesmophytosis
Discitis	"Erosive" abnormalities of the discovertebral junction related to several mechanisms (see Table 28–3)
Discal ballooning	Biconvex shape of the intervertebral disc related to osteoporotic deformity of the vertebral body
Trolley-track sign	Three vertical radiodense lines on frontal radiographs related to ossification of supraspinous and interspinous ligaments and apophyseal joint capsules
Dagger sign	Single central radiodense line on frontal radiographs related to ossification of supraspinous and interspinous ligaments

of the disease when the sacroiliac joints appear grossly unremarkable.

Abnormalities of paraspinal musculature have been observed in patients with ankylosing spondylitis. Elevated serum enzyme levels[254] and abnormal electromyographic and biopsy studies[255] suggest direct muscle involvement as a feature of the disease. Muscle atrophy is well recognized on clinical examination and can be visualized with CT[256, 301] (see Fig. 28–48).

Discovertebral Junction. Lesions affecting the discovertebral junction include osteitis, syndesmophytosis, erosions, discal calcification, and osteoporosis and discal ballooning.

Osteitis (Fig. 28–8). Focal destructive areas along the anterior margin of the discovertebral junction at the superior and inferior portions of the vertebral body have been termed "Romanus lesions."[84] They are an early and significant feature of ankylosing spondylitis. Osseous erosion (osteitis) of the corners of the vertebral body, when combined with bone formation, results in loss of the normal concavity of the anterior vertebral surface, creating a squared or planed-down contour.[330] This change in vertebral configuration is much easier to assess in the lumbar spine, owing to the normal exaggerated concavity of the vertebral bodies, and more difficult to detect in the thoracic spine, at which site the vertebral bodies may have a relatively straight configuration normally. As the erosions heal, reactive sclerosis produces highlighting, "whitening," or a "shiny corner" configuration. The increased radiodensity at the vertebral margins is accentuated by adjacent osteoporosis, which increases in severity as the disease progresses.

Syndesmophytosis (Fig. 28–9). The erosive vertebral abnormalities are associated with bone formation, which extends across the margin of the intervertebral disc. Thin

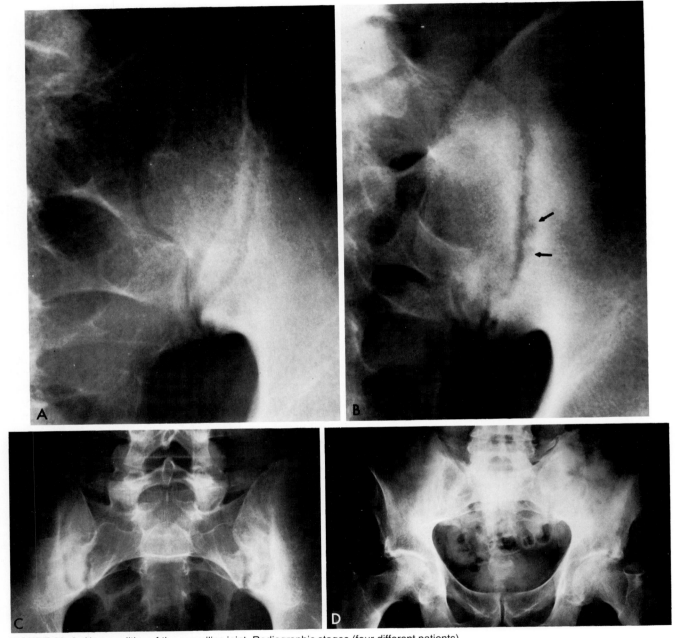

FIGURE 28–6. Abnormalities of the sacroiliac joint. Radiographic stages (four different patients).
  A Initial abnormalities consist of superficial bony erosion and eburnation, predominantly in the ilium.
  B At a slightly later stage, note larger erosions (arrows), progressive sclerosis, and focal narrowing of the articular space.
  C At a more advanced stage, bilateral symmetric changes consist of extensive sclerosis and focal ankylosis.
  D Eventually, complete ankylosis of the synovial and ligamentous portions of the sacroiliac space on both sides is evident. Sclerosis has diminished.

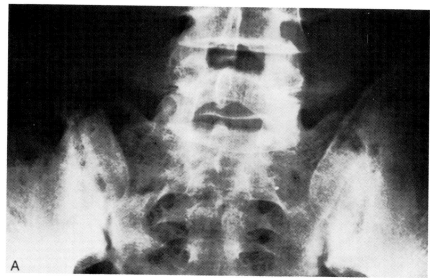

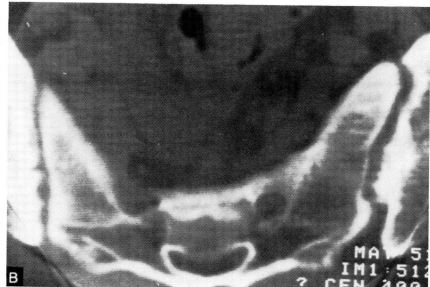

FIGURE 28–7. Abnormalities of the sacroiliac joint: Use of CT scanning.

A The routine radiograph documents bilateral, symmetric abnormalities consisting of bone erosion and sclerosis.

B With CT, a transverse section of the lower portion of the synovium-lined area of the joint confirms the presence of bilateral alterations and the predominant involvement of the ilium.

vertical outgrowths are termed syndesmophytes and represent ossification of the anulus fibrosus itself.[37, 69] As the syndesmophytes enlarge, ossification can involve the adjacent anterior longitudinal ligament and paravertebral connective tissue. Syndesmophytes predominate on the anterior and lateral aspects of the spine, particularly near the thoracolumbar junction. Eventually they bridge the intervertebral disc space, connecting one vertebral body with its neighbor, merging with the vertebral margins on either side. Even in later stages of the disease, the vertical nature of the outgrowths and their connection to the vertebral edges allow their differentiation from spinal osteophytes (which are triangular in shape and arise several millimeters from the discovertebral junction), and the paravertebral ossification of psoriasis and Reiter's syndrome (which begins at a distance from the vertebral body and intervertebral disc). In the later phases of ankylosing spondylitis, extensive syndesmophytes produce the undulating vertebral contour that is termed bamboo spine.

Discovertebral Erosions and Destruction (Table 28–3). Destructive foci that appear throughout the discovertebral

junction in ankylosing spondylitis are frequently termed Andersson lesions after the investigator who first noted them in two patients with the disease in 1937.[86] In 1940, Edstrom[87] further delineated the radiographic abnormalities

TABLE 28–3. Types of Discovertebral Erosions in Ankylosing Spondylitis

Type	Probable Mechanism
Localized central lesions	Cartilaginous node formation aggravated by a. Osteoporosis b. Instability due to apophyseal joint disease c. Intraosseous inflammatory changes
Localized peripheral lesions	
1. Anterior	Enthesopathy, cartilaginous node formation, or intervertebral disc changes related to kyphosis
2. Posterior	Enthesopathy or cartilaginous node formation
Extensive central and peripheral lesions	Fracture with "pseudarthrosis," or segmental spinal ankylosis with abnormal motion at unfused levels

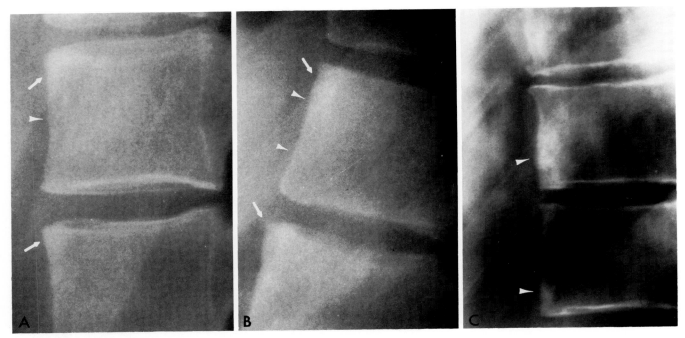

FIGURE 28–8. Osteitis: Radiographic abnormalities (three different patients).
  A Osseous erosion and sclerosis have produced whitening of the corners and margins along the anterior surfaces of the vertebrae (arrows). Note the straightening of the vertebral surface (arrowhead).
  B Considerable straightening (arrowheads) and bone formation (arrows) along the anterior vertebral surface are observed.
  C A convex anterior margin (arrowheads) of the vertebral bodies is associated with eburnation.

of these lesions in an investigation of a male patient with ankylosing spondylitis. Since that report, numerous articles have emphasized destructive abnormalities of the discovertebral junction in this disorder.[21, 86, 88–106, 195–197, 313, 331–333] In previous investigations, these abnormalities had been attributed to various factors, including inflammatory lesions, infections, discal displacements, and fractures with improper healing or pseudarthroses. It is evident from these prior reports that the lesions are not identical, some being localized to a segment of the discovertebral junction and others involving the entire intervertebral disc–bony margin; in addition, they have been observed during early and late phases of disease, and they have occurred in traumatized and nontraumatized spines.

Cawley and collaborators[195] classified the lesions into three types: those that involve the central portions of the discovertebral junction, which are covered by the cartilaginous endplate (type I); those that involve the peripheral portions of the discovertebral junction, which are not covered by the cartilaginous endplate (type II); and those that involve both peripheral and central portions of the discovertebral junction (type III) (Fig. 28–10). From a review of available literature, these investigators noted that radiographically evident destructive lesions had been reported in 1 to 28 per cent of patients and that localized lesions (types I and II) occurred in early or late stages of the disease, whereas extensive lesions (type III) rarely were observed without widespread spinal ankylosis. Furthermore, the severely destructive discovertebral lesions were relatively uncommon and showed predilection for the thoracic or lumbar segments. The comprehensive study of the clinical, radiologic, and pathologic characteristics of localized and generalized lesions of the discovertebral junction that was un-

dertaken by these investigators represents the most accurate analysis to date. In the following paragraphs, each of these three types of discovertebral destruction is summarized. Subsequently, problems relating to this classification system are addressed.

Localized, Central Discovertebral Lesions (Type I) (Fig. 28–11). Lesions localized to the central subchondral portions of the discovertebral junction can be observed in ankylosed and nonankylosed spines. Histologic evaluation confirms the presence of intraosseous discal displacement (Schmorl's or cartilaginous nodes) in many of the cases. Although such displacements can occur in association with many disease processes or as an incidental finding during postmortem examination,[107] there are three factors in ankylosing spondylitis, which, working independently or together, can contribute to their production. First, osteoporosis of the vertebrae, which may be marked in patients with this disease, leads to osseous weakening, allowing displacement of discal contents through the cartilaginous endplate into the vertebral body. Second, abnormalities at the apophyseal joints in ankylosing spondylitis alter the forces across the discovertebral junction and can result in recurrent traumatic insults to the intervertebral disc–bone interface. These insults eventually can produce infractions of the cartilaginous endplate or subchondral bone plate, facilitating the protrusion of discal material into the vertebral body. A third factor, inflammatory changes in the subchondral bone leading to osseous weakening and discal displacement, has not been verified by most available pathologic data,[69] although Sutherland and Matheson[98] observed granulomatous lesions without obvious changes in the cartilaginous endplate.

Radiographic examination outlines irregularity of the

central portion of the superior and inferior vertebral margins, and radiolucent areas with surrounding sclerosis in the vertebral bodies are present. The appearance is similar or identical to that associated with cartilaginous nodes from any cause, the discovertebral lesions of rheumatoid arthritis, and infection.

Localized, Peripheral Discovertebral Lesions (Type II) (Fig. 28–11). Although discal displacement can lead to eccentric irregularities of the discovertebral junction, other mechanisms may be important in the production of peripheral discovertebral lesions in ankylosing spondylitis. The resemblance of anterior discovertebral lesions in the spondylitic thoracic spine to those seen in senile kyphosis may be striking[108] (see Chapter 51). Progressive kyphosis in elderly, nonspondylitic persons may lead to injury to the anterior fibers of the anulus fibrosus and to invasion and replacement of the discal material by vascular fibrous tissue, which ultimately ossifies (senile kyphosis). Alternatively, collapse of osteoporotic anterior vertebral margins (osteoporotic kyphosis) can be encountered in these persons. As thoracic kyphosis is common in patients with ankylosing spondylitis, a similar sequence of abnormalities may occur, producing anterior discovertebral lesions.

Although the pathogenesis of localized lesions of the posterior portion of the discovertebral junction in the thoracic spine and the anterior and posterior portions of the discovertebral junction in the lumbar spine in patients with ankylosing spondylitis is not clear, osteoporotic collapse or cartilaginous (Schmorl's) nodes could be important. Furthermore, inflammation in the outer fibers of the anulus fibrosus related to the spondylitic process may play a role in the development of these lesions; such inflammatory lesions may heal spontaneously, with the development of bony ankylosis.[99]

Extensive Central and Peripheral Discovertebral Lesions (Type III) (Fig. 28–12). Destruction of the entire discovertebral junction of two neighboring vertebral bodies occurs almost exclusively in patients with advanced ankylosis. Narrowing of the intervertebral disc space and reactive sclerosis of the subjacent bone can be observed. Many patients relate a history of significant trauma, and radiographs (or conventional tomograms) obtained at the time of injury may reveal an associated fracture through the ankylosed apophyseal articulations, the neighboring articular processes, or, rarely, the laminae or spinous process. Histologic data[86, 96, 241, 334] are consistent with improper healing following a fracture of the discovertebral junction. Callus and hemorrhage have been observed, and, although inflammatory changes with cellular infiltration can be seen, these latter abnormalities generally are mild, suggesting that trauma rather than inflammation is the major factor in the production of these lesions. Epidural hematomas are seen in approximately 20 per cent of cases.[243, 314, 339] The bleeding may arise from lacerated vessels or from the diploe of the pathologic bone or, rarely, from aortic disruption.[333] Damage to the aorta may relate to its adherence to the anterior longitudinal ligament or to the unstable nature of the fracture, or both.[333] The importance of a traumatic pathogenesis in the production of generalized discovertebral abnormalities is underscored by serial radiographs that indicate an initial fracture of the spine and the subsequent development of bone destruction and sclerosis.

The ankylosed spine in later stages of this disease is

vulnerable to fracture, a vulnerability that is accentuated by adjacent vertebral osteoporosis (Fig. 28–13). The cervical spine is especially susceptible to fracture, and neurologic complications with death may result.[109, 110, 198, 335, 336] The fracture usually results from a hyperextension injury, which may be mild, and typically affects the lower cervical segments; it generally extends through what was formerly an intervertebral disc and is unstable.[242, 302–304] Rarely, higher segments of the cervical spine, including the odontoid process, may be affected.[337, 338] Conversely, fractures in the thoracic and lumbar spine in ankylosing spondylitis often are unrecognized clinically.[100, 244, 340, 341] Biomechanically, these latter fractures resemble the "seat-belt" or Chance fracture, presumably because of a shift of the axis of flexion and extension in the ankylosed spine from its normal location in the center of the nucleus pulposus.[102] Hyperextension injuries lead to spinal fractures that begin anteriorly in the vertebral body or, more commonly, the intervertebral disc; hyperflexion injuries produce spinal fractures that commence in the posterior osseous elements of the vertebra.[342, 345] Many of the resulting fractures become displaced, although healing frequently occurs satisfactorily with suitable immobilization. With continued movement at the fracture site, however, fibrous union, resulting in what has been labeled a "pseudarthrosis," can occur.[342, 343] In these latter cases, spinal fusion may be required.

The radiographic appearance of improper fracture union of the spine resembles that observed in infection or neuropathic osteoarthropathy, although a soft tissue mass is common in infective spondylitis and rare in delayed union or nonunion of a fracture.[245, 332] Detection of bony ankylosis of adjacent vertebral segments and a fracture of the posterior elements ensures accurate diagnosis.

Other Types of Discovertebral Lesions. The classification system outlined by Cawley and collaborators[195] just described is useful, but other varieties of discovertebral lesions are encountered in ankylosing spondylitis. In some cases, focal areas of bone erosion and sclerosis involve both the central and the peripheral portions of the discovertebral junction. The lesions, which often are referred to as spondylodiscitis, appear to be inflammatory in pathogenesis and may occur at a very early stage of the disease.[236–238, 313] Single or multiple levels in the thoracic and lumbar segments of the spine are affected. Loss of intervertebral disc height and extensive new bone formation resemble the findings of infection, although there is no clinical or laboratory evidence to support the latter diagnosis. When the discovertebral lesions are unaccompanied by sacroiliac joint changes, the presence of ankylosing spondylitis is difficult to establish.[299] Later, with the appearance of sacroiliitis and more typical spinal abnormalities, the diagnostic dilemma is resolved. In some cases, spondylodiscitis remains an isolated phenomenon and, in fact, the discovertebral destruction disappears.[238–240] The term erosive spondylopathy is commonly applied to these latter cases, and their relationship to ankylosing spondylitis appears distant or nonexistent (Fig. 28–14).

Extensive central and peripheral discovertebral destruction (type III lesion) is seen in some patients with ankylosing spondylitis who have not had a spinal fracture. In these persons, uneven or segmental involvement of the vertebral column leads to ankylosed portions separated by a relatively mobile region. Abnormal motion at the latter site

Text continued on page 1031

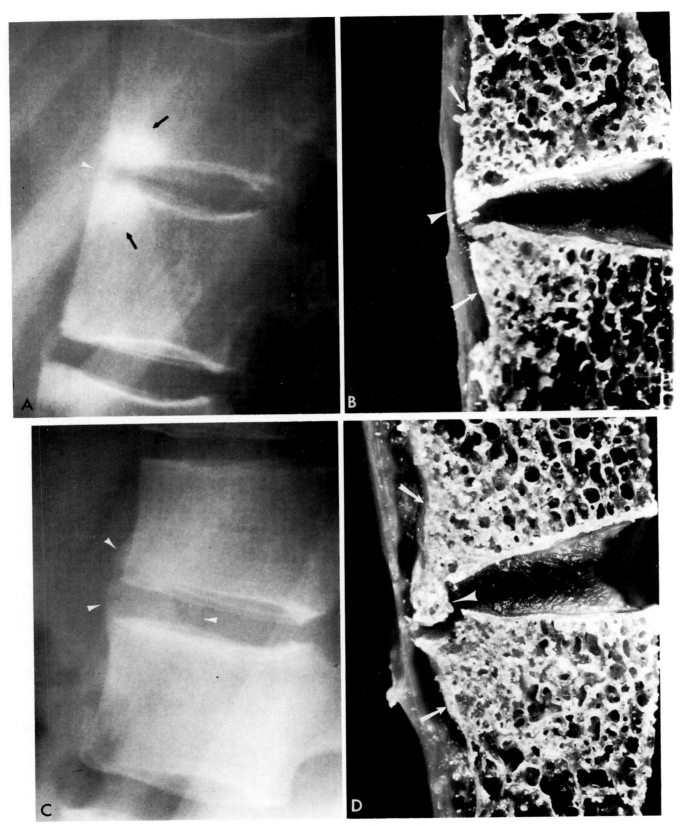

FIGURE 28–9. *See legend on opposite page*

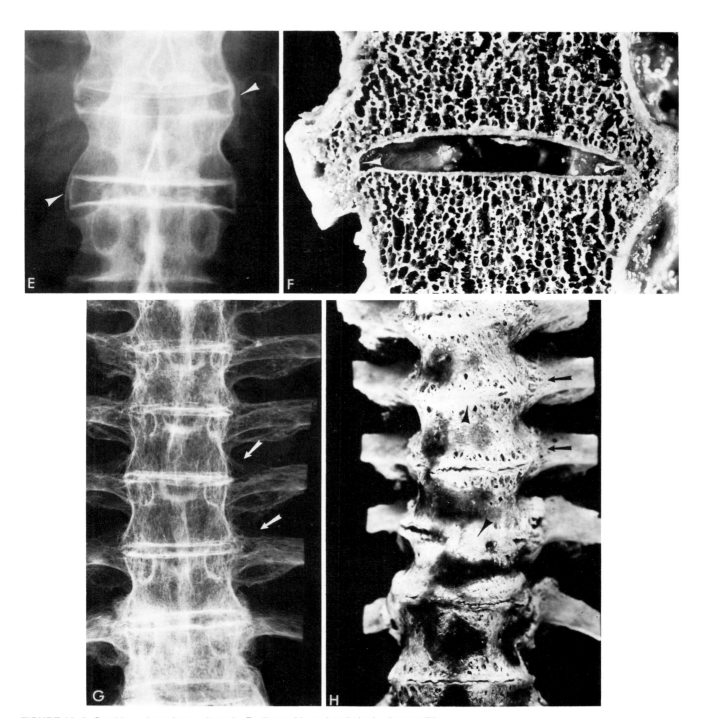

FIGURE 28–9. Osteitis and syndesmophytosis: Radiographic and pathologic abnormalities.

A In association with osteitis of the corners of the vertebral bodies (arrows), early syndesmophyte formation has produced blurring of the margin of the intervertebral disc (arrowhead).

B A photograph of a sagittal section of two vertebral bodies reveals osteitis (arrows) and syndesmophytosis (arrowhead), representing ossification of the intervertebral disc.

C In a different patient, more extensive syndesmophyte formation (arrowheads) is apparent.

D An additional photograph of a macerated sagittal section of two vertebral bodies indicates progressive osteitis (arrows) and syndesmophyte formation (arrowhead).

E A frontal radiograph reveals typical syndesmophytes (arrowheads). They extend in a vertical fashion from one vertebral body to the next.

F These outgrowths (arrowheads) are well shown on a macerated coronal section of the spine. Note that with growth, the syndesmophytes may extend into the adjacent soft tissues.

G, H Bamboo spine. An anteroposterior radiograph and photograph (anterior view) of a macerated whole spine reveal widespread syndesmophytosis, leading to ossification of multiple intervertebral discs (arrowheads). An undulating spinal contour has been produced. Observe costovertebral joint ankylosis (arrows).

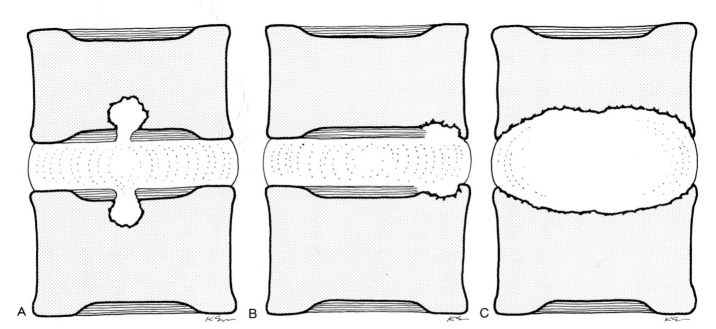

FIGURE 28–10. Discovertebral erosion and destruction: Types of lesions.

A Localized central discovertebral lesions. Defects with surrounding eburnation in the central portion of the discovertebral junction may reflect intraosseous displacement of disc material (cartilaginous nodes).

B Localized peripheral discovertebral lesions. Defects may occur on the anterior or posterior aspect of the discovertebral junction. Their cause is obscure; they may relate to kyphosis with discal injury, cartilaginous node formation, or enthesopathy.

C Extensive central and peripheral discovertebral lesions. Destruction of the entire discovertebral junction frequently is the result of improper fracture healing.

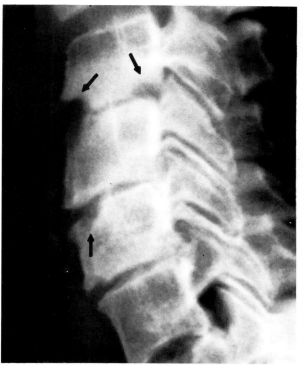

A

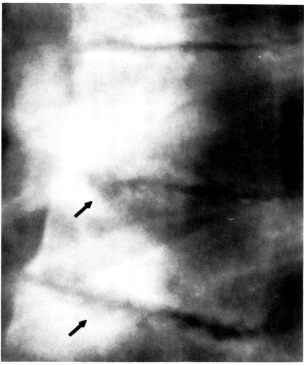

B

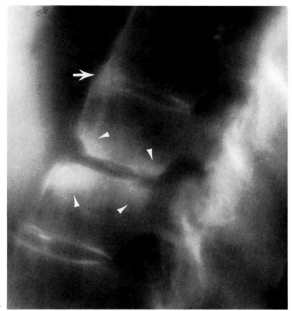

C

FIGURE 28–11. Discovertebral erosions and destruction: Localized peripheral and localized central lesions.

A Localized anterior and posterior defects (arrows) are apparent at multiple levels. Considerable intervertebral disc space narrowing and bony sclerosis are accompanying findings, and the apophyseal joints are relatively intact. The appearance of some of the localized lesions is reminiscent of that associated with cartilaginous nodes.

B Localized central and peripheral defects (arrows) are recognized. They have produced slight irregularity of the entire discovertebral junction, although extensive resorption and sclerosis, as seen in a so-called pseudarthrosis, are not evident. The precise cause of the findings is obscure, although some of the lesions may be produced by discal displacements (cartilaginous nodes).

C Localized central and peripheral defects with bone sclerosis (arrowheads) are observed on a lateral conventional tomogram of the thoracolumbar junction. Syndesmophytosis (arrow) also is seen. The apophyseal joint at this level is only partially ossified. (**C,** Courtesy of V. Vint, M.D., San Diego, California.)

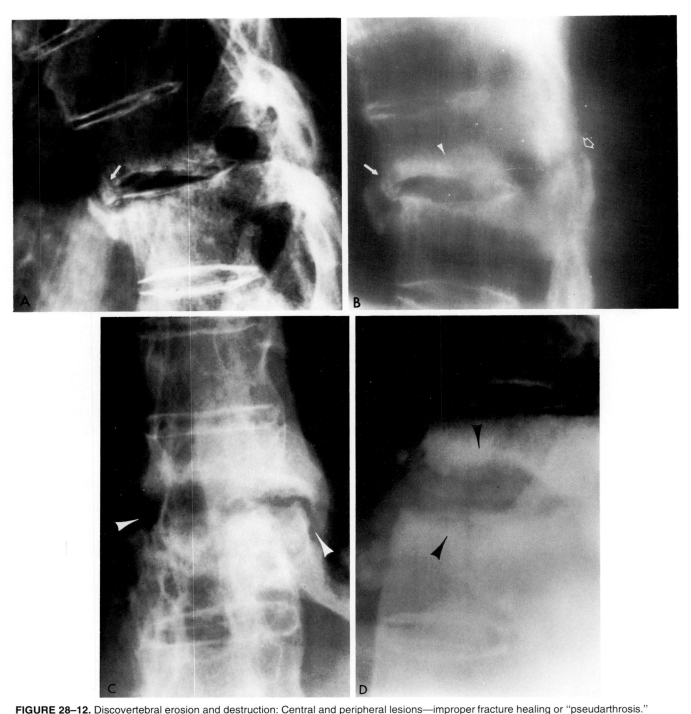

FIGURE 28–12. Discovertebral erosion and destruction: Central and peripheral lesions—improper fracture healing or "pseudarthrosis."

A, B The radiograph and conventional tomogram were obtained several weeks after this spondylitic patient suffered a fall. Observe the anterior subluxation (solid arrows) of the superiorly located vertebra, fragmentation, and mild subchondral sclerosis at the discovertebral junction. The subluxation (solid arrow) and sclerosis (arrowhead) are better seen on the tomogram. A fracture through the posterior elements (open arrow) also is evident.

C, D Frontal and lateral radiographs reveal a typical "pseudarthrosis" of the lower thoracic spine characterized by extensive osseous resorption and sclerosis (arrowheads). The appearance simulates that of an infection.

Illustration continued on opposite page

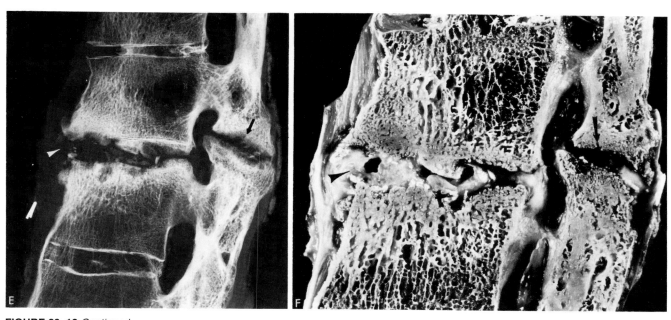

FIGURE 28–12 *Continued*

E, F A radiograph and photograph of a sagittal section of a spondylitic spine demonstrate a classic "pseudarthrosis." Findings include resorption and sclerosis of bone about the discovertebral junction (arrowheads), a fracture through the fused posterior elements (arrows), and syndesmophytosis at other levels. The presence of surgical clips reflects a previous attempt at anterior spinal fusion.

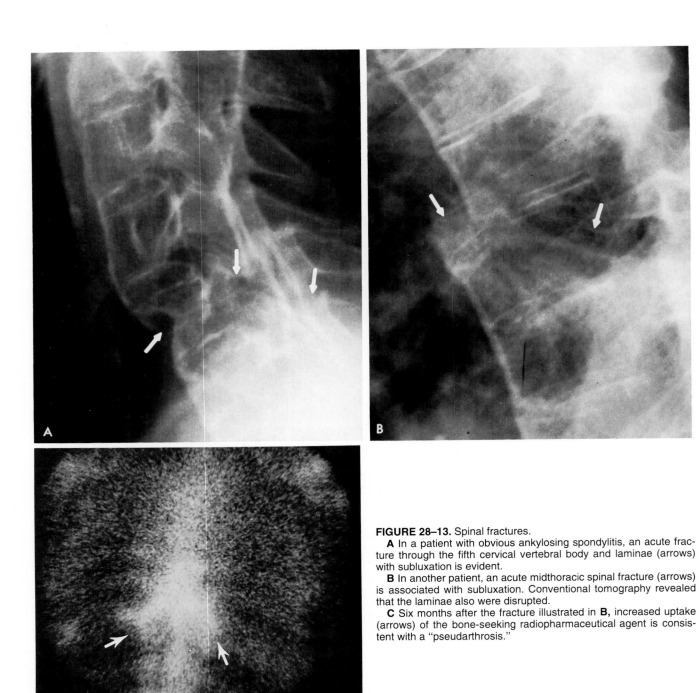

FIGURE 28–13. Spinal fractures.

A In a patient with obvious ankylosing spondylitis, an acute fracture through the fifth cervical vertebral body and laminae (arrows) with subluxation is evident.

B In another patient, an acute midthoracic spinal fracture (arrows) is associated with subluxation. Conventional tomography revealed that the laminae also were disrupted.

C Six months after the fracture illustrated in **B**, increased uptake (arrows) of the bone-seeking radiopharmaceutical agent is consistent with a "pseudarthrosis."

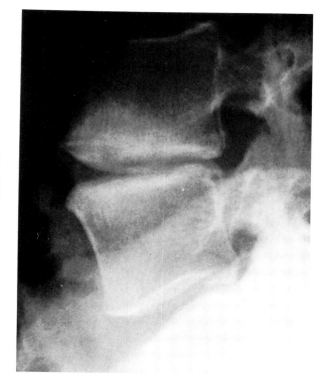

FIGURE 28–14. Idiopathic erosive spondylopathy. A 28 year old woman had had pain in her lower back for 8 years, which had increased in intensity during the last 3 years. A radiograph shows narrowing of the intervertebral disc and adjacent bone sclerosis in the lumbar spine. The abnormalities had progressed slightly compared with those on a radiograph obtained 9 months earlier. No clinical or laboratory evidence of infection was present. (Courtesy of J. Scavulli, M.D., San Diego, California.)

creates radiographic alterations that resemble those of a "pseudarthrosis"—alterations that have been called "pseudopseudarthroses"[344] (Fig. 28–15).

Although most cases of extensive discovertebral destruction in ankylosing spondylitis are aseptic, infectious spondylodiscitis in this disorder does occur, may involve single or multiple spinal segments, predominates in the thoracic and lumbar regions, and produces radiographic changes similar to those of a "pseudarthrosis."[346]

Discal Calcification (Fig. 28–16). Central or eccentric circular or linear calcific collections may appear within the intervertebral disc at single or multiple sites in the spinal column. These deposits usually are associated with apophyseal joint ankylosis at the same vertebral level and with adjacent syndesmophytes. Calcifications are accentuated by osteoporosis of surrounding vertebral bodies. Similar deposits accompany other conditions of the vertebral column that are characterized by ankylosis, such as diffuse idiopathic skeletal hyperostosis and juvenile chronic arthritis, suggesting that immobilization of a segment of the spine may interfere with discal nutrition, leading to degeneration and calcification.

Osteoporosis and Discal Ballooning (Fig. 28–16). In many patients with ankylosing spondylitis, especially when the disease is of long duration, osteoporosis of vertebral bodies becomes apparent and in some instances may reach severe proportions.[37, 190] In some persons, typical biconcave deformities of the vertebral bodies ("fish vertebrae") lead to biconvex or ballooned intervertebral discs.

Apophyseal Joint. Some investigators regard inflammation in the apophyseal joints as the essential abnormality of ankylosing spondylitis, leading to flattening of the lumbar spinal curve, exaggeration of the normal thoracic kyphosis,

and straightening and eventual flexion of the cervical spine.[347] On radiographs, lesions affecting the apophyseal joint include erosion, sclerosis, and bony ankylosis.

Erosion and Sclerosis. Poorly defined erosions of apophyseal joints in the lumbar, thoracic, and cervical segments of the spine are accompanied by reactive subchondral bone formation. These changes can be difficult to detect radiographically in the thoracic and lumbar spine, requiring oblique projections and even conventional tomography or CT scanning. In the cervical spine, such abnormalities are readily apparent on lateral radiographs. In this area, changes predominate in the upper cervical region, although in some patients, significant alterations are evident in the lower cervical spine. In any segment of the spine, apophyseal joint space narrowing is common as the disease process continues.

Bony Ankylosis. Apophyseal joint osseous fusion and capsular ossification are frequent in the lumbar, thoracic, and cervical spine in this disease (Fig. 28–17). These findings, which are less common in psoriatic spondylitis and Reiter's syndrome, eventually can extend throughout the vertebral column. In this situation, frontal radiographs of the thoracic and lumbar segments reveal two vertical radiodense bands representing intra- and extra-articular ossification about the apophyseal joints, which, when combined with a third central band (resulting from ossification of supraspinous and interspinous ligaments), lead to the "trolley-track" sign.

Apophyseal joint ankylosis can be very striking in the cervical spine. Complete obliteration of the articular spaces between the posterior elements of the second through seventh vertebrae results in a true column or pillar of bone. The appearance is reminiscent of that in juvenile chronic

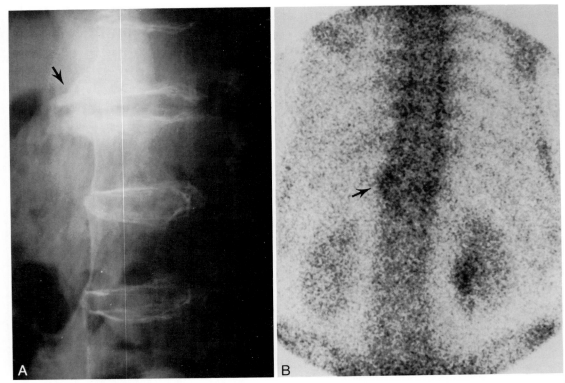

FIGURE 28–15. Abnormal spinal motion without fracture. In an 82 year old man with long-standing ankylosing spondylitis, a lateral radiograph **(A)** documents exuberant new bone formation (arrow), indicating a site of abnormal motion between two ankylosed segments of the spine. The bone scan **(B)** reveals slightly increased accumulation of the radiopharmaceutical agent at the site of motion (arrow). (Courtesy of V. Vint, M.D., San Diego, California.)

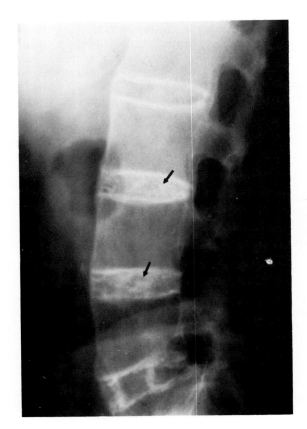

FIGURE 28–16. Discal calcification and ballooning. Long-standing ankylosing spondylitis is characterized by syndesmophytosis, apophyseal joint ankylosis, discal calcification (arrows), osteoporosis, and ballooning or biconvexity of the intervertebral disc.

CHAPTER 28—Ankylosing Spondylitis

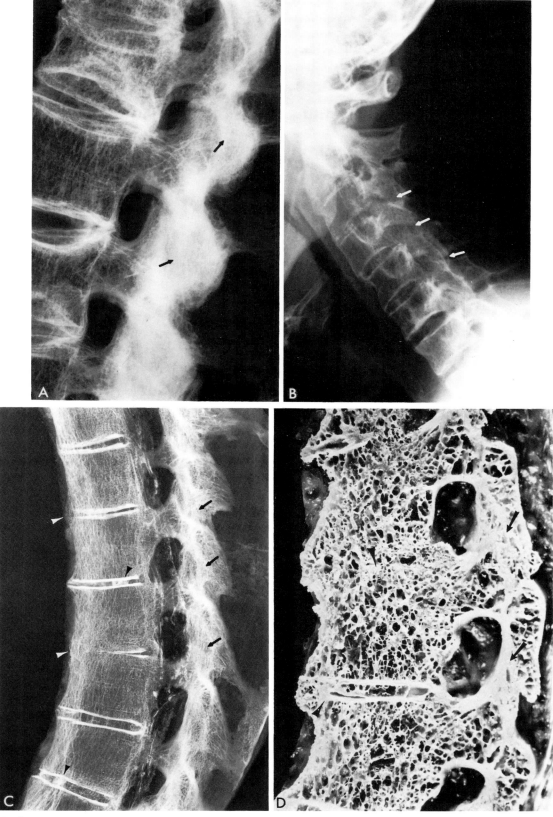

FIGURE 28–17. Apophyseal joint ankylosis.
   A In the lumbar spine, osseous fusion (arrows) of multiple apophyseal articulations is evident (specimen radiograph).
   B In the cervical spine, note apophyseal joint narrowing and fusion (arrows) extending from C2 to C7. Syndesmophytes, osteoporosis, and mild subluxation at C4-C5 are seen.
   C, D In the thoracic spine, a radiograph and photograph of a parasagittal section indicate extensive apophyseal joint bony fusion (arrows) with syndesmophytosis and discal ossification (arrowheads). A previous myelogram had been obtained.

Illustration continued on following page

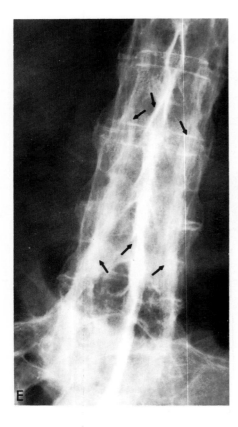

FIGURE 28–17 *Continued*
E Trolley-track sign. Observe three radiodense lines (arrows) extending vertically along the spine. The lateral lines represent capsular ossification about the apophyseal joints, whereas the central line represents ossification of the interspinous and supraspinous ligaments.

arthritis, although hypoplasia of vertebral bodies and intervertebral disc spaces, a prominent finding in juvenile chronic arthritis, is not observed in ankylosing spondylitis.

Costovertebral Joints. The costovertebral joints may demonstrate erosion, sclerosis, and ankylosis.[315, 379]

Erosion, Sclerosis, and Ankylosis (Figs. 28–18 and 28–19). Although pathologic evidence of intra-articular inflammation in costovertebral joints is well documented in ankylosing spondylitis, radiographic demonstration of changes in these locations is difficult. Tomographic techniques may indicate indistinctness and erosion of subchondral bone, sclerosis or eburnation, and partial or complete osseous fusion. It is the presence of significant ankylosis at costovertebral joints that is responsible for reduced chest expansion in this disease. Furthermore, in the presence of partial or complete bone ankylosis at the costovertebral

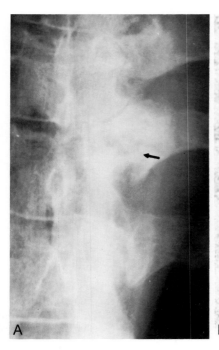

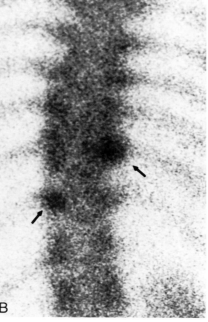

FIGURE 28–18. Costovertebral joint erosion. This 60 year old man had a long history of ankylosing spondylitis.

A A frontal radiograph of the thoracic spine with the patient turned slightly shows bone erosions about many costovertebral joints, especially prominent at one level (arrow).

B Abnormal uptake of the bone-seeking radiopharmaceutical agent is evident at multiple costovertebral joints (arrows).

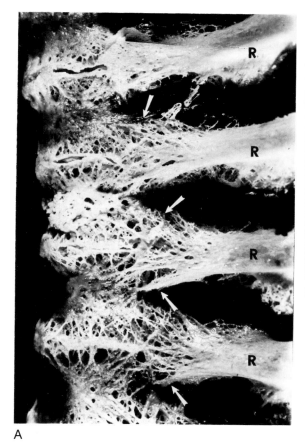

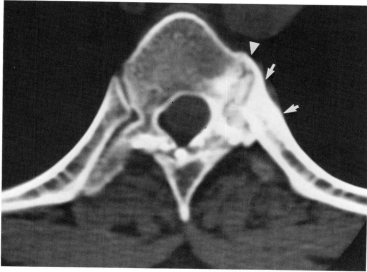

FIGURE 28–19. Costovertebral joint ankylosis.

A A photograph of the lateral aspect of a macerated thoracic spine of a spondylitic cadaver demonstrates extensive bony ankylosis (arrows) of the heads of the ribs (R) and vertebral bodies. Discal ossification also is seen.

B Transaxial CT scan of a thoracic vertebra in a patient with ankylosing spondylitis reveals bone erosions and partial ankylosis (arrowhead) of the costovertebral joints on one side. Note involvement of the ipsilateral rib with cortical thickening (arrows).

joint, sclerosis and thickening of the posterior portion of the adjacent rib may be evident.[386] The precise cause for this is not clear.

Posterior Ligamentous Attachments. Lesions affecting the posterior ligamentous attachments include calcification, ossification, and subligamentous erosion.

Ligamentous Calcification and Ossification (Fig. 28–20). Calcification and ossification of interspinous and supraspinous ligaments represent prominent features of ankylosing spondylitis. These changes usually become more evident as the disease progresses. In later stages, a central radiodense stripe can be identified on frontal radiographs of

FIGURE 28–20. Posterior spinal ligamentous ossification.

A A frontal radiograph of the lumbar spine reveals ossification of the interspinous and supraspinous ligaments, producing a vertical central radiodense shadow (arrows), the dagger sign.

B On a photograph of the posterior aspect of a macerated spine in a cadaver with ankylosing spondylitis, the ossification of the supra- and interspinous ligaments (arrows) is well seen.

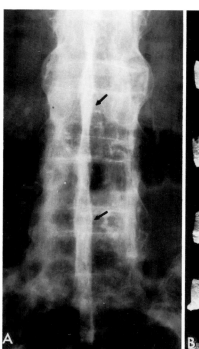

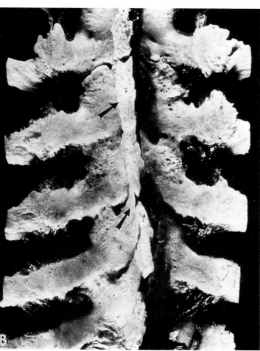

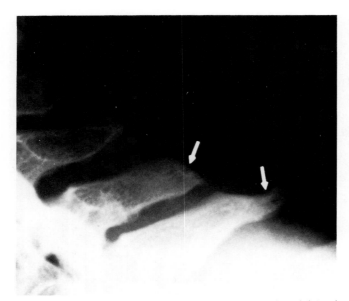

FIGURE 28–21. Posterior spinal subligamentous erosion. A lateral radiograph of the cervical spine reveals erosions of the spinous processes of the lower cervical vertebrae (arrows). The erosions are associated with apophyseal joint ankylosis.

the thoracic and lumbar spine, the dagger sign, corresponding to the calcified and ossified ligamentous structures.

Ossification of the posterior longitudinal ligament (see Chapter 42) also has been described in patients with ankylosing spondylitis,[333, 348, 349] although a meaningful association of the two disorders is not yet clear. In reported cases, predilection for the cervical spine and traumatic quadriplegia after injury have been observed.

Calcification of the ligamenta flava in the lumbosacral spine in patients with ankylosing spondylitis has been accompanied by spinal stenosis.[350]

Subligamentous Erosion (Fig. 28–21). Erosion of the tips of spinous processes is encountered most commonly in the lower cervical and upper thoracic regions. A poorly defined and sclerotic osseous outline becomes evident. With extensive whittling, the spinous processes appear pointed or sharpened.[111] A similar appearance can be encountered in rheumatoid arthritis.

Atlantoaxial Articulations. The atlantoaxial joints may be involved by erosions and subluxation.

Erosions (Fig. 28–22). Synovial tissue surrounds the odontoid process both anteriorly and posteriorly, corresponding to the location of the joint cavity between the anterior arch of the atlas and the anterior surface of the odontoid process (dens) and the joint cavity between the transverse ligament of the atlas and the posterior surface of the odontoid. Inflammatory changes of the synovial and adjacent ligamentous structures can lead to erosion of the dens.[112] In long-standing and severe ankylosing spondylitis, this osseous peg may become extremely short and irregular in shape, or it may disappear completely. Similar abnormalities can be evident in rheumatoid arthritis (and psoriatic arthritis), although surrounding bony proliferation is more characteristic of ankylosing spondylitis than of rheumatoid arthritis.

Subluxation. Although atlantoaxial subluxation can be observed in patients with ankylosing spondylitis,[111–119, 246]

the frequency of this complication appears to be less than that in rheumatoid arthritis. Of the over 200 spondylitic patients followed by Wilkinson and Bywaters,[21] only one patient (less than 1 per cent) complaining of neck pain revealed such subluxation; Sharp and Purser noted atlantoaxial subluxation in approximately 2 per cent of a large number of patients with ankylosing spondylitis.[113] A higher frequency of peripheral joint disease in patients with ankylosing spondylitis who have atlantoaxial subluxation has been observed.[351] When present, atlantoaxial subluxation generally is observed in the later stages of the disease, although, rarely, it may be an early complication.[120] Forward subluxation of the atlas with respect to the odontoid process exaggerated on lateral views of the cervical spine obtained during flexion of the neck is most typical, although cranial settling and atlantoaxial rotary subluxation also may be observed.[121, 215, 352] The spine may become "reankylosed" in the subluxed position, providing some degree of stability. Subaxial subluxation in the cervical spine is much less characteristic of ankylosing spondylitis than of rheumatoid arthritis.[353]

Miscellaneous Spinal Sites. Resorption of the cervical vertebral bodies, fractures, and abnormalities of spinal curvature also may be seen.

Cervical Vertebral Body Resorption (Fig. 28–23). Extensive bony resorption of the anterior surface of the lower cervical vertebrae may be a late manifestation of the disease.[111] This finding, which almost invariably is associated

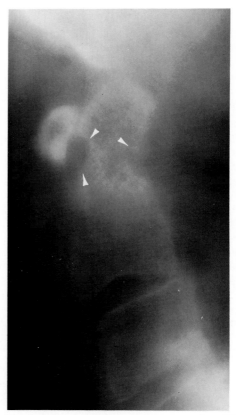

FIGURE 28–22. Erosion of the odontoid process. In a 59 year old man with ankylosing spondylitis, a lateral conventional tomogram of the cervical spine reveals erosions of the anterior and posterior surfaces of the odontoid process (arrowheads). Mild vertical translocation at the atlantoaxial joint is apparent.

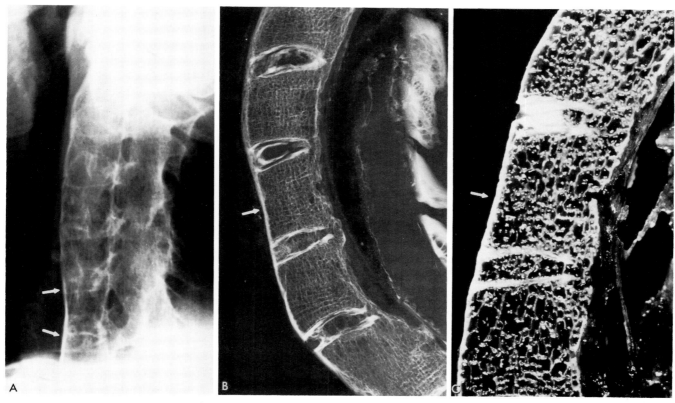

FIGURE 28–23. Cervical vertebral body resorption.

A In addition to other severe abnormalities of ankylosing spondylitis (apophyseal joint ankylosis, syndesmophytosis), note the osseous resorption along the anterior aspect of the lower cervical vertebral bodies (arrows).

B, C A radiograph and photograph of a sagittal section of the cervical spine in a spondylitic cadaver reveal similar resorption of the vertebral bodies (arrows) associated with syndesmophytes. This change may be due to bony atrophy related to immobilization of the adjacent spinal segment.

with syndesmophytes and complete ankylosis of the apophyseal joints in the cervical spine and extensive dorsal kyphosis, results in a decrease in the anteroposterior diameter of the involved cervical segment. The resulting osseous contour frequently is smooth. Bony atrophy due to disuse may be one factor in the pathogenesis of this finding.

Fractures. This well-known complication of ankylosing spondylitis has been discussed already. Fractures may involve a single level or multiple levels of the vertebral column. They predominate in the cervical spine, although they may be detected at any level of the vertebral column including the sacrum[380] and, when clinically silent, they eventually may be associated with improper fracture healing.

Abnormalities of Spinal Curvature. As the disease progresses, straightening of the normal lumbar lordosis and exaggeration of the normal thoracic kyphosis are seen. Straightening of the normal cervical lordosis and forward flexion also are common.

Complications of Spinal Involvement. Neurospinal complications, including spinal cord compression and even death, are a recognized, although infrequent, manifestation of ankylosing spondylitis. Vertebral fractures, especially in the cervical region, are associated with significant morbidity and mortality, related to deformity of the cord produced by osseous surfaces as well as hematomas. Atlantoaxial instability, in either a horizontal or a vertical direction, can produce neurologic deficit and may be fatal.[121] Spondylo-

discitis has been associated with compression of the cord or nerve roots, especially in the lumbar segment.[247] In this situation, meningeal disease and a potential for an extradural mass of fibroadipose tissue have been suggested as pathogenetic factors.[247] Posttraumatic contusion of the cord, in the absence of spinal fracture, in ankylosing spondylitis may reflect a vulnerability produced by a rigid vertebral column that cannot bend or rotate on impact to absorb traumatic stress.[246]

Although the mechanism is not clear, spinal stenosis is being recognized with increasing frequency in patients with ankylosing spondylitis.[246, 248, 333] This complication, which is best identified with CT scanning or MR imaging, is not unexpected in the presence of a disease that leads to ossification of the intervertebral disc, apophyseal joints, and vertebral ligaments. Stenosis of the central spinal canal, lateral recesses, and intervertebral foramina can be explained on the basis of the pathology of the disease.

As indicated previously, the cauda equina syndrome is observed in some patients with ankylosing spondylitis.[39–42, 249–253, 354, 355] This syndrome occurs late in the course of the disease and in persons with marked spinal ankylosis. Typical clinical findings include cutaneous sensory impairment of the lower limbs and perineum with sphincter disturbances; motor impairment occurs less commonly, and associated pain is an inconstant feature.[354] Widening of the neural canal in the lumbar segment, dilation of the dural

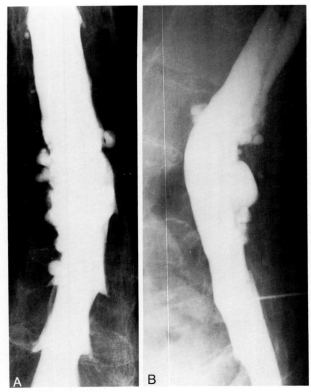

FIGURE 28–24. Thecal diverticula. An elderly man with ankylosing spondylitis developed a cauda equina syndrome, manifested as loss of sphincter tone and perineal dysesthesia. Frontal (supine) **(A)** and lateral **(B)** radiographs during myelography outline multiple arachnoid diverticula. (Courtesy of D. Moody, M.D., Winston-Salem, North Carolina.)

sac, and thecal diverticula are the associated pathologic aberrations. Myelography reveals contrast opacification of the saccular diverticula (Fig. 28–24), and CT scans demonstrate scalloped erosions of the laminae (Fig. 28–25).[354, 356, 357] Similar erosions may involve the pedicles, spinous process or, rarely, vertebral body. Asymmetric abnormalities at multiple spinal levels or, less commonly, unilateral involvement at multiple levels or single level involvement is seen.[354] MR imaging reveals widening of the dural sac with signal intensity corresponding to that of fluid.[355, 357, 358] It is possible that atrophy of the peridural tissues and adherence of the dura to adjacent structures in ankylosing spondylitis reduce the compliance and the elasticity of the caudal sac and its ability to diminish fluctuations in the pressure of the cerebrospinal fluid, resulting in slowly enlarging arachnoid diverticula and bone erosions.[250] Arachnoiditis and postirradiation ischemia may be additional important factors.[251, 354]

Symphysis Pubis (Fig. 28–26)

Alterations of the symphysis pubis have been described in 16 to 23 per cent of patients with ankylosing spondylitis.[36] They may be more frequent and more prominent in women than in men.[68, 122] Erosion and blurring of the subchondral bone on both sides of the joint are combined with adjacent eburnation.[70, 202] Articular space narrowing and bony ankylosis can be noted. With complete intra-articular osseous fusion, the sclerosis subsequently may decrease or disappear.

Additional Pelvic Sites (Fig. 28–27)

Enthesopathy is especially prominent in certain pelvic sites, such as the ischial tuberosities, the iliac crests, and the sacroiliac spaces above the true synovial joints; similar abnormalities occur at extrapelvic sites, such as the femoral trochanters, humeral tuberosities, inferior clavicular margin at the site of attachment of the coracoclavicular ligament, anterior surface of the patella, and plantar aspect of the calcaneus. Abnormalities usually are bilateral and symmet-

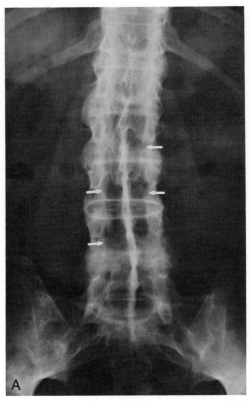

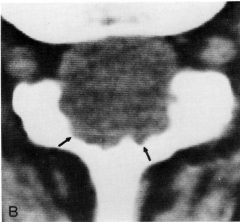

FIGURE 28–25. Thecal diverticula. This 48 year old man had had ankylosing spondylitis for 19 years. Current findings included hip and knee pain and numbness and muscle weakness in the feet.

A Anteroposterior radiograph reveals spinal and sacroiliac joint ankylosis. Note extensive erosions of the laminae at multiple levels (arrows).

B Transaxial CT scan at the level of the third lumbar vertebra demonstrates asymmetric erosion of the lamina and spinous process (arrows).

(From Mitchell MJ, et al, Radiology *175:* 521, 1990.)

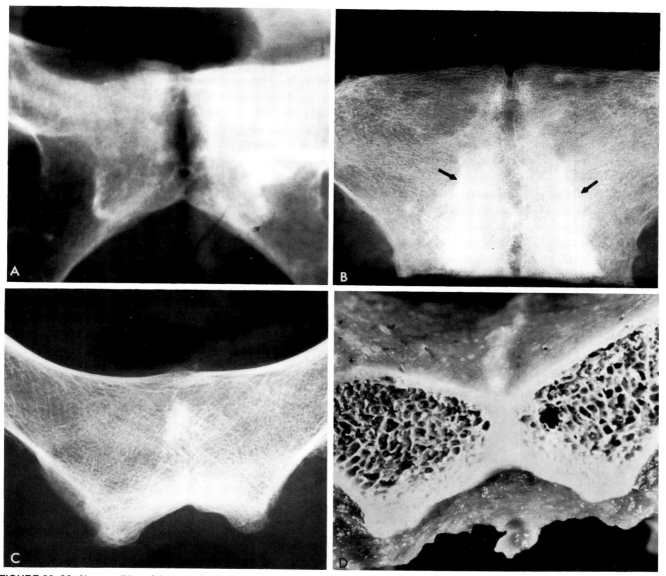

FIGURE 28–26. Abnormalities of the symphysis pubis.
   A Note narrowing, osseous fusion, and sclerosis of the symphysis pubis.
   B In a spondylitic cadaver, a radiograph of a coronal section through the symphysis pubis demonstrates focal bony ankylosis with surrounding eburnation (arrows).
   C, D A radiograph and photograph of a coronal section of the symphysis pubis in another cadaver with ankylosing spondylitis indicate complete osseous fusion and absence of sclerosis.

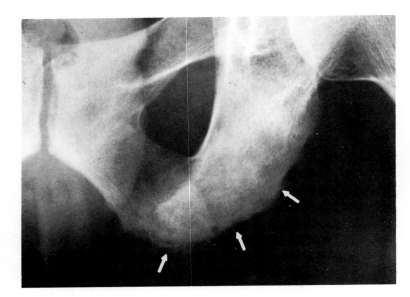

FIGURE 28–27. Abnormalities of the ischial tuberosity. Observe slight contour irregularity and sclerosis of the ischial tuberosity (arrows).

ric in distribution, although asymmetric and unilateral findings occasionally can be evident. Osteoporosis, osseous erosion with poorly defined subchondral bony margins, and reactive sclerosis are the observed radiographic alterations. Although the resulting radiographic picture is reminiscent of that occurring in diffuse idiopathic skeletal hyperostosis, the degree of sclerosis and surface irregularity is more prominent in ankylosing spondylitis. Similar abnormalities are apparent in psoriatic arthritis, Reiter's syndrome, and inflammatory bowel disorders.

Manubriosternal Joint (Fig. 28–28)

Involvement of the manubriosternal joint can lead to significant clinical findings in patients with ankylosing spondylitis.[123] In some persons, the abnormalities in this location represent a dominant part of the disease.[306] They generally occur in patients with long-standing disease and severe sacroiliitis.[360] Osteoporosis of the subchondral bone is associated with subacute osteitis, osteoclastosis, and infiltration with chronic inflammatory cells.[70, 124] Osseous erosion reflects extensive replacement of fibrocartilage and bone by granulation tissue. Bony proliferation leads to sclerosis and intra-articular ankylosis.[257] Soft tissue masses about the affected joint have been described.[359]

The radiographic and pathologic changes in the manubriosternal articulation are similar to those that are observed at the discovertebral junction and symphysis pubis. Identical abnormalities are evident in other seronegative spondyloarthropathies, particularly psoriatic arthritis.

It should be noted that difficulty in defining the prevalence of involvement of the manubriosternal joint precisely in ankylosing spondylitis, as well as in other rheumatic disorders, is related to the occurrence of spontaneous bone fusion at this site in a significant number of normal adult persons. In this regard, the finding of complete intra-articular osseous ankylosis must be interpreted cautiously. Partial ankylosis, in the form of a bone bar resembling a syndesmophyte, may be a more specific abnormality of the manubriosternal joint in ankylosing spondylitis.[227] In gen-

eral, such involvement is neither an early nor an isolated manifestation of the disease.

Hip (Table 28–4)

General Abnormalities. Clinical and radiologic involvement of the hip is an important feature of ankylosing

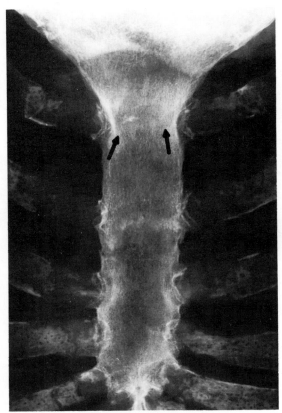

FIGURE 28–28. Abnormalities of the manubriosternal joint. On a radiograph of a coronal section of the sternum, complete osseous fusion of the manubriosternal joint is apparent (arrows), with minor surrounding bony sclerosis.

TABLE 28–4. Differential Diagnosis of Hip Involvement

Disease	Typical Distribution	Femoral Head Migration	Osteophytosis	Miscellaneous Findings
Ankylosing spondylitis	Bilateral, symmetric	Axial	Lateral aspect of femur; collar at femoral head-femoral neck junction	Cysts, bony ankylosis, protrusion deformity, postoperative heterotopic ossification
Rheumatoid arthritis	Bilateral, symmetric	Axial	Rare	Osteoporosis, erosions, protrusion deformity
Osteoarthritis	Unilateral or bilateral	Superior or Medial	Lateral and medial Femoral and acetabular	Sclerosis, cysts, buttressing
Calcium pyrophosphate dihydrate crystal deposition disease	Bilateral, symmetric or asymmetric	Axial	Lateral and medial Femoral and acetabular	Sclerosis, cysts, collapse, fragmentation, calcification

spondylitis.[46, 305] A bilateral (93 per cent) and symmetric (73 per cent) distribution with concentric joint space narrowing (50 per cent) and osteophytosis (58 per cent) is characteristic.

Osteophytosis (Fig. 28–29). An early and distinctive abnormality is an osteophyte or "bump" on the lateral aspect of the femoral head. Osteophytes subsequently progress, creating a collar around the femoral neck at the margin of the articular surface.[46, 125]

Joint Space Narrowing (Fig. 28–30). Diffuse or concentric joint space narrowing producing axial migration of the femoral head with respect to the acetabulum is a frequent but not invariable feature of hip involvement in ankylosing spondylitis. Although such an appearance classically is related to superficial erosion of cartilage from inflammatory synovial tissue or pannus,[70] subchondral extension of inflamed synovium also has been observed.[126, 127] Granulation tissue deep to the cartilage can erode the bony plate and invade the calcified zone of cartilage. As the nutrition of mature articular cartilage is derived from the synovial surface, subchondral infiltration does not necessarily destroy the overlying cartilage or produce cartilaginous proliferation. It may disrupt the normal attachment of the articular cartilage to the subchondral bone, however, allowing it to break free. Denudation of large segments of the bony surface thus could be associated with diffuse joint space loss. Protrusio acetabuli eventually can occur. The combination of concentric diminution of the articular space and osteophytosis is characteristic of the hip disease in ankylosing spondylitis, although it also may be observed in calcium pyrophosphate dihydrate crystal deposition disease, Paget's disease, and, rarely, uncomplicated osteoarthritis. Although concentric joint space narrowing also is seen in rheumatoid arthritis, osteophytosis generally is not a prominent feature of this disease.

Loss of the articular space in the upper portion of the joint resulting in superior migration of the femoral head with respect to the acetabulum may be seen in 5 to 6 per cent of patients with ankylosing spondylitis, although this pattern may reflect the incidental occurrence of degenerative joint disease in these persons.[46]

Bony Ankylosis (Fig. 28–31). Intra-articular bony ankylosis has been emphasized as a complication of spondylitic hip disease. Although Rutishauser and Jacqueline[47] have stated that ankylosis always is generalized, Dürrigl and coworkers[128] have reported a case that on conventional tomography demonstrated only capsular ankylosis, with spar-

ing of the joint space. In this situation, trabeculae can be traced from the femoral head to the acetabulum across a relatively intact articular cavity. Some investigators note that bony ankylosis of the hip appears to be a feature of ankylosing spondylitis in women.[199]

Cysts (Fig. 28–29B). Subchondral cysts also can be observed.[361] These generally are multiple and of variable size and predominate in the acetabulum.

Progression of Hip Disease. The radiographic course of spondylitic hip disease is variable. Forestier and associates[37] reported two types of hip involvement: One was a nondestructive, ankylosing form that occurred in patients less than 40 years of age, which was bilateral and unassociated with joint space loss, and which led to rapid loss in motion; the second type occurred in older persons, was unilateral and destructive, and had a slower course, with eventual joint space loss, femoral head irregularity, osteophytosis, and ankylosis. Dwosh and colleagues[46] observed that, in their patients with ankylosing spondylitis, hip disease began in young patients, was often very destructive, and progressed to severe protrusion deformity and new bone formation. Bony ankylosis was found rarely (approximately 2 to 3 per cent of cases).

Postoperative Abnormalities (Fig. 28–32). A survey of available literature indicates that some patients with ankylosing spondylitis who require arthroplasty for hip disease will develop restricted motion and periarticular bone formation in the postoperative period. In a long-term follow-up study of cup arthroplasties in patients with rheumatoid diseases (with either ankylosing spondylitis or rheumatoid arthritis), Edstrom and Fellander[129] noted that although the range of motion was definitely improved after surgery, marked new bone formation occurred in 9 of 37 hips. Freeman[130] studied the results of McKee-Farrar total hip arthroplasties in patients with rheumatic diseases, including four patients with ankylosing spondylitis, and noted one person with "ectopic calcification." In a report of 33 total hip arthroplasties in patients with ankylosing spondylitis, Welch and Charnley[131] occasionally detected ectopic bone formation, although clinical "reankylosis" was not evident. In an evaluation of total hip replacements in patients with ankylosing spondylitis or juvenile chronic arthritis, Arden and coworkers[132] reported only fair results regarding increased range of motion after surgery in some persons. Wilde and associates[133] reported complete reankylosis after total hip replacement in a 57 year old man with ankylosing spondylitis. In a study of 11 patients with this disease who

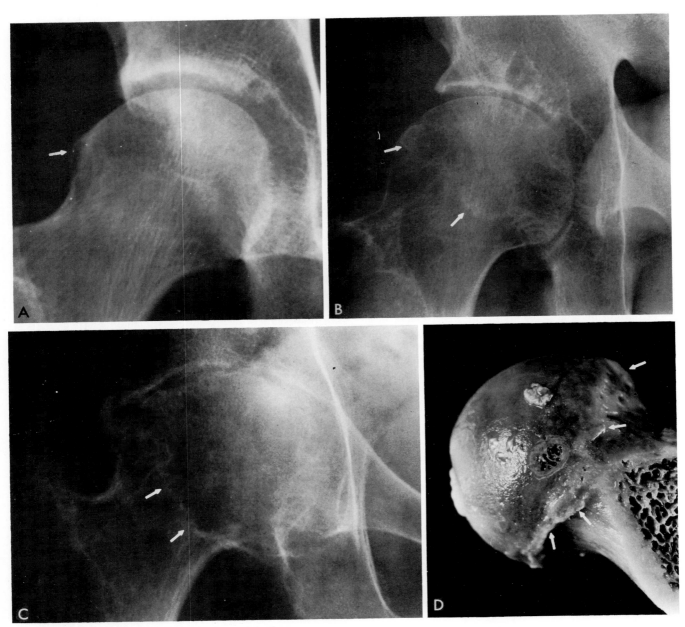

FIGURE 28–29. Abnormalities of the hip: Osteophytosis.

  A Observe bone formation on the lateral margin of the femoral head (arrow), which has resulted in a bumpy contour.

  B More extensive osteophyte formation can be seen on the lateral margin of the femoral head with progression over a portion of the femoral neck (arrows). Note subchondral cysts in the acetabulum.

  C The osteophytes have formed a collar about the femoral neck (arrows). Extensive concentric joint space narrowing has occurred.

  D A photograph of a macerated femoral head from a cadaver with ankylosing spondylitis indicates the ringlike osteophytes extending around the femoral head (arrows).

  (**A–C,** From Dwosh I, et al: Arthritis Rheum *19:* 683, 1976.)

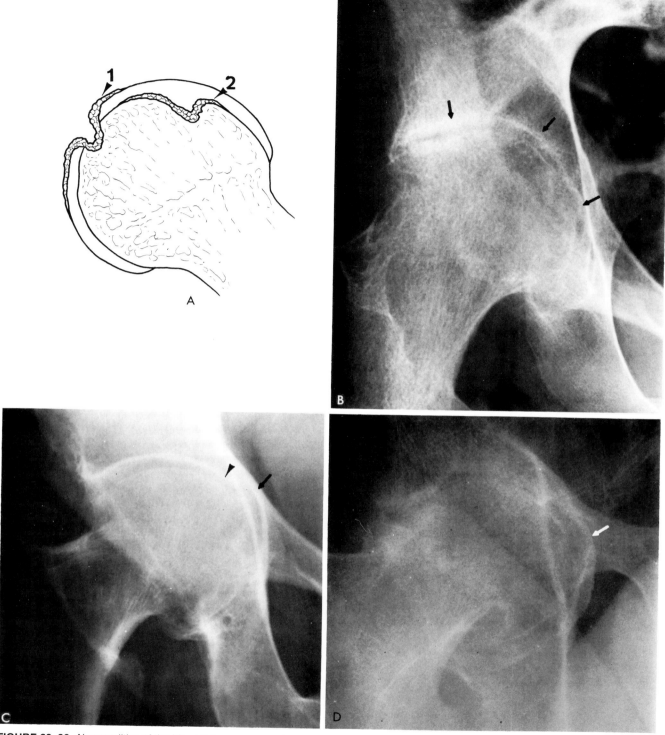

FIGURE 28–30. Abnormalities of the hip: Joint space narrowing.

A Pannus can extend across the surface of the cartilage *(1)* or subchondrally *(2)*. The latter route may be associated with defective chondral nutrition and separation or fragmentation of the cartilaginous surface.

B Concentric loss of joint space (arrows) with axial migration of the femoral head with respect to the acetabulum is common in ankylosing spondylitis.

C Minimal protrusio acetabuli deformity (arrow) is associated with axial migration of the femoral head and mild joint space narrowing (arrowhead).

D Severe protrusio acetabuli deformity (arrow) with obliteration of articular space is evident in another patient with ankylosing spondylitis.

(C, D, From Dwosh I, et al: Arthritis Rheum *19:* 683, 1976.)

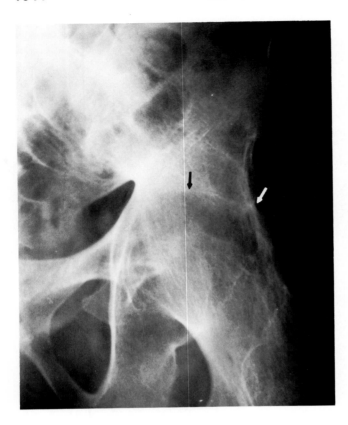

FIGURE 28–31. Abnormalities of the hip: Intra-articular bony ankylosis. Note the extensive capsular and interior bony ankylosis (arrows). The medial aspect of the articulation still is visible.

underwent hip arthroplasty, Resnick and collaborators[134] detected clinical reankylosis in 6 of 20 hips (30 per cent) followed postoperatively for longer than 6 months and radiographic reankylosis in 9 of 16 hips (56 per cent) followed for a similar length of time. Bisla and colleagues[135] evaluated 34 total hip arthroplasties in 23 patients with ankylosing spondylitis, and noted postoperative heterotopic bone formation in 62 per cent of articulations, which was of severe proportions in 27 per cent. More recently, Williams and coworkers,[136] Walker and Sledge,[362] and Kilgus and associates[363] also have observed para-articular ossification leading to bony ankylosis in the postoperative period in some patients with ankylosing spondylitis who had undergone hip arthroplasty.

Although some reports do not confirm a high frequency of new bone formation or significant postoperative disability[258, 364] after hip surgery in patients with ankylosing spondylitis,[137] and others note a disturbing prevalence of these complications in patients who do not have ankylosing spondylitis, particularly if prior surgical procedures have been performed or postoperative infection has appeared,[138] it is difficult to ignore a possible relationship between ankylosing spondylitis and postoperative heterotopic ossification in view of the many reports cited previously. The cause of this apparently high frequency of bone formation after hip surgery in spondylitic patients is obscure, although it is particularly common after multiple surgical procedures.[316] As bone proliferation leading to intra-articular ankylosis and "whiskering" at sites of tendon and ligament attachment is frequent in this disorder, perhaps surgical intervention in this ossifying diathesis, by changing the local environment around the joint, accentuates osteoblastic activity, leading to excess ossification. Whether or not such heterotopic ossification is important clinically is another issue;

however, if future reports confirm that heterotopic ossification is a clinically significant problem postoperatively in ankylosing spondylitis, hip arthroplasty may be judged not to be a useful procedure in this disorder when the prime indication for such surgery is restricted motion of the joint.

Shoulder (Fig. 28–33)

Patients with ankylosing spondylitis may reveal abnormalities of the glenohumeral or acromioclavicular joint or along the undersurface of the distal end of the clavicle at the attachment site of the coracoclavicular ligament.[64, 72]

Glenohumeral Joint Abnormalities. With the exception of the hip, the glenohumeral joint is the peripheral articular site most frequently affected in patients with long-standing ankylosing spondylitis (32 per cent of patients).[72] The abnormalities more commonly are bilateral than unilateral and may appear without changes in any other appendicular skeletal site. Osteoporosis, diffuse joint space narrowing, and erosive changes predominantly in the superolateral aspect of the humeral head simulate the changes in rheumatoid arthritis. In some spondylitic patients, the entire outer aspect of the humerus may be destroyed, the "hatchet" sign.[200, 259] Atrophy or disruption of the rotator cuff can lead to elevation of the humeral head with respect to the glenoid cavity. Synovial cysts are seen in rare instances.

Acromioclavicular Joint Abnormalities. Destructive articular changes in this location, which commonly are bilateral in distribution, are identical to those in rheumatoid arthritis.[365] Resorption of the distal end of the clavicle can be seen.

Coracoclavicular Joint Abnormalities. Scalloped clavicular erosion beneath the coracoclavicular ligament occurs not only in ankylosing spondylitis but also in other synovial disorders, as well as in hyperparathyroidism.[139]

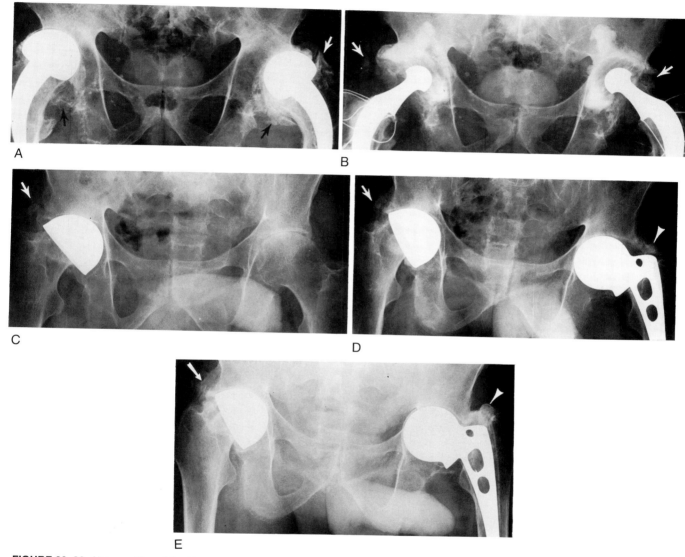

FIGURE 28–32. Abnormalities of the hip: Postoperative heterotopic ossification.

A, B A 61 year old man with a 20 year history of ankylosing spondylitis underwent bilateral femoral prosthetic replacements. After the procedures **(A),** moderate to extensive new bone formation is apparent about the femoral prostheses on both sides (arrows). An evaluation 2 years after bilateral total hip replacements **(B)** shows mild (right side) and moderate (left side) heterotopic ossification about the arthroplasties (arrows).

C–E A 38 year old man with a 16 year history of disease underwent a cup arthroplasty of the right hip. After the operation **(C),** mild to moderate bone formation has appeared about the femoral cup (arrow). Three months after replacement of the left femoral head with an Austin-Moore prosthesis **(D),** moderate new bone formation (arrowhead) can be identified. Tilting of the right femoral cup and adjacent new bone formation (arrow) also are seen. Four and one half years later **(E),** apparent ankylosis about the femoral cup arthroplasty (arrow) and a protruded and loosened Austin-Moore prosthesis (arrowhead) are seen.

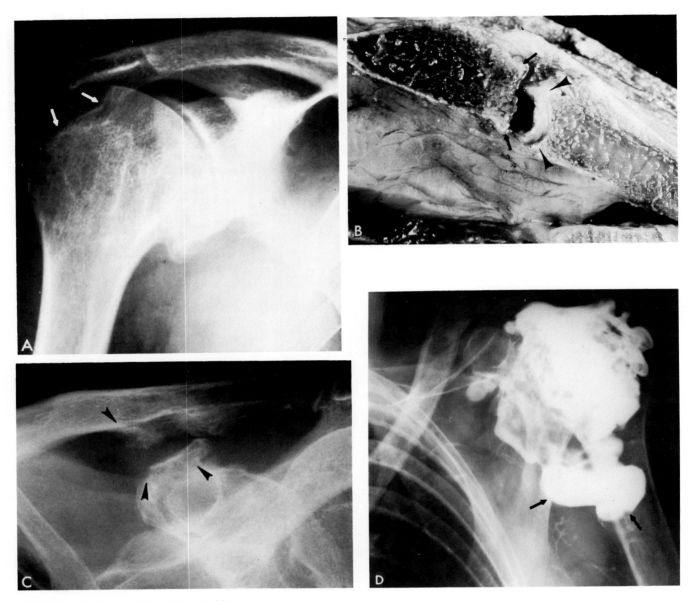

FIGURE 28–33. Abnormalities of the shoulder.
   A Glenohumeral joint. Observe joint space narrowing, mild osteoporosis, and a large erosive abnormality along the lateral aspect of the humeral head (arrows).
   B Acromioclavicular joint. A photograph of a coronal section of the acromioclavicular joint in a cadaver with ankylosing spondylitis reveals erosion of the distal end of the clavicle (arrows) and medial end of the acromion (arrowheads).
   C Coracoclavicular ligamentous attachments. Bony proliferation and irregularity on the inferior surface of the clavicle and coracoid process (arrowheads) are seen in this patient with ankylosing spondylitis.
   D Synovial cyst formation. In a 59 year old man with ankylosing spondylitis, single contrast glenohumeral joint arthrography delineates nodular proliferation of the synovial membrane leading to radiolucent filling defects, a synovial cyst (arrows), irregularities of the undersurface of the rotator cuff, and opacification of lymphatic channels.

Factors responsible for this erosion may include an enthe-sopathy related to the ligamentous attachment site itself, synovial inflammation within an adjacent bursa or aberrant coracoclavicular joint, or pressure resorption owing to con-tact of the coracoid process and clavicle. In ankylosing spondylitis, proliferative alterations may accompany the erosive process, providing a clue to accurate diagnosis. Progressive ossification of the coroclavicular ligaments also has been reported.[260, 261]

Sternoclavicular Joint (Fig. 28–34)

Bilateral or, less commonly, unilateral abnormalities of the sternoclavicular joint in ankylosing spondylitis[140] con-sist of erosion and sclerosis of the sternum and the medial end of the clavicle, which mimic the findings in rheumatoid arthritis[141] or infection. Intra-articular osseous fusion even-tually may occur.[201] Referred pain in association with ster-noclavicular joint disease may lead to a confusing clinical presentation.

Elbow (Fig. 28–35)

Radiographic elbow abnormalities are relatively uncom-mon in ankylosing spondylitis, having been observed in 12 per cent of patients with long-standing disease.[72] Effusions, osteoporosis, joint space narrowing, and bony proliferation are detected in a unilateral or bilateral distribution.

Hand and Wrist (Fig. 28–36)

Asymmetrically distributed abnormalities of the small joints of the hands and the wrists in ankylosing spondylitis are not infrequent (approximately 30 per cent of patients with severe disease).[72] Periarticular swelling, juxta-articular osteoporosis, joint space narrowing, and osseous erosions are observed. Metacarpophalangeal, proximal interphalan-geal, and distal interphalangeal joints, all the compartments of the wrist, and the ulnar styloid can be affected. In gen-eral, erosive abnormalities are less prominent than in rheu-matoid arthritis and are associated with adjacent periarticu-lar bone proliferation, producing a poorly defined and fuzzy osseous contour. The degree of joint diminution is variable, although intra-articular bony ankylosis can appear in a rel-atively short period of time. Somewhat infrequently, defor-mity, such as ulnar subluxation of the carpus with respect to the distal portions of the radius and ulna, and ulnar deviation of the digits at the metacarpophalangeal joints, is seen.

Knee (Fig. 28–37)

In approximately 30 per cent of patients with ankylosing spondylitis of long duration, radiographic abnormalities ap-pear in the knees.[72] Typically, bilateral and symmetric changes in the three compartments of the knee (medial femorotibial, lateral femorotibial, patellofemoral compart-ments) include effusions, osteoporosis, and joint space nar-rowing. Additional manifestations are marginal erosions, subchondral cysts, and juxta-articular periostitis. Intra-artic-ular bone fusion also is reported.[366] Similar abnormalities can be evident in the proximal tibiofibular joint. Hyperos-tosis on the anterior aspect of the patella at the quadriceps attachment can be noted. Rarely, in the knee as in other joints, a more aggressive pattern of synovial inflammation is apparent. Extensive soft tissue swelling and a massive

synovial effusion simulate the findings of septic arthritis or pigmented villonodular synovitis, especially if the involve-ment of the peripheral skeleton is monoarticular in distri-bution (Fig. 28–38).

Ankle

Rarely, changes in the ankle can be noted in ankylosing spondylitis.[72, 142] They resemble findings in other articula-tions. Periostitis is particularly characteristic in the distal and medial portions of the tibia. An adjacent soft tissue mass due to hypertrophic synovitis can be associated with the tarsal tunnel syndrome.[143]

Forefoot and Midfoot (Fig. 28–39)

Bilateral symmetric or asymmetric abnormalities of the feet, which can be evident in approximately 15 per cent of patients with long-standing ankylosing spondylitis,[72] show predilection for the metatarsophalangeal and first tarsometa-tarsal joints and for the interphalangeal joint of the great toe. Soft tissue swelling, diffuse joint space narrowing, ero-sions with adjacent bony proliferation predominantly on the medial aspect of the metatarsal heads, periostitis of phalan-geal and metatarsal shafts, and intra-articular bony anky-losis can be detected. Subluxation at metatarsophalangeal joints consisting of fibular deviation of the toes is less frequent and severe than in rheumatoid arthritis.

Calcaneus (Fig. 28–40)

Although clinically manifest heel abnormalities are infre-quent in ankylosing spondylitis, radiographic changes of the calcaneus are common. In an investigation of 40 pa-tients with ankylosing spondylitis who had heel radiographs obtained, Resnick and coworkers[144] observed alterations in 15 (38 per cent). Bilateral abnormalities predominate. Well-defined plantar or posterior calcaneal enthesophytes, or both, are a common manifestation but are similar in appear-ance to those in a "normal" population. Retrocalcaneal swelling (related to bursitis), posterior calcaneal erosion, and Achilles tendon thickening also are frequent. Bony erosion and proliferation resulting in poorly defined enthe-sophytes at the site of ligamentous attachment to bone on the inferior surface of the calcaneus are identical to the findings of psoriatic arthritis and Reiter's syndrome.[262] Peri-osteal proliferation along the entire undersurface of the bone also is evident in a few patients.

Temporomandibular Joint (Fig. 28–41)

Clinical and radiologic manifestations resulting from temporomandibular joint arthritis in patients with ankylos-ing spondylitis have been recorded. Estimates of the preva-lence of such manifestations generally are in the range of 4 to 8 per cent.[145] Maes and Dihlmann[146] reported right tem-poromandibular joint involvement in 4 per cent of 100 unselected cases of ankylosing spondylitis, characterized by narrowing of the articular space, irregularities of the con-dylar head, and periostitis of the adjacent coronoid process at the attachment of the temporal muscle. Resnick[147] ob-served similar involvement in 32 per cent of 25 patients with relatively long-standing disease. In this latter series, the findings of joint space narrowing, erosions, decreased range of motion, beaking, and osteophytic alterations at the joint margins were similar to those accompanying psoriatic

Text continued on page 1054

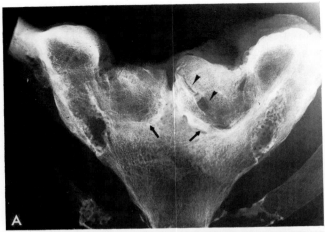

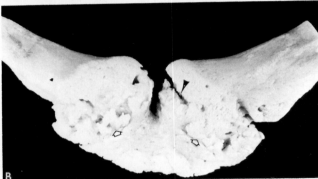

FIGURE 28–34. Abnormalities of the sternoclavicular joint.
  A A radiograph of a coronal section of the sternoclavicular joints indicates intra-articular osseous fusion (arrows) between the medial end of each clavicle and the sternum. A remnant of the articular space on one side can be identified (arrowheads).
  B Photograph of the anterior aspect of the coronal section in **A** demonstrates the extent of intra-articular ankylosis. Note an identifiable segment of the articular space (arrowhead) and the irregular anterior bony excrescences (open arrows).

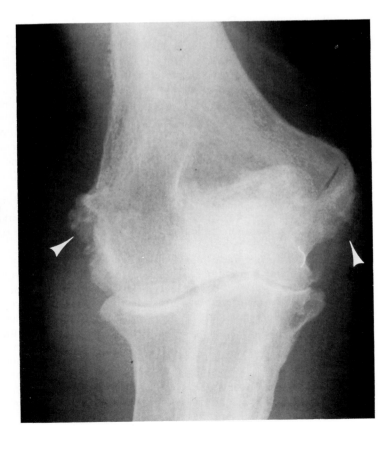

FIGURE 28–35. Abnormalities of the elbow. Findings include joint space narrowing and periosteal irregularity at the articular margins (arrowheads). (From Resnick D: Radiology *110:* 523, 1974.)

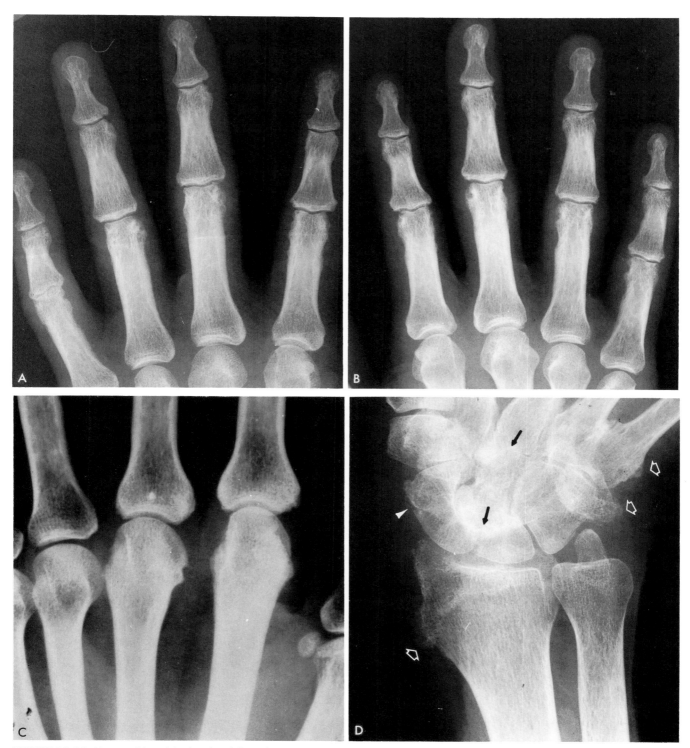

FIGURE 28–36. Abnormalities of the hand and the wrist.

A, B Bilateral abnormalities consist of fusiform periarticular soft tissue swelling, mild joint space diminution, and marginal erosion of proximal interphalangeal and distal interphalangeal joints.

C At the metacarpophalangeal joints, erosions on both the ulnar and radial aspects can be seen. Mild osteoporosis and joint space narrowing are evident.

D In the wrist, findings include narrowing of the midcarpal and common carpometacarpal compartments (solid arrows), erosions (arrowhead), and marginal irregular new bone formation (open arrows).

(**A, C, D,** From Resnick D: Radiology *110:* 523, 1974.)

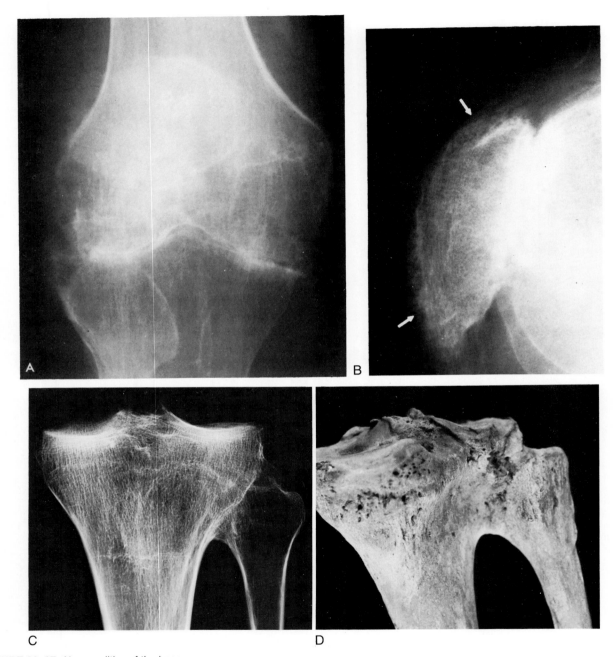

FIGURE 28–37. Abnormalities of the knee.
 A Anteroposterior radiograph demonstrates narrowing of the medial femorotibial and lateral femorotibial spaces.
 B Poorly defined hyperostosis on the anterior surface of the patella (arrows) is indicative of spondylitic enthesopathy. Patellofemoral space narrowing also is apparent.
 C, D Complete bone ankylosis of the proximal tibiofibular joint is observed on this radiograph and corresponding photograph of a macerated specimen.
 (**A,** From Resnick D: Radiology *110:* 523, 1974.)

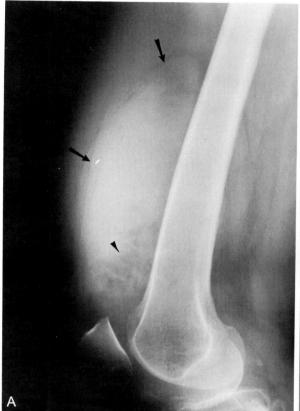

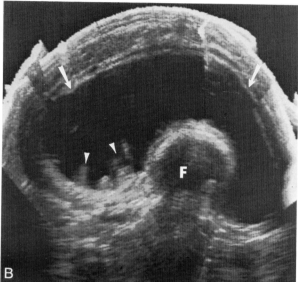

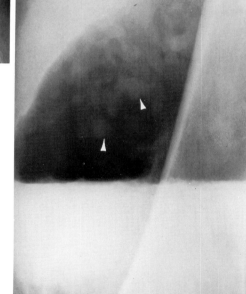

FIGURE 28–38. Abnormalities of the knee. This 54 year old man had had ankylosing spondylitis for approximately 25 years. Multiple episodes of painless swelling of the supra-patellar region were followed by spontaneous resolution. At the time of the imaging studies illustrated, an aspiration of the fluid in the distended suprapatellar pouch revealed 3000 cells per cu mm and, subsequently, no growth of organisms. Over a period of several weeks, the swelling resolved.

A The lateral radiograph demonstrates massive distention of the suprapatellar pouch (arrows) and multiple nodular radiolucent shadows (arrowhead).

B On a transverse sonogram, note the distended bursa (arrows) containing nodular synovial excrescences (arrow-heads). F, Femur.

C An upright frontal image during double contrast arthrog-raphy documents the nodular synovial hyperplasia (arrow-heads) in the distended suprapatellar pouch.

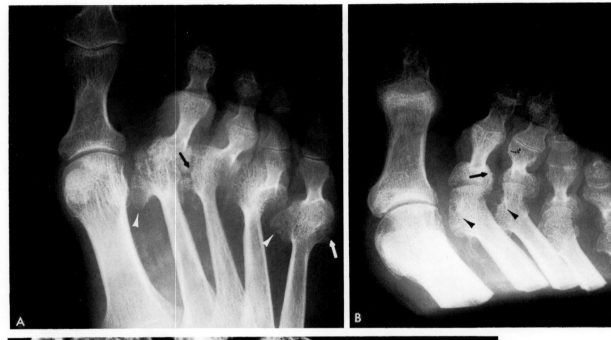

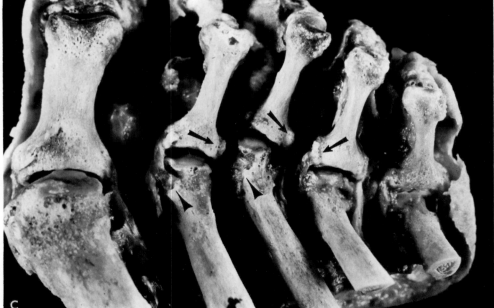

FIGURE 28–39. Abnormalities of the forefoot.

A Observe extensive bony proliferation of the metatarsal heads of the second to fifth digits (arrowheads). Superficial erosions (arrows) and subluxations are evident.

B, C On a radiograph and photograph of a macerated forefoot in a cadaver with ankylosing spondylitis, note osseous erosion with proliferation, predominantly on the medial aspect of the metatarsal heads (arrowheads) and the medial and lateral aspects of the proximal phalanges (arrows). Dorsiflexion and fibular deviation of the toes can be appreciated.

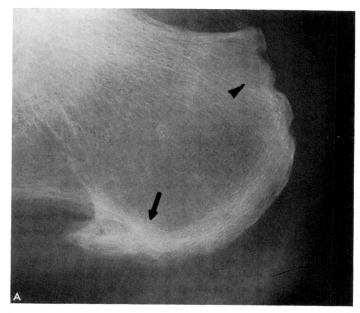

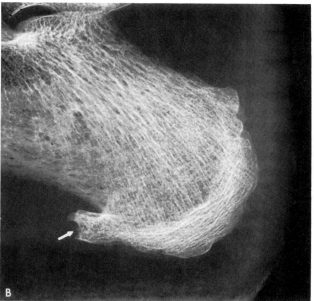

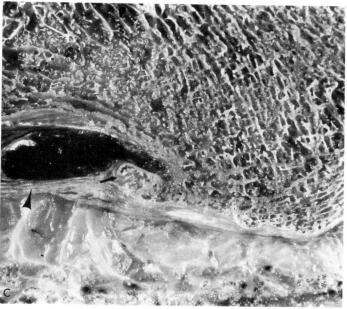

FIGURE 28–40. Abnormalities of the calcaneus.

A Findings include erosion of the posterosuperior aspect of the bone (arrowhead), related to retrocalcaneal bursitis, and erosive and proliferative changes of the plantar aspect of the bone (arrow), related to an enthesopathy at the ligamentous attachments.

B, C On a radiograph and photograph of a sagittal section of the calcaneus, the nature of the proliferative enthesophyte (arrows) on the plantar aspect of the bone is evident. Note its relationship to the plantar aponeurosis (arrowhead).

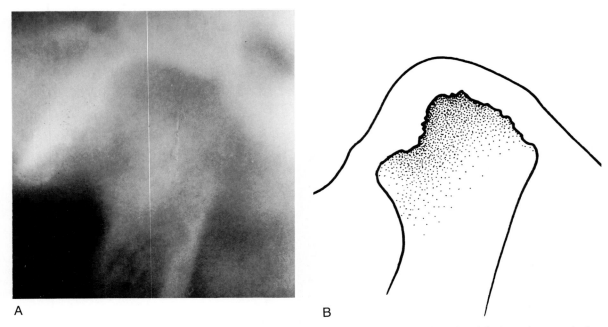

FIGURE 28–41. Abnormalities of the temporomandibular joint. Erosive abnormalities. A large irregular defect can be seen in the anterior portion of the mandibular condyle with smaller defects along the posterosuperior aspect of the condyle and the anterior margin of the temporal fossa and tubercle. Mild sclerosis is present. (From Resnick D: Radiology *112:* 587, 1974.)

arthritis and rheumatoid arthritis. Asymmetric or unilateral involvement is frequent. Erosions predominate on the mandibular condyle, either at its anterior margin or superiorly at the junction of its middle and posterior thirds. Because of the thickness of the temporal fossa, erosions in that area are difficult to identify. Davidson and associates[148] studied 79 patients with ankylosing spondylitis and detected clinical abnormalities of the temporomandibular joints in 16 persons (21 per cent). These abnormalities consisted of pain or limitation of motion, or both, malocclusion of teeth, and "clicking." In some of their patients, radiographs revealed flattening or erosion of the condylar heads and asymmetry or restricted movement on open-mouth and closed-mouth projections. Histologic evaluation of a joint in one patient demonstrated an inflammatory synovial process, meniscal and articular cartilaginous damage, and "degenerative" features.

As in other processes that involve this joint, CT scanning and MR imaging can be used effectively to study temporomandibular joint abnormalities in ankylosing spondylitis.

COEXISTENCE WITH OTHER DISORDERS

Rheumatoid Arthritis (Fig. 28–42)

The concept that ankylosing spondylitis and rheumatoid arthritis are separate and distinct diseases rarely is challenged today. The accurate diagnosis of one or the other is facilitated by characteristic clinical, radiologic, and laboratory features. In some instances, however, difficulty arises in the differentiation of these two disorders—for example, in the patient with ankylosing spondylitis who develops peripheral joint involvement or in the patient with rheumatoid arthritis who develops sacroiliitis.

Rarely, both ankylosing spondylitis and rheumatoid arthritis appear to develop in the same person.[149–154, 265, 266,]

[311, 367–369] In this situation, the two disorders commonly do not have any unusual features. Typically, a male patient will develop ankylosing spondylitis at a young age and subsequently, at a time when his spondylitic process largely is inactive, he will develop rheumatoid arthritis.[154] Furthermore, there appears to be little interaction between the disorders, the clinical and radiographic manifestations of one disease not being significantly modified by the second disease.[214]

In these persons, the diagnosis of rheumatoid arthritis is firmly established by the presence of a high-titer seropositive (for rheumatoid factor), symmetrically distributed erosive arthritis of the joints of the appendicular skeleton, with or without rheumatoid nodules, and, frequently, with seropositivity for the histocompatibility antigen HLA-DR4; the diagnosis of ankylosing spondylitis is documented by the presence of typical sacroiliitis and spondylitis in a patient who possesses the histocompatibility antigen HLA-B27. In this fashion, the diagnostic criteria for both rheumatoid arthritis and ankylosing spondylitis are fulfilled.

Although certain authors have established that the two diseases should coexist in approximately 1 in 238,000 persons,[151] only a relatively few patients have been reported who have both rheumatoid arthritis and ankylosing spondylitis. It is probable that the clinical and radiologic manifestations of one of these disorders obscure many of the features of the second, so that the single more appropriate diagnosis is applied to many patients who have both ankylosing spondylitis and rheumatoid arthritis: in patients in whom spondylitis has long dominated, the possibility might easily be overlooked that a newly acquired peripheral joint disease is rheumatoid arthritis; or in those in whom rheumatoid arthritis has been active and severe, the low back pain of ankylosing spondylitis easily might be attributed to the rheumatoid process.[152] On the other hand, the possibility

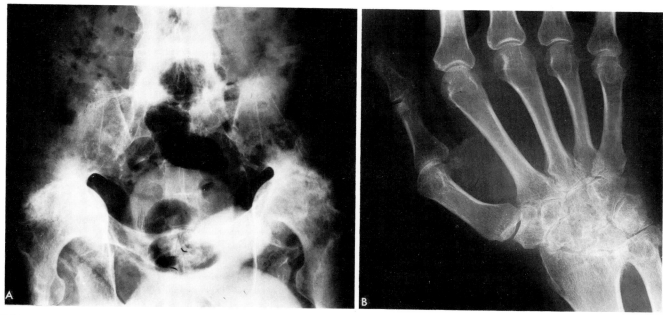

FIGURE 28–42. Coexistent ankylosing spondylitis and rheumatoid arthritis. A 61 year old man had had documented HLA-B27–positive ankylosing spondylitis for over 20 years and high titer seropositive rheumatoid arthritis for 10 years.

A The radiograph of the pelvis indicates complete ankylosis of both sacroiliac joints, spinal syndesmophytes, and bilateral protrusio acetabuli deformities.

B The hand and wrist abnormalities are those of rheumatoid arthritis. They include diffuse involvement of the wrist with joint space narrowing and osseous erosion and, at the metacarpophalangeal joints, osteoporosis, diminution of interosseous space, and marginal erosions of the metacarpal heads.

that one of these diseases interferes with the expression of the second, explaining the rarity of the reported patients with this combination of diseases, has not been verified.[155]

Diffuse Idiopathic Skeletal Hyperostosis (DISH)

During the radiographic examination of older persons with long-standing ankylosing spondylitis, it is not unusual to document the presence of both ankylosing spondylitis and DISH.[267, 381] In this situation, widespread intra-articular bony ankylosis of both sacroiliac joints, syndesmophytosis, and apophyseal joint space narrowing or osseous fusion are combined with "flowing" ossification along the anterior aspect of a portion of the spine, particularly in the thoracic segment. Although there is a natural tendency to attribute all the radiographic findings to one disease, careful analysis ensures the accurate diagnosis of both disorders. The anteriorly distributed broad osseous excrescences of DISH differ considerably from the thin vertical syndesmophytes of ankylosing spondylitis, which hug the outer portion of the intervertebral disc; and the intra-articular bony ankylosis of the sacroiliac and apophyseal joints, which is typical of ankylosing spondylitis, is easily differentiated from the para-articular osteophytic changes of DISH. Considering the frequency of DISH in middle-aged and elderly persons, the clinician should not be surprised by its appearance in patients with ankylosing spondylitis.

Inflammatory Bowel Disorders

The well-documented association of ankylosing spondylitis and certain inflammatory bowel disorders such as ul-

cerative colitis and Crohn's disease is discussed in Chapter 31.

Paget's Disease

The difficulty in assessing radiographs of the sacroiliac joints in patients with Paget's disease and the possible association of ankylosing spondylitis and Paget's disease are discussed in Chapter 54.

Other Articular Disorders

Some persons with ankylosing spondylitis reveal clinical and radiographic manifestations of additional articular disorders, such as crystal-induced arthropathies (gout, calcium pyrophosphate dihydrate crystal deposition disease) or septic arthritis. The accurate diagnosis of the superimposed condition generally is not difficult. Occasionally, rapidly appearing and progressive abnormalities in a joint of the peripheral skeleton due to the spondylitic process itself can stimulate an unrewarding search for a causative crystalline or infective agent (Fig. 28–43).

OTHER DIAGNOSTIC TECHNIQUES

Scintigraphy

The evaluation of sacroiliac and spinal abnormalities in ankylosing spondylitis using radionuclide techniques has been attempted with varying degrees of success.[156–169, 191–193, 206–208, 213, 307, 370, 382, 387] Application of such techniques to the detection of sacroiliitis has been stimulated by the difficulty in recognizing early sacroiliac joint abnormalities on rou-

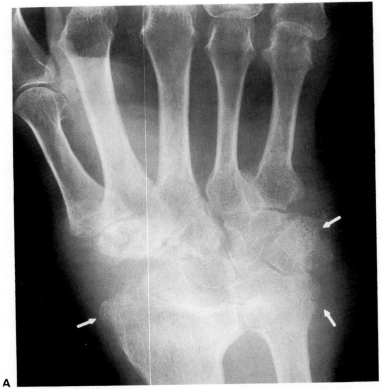

FIGURE 28–43. Rapidly progressive wrist abnormalities in ankylosing spondylitis.

A In this patient, increasing soft tissue swelling and bony destruction suggested the possibility of infectious arthritis superimposed on the spondylitic process. Multiple aspirations and biopsies failed to document the presence of an infection. The proliferative osseous abnormalities (arrows) are consistent with ankylosing spondylitis alone.

B, C A routine radiograph and arthrogram document severe disease of the wrist in a 60 year old man with ankylosing spondylitis. In **B,** observe soft tissue swelling, bone destruction throughout the carpus, and joint space narrowing, especially in the radiocarpal compartment. In **C,** the radiopaque contrast material outlines irregular synovium in the radiocarpal compartment (arrow) and communication of this compartment with the inferior radioulnar compartment (arrowhead) through a defect in the triangular fibrocartilage. Contrast material adjacent to the styloid process of the ulna may be within the extensor carpi ulnaris tendon sheath and soft tissues.

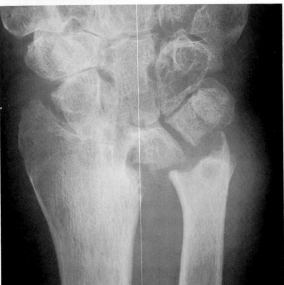

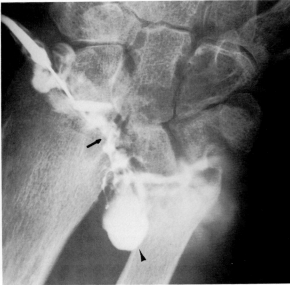

tine radiographic examination. Qualitative analysis of the accumulation of bone-seeking radiopharmaceutical preparations in the sacroiliac region is difficult, however, because of the normal radionuclide activity in this location. Visual comparison of sacroiliac joint to sacral activity occasionally can provide helpful information regarding the presence and distribution of articular inflammation, although quantitative analysis is far superior.[159-165, 269-278] Such analysis appears most useful in those patients with early disease whose radiographs are normal or questionably abnormal.[212] Quantitative analysis is accomplished by delineating an "area of interest" cursor along a line that encompasses the joints and the sacrum. The ratio of sacroiliac joint to sacral radionuclide activity is calculated and the result is compared to normal values for each individual x-ray department. Generally, ratios greater than 1.3 to 1 or 1.45 to 1 are considered abnormal.[268] It is obvious that any increase in sacral scintigraphic activity can lower this ratio and obscure the diagnosis of sacroiliitis; anatomic variations, such as a prominent sacral tubercle, can produce an elevation of radionuclide activity in the sacrum. Furthermore, uptake of the radionuclide in the sacrum and the joint is influenced by age and sex of the patient, and ratios are not always uniform for the two sides of the body in normal persons.[270, 274, 276] Some investigators believe that the sacrum is not an ideal reference point in the assessment of radionuclide activity in the sacroiliac joints as accumulation of the radiopharmaceutical agent by the sacrum may increase in the presence of nearby inflammation.[277] Other reference areas, such as the paraspinal soft tissues and proximal end of the femur, have been advocated. In patients with advanced disease, radionuclide uptake in the sacroiliac joints (as well as the spine) may not be abnormal[162, 166, 167] (Fig. 28–44A, B). Unilateral alterations frequently are easier to interpret both qualitatively and quantitatively (particularly if the ratio of the activity of the involved sacroiliac joint to that of the sacrum is used, rather than averaging the activity of both sides).

Increased accumulation of radionuclide in spinal and peripheral articulations and at entheses also can be observed in patients with ankylosing spondylitis, especially in the presence of active disease.[166, 206, 383] At any location, an abnormal scintigraphic examination is not specific, accurate diagnosis necessitating its correlation with clinical and radiologic investigations. Such correlation is especially important in the evaluation of patients with long-standing ankylosing spondylitis who develop new back pain with or without a history of trauma. Focal areas of augmented radionuclide accumulation in the spine may indicate the site of an acute fracture or chronic "pseudarthrosis," and the exact diagnosis then can be substantiated by plain films and conventional tomograms or CT scans (Fig. 28–44C–F).[279, 280] Other spinal abnormalities can be detected in a similar fashion (Fig. 28–44G–I).

Computed Tomography

Owing to the difficulty in detecting sacroiliitis by conventional radiography and to the controversy regarding the role of scintigraphy in this detection, CT scanning has been employed by some investigators in an effort to delineate early abnormalities of the sacroiliac joint in ankylosing spondylitis. The results have been conflicting. Some reports

indicate clear superiority of CT over routine radiography,[281, 282, 308] whereas others question this superiority.[283, 284] Most investigators would agree that careful analysis of high quality radiographs of the sacroiliac joint remains the fundamental method of examination, and that CT should be reserved for cases in which results of the initial radiographs are equivocal or normal, especially in those patients in whom clinical or laboratory parameters indicate a high index of suspicion for sacroiliitis.[285] Interpretation of the CT scans must be accomplished by those knowledgeable in the normal variations of the sacroiliac joint that can simulate the findings of inflammation.[286] In this regard, severe joint space loss, subchondral bone sclerosis in subjects under the age of 40 years, osseous erosions, and intra-articular bone ankylosis are more valuable CT indicators of sacroiliitis than are nonuniform iliac sclerosis and focal joint space narrowing in patients over the age of 30 years.[286] Although CT would appear superior to conventional tomography, especially in view of the relatively high radiation exposure of the latter method,[287, 288] meticulous technique is required. The authors prefer to obtain coronal images of the sacroiliac joint, as well as to examine the patient in the supine position and also to angle the gantry approximately 10 degrees toward the head, enabling them to obtain transverse images of the sacroiliac joint (Fig. 28–45). Others prefer using a coronal display alone.

Additional indications for CT scanning in patients with ankylosing spondylitis are variable and include the detection of spinal fractures, spinal stenosis, thecal diverticula (Figs. 28–46 and 28–47), atlantoaxial instability, and manubriosternal and costovertebral disease.[317, 339, 341, 354, 356, 357, 388] Reformation of original transaxial data into coronal and sagittal planes can be useful, especially in the analysis of spinal fractures.[371, 372] Paraspinal muscle atrophy also can be documented (Fig. 28–48).[301]

Magnetic Resonance Imaging

Certain manifestations and complications of ankylosing spondylitis exist for which MR imaging may prove useful. Although the technique has been applied to the assessment of activity of discovertebral disease in a relatively early stage of ankylosing spondylitis,[373] at present this appears to represent a minor indication for MR imaging. Increased signal intensity within the vertebral body marrow, adjacent to abnormal intervertebral discs, in T2-weighted spin echo sequences is consistent with the presence of edema (Fig. 28–49). This finding is not unexpected with active spondylodiscitis. More important, however, may be the role of MR imaging in the assessment of chronic discovertebral destruction, particularly in the differentiation of improper fracture healing and infection. The characteristic features of infective spondylitis as shown with MR imaging are well documented (see Chapter 65); those of a "pseudarthrosis" are not yet clear.[384] Fibrous tissue, however, which may be present in abundance at the fracture site, would be expected to have different signal characteristics than those of infective tissue.

MR imaging has been applied successfully to the evaluation of spondylitic patients with the cauda equina syndrome.[357, 358] Dorsally situated arachnoid diverticula are visualized directly with this method. The fluid contents of the diverticula are well demonstrated, as are the accompa-

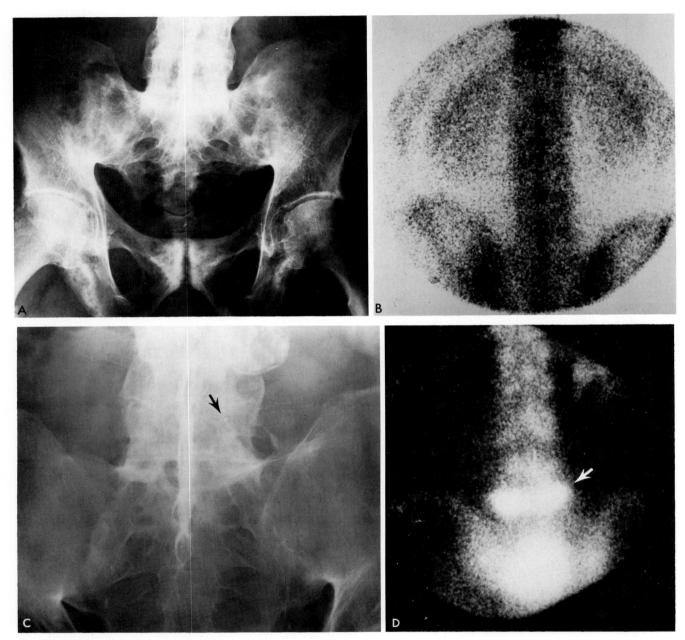

FIGURE 28–44. Scintigraphic abnormalities in ankylosing spondylitis.

A, B In this patient with typical spondylitic radiographic changes in the sacroiliac joints, spine, hips, and symphysis pubis, a radionuclide study using ^{99m}Tc pyrophosphate reveals no abnormal uptake within the vertebral column. Lack of uptake is thought to indicate "burned-out" disease.

C, D In this patient with long-standing ankylosing spondylitis who had sustained a fall, a focal area of augmented activity on bone scan (arrow) corresponds to the site of a subtle fracture of the fifth lumbar vertebra on radiographic examination (arrow).

Illustration continued on opposite page

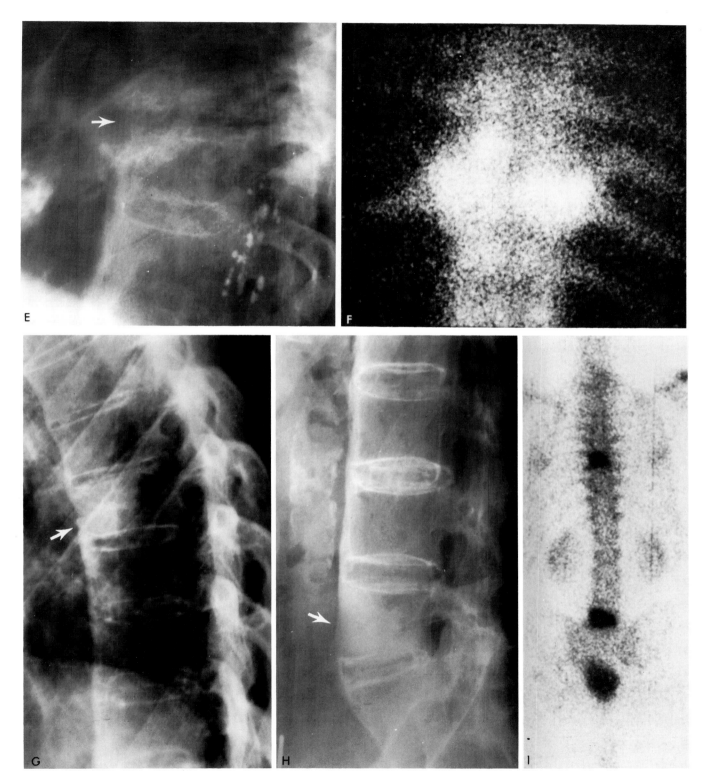

FIGURE 28–44 *Continued*

E, F In a different patient with ankylosing spondylitis, abnormal radionuclide uptake in the midthoracic spine indicates the presence of a "pseudarthrosis" at the site of a previous fracture (arrow).

G–I In this patient with ankylosing spondylitis, new back pain resulted from spinal metastases originating from a carcinoma of the prostate. The lateral radiographs of the thoracic and lumbar spine reveal subtle osteoblastic lesions (arrows), superimposed on the changes of ankylosing spondylitis. The radionuclide study demonstrates two areas of augmented isotopic activity, corresponding to the sites of metastasis.

(**A, B,** From Weissberg D, et al: AJR *131:* 665, 1978. Copyright 1978, American Roentgen Ray Society.)

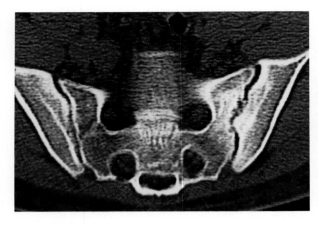

FIGURE 28–45. CT scanning in ankylosing spondylitis: Sacroiliitis. A transaxial image through the lower portion of the sacroiliac joint shows bilateral articular abnormalities, greater on the left side, consisting of joint surface irregularity and erosion in both the ilium and the sacrum, with associated new bone formation.

nying osseous erosions of the posterior elements of affected vertebrae. Although CT probably is superior to MR imaging in the demonstration of the bone abnormalities, the usefulness of the latter method in the exclusion of an intraspinal tumor should be emphasized.

Several investigations have focused on the role of MR imaging in the analysis of sacroiliac joint inflammation. Ahlström and coworkers[374] used this method to evaluate 27 consecutive patients with symptoms suggestive of sacroiliitis. These investigators found that the diagnostic sensitivity of MR imaging was similar to that of CT; however, they also emphasized that MR imaging provided insight into the pathologic events that accompany sacroiliitis. Indeed, two different patterns of altered signal intensity were observed. In the first, low signal intensity in the subchondral bone marrow on the more T1-weighted spin echo images was associated with high signal intensity on the more T2-weighted spin echo images (Fig. 28–50A, B). In the second, which was more frequent, low signal intensity was evident in all sequences (Fig. 28–50C, D). The authors postulated that the first type of abnormality was consistent with inflammatory edema in the bone marrow and the second, with fibrosis or bone sclerosis.

Murphey and collaborators,[375] in a study of 17 patients with clinical and radiologic evidence of sacroiliitis, found MR imaging superior to CT scanning in the evaluation of cartilage and the detection of bone erosions. Standard spin echo sequences and coronal imaging were employed. With

MR, findings of sacroiliitis were abnormal signal intensity of cartilage and bone erosions on T1-weighted images, and increased signal intensity in the joint or in erosions on T2-weighted images. Docherty and coworkers[376] studied 20 patients with established or suspected sacroiliitis on the basis of conventional radiography. As in the investigation of Murphey and coworkers, these investigators stressed the sensitivity of MR imaging, which they believed was superior to routine radiography, and they indicated that interobserver and intraobserver variability was no poorer than that encountered with routine radiography. MR imaging proved useful in the analysis of articular cartilage and subchondral bone marrow.

Because of these results, it appears that MR imaging may play a role in the early diagnosis of sacroiliitis. How MR compares with other methods, including quantitative scintigraphy, in the assessment of sacroiliitis, and the clinical impact of such early diagnosis, require further investigation.

Other potential applications of MR imaging in patients with ankylosing spondylitis include assessment of spinal stenosis and of peripheral joint involvement (Fig. 28–51).

ETIOLOGY AND PATHOGENESIS

Early studies of spondylitic patients implicated a variety of etiologic factors in the disease, such as trauma,[170] pulmonary tuberculosis,[171] parathyroid disease,[172] sepsis, lead

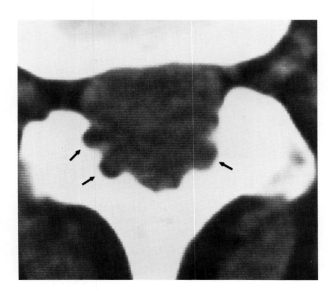

FIGURE 28–46. CT scanning in ankylosing spondylitis: Thecal diverticula. In this transaxial image through the lower portion of the lumbar spine, scalloped erosions (arrows) of the laminae are diagnostic of thecal diverticula, a known complication of ankylosing spondylitis. (Courtesy of A. Brower, M.D., Washington, D.C.)

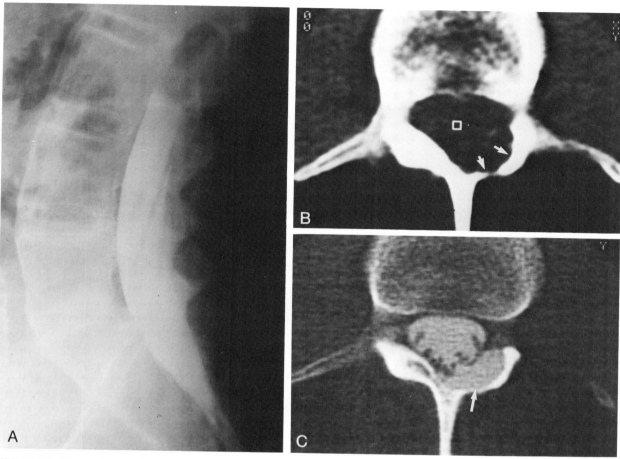

FIGURE 28–47. CT scanning in ankylosing spondylitis: Thecal diverticula.
   A A lateral view obtained during lumbar myelography with the patient prone shows no abnormality.
   B A transaxial CT scan at the level of the third lumbar vertebra demonstrates smooth erosion of the left lamina (arrows).
   C A transaxial CT scan at a more caudal level than that in **B**, obtained after myelography, reveals a diverticulum (arrow) extending dorsolaterally from the dural sac and filling the osseous defect within the lamina. (From Mitchell MJ, et al: Radiology *175:* 521, 1990.)

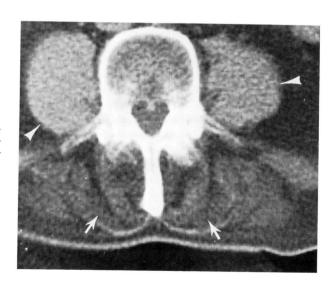

FIGURE 28–48. CT scanning in ankylosing spondylitis: Paraspinal muscle atrophy. Observe atrophy of paraspinal musculature (arrows). Compare the appearance to that of the psoas muscles (arrowheads). (Courtesy of M. Sage, M.D., Bedford Park, South Australia.)

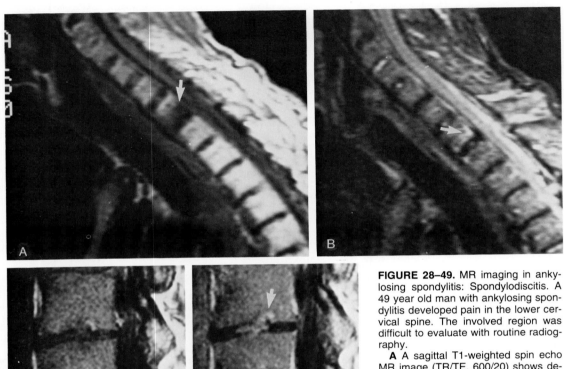

FIGURE 28–49. MR imaging in ankylosing spondylitis: Spondylodiscitis. A 49 year old man with ankylosing spondylitis developed pain in the lower cervical spine. The involved region was difficult to evaluate with routine radiography.

A A sagittal T1-weighted spin echo MR image (TR/TE, 600/20) shows decreased signal intensity (arrow) in the lower portion of the seventh cervical vertebral body. The anterior longitudinal ligament appears slightly displaced.

B On a sagittal T2-weighted spin echo MR image (TR/TE, 2182/70), an increase in signal intensity occurs in this region (arrow). The findings are compatible with edema, which may accompany enthesitis or previous fracture. The posterior osseous elements and soft tissues are not well evaluated on these images.

C, D Sagittal T1-weighted (TR/TE, 650/20) spin echo MR images obtained before (**C**) and after (**D**) intravenous injection of gadolinium contrast agent reveal irregular discovertebral junctions with enhancement of signal intensity (arrows) in **D.**

(**C, D,** Courtesy of J. Hodler, M.D., Zurich, Switzerland.)

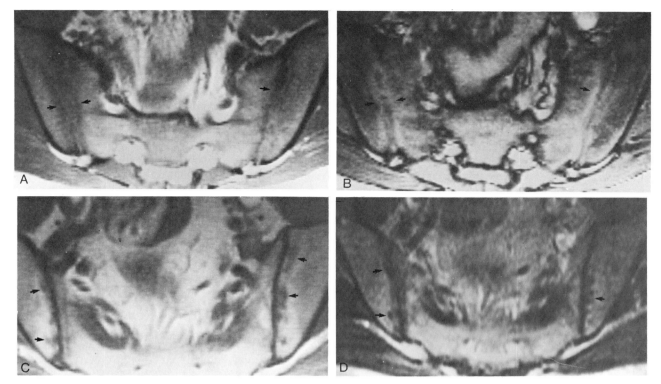

FIGURE 28–50. MR imaging in ankylosing spondylitis: Sacroiliitis.

A, B In this 17 year old patient with suspected sacroiliitis, conventional radiography and CT failed to reveal any abnormalities. In a transaxial T1-weighted spin echo MR image (TR/TE, 500/22) **(A)** regions of low signal intensity are seen about both sacroiliac joints (arrows). In a transaxial proton density weighted spin echo MR image (TR/TE, 1500/37) **(B)**, the signal intensity in the periarticular bone marrow is increased (arrows).

C, D In a different patient with confirmed ankylosing spondylitis, a transaxial T1-weighted spin echo MR image (TR/TE, 500/22) **(C)** reveals low signal intensity within periarticular bone marrow (arrows). A similar image with T2 weighting (TR/TE, 2000/90) **(D)** shows persistent low signal intensity in these regions (arrows)

(From Ahlstrom H, et al: Arthritis Rheum *33:* 1763, 1990.)

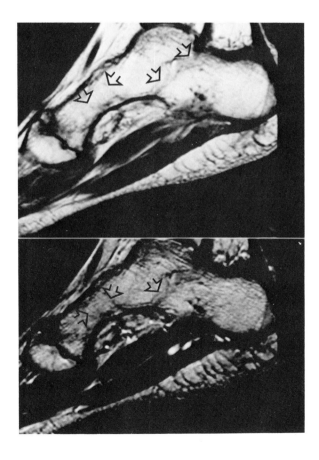

FIGURE 28–51. MR imaging in ankylosing spondylitis: Peripheral joint involvement. On parasagittal proton density (TR/TE, 1500/25) (top) and T2-weighted (TR/TE, 1500/80) (bottom) MR images, intra-articular bone fusion is evident in the subtalar and intertarsal joints (arrows). Small fluid collections are visible in the plantar soft tissues.

(Courtesy of S. Fernandez, M.D., Mexico City, Mexico.)

intoxication, allergy, and endocrine and metabolic defects.[1] These theories now are outdated, and many of the current investigations cite the importance of genetic factors.

A strikingly high frequency of the HLA-B27 antigen in patients with ankylosing spondylitis now has been observed all over the world.[173, 174, 290, 292, 377, 389] In most reports, more than 90 per cent of white spondylitic patients possess the B27 gene; the frequency of this gene among whites who do not have ankylosing spondylitis is approximately 6 to 8 per cent. To date, this remains the most significant association between a readily detectable HLA antigen and a well-defined disease, underscoring the importance of genetics in the causation of ankylosing spondylitis. It appears that the B27 gene interacts with other, as yet unidentified genes as well as environmental factors to lead to the development of this disease.[377]

A high prevalence of ankylosing spondylitis or asymptomatic sacroiliitis has been observed within the families of spondylitic patients[175–179]; it has been estimated that approximately 50 per cent of family members of patients with ankylosing spondylitis who inherit the B27-containing haplotype will themselves develop the disease.[174] The mode of inheritance is not clear. Some investigators conclude that ankylosing spondylitis is due to an autosomal dominant factor with variable penetrance,[180, 181] although multiple factors may be operational,[182] perhaps explaining why some studies note a lower prevalence (less than 20 per cent) of ankylosing spondylitis among B27-positive persons.[209]

Ankylosing spondylitis can develop in the absence of the HLA-B27 antigen,[183, 184] although it has been suggested by some investigators that B27-positive patients have more severe clinical and radiologic manifestations than do B27-negative patients.[185, 189, 194, 291] Other authors have not confirmed specific differences between these two groups of patients,[67, 186, 378] although additional genetic markers, such as HLA-DR4, have been associated with characteristic clinical features in patients with ankylosing spondylitis in some reports.[309]

These results and others now indicate that additional genetic or environmental factors are important in disease expression. Pelvic inflammation may represent one such factor, acting as an environmental trigger in genetically predisposed persons.[1, 210, 293] The importance of genitourinary tract infection as a cause of ankylosing spondylitis was stressed by Romanus in 1953.[187] After observing such infection in nearly 90 per cent of men with ankylosing spondylitis, this investigator suggested that spinal and sacroiliac joint contamination occurring after pelvic sepsis resulted from spread via lymphatic routes or Batson's vertebral venous plexus. Mason and coworkers[188] noted chronic prostatitis in 83 per cent of patients with spondylitis, further substantiating a relationship between ankylosing spondylitis and genitourinary tract infection. Although this relationship has not been definitely verified, the appearance of sacroiliac joint and spinal abnormalities in patients with chronic bowel disease or paralysis, conditions that are associated with pelvic infection, is of particular interest. Similarly, it is interesting to note that a relationship between sacroiliitis and salpingitis has been recorded in some reports.[210, 289]

DIFFERENTIAL DIAGNOSIS

Sacroiliitis

The sacroiliac joint abnormalities in ankylosing spondylitis must be differentiated from those accompanying other disorders (Table 28–5). This can be accomplished by analysis of both distribution and morphology of the articular changes. Classically, a bilateral and symmetric distribution is observed in ankylosing spondylitis. Although a similar pattern can be evident in other seronegative spondyloarthropathies, such as psoriasis and Reiter's syndrome, asymmetric or, rarely, unilateral alterations may accompany these latter disorders (Fig. 28–52). A bilateral and symmetric distribution also is associated with the sacroiliitis of inflammatory bowel disease (ulcerative colitis, Crohn's disease, Whipple's disease), which is identical in every regard to that of classic ankylosing spondylitis. In rheumatoid arthritis, minor sacroiliac articular abnormalities commonly are bilateral but may be asymmetric in appearance. Bilateral and symmetric alterations of the sacroiliac joint also are noted in hyperparathyroidism (and renal osteodystrophy), osteitis condensans ilii, gouty arthritis, and degenerative joint disease, although in the last two conditions, an asym-

TABLE 28–5. Distribution of Sacroiliac Joint Abnormalities in Various Disorders*

Disorder	Bilateral, Symmetric Distribution	Bilateral, Asymmetric Distribution	Unilateral Distribution
Ankylosing spondylitis	+	−	−
Psoriatic spondylitis	+	+	+
Reiter's syndrome	+	+	+
Sacroiliitis of inflammatory bowel disease	+	−	−
Rheumatoid arthritis	−	+	+
Osteitis condensans ilii	+	−	−
Hyperparathyroidism	+	−	−
Gouty arthritis	+	+	+
Osteoarthritis	+	+	+
Infection	−	−	+

*Only most typical patterns of distribution are indicated.

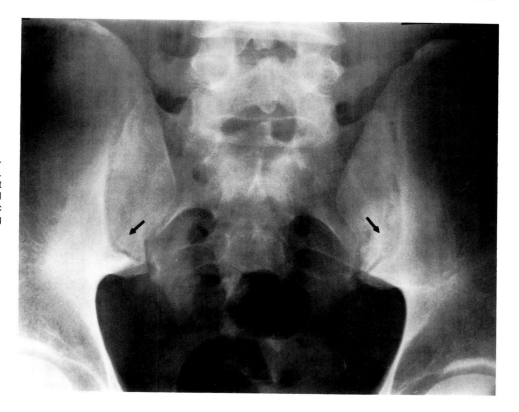

FIGURE 28–52. Sacroiliac joint abnormalities in Reiter's syndrome. Bilateral asymmetric sacroiliac joint changes (arrows) are more typical of Reiter's syndrome and psoriatic arthritis than of classic ankylosing spondylitis.

metric or unilateral distribution is not uncommon. Unilateral abnormalities are most typical in infection and may accompany contralateral hip disease and ipsilateral paralysis or disuse (cartilage atrophy).

Poorly defined erosive abnormality with adjacent sclerosis, particularly in the ilium, with associated joint space narrowing, intra-articular osseous fusion, and ligamentous ossification is the characteristic appearance of sacroiliac joint disease in classic ankylosing spondylitis and in the sacroiliitis of inflammatory bowel disease. In psoriasis and Reiter's syndrome, extensive bony eburnation may be unaccompanied by intra-articular osseous fusion. Sacroiliac joint involvement in rheumatoid arthritis usually is manifested as superficial erosions, minimal sclerosis, and absence of significant bony ankylosis. Subchondral resorption of bone, predominantly in the ilium, in conjunction with primary or secondary hyperparathyroidism leads to irregularity of the osseous surface, adjacent sclerosis, and widening of the interosseous joint space; articular space diminution and bony fusion are not seen. In osteitis condensans ilii, a triangular segment of bone sclerosis is evident in the inferior aspect of the ilium. The joint surface is well defined, and the articular space is not diminished. Sacral alterations indeed are unusual. In chronic tophaceous gouty arthritis, large, gouged-out defects with surrounding sclerosis are observed, whereas in degenerative arthritis, joint space narrowing, bony sclerosis, and anterior osteophytes are associated with a noneroded, smooth subchondral bony margin. Calcification and ossification of the interosseous ligament above the synovial sacroiliac joint can be encountered in degenerative joint disease, but widespread ossification of this structure, as noted in ankylosing spondylitis, is not common. Cartilage atrophy accompanying paralysis or

disuse produces diffuse loss of articular space with surrounding osteoporosis. In some patients with long-standing paralysis, intra-articular osseous fusion is seen, perhaps related to chronic low-grade inflammation.

Spondylitis

Spinal abnormalities in classic ankylosing spondylitis initially appear in the thoracolumbar and lumbosacral junctions and subsequently may extend throughout the thoracic and lumbar spine and into the cervical region. An identical distribution is encountered in the spondylitis of inflammatory bowel disease. Although the entire vertebral column may be altered in psoriasis and Reiter's syndrome, spotty involvement and absence of severe cervical spinal changes are typical of the latter disorder. In some women with classic ankylosing spondylitis, significant sacroiliac joint and cervical spine abnormalities may appear without obvious thoracic and lumbar spinal changes. This same distribution can be encountered in patients with psoriasis. Spondylitis without sacroiliitis is relatively rare in classic ankylosing spondylitis, although it may be observed in both psoriasis and Reiter's syndrome. Spinal involvement in rheumatoid arthritis has predilection for the cervical spine, with relative sparing of the thoracic and lumbar segments.

The thin vertically oriented syndesmophytes that are evident in classic ankylosing spondylitis and the spondylitis of inflammatory bowel disease differ considerably in appearance from the broad asymmetric bony outgrowths of psoriasis and Reiter's syndrome (Fig. 28–53), the triangular outgrowths of spondylosis deformans, and the flowing anterolateral ossification of diffuse idiopathic skeletal hyperostosis (Table 28–6). Some patients who develop ankylos-

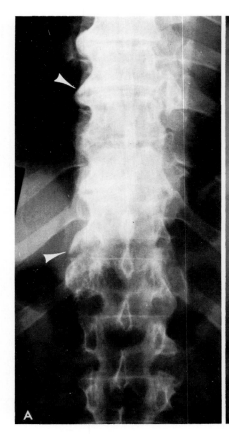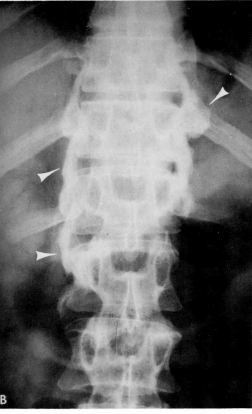

FIGURE 28–53. Spinal abnormalities in Reiter's syndrome and psoriatic spondylitis. In the spondylitis of both Reiter's syndrome **(A)** and psoriatic spondylitis **(B)**, large, bulky irregular, asymmetrically distributed excrescences (arrowheads) are more typical than in classic ankylosing spondylitis. (**B,** Courtesy of E. G. L. Bywaters, M.D., Taplow, Buckinghamshire, England.)

ing spondylitis at an advanced age reveal more laterally displaced excrescences (due to the location of the bulging fibers of the anulus fibrosus), however, which resemble osteophytes accompanying spondylosis deformans, and some patients with psoriasis and Reiter's syndrome demonstrate typical syndesmophytes. The bony excrescences accompanying neuropathic osteoarthropathy, acromegaly, and fluorosis realistically are not confused with the syndesmophytes of ankylosing spondylitis. Syndesmophytes may be seen in patients with alkaptonuria, but additional radiographic manifestations (such as discal calcification and loss of height of the intervertebral disc spaces) ensure accurate differential diagnosis. Vertebral (and sacroiliac joint) abnor-

malities in X-linked hypophosphatemic vitamin D–resistant osteomalacia (Fig. 28–54) may simulate those in ankylosing spondylitis (see Chapter 53).

Osteitis with sclerosis and erosion of the anterior corners of the vertebral bodies and squaring are encountered much more commonly in classic ankylosing spondylitis and the spondylitis of inflammatory bowel disease than in psoriasis and Reiter's syndrome. Similarly, apophyseal joint sclerosis and osseous fusion are more typical of classic ankylosing spondylitis and the spondylitis of inflammatory bowel disease than of the other seronegative spondyloarthropathies.

Discovertebral erosions and sclerosis, which are seen in ankylosing spondylitis, also are observed in psoriasis. Sim-

TABLE 28–6. Bony Outgrowths of the Spine

Outgrowth	Definition	Representative Disorders	Appearance
Syndesmophyte	Ossification of the anulus fibrosus	Ankylosing spondylitis Alkaptonuria	Vertical outgrowth extending from edge of one vertebral body to the next
Osteophyte	Hyperostosis at attachment of annular fibers	Spondylosis deformans	Triangular outgrowth located several millimeters from edge of the vertebral body
Flowing anterior ossification	Ossification of the intervertebral disc, anterior longitudinal ligament, and paravertebral connective tissue	Diffuse idiopathic skeletal hyperostosis	Undulating outgrowth along the anterior aspect of the spine
Paravertebral ossification	Ossification of paravertebral connective tissue	Psoriatic spondylitis Reiter's syndrome	Poorly defined or well-defined outgrowth separated from the edge of the vertebral body and the intervertebral disc

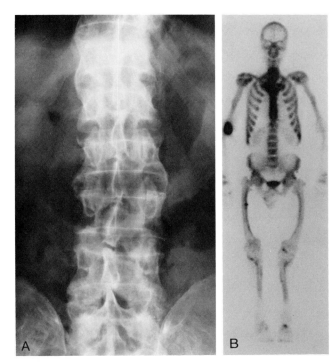

FIGURE 28–54. Spinal abnormalities in X-linked hypophosphatemic vitamin D–resistant osteomalacia.

A Note syndesmophyte formation at multiple spinal levels. Radiographs of the pelvis (not shown) revealed bilateral sacroiliac joint fusion, widespread enthesopathy, and insufficiency fractures of the femoral necks.

B A bone scan shows femoral and tibial bowing and regions of increased accumulation of the radionuclide in the femora that corresponded to sites of insufficiency fracture.

ilar lesions are evident in the cervical spine in patients with rheumatoid arthritis and throughout the spine in many disorders that are associated with cartilaginous nodes (Schmorl's nodes). When severe, spondylitic erosions can simulate the findings in infection, although more widespread osseous destruction and rapid disc space loss are more characteristic of infectious lesions of the spine. Spinal "pseudarthrosis" accompanying ankylosing spondylitis also resembles osteomyelitis, although the detection of fractures of the posterior elements is an important clue to the traumatic nature of the vertebral body and discal destruction.

Odontoid erosion and atlantoaxial subluxation are encountered in ankylosing spondylitis, usually in patients with long-standing disease. Similar findings are observed in psoriasis and, less commonly, in Reiter's syndrome. In rheumatoid arthritis, these findings are combined with other diagnostic features in the cervical spine, such as extensive discovertebral erosions, disc space narrowing, subluxation at subaxial levels, and absence of osteophytes.

In the cervical spine, widespread apophyseal joint ankylosis accompanying ankylosing spondylitis resembles the findings in juvenile chronic arthritis. In this latter disorder, associated hypoplasia of vertebral bodies and intervertebral discs is distinctive. Abnormalities of the cervical spine in other diseases as well generally can be differentiated from those in ankylosing spondylitis (Fig. 28–55).

Abnormalities of Extraspinal Synovial Articulations

The absence of symmetric changes and osteoporosis, and the presence of bony proliferation and intra-articular osseous fusion, are features that are common to all three seronegative spondyloarthropathies (ankylosing spondylitis, psoriasis, and Reiter's syndrome), differing from the characteristics of rheumatoid arthritis (symmetry, osteoporosis, fibrous ankylosis, and absence of bony proliferation) (Table 28–7). Differentiating among the seronegative spondyloarthropathies on the basis of abnormalities of synovial joints in the appendicular skeleton can be difficult. Alterations in ankylosing spondylitis most commonly are located in the hip, the glenohumeral joint, and the knee, although changes in the small joints of the hand and the foot can be observed. In psoriasis, predilection for the interphalangeal, metacarpophalangeal, and metatarsophalangeal joints may be marked, whereas in Reiter's syndrome, involvement of the joints of the lower extremities, such as the knee and the metatarsophalangeal and interphalangeal joints, is noted. In both psoriasis and Reiter's syndrome, hip involvement is relatively unusual, whereas in ankylosing spondylitis, such involvement is common and leads to a typical radiographic picture consisting of concentric joint space narrowing and osteophytes at the junction of the femoral head and neck.

Abnormalities of Extraspinal Cartilaginous Articulations

The seronegative spondyloarthropathies frequently are associated with significant abnormalities of the symphysis pubis and the manubriosternal joint. Although similar changes appear in rheumatoid arthritis, their frequency and severity are less striking.

TABLE 28–7. Abnormalities of Synovial Articulations

Disease	Symmetric Involvement	Soft Tissue Swelling	Osteoporosis	Joint Space Narrowing	Bony Ankylosis	Erosions, Cysts	Bony Proliferation or "Whiskering"
Ankylosing spondylitis	±	+	±	+	+	+	+
Rheumatoid arthritis	+	+	+	+	±	+	−
Psoriatic arthritis	±	+	−	+	+	+	+
Reiter's syndrome	−	+	±	+	+	+	+
Gouty arthritis	±	+	−	±	−	+	+ *
Septic arthritis	−	+	+	+	+	+	+ †

*Irregular lips of bone are apparent.
†Poorly defined "fraying" of bone is seen.

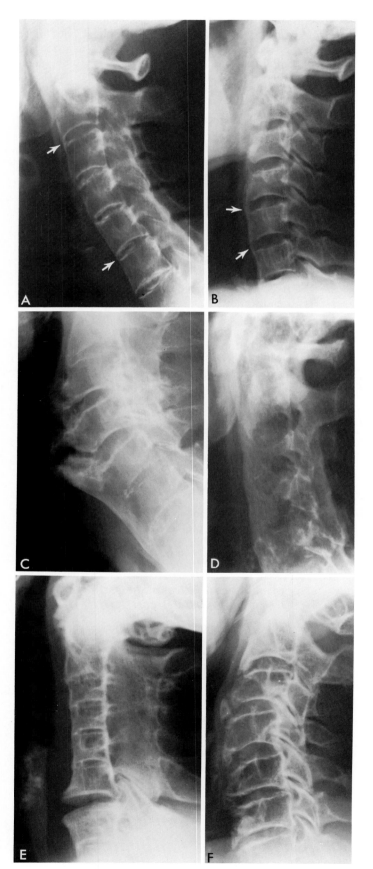

FIGURE 28–55. Differential diagnosis of cervical spine abnormalities.

A Ankylosing spondylitis is characterized by syndesmophytes (arrows) and apophyseal joint ankylosis.

B Psoriatic spondylitis leads to bone outgrowths (arrows) that predominate in the lower cervical spine. Apophyseal joints appear normal.

C Diffuse idiopathic skeletal hyperostosis is accompanied by extensive bone deposition on the anterior portion of the vertebral column.

D Sternocostoclavicular hyperostosis is characterized by exuberant bone formation anteriorly and centrally that obliterates the interface between vertebral bodies and intervertebral discs and by apophyseal joint ankylosis.

E Juvenile chronic arthritis is associated with hypoplasia of the vertebral bodies and intervertebral discs, apophyseal joint ankylosis, and predilection for the upper cervical region.

F Acromegaly leads to bone deposition that resembles that of spondylosis deformans and an increase in the anteroposterior dimension of the vertebral bodies.

Enthesopathy

Bony erosion with proliferation at the site of osseous attachment of ligaments and tendons represents a typical lesion of ankylosing spondylitis, psoriasis, and Reiter's syndrome.[211] Abnormalities may be encountered in the iliac crest, the ischial tuberosity, the femoral trochanters, the humeral tuberosities, the plantar aspect of the calcaneus, the malleoli about the ankle, the inferior aspect of the distal end of the clavicle, the spinous processes of the vertebrae, and the patella. In all locations, an irregular frayed surface may be created, which is virtually diagnostic of one of these three conditions. Enthesopathic alterations are less prominent in rheumatoid arthritis, and when present they commonly are unassociated with severe bony proliferation.

SUMMARY

Ankylosing spondylitis is a disease with widespread musculoskeletal manifestations. Abnormalities are detected at synovial and cartilaginous joints and at sites of tendinous and ligamentous attachment to bone in spinal and extraspinal locations. The hallmark of the disorder is sacroiliitis, which typically is bilateral and symmetric in distribution. Spondylitis leads to significant abnormalities at the discovertebral junction, apophyseal and costovertebral joints, and posterior ligamentous attachments. The earliest spinal changes commonly are detected at the thoracolumbar and lumbosacral junctions, although with disease progression, the entire spine can be affected, including the cervical region. Accurate differentiation of ankylosing spondylitis from rheumatoid arthritis is not difficult, although distinguishing the articular abnormalities of ankylosing spondylitis from those in psoriasis and Reiter's syndrome is more troublesome.

References

1. Moll JMH: Ankylosing spondylitis. In JT Scott (Ed): Copeman's Textbook of the Rheumatic Diseases. 5th Ed. Edinburgh, Churchill Livingstone, 1978, p 511.
2. Ogryzlo MA: Ankylosing spondylitis. In JL Hollander, DJ McCarty Jr (Eds): Arthritis and Allied Conditions. 8th Ed. Philadelphia, Lea & Febiger, 1972, p 699.
3. Blumberg B, Ragan C: The natural history of rheumatoid spondylitis. Medicine 35:1, 1956.
4. Connor B: Sur la continuité de plusieurs os, à l'occasion d'un tron de squelette humain, ou les vertébres, les côtes, l'os sacrum, et les os des iles, qui naturellements son distincts et separés, ne font qu'un seul os continu et inseparable. MD Thesis, University of Rheims, France, 1691.
5. Dunham CL, Kautz FG: Spondylarthritis ankylopoietica. Review and report of twenty cases. Am J Med Sci 201:232, 1941.
6. von Bechterew W: Steifigkeit der Wirbelsäule und ihre Verkrümmung als besondere Erkrankungsform. Neurologisches Zentralblatt 12:426, 1893.
7. Strumpell A: Bemerkungen über die chronische ankylosierende Entzündung der Wirbelsäule und der Hüftgelenke. Dtsch Z Nervenheilkd 11:338, 1897.
8. Marie P: Sur la spondylose rhizomélique. Rev Méd 18:285, 1898.
9. Fraenkel E: Über chronische ankylosierende Wirbelsaulenversteifung. ROFO 7:62, 1904.
10. Simmonds M: Über Spondylitis deformans und ankylosierende Spondylitis. ROFO 7:51, 1904.
11. Kellgren JH, Jeffrey MR, Ball J: The Epidemiology of Chronic Rheumatism. Vol 1. Oxford, England, Blackwell, 1963, p 326.
12. Bennet PH, Wood PHN: Population Studies of the Rheumatic Diseases. Proceedings of the 3rd International Symposium, New York, 1966. Amsterdam, Excerpta Medica Foundation, 1968, p 456.
13. Moll JMH, Wright V: New York clinical criteria for ankylosing spondylitis: A statistical evaluation. Ann Rheum Dis 32:354, 1973.
14. Savage O: Management of rheumatic diseases in the forces. Br Med J 2:336, 1942.
15. Boland EW, Shebesta EM: Rheumatoid spondylitis: Correlation of clinical and roentgenographic features. Radiology 47:551, 1946.
16. Kellgren JH: The epidemiology of rheumatic diseases. Ann Rheum Dis 23:109, 1964.
17. Blecourt JJ de: 533 patients with ankylosing spondylitis seen and followed in the period 1948–1971. Ann Rheum Dis 32:383, 1973.
18. Holst H, Iversen PF: On the incidence of spondylarthritis ankylopoetica in a Norwegian county. Acta Med Scand 142:333, 1952.
19. Baum J, Ziff M: The rarity of ankylosing spondylitis in the black race. Arthritis Rheum 14:12, 1971.
20. Gofton JP, Lawrence JS, Bennett PH, et al: Sacro-iliitis in eight populations. Ann Rheum Dis 25:528, 1966.
21. Wilkinson M, Bywaters EGL: Clinical features and course of ankylosing spondylitis as seen in a follow up of 222 hospital referred cases. Ann Rheum Dis 17:209, 1958.
22. West HF: The aetiology of ankylosing spondylitis. Ann Rheum Dis 8:143, 1949.
23. Polley HF, Slocumb CH: Rheumatoid spondylitis. A study of 1035 cases. Ann Intern Med 26:240, 1947.
24. Lawrence JS: The prevalence of arthritis. Br J Clin Pract 17:699, 1963.
25. Hill HFH, Hill AGS, Bodmer JG: Clinical diagnosis of ankylosing spondylitis in women and relation to presence of HLA-B27. Ann Rheum Dis 35:267, 1976.
26. Tyson TL, Thompson WAL, Ragan C: Marie-Strumpell spondylitis in women. Ann Rheum Dis 12:40, 1953.
27. Hart FD, Robinson KC: Ankylosing spondylitis in women. Ann Rheum Dis 18:15, 1959.
28. Boland EW: Rheumatoid spondylitis: Clinical features and current methods of treatment. Bull Rheum Dis 2:11, 1952.
29. McBryde AMJ, McCollum DE: Ankylosing spondylitis in women. The disease and its prognosis. NC Med J 34:34, 1973.
30. Riley MJ, Ansell BM, Bywaters EGL: Radiological manifestations of ankylosing spondylitis according to age at onset. Ann Rheum Dis 30:138, 1971.
31. Hart FD, Robinson KC, Allchin FM, et al: Ankylosing spondylitis. Q J Med 18:217, 1949.
32. Cheshire DJE, Nichols PJR: The early stages of ankylosing spondylitis. Rheumatism 11:79, 1955.
33. Sharp J: Ankylosing spondylitis, a review. In AS Dixon (Ed): Progress in Clinical Rheumatology. London, Churchill Livingstone, 1965, p 180.
34. Good AE: The chest pain of ankylosing spondylitis. Its place in the differential diagnosis of heart pain. Ann Intern Med 58:926, 1963.
35. Kinsella TD, MacDonald FR, Johnson LG: Ankylosing spondylitis: A late re-evaluation of 92 cases. Can Med Assoc J 95:1, 1966.
36. Rosen PS, Graham DC: Ankylosing (Strumpell-Marie) spondylitis (a clinical review of 128 cases). AIR 5:158, 1962.
37. Forestier J, Jacqueline F, Rotes-Querol J: Ankylosing Spondylitis. Springfield, Ill, Charles C Thomas, 1956.
38. Simmons EH: Kyphotic deformity of the spine in ankylosing spondylitis. Clin Orthop 128:65, 1977.
39. Hauge T: Chronic rheumatoid polyarthritis and spondylarthritis associated with neurological symptoms and signs occasionally simulating an intraspinal expansive process. Acta Chir Scand 120:395, 1961.
40. Bowie EA, Glasgow GL: Cauda-equina lesions associated with ankylosing spondylitis. Report of three cases. Br Med J 2:24, 1961.
41. Milde E-J, Aarli J, Larsen JL: Cauda equina lesions in ankylosing spondylitis. Scand J Rheumatol 6:118, 1977.
42. Rosenkranz W: Ankylosing spondylitis: Cauda equina syndrome with multiple spinal arachnoid cysts. J Neurosurg 34:241, 1971.
43. Dilsen N, McEwen C, Poppel M, et al: A comparative roentgenographic study of rheumatoid arthritis and rheumatoid (ankylosing) spondylitis. Arthritis Rheum 5:341, 1962.
44. Simpson NRW, Stephenson CJ: An analysis of 200 cases of ankylosing spondylitis. Br Med J 1:214, 1949.
45. Adler E, Carmon A: Ankylosing spondylitis—a review of 115 cases. Acta Rheumatol Scand 7:219, 1961.
46. Dwosh IL, Resnick D, Becker MA: Hip involvement in ankylosing spondylitis. Arthritis Rheum 19:683, 1976.
47. Rutishauser E, Jacqueline F: Involvement of the hip in ankylosing spondylitis and rheumatoid arthritis. Doc Geigy Acta Rheumatol 16:9, 1964.
48. Birkbeck MQ, Buckler WS, Mason RM, Tegner WS: Iritis as the presenting symptom in ankylosing spondylitis. Lancet 2:802, 1951.
49. Clark WS, Kulka JP, Bauer W: Rheumatoid arthritis with aortic regurgitation: Unusual manifestation of rheumatoid arthritis (including spondylitis). Am J Med 22:580, 1957.
50. Ansell BM, Bywaters EGL, Doniach I: The aortic lesion of ankylosing spondylitis. Br Heart J 20:507, 1958.
51. Sobin LH, Hagstrom JWC: Lesions of cardiac conduction tissue in rheumatoid aortitis. JAMA 180:1, 1962.
52. Campbell AH, MacDonald CB: Upper lobe fibrosis associated with ankylosing spondylitis. Br J Dis Chest 59:90, 1965.
53. Davies D: Ankylosing spondylitis and lung fibrosis. Q J Med 41:395, 1972.
54. Rosenow EC, Strimlan CV, Muhm JR, Ferguson RH: Pleuropulmonary manifestations of ankylosing spondylitis. Mayo Clin Proc 52:641, 1977.
55. Cruickshank B: Pathology of ankylosing spondylitis. Bull Rheum Dis 10:211, 1960.
56. Villiaumey J, Lejeune E, Avouac B, Horreard P: Spondylarthrite ankylosante et amylose. Ann Med Intern 129:67, 1978.
57. Arroyo H, Bourdais A, Joly R, et al: Amylose au décours d'une spondylarthrite ankylosante. Mars Med 108:465, 1971.

58. Ennevaara K, Oka M: Amyloidosis in ankylosing spondylitis. Ann Rheum Dis 22:336, 1963.
59. Halford ME, Clark CJ: Amyloid disease complicating ankylosing spondylitis. Ann Rheum Dis 16:460, 1957.
60. Court Brown WM, Doll R: Mortality from cancer and other causes after radiotherapy for ankylosing spondylitis. Br Med J 2:1327, 1965.
61. Court Brown WM, Abbott JD: The incidence of leukaemia in ankylosing spondylitis treated with x-rays. A preliminary report. Lancet 1:1283, 1955.
62. Edgar MA, Robinson MP: Post-irradiation sarcoma in ankylosing spondylitis. J Bone Joint Surg [Br] 55:183, 1973.
63. Bentley SJ, Davis P, Jayson MIV: Neurofibrosarcoma following radiotherapy for ankylosing spondylitis. Ann Rheum Dis 34:536, 1975.
64. Berens DL: Roentgen features of ankylosing spondylitis. Clin Orthop 74:20, 1971.
65. McEwen C, DiTata D, Longg C, et al: Ankylosing spondylitis and the spondylitis accompanying ulcerative colitis, regional enteritis, psoriasis, and Reiter's disease. A comparative study. Arthritis Rheum 14:291, 1971.
66. Moll JMH, Haslock I, Macrae IF, et al: Associations between ankylosing spondylitis, psoriatic arthritis, Reiter's disease, the intestinal arthropathies and Behçet's syndrome. Medicine 53:343, 1974.
67. Schumacher TM, Genant HK, Kellet MJ, et al: HLA-B27 associated arthropathies. Radiology 126:289, 1978.
68. Resnick D, Dwosh IL, Goergen TG, et al: Clinical and radiographic abnormalities in ankylosing spondylitis: A comparison of men and women. Radiology 119:293, 1976.
69. Ball J: Enthesopathy of rheumatoid and ankylosing spondylitis. Ann Rheum Dis 30:213, 1971.
70. Cruickshank B: Pathology of ankylosing spondylitis. Clin Orthop 74:43, 1971.
71. Fassbender HG: Pathology of Rheumatic Diseases. New York, Springer-Verlag, 1975, p 221.
72. Resnick D: Patterns of peripheral joint disease in ankylosing spondylitis. Radiology 110:523, 1974.
73. Cruickshank B: Histopathology of diarthrodial joints in ankylosing spondylitis. Ann Rheum Dis 10:393, 1951.
74. Van Swaay H: Spondylosis ankylopoietica. En pathogenetische Studie. Medical Dissertation, University of Leiden, Netherlands, 1950.
75. Aufdermaur M: Die pathologische Anatomie der Spondylitis ankylopoietica. I. Pathologische anatomie. Documenta Rheumatologica, Basel, Geigy, No. 2, 1953.
76. Resnick D, Niwayama G: On the nature and significance of bony proliferation in "rheumatoid variant" disorders. AJR 129:275, 1977.
77. Ott R, Wurm H: Spondylitis ankylopoetica. In R Schoen (Ed): Der Rheumatismus. Darmstadt, Germany, Dietrich Steinkopff Verlag, 1957.
78. Resnick D, Niwayama G, Goergen TG: Comparison of radiographic abnormalities of the sacro-iliac joint in degenerative disease and ankylosing spondylitis. AJR 128:189, 1977.
79. Macrae IF, Haslock DI, Wright V: Grading of films for sacro-iliitis in population studies. Ann Rheum Dis 30:58, 1971.
80. Dihlmann W: Das "bunte Sakroiliakalbild"—das roentgenologische Frühkriterium der ankylosierenden Spondylitis. ROFO 121:564, 1974.
81. Dihlmann W, Lindenfelser R, Selberg W: Sakroiliakale histomorphologie der ankylosierende Spondylitis als Beitrag zu Therapie. Dtsch Med Wochenschr 102:129, 1977.
82. Resnick D, Niwayama G, Goergen TG: Degenerative disease of the sacroiliac joint. Invest Radiol 10:608, 1975.
83. Carter ME, Loewi G: Anatomical changes in normal sacro-iliac joints during childhood and comparison with the changes in Still's disease. Ann Rheum Dis 21:121, 1965.
84. Romanus R, Yden S: Pelvo-spondylitis ossificans, rheumatoid or ankylosing spondylitis. A roentgenological and clinical guide to its early diagnosis (especially anterior spondylitis). Copenhagen, Munksgaard, 1955, p 22.
85. Cheatum DE: "Ankylosing spondylitis" without sacroiliitis in a woman without the HLA B27 antigen. J Rheumatol 3:420, 1976.
86. Andersson O: Röntgenbilden vid spondylarthritis ankylopoetica. Nord Med Tidskr 14:2000, 1937.
87. Edstrom G: Is spondylarthritis ankylopoietica an independent disease or a rheumatic syndrome? Acta Med Scand 104:396, 1940.
88. Guest CM, Jacobson HG: Pelvic and extrapelvic osteopathy in rheumatoid spondylitis. A clinical and roentgenographic study of ninety cases. AJR 65:760, 1951.
89. Jacqueline F: Troubles de la structure osseuse et lésions destructives au cours de la spondylarthrite ankylosante. J Radiol Electrol Med Nucl 37:887, 1956.
90. Jacqueline F; Destructions du rachis antérieur lombo-dorsal au cours de la spondylarthrite ankylosante (classification, interprétation). Rhumatologie 17:223, 1965.
91. Seaman WB, Wells J: Destructive lesions of the vertebral bodies in rheumatoid disease. AJR 86:241, 1961.
92. Louyot P, Gaucher A, Mathieu J, et al: La spondylodiscite de la spondylarthrite ankylosante. Rev Rhum Mal Osteoartic 30:263, 1963.
93. Coste F, Delbarre F, Cayla J, et al: Spondylites destructives dans la spondylarthrite ankylosante. Presse Med 71:1013, 1963.
94. Serre H, Simon L, Claustre J: Les lésions destructrices des disques et des corps vertébraux au cours de la spondylarthrite ankylosante. J Radiol Electrol Med Nucl 46:538, 1965.
95. Schultiz K-P: Spondylodiszitis bei Morbus Bechterew. Med Klin 64:593, 1969.

96. Rivelis M, Freiberger RH: Vertebral destruction at unfused segments in late ankylosing spondylitis. Radiology 93:251, 1969.
97. Daneo V, DiVittorio S: La spondylodiscite de la spondylarthrite ankylosante. Rev Rhum Mal Osteoartic 37:155, 1970.
98. Sutherland RIL, Matheson D: Inflammatory involvement of vertebrae in ankylosing spondylitis. J Rheumatol 2:296, 1975.
99. Dihlmann W, Delling G: Disco-vertebral destructive lesions (so-called Andersson lesions) associated with ankylosing spondylitis. Skel Radiol 3:10, 1978.
100. Little H, Urowtiz MB, Smythe HA, et al: Asymptomatic spondylodiscitis. An unusual feature of ankylosing spondylitis. Arthritis Rheum 17:487, 1974.
101. Gougeon J, Rampon S, Deshayes P, et al: Discopathies post-fracturaires et lésions vertébrales destructices au cours de la pelvispondylite rhumatismale. Rev Rhum Mal Osteoartic 44:17, 1977.
102. Gelman MI, Umber JS: Fractures of the thoracolumbar spine in ankylosing spondylitis. AJR 130:485, 1978.
103. Martel W: Spinal pseudoarthrosis. A complication of ankylosing spondylitis. Arthritis Rheum 21:485, 1978.
104. Kanefield DG, Mullins BP, Freehafer AA, et al: Destructive lesions of the spine in rheumatoid ankylosing spondylitis. J Bone Joint Surg [Am] 51:1369, 1969.
105. Good AE: Non-traumatic fracture of the thoracic spine in ankylosing spondylitis. Arthritis Rheum 10:467, 1967.
106. Yau ACMC, Chan RNW: Stress fracture of the fused lumbo-dorsal spine in ankylosing spondylitis. A report of three cases. J Bone Joint Surg [Br] 56:681, 1974.
107. Resnick D, Niwayama G: Intravertebral disc herniations: Cartilaginous nodes. Radiology 126:57, 1978.
108. Schmorl G, Junghanns H: The Human Spine in Health and Disease. New York, Grune & Stratton, 1959.
109. Woodruff FB, Dewing SB: Fracture of the cervical spine in patients with ankylosing spondylitis. Radiology 80:17, 1963.
110. Kewalramani LS, Taylor RG, Albrand OW: Cervical spine injury in patients with ankylosing spondylitis. J Trauma 15:931, 1975.
111. Martel W: Radiology of the rheumatic diseases. In JL Hollander, DJ McCarty Jr (Eds): Arthritis and Allied Conditions. 8th Ed. Philadelphia, Lea & Febiger, 1972, p 82.
112. Martel W: The occipito-atlanto-axial joints in rheumatoid arthritis and ankylosing spondylitis. AJR 86:223, 1961.
113. Sharp J, Purser DW: Spontaneous atlanto-axial dislocation in ankylosing spondylitis and rheumatoid arthritis. Ann Rheum Dis 20:47, 1961.
114. Martel W, Page JW: Cervical vertebral erosions and subluxations in rheumatoid arthritis and ankylosing spondylitis. Arthritis Rheum 3:546, 1960.
115. Kornblum D, Clayton M, Nash HH: Non-traumatic cervical dislocations in rheumatoid spondylitis. JAMA 149:431, 1952.
116. Margulies ME, Katz I, Rosenberg M: Spontaneous dislocation of the atlanto-axial joint in rheumatoid spondylitis. Neurology 5:290, 1955.
117. Pratt TLC: Spontaneous dislocation of the atlanto-axial articulation occurring in ankylosing spondylitis and rheumatoid arthritis. J Fac Radiologists 10:40, 1959.
118. Lourie H, Stewart WA: Spontaneous atlanto-axial dislocation. N Engl J Med 265:677, 1961.
119. Coutts MB: Atlanto-epistropheal subluxations. Arch Surg 29:297, 1934.
120. Sorin S, Askari A, Moskowitz RW: Atlanto-axial subluxation as a complication of early ankylosing spondylitis. Two case reports and a review of the literature. Arthritis Rheum 22:273, 1979.
121. Little H, Swinson DR, Cruickshank B: Upward subluxation of the axis in ankylosing spondylitis. Am J Med 60:279, 1976.
122. Hart FD, Robinson KC: Ankylosing spondylitis in women. Ann Rheum Dis 18:15, 1959.
123. Savill DL: The manubrio-sternal joint in ankylosing spondylitis. J Bone Joint Surg [Br] 33:56, 1951.
124. Candardjis G, Saudan Y, DeBosset PH: Etude radiologique de l'articulation manubrio-sternale dans la pelvispondylite rhumatismale et le syndrome de Reiter. J Radiol Electrol Med Nucl 59:93, 1978.
125. Glick EN: A radiological comparison of the hip-joint in rheumatoid arthritis and ankylosing spondylitis. Proc R Soc Med 59:1229, 1966.
126. Bywaters EGL: A case of early ankylosing spondylitis with fatal secondary amyloidosis. Br Med J 2:412, 1968.
127. Pasion EG, Goodfellow JW: Pre-ankylosing spondylitis. Histopathological report. Ann Rheum Dis 58:677, 1961.
128. Dürrigl TH, Hausler Z, Kriz L: A propos d'une coxite dans la spondylite ankylosante. Rev Rhum Mal Osteoartic 32:623, 1965.
129. Edstrom B, Fellander M: Cup arthroplasty of the hip in rheumatic patients. A follow-up study. Acta Orthop Belg 40:113, 1974.
130. Freeman PA: McKee-Farrar total replacement of the hip joint in rheumatoid arthritis and allied conditions. Clin Orthop 72:106, 1970.
131. Welch RB, Charnley J: Low-friction arthroplasty of the hip in rheumatoid arthritis and ankylosing spondylitis. Clin Orthop 72:22, 1970.
132. Arden GP, Ansell BM, Hunter MJ: Total hip replacement in juvenile chronic polyarthritis and ankylosing spondylitis. Clin Orthop 84:130, 1972.
133. Wilde AH, Collins R, Mackenzie AH: Reankylosis of the hip joint in ankylosing spondylitis after total hip replacement. Arthritis Rheum 15:493, 1972.
134. Resnick D, Dwosh IL, Goergen TG, et al: Clinical and radiographic "reankylosis" following hip surgery in ankylosing spondylitis. AJR 126:1181, 1976.
135. Bisla RS, Ranawat CS, Inglis AE: Total hip replacement in patients with ankylosing spondylitis with involvement of the hip. J Bone Joint Surg [Am] 58:233, 1976.

136. Williams E, Taylor AR, Arden GP, et al: Arthroplasty of the hip in ankylosing spondylitis. J Bone Joint Surg [Br] 59:393, 1977.
137. Baldursson H, Brattstrom H, Olsson TH: Total hip replacement in ankylosing spondylitis. Acta Orthop Scand 48:499, 1977.
138. Brooker AF, Bowerman JW, Robinson RA, et al: Ectopic ossification following total hip replacement. Incidence and a method of classification. J Bone Joint Surg [Am] 55:1629, 1973.
139. Resnick D, Niwayama G: Resorption of the undersurface of the distal clavicle in rheumatoid arthritis. Radiology 120:75, 1976.
140. Reuler JB, Girard DE, Nardone DA: Sternoclavicular joint involvement in ankylosing spondylitis. South Med J 71:1480, 1978.
141. Kalliomaki JL, Viitanen SM, Virtama P: Radiological findings of sternoclavicular joints in rheumatoid arthritis. Acta Rheumatol Scand 14:233, 1968.
142. Pohl W, Schöffel J: Ankylosen an den unteren Gliedmassen bei Spondylitis ankylosans. Z Rheumatol 36:84, 1977.
143. Enright T, Liang GC, Fox TA, et al: Tarsal tunnel syndrome with ankylosing spondylitis. Arthritis Rheum 22:77, 1979.
144. Resnick D, Feingold ML, Curd J, et al: Calcaneal abnormalities in articular disorders. Rheumatoid arthritis, ankylosing spondylitis, psoriatic arthritis, and Reiter's syndrome. Radiology 125:355, 1977.
145. Einaudi G, Viara M: Ricerche sul comportamento dell'articolazione temporomandibolare nei pazienti affetti da spondilite anchilosante. Reumatismo 16:351, 1964.
146. Maes HJ, Dihlmann W: Befall der Temporomandibulargelenke bei der Spondylitis ankylopoetica. ROFO 109:513, 1968.
147. Resnick D: Temporomandibular joint involvement in ankylosing spondylitis. Comparison with rheumatoid arthritis and psoriasis. Radiology 112:587, 1974.
148. Davidson C, Wojtulewski JA, Bacon PA, et al: Temporomandibular joint disease in ankylosing spondylitis. Ann Rheum Dis 34:87, 1975.
149. Fallet GH, Mason M, Berry H, et al: Coexistence of rheumatoid arthritis and ankylosing spondylitis—report of 10 cases. J Rheumatol (Suppl 3) 4:70, 1977.
150. Fallet GH, Mason M, Berry H, et al: Rheumatoid arthritis and ankylosing spondylitis occurring together. Br Med J 1:804, 1976.
151. Luthra HS, Ferguson RH, Conn DL: Coexistence of ankylosing spondylitis and rheumatoid arthritis. Arthritis Rheum 19:111, 1976.
152. Good AE, Hyla JF, Rapp R: Ankylosing spondylitis with rheumatoid arthritis and subcutaneous nodules. Arthritis Rheum 20:1434, 1977.
153. Rosenthal SH, Lidsky MD, Sharp JT: Arthritis with nodules following ankylosing spondylitis. JAMA 206:2893, 1968.
154. Chapman MD, Reinertsen JL: Ankylosing spondylitis with subsequent development of rheumatoid arthritis, Sjögren's syndrome, and rheumatoid vasculitis. Arthritis Rheum 21:383, 1978.
155. Bywaters EGL: Discussion. Arthritis Rheum 21:388, 1978.
156. Dihlmann W, Klemm C, Stockberg H, et al: Sakroiliakale 85Sr-Profilographic bei der ankylosierenden Spondylitis. ROFO 115:42, 1971.
157. Bull U, Schattenkirchner M, Frey KW: Vergleich röntgenologischer und szintigraphischer Befunde bei der Spondylitis ankylopoetica. ROFO 121:369, 1974.
158. Szanto E, Ruden B-I: 99mTc in evaluation of sacro-iliac arthritis. Scand J Rheumatol 5:11, 1976.
159. Russell AS, Lentle BC, Percy JS: Investigation of sacro-iliac disease: Comparative evaluation of radiological and radionuclide techniques. J Rheumatol 2:45, 1975.
160. Lentle BC, Russell AS, Percy JS, et al: Scintigraphic findings in ankylosing spondylitis. J Nucl Med 18:524, 1977.
161. Lentle BC, Russell AS, Percy JS, et al: The scintigraphic investigation of sacroiliac disease. J Nucl Med 18:529, 1977.
162. Goldberg RP, Genant HK, Shimshak R, et al: Applications and limitations of quantitative sacroiliac joint scintigraphy. Radiology 128:683, 1978.
163. Namey TC, McIntyre J, Buse M, et al: Nucleographic studies of axial spondarthritides. I. Quantitative sacroiliac scintigraphy in early HLA-B27-associated sacroiliitis. Arthritis Rheum 20:1058, 1977.
164. Dequeker J, Goddeeris T, Walravens M, et al: Evaluation of sacroiliitis: Comparison of radiological and radionuclide techniques. Radiology 128:687, 1978.
165. Berghs H, Remans J, Drieskens L, et al: Diagnostic value of sacroiliac joint scintigraphy with 99m-technetium pyrophosphate in sacroiliitis. Ann Rheum Dis 37:190, 1978.
166. Weissberg DL, Resnick D, Taylor A, et al: Rheumatoid arthritis and its variants: Analysis of scintigraphic, radiographic, and clinical examinations. AJR 131:665, 1978.
167. VanLaere M, Veys EM, Mielants H: Strontium 87m scanning of the sacroiliac joints in ankylosing spondylitis. Ann Rheum Dis 31:201, 1972.
168. Sonnemaker RE, Ferguson RH, Tauxe WN: 87mSr scintiphotography of the sacro-iliac joints: A new criterion for the diagnosis of ankylosing spondylitis. J Nucl Med 13:467, 1972.
169. Ranawat NS, Rivelis M: Strontium 85 scintimetry in ankylosing spondylitis. JAMA 222:553, 1972.
170. Erhardt O: Über chronische ankylosierende Wirbelsaulenversteifung. Mitt aus den Grenzgebieten der Medizin und Chirurgie 14:726, 1905.
171. Scott SG: Chronic infection of sacro-iliac joints as possible cause of spondylitis adolescens. Br J Radiol 9:126, 1936.
172. Junghanns H: In H Henke, O Lubarsch (Eds): Handbuch der speziellen pathologische Anatomie. Berlin, Springer Verlag, 1939.
173. Bluestone R, Pearson CM: Ankylosing spondylitis and Reiter's syndrome. Their interrelationship and association with HL-A-B27. Adv Intern Med 22:1, 1977.
174. Bluestone R: Histocompatibility antigens and rheumatic disease. In Current Concepts. Kalamazoo, Michigan, Upjohn Co, 1978, p 17.
175. Rogoff B, Freyberg RH: The familial incidence of rheumatoid spondylitis. Ann Rheum Dis 8:139, 1949.
176. Hersh AH, Stecher RM, Solomon WM, et al: Heredity in ankylosing spondylitis; study of 50 families. Am J Hum Genet 2:391, 1950.
177. Espinoza L, Oh JH, Kinsella TD, et al: Ankylosing spondylitis. Family studies and HL-A 27 antigen distribution. J Rheumatol 1:254, 1974.
178. Daneo V, Migone N, Modena V, et al: Family studies and HLA typing in ankylosing spondylitis and sacroiliitis. J Rheumatol (Suppl 3) 4:5, 1977.
179. Arnett FC Jr, Schacter BZ, Hochberg MC, et al: Homozygosity for HLA-B27. Impact on rheumatic disease expression in two families. Arthritis Rheum 20:797, 1977.
180. Stecher RM: Heredity in Joint Diseases. Documenta Rheumatologica. Basle, Geigy, 1957, No 12, p 41.
181. Graham W, Uchida IA: Heredity in ankylosing spondylitis. Ann Rheum Dis 16:334, 1957.
182. Emery AE, Lawrence JS: Genetics of ankylosing spondylitis. J Med Genet 4:239, 1967.
183. Brewerton DA, Caffrey M, Hart FD, et al: Ankylosing spondylitis and HLA-B27. Lancet 1:904, 1973.
184. Khan MA, Braun WE, Kushner I: Low frequency of HLA-B27 in American blacks with ankylosing spondylitis. Clin Res 24:331A, 1976.
185. Russell AS, Lentle BC, Schlaut J: Radiologic and scintiscan findings in HLA-B27 negative patients with ankylosing spondylitis. J Rheumatol 3:321, 1976.
186. Khan MA, Kushner I, Braun WE: Comparison of clinical features in HLA-B27 positive and negative patients with ankylosing spondylitis. Arthritis Rheum 20:909, 1977.
187. Romanus R: Pelvo-spondylitis ossificans in the male (ankylosing spondylitis, morbus Bechterew-Marie-Strumpell) and genito-urinary infection; the aetiological significance of the latter and the nature of disease based on a study of 117 male patients. Acta Med Scand Suppl 280:7, 1953.
188. Mason RM, Murray RS, Oates JK, et al: Prostatitis and ankylosing spondylitis. Br Med J 1:748, 1958.
189. Inman RD, Mani VJ: Subluxation of the sacroiliac joints in a Black female with ankylosing spondylitis. J Rheumatol 6:300, 1979.
190. Spencer DG, Park WM, Dick HM, et al: Radiological manifestations in 200 patients with ankylosing spondylitis: Correlation with clinical features and HLA B27. J Rheumatol 6:305, 1979.
191. Chalmers IM, Lentle BC, Percy JS, et al: Sacroiliitis detected by bone scintiscanning: A clinical, radiological, and scintigraphic follow-up study. Ann Rheum Dis 38:112, 1979.
192. Szanto E, Lindvall N: Quantitative 99mTc pertechnetate scanning of the sacroiliac joints. A follow-up study of patients with suspected sacroiliitis. Scand J Rheumatol 7:93, 1978.
193. Davis P: Quantitative sacroiliac scintigraphy in ankylosing spondylitis and Crohn's disease: A single family study. Ann Rheum Dis 38:241, 1979.
194. Calin A, Fries JF, Schurman D, et al: The close correlation between symptoms and disease expression in HLA B27 positive individuals. J Rheumatol 4:277, 1977.
195. Cawley MID, Chalmers TM, Kellgren JH, et al: Destructive lesions of vertebral bodies in ankylosing spondylitis. Ann Rheum Dis 31:345, 1972.
196. Dihlmann W, Lindenfelser R: Polysegmentare Anderssonlasion bei ankylosierender Spondylitis (röntgenologisch-histologische Synopsis). ROFO 130:454, 1979.
197. Bouvier M, Lejeune E, Rouillat M, et al: Les formes pseudo-pottiques et pseudo-dystrophiques des spondylodiscites de la spondylarthrite ankylosante. A propos de quatre observations personnelles et de vingt observations de la literature. Rev Rhum Mal Osteoartic 47:21, 1980.
198. Surin VV: Fractures of the cervical spine in patients with ankylosing spondylitis. Acta Orthop Scand 51:79, 1980.
199. Marks JS, Hardinge K: Clinical and radiographic features of spondylitic hip disease. Ann Rheum Dis 38:332, 1979.
200. Rosen PS: A unique shoulder lesion in ankylosing spondylitis: Clinical comment. J Rheumatol 7:109, 1980.
201. Yood RA, Goldenberg DL: Sternoclavicular joint arthritis. Arthritis Rheum 23:232, 1980.
202. Scott DL, Eastmond CJ, Wright V: A comparative radiological study of the pubic symphysis in rheumatic disorders. Ann Rheum Dis 38:529, 1979.
203. Resnick D: Radiology of seronegative spondyloarthropathies. Clin Orthop 143:38, 1979.
204. Ball J: Articular pathology of ankylosing spondylitis. Clin Orthop 143:30, 1979.
205. Dihlmann W: Current radiodiagnostic concept of ankylosing spondylitis. Skel Radiol 4:179, 1979.
206. Esdaile J, Hawkins D, Rosenthall L: Radionuclide joint imaging in the seronegative spondyloarthropathies. Clin Orthop 143:46, 1979.
207. Spencer DG, Adams FG, Horton PW, et al: Scintiscanning in ankylosing spondylitis: A clinical, radiological and quantitative radio-isotopic study. J Rheumatol 6:426, 1979.
208. Ho G Jr, Sadovnikoff N, Malhotra C, et al: Quantitative sacroiliac joint scintigraphy. A critical assessment. Arthritis Rheum 22:837, 1979.
209. Christiansen FT, Hawkins BR, Dawkins RL, et al: The prevalence of ankylosing spondylitis among B27 positive normal individuals—a reassessment. J Rheumatol 6:713, 1979.
210. Szanto E, Hagenfeldt K: Sacro-iliitis and salpingitis. Quantitative 99mTC pertechnetate scanning in the study of sacro-illitis in women. Scand J Rheumatol 8:129, 1979.
211. Niepel GA, Sitaj S: Enthesopathy. Clin Rheum Dis 5:857, 1979.

212. Dunn EC, Ebringer RW, Ell PJ: Quantitative scintigraphy in the early diagnosis of sacro-iliitis. Rheumatol Rehabil 19:69, 1980.

213. Esdaile JM, Rosenthall L, Terkeltaub R, et al: Prospective evaluation of sacroiliac scintigraphy in chronic inflammatory back pain. Arthritis Rheum 23:998, 1980.

214. Major P, Resnick D, Dalinka M, et al: Coexisting rheumatoid arthritis and ankylosing spondylitis. AJR 134:1076, 1980.

215. Baron M, Tator CH, Little H: Hangman's fracture in ankylosing spondylitis preceded by vertical subluxation of the axis. Arthritis Rheum 23:850, 1980.

216. Benedek TG, Rodnan GD: A brief history of the rheumatic diseases. Bull Rheum Dis 32:59, 1982.

217. Francois RJ: Bechterew and ankylosing spondylitis. Clin Orthop 154:299, 1981.

218. Van der Linden S, Valkenburg HA, Cats A: Evaluation of diagnostic criteria for ankylosing spondylitis. A proposal for modification of the New York Criteria. Arthritis Rheum 27:361, 1984.

219. Marks SH, Barnett M, Calin A: Ankylosing spondylitis in women and men: A case-control study. J Rheumatol 10:624, 1983.

220. Marks SH, Barnett M, Calin A: A case-control study of juvenile- and adult-onset ankylosing spondylitis. J Rheumatol 9:739, 1982.

221. Garcia-Morteo O, Maldonado-Cocco A, Suarez-Almazor ME, et al: Ankylosing spondylitis of juvenile onset: Comparison with adult onset disease. Scand J Rheumatol 12:246, 1983.

222. Pastershank SP: Ankylosing spondylitis in women. J Can Assoc Radiol 32:93, 1981.

223. Braunstein EM, Martel W, Moidel R: Ankylosing spondylitis in men and women: A clinical and radiographic comparison. Radiology 144:91, 1982.

224. Carette S, Graham D, Little H, et al: The natural disease course of ankylosing spondylitis. Arthritis Rheum 26:186, 1983.

225. Revell PA, Mayston V: Histopathology of the synovial membrane of peripheral joints in ankylosing spondylitis. Ann Rheum Dis 41:579, 1982.

226. Francois RJ: Some pathological features of ankylosing spondylitis as revealed by microradiography and tetracycline labelling. Clin Rheumatol 1:23, 1982.

227. Ball J: Pathology and pathogenesis. In JMH Moll (Ed): Ankylosing Spondylitis. Edinburgh, Churchill Livingstone, 1980, p 96.

228. Albert J, Lagier R: Enthesopathic erosive lesions of patella and tibial tuberosity in juvenile ankylosing spondylitis. ROFO 139:544, 1983.

229. Prohaska E: Isolated sacroiliitis as monosymptomatic form of ankylosing spondylitis—a possible cause of chronic back pain. Clin Rheumatol 3:33, 1984.

230. Cone RO, Resnick D: Roentgenographic evaluation of the sacroiliac joints. Orthop Rev 12:95, 1983.

231. Greenway GD, Resnick D: Problems in radiographic technique and in radiologic assessment of the sacroiliac joints. In JMH Moll (Ed): Ankylosing Spondylitis. Edinburgh, Churchill Livingstone, 1980, p 87.

232. Ryan LM, Carrera GF, Lightfoot RW Jr, et al: The radiographic diagnosis of sacroiliitis. Arthritis Rheum 26:760, 1983.

233. Hollingsworth PN, Cheah PS, Dawkins RL, et al: Observer variation in grading sacroiliac radiographs in HLA-B27 positive individuals. J Rheumatol 10:247, 1983.

234. Russell AS: Comments on Ryan article. Arthritis Rheum 27:596, 1984.

235. Resnick D: Comment on Sienknecht letter. Arthritis Rheum 27:357, 1984.

236. Mau G, Helbig B, Mann M: Discitis—a rare early symptom of ankylosing spondylitis. Eur J Pediatr 137:85, 1981.

237. Wise CM, Irby WR: Spondylodiscitis in ankylosing spondylitis: Variable presentations. J Rheumatol 10:1004, 1983.

238. Jajic I, Furst Z, Vuksic B: Spondylitis erosiva: Report on 9 patients. Ann Rheum Dis 41:237, 1982.

239. Courtois C, Fallet GH, Vischer TL, et al: Erosive spondylopathy. Ann Rheum Dis 39:462, 1980.

240. Fallet GH, Courtois C, Vischer TL, et al: Erosive spondylopathy. Scand J Rheumatol (Suppl) 32:110, 1980.

241. Resnick D, Niwayama G: Discovertebral destruction in a man with chronic back problems. Invest Radiol 16:89, 1981.

242. Murray GC, Persellin RH: Cervical fracture complicating ankylosing spondylitis. Am J Med 70:1033, 1981.

243. Hunter T, Dubo HIC: Spinal fractures complicating ankylosing spondylitis. Arthritis Rheum 26:751, 1983.

244. Thorngren K-G, Liedberg E, Aspelin P: Fractures of the thoracic and lumbar spine in ankylosing spondylitis. Arch Orthop Trauma Surg 98:101, 1981.

245. Karlstrom G, Olerud S: Spinal pseudarthrosis with paraplegia in ankylosing spondylitis. Arch Orthop Trauma Surg 98:297, 1981.

246. Weinstein PR, Karpman RR, Gall EP, et al: Spinal cord injury, spinal fracture, and spinal stenosis in ankylosing spondylitis. J Neurosurg 57:609, 1982.

247. Good AE, Keller TS, Weatherbee L, et al: Spinal cord block with a destructive lesion of the dorsal spine in ankylosing spondylitis. Arthritis Rheum 25:218, 1982.

248. Leuken MG III, Patel DV, Ellman MH: Symptomatic spinal stenosis associated with ankylosing spondylitis. Neurosurgery 11:703, 1982.

249. Young A, Dixon A, Getty J, et al: Cauda equina syndrome complicating ankylosing spondylitis: Use of electromyography and computerized tomography in diagnosis. Ann Rheum Dis 40:317, 1981.

250. Bartleson JD, Cohen MD, Harrington TM, et al: Cauda equina syndrome secondary to long-standing ankylosing spondylitis. Ann Neurol 14:662, 1983.

251. Grossman H, Gray R, St Louis EL: CT of long-standing ankylosing spondylitis with cauda equina syndrome. Am J Neuroradiol 4:1077, 1983.

252. Contamin F, Doubrere JF, Struz PH, et al: Sur l'association spondylarthrite ankylosante syndrome de la queue de cheval et dilatation du cul-de-sac lombaire avec volumineux diverticule arachnoidien. Sem Hop Paris 59:1401, 1983.

253. Scheines E, Cocco JAM, Porrini AA, et al: Manifestaciones neurologicas en espondilitis anquilosante. Medicina 43:369, 1983.

254. Calin A: Raised serum creatinine phosphokinase activity in ankylosing spondylitis. Ann Rheum Dis 34:244, 1975.

255. McDougall J, Mills K, Isenberg D, et al: Muscle involvement in ankylosing spondylitis. Ann Rheum Dis 41:316, 1982.

256. Sage MR, Gordon TP: Muscle atrophy in ankylosing spondylitis: CT demonstration. Radiology 149:780, 1983.

257. Grosbois B, Paxlotsky Y, Chales G, et al: Clinical and radiological study of the manubrio-sternal joint. Rev Rhum Mal Osteoartic 49:232, 1982.

258. Shanahan WR Jr, Kaprove RE, Major PA, et al: Assessment of longterm benefit of total hip replacement in patients with ankylosing spondylitis. J Rheumatol 9:101, 1982.

259. Hill JA, Lombardo SJ: Ankylosing spondylitis presenting as shoulder pain in an athlete. A case report. Am J Sports Med 9:262, 1981.

260. Pritchett JW: Ossification of the coracoclavicular ligaments in ankylosing spondylitis. A case report. J Bone Joint Surg [Am] 65:1017, 1983.

261. Resnick D: Letter to the editor. J Bone Joint Surg [Am] 65:1356, 1983.

262. Albert J, Lagier R, Ott H: Erosions enthesopathiques extra-rachidiennes dans la spondylarthrite ankylosante. Rev Rhum Mal Osteoartic 50:573, 1983.

263. Cohen MD, Ginsburg WW: Late-onset peripheral joint disease in ankylosing spondylitis. Ann Rheum Dis 41:574, 1982.

264. Ginsburg WW, Cohen MD: Peripheral arthritis in ankylosing spondylitis. Mayo Clin Proc 58:583, 1983.

265. Lemmer JP, Irby WR: Coexistence of HLA-B27 ankylosing spondylitis and DR4 seropositive nodular rheumatoid arthritis in a patient with membranous nephropathy. J Rheumatol 8:661, 1981.

266. Alexander EL, Bias WB, Arnett FC: The coexistence of rheumatoid arthritis with Reiter's syndrome and/or ankylosing spondylitis: A model of dual HLA-associated disease susceptibility and expression. J Rheumatol 8:398, 1981.

267. Williamson PK, Reginato AJ: Diffuse idiopathic skeletal hyperostosis of the cervical spine in a patient with ankylosing spondylitis. Arthritis Rheum 27:570, 1984.

268. Matin P: Bone scintigraphy in the diagnosis and management of traumatic injury. Semin Nucl Med 13:104, 1983.

269. Rothwell RS, Davis P, Lentle BC: Radionuclide bone scanning in females with chronic low back pain. Ann Rheum Dis 40:79, 1981.

270. Vyas K, Eklem M, Seto H, et al: Quantitative scintigraphy of sacroiliac joints: Effect of age, gender, and laterality. AJR 136:589, 1981.

271. Ayres J, Hilson AJW, Maisey MN, et al: An improved method for sacroiliac joint imaging: A study of normal subjects, patients with sacroiliitis, and patients with low back pain. Clin Radiol 32:441, 1981.

272. Schorner W, Haubold W: Die szintigraphische untersuchung der iliosakralgelenke bei patienten mit spondylitis ankylopoetica. ROFO 135:41, 1981.

273. Snaith ML, Galvin SEJ, Short MD: The value of quantitative radioisotope scanning in the differential diagnosis of low back pain and sacroiliac disease. J Rheumatol 9:435, 1982.

274. Pitkanen M, Lahtinen T, Hyodynmaa S, et al: Quantitative sacro-iliac scintigraphy. Scand J Rheumatol 11:199, 1982.

275. Chase WF, Houk RW, Winn RE, et al: The clinical usefulness of radionuclide scintigraphy in suspected sacroiliitis: A prospective study. Br J Rheumatol 22:67, 1983.

276. Miron SD, Khan MA, Wiesen EJ, et al: The value of quantitative sacroiliac scintigraphy in detection of sacroiliitis. Clin Rheumatol 2:407, 1983.

277. Paquin J, Rosenthall L, Esdaile J, et al: Elevated uptake of ^{99m}-technetium methylene diphosphonate in the axial skeleton in ankylosing spondylitis and Reiter's disease: Implications for quantitative sacroiliac scintigraphy. Arthritis Rheum 26:217, 1983.

278. Dunn NA, Mahida BH, Merrick MV, et al: Quantitative sacroiliac scintiscanning: A sensitive and objective method for assessing efficacy of nonsteroidal, anti-inflammatory drugs in patients with sacroiliitis. Ann Rheum Dis 43:157, 1984.

279. Park WM, Spencer DG, McCall IW, et al: The detection of spinal pseudarthrosis in ankylosing spondylitis. Br J Radiol 54:467, 1981.

280. Resnick D, Williamson S, Alazraki N: Focal spinal abnormalities on bone scans in ankylosing spondylitis: A clue to the presence of fracture or pseudarthrosis. Clin Nucl Med 5:213, 1981.

281. Kozin F, Carrera GF, Ryan LM, et al: Computed tomography in the diagnosis of sacroiliitis. Arthritis Rheum 24:1479, 1981.

282. Carrera GF, Foley WD, Kozin F, et al: CT of sacroiliitis. AJR 136:41, 1981.

283. Borlaza GS, Seigel R, Kuhns LR, et al: Computed tomography in the evaluation of sacroiliac arthritis. Radiology 139:437, 1981.

284. Calin A: Abuse of computed tomography. Arthritis Rheum 25:1147, 1982.

285. Ryan LM, Carrera GF, Lightfoot RW Jr, et al: The radiographic diagnosis of sacroiliitis. Arthritis Rheum 26:760, 1983.

286. Volger JB III, Brown WH, et al: The normal sacroiliac joint: A CT study of asymptomatic patients. Radiology 151:433, 1984.

287. DeSmet AA, Gardner JD, Lindsley HB, et al: Tomography for evalution of sacroiliitis. AJR 139:577, 1982.

288. Dihlmann W: Kritik der Sacroiliitis-Stadieneinteilung (''grading,'' ''staging'') bei Spondylitis ankylosans. Z Rheumatol 42:49, 1983.

289. Szanto E, Hagenfeldt K: Sacro-iliitis in women—a sequela to acute salpingitis. Scand J Rheumatol 12:89, 1983.

290. Calin A: Spondyloarthropathy in Caucasians and non-Caucasians. J Rheumatol 10:16, 1983.
291. Zeidler H, Wagener P, Eckert G, et al: HLA-B27 in possible ankylosing spondylitis with peripheral arthritis. Rheumatol Int 2:35, 1982.
292. Armstrong RD, Panayi GS, Welsh KI: Histocompatibility antigens in psoriasis, psoriatic arthropathy, and ankylosing spondylitis. Ann Rheum Dis 42:142, 1983.
293. Kinsella TD, Fritzler MJ, McNeil DJ: Ankylosing spondylitis. A disease in search of microbes. J Rheumatol 10:2, 1983.
294. Russell ML: Ankylosing spondylitis: The case for the underestimated female. J Rheumatol 12:4, 1985.
295. Gran JT, Ostensen M, Husby G: A clinical comparison between males and females with ankylosing spondylitis. J Rheumatol 12:126, 1985.
296. Maldonado-Cocco JA, Babini S, Garcia-Morteo O: Clinical features of ankylosing spondylitis in women and men and its relationship with age of onset. J Rheumatol 12:179, 1985.
297. Diaz MR, Lopez AG: Manifestaciones clinicorradiologicas de la espondilitis anquilosante en la mujer. Estudio de 22 casos. Rev Clin Esp 176:460, 1985.
298. Gran JT, Husby G, Hordvik M, et al: Radiological changes in men and women with ankylosing spondylitis. Ann Rheum Dis 43:570, 1984.
299. Gran JT, Husby G, Hordvik M: Spinal ankylosing spondylitis: A variant form of ankylosing spondylitis or a distinct disease entity? Ann Rheum Dis 44:368, 1985.
300. Kerr R, Resnick D: Radiology of the seronegative spondyloarthropathies. Clin Rheum Dis 11:113, 1985.
301. Gordon TP, Sage MR, Bertouch JV, Brooks PM: Computed tomography of paraspinal musculature in ankylosing spondylitis. J Rheumatol 11:794, 1984.
302. Kiwerski J, Wieclawek H, Garwacka I: Fractures of the cervical spine in ankylosing spondylitis. Int Orthop (SICOT) 8:243, 1985.
303. Harding JR, McCall IW, Park WM, et al: Fracture of the cervical spine in ankylosing spondylitis. Br J Radiol 58:3, 1985.
304. McCall I, El Masri W, Jaffray D: Hangman's fracture in ankylosing spondylitis. Injury 16:483, 1985.
305. Vinje O, Dale K, Moller P: Radiographic evaluation of patients with Bechterew's syndrome (ankylosing spondylitis). Findings in peripheral joints, tendon insertions and the pubic symphysis and relations to nonradiographic findings. Scand J Rheumatol 14:279, 1985.
306. The HSG, Lemmens AJ, Goedhard G, et al: Radiological and scintigraphic findings in patients with a clinical history of chronic inflammatory back pain. Skel Radiol 14:243, 1985.
307. Diffey BL, Pal B, Gibson CJ, et al: Application of Bayes' theorem to the diagnosis of ankylosing spondylitis from radio-isotope bone scans. Ann Rheum Dis 44:667, 1985.
308. Fam AG, Rubenstein JD, Chin-Sang H, et al: Computed tomography in the diagnosis of early ankylosing spondylitis. Arthritis Rheum 28:930, 1985.
309. Miehle W, Schattenkirchner M, Albert D, et al: HLA-DR4 in ankylosing spondylitis with different patterns of joint involvement. Ann Rheum Dis 44:39, 1985.
310. Lampman JH: Origin of enthesopathy. J Rheumatol 12:1030, 1985.
311. Streilein KF, Rosenberg AM: Coexistent rheumatoid arthritis and ankylosing spondylitis in a child. J. Rheumatol 12:1216, 1985.
312. Cunningham TJ, Cumber PM, Evison G, et al: Unusual radiographic features in a female patient with ankylosing spondylitis. Ann Rheum Dis 45:776, 1986.
313. Bourqui M, Gerster JC: Ankylosing spondylitis presenting as spondylodiscitis. Clin Rheumatol 4:458, 1985.
314. Hissa E, Boumphrey F, Bay J: Spinal epidural hematoma and ankylosing spondylitis. Clin Orthop 208:225, 1986.
315. Ellrodt A, Goldberg D, Oberlin F, et al: Erosive arthritis of the costovertebral joint in seronegative spondyloarthropathy. J Rheumatol 13:452, 1986.
316. Sunderam NA, Murphy JCM: Heterotopic bone formation following total hip arthroplasty in ankylosing spondylitis. Clin Orthop 207:223, 1986.
317. Russell AS, Jackson F: Computer assisted tomography of the apophyseal changes in patients with ankylosing spondylitis. J Rheumatol 13:581, 1986.
318. Dougados M, van der Linden S, Juhlin R, et al: The European spondyloarthropathy study group preliminary criteria for the classification of spondyloarthropathy. Arthritis Rheum 34:1218, 1991.
319. Gran JT, Husby G: Ankylosing spondylitis in women. Semin Arthritis Rheum 19:303, 1990.
320. Kidd B, Mullee M, Frank A, et al: Disease expression of ankylosing spondylitis in males and females. J Rheumatol 15:1407, 1988.
321. Calin A, Elswood J, Rigg S, et al: Ankylosing spondylitis—an analytical review of 1500 patients: The changing pattern of disease. J Rheumatol 15:1234, 1988.
322. Little H: The natural history of ankylosing spondylitis. J Rheumatol 15:1179, 1988.
323. Burkus JK: Herniated nucleus pulposus in a patient with ankylosing spondylitis. A case report. Spine 13:103, 1988.
324. Mander M, Simpson JM, McLellan A, et al: Studies with an enthesis index as a method of clinical assessment in ankylosing spondylitis. Ann Rheum Dis 46:197, 1987.
325. Will R, Edmunds L, Elswood J, et al: Is there sexual inequality in ankylosing spondylitis? A study of 498 women and 1202 men. J Rheumatol 17:1649, 1990.
326. Resnick D: Inflammatory disorders of the vertebral column: Seronegative spondyloarthropathies, adult-onset rheumatoid arthritis, and juvenile chronic arthritis. Clin Imaging 13:253, 1989.
327. Forrester DM: Imaging of the sacroiliac joints. Radiol Clin North Am 28:1055, 1990.
328. Olivieri I, Gemignani G, Pasero G: Ankylosing spondylitis with exuberant sclerosis in the sacroiliac joints, symphysis pubis and spine. J Rheumatol 17:1515, 1990.
329. Dihlmann W: Osteitis condensans ilii and sacroiliitis. J Rheumatol 18:1430, 1991.
330. Aufdermaur M: Pathogenesis of square bodies in ankylosing spondylitis. Ann Rheum Dis 48:628, 1989.
331. Agarwal AK, Reidbord HE, Kraus DR, et al: Variable histopathology of discovertebral lesion (spondylodiscitis) of ankylosing spondylitis. Clin Exp Rheumatol 8:67, 1990.
332. Jobanputra P, Kirkham B, Duke O, et al: Discovertebral destruction in ankylosing spondylitis complicated by spinal cord compression. Ann Rheum Dis 47:344, 1988.
333. Hunter T: The spinal complications of ankylosing spondylitis. Semin Arthritis Rheum 19:172, 1989.
334. Wu PC, Fang D, Ho EKW, et al: The pathogenesis of extensive discovertebral destruction in ankylosing spondylitis. Clin Orthop 230:154, 1988.
335. Broom MJ, Raycroft JF: Complications of fractures of the cervical spine in ankylosing spondylitis. Spine 13:763, 1988.
336. Amamilo SC: Fractures of the cervical spine in patients with ankylosing spondylitis. Orthop Rev 18:339, 1989.
337. Govender S, Charles RW: Fracture of the dens in ankylosing spondylitis. Injury 18:213, 1987.
338. Miller FH, Rogers LF: Fractures of the dens complicating ankylosing spondylitis with atlantooccipital fusion. J Rheumatol 18:771, 1991.
339. Fitt G, Hennessy O, Thomas D: Case report 709. Skel Radiol 21:61, 1992.
340. Trent G, Armstrong GWD, O'Neil J: Thoracolumbar fractures in ankylosing spondylitis. High-risk injuries. Clin Orthop 227:61, 1988.
341. Gelineck J, De Carvalho A: Fractures of the spine in ankylosing spondylitis. ROFO 152:307, 1990.
342. Fang D, Leong JCY, Ho EKW, et al: Spinal pseudarthrosis in ankylosing spondylitis. J Bone Joint Surg [Br] 70:443, 1988.
343. Chan FL, Ho EKW, Fang D, et al: Spinal pseudarthrosis in ankylosing spondylitis. Acta Radiol 28:383, 1987.
344. Furst SR, Kyndynis P, Gundry C, et al: Pseudopseudarthrosis in a patient with ankylosing spondylitis. J Rheumatol 17:258, 1990.
345. Ho EKW, Chan FL, Leong JCY: Postsurgical recurrent stress fracture in the spine affected by ankylosing spondylitis. Clin Orthop 247:87, 1989.
346. Lohr KM, Barthelemy CR, Schwab JP, et al: Septic spondylodiscitis in ankylosing spondylitis. J Rheumatol 14:616, 1987.
347. Simkin PA, Downey DJ, Kilcoyne RF: Apophyseal arthritis limits lumbar motion in patients with ankylosing spondylitis. Arthritis Rheum 31:798, 1988.
348. Olivieri I, Trippi D, Gemignani G, et al: Ossification of the posterior longitudinal ligament in ankylosing spondylitis. Arthritis Rheum 31:452, 1988.
349. Ho EKW, Leong JCY: Traumatic teraparesis: A rare neurologic complication in ankylosing spondylitis with ossification of posterior longitudinal ligament of the cervical spine. Spine 12:403, 1987.
350. Avrahami E, Wigler I, Stern D, et al: Computed tomographic demonstration of calcification of the ligamenta flava of the lumbosacral spine in ankylosing spondylitis. Ann Rheum Dis 47:62, 1988.
351. Suarez-Almazor ME, Russell AS: Anterior atlantoaxial subluxation in patients with spondyloarthropathies: Association with peripheral disease. J Rheumatol 15:973, 1988.
352. Leventhal MR, Maguire JK Jr, Christian CA: Atlantoaxial rotary subluxation in ankylosing spondylitis. A case report. Spine 15:1374, 1990.
353. Santavirta S, Konttinen YT, Sandelin J, et al: Cervical spine subluxation in ankylosing spondylitis treated surgically. J Orthop Rheumatol 3:57, 1990.
354. Mitchell MJ, Sartoris DJ, Moody D, et al: Cauda equina syndrome complicating ankylosing spondylitis. Radiology 175:521, 1990.
355. Paul G, Engelbeen JP, Malghem J, et al: Spondylarthrite ankylosante et syndrome partiel de la queue de cheval. Rev Rhum Mal Osteoartic 58:527, 1991.
356. Rubenstein DJ, Ghelman B: Case report 477. Skel Radiol 17:212, 1988.
357. Abelló R, Rovira M, Sanz MP, et al: MRI and CT of ankylosing spondylitis with vertebral scalloping. Neuroradiology 30:272, 1988.
358. Sparling MJ, Bartleson JD, McLeod RA, et al: Magnetic resonance imaging of arachnoid diverticula associated with cauda equina syndrome in ankylosing spondylitis. J Rheumatol 16:1335, 1989.
359. Lindsley HB, DeSmet AA, Neff JR: Ankylosing spondylitis presenting as juxta-articular masses in females. Skel Radiol 16:142, 1987.
360. Jurik AG: Anterior chest wall involvement in seronegative arthritides. A study of the frequency of changes at radiography. Rheumatol Int 12:7, 1992.
361. Doury P, Pattin S, Eulry F, et al: La coxite macrogéodique au cours de la spondylarthrite ankylosante. Rev Rhum Mal Osteoartic 54:197, 1987.
362. Walker LG, Sledge CB: Total hip arthroplasty in ankylosing spondylitis. Clin Orthop 262:198, 1991.
363. Kilgus DJ, Namba RS, Gorek JE, et al: Total hip replacement for patients who have ankylosing spondylitis. J Bone Joint Surg [Am] 72:834, 1990.
364. Calin A, Elswood J: The outcome of 138 total hip replacements and 12 revisions in ankylosing spondylitis: High success rate after a mean followup of 7.5 years. J Rheumatol 16:955, 1989.
365. Emery RJH, Ho EKW, Leong JCY: The shoulder girdle in ankylosing spondylitis. J Bone Joint Surg [Am] 73:1526, 1991.
366. Schurman JR II, Wilde AH: Total knee replacement after spontaneous osseous ankylosis. A report of three cases. J Bone Joint Surg [Am] 72:455, 1990.

367. Fallet GH, Barnes CG, Berry H, et al: Coexisting rheumatoid arthritis and ankylosing spondylitis. J Rheumatol 14:1135, 1987.
368. Helfgott SM, La Zarides G, Sandberg-Cook J: Cooccurrence of rheumatoid arthritis and ankylosing spondylitis. J Rheumatol 15:1451, 1988.
369. Hart FD, Lipner AE: Co-existent ankylosing spondylitis and seropositive rheumatoid arthritis. J Orthop Rheumatol 4:56, 1991.
370. Kjällman M, Nylén O, Hansén M: Evaluation of quantitative sacro-iliac scintigraphy in the early diagnosis of ankylosing spondylitis. Scand J Rheumatol 15:265, 1986.
371. Fishman EK, Magid D: Cervical fracture in ankylosing spondylitis: Value of multidimensional imaging. Clin Imaging 16:31, 1992.
372. Chan F-L, Ho EKW, Chau EMT: Spinal pseudarthrosis complicating ankylosing spondylitis: Comparison of CT and conventional tomography. AJR 150:611, 1988.
373. Wienands K, Lukas P, Albrecht HJ: Klinische Bedeutung der MR-Tomographie von Spondylodiscitiden bei Spondylitis ankylopoetica. Z Rheumatol 49:356, 1990.
374. Ahlström H, Feltelius N, Nyman R, et al: Magnetic resonance imaging of sacroiliac joint inflammation. Arthritis Rheum 33:1763, 1990.
375. Murphey MD, Wetzel LH, Bramble JM, et al: Sacroiliitis: MR imaging findings. Radiology 180:239, 1991.
376. Docherty P, Mitchell MJ, MacMillan L, et al: Magnetic resonance imaging of sacroiliitis. J Rheumatol 19:393, 1992.
377. Khan MA: Ankylosing spondylitis and heterogeneity of HLA-B27. Semin Arthritis Rheum 18:134, 1988.
378. Linssen A, Feltkamp TEW: B27 positive diseases versus B27 negative diseases. Ann Rheum Dis 47:431, 1988.
379. Pascual E, Castellano JA, Lopez E: Costovertebral joint changes in ankylosing spondylitis with thoracic pain. Br J Rheumatol 31:413, 1992.
380. Markel DC, Graziano GP: Fracture of the S1 vertebral body in a patient with ankylosing spondylitis. J Spinal Dis 5:222, 1992.
381. Maertens M, Meilants H, Verstraete K, et al: Simultaneous occurrence of diffuse idiopathic skeletal hyperostosis and ankylosing spondylitis in the same patient. J Rheumatol 19:1978, 1992.
382. Verlooy H, Mortelmans L, Vleugels S, et al: Quantitative scintigraphy of the sacroiliac joints. Clin Imag 16:230, 1992.
383. Baumgarten DA, Taylor AT Jr: Enthesopathy associated with seronegative spondyloarthropathy: 99mTc-methylene diphosphonate scintigraphic findings. AJR 160:1249, 1993.
384. Peh WCG, Ho TK, Chan FL: Case report: Pseudoarthrosis complicating ankylosing spondylitis—appearances on magnetic resonance imaging. Clin Radiol 47:359, 1993.
385. Jiménez-Balderas FJ, Mintz G: Ankylosing spondylitis: Clinical course in women and men. J Rheumatol 20:2069, 1993.
386. Huang G-S, Park Y-H, Taylor JAM, et al: Hyperostosis of ribs: Association with vertebral ossification. J Rheumatol 20:2073, 1993.
387. Hanly JG, Barnes DC, Mitchell MJ, et al: Single photon emission computed tomography in the diagnosis of inflammatory spondyloarthropathies. J Rheumatol 20:2062, 1993.
388. Goldberg AL, Keaton NL, Rothfus WE, et al: Ankylosing spondylitis complicated by trauma: MR findings correlated with plain radiographs and CT. Skeletal Radiol 22:333, 1993.
389. Kahn MS: Pathogenesis of ankylosing spondylitis. J Rheumatol 20:1273, 1993.

29

Psoriatic Arthritis

Donald Resnick, M.D., and Gen Niwayama, M.D.

With the accumulation of an increasing amount of clinical, laboratory, and radiologic data, psoriatic arthritis has been identified as a separate and distinct articular disorder. For many years after the original descriptions of the disease in the late nineteenth century,[1–3] however, the joint abnormalities associated with psoriasis were considered to be part of the spectrum of rheumatoid arthritis. Through the investigations of Hench (1935, Rochester, Minnesota) and Wright (1956–1959, Leeds) as well as others, the distinctive alterations of psoriatic arthritis gradually were recog-

nized.[107] Currently, the concept of a specific type of arthritis in psoriasis rarely is challenged, but the definition of this arthritis frequently varies from one report to another. Descriptions that use the finding of polyarticular abnormalities with predilection for the distal interphalangeal joints as the sine qua non of psoriatic arthritis are too limited. This articular disorder has a wide clinical and radiologic spectrum, and placing undue emphasis on any one of its many manifestations may lead to misdiagnosis of others.

This chapter is not meant to compete with some of the excellent clinical reviews of psoriatic arthritis that are available to the interested reader.[4–7] Rather, emphasis is given to the varied radiographic manifestations that are part of this important articular disorder.

PREVALENCE AND SPECTRUM OF PSORIATIC ARTHRITIS

The reported frequency of articular abnormalities in patients with psoriasis has varied from less than 0.5 per cent to greater than 40 per cent.[8–10, 110] Much of this variation is related to methods of patient selection. For example, studies based on hospital populations have a tendency to include only those persons with relatively severe psoriatic skin disease or joint abnormalities; many persons with trivial cutaneous or articular abnormalities never seek the aid of a physician. Estimates of the frequency of arthritis in patients with psoriasis in the range of 2 to 6 per cent appear most accurate.[11–14] Conversely, the reported prevalence of psoriasis among patients with polyarticular arthritis has ranged from 3 to 5 per cent.[11, 15, 16] In many series, men have been affected two or three times more frequently than women,[17, 18] although in some series, a predilection for female involvement has been noted.[14, 19] Earlier descriptions of psoriatic arthritis frequently stressed one aspect of the disease.[6] To some investigators, psoriatic arthritis was a type of joint disease confined to distal interphalangeal joints,[20, 21] whereas others regarded it as a severely destructive and mutilating process.[10, 22] Additional reports emphasized its atypical[23] or fluctuating nature,[24, 25] its associated laboratory manifestations,[26] or its relationship to rheuma-

TABLE 29–1. Varied Patterns of Psoriatic Arthritis*

Polyarthritis with distal interphalangeal joint involvement
Symmetric seronegative polyarthritis simulating rheumatoid arthritis
Monoarthritis or asymmetric oligoarthritis
Sacroiliitis and spondylitis
Arthritis mutilans

*In addition, patients with psoriasis may have coincidental rheumatoid arthritis.

toid arthritis. With the publication of comprehensive analyses by Wright and Moll,[4, 6, 27] five broad clinical varieties of psoriatic arthritis have been recognized: polyarthritis characterized by distal interphalangeal joint involvement; a deforming type of arthritis characterized by widespread ankylosis and, occasionally, arthritis mutilans; a symmetric seronegative polyarthritis simulating rheumatoid arthritis but without its laboratory parameters; monoarthritis or asymmetric oligoarthritis; and sacroiliitis and spondylitis resembling ankylosing spondylitis (Table 29–1). Although radiographic abnormalities accompany these five types of disease, features in certain groups are much more specific than those in other groups, and in some patients, a single diagnosis of psoriatic arthritis on the basis of radiographic changes cannot be accomplished. Indeed, some of these latter patients have rheumatoid arthritis with typical clinical, serologic, and radiologic findings.

CLINICAL ABNORMALITIES

The age of onset of psoriatic arthritis does not differ significantly from that of rheumatoid arthritis, although children with psoriatic arthritis increasingly are being recognized.[28–30, 104, 162] In children, initial skin changes frequently are mild, intermittent, and easily missed; a monoarticular presentation, especially of the knee, is common; and an asymmetric pattern of polyarthritis ultimately develops in most instances.[108] In most adult patients, a long history of psoriatic skin disease is evident, although in a few persons, the articular abnormalities coincide with or antedate the appearance of the skin lesions.[31] In some reports, the appearance of arthritis prior to the identification of cutaneous abnormalities has occurred in as many as 20 per cent of patients with psoriatic arthritis.[149] Uncommonly, exacerbations and remissions of both cutaneous and articular manifestations occur simultaneously.

Articular disease is much more prevalent in patients with moderate or severe skin abnormalities.[14] Furthermore, the severe deforming arthropathy of psoriasis commonly is associated with extensive and exfoliative cutaneous changes.[6] Other than these associations between skin and joint manifestations, it is the nail abnormalities that appear to correlate most closely with articular disease.[32, 110] These nail changes, which include pitting, discoloration, ridging, splintering, erosion, thickening, and detachment,[40] are common at the onset of articular disease and generally are apparent in the same digit that has a significant distal interphalangeal articular abnormality.

The clinical nature of the articular disease is variable. A monoarticular, pauciarticular, or polyarticular distribution can be encountered, and virtually any joint can be affected, although the small joints of the hands and feet reportedly are involved in 25 to 75 per cent of patients with arthritis, the frequency increasing with the duration of the disease.[33]

In some patients, low back complaints predominate, related to involvement of the spine and the sacroiliac joints. The articular symptoms may be acute or insidious in nature. Soft tissue swelling can be prominent, and in some patients an entire digit is enlarged (sausage digit) owing to abnormality of the distal interphalangeal and proximal interphalangeal joints and tendon sheath. Subcutaneous nodules characteristically are not evident. Additional clinical manifestations may include fatigue, fever, stiffness, and ocular problems, such as conjunctivitis, iritis, and scleritis. In rare instances, myopathy may be evident.[163]

Laboratory analysis confirms the absence of serologically detectable rheumatoid factor in the majority of patients (in certain cases, clinically apparent rheumatoid arthritis in patients with psoriasis is accompanied by positive test results for rheumatoid factor).[34] Additional laboratory parameters may include a mild anemia, elevated erythrocyte sedimentation rate, occasionally elevated serum uric acid levels (related to cellular turnover in psoriatic cutaneous lesions), and raised concentrations of IgG antiglobulins.[35–39] Some reports have indicated differences in serum immunoglobulin concentrations between those psoriatic patients with arthropathy and those without arthropathy, suggesting that psoriatic arthritis is not a single uniform joint disease.[109] The histocompatibility antigen HLA-B27 frequently is present in patients with psoriasis and sacroiliitis (see discussion later in this chapter).

Synovial fluid examination reveals an inflammatory exudate.[7] The fluid appears yellow in color and demonstrates total leukocyte counts between 5000 and 40,000 cells per cu mm, predominantly neutrophils.

RADIOGRAPHIC ABNORMALITIES

Many reviews of the radiographic features of psoriatic arthritis are available[21, 22, 41–44, 99, 102] (Table 29–2). From these descriptions, it is evident that the disorder shares certain features with other seronegative spondyloarthropathies, such as Reiter's syndrome and ankylosing spondylitis, although its articular distribution is different from the distribution in these other disorders.

Prevalence of Radiographic Abnormalities

No reliable figures appear to exist regarding the prevalence of radiographic manifestations in psoriatic patients with either skin lesions alone or both cutaneous and articular manifestations of the disease. The former situation would require careful radiographic monitoring of all patients with skin changes of any magnitude, whereas the latter situation would necessitate radiographic analysis of all persons with clinically detectable articular findings, no matter what their extent and severity. What appears obvious

TABLE 29–2. Characteristics of Psoriatic Arthritis

Involvement of synovial and cartilaginous joints and entheses
Asymmetric distribution more common than symmetric distribution
Involvement of interphalangeal joints of the hands and feet
Sacroiliitis and spondylitis with paravertebral ossification
Bony erosion with adjacent proliferation
Intra-articular bony ankylosis
Destruction of phalangeal tufts

is that in the initial phase of psoriatic arthritis, radiographs may be entirely normal. Early radiographic abnormalities, which may include soft tissue swelling and some degree of osteoporosis, can resolve without any permanent sequelae. With clinical progression of articular problems, more extensive radiographic abnormalities appear, and these may worsen at a variable rate.[156] Significant joint destruction and deformity are more characteristic of psoriatic arthritis than of Reiter's syndrome.

Distribution of Radiographic Abnormalities
(Fig. 29–1)

Psoriatic arthritis can affect synovial and cartilaginous joints and sites of tendon and ligament attachment to bone in both the appendicular and the axial skeleton. In this regard, it is similar to Reiter's syndrome and ankylosing spondylitis and differs from rheumatoid arthritis, in which significant alterations of cartilaginous joints and tendinous attachments are less frequent.

Although the articular distribution of psoriatic arthritis is somewhat variable, certain characteristics deserve emphasis. An asymmetric or even unilateral appearance is much more common in psoriatic arthritis than in rheumatoid ar-

thritis, although widespread involvement of one side of the body almost invariably is associated with changes on the other side. An exception to this rule occurs in the presence of hemiplegia, in which abnormalities of psoriatic arthritis may appear only in the nonparalyzed side of the body.[150] Both upper extremity and lower extremity joints are affected in psoriatic arthritis. (This differs from the distribution of Reiter's syndrome, which involves predominantly the joints of the lower extremity.) Distal interphalangeal and proximal interphalangeal joints (as well as metacarpophalangeal and metatarsophalangeal joints) of the hand and the foot commonly are affected (including the interphalangeal joints of the thumb and great toe). Abnormalities of the phalangeal tufts and calcaneus also are characteristic.

Generally the larger joints of the upper and lower extremities in psoriatic arthritis show fewer changes than the small joints of the hand and foot. Significant abnormalities of the hip and shoulder are relatively uncommon. In the axial skeleton, sacroiliac joint and spinal abnormalities predominate. Any segment of the vertebral column, including the cervical spine, may be affected. Elsewhere in the axial skeleton, the manubriosternal, sternoclavicular, and costovertebral joints, the symphysis pubis, and the tendinous connections of the pelvis may demonstrate significant changes.

General Radiographic Abnormalities
(Fig. 29–2)

Soft Tissue Swelling. Fusiform or symmetric soft tissue swelling frequently is evident about involved joints, reflecting the presence of synovial effusions of variable size[111] and soft tissue edema. Sausage-like swelling of entire digits also may be encountered.[112]

Osteoporosis. Osteoporosis is not a prominent feature of psoriatic arthritis, although it may be demonstrated in early phases of the disease. In fact, the radiodensity of the bone may be remarkably well preserved, even in patients with severely destructive arthritis. This lack of osteoporosis is a reliable sign in the differentiation of psoriatic arthritis from rheumatoid arthritis, although the presence of osteoporosis does not eliminate the diagnosis of psoriatic arthritis.

Joint Space Narrowing and Widening. The articular space may be narrowed or widened. In large joints, such as the knee, the ankle, the elbow, and the hip, diffuse loss of interosseous space is identical to that observed in rheumatoid arthritis. In the small joints of the fingers and toes, severe destruction of marginal and subchondral bone can lead to considerable widening of the articular space. This finding is uncommon in rheumatoid arthritis but may be seen in other articular disorders characterized by extensive osseous destruction, such as gout and multicentric reticulohistiocytosis. The adjacent bony surfaces may reveal well-defined and angulated margins.

Bone Erosion. Erosive abnormalities are prominent in psoriatic arthritis. Initially, erosions predominate in the marginal areas of the articulation, but as they progress, central areas also are affected. Over a period of time, it appears as if the bones are being gnawed away[45] or have been whittled by a pencil sharpener.[40] The remaining osseous surfaces in the central aspect of the joint frequently are irregular or jagged but sharply delineated, whereas peripherally, irregular new bone formation may create a poorly

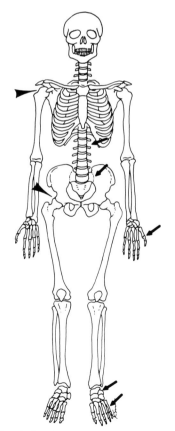

FIGURE 29–1. Psoriatic arthritis: Distribution of radiographic abnormalities. The most typical sites of abnormality are the interphalangeal joints of the hand and the foot, the metacarpophalangeal and metatarsophalangeal joints, the calcaneus, the sacroiliac joint, and the spine (arrows). Changes in the knee, ankle, manubriosternal, sternoclavicular, acromioclavicular, and costovertebral joints, symphysis pubis, tendinous connections of the pelvis, elbow, and wrist are not uncommon. Significant alterations of the hip and the glenohumeral joint are relatively unusual (arrowheads).

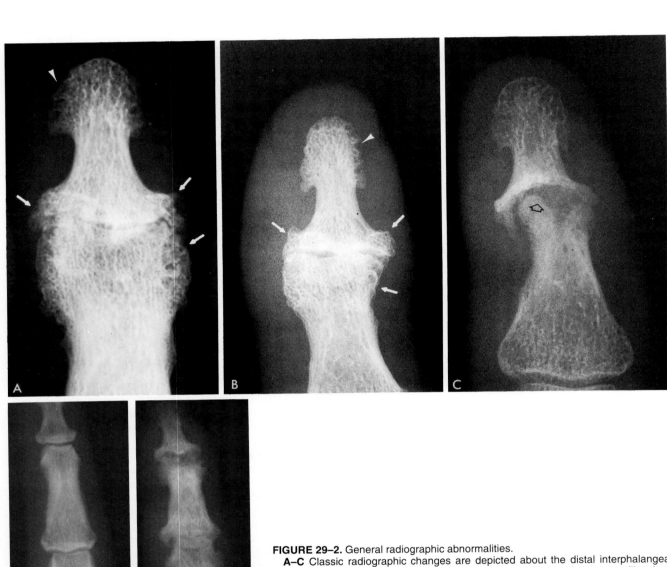

FIGURE 29–2. General radiographic abnormalities.

A–C Classic radiographic changes are depicted about the distal interphalangeal joints in three patients with psoriasis. These changes include soft tissue swelling, lack of osteoporosis, joint space narrowing, osseous erosions with accompanying proliferation (solid arrows), osteolysis with a "pencil and cup" appearance (open arrow), and tuftal resorption (arrowheads).

D, E These two radiographs of the third finger, obtained 4 years apart, indicate that psoriasis may appear initially as soft tissue swelling and periostitis (arrows).

defined or "whiskered" appearance (see discussion later in this chapter). In the small joints of the hands and feet, destruction or whittling of the head of one phalanx may produce a small blunt osseous surface which projects into the expanded base of a neighboring phalanx, resembling a pencil-and-cup or cup-and-saucer appearance. Similar changes are encountered at metacarpophalangeal and metatarsophalangeal locations. In some patients with psoriatic arthritis, complete dissolution of large segments of apposing bones, fragmentation with osseous debris, and disorganization of the joint resemble the changes of neuropathic osteoarthropathy.

Bone Proliferation. As in the other seronegative spondyloarthropathies, proliferation of bone is a striking feature of psoriatic arthritis. This proliferation about the erosions may take several forms. Irregular excrescences create a spiculated, frayed, or "paintbrush" appearance. Pathologically, subperiosteal deposition of bone is accompanied by subchondral sclerosis. Bone proliferation, which cannot be overemphasized as a diagnostic sign of psoriatic arthritis (or other spondyloarthropathies), probably relates to an exaggerated healing response of the injured bone.[46] Osseous erosion in rheumatoid arthritis generally is not associated with adjacent bony deposition. Although bone proliferation may accompany erosions in gouty arthritis, the resulting excrescences generally are well defined.

Periostitis in the metaphyses and diaphyses of bones is not uncommon in psoriatic arthritis, particularly in the hands and the feet.[47, 48] In these locations, periosteal bone formation may lead to significant "cloaking" of an entire phalanx or a portion of a metacarpal or metatarsal bone. This change may appear early in the disease course, associated with soft tissue swelling, before significant abnormalities occur in the adjacent articulations. A similar abnormality accompanies Reiter's syndrome, juvenile chronic arthritis, and infection. Condensation of bone on the periosteal and endosteal surfaces of the cortex and trabecular thickening in the spongiosa can cause an entire phalanx to appear radiodense. This latter appearance, which is termed the ivory phalanx, is most frequent in the terminal phalanges of toes (particularly the first), can occur as an early radiographic manifestation of the disease, can be evident without obvious articular abnormality or spiculated bone proliferation, and almost invariably is associated with soft tissue swelling and nail disease of the same digit.[48, 106]

Intra-articular osseous fusion is another manifestation of bone proliferation in psoriatic arthritis. Although such fusion may be observed in large joints such as the knee,[166] it is particularly prominent in the hands and feet and usually affects proximal interphalangeal and distal interphalangeal joints; as the ankylosis becomes complete, the adjacent erosions and bone proliferation may become less evident. Although intra-articular osseous fusion also is observed in inflammatory (erosive) osteoarthritis, septic arthritis, and even rheumatoid arthritis (carpal and tarsal areas), it should be stressed as an important radiographic sign of the seronegative spondyloarthropathies (psoriatic arthritis, ankylosing spondylitis, and Reiter's syndrome).

Bone proliferation occurs at sites at which tendons and ligaments insert on bones. These include the posterior and inferior surfaces of the calcaneus, the femoral trochanters, the ischial tuberosities, the medial and lateral malleoli, the ulnar olecranon, the anterior surface of the patella, the ra-

dial tuberosity, and the condyles of the distal portion of the femur and proximal part of the tibia. In some patients, the resulting abnormalities overshadow less prominent or subtle intra-articular changes. Indeed, the term tumoral enthesopathy has been applied to these changes, indicating how prominent they may become.[164]

Tuftal Resorption. Resorption of the tufts of the distal phalanges of the hands and feet is characteristic of psoriatic arthritis.[100] Progressive osteolysis or whittling of the bone eventually may lead to destruction of the majority of the phalanx. The eroded bone may be smoothly tapered or irregular in outline. Soft tissue swelling and adjacent interphalangeal joint abnormalities are frequent. The nail of the involved digit almost always is involved. Subungual calcification also has been observed.[113]

Malalignment and Subluxation. Deformities of the hands and the feet can be encountered in some patients with psoriatic arthritis.[114] Telescoping of one bone on its neighbor reflects the severity of osseous destruction and may lead to the "opera-glass hand." In this situation, excess skin may be folded over the involved joints, producing a concertina-like appearance. Ulnar deviation at the metacarpophalangeal joints, fibular deviation at the metatarsophalangeal joints, and boutonnière and swan-neck deformities are not as common in psoriatic arthritis as in rheumatoid arthritis.

Radiographic Abnormalities at Specific Sites

Hand (Figs. 29–3 and 29–4). It is the destructive arthritis of distal interphalangeal joints of the hand that is the best-known manifestation of psoriasis.[115] At these sites, bilateral, symmetric or asymmetric, or unilateral changes are observed. Initial erosions occur at the margins of the articulation and proceed centrally. The resulting irregular osseous surfaces may become separated from each other, indicating the extensive nature of the erosive process. It is this lack of apposition of adjacent bony margins that distinguishes the radiographic picture of psoriatic arthritis from that of osteoarthritis, in which closely applied undulating osseous surfaces are the rule. Adjacent proximal interphalangeal joints frequently are affected, although an asymmetric or spotty involvement is common. Severe abnormalities may be encountered at the interphalangeal joint of the thumb with dorsal subluxation of the distal phalanx. The metacarpophalangeal joints may be relatively spared, although occasionally severe destruction, resorption, and proliferation at these sites also are encountered. At the first metacarpophalangeal joint, sesamoid destruction can accompany other articular abnormalities.

At any altered interphalangeal site, radiographic findings may include separated and eroded, well-demarcated bone margins, protrusion of a blunted and distorted osseous surface into an adjacent expanded one (pencil-and-cup appearance), irregular periosteal bone proliferation (whiskering), and intra-articular osseous fusion.

Tuftal resorption can be evident in one or more terminal phalanges. Whittling or penciling of the tufts can result in a peg-shaped phalanx. When severe, tuftal resorption almost inevitably is associated with destructive articular findings, although minor degrees of osseous resorption can be seen in the absence of obvious joint abnormality.[49] In these latter instances, the changes simulate those in various col-

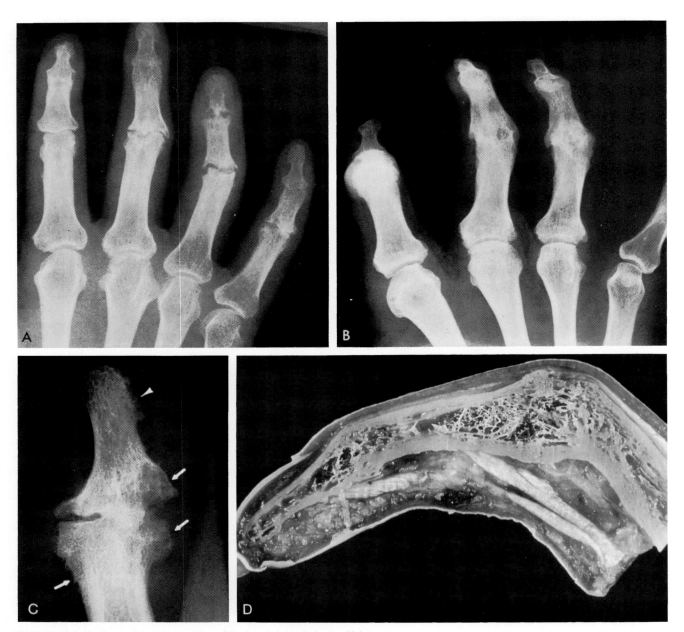

FIGURE 29–3. Radiographic abnormalities of the hand. Interphalangeal joints.

A, B Interphalangeal joint changes in two persons consist of articular space narrowing, intra-articular bony ankylosis, marginal and central erosions, flexion contractures, and osteolysis of phalangeal tufts. Metacarpophalangeal joint abnormalities, although less marked, include joint space narrowing, marginal erosions, and bony proliferation.

C Prominent abnormalities at the interphalangeal joint of the thumb include joint space narrowing, marginal erosions with adjacent proliferation (arrows), and tuftal resorption (arrowhead).

D A sagittal sectional photograph of a finger in this cadaver with psoriatic arthritis shows solid fusion of both interphalangeal joints.

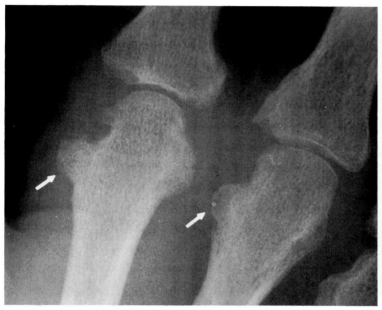

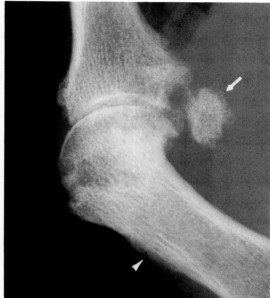

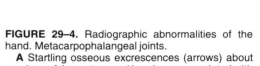

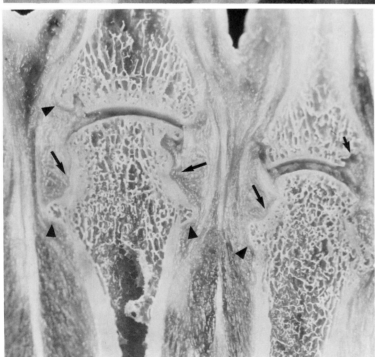

FIGURE 29–4. Radiographic abnormalities of the hand. Metacarpophalangeal joints.

A Startling osseous excrescences (arrows) about erosions of the metacarpal heads are associated with soft tissue swelling, joint space narrowing, and bony erosion and proliferation in the phalanges. (Courtesy of A. Brower, M.D., Norfolk, Virginia.)

B At the first metacarpophalangeal joint, irregular bone formation on the metacarpal head, proximal phalanx, and adjacent sesamoid (arrow) can be seen. Periostitis of the metacarpal diaphysis also is evident (arrowhead).

C In this photograph of a coronal section of the third and fourth metacarpophalangeal joints in a cadaver with psoriatic arthritis, observe marginal erosions (arrows) and bone proliferation (arrowheads).

lagen vascular disorders, particularly scleroderma, or those occurring after thermal injuries. More extensive osteolysis can be encountered in the proximal segments of the hand, although this mutilating variety of bone and joint disease in psoriasis is relatively uncommon. Both phalangeal resorption and destructive arthritis of distal interphalangeal joints generally are associated with significant nail changes in the same digit, which can lead to recognizable radiographic alterations in the soft tissues.

Wrist (Fig. 29–5). Abnormalities in the wrist in psoriatic arthritis are not so frequent as those in the fingers and rarely are encountered without more typical distal changes. Any compartment may be altered in one or both wrists.[50, 100] Occasionally, the changes in the inferior radioulnar compartment may be extensive, leading to osteolysis and dorsal subluxation of the distal ulna.[41]

Other Upper Extremity Sites (Figs. 29–6 and 29–7). Psoriatic arthritis can lead to changes in the elbow and glenohumeral, acromioclavicular, and sternoclavicular joints.[103] As at other sites, findings may vary from minor degrees of osseous erosion to extensive osteolysis. Adjacent bone eburnation is characteristic in any of these sites.

Forefoot (Fig. 29–8). The forefoot commonly is affected in psoriatic arthritis. Bilateral, asymmetric changes predominate in the interphalangeal and metatarsophalangeal joints and are characterized by the appearance of marginal erosions, bone proliferation, alterations in joint space (narrow or wide), and lack of osteoporosis. Extensive destruction of the interphalangeal joint of the great toe is more characteristic of this articular disorder than of any other disease, although Reiter's syndrome occasionally produces similar but less marked changes at this site. Osteolysis of tufts and of phalangeal and metatarsal shafts can be encountered. In the terminal phalanges, particularly that of the great toe, extensive new bone formation may lead to increased osseous density of the entire bone, the ivory phalanx.[48] Sesamoid involvement also is common. Involvement of the tibialis posterior tendon can lead to pes planus with talonavicular malalignment.[165]

Calcaneus (Fig. 29–9). As in other seronegative spondyloarthropathies (Reiter's syndrome, ankylosing spondylitis), erosion and proliferation of the posterior or inferior surface of the calcaneus, or of both surfaces, may be prominent in psoriatic arthritis.[51] Retrocalcaneal bursitis creates a radiodense area adjacent to the posterosuperior aspect of the bone, which may extend into the preachilles fat pad. Subjacent erosion of the calcaneus is associated with surrounding bony proliferation. The neighboring Achilles tendon may be thickened, and irregular excrescences may develop at its site of attachment to the calcaneus. Inferiorly, erosions of the plantar aspect of the calcaneus frequently evoke extensive sclerosis of the surrounding bone, creating irregular and poorly defined enthesophytes at the attachment sites of the plantar ligaments and aponeurosis. With time, the enthesophytes may become more sharply delineated in outline. Occasionally the entire inferior surface of the calcaneus becomes eburnated.

Other Lower Extremity Sites (Figs. 29–10 and 29–11). Articular involvement in psoriasis may be apparent in the midfoot or hindfoot, the ankle, or the knee. Abnormality of the hip is relatively unusual. Concentric loss of joint space in one or both hips may occur in association with sacroili-

itis; rarely, destructive neuropathic-like findings are encountered.

Sacroiliac Joint (Fig. 29–12). In 1961, Dixon and Lience[52] were the first to emphasize changes in the sacroiliac joint in psoriatic arthritis. Subsequent reports have frequently conflicted regarding the prevalence and the pattern of such sacroiliac joint abnormalities.[33, 53–60] Much of the discrepancy in the reported prevalence of sacroiliitis in psoriasis has been related to methods of patient selection. Some investigators have evaluated patients with skin disease alone, whereas others have included patients with moderate or severe psoriatic arthritis. Furthermore, the technique of radiographic examination of the sacroiliac joints has varied considerably. Some reports used abdominal radiographs, whereas others required specific sacroiliac joint radiographs with or without conventional tomography. Finally, the expertise of the observers also influenced the results.

It appears that approximately 10 to 25 per cent of patients with moderate or severe psoriatic skin disease will reveal sacroiliac joint changes on radiographic examination.[56, 58, 116] It also appears that approximately 30 to 50 per cent of patients with psoriatic arthritis will develop such changes,[55, 56] although estimates as low as 14 per cent[53] and as high as 84 per cent[54, 59] have appeared. The prevalence may be increased if radionuclide examination also is used.[57]

Nearly all observers would agree that bilateral abnormalities of the sacroiliac joint are much more frequent than unilateral changes in psoriatic arthritis. Although asymmetric findings may be apparent, in the authors' experience and that of others,[33, 54, 55] symmetric abnormalities predominate. Sacroiliitis can appear without spondylitis (in fact, spondylitis may appear without sacroiliitis). Radiographic sacroiliac joint changes include erosions and sclerosis, predominantly in the ilium, and widening of the articular space. Although significant joint space diminution and bony ankylosis can occur, the prevalence of these findings, particularly ankylosis, is less than that in classic ankylosing spondylitis or the spondylitis associated with inflammatory bowel disease. Thus, some patients with psoriatic sacroiliitis demonstrate considerably eroded and eburnated subchondral bony surfaces at these joints without narrowing of the interosseous space. Above the true articulation, interosseous ligament calcification and ossification, as well as hyperostosis with blurring of the adjacent sacrum and ilium, can be noted. Bone proliferation also is apparent in the pelvis at tendo-osseous junctions, such as the iliac crest and ischial tuberosities,[117] and may be associated with similar changes of the trochanters and osteitis pubis.

Spine (Figs. 29–13 and 29–14). As in Reiter's syndrome, paravertebral ossification about the lower thoracic and upper lumbar segments can occur in psoriatic arthritis, and it may represent an early manifestation of the disease. As reported by Sundarim and Patton,[61] such ossification was noted in 17 per cent of 122 psoriatic patients with spinal radiographs: In 62 per cent of patients with paravertebral ossification, the sacroiliac joints were considered radiographically within normal limits; in 81 per cent of patients with paravertebral ossification, the peripheral joints were without abnormality. Initially, ossification appears as a thick and fluffy or thin and curvilinear radiodense region on one side of the spine, paralleling the lateral surface of the vertebral bodies and the intervertebral discs. It extends

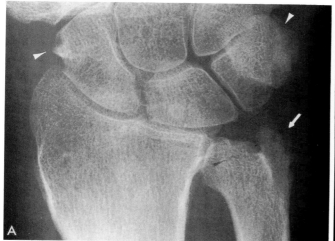

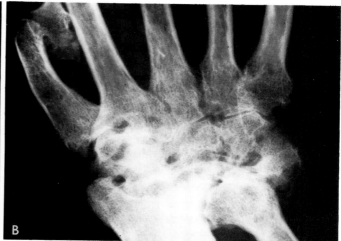

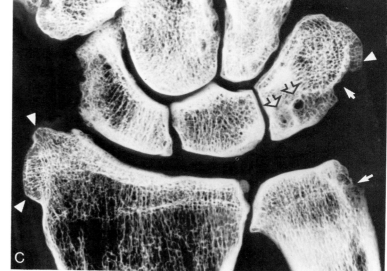

FIGURE 29–5. Radiographic abnormalities of the wrist.

A Note the poorly defined new bone formation on the distal portion of the ulna with adjacent soft tissue swelling (arrow). Osseous erosion and proliferation of carpal bones also are evident (arrowheads).

B Severe pancompartmental involvement of the wrist is characterized by joint space narrowing, intra-articular osseous fusion, erosions, bony proliferation, and the absence of osteoporosis. Considerable destruction about the first metacarpophalangeal joint also is seen.

C–E On a radiograph **(C)** and photographs **(D, E)** of a coronal section of a cadaveric wrist, important findings include bone erosions (closed arrows), intraosseous cysts (open arrows), and bone proliferation (arrowheads).

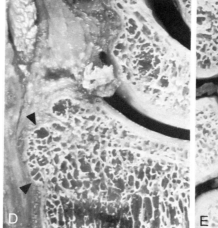

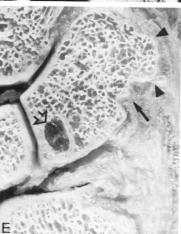

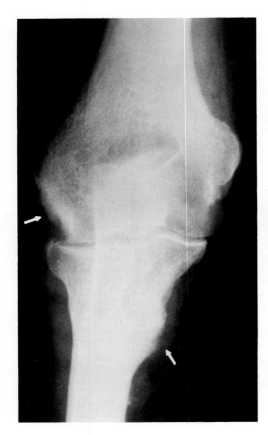

FIGURE 29–6. Radiographic abnormalities of the elbow. A frontal radiograph delineates irregular erosion and proliferation of the distal end of the humerus and proximal end of the ulna (arrows). The joint space is narrowed.

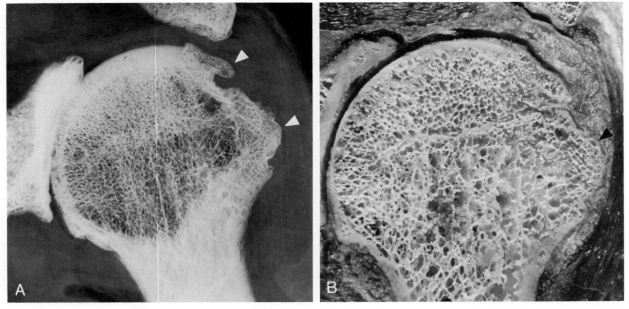

FIGURE 29–7. Radiographic abnormalities of the shoulder. In a cadaver with psoriatic arthritis, a radiograph **(A)** and photograph **(B)** of a coronal section of the shoulder reveal narrowing of the glenohumeral joint and bone proliferation of the greater tuberosity (arrowheads).

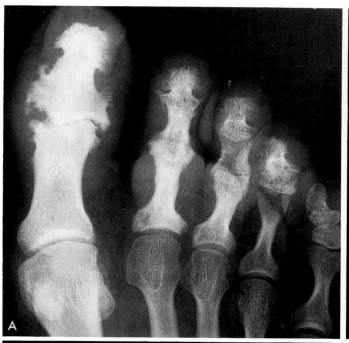
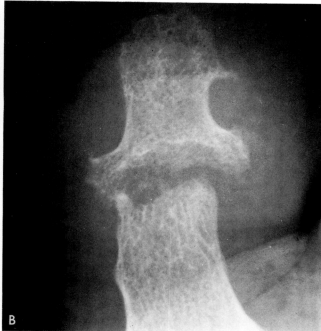
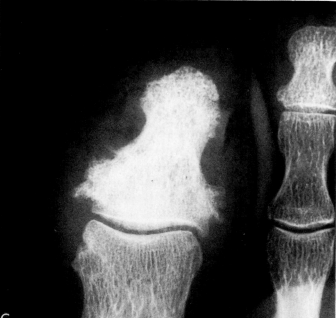

FIGURE 29–8. Radiographic abnormalities of the forefoot.

A Findings include joint space narrowing and bony ankylosis of multiple interphalangeal joints and osseous erosion and proliferation, particularly about the interphalangeal joint of the great toe. Note tuftal osteolysis and sclerosis of bone in multiple digits.

B Considerable bony destruction about the interphalangeal joint of the great toe is associated with widening of the interosseous space, an expanded phalangeal base, and soft tissue swelling.

C Sclerosis of the entire terminal phalanx of the great toe (ivory phalanx) is accompanied by erosion and proliferation of its base and soft tissue swelling. Soft tissue fullness also is apparent in the second digit.

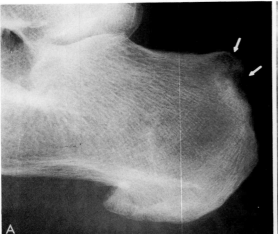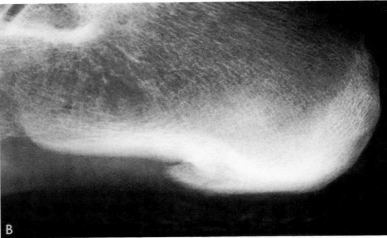

FIGURE 29–9. Abnormalities of the calcaneus.
   A Retrocalcaneal bursitis is manifested as erosion of the posterosuperior aspect of the calcaneus (arrows). A large plantar calcaneal enthesophyte is identified.
   B Extreme sclerosis along the entire undersurface of the calcaneus is associated with a poorly defined plantar excrescence.

progressively at a variable rate, and eventually it may produce a large and bulky outgrowth that merges with the underlying osseous and discal tissue. Its greater size, its unilateral or asymmetric distribution, and its location farther away from the vertebral column are features that distinguish paravertebral ossification from typical syndesmophytosis of ankylosing spondylitis and of spondylitis in inflammatory bowel disease. Occasionally, however, slender, centrally located, and symmetric spinal outgrowths in psoriasis are identical to the syndesmophytes of ankylosing spondylitis.

In addition to the pattern and distribution of bony outgrowths, there are other features of psoriatic spondylitis that differ from those in classic ankylosing spondylitis.[33, 55, 56] Osteitis and squaring of the anterior surfaces of the vertebral bodies are relatively infrequent in psoriasis. Although apophyseal joint space narrowing, sclerosis, and bony ankylosis may be seen, the frequency of these findings is much less than that in ankylosing spondylitis.

Cervical spine abnormalities may become striking in patients with psoriasis.[55, 62] These abnormalities, which occasionally may be combined with sacroiliac joint alterations with relatively minor changes in the thoracolumbar spine, include apophyseal joint space narrowing and sclerosis,[151] osseous irregularity at the discovertebral joint, and extensive proliferation along the anterior surface of the spine. Atlantoaxial subluxation also can be evident; Killebrew and collaborators noted such subluxation in 45 per cent of 20 patients with psoriatic spondylitis.[55] Although anterior subluxation predominates,[167] lateral instability, as observed in rheumatoid arthritis, also is encountered.[118] Associated erosive and sclerotic abnormalities of the odontoid process are frequent in patients demonstrating atlantoaxial subluxation. Spontaneous fusion of the subluxed spine has been observed.[155] Rarely, subaxial cervical instability with cord compression is evident in psoriatic spondylitis.[119, 169, 170] This finding, when combined with discovertebral erosion, resembles changes observed in rheumatoid arthritis.[168] Histologic evidence has suggested that the latter erosion results from a destructive inflammatory process characterized by

the presence of vascular granulation tissue containing plasma cells and lymphocytes.[119]

Other Sites (Fig. 29–15). The manubriosternal joint can reveal severe alterations, almost invariably in association with changes in other skeletal sites.[63, 157, 171] Osteoporosis, subchondral erosion, eburnation, and synostosis are seen. Adjacent soft tissue swelling can be a prominent clinical and radiologic finding, and it may be accompanied by significant sternal pain and tenderness. The radiographic changes at this site in psoriatic arthritis are similar to those that may be observed in rheumatoid arthritis and ankylosing spondylitis.[64, 65]

The temporomandibular joint also can be significantly affected in psoriatic arthritis.[66–69, 120, 172] The changes, which resemble those of rheumatoid arthritis and ankylosing spondylitis, include erosion of the mandible and temporal bone, sclerosis, malposition, and limited mobility. Intra-articular bony ankylosis has been recorded.[121] CT scanning is well suited to the evaluation of psoriatic involvement of the temporomandibular joint.[173, 174]

Involvement of the sternoclavicular joint is evident in some patients with psoriatic arthritis. Conventional tomography and CT scanning are useful in delineating abnormalities at this site.

RADIONUCLIDE ABNORMALITIES

Scintigraphy with bone-seeking radiopharmaceutical agents can delineate articular abnormality of psoriatic arthritis prior to its appearance on radiographic examination.[70, 71] Although the scintigraphic pattern will vary from one patient to another, increased radionuclide accumulation predominates at interphalangeal, metacarpophalangeal, and metatarsophalangeal joints of the hands and feet; however, calcaneal, sacroiliac joint, and spinal uptake can be considerable (Fig. 29–16). The asymmetric nature of the scintigraphic alterations in psoriasis frequently permit its differentiation from rheumatoid arthritis, although radiographic correlation generally is required.

Usually it is assumed that the accumulation of bone-

Text continued on page 1094

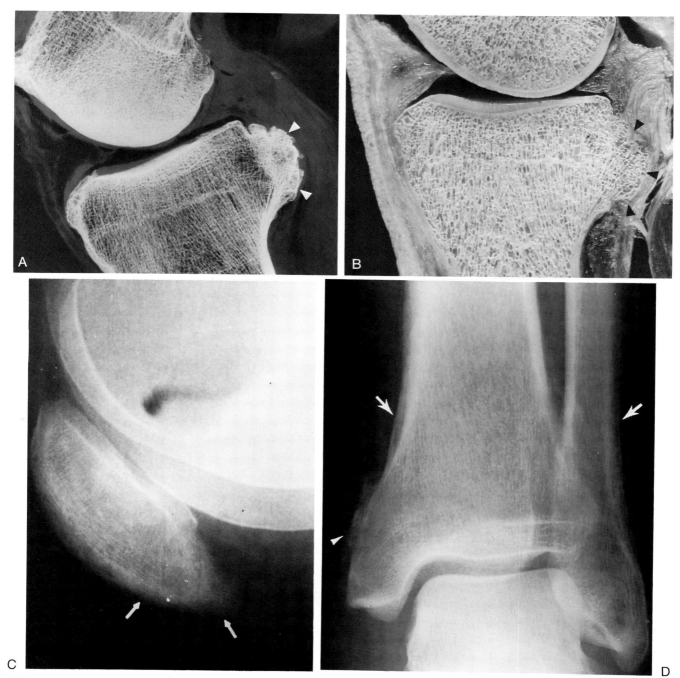

FIGURE 29–10. Abnormalities of the knee and ankle.

A, B A radiograph and photograph of a sagittal section of a cadaveric knee are shown in which psoriatic arthritis has led to dramatic bone proliferation (arrowheads) in the posterior surface of the tibia.

C Hyperostosis on the anterior and inferior surfaces of the patella is observed (arrows). (Courtesy of A. Brower, M.D., Norfolk, Virginia.)

D Although the tibiotalar joint is normal, observe periostitis in the tibia and fibula (arrows). The irregular excrescence arising from the medial malleolus (arrowhead) is particularly characteristic of psoriasis. (Courtesy of T. Marklund, M.D., Linkoping, Sweden.)

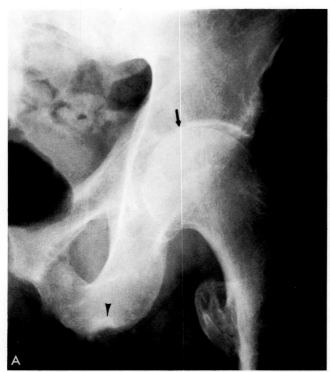

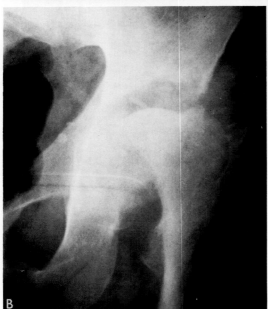

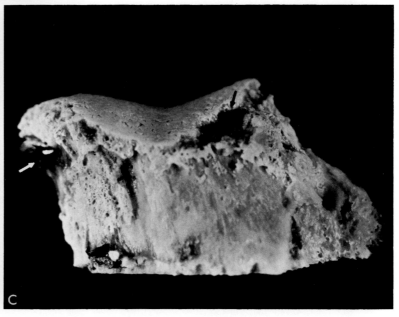

FIGURE 29–11. Abnormalities of the hip.

A Observe concentric joint space narrowing of the hip (arrow) associated with erosion and sclerosis of the ischial tuberosity (arrowhead). The sacroiliac joints and spine also were involved. The changes of the lesser trochanter include bone proliferation.

B, C This 55 year old man with psoriasis developed rapidly progressive hip destruction, which required an arthroplasty. Histologic findings were typical of severe psoriatic arthritis. On the preoperative radiograph **(B),** the considerable destruction of the femoral head is identified. The proximal end of the femur has been reduced to a blunt peg. Fragmentation is evident. On a photograph of the intact specimen **(C),** the flattened and deformed femoral head is obvious. Eroded areas are detected (arrows).

FIGURE 29–12. Abnormalities of the sacroiliac joint.

A Bilateral and symmetric changes consist of erosions and sclerosis, predominantly in the ilium. Intra-articular bony ankylosis is not seen.

B In this patient, asymmetric abnormalities are present. The right sacroiliac joint reveals joint space narrowing and sclerosis with blurring of the interosseous space above the true joint. Minimal changes are present on the left side.

C Observe bilateral symmetric abnormalities with ilial erosion and sclerosis. Although bony ankylosis can be observed in segments of the joints and in the interosseous space above the joints, the articular space still can be identified.

D In a fourth patient, intra-articular osseous fusion of both sacroiliac joints is more complete. The sclerosis has disappeared.

E, F In a psoriatic cadaver, a coronal sectional radiograph **(E)** and photograph **(F)** reveal extensive intra-articular bone ankylosis (straight arrows). In **F,** note remnants of the articular space (lower curved arrow) and lack of ossification in the interosseous space (upper curved arrow) above the true synovial portion of the joint.

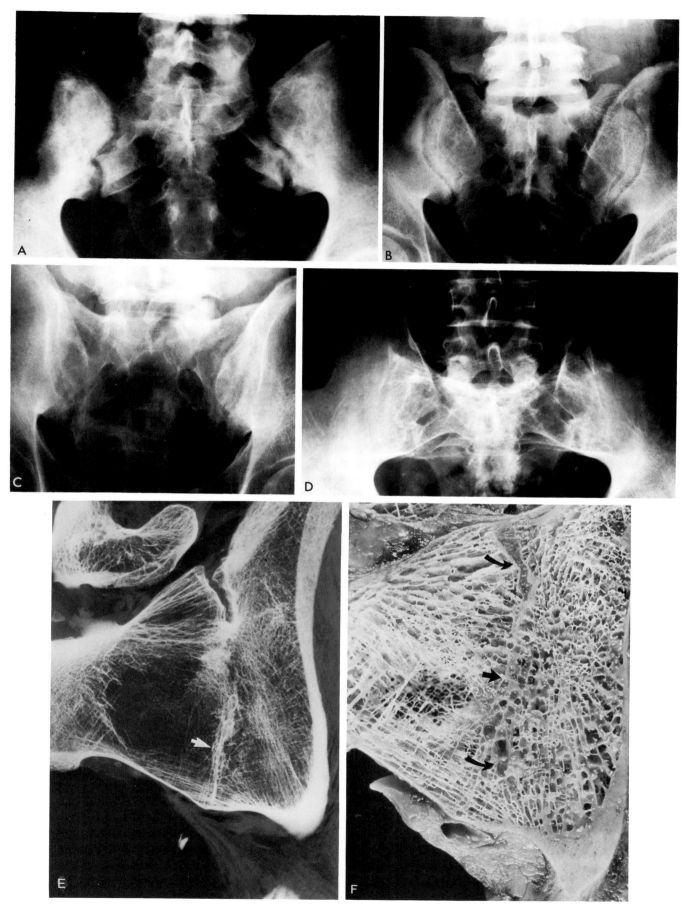

FIGURE 29–12 *See legend on opposite page*

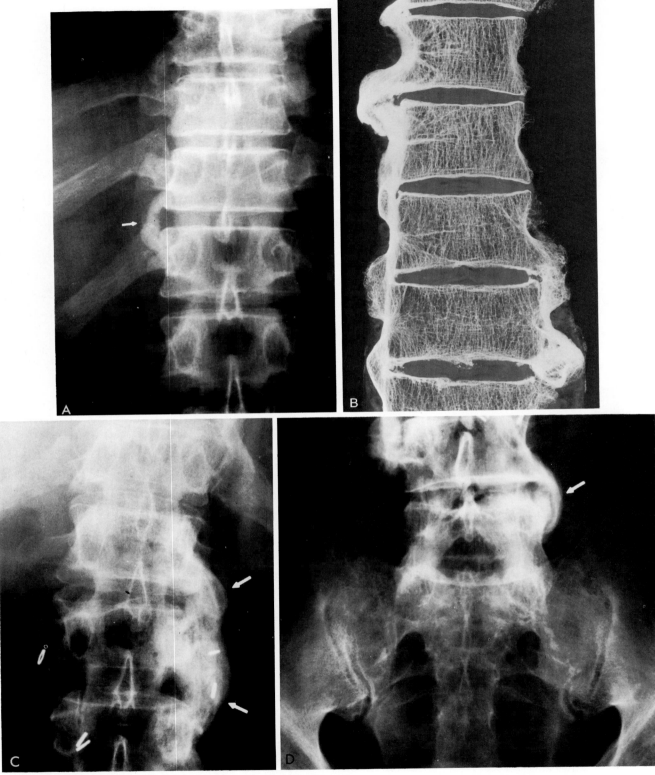

FIGURE 29–13. Radiographic abnormalities of the thoracic and lumbar spine.

A Early findings consist of irregular, asymmetrically distributed, paravertebral bony excrescences (arrow), particularly at the thoracolumbar junction.

B In this radiograph of a coronal section of a thoracic spine, the pattern of paravertebral ossification is characteristic of psoriasis (as well as Reiter's syndrome). Note its asymmetric distribution.

C, D With progression (in a different patient), bulky outgrowths appear (arrows), which merge with the underlying vertebral bodies and intervertebral discs. Note the asymmetric distribution and the absence of significant sacroiliac joint disease. Surgical clips are evident.

Illustration continued on opposite page

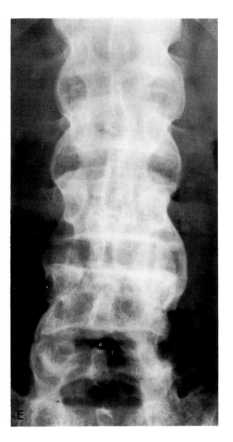

FIGURE 29–13 *Continued*

E In some patients with psoriasis, the excrescences resemble the syndesmophytes seen in classic ankylosing spondylitis, although they may be larger, asymmetric in distribution, and located farther from the spine.

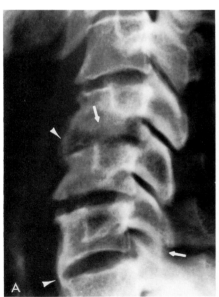

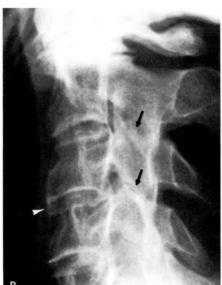

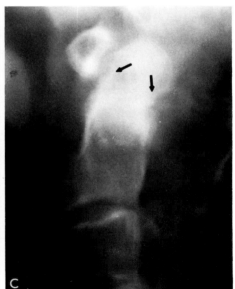

FIGURE 29–14. Radiographic abnormalities of the cervical spine.

A Note erosions at the discovertebral junction and apophyseal joints (arrows) and syndesmophytes (arrowheads).

B Findings include apophyseal joint space narrowing and bony ankylosis (arrows), syndesmophytosis (arrowhead), and proliferation at the atlantoaxial articulations.

C Odontoid erosions predominate on both the anterior and posterior surfaces of the bone (arrows).

D, E Prominent bone proliferation (arrows) about the odontoid process is evident on this radiograph **(D)** and photograph **(E)** of a sagittal section of a psoriatic spine. Note narrowing and irregularity of the anterior median atlantoaxial joint, ossification of the transverse ligament of the atlas (arrowheads), and syndesmophytes.

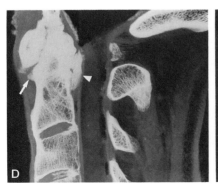

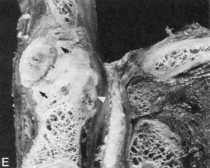

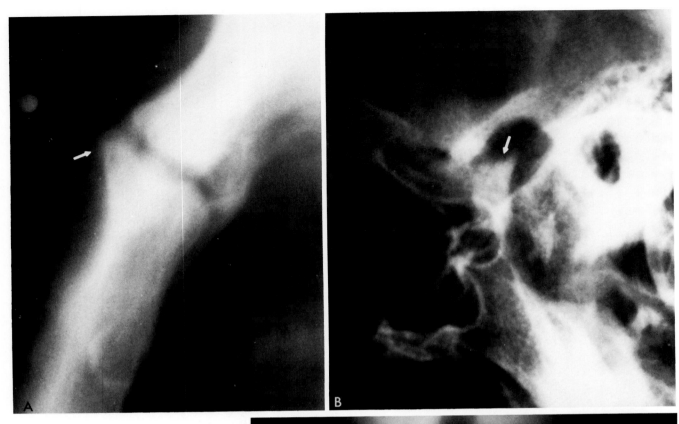

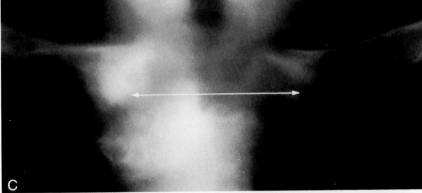

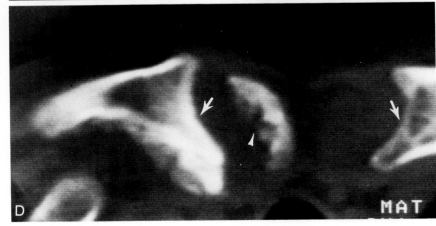

FIGURE 29–15. Radiographic abnormalities at other sites.

A Manubriosternal joint. A conventional tomogram outlines severe sclerosis and bone proliferation, particularly anteriorly (arrow).

B Temporomandibular joint. Considerable erosion and sclerosis of the condylar process of the mandible are recognized (arrow).

C, D Sternoclavicular joint. In a 50 year old man with psoriasis, pain, swelling, and a bony prominence developed about both sternoclavicular joints. Conventional tomography **(C)** indicates considerable bone erosion and eburnation involving the medial end of the clavicles and the sternum, especially on the right side. A transaxial image with CT scanning **(D)** at the level indicated in **C** confirms the erosion of the clavicles (arrows) and sternum (arrowhead).

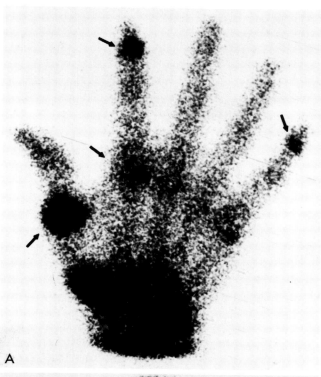

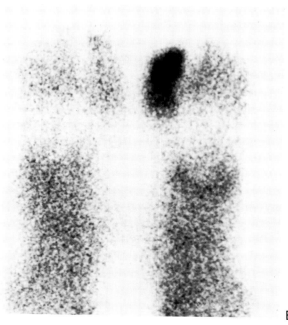

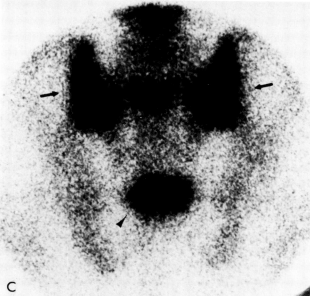

FIGURE 29–16. Scintigraphic abnormalities.

A Radionuclide imaging using a bone-seeking pharmaceutical preparation in a patient with psoriatic arthritis outlines uptake in the metacarpophalangeal and interphalangeal joints of the hand (arrows). Although the other side was involved, the distribution of abnormalities was asymmetric.

B Intense uptake of the bone-seeking radiopharmaceutical agent in the great toe of a patient with psoriatic arthritis corresponded to a radiographically abnormal site in which soft tissue swelling and an ivory terminal phalanx were seen.

C In a different patient with psoriatic arthritis, symmetric uptake of radionuclide in the sacroiliac joints is evident (arrows). This activity is much greater than that in the sacrum. Radioactive tracer also is observed in the bladder (arrowhead).

(**A, C** From Weissberg D, et al: AJR *131*:665, 1978. Copyright 1978, American Roentgen Ray Society.)

seeking radiopharmaceutical preparations in psoriatic arthritis (as in other arthritides) is based on increased blood flow and osteogenesis. However, published evidence supporting preferential binding of certain agents in immature collagen[72, 73] has suggested to some observers[71] that radionuclide abnormalities in psoriasis may be related to periarticular synthesis of immature collagen or breakdown of existing collagen rather than to synovial or osseous alterations. The documentation that radionuclide changes in psoriasis may correlate with cutaneous activity and occur without clinically apparent joint disease makes this hypothesis more plausible.[71]

As has been noted in rheumatoid arthritis, whole-body scintigraphy, using ^{99m}Tc-methylene diphosphonate (MDP), in psoriatic arthritis reportedly has demonstrated increased accumulation of the radiopharmaceutical agent in extra-articular structures, including the thorax and the skull, suggesting the presence of a diffuse osteopathy.[122]

PATHOLOGIC ABNORMALITIES

Synovial Articulations (Fig. 29–17)

Although the pathologic changes of psoriatic arthritis basically are similar to those of rheumatoid arthritis, there also are some pathologic characteristics of psoriasis that are distinctive.[4, 74–76, 123, 124]

1. Synovial inflammation is encountered, but the degree of cellular infiltration with lymphocytes and plasma cells is much less marked than in rheumatoid arthritis. Small aggregates of lymphocytes are observed in scar tissue. Polymorphonuclear leukocytes may be noted in joint effusions accompanying the synovitis. Early fibrosis of the proliferating synovium is typical of psoriatic arthritis. Regressive changes of the small and medium-sized blood vessels are pronounced in this disease.

2. Inflammatory synovial tissue, or pannus, is prominent only on the surface of the cartilage, whereas in rheumatoid arthritis, hyperplastic synovium is seen in both superficial and deep layers of the cartilage. In psoriatic arthritis, remnants of the cartilaginous surface can be evident for considerable periods of time, although eventual destruction of cartilage with formation of fibrous scar tissue may lead to synovial invasion of subchondral bone.

3. Bone proliferation is evident in periarticular regions.[48, 76] This may take the form of subchondral trabecular thickening and periosteal bone formation.

4. Fibrous ankylosis of the articulation may be noted, as in rheumatoid arthritis. In psoriatic arthritis, however, bony ankylosis also is prominent. Metaplastic bone formation originates from isolated cartilaginous foci within the fibrous scar tissue.

These pathologic aberrations explain some of the more characteristic radiographic features of psoriatic arthritis. The lack of both intense synovial inflammation and severe synovial hyperemia in this disease may account for the absence of significant periarticular osteoporosis. Synovial villi do not reveal a great increase in number or size, and stromal cells are only slightly increased in number. What is evident is prominent synovial fibrosis with an unusual degree of thickening of the wall of adjacent small and medium

sized arteries.[76] This vascular sclerosis is less marked in rheumatoid arthritis.

Articular space loss, which almost is universal in rheumatoid arthritis, is much less constant in psoriatic arthritis. In the latter disease, the degree of chondrolysis by the inflamed synovium is variable. In some patients, progressive osteolysis of the supporting subchondral bone may lead to articular space widening before the entire cartilaginous coat has been lost.

A tendency to new bone formation in psoriatic arthritis can be profound. Cellular proliferation in the surrounding periosteal membrane is associated with significant osteoblastosis. Subjacent bone formation frequently creates poorly defined spiculation of the adjacent cortex. Within the articulation, metaplastic bone can produce partial or complete osseous fusion.

Discovertebral Junction (Fig. 29–18)

Details of the histologic findings related to paravertebral ossification in psoriasis (and Reiter's syndrome) are lacking. An inflammatory process in the paravertebral connective tissue or periosteal reaction at the site of osseous attachment of the ligaments and tendons may be significant in this regard.[77, 78] The anulus fibrosus itself is not ossified.[77]

Osteolysis

Tapering and dissolution of terminal phalanges are characteristic alterations in psoriasis.[79] Initially, thinning or loss of the cortex is related to irregular rapid removal and synthesis of bone. The surrounding periosteal membrane demonstrates noninflammatory cellular proliferation with an inner layer of osteoblasts and outer layers of fibroblasts. Bone removal by periosteal cells and bone formation by osteoblasts are encountered. The periosteal process ceases with time, the fibroblasts being transformed into fibrocytes.[76] The osteolytic process usually predominates over the osteoblastic process in this disease.

ETIOLOGY AND PATHOGENESIS

Hereditary factors appear to be important in the pathogenesis of uncomplicated psoriasis, but the exact mode of inheritance is not known. Both dominant[80] and recessive[81] mechanisms of transmission have been suggested, although psoriatic pedigrees reveal considerable variability, which at times does not conform to mendelian modes of inheritance, suggesting that the cause of psoriasis may be multifactorial.[6] Histocompatibility typing among patients with cutaneous disease has revealed an increased frequency of HLA-BW17, HLA-B13, and, more recently, HLA-BW16,[82–85, 126] indicating that these antigens may be an important genetic marker for the inherited skin manifestations of psoriasis.

The role of heredity in the articular manifestations of this disease also has been emphasized.[105] Family studies have indicated that rheumatic complaints are common in relatives of patients with psoriatic arthritis.[86–88] Histocompatibility typing in patients with psoriatic arthritis has revealed a high frequency (approximately 25 to 60 per cent) of HLA-B27 antigen,[89–92] particularly in patients with sacroiliitis[176] or spondylitis,[177] or both,[178] but also in those with distal interphalangeal joint involvement.[93] The presence of

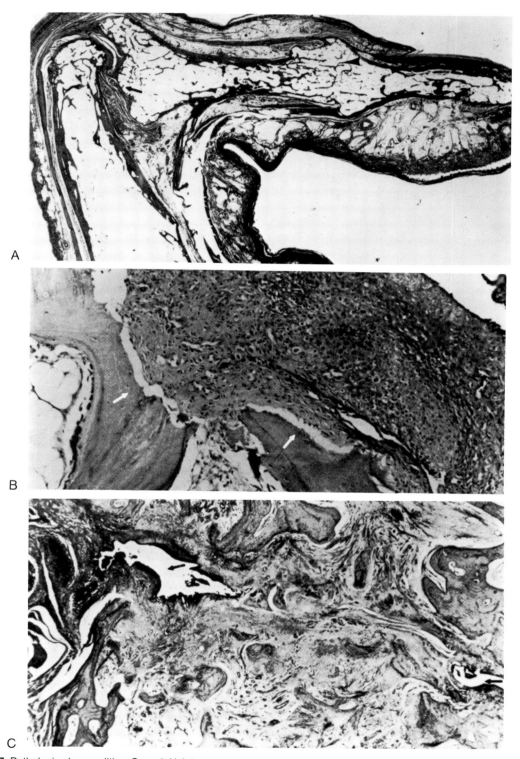

FIGURE 29–17. Pathologic abnormalities: Synovial joints.

A Fibrous ankylosis of the proximal interphalangeal joint (arrow) and bony ankylosis of the distal interphalangeal joint (arrowhead) can be identified. Observe cortical changes with periosteal fibrosis and osteoporosis.

B Articular cartilage and subchondral bone (arrows) are being destroyed by cellular, fibrous, inflammatory synovial tissue (pannus). This stage may precede fibrous ankylosis of the joint.

C In a different joint of the same finger, fibrous ankylosis is observed. Remnants of the joint space can be identified (arrows).

(From Fassbender HG: Pathology of Rheumatoid Diseases. New York, Springer-Verlag, 1975.)

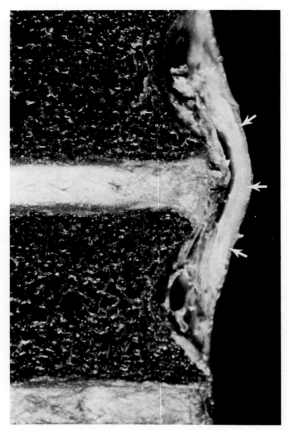

FIGURE 29–18. Pathologic abnormalities: Discovertebral junction. A photograph of a coronal section of the thoracolumbar spine in a cadaver with psoriatic spondylitis reveals paravertebral ossification (arrows). Note that the ossified bridge is separate from the outer fibers of the anulus fibrosus.

this histocompatibility antigen in a patient with psoriasis apparently increases his or her susceptibility to axial (and perhaps appendicular) skeletal disease. Similarly, elevation of HLA-BW38, CW6, and DR4 antigens has been observed in patients with psoriatic arthritis and, in some cases, linked to specific varieties of the articular disease.[125, 158] For example, HLA-CW6 is seen with increased frequency in all forms of psoriatic arthritis, HLA-BW38 in all types and all classes of severity, and HLA-DR4 with severe psoriatic articular destruction.[125] HLA-BW38 and HLA-BW39 have been associated with peripheral joint involvement in psoriatic arthritis,[175] and HLA-DR7, with peripheral arthritis alone.[177]

Environmental factors also may be influential in the development of psoriatic arthritis, perhaps by triggering articular manifestations in patients who are genetically predisposed to the disease. Proposed environmental events have included trauma,[94, 95, 179] capillary changes,[96] neurotrophic effects,[97] and infection.[98]

ADDITIONAL DISEASES OF SKIN AND JOINTS

Certain cutaneous disorders are associated with clinical and radiologic findings of arthritis, which in some cases simulate those of psoriasis. *Acne fulminans,* in which acute activation of chronic acne in the form of acute ulceration

and hemorrhage in the dermis is seen, is associated with systemic manifestations that include fever, weight loss, an increase in erythrocyte sedimentation rate, microscopic hematuria, and myalgias and polyarthralgias. Musculoskeletal symptoms typically begin at the same time as the skin abnormalities. Although the joint involvement usually is asymptomatic, self-limited, and nondeforming in nature,[127–130] more significant articular disease, in both the appendicular and the axial skeleton, can become apparent.[127, 131, 132, 154] Findings have included sacroiliitis,[131, 133] synovitis in peripheral joints[131, 134] associated with osteopenia and periostitis,[135] destructive lesions of cervical vertebral bodies and intervertebral discs,[127] and even osteolytic foci in periarticular locations.[132, 181] The osteolytic lesions may be multiple in about 50 per cent of patients, and commonly they are accompanied by periosteal reaction. The clavicle, sternum, and tubular bones are frequent sites of involvement.[180] An increased prevalence of HLA-B27 in those patients with sacroiliitis has not been evident.[131]

Acne conglobata is characterized by large, inflamed cystic lesions in the skin and few constitutional symptoms and signs. In this disease as well as in *hidradenitis suppurativa,* only a few reports of arthritis have appeared.[136, 152, 153, 180, 185] As opposed to the situation in acne fulminans, in which arthritis typically occurs in male adolescents, in acne conglobata and hidradenitis suppurativa articular disease is seen in mature adults. Bone erosion about the small joints of the hand, wrist, and foot, periostitis, soft tissue swelling, and osteoporosis are noted. Periosteal bone formation occurs beneath skin ulcerations in the lower leg. In the axial skeleton, unilateral or, less commonly, bilateral sacroiliitis and syndesmophytosis, particularly in an asymmetric distribution in the lumbar and thoracic segments, are the reported manifestations (Fig. 29–19).[136] Additional findings include squaring of the vertebral bodies and calcification in the anterior longitudinal ligament.

Although the precise mechanism responsible for these articular abnormalities is not known, the possibility exists that the arthropathy is a reaction to the chronic cutaneous infection that characterizes these disorders (as well as pustular psoriasis).[136] Reactive arthritis is a known complication of a variety of nonarticular infections. Furthermore, arthropathy and dermatitis may complicate intestinal bypass surgery, in which evidence has been accumulated that the articular manifestations are caused by circulating immune complexes containing antibody against *Escherichia coli* and *Bacteroides fragilis.*[131] Enteric infections also may be operative in the pathogenesis of ankylosing spondylitis.[137] On the basis of the finding of decreased serum complement levels, an immune complex-mediated mechanism has been postulated for the arthritis accompanying acne skin disease.[129]

Pyoderma gangrenosum is characterized by painful ulcers in the skin and occurs as an isolated event or in combination with ulcerative colitis, Crohn's disease, myeloproliferative disorders, and paraproteinemias. Approximately 30 per cent of patients with this skin disease develop articular manifestations.[138] Although variable in its joint alterations, pyoderma gangrenosum may be accompanied by a seronegative polyarthritis. In some cases, bone erosions are seen in periarticular regions in the hands,[159] elbows, hips, and knees, as well as in the odontoid process; subluxation of cervical vertebrae also has been recorded.[139] In other

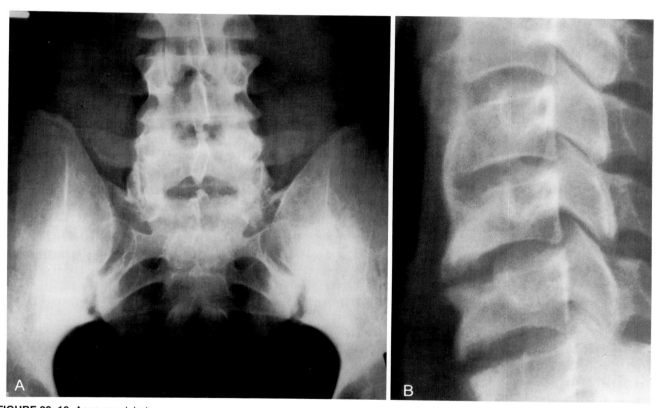

FIGURE 29–19. Acne conglobata.
A In a 20 year old man with acne conglobata, observe bilateral symmetric sacroiliitis. (Courtesy of A. Brower, M.D., Norfolk, Virginia.)
B In a different patient with the same disease, bone proliferation involves the anterior surface of the cervical vertebral bodies. Syndesmo-phytes are seen. The apophyseal joints are normal. (Courtesy of N. Kinnis, M.D., Chicago, Ill.)

instances, especially those in which ulcerative colitis also is present, an acute nonerosive oligoarthritis of the lower limbs is seen.[140] Pyoderma gangrenosum also is accompanied by an articular disease that is similar or identical to rheumatoid arthritis.[141]

Pustular lesions of the skin in the hand and foot *(pustulosis palmaris et plantaris)* are observed in some persons who develop hyperostosis in the clavicles, upper ribs, and sternum. The syndrome, which is termed sternocostoclavicular hyperostosis, and related syndromes, including chronic recurrent multifocal osteomyelitis (CRMO) and synovitis, acne, pustulosis, hyperostosis, and osteitis (SAPHO syndrome), are discussed in Chapters 41 and 93. Of interest, a patient with psoriasis and sternocostoclavicular hyperostosis has been described.[142]

Sweet's syndrome, or acute febrile neutrophilic dermatosis, is an uncommon disorder that is characterized clinically by fever, leukocytosis, and raised tender plaques or nodules on the face, neck, and limbs; and, histologically, by a dense neutrophilic infiltration in the dermis.[143, 182] It usually is observed in middle-aged women and may be complicated by myalgias, arthralgias, and even arthritis.[144, 145] Acute or transient polyarticular involvement of large and small joints is seen.[146] Knees and wrists are involved most frequently. Histologic studies indicate vascular congestion and mild inflammation in the synovial membrane.[144] Radiographic findings are generally confined to soft tissue swelling and a joint effusion. Sterile osteomyelitis has been described.[160]

Additional skin disorders associated with musculoskeletal abnormalities include *papular mucinosis* (scleromyxedema or lichen myxedematosus), in which clinical manifestations, such as sclerodactyly, acrolysis, and stiffness, resemble those of scleroderma[147, 161]; and *Mucha-Habermann disease* (pityriasis lichenoides et varioliformis acuta), in which an allergic vasculitis–like disorder affects adolescents and young adults and, in rare instances, is associated with articular abnormalities that resemble juvenile chronic arthritis or adult-onset rheumatoid arthritis.[148]

Acro-osteolysis may accompany a variety of dermatologic conditions, in addition to psoriasis, such as mycosis fungoides, pityriasis rubra pilaris, epidermolysis bullosa, and ichthyosiform erythroderma.[183, 184]

DIFFERENTIAL DIAGNOSIS (Table 29–3)

Other Seronegative Spondyloarthropathies (Ankylosing Spondylitis, Reiter's Syndrome)

The radiographic findings in psoriatic arthritis are fundamentally similar to those in the other two seronegative spondyloarthropathies, ankylosing spondylitis and Reiter's syndrome. In all three disorders, synovial joint involvement is characterized by the absence of osteoporosis and the presence of soft tissue swelling, joint space abnormality, osseous erosion, and bony proliferation. In psoriatic arthritis and ankylosing spondylitis, intra-articular bony ankylosis is not uncommon; in Reiter's syndrome, such ankylosis is less frequent. In psoriatic arthritis, the extent of osteolysis of juxta-articular bone is greater than in Reiter's syndrome and ankylosing spondylitis.

In each of these seronegative spondyloarthropathies, abnormalities of cartilaginous joints (discovertebral junction, symphysis pubis, manubriosternal joint), consisting of ero-

sion and bone proliferation, may be observed. Similarly, each of these diseases may be associated with abnormalities at tendon and ligament attachments to bone (calcaneus, femoral trochanters, ischial tuberosities). In psoriasis, osteolysis of terminal phalanges is characteristic.

The distribution of articular abnormalities differs among psoriatic arthritis, Reiter's syndrome, and ankylosing spondylitis. In psoriatic arthritis, an asymmetric polyarticular disorder involving upper and lower extremities with predilection for interphalangeal joints of the hands and metatarsophalangeal and interphalangeal joints of the feet is observed. In Reiter's syndrome, asymmetric disease of the articulations of the lower extremity is most characteristic, whereas in ankylosing spondylitis, appendicular skeletal involvement is less prominent than axial skeletal involvement.

Spinal and sacroiliac joint alterations occur in psoriatic arthritis, Reiter's syndrome, and ankylosing spondylitis. In the former two disorders, symmetric or asymmetric abnormalities of the sacroiliac joints and large broad excrescences of the spine may be seen; however, the prevalence and severity of spinal changes, particularly in the cervical spine, are less in Reiter's syndrome than in psoriatic arthritis. In ankylosing spondylitis (as well as in the sacroiliitis and spondylitis of inflammatory bowel disease), bilateral, symmetric sacroiliac joint abnormalities are almost universal, and spinal changes typically consist of thin, linear, and symmetrically distributed outgrowths. In ankylosing spondylitis, apophyseal joint involvement and osteitis with squaring of vertebral bodies are more frequent than in either psoriatic arthritis or Reiter's syndrome.

Rheumatoid Arthritis

In some patients with psoriatic arthritis, the distribution of articular abnormalities in the appendicular skeleton is similar to that in rheumatoid arthritis, whereas in others, asymmetry and extensive distal interphalangeal articular alterations facilitate differentiation from rheumatoid arthritis. In the latter disease, osteoporosis, diffuse joint space narrowing, marginal erosions, and fibrous ankylosis are most characteristic. In psoriatic arthritis, severe marginal and central erosions, bony ankylosis, and the absence of osteoporosis are typical. Furthermore, in psoriatic arthritis, bony proliferation leads to fraying or irregularity of periarticular bony surfaces, a finding not evident in rheumatoid arthritis.

Rheumatoid involvement of the vertebral column is characterized by severe cervical spinal changes with minor or absent changes in the thoracic and lumbar segments. Paravertebral ossification is not observed. Furthermore, sacroiliac joint abnormalities are a minor feature of rheumatoid arthritis and, when present, consist of superficial erosions with little adjacent bony eburnation.

Other Disorders

A variety of patterns of vertebral ossification are observed in patients with quadriplegia or paraplegia.[186] Spinal abnormalities in these patients may simulate those of psoriatic spondylitis, ankylosing spondylitis, diffuse idiopathic skeletal hyperostosis, or spondylosis deformans (see Chapter 77).

A painful, diffusely swollen digit of the hand or foot, the

TABLE 29–3. Differential Diagnosis of Psoriatic Arthritis

	Psoriatic Arthritis	Reiter's Syndrome	Rheumatoid Arthritis
Types of involved articulations	Synovial joints	Synovial joints	Synovial joints*
	Symphyses	Symphyses	
	Entheses	Entheses	
Distribution of arthritis	Appendicular and axial skeleton	Appendicular and axial skeleton	Appendicular and axial skeleton
	Polyarticular or pauciarticular	Polyarticular or pauciarticular	Polyarticular
	Symmetric, asymmetric, or unilateral	Asymmetric	Symmetric
	Upper and lower extremities	Lower extremities	Upper and lower extremities
	Sacroiliac joints and entire spine	Sacroiliac joints and, less commonly, spine	Cervical spine
Nature of lesions†			
Osteoporosis	+	+	+ +
Soft tissue swelling	+ +	+ +	+ +
Joint space narrowing	+	+	+ +
Severe periarticular osteolysis	+ +	+	+
Intra-articular bony ankylosis	+ +	+ +‡	+
Bone proliferation and periostitis	+ +	+ +	− §
Tuftal resorption	+ +	−	−

*Symphyses and entheses are less commonly and less extensively involved in rheumatoid arthritis than in psoriatic arthritis or Reiter's syndrome.
†− = absent; + = occasionally present; + + = commonly present.
‡Less frequent than in psoriatic arthritis.
§Occasionally seen in male patients with rheumatoid arthritis and in those with both rheumatoid arthritis and diffuse idiopathic skeletal hyperostosis.

"cocktail sausage" digit, is seen not only in psoriasis but also in other seronegative spondyloarthropathies, gout, and infectious and traumatic disorders.[112] As these conditions also are associated with periosteal bone formation and osseous or articular destruction, accurate differentiation among them solely on the basis of radiographic abnormalities in the digit is difficult, and clinical information as well as additional radiographic data commonly is required.

Erosive arthritis of distal interphalangeal joints can be observed in many disease processes, including inflammatory (erosive) osteoarthritis, multicentric reticulohistiocytosis, gout, and scleroderma, and after thermal injuries.[115] In most of these disorders, obvious clinical findings allow differentiation from psoriatic arthritis. In addition, in inflammatory (erosive) osteoarthritis, osteophytes are evident, and the erosions may predominate in the central regions of the joint. In gout, asymmetric soft tissue masses, eccentric erosive changes, preservation of joint space, and osseous proliferation in the form of bony spicules (overhanging edges) are frequent. In scleroderma, soft tissue tuftal calcification is a helpful diagnostic clue. Differentiation of multicentric reticulohistiocytosis and psoriasis on the basis of interphalangeal joint abnormalities can be extremely difficult.

Martel and coworkers[100] have emphasized several features of hand and wrist involvement in psoriatic arthritis that allow its differentiation from other disorders, especially inflammatory (erosive) osteoarthritis. These include a tendency to involve articulations of a single ray (ray pattern) or to affect many joints of one hand with sparing of the other (polyarticular unilateral pattern), marginal osseous erosions resembling mouse ears, and the presence or absence of soft tissue swelling.

SUMMARY

Psoriatic arthritis produces distinctive abnormalities of synovial and cartilaginous joints as well as tendon and ligament attachments to the bone. Although the classic presentation is that of a polyarticular disorder with predilection for the distal interphalangeal joints of the fingers, a variety of additional clinical patterns may be observed, including a symmetric seronegative polyarthritis identical in distribution to rheumatoid arthritis; arthritis mutilans; oligoarthritis or monoarthritis; and sacroiliitis and spondylitis. In most instances, the diagnosis is not difficult and is based on the characteristic radiographic features, which include some degree of asymmetry, progressive intra-articular erosive changes with separation of the subchondral margins of adjacent bones, periosteal proliferation, intra-articular osseous fusion, and absence of osteoporosis in synovial articulations; bilateral symmetric or asymmetric sacroiliac joint abnormalities and paravertebral ossification; erosion and sclerosis in cartilaginous articulations; erosion and bone proliferation at sites of tendon and ligament attachment to bone; and osteolysis of terminal phalanges.

References

1. Alibert JL: Precis théorique et pratique sur les maladies de la peau. 2nd Ed. Paris, Caille et Ravier, 1822, p 21.
2. Bazin P: Leçons théoriques et cliniques sur les affections cutanées de nature arthritique et dartreu. Paris, Delahaye, 1860, p 154.
3. Bourdillon C: Psoriasis et arthropathies. Thèse, University of Paris, 1888.
4. Moll JMH, Wright V: Psoriatic arthritis. Semin Arthritis Rheum 3:55, 1973.
5. Wright V: Rheumatism and psoriasis: A re-evaluation. Am J Med 27:454, 1959.
6. Wright V: Psoriatic arthritis. In JT Scott (Ed): Copeman's Textbook of the Rheumatic Diseases. 5th Ed. Edinburgh, Churchill Livingstone, 1978, p 537.
7. Sigler JW: Psoriatic arthritis. In JL Hollander, DJ McCarty Jr (Eds): Arthritis and Allied Conditions. 8th Ed. Philadelphia, Lea & Febiger, 1972, p 724.
8. Baker H, Golding DN, Thompson M: Psoriasis and arthritis. Ann Intern Med 58:909, 1963.
9. Reed WB, Becker SW: Psoriasis and arthritis. Arch Dermatol 81:577, 1960.
10. Sterne EH Jr, Schneider B: Psoriatic arthritis. Ann Intern Med 38:512, 1953.
11. Hellgren L: Association between rheumatoid arthritis and psoriasis in total populations. Acta Rheumatol Scand 15:316, 1969.
12. Church R: The prospect of psoriasis. Br J Dermatol 70:139, 1958.
13. Tiedemann G: Symptomatologie und Aetiologie der Psoriasis arthropathica im Blickpunkt der Vererbung und Umweltbeeinflussung. Ztschr Menschl Vererb-u Konstitutionslehre 30:248, 1951.
14. Leczinsky CG: The incidence of arthropathy in a ten-year series of psoriasis cases. Acta Derm Venereol 28:483, 1948.
15. Gribble M de G: Rheumatoid arthritis and psoriasis. Ann Rheum Dis 14:198, 1955.
16. Wassmann K: Rheumatoid arthritis and psoriasis—statistical statement. Ann Rheum Dis 8:70, 1949.
17. Reed WB, Heiskell CL, Becker SW: Negative latex-fixation test in psoriasis arthritis. Arch Dermatol 83:653, 1961.
18. Bollet AJ, Turner RE: Psoriatic arthritis. Ann NY Acad Sci 73:1013, 1958.
19. Wright V: Psoriatic arthritis: A comparative study of rheumatoid arthritis, psoriasis, and arthritis associated with psoriasis. Arch Dermatol 80:27, 1959.
20. Bauer W, Bennett GA, Zeller JW: Pathology of joint lesions in patients with psoriasis and arthritis. Trans Assoc Am Physicians 56:349, 1941.
21. Meaney TF, Hays RA: Roentgen manifestations of psoriatic arthritis. Radiology 68:403, 1957.
22. Fawcitt J: Bone and joint changes associated with psoriasis. Br J Radiol 23:440, 1950.
23. Dawson MH, Tyson TL: Psoriasis arthropathica with observations on certain features common to psoriasis and rheumatoid arthritis. Trans Assoc Am Physicians 53:303, 1938.
24. Epstein E: Differential diagnosis of keratosis blennorrhagica and psoriatic arthropathica. Arch Dermatol 40:547, 1939.
25. Jeghers H, Robinson LJ: Arthropathia psoriatica—report of a case and discussion of the pathogenesis, diagnosis and treatment. JAMA 108:949, 1937.
26. Wright V: Psoriasis and arthritis. Ann Rheum Dis 15:348, 1956.
27. Moll JMH, Wright V: Family occurrence of psoriatic arthritis. Ann Rheum Dis 32:181, 1973.
28. Angevine CD, Pless, IB, Baum J, et al: Psoriatic arthritis in a child. Arthritis Rheum 16:278, 1973.
29. Beylot C, Bioulac P, Julien B, et al: Psoriasis pustuleux généralisé du nourrisson et de l'enfant. Ann Dermatol Syphiligr 100:121, 1973.
30. Lambert JR, Ansell BM, Stephenson E, et al: Psoriatic arthritis in childhood. Clin Rheum Dis 2:339, 1976.
31. Dixon AS: Rheumatoid polyarthritis associated with a negative sheep cell agglutination test. Ann Rheum Dis 17:252, 1958.
32. Wright V: Psoriasis and arthritis. Br J Dermatol 69:1, 1957.
33. McEwen C, Ditata D, Lingg C, et al: Ankylosing spondylitis and spondylitis accompanying ulcerative colitis, regional enteritis, psoriasis, and Reiter's disease. Arthritis Rheum 14:291, 1971.
34. Roberts MET, Wright V, Hill AGS, et al: Psoriatic arthritis: Follow-up study. Ann Rheum Dis 35:206, 1976.
35. Howell FA, Chamberlain MA, Perry RA, et al: IgG antiglobulin levels in patients with psoriatic arthropathy, ankylosing spondylitis and gout. Ann Rheum Dis 31:129, 1972.
36. Bremner JM, Lawrence JS: Population studies of serum uric acid. Proc R Soc Med 59:319, 1966.
37. Walton R, Block WD, Heyde J: A comparative study of uric acid values of whole blood in patients with psoriasis and other dermatoses. J Invest Dermatol 37:125, 1961.
38. Eisen AZ, Seegmiller JE: Uremic acid metabolism in psoriasis. J Clin Invest 40:1486, 1961.
39. Lodin A, Gentele H, Lagerholm B, et al: Psoriatic arthritis and elevated ESR. Acta Derm Venereol 37:459, 1957.
40. Zaias N: Psoriasis of the nail: A clinico-pathological study. Arch Dermatol 99:567, 1969.
41. Sherman MS: Psoriatic arthritis. Observations on the clinical, roentgenographic, and pathological changes. J Bone Joint Surg [Am] 34:831, 1952.
42. Avila R, Pugh D, Slocumb CH, et al: Psoriatic arthritis: A roentgenologic study. Radiology 75:691, 1960.
43. Wright V: Psoriatic arthritis. A comparative radiographic study of rheumatoid arthritis and arthritis associated with psoriasis. Ann Rheum Dis 20:123, 1961.
44. Peterson CC Jr, Silbiger ML: Reiter's syndrome and psoriatic arthritis. Their roentgen spectra and some interesting similarities. AJR 101:860, 1967.
45. Zellner E: Arthropathia psoriatica und Arthritis bei Psoriatikern. Wien Arch Inn Med 15:435, 1928.
46. Resnick D, Niwayama G: On the nature and significance of bony proliferation in "rheumatoid variant" disorders. AJR 129:275, 1977.
47. Forrester DM, Kirkpatrick J.: Periostitis and pseudoperiostitis. Radiology 118:597, 1976.
48. Resnick D, Broderick RW: Bony proliferation of terminal phalanges in psoriasis. The "ivory" phalanx. J Can Assoc Radiol 28:187, 1977.

49. Miller JL, Soltani K, Tourtellotte CD: Psoriatic acro-osteolysis without arthritis. A case study. J Bone Joint Surg [Am] 53:371, 1971.
50. Resnick D: Rheumatoid arthritis of the wrist. The compartmental approach. Med Radiol Photogr 52:50, 1976.
51. Resnick D: Radiology of the talocalcaneal articulations. Anatomic considerations and arthrography. Radiology 111:581, 1974.
52. Dixon AS, Lience E: Sacroiliac joint in adult rheumatoid arthritis and psoriatic arthropathy. Ann Rheum Dis 20:247, 1961.
53. Lassus A, Mustakallio KK, Laine V: Psoriatic arthropathy and rheumatoid arthritis: A roentgenological comparison. Acta Rheumatol Scand 10:62, 1964.
54. Jajic I: Radiological changes in the sacroiliac joints and spine of patients with psoriatic arthritis and psoriasis. Ann Rheum Dis 27:1, 1968.
55. Killebrew K, Gold RH, Sholkoff SD: Psoriatic spondylitis. Radiology 108:9, 1973.
56. Harvie JN, Lester RS, Little AH: Sacroiliitis in severe psoriasis. AJR 127:579, 1976.
57. Barraclough D, Russell AS, Percy JS: Psoriatic spondylitis: A clinical, radiological, and scintiscan survey. J Rheumatol 4:282, 1977.
58. Maldonado-Cocco JA, Porrini A, Garcia-Morteo O: Prevalence of sacroiliitis and ankylosing spondylitis in psoriasis patients. J Rheumatol 5:311, 1978.
59. Sváb V, Tesárek B: Arthropathien an den Sakroiliakalgelenken bei Psoriasis. Radiologe 18:194, 1978.
60. Moll JMH: Psoriatic spondylitis: Clinical, radiological and familial aspects. Proc R Soc Med 67:46, 1974.
61. Sundaram M, Patton JT: Paravertebral ossification in psoriasis and Reiter's disease. Br J Radiol 48:628, 1975.
62. Kaplan D, Plotz CM, Nathanson L, et al: Cervical spine in psoriasis and in psoriatic arthritis. Ann Rheum Dis 23:50, 1964.
63. Kormano M, Karvonen J, Lassus A: Psoriatic lesion of the sternal synchondrosis. Acta Radiol 16:463, 1975.
64. Kormano M.: A microradiographic and histologic study of the manubriosternal joint in rheumatoid arthritis. Acta Rheumatol Scand 16:47, 1970.
65. Solovay J, Gardner C: Involvement of the manubriosternal joint in Marie-Strumpell disease. AJR 65:749, 1951.
66. Resnick D: Temporomandibular joint involvement in ankylosing spondylitis. Comparison with rheumatoid arthritis and psoriasis. Radiology 112:587, 1974.
67. Lundberg M, Ericson S: Changes in the temporomandibular joint in psoriasis arthropathica. Acta Derm Venereol 47:354, 1967.
68. Blair GS: Psoriatic arthritis and the temporomandibular joint. J Dent 4:123, 1976.
69. Franks AST: Temporomandibular joint arthrosis associated with psoriasis. Oral Surg 19:301, 1965.
70. Weissberg D, Resnick D, Taylor A, et al: Rheumatoid arthritis and its variants: Analysis of scintiphotographic, radiographic, and clinical examinations. AJR 131:665, 1978.
71. Namey TC, Rosenthall L: Periarticular uptake of 99mtechnetium diphosphonate in psoriatics. Correlation with cutaneous activity. Arthritis Rheum 19:607, 1976.
72. Kaye M, Silverton S, Rosenthall L: Technetium-99m-pyrophosphate: Studies in vivo and in vitro. J Nucl Med 16:40, 1975.
73. Rosenthall L, Kaye M: Technetium-99m-pyrophosphate kinetics and imaging in metabolic bone disease. J Nucl Med 16:33, 1975.
74. Bauer W, Bennett GA, Zeller JW: The pathology of joint lesions in patients with psoriasis and arthritis. Trans Assoc Am Physicians 56:349, 1941.
75. Coste F: La polyarthrite psoriasique. Z Rheumaforsch 17:90, 1958.
76. Fassbender HG: Pathology of Rheumatic Diseases. Translated by G. Loewi. Heidelberg, Springer-Verlag, 1975, p 245.
77. Bywaters EGL, Dixon AS: Paravertebral ossification in psoriatic arthritis. Ann Rheum Dis 23:313, 1965.
78. Schacherl M, Schilling F: Röntgenbefunde an den Gliedmassengelenken bei Polyarthritis psoriatica. Z Rheumaforsch 26:442, 1967.
79. Fassbender HG: Pathomechanismen der Arthritis psoriatica. Z Rheumaforsch 33(Suppl 3):286, 1974.
80. Hoede K: Zur Frage der Erblichkeit der Psoriasis. Hautarzt 8:433, 1957.
81. Steinberg AG, Becker SW, Fitzpatrick TB, et al: A genetic and statistical study of psoriasis. Am J Hum Genet 3:267, 1951.
82. White S, Newcomer V, Mickey M, et al: Disturbances of HL-A antigen frequency in psoriasis. N Engl J Med 287:740, 1972.
83. Russell TJ, Schultes LM, Kuban D: Histocompatibility (HL-A) antigens associated with psoriasis. N Engl J Med 287:738, 1972.
84. Karvonen J, Lassus A, Sievers U, et al: HL-A antigens in psoriatic arthritis. Ann Clin Res 6:304, 1974.
85. Krulig L, Farber EM, Grumet C, et al: Histocompatibility (HL-A) antigens in psoriasis. Arch Dermatol 111:857, 1975.
86. Baker H, Golding DN, Thompson M: Atypical polyarthritis in psoriatic families. Br Med J 2:348, 1963.
87. Moll JMH: A family study of psoriatic arthritis. DM Thesis, University of Oxford, England, 1971.
88. Moll JMH, Wright V: Family occurrence of psoriatic arthritis. Ann Rheum Dis 32:181, 1973.
89. Metzger AL, Morris RI, Bluestone R, et al: HL-A W27 in psoriatic arthropathy. Arthritis Rheum 18:111, 1975.
90. Lambert JR, Wright V, Rajah SM, et al: Histocompatibility antigens in psoriatic arthritis. Ann Rheum Dis 35:526, 1976.
91. Brewerton DA, Walters D, Caffrey MJ, et al: HL-A 27 and the arthropathies associated with ulcerative colitis and psoriasis. Lancet 1:956, 1974.
92. Bluestone R, Morris RI, Metzger AL, et al: (HL-A) W27 and the spondylitis of chronic inflammatory bowel disease and psoriasis. Ann Rheum Dis 34(Suppl 1):31, 1975.
93. Eastmond CJ, Woodrow JC: The HLA system and the arthropathies associated with psoriasis. Ann Rheum Dis 36:112, 1977.
94. Buckley WR, Raleigh RL: Psoriasis with acro-osteolysis. N Engl J Med 261:539, 1959.
95. Williams KA, Scott JT: Influence of trauma on the development of chronic inflammatory polyarthritis. Ann Rheum Dis 26:532, 1967.
96. Ross JB: The psoriatic capillary: Its nature and value in the identification of the unaffected psoriatic patient. Br J Dermatol 76:511, 1964.
97. Weddell G, Cowan MA, Palmer E, et al: Psoriatic skin. Arch Dermatol 91:252, 1965.
98. Mustakallio KK, Lassus A: Staphylococcal alpha-antitoxin in psoriatic arthropathy. Br J Dermatol 76:544, 1964.
99. Latulippe L, Azouz EM: Arthrite psoriasique: Analyse de 69 cas et revue de la litérature. Can Med Assoc J 120:1515, 1979.
100. Martel W, Stuck KJ, Dworin AM, et al: Erosive osteoarthritis and psoriatic arthritis: A radiologic comparison in the hand, wrist, and foot. AJR 134:125, 1980.
101. Fassbender HG: Extra-articular processes in osteoarthropathia psoriatica. Arch Orthop Trauma Surg 95:37, 1979.
102. Loebl DH, Kirby S, Stephenson R, et al: Psoriatic arthritis. JAMA 242:2447, 1979.
103. Yood RA, Goldenberg DL: Sternoclavicular joint arthritis. Arthritis Rheum 23:232, 1980.
104. Ghozlan R, Guillon C, Grupper C, et al: Le rhumatisme psoriasique infantile. A propos d'un cas avec revue de la littérature. Rev Rhum Mal Osteoartic 47:187, 1980.
105. Arnett FC, Blas WB: HLA-Bw 38 and Bw 39 in psoriatic arthritis: Relationships and implications for peripheral and axial involvement (Abstr). Arthritis Rheum 23:649, 1950.
106. Ayerbe E, Echeverria F, DeOrbe GG, et al: Falange esclerosa como manifestación de artropatía psoriásica. Radiologia 21:459, 1979.
107. Benedek TG, Rodnan GP: A brief history of the rheumatic diseases. Bull Rheum Dis 32:59, 1982.
108. Shore A, Ansell BM: Juvenile psoriatic arthritis—an analysis of 60 cases. J Pediatr 100:529, 1982.
109. Vinje O, Moller P, Mellbye OJ: Laboratory findings in patients with psoriases, with special reference to immunological parameters, associated with arthropathy and sacro-iliitis. Scand J Rheumatol 9:97, 1980.
110. Green L, Meyers OL, Gordon W, et al: Arthritis in psoriasis. Ann Rheum Dis 40:366, 1981.
111. Yunus M: Huge knee effusion: A record? Arthritis Rheum 24:109, 1981.
112. Forrester DM: The "cocktail sausage" digit. Arthritis Rheum 26:664, 1983.
113. Fischer E: Subunguale verkalkungen. ROFU 137:580, 1982.
114. Belsky MR, Feldon P, Mullender LH, et al: Hand involvement in psoriatic arthritis. J Hand Surg 7:203, 1982.
115. Gold RH, Bassett LW, Theros EG: Radiologic comparison of erosive polyarthritides with prominent interphalangeal involvement. Skel Radiol 8:89, 1982.
116. Moller P, Vinge O: Arthropathy and sacro-iliitis in severe psoriasis. Scand J Rheumatol 9:113, 1980.
117. Heuck F: Ungewohnliche form der osteoarthropathie bei einer psoriasis—erythroderme. Radiologe 22:572, 1982.
118. Yeadon C, Dumas J-M, Karsh J: Lateral subluxation of the cervical spine in psoriatic arthritis: A proposed mechanism. Arthritis Rheum 26:109, 1983.
119. Fam AG, Cruicksank B: Subaxial cervical subluxation and cord compression in psoriatic spondylitis. Arthritis Rheum 25:101, 1982.
120. Rasmussen OC, Bakke M: Psoriatic arthritis of the temporomandibular joint. Oral Surg 53:351, 1982.
121. Stimson CW, Leban SG: Recurrent ankylosis of the temporomandibular joint in a patient with chronic psoriasis. J Oral Maxillofac Surg 40:678, 1982.
122. Hahn K, Thiers G, Eibner D, et al: Skelettszintigraphische befunde bei der psoriasis. Nuklearmedizin 19:178, 1980.
123. Soren A, Waugh ThR: The synovial changes in psoriatic arthritis. Rev Rhum Mal Osteoartic 50:390, 1983.
124. Fassbender HG: Pathological aspects and findings of Bechterew's syndrome and osteoarthropathia psoriatica. Scand J Rheumatol 32:50, 1980.
125. Gerber LH, Murray CL, Perlman SG, et al: Human lymphocyte antigens characterizing psoriatic arthritis and its subtypes. J Rheumatol 9:703, 1982.
126. Espinoza LR, Bombardier C, Gaylord SW, et al: Histocompatibility studies in psoriasis vulgaris: Family studies. J Rheumatol 7:445, 1980.
127. Hunter LY, Hensinger RN: Destructive arthritis associated with acne fulminans: A case report. Ann Rheum Dis 39:403, 1980.
128. Kelly A, Burns R: Acute febrile acne conglobata with polyarthralgia. Arch Dermatol 104:182, 1972.
129. Lane J, Leyden J, Spiegel R: Acne arthralgia. J Bone Joint Surg [Am] 45:672, 1974.
130. Windom R, Sanford J, Ziff M: Acne conglobata and arthritis. Arthritis Rheum 4:632, 1961.
131. McKendry RJR, Hamdy H: Acne, arthritis, and sacroiliitis. Can Med Assoc J 128:156, 1983.
132. Siegel D, Strosberg JM, Wiese F, et al: Acne fulminans with a lytic bone lesion responsive to dapsone. J Rheumatol 9:344, 1982.
133. Davis DE, Viozzi FJ, Miller OF, et al: The musculoskeletal manifestations of acne fulminans. J Rheumatol 8:317, 1981.

134. Engber PB, Marino CT: Acne fulminans with prolonged polyarthralgia. Int J Dermatol 19:567, 1980.

135. Cros D, Gamby T, Serratrice G: Acne rheumatism. Report of a case. J Rheumatol 8:336, 1981.

136. Rosner IA, Richter DE, Huettner TL, et al: Spondyloarthropathy associated with hidradenitis suppurativa and acne conglobata. Ann Intern Med 97:520, 1982.

137. Cowling P, Ebringer R, Cawdell D, et al: C-reactive protein, ESR, and klebsiella in ankylosing spondylitis. Ann Rheum Dis 39:45, 1980.

138. Van der Sluis I: Two cases of pyoderma (ecthyma) gangrenosum associated with the presence of abnormal serum protein (b₂ A-paraprotein). Dermatologica 132:409, 1966.

139. Palferman T, Colver G, Doyle D, et al: Pyoderma gangrenosum and seronegative erosive polyarthritis. Arthritis Rheum 26:813, 1983.

140. Wright V, Watkinson G: The arthritis of ulcerative colitis. Br Med J 3:670, 1965.

141. Holt P, Davies MG, Saunders KC, et al: Pyoderma gangrenosum: Clinical and laboratory findings in 15 patients with special reference to polyarthritis. Medicine 59:114, 1980.

142. Fallet GH, Arroyo J, Vischer TL: Sternocostoclavicular hyperostosis: Case report with a 31-year follow-up. Arthritis Rheum 26:784, 1983.

143. Sweet RD: Acute febrile neutrophilic dermatosis. Br J Dermatol 76:349, 1964.

144. Krauser RE, Schumacher HR: The arthritis of Sweet's syndrome. Arthritis Rheum 18:35, 1975.

145. Trentham DE, Masi AT, Bale GF: Arthritis with an inflammatory dermatosis resembling Sweet's syndrome. Am J Med 61:424, 1976.

146. Crow KD, Kerdel-Vegas F, Rook A: Acute febrile neutrophilic dermatosis. Dermatologica 139:123, 1969.

147. Frayha RA: Papular mucinosis, destructive arthropathy, median neuropathy, and sicca complex. Clin Rheumatol 2:277, 1983.

148. Ellsworth JE, Cassidy JT, Ragsdale CG, et al: Mucha-Habermann disease in children—the association with rheumatic diseases. J Rheumatol 9:319, 1982.

149. Scarpa R, Oriente P, Pucino A, et al: Psoriatic arthritis in psoriatic patients. Br J Rheumatol 23:246, 1984.

150. Weiner SR, Bassett LW, Reichman RP: Protective effect of poliomyelitis on psoriatic arthritis. Arthritis Rheum 28:703, 1985.

151. Dzioba RB, Benjamin J: Spontaneous atlantoaxial fusion in psoriatic arthritis. Spine 10:102, 1985.

152. Kenik J, Hurley J: Arthritis occurring with hidradenitis suppurativa. J Rheumatol 12:183, 1985.

153. Houben HHML, Lemmens JAM, Boerbooms AMT: Sacroiliitis and acne conglobata. Clin Rheumatol 4:86, 1985.

154. Gonzalex T, Gantes M, Bustabad S, et al: Acne fulminans associated with arthritis in monozygotic twins. J Rheumatol 12:389, 1985.

155. Däunt SON, Robertson JC: Spontaneous fusion of atlanto-axial dislocation in psoriatic spondylitis. Clin Rheumatol 4:465, 1985.

156. Juozevicius JL, Parhami N: Psoriatic arthritis rapidly progressing to arthritis mutilans. J Rheumatol 13:654, 1986.

157. Becker NJ, De Smet AA, Cathcart-Rake W, et al: Psoriatic arthritis affecting the manubriosternal joint. Arthritis Rheum 29:1029, 1986.

158. Gladman DD, Anhorn KAB, Schachter RK, et al: HLA antigens in psoriatic arthritis. J Rheumatol 13:586, 1986.

159. Griffiths HJ, Sundaram M: Pyoderma gangrenosum and erosive peripheral arthritis. J Can Assoc Radiol 37:125, 1986.

160. Edwards TC, Stapleton FB, Bond MJ, et al: Sweet's syndrome with multifocal sterile osteomyelitis. Am J Dis Child 140:817, 1986.

161. Dufour JP, Lachapelle JM, de Deuxchaisnes CN, et al: Cutaneous mucinosis associated with multiple frozen joints and bony heterotopic deposits around the hips. Clin Rheumatol 5:245, 1986.

162. Southwood TR, Petty RE, Malleson PN, et al: Psoriatic arthritis in children. Arthritis Rheum 32:1007, 1989.

163. Thomson GTD, Johnston JL, Baragar FD, et al: Psoriatic arthritis and myopathy. J Rheumatol 17:395, 1990.

164. Smith DL, Campbell SM, Wernick R: "Tumoral" enthesopathy: A juxtacortical osteosarcoma simulation. J Rheumatol 18:1631, 1991.

165. Myerson M, Solomon G, Shereff M: Posterior tibial tendon dysfunction: Its association with seronegative inflammatory disease. Foot Ankle 9:219, 1989.

166. Schurman JR III, Wilde AH: Total knee replacement for spontaneous osseous ankylosis. A report of three cases. J Bone Joint Surg [Am] 72:455, 1990.

167. Buskila D, Gladman D: Atlantoaxial subluxation in a patient with psoriatic arthritis. Arthritis Rheum 32:1338, 1989.

168. Lassoued S, Hamidou M, Fournie A, et al: Cervical spine involvement in psoriatic arthritis. J Rheumatol 16:251, 1989.

169. Blau RH, Kaufman RL: Erosive and subluxing cervical spine disease in patients with psoriatic arthritis. J Rheumatol 14:111, 1987.

170. Pease CT, Pozo JL: Atlantoaxial subluxation and spinal cord compression in psoriatic arthropathy. Ann Rheum Dis 46:717, 1987.

171. Jurik AG: Anterior chest wall involvement in seronegative arthritides. A study of the frequency of changes at radiography. Rheumatol Int 12:7, 1992.

172. Könönen M: Radiographic changes in the condyle of the temporomandibular joint in psoriatic arthritis. Acta Radiol 28:185, 1987.

173. Avrahami E, Garti A, Weiss-Peretz J, et al: Computerized tomographic findings in the temporomandibular joint in patients with psoriatic arthritis. J Rheumatol 13:1096, 1986.

174. Koorbusch GF, Zeitler DL, Fotos PG, et al: Psoriatic arthritis of the temporomandibular joint with ankylosis. Oral Surg 71:267, 1991.

175. Arnett FC: Seronegative spondyloarthropathies. Bull Rheum Dis 37:1, 1987.

176. Fournié B, Granel J, Heraud A, et al: HLA-B et rhumatisme psoriasique. Étude de 193 cas. Rev Rhum Mal Osteoartic 58:269, 1991.

177. McHugh NJ, Laurent MR, Treadwell BLJ, et al: Psoriatic arthritis: Clinical subgroups and histocompatibility antigens. Ann Rheum Dis 46:184, 1987.

178. Russell AS, Suarez-Almazor ME: Sacroiliitis in psoriasis: Relationship to peripheral arthritis and HLA-B27. J Rheumatol 17:804, 1990.

179. Goupille P, Soutif D, Valat J-P: Psoriatic arthritis precipitated by physical trauma. J Rheumatol 18:633, 1991.

180. Knitzer RH, Needleman BW: Musculoskeletal syndromes associated with acne. Semin Arthritis Rheum 20:247, 1991.

181. Falcini F, Trapani S, Taccetti G, et al: Musculoskeletal syndromes associated with acne. J Rheumatol 18:1770, 1991.

182. Moreland LW, Brick JE, Kovach RE, et al: Acute febrile neutrophilic dermatosis (Sweet syndrome): A review of the literature with emphasis on musculoskeletal manifestations. Semin Arthritis Rheum 17:143, 1988.

183. Duke RA, Barrett MR, Salazar JE, et al: Acro-osteolysis secondary to pityriasis rubra pilaris. AJR 149:1082, 1987.

184. Vidal JJ, Ruiz J, Sanjuro P, et al: Case report 106. Skel Radiol 4:251, 1979.

185. Rosner IA, Burg CG, Wisnieski JJ, et al: The clinical spectrum of the arthropathy associated with hidradenitis suppurativa and acne conglobata. J Rheumatol 20:684, 1993.

186. Park Y-H, Huang G-S, Taylor JAM, et al: Patterns of vertebral ossification and pelvic abnormalities in paralysis: A study of 200 patients. Radiology 188:561, 1993.

Reiter's Syndrome

Donald Resnick, M.D.

An association of arthritis and urethritis was first recognized over 300 years ago.[1] In 1818, Brodie[2] added a third component, conjunctivitis, completing the classic triad of Reiter's syndrome—urethritis, arthritis, and conjunctivitis. In 1916, Reiter[3] linked this same triad with an acute dysenteric illness in a cavalry officer serving on the Balkan front,[4] although he falsely attributed the abnormalities to syphilis. In the same year, Fiessinger and LeRoy[5] noted four patients with mild diarrhea associated with a conjunctivo-urethrosynovial syndrome. The first American description of the disease occurred in 1942.[6] In the last five decades, numerous accounts of Reiter's syndrome have appeared, firmly

establishing its place in the spectrum of rheumatic disorders.[7–11]

Any historical review of Reiter's syndrome is complicated by the undoubted inclusion of patients with gonococcal arthritis in some reports of clinical and radiologic manifestations of the disease.[99] In 1963, Wright defined characteristics of both Reiter's syndrome and the arthritis of gonococcal infection, establishing the spectrum of the two disorders.[12] Currently, it is recognized that many patients who apparently have Reiter's syndrome will not demonstrate the entire clinical triad. Until the cause of Reiter's syndrome is firmly established, however, it cannot be said with certainty that patients with an incomplete syndrome suffer from the same disorder as patients with a classic triad of urethritis, arthritis, and conjunctivitis.[1] This uncertainty has led to the introduction of preliminary criteria that can be used in the diagnosis of definite Reiter's syndrome.[104] Although radiographic findings may not be an essential part of these criteria, few investigators would dispute that radiographs are important in the evaluation of patients with this syndrome.

Reiter's syndrome is accompanied by typical radiographic features, which it shares with other seronegative spondyloarthropathies, such as psoriatic arthritis and ankylosing spondylitis. It is the distribution of articular abnormalities that allows a firm radiographic diagnosis in many patients with Reiter's syndrome. This chapter delineates the radiographic characteristics and distribution of the syndrome.

CLINICAL ABNORMALITIES

Age and Sex

Reiter's syndrome is a relatively uncommon articular disorder. It has greater prevalence in military personnel. It appears likely that the disease can be transmitted in association with either epidemic dysentery[13–21] or sexual intercourse.[22] Indeed, the majority of patients acknowledge themselves to be sexually promiscuous,[7] the disease may follow shortly the first sexual experience, and many patients reveal clinical manifestations of other venereal disorders,[7, 23, 24] facts that support a close relationship between Reiter's syndrome and sexual activity.

Most patients with Reiter's syndrome are between 15 and 35 years of age.[4] Occasional reports document its occurrence in children,[15, 25–29, 100, 118] even before the age of 3 years,[30] and in persons over the age of 50 years.[31] In childhood, boys are affected almost exclusively, and diarrhea may be particularly prominent.[28, 95] At any age, the disease is much more common in men than in women, the cited ratio of males to females ranging between 5 to 1 and 50 to 1.[4, 31] Reiter's syndrome in female patients is especially common after dysentery and may consist of arthritis, conjunctivitis, and cystitis[1, 94, 96]; involvement of the joints of the upper extremity appears to be more frequent in women.[101] The intestinal variety of the disease usually follows bacillary dysentery,[13] although the syndrome may occur after amebic dysentery,[32] shigellosis,[103] and additional gastrointestinal disorders.[21, 33, 97, 98, 102] Reiter's syndrome also may coexist with human immunodeficiency virus (HIV) infection (see Chapter 66), and infection with *Borrelia burgdorferi,* implicated in cases of Lyme disease, may be accompanied by Reiter's syndrome.[119, 120]

General Symptoms and Signs

Urethritis frequently is the initial manifestation of the disease. Although it may be asymptomatic, detected only by careful examination of the urine, symptoms and signs may develop shortly after a sexual encounter, with accompanying cystitis and prostatitis. Mucopurulent or mucoid urethral discharge, dysuria, urinary frequency, and local pain can be associated with an enlarged, soft, and tender prostate gland on physical examination. Bits of mucoid material, pyuria, and gross or microscopic hematuria can be apparent. In severe cases the patient may suffer scarring and shrinkage of the bladder, secondary urinary tract obstruction, and hydronephrosis.

Circinate balanitis has been noted in 20 to 80 per cent of patients with dysenteric and venereal forms of Reiter's syndrome.[34] This penile lesion may be the initial mucocutaneous manifestation of the disease.[11, 35] The appearance of this skin lesion varies from a localized superficial ulceration to scaly cutaneous patches.[36]

Early and transient conjunctivitis frequently accompanies the acute attack. Mild bilateral involvement is characteristic, leading to burning and itching of the eyes. Later and more severe ocular involvement may include episcleritis, keratitis, uveitis, iritis, retrobulbar neuritis, corneal ulceration, and intraocular hemorrhage.[37–40]

The characteristic skin lesion, which occurs in 5 to 30 per cent of patients, is termed keratoderma blenorrhagicum. It most commonly is noted on the soles of the feet and the palms of the hands, although a more widespread distribution may be encountered, including involvement of the extremities, the trunk, and the scalp. The skin lesions pass through various stages: macular, papular, vesicular, and pustular. They may begin as focal abnormalities and become confluent, producing a thick keratotic crust. Keratosis of the nails also may be observed, simulating the findings of psoriasis.[41, 42] With extensive involvement, the nail may separate from the nail bed. The skin abnormalities frequently are self-limited, persisting for several weeks and then peeling, leaving no residual scar.[1] They commonly are seen in patients who also reveal lesions on the genitalia and oral mucosa.

On the buccal mucosa and the tongue, superficial erythematous ulcerations may be evident in 5 to 10 per cent of patients. They also may affect the lips, the palate, the tonsils, and the uvula.[4] Reiter's syndrome may involve other organ systems, including the gastrointestinal tract (diarrhea, dysentery) and the cardiovascular (palpitations, valvular damage), neurologic (encephalitis, peripheral neuropathy), and pulmonary (pneumonia, fibrosis, pleurisy) systems.[43, 44]

Additional clinical findings in Reiter's syndrome include fever, weight loss, thrombophlebitis, amyloidosis, and rheumatoid arthritis.[1, 4, 45–49] Characteristic laboratory findings can include leukocytosis, anemia, and elevation of the erythrocyte sedimentation rate. The serum histocompatibility antigen HLA-B27 may be present in as many as 75 per cent of patients (see discussion later in this chapter).

Articular Symptoms and Signs

Characteristically, an asymmetric arthritis of the lower extremity becomes evident in Reiter's syndrome. Initially, the most commonly affected joints are the knee and the ankle,[104] followed in descending order of frequency by the metatarsophalangeal joints, the heel, the shoulder, the wrist, the hip, and the lumbar spine.[4] Monoarticular arthritis predominates in the early phase of the disease. Subsequently, more widespread articular changes occur, with predilection for, in descending order of frequency, the knee, the ankle, the shoulder, the wrist, and the metatarsophalangeal joints.[4]

The occurrence of heel pain and tenderness should be stressed as a common manifestation of Reiter's syndrome.[50, 51] Similarly, these clinical findings may be observed in ankylosing spondylitis and psoriatic arthritis, but they are uncommon in rheumatoid arthritis. The pain, which may be located posteriorly (in the region of the retrocalcaneal bursa or Achilles tendon) or inferiorly (at the site of attachment of the aponeurosis on the plantar surface of the calcaneus), can be the initial symptom of the disease, preceding even the ocular and urethral findings, and can persist for a period of years, even after remission of other clinical manifestations. Heel pain, which may vary from mild to incapacitating, can be associated with thickening of the Achilles tendon, skin erythema, and plantar swelling.

The arthritic attacks of Reiter's syndrome usually are self-limited and of short duration, although recurrences are frequent.[52] Residual disability and deformity occur in approximately 5 per cent of patients. These chronic changes are most frequent in the metatarsophalangeal joints, the heel, the lumbar spine, the knee, and the ankle.[4]

On joint aspiration, inflammatory synovial fluid is recovered.[36, 53] Occasionally the degree of polymorphonuclear leukocytosis within the fluid is so great as to resemble a purulent arthritis.[4] Some observers have noted large macrophages engulfing one or more of the polymorphonuclear leukocytes,[91] although this appears to be a nonspecific finding.[92] The characteristics of fluid removed from inflamed bursae are similar to those of the joint effusion.[105]

RADIOGRAPHIC ABNORMALITIES

The radiographic features of Reiter's syndrome have received considerable emphasis in the literature[54-59] (Table 30–1).

Frequency of Radiographic Abnormalities

Some observers have estimated that 60 to 80 per cent of patients with Reiter's syndrome will develop radiographic alterations,[57, 58] although this rate will vary according to the criteria used to diagnose the disease, the chronicity of the disorder, and the method and extent of radiographic examination.

In the early phases of the disease, radiographs may be entirely normal. Acute attacks of arthritis may be accompanied by soft tissue swelling and osteoporosis, but these findings then can disappear completely, without residual abnormalities. With repeated episodes of arthritis, however, permanent radiographic abnormalities are very common.

Distribution of Radiographic Abnormalities

Synovial joints, symphyses, and entheses are affected. Typically, an asymmetric distribution with predilection for articulations of the lower extremity is seen (Fig. 30–1). The most characteristic sites of abnormality are the small articulations of the foot, the calcaneus, the ankle, and the knee. Joint alterations in the upper extremity are less frequent, and abnormalities of the hip are uncommon. In the axial skeleton, the sacroiliac joints, the spine, the symphysis pubis, and the manubriosternal articulation are frequent target areas.

General Radiographic Abnormalities

The general radiographic characteristics of articular involvement in Reiter's syndrome are similar to those in the other seronegative spondyloarthropathies (ankylosing spondylitis and psoriatic arthritis) and differ from the findings of rheumatoid arthritis (Fig. 30–2).

Soft Tissue Swelling. Soft tissue prominence is related to intra-articular effusion, periarticular edema, and inflammation of bursal and tendinous structures. This finding, which is not specific, is frequent in the interphalangeal joints of the toes and the fingers and may result in sausage-like swelling of an entire digit.[104] Large effusions may be encountered in the knee and the ankle.

Osteoporosis. Regional or periarticular osteoporosis accompanies acute episodes of arthritis. With recurrent or prolonged bouts of articular disease, osteoporosis may de-

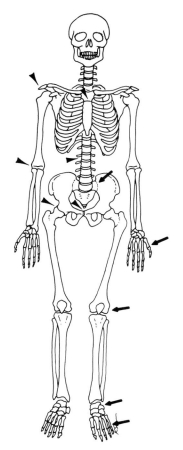

FIGURE 30–1. Reiter's syndrome: Distribution of articular abnormalities. The most characteristic sites of involvement are the small articulations of the foot, calcaneus, ankle, knee, hand, and sacroiliac joint (arrows). Less commonly, the shoulder, elbow, hip, spine, symphysis pubis, and manubriosternal joint are affected (arrowheads).

TABLE 30–1. Characteristics of Arthritis in Reiter's Syndrome

Involvement of synovial joints, symphyses, and entheses
Asymmetric arthritis of the lower extremities
Predilection for the small articulations of the foot, the calcaneus, the ankle, the knee, and the sacroiliac joint
Bony erosion with adjacent proliferation
Paravertebral ossification

crease in extent and severity, and it is not uncommon to detect severe cartilaginous and osseous lesions without adjacent osteoporosis.

Joint Space Narrowing. Loss of the interosseous space is more frequent in the small articulations of the foot, hand, and wrist than in the knee and the ankle. This finding may be observed in the acute or chronic phases of the disease. Diffuse or symmetric loss of articular space is more characteristic than is asymmetric joint space diminution.

Bone Erosion. Erosion of articular surfaces may be noted in both the appendicular and the axial skeleton. The most frequent sites of osseous erosion are the small joints of the foot, hand, and wrist, the knee, and the sacroiliac joint. Erosions initially appear at the joint margins and later may progress to involve the subchondral bone in the central portion of the articulation. Associated loss of interosseous space is common but not invariable. Superficial resorption of the osseous surface also may occur beneath inflamed bursae and tendon sheaths, particularly in the forefoot, the posterior surface of the calcaneus, and the wrist. The osseous erosions are not discrete or distinct in outline. Rather, adjacent bony proliferation produces an irregular osseous surface (see later discussion).

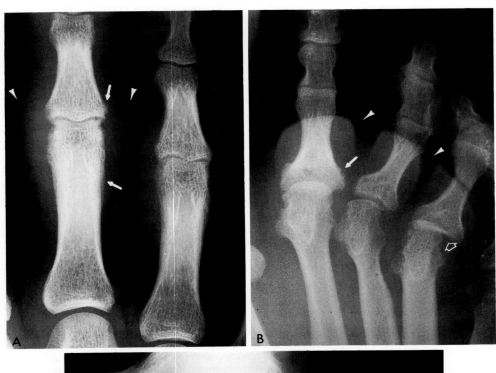

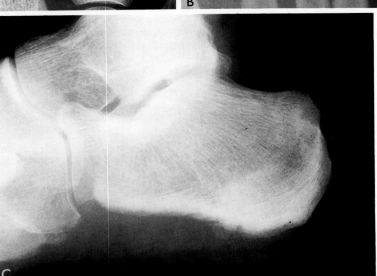

FIGURE 30–2. General radiographic abnormalities. In three different patients, the general radiographic characteristics of Reiter's syndrome are indicated. Note the absence of osteoporosis and the presence of soft tissue swelling (arrowheads), periostitis and "whiskering" (solid arrows) **(A, B),** osseous erosions, subluxation (open arrow) **(B),** and bone production along the plantar aspect of the calcaneus **(C).**

Bone Proliferation. Bone proliferation is particularly characteristic of all three seronegative spondyloarthropathies—Reiter's syndrome, ankylosing spondylitis, and psoriasis—and is the most helpful radiographic feature in distinguishing these conditions from rheumatoid arthritis.[60] Bone proliferation may take several forms. Linear or fluffy periosteal bone proliferation is not uncommon in Reiter's syndrome, especially in the metacarpal, metatarsal, and phalangeal shafts, the malleolar region, and the knee. The adjacent articulations may be affected, but periostitis can occur without articular abnormality. Its appearance is not unlike that of hypertrophic osteoarthropathy.

A second variety of bone proliferation occurs at sites of tendon and ligament attachment to bone. These sites include the plantar aspect of the calcaneus, the ischial tuberosity, the trochanters, and the apposing portions of sacrum and ilium about the true sacroiliac articulation. The osseous surfaces frequently appear poorly defined or frayed.

Intra-articular bone production occurs about sites of osseous erosion. The eroded bony surfaces appear irregular, fuzzy, or blurred in outline, and the articular bone may be enlarged. Subchondral sclerosis and eburnation and adjacent periostitis are associated radiographic findings. Intra-articular bony ankylosis has been recorded in the small joints of the hands and feet in patients with Reiter's syndrome, but this complication is far less frequent in this disease than in ankylosing spondylitis and psoriatic arthritis.[56, 57] Osseous fusion is not uncommon in the sacroiliac joint and it is somewhat less frequent in the apophyseal joints in Reiter's syndrome.

Tendinous Calcification and Ossification. Tendinous calcification and ossification have been observed in patients with Reiter's syndrome.[56, 57] These manifestations are frequent about the knee, at which site the findings can resemble Pellegrini-Stieda syndrome (posttraumatic calcification of the medial collateral ligament). In some instances, the abnormalities probably are related to bony proliferation at the site of attachment of the tendon to the underlying bone rather than to true tendinous calcification or ossification. More widespread calcification involving the collateral ligaments of metacarpophalangeal and proximal interphalangeal joints has been noted in a patient with both Reiter's syndrome and amyloidosis.[106]

Specific Sites of Abnormality

Forefoot (Fig. 30–3). Radiographs of the feet frequently reveal asymmetric involvement of the metatarsophalangeal and interphalangeal joints, the reported prevalence of the findings varying from 40 to 55 per cent.[57, 58] Any of the joints may be affected, although the metatarsophalangeal articulations and the interphalangeal joint of the great toe are especially vulnerable. In fact, selective and severe involvement of the interphalangeal joint of the great toe suggests the diagnosis of Reiter's syndrome or psoriasis, although gout and rheumatoid arthritis occasionally may produce similar abnormalities.[61] At any location in the foot, osteoporosis, joint space loss, and marginal erosions with adjacent proliferation can be observed, as can periostitis of neighboring diaphyses of metatarsals and phalanges. The sesamoid bones can demonstrate significant erosion and proliferation, creating enlarged and irregular osseous outlines.[62]

Subluxation and deformity of the metatarsophalangeal articulations may be evident, an appearance that has been termed Launois's deformity.[35] In these cases, the degree of articular mutilation (arthritis mutilans) may resemble that in psoriatic or rheumatoid arthritis.

Calcaneus (Figs. 30–4 and 30–5). Calcaneal alterations are characteristic of Reiter's syndrome (25 to 50 per cent). They may represent the sole or predominant radiographic manifestation of the disease and commonly are associated with significant symptoms and signs. Both the posterior and the plantar aspects of the bone are affected.[50, 107] Bilateral changes are frequent. Retrocalcaneal bursitis with fluid accumulation creates a radiodense shadow that, on lateral radiographs, obliterates the normal lucent area that exists between the top of the calcaneus and the adjacent Achilles tendon and projects into the preachilles fat pad.[105] Subsequently, poorly defined calcaneal erosions appear on the posterior and posterosuperior aspects of the bone.[63] The Achilles tendon frequently is thickened, and the adjacent soft tissues appear prominent. Posterior calcaneal enthesophytes at the site of attachment of the Achilles tendon to the calcaneus are rare in Reiter's syndrome compared with their frequency in rheumatoid arthritis, psoriatic arthritis, and ankylosing spondylitis, perhaps reflecting the younger ages of the patients.

On the plantar surface of the bone, osseous erosion, hyperostosis, and poorly defined enthesophytes may develop. These latter excrescences, which occur at sites of ligamentous and aponeurotic attachment to the calcaneus, are similar to those occurring in psoriatic arthritis and ankylosing spondylitis. Initially these enthesophytes, which represent an exaggerated reparative response of the eroded bone, appear irregular in outline. They may become better defined on follow-up radiographs, simulating the outgrowths in normal patients and in those with rheumatoid arthritis.

Other Tarsal Areas (Fig. 30–6). In approximately 25 per cent of patients, erosive and proliferative changes are evident in other tarsal areas. The osseous contours, particularly on the dorsal and medial aspects of the midfoot, commonly are irregular or fluffy, again reflecting exuberant new bone formation in response to erosion.

Ankle (Fig. 30–7). Radiographic abnormalities about one or both ankles can be recognized in 30 to 50 per cent of patients.[54, 57, 58] Changes include soft tissue swelling, linear or fluffy periostitis of the distal tibial and fibular diaphyses and metaphyses, articular space loss, and, less frequently, marginal erosions.

Knee (Fig. 30–8). Radiographic abnormalities of the knee are apparent in 25 to 40 per cent of patients. The most common abnormality is a joint effusion, although osteoporosis, periostitis of the distal femur or proximal tibia, and erosive changes can be detected. Periarticular tendinous calcification has been described.[57]

Hand and Wrist (Figs. 30–9 and 30–10). Severe and widespread radiographic abnormalities of the upper extremity are distinctly unusual in Reiter's syndrome. In 10 to 30 per cent of patients, however, one or more fingers of one or both hands reveal significant radiographic changes. Proximal interphalangeal joint abnormalities are more frequent than metacarpophalangeal or distal interphalangeal joint alterations, although the metacarpophalangeal and interphalangeal joints of the thumb may be affected. Fusiform or sausage-like soft tissue swelling, regional or periarticular

Text continued on page 1112

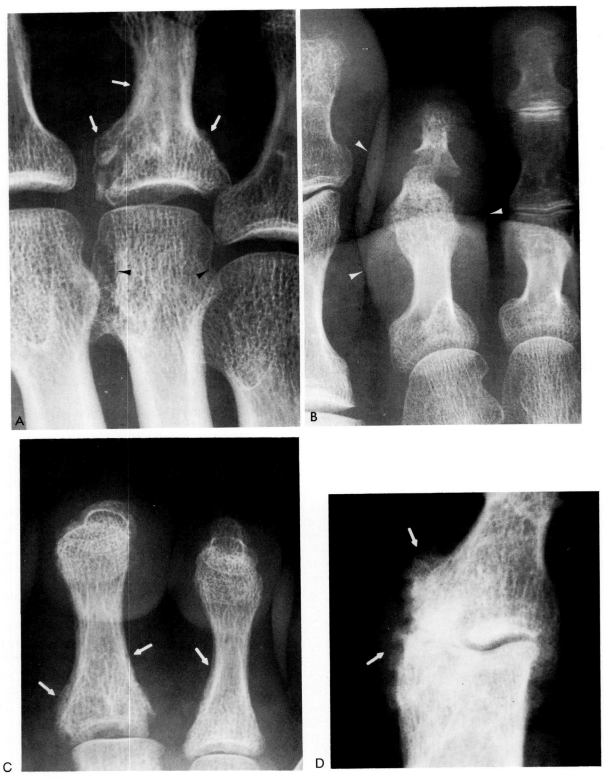

FIGURE 30–3. Abnormalities of the forefoot.

  A A magnification radiograph of the third metatarsophalangeal joint outlines erosions of the metatarsal head (arrowheads) and adjacent bony proliferation (arrows). The joint space is not narrowed.

  B A radiograph of the forefoot reveals soft tissue swelling of the second digit (arrowheads), destruction of the distal interphalangeal joint, and intra-articular bony ankylosis of the proximal interphalangeal joint. Note the absence of osteoporosis.

  C In addition to soft tissue swelling, observe periostitis of the phalangeal shafts and irregular periarticular osseous surfaces (arrows). There is no significant osteoporosis. Flexion of the digit has obscured the interphalangeal articulations.

  D An example is shown of the type of abnormality that can be encountered about the interphalangeal joint of the great toe. Note erosions and bony proliferation (arrows).

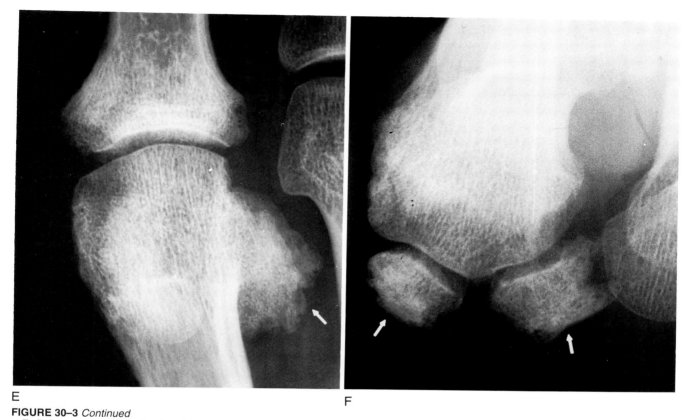

E

F

FIGURE 30–3 *Continued*
E, F Sesamoid participation is evidenced by considerable bony proliferation, leading to a poorly defined osseous outline (arrows). The adjacent articulation also is abnormal.

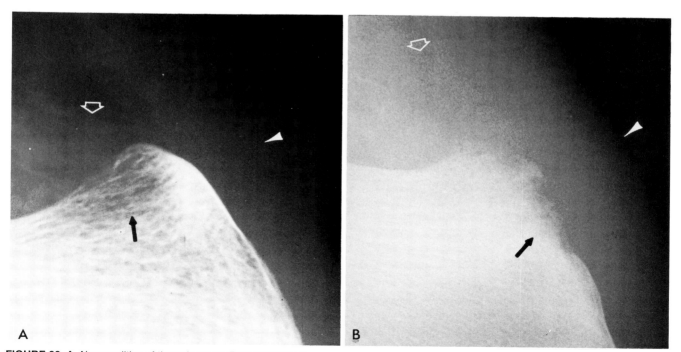

A

B

FIGURE 30–4. Abnormalities of the calcaneus: Posterior aspect.
A Note soft tissue swelling about the Achilles tendon (arrowhead), an effusion in the retrocalcaneal bursa (open arrow), and subjacent erosion of the top of the calcaneus (solid arrow).
B In a different patient, soft tissue swelling (arrowhead), retrocalcaneal bursitis (open arrow), and irregular osseous erosion and proliferation (solid arrow) are apparent.

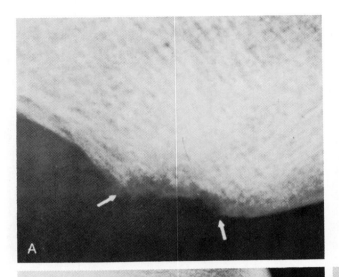

FIGURE 30–5. Abnormalities of the calcaneus: Plantar aspect.

A A magnification radiograph delineates erosion of the inferior surface of the calcaneus (between arrows).

B, C Radiographs of the plantar aspect of the calcaneus obtained 2 years apart reveal striking progression of osseous proliferation (arrows). Note the poorly defined nature of the developing outgrowth.

D, E Radiographs of the plantar aspect of the calcaneus obtained 1 year apart demonstrate healing of a poorly defined plantar enthesophyte (arrow). Observe the well-defined outgrowth on the later film (arrowhead).

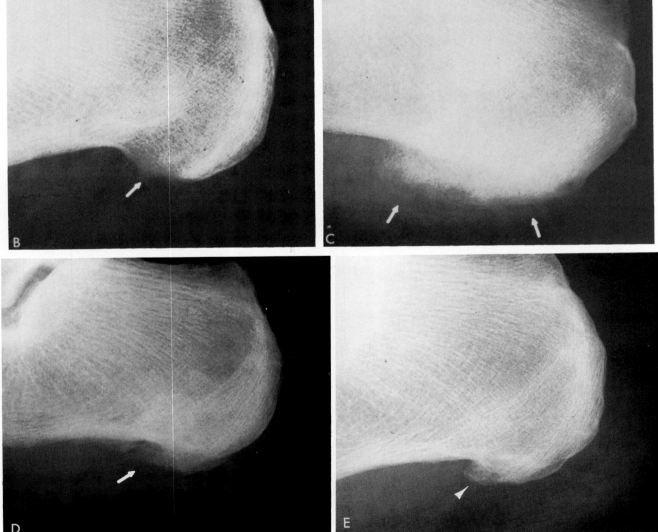

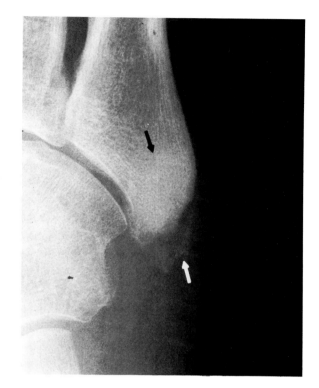

FIGURE 30–6. Abnormalities of other tarsal areas. Hyperostosis and bone fragmentation are evident at the base of the fifth metatarsal (arrows). The lateral tarsometatarsal joint appears normal. The patient denied a history of trauma to this area.

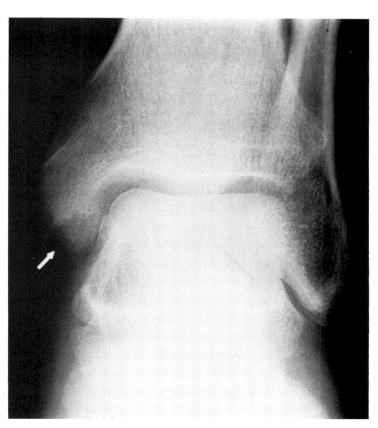

FIGURE 30–7. Abnormalities of the ankle. Irregular bony proliferation of the medial malleolus (arrow) is associated with soft tissue swelling.

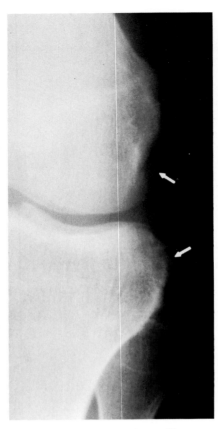

FIGURE 30–8. Abnormalities of the knee. Observe erosions and bony reaction on the lateral aspect of the distal end of the femur and proximal portion of the tibia (arrows).

osteoporosis, and joint space narrowing can be evident. The erosive changes are accompanied by fluffy new bone formation. Such proliferation also can involve adjacent sesamoids, producing an enlarged bony contour.[64]

Abnormalities also may be apparent in one or both wrists. Involvement usually is asymmetric, although any compartment can be affected. Rarely, severe bone destruction and inflammation of adjacent tendons and tendon sheaths are encountered.[108]

Manubriosternal Joint and Symphysis Pubis. Osseous erosion and adjacent bony proliferation at the manubriosternal articulation are not rare in Reiter's disease.[65] These changes also are seen in the other seronegative spondyloarthropathies (ankylosing spondylitis and psoriatic arthritis) and less commonly in rheumatoid arthritis. They may be associated with local pain and tenderness.

Similar abnormalities occur at the symphysis pubis in Reiter's syndrome and the other spondyloarthropathies. At this location, apposing margins of the pubic bones may appear eroded and sclerotic. The radiographic findings are identical to those of osteitis pubis, the latter condition being encountered in multiparous women, in athletes, and in men who have undergone genitourinary surgical procedures.

Sacroiliac Joint (Fig. 30–11). Sacroiliitis is common in Reiter's syndrome. The frequency of this finding increases dramatically with disease chronicity. Initially, abnormalities may be detected in 5 to 10 per cent of patients, whereas after several years, the occurrence of sacroiliac joint alterations may reach 40 to 60 per cent.[54, 57, 59] This prevalence can be even more startling if radiographic examination is supplemented with radionuclide investigation, and in these circumstances it may reach 75 per cent of patients.[66]

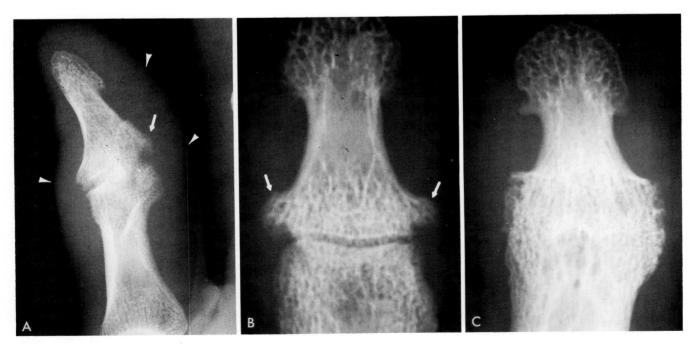

FIGURE 30–9. Abnormalities of the hand.
A Soft tissue swelling (arrowheads), erosion, and bony proliferation (arrow) are the radiographic findings.
B Note joint space narrowing and irregular excrescences or "whiskers" (arrows) at the margins of the distal interphalangeal joint.
C In another patient, intra-articular bony ankylosis is evident.

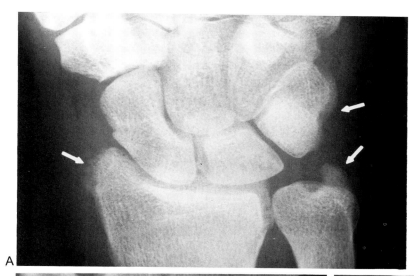

FIGURE 30–10. Abnormalities of the wrist.

A The major radiographic abnormality consists of bony proliferation (arrows) about several compartments of the wrist. Soft tissue swelling also is evident.

B, C Radiographs obtained 3 years apart in a different patient with Reiter's syndrome reveal marked progression of the disease. Findings in **C** include soft tissue swelling, bone erosions, bone proliferation (particularly in the radial styloid process), osteoporosis, and ulnar translocation at the radiocarpal joint.

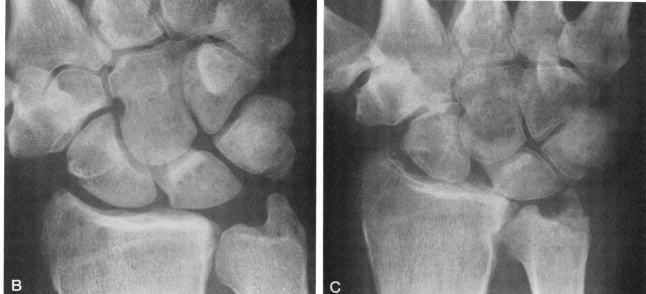

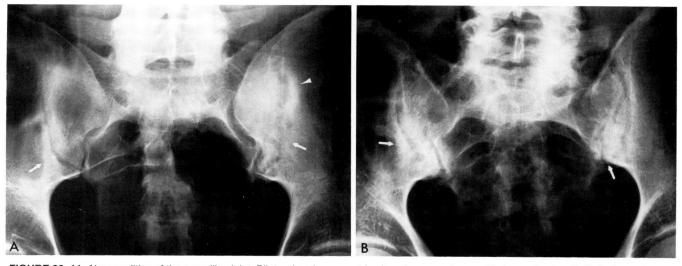

FIGURE 30–11. Abnormalities of the sacroiliac joint. Bilateral and asymmetric alterations are observed in two patients with Reiter's syndrome. Erosions and reactive eburnation predominate in the ilium (arrows). Also, hyperostosis can be seen at the superior aspect of the joint in one of the patients (arrowhead).

A common misconception is that Reiter's syndrome more typically is associated with unilateral sacroiliac joint changes than with bilateral changes. This is not true. In the author's experience and that of others, bilateral symmetric or asymmetric changes are most typical. As opposed to the situation in classic ankylosing spondylitis, however, in which bilateral and symmetric changes are the rule, asymmetric and, less commonly, unilateral sacroiliac joint abnormalities in Reiter's syndrome do occur, particularly early in the disease process.[67] Thus, faced with a radiograph that demonstrates asymmetric alterations of these joints, the radiologist should suggest the diagnosis of Reiter's syndrome (or psoriatic arthritis) rather than classic ankylosing spondylitis.

Osseous erosion on the iliac surface predominates over that on the sacral surface. Adjacent sclerosis varies from mild to severe. Early joint space widening may later be replaced by narrowing of the space between sacrum and ilium. Although intra-articular osseous fusion eventually may appear, this finding is less frequent in Reiter's syndrome (and psoriatic arthritis) than in classic ankylosing spondylitis and the sacroiliitis of inflammatory bowel disease. A prominent finding in both Reiter's syndrome and psoriasis may be blurring and eburnation of apposing sacral and iliac surfaces above the true joint in the region of the interosseous ligament.[93]

Spine (Fig. 30–12). Although abnormalities of the spine occur in Reiter's syndrome, their frequency and extent are less than in classic ankylosing spondylitis and psoriatic arthritis. When present, the changes may resemble those of ankylosing spondylitis, although specific radiographic features frequently allow accurate differentiation of the two conditions.

An early finding in Reiter's syndrome (and psoriatic arthritis) is the appearance of paravertebral ossification about the lower three thoracic and upper three lumbar vertebrae.[68] Sundaram and Patton[69] noted this abnormality in 5 of 35 radiographed patients (14 per cent) with Reiter's syndrome and emphasized that this change could be the only manifestation of the disease, antedating the more widely recognized sacroiliac and peripheral articular alterations. On frontal radiographs, elongated vertical osseous bridges extend across the intervertebral disc but are separated by a clear space from the lateral margins of both the disc and the vertebral body. The outgrowths may be either well defined and linear or thick and fluffy. Their variable appearance has led to a variety of designations, including teardrop, comma-shaped, or bagpipe excrescences and nonmarginal syndesmophytes.[70, 71] Their course also is variable, although many of the ossifications eventually fuse with the underlying intervertebral disc and vertebral body, simulating the appearance of bulky osteophytes (spondylosis deformans). Involvement of large segments of the thoracic and lumbar spine as well as the cervical spine eventually may be noted. Although the pathologic process related to these paravertebral ossifications has not been clearly delineated, they may represent the result of inflammatory changes in the paravertebral connective tissue or of ligamentous and tendinous traction that stimulates periosteal bone formation.[72, 73]

The importance of recognizing paravertebral ossification is twofold: The finding may be an initial manifestation of the disease; and the abnormality is diagnostic of Reiter's syndrome or psoriatic arthritis rather than of classic ankylosing spondylitis or the spondylitis associated with inflammatory bowel disease. In this latter regard, the asymmetric distribution (right and left sides), the broader or bulkier

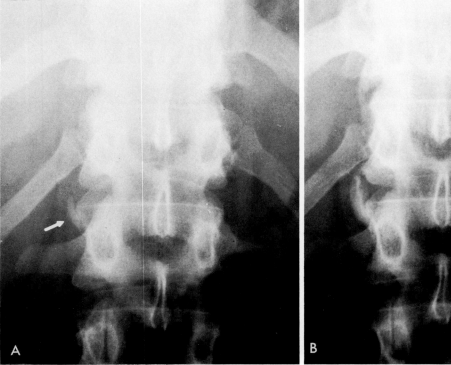
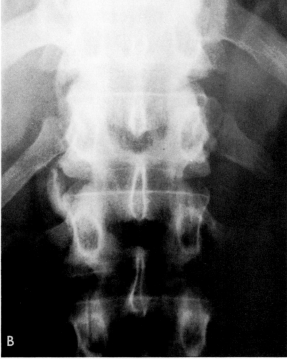

FIGURE 30–12. Abnormalities of the spine. In radiographs of the thoracolumbar spine obtained approximately 1 year apart, progressive paravertebral ossification can be delineated (arrow). Note the asymmetric nature and lateral location of the outgrowths.

nature of the radiodense areas, and their relatively distant position from the spine are characteristic of paravertebral ossification. It must be stressed, however, that some patients with Reiter's syndrome and psoriatic arthritis develop typical syndesmophytes of the spine, which may progress to a bamboo spine appearance. In these patients, accurate differentiation among the seronegative spondyloarthropathies cannot be accomplished. Furthermore, apophyseal joint erosion, sclerosis, and osseous fusion may be apparent in Reiter's syndrome,[74] although the frequency of these findings is less than in classic ankylosing spondylitis. Erosion or "osteitis" along the anterior corners of vertebral bodies also is uncommon in Reiter's syndrome.

Cervical spine abnormalities are not frequent in Reiter's syndrome. Occasionally, paravertebral ossification and irregularity at discovertebral junctions and apophyseal joints can be seen.[115] Atlantoaxial subluxation and odontoid erosion, although rare, have been observed in patients with Reiter's syndrome.[75, 121, 122] Such subluxation may be a presenting manifestation of the disease or occur early in its course. Craniocervical involvement in Reiter's syndrome also can produce nonreducible head tilt identical to that occurring in rheumatoid arthritis.[123]

Other Sites. Infrequently, Reiter's syndrome leads to radiographic abnormalities in the temporomandibular joint.[109] Reported findings have included bone erosion and sclerosis, resembling the changes in ankylosing spondylitis and rheumatoid arthritis.

RADIONUCLIDE ABNORMALITIES

Scintigraphy with bone-seeking radiopharmaceutical agents may allow early diagnosis of Reiter's syndrome and provide a more accurate appraisal of the extent of disease.[76, 77] The distribution of abnormal radionuclide accumulation parallels that obtained by radiographic examination, although such accumulation may occur prior to radiographic (and clinical) alterations. Asymmetric involvement of the articulations of the lower extremity again is revealed (Fig. 30–13). Increasing radioactivity related to the plantar and posterior aspects of the calcaneus may be striking.[78] As prominent uptake of bone-seeking radiopharmaceutical agents about the sacroiliac joints is a normal finding, interpretation of scintigraphic abnormalities in this location may be difficult. Application of quantitative digital analysis and sacroiliac-to-sacrum ratios can allow differentiation between normal and abnormal activity.[66, 79] Asymmetric accumulation about the sacroiliac joints also facilitates the diagnosis of sacroiliitis (Fig. 30–14).

PATHOLOGIC ABNORMALITIES

Synovial biopsy findings in the initial phase of the disease indicate edema, vascular congestion, moderate cellular infiltration with neutrophils, lymphocytes, and occasional plasma cells, and synoviocytic and fibroblastic proliferation.[4, 124] Subsequent changes include perivenular infiltration with lymphocytes and plasma cells and formation of lymphocytic nodules that are indistinguishable from those of rheumatoid arthritis.[36] Extensive pannus formation is unusual.

Bony proliferation results from subchondral osseous hyperplasia and periosteal new bone formation.[60]

ETIOLOGY AND PATHOGENESIS

Of all of the rheumatic diseases, Reiter's syndrome is most suspect for an infectious cause.[80, 81] The syndrome frequently follows an infection of the bowel or lower genitourinary tract, and it seems likely that these sites are the portals of entry for the causative agent. It has been suggested that the abnormalities of the vertebral column may be related to organisms extending directly to the sacroiliac joints and spine via the prostatic venous plexus[82] or the venous plexus of Batson.[83] A similar mechanism may explain the occurrence of sacroiliac joint abnormalities in ankylosing spondylitis and following paraplegia.[84] Considerable difficulty has been encountered in attempting to isolate a specific infective agent in Reiter's syndrome, however.[4, 85] Implicated species have included pleuropneumonia-like organisms (PPLO),[86] the Bedsonia group of organisms,[4] Chlamydia,[124] and viruses,[80] although to date no single agent has been definitely incriminated in this disease.[116]

An alternative explanation for the association of Reiter's syndrome and bowel or genitourinary infection is that Reiter's syndrome is related not to purulent arthritis but rather to a reaction of a joint (or other target site) to infection elsewhere in the body. The concept of reactive arthritis, which is discussed in Chapters 31 and 64, is not without example. Rheumatic fever, initiated by a beta-hemolytic streptococcal infection in the throat, is a classic example of reactive arthritis; other examples include the arthritis associated with Shigella, Salmonella, Yersinia, Campylobacter, gonococcal, and Chlamydia infections.[110] Such reactive arthritis generally is not associated with a full Reiter's-like syndrome. It is not clear, therefore, if Reiter's syndrome and reactive arthritis are the same disease. It seems reasonable to suggest that both are related to the release of mediators—immunologic or otherwise—into the circulation at the site of the primary infection.[111] The term reactive arthritis could be applied to the entire spectrum of infection-triggered arthritis, and the term Reiter's syndrome could be given to cases in which the classic clinical triad is evident.[111]

As the clinical expression of disease may be influenced to a great degree by genetic factors, the immunologic nature of Reiter's syndrome has been stressed.[110, 114] The increased frequency of the histocompatibility antigen HLA-B27 in this disorder is well recognized,[87–89, 113, 117, 125] a frequency that may reach 96 per cent.[90] Possession of this antigen may predispose patients to Reiter's syndrome after exposure to an infectious agent. Furthermore, testing for the presence of HLA-B27 in male patients with urethritis and arthritis may help distinguish between those with Reiter's syndrome and those with acute gonococcal arthritis.[90, 112] It may be best to divide reactive arthritis into two categories, those cases that are associated with HLA-B27 and those that are not.[111] Further division of the former category into diseases that are sexually acquired, enterocolitic, and of unknown origin then could be accomplished.

DIFFERENTIAL DIAGNOSIS

Other Seronegative Spondyloarthropathies

Although its general features resemble those of the other two seronegative spondyloarthropathies (ankylosing spon-

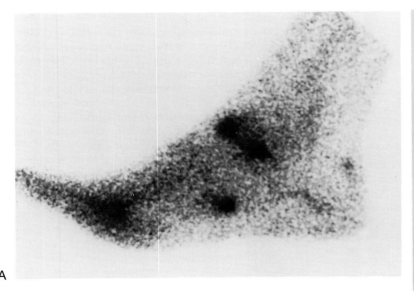
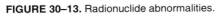
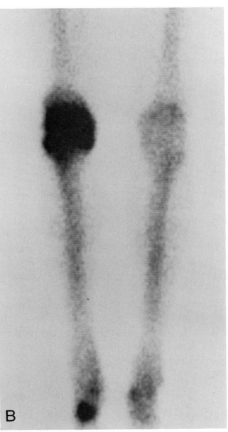

FIGURE 30–13. Radionuclide abnormalities.
 A After the injection of a bone-seeking radiopharmaceutical agent in this 60 year old man with Reiter's syndrome, a lateral image of the foot reveals intense radionuclide activity about multiple articulations and in the base of the fifth metatarsal bone.
 B In a different patient the bone scan shows intense uptake in the right foot and about the right knee; the opposite side appears normal.

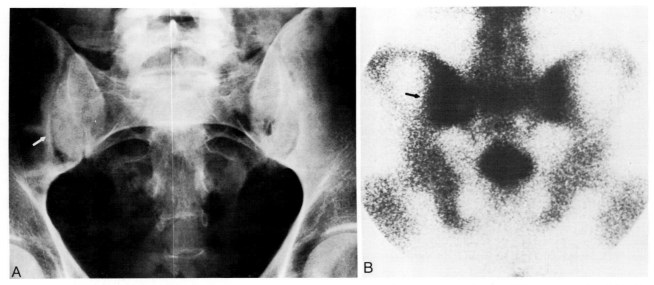

FIGURE 30–14. Radionuclide abnormalities. In a 36 year old man with Reiter's syndrome, asymmetric sacroiliitis, greater on the right side, is evident on both radiographic examination and scintigraphy (arrows).

dylitis and psoriatic arthritis), Reiter's syndrome possesses a sufficiently characteristic articular distribution to allow accurate diagnosis (see Chapters 28 and 29). This syndrome is associated with an asymmetric arthritis of the lower extremity, sacroiliitis, and, less commonly, spondylitis. Ankylosing spondylitis has a similar axial skeletal distribution (although cervical spine changes are more frequent in ankylosing spondylitis than in Reiter's syndrome), but significant peripheral articular changes are less frequent. Psoriatic arthritis may lead to considerable alterations in the articulations of both the appendicular and the axial skeleton. In psoriasis, however, widespread involvement of the upper extremity may be apparent, and distal interphalangeal joint abnormalities in both upper and lower extremities are common.

In all three spondyloarthropathies, the presence of soft tissue swelling, joint space narrowing, erosions, and bony proliferation in synovial articulations is typical. In Reiter's syndrome, the frequency of osteoporosis in the acute phase of the disease appears to be greater than in psoriatic arthritis and ankylosing spondylitis, and the frequency of intra-articular bony ankylosis is less than in the other two diseases. In addition, the resolving nature of some of the lesions of Reiter's syndrome is distinctive, differing from the progressive and severe alterations that may accompany psoriatic arthritis. Each of the three spondyloarthropathies is associated with abnormalities of cartilaginous joints (symphysis pubis, manubriosternal joint) and of sites of tendon and ligament attachment to bone.

The sacroiliac and spinal changes of Reiter's syndrome are virtually identical to those of psoriasis, although the prevalence and severity of these abnormalities and the tendency to involve the cervical spine are greater in psoriasis. Symmetric, asymmetric, or unilateral sacroiliac articular changes and broad asymmetric spinal outgrowths occur in both Reiter's syndrome and psoriatic arthritis. In classic ankylosing spondylitis, symmetric sacroiliac joint changes and symmetric slender bony outgrowths of the spine are typical. Furthermore, in ankylosing spondylitis, vertebral body osteitis, apophyseal joint ankylosis, and intra-articular osseous fusion of the sacroiliac joint are more frequent than in Reiter's syndrome or psoriatic arthritis. The spondylitis and sacroiliitis of inflammatory bowel disease are identical to those of classic ankylosing spondylitis.

Rheumatoid Arthritis

The radiographic features of rheumatoid arthritis differ considerably from those of Reiter's syndrome. In the synovial joints of the appendicular skeleton, rheumatoid arthritis is associated with bilateral and symmetric alterations. Osteoporosis, early joint space narrowing, and marginal erosions are observed. Bony proliferation is unusual, and the irregular proliferative erosive changes of the spondyloarthropathies are not seen in rheumatoid arthritis.

Widespread and severe sacroiliac and thoracolumbar spinal changes are very uncommon in rheumatoid arthritis. Occasionally, unilateral sacroiliac articular abnormalities are encountered that are mild in nature. In the cervical spine, rheumatoid arthritis is associated with characteristic osseous and articular alterations.

Septic Arthritis and Osteomyelitis

The early localized abnormalities of Reiter's syndrome may resemble the findings of osseous and articular infection. Soft tissue swelling, osteoporosis, bony and cartilaginous destruction, and periostitis are evident in both Reiter's syndrome and infectious disease. Eventually, the polyarticular nature of Reiter's syndrome will allow its accurate differentiation from infectious disease.

SUMMARY

Reiter's syndrome has a distinctive radiographic appearance. Involvement of synovial and cartilaginous joints as well as of sites of tendon and ligament attachment to bone is observed. In the appendicular skeleton, an asymmetric arthritis of the articulations of the lower extremity distal to the hip is most typical. Extensive changes may be observed in the foot, particularly at the metatarsophalangeal articulations, the interphalangeal joint of the great toe, and the posterior and plantar aspects of the calcaneus. Widespread and severe changes in the upper extremity are unusual. In the axial skeleton, bilateral symmetric or asymmetric (or even unilateral) sacroiliac joint abnormalities are seen. Paravertebral ossification may produce bulky outgrowths, particularly in the thoracolumbar region. The symphysis pubis and manubriosternal joint can reveal significant erosion and sclerosis.

The findings of Reiter's syndrome are similar to those of the other two seronegative spondyloarthropathies, ankylosing spondylitis and psoriatic arthritis, although their distribution usually allows accurate diagnosis. At times, however, differentiation between Reiter's syndrome and psoriatic arthritis can be exceedingly difficult.

References

1. Sharp JT: Reiter's syndrome. *In* JL Hollander, DJ McCarty Jr (Eds): Arthritis and Allied Conditions. 8th Ed. Philadelphia, Lea & Febiger, 1972, p 1229.
2. Brodie BC: Pathological and Surgical Observations of Diseases of Joints. London, Longman, 1818, p 54.
3. Reiter H: Über eine bisher unerkannte Spirochäteninfektion (Spirochaetosis arthritica). Dtsch Med Wochenschr *42:*1535, 1916.
4. Wright V: Reiter's disease. *In* JT Scott (Ed): Copeman's Textbook of the Rheumatic Diseases. 5th Ed. Edinburgh, Churchill Livingstone, 1978, p 549.
5. Fiessinger N, Leroy E: Contribution á l'étude d'une épidémie de dysenterie dans la Somme. Bull Mem Soc Med Hop Paris *40:*2030, 1916.
6. Bauer W, Engleman EP: Syndrome of unknown aetiology characterized by urethritis, conjunctivitis, and arthritis (so-called Reiter's disease). Trans Assoc Am Physicians *57:*307, 1942.
7. Csonka GW: The course of Reiter's syndrome. Br Med J *1:*1088, 1958.
8. Csonka GW: Recurrent attacks in Reiter's disease. Arthritis Rheum *3:*164, 1960.
9. Murray RS, Oates JK, Young AC: Radiological changes in Reiter's syndrome and arthritis associated with urethritis. J Fac Radiologists *9:*37, 1958.
10. Gates JK, Csonka GW: Reiter's disease in the female. Ann Rheum Dis *18:*37, 1959.
11. Hancock JAH: Surface manifestations of Reiter's disease in the male. Br J Vener Dis *36:*36, 1960.
12. Wright V: Arthritis associated with venereal disease. Ann Rheum Dis *22:*77, 1963.
13. Noer HR: An "experimental" epidemic of Reiter's syndrome. JAMA *198:*693, 1966.
14. Young RH, McEwen EG: Bacillary dysentery as the cause of Reiter's syndrome. JAMA *134:*1456, 1947.
15. Paronen I: Reiter's disease. A study of 344 cases observed in Finland. Acta Med Scand (Suppl) *212:*1, 1948.
16. Schittenhelm A, Schlecht H: Über Polyarthritis enterica. Dtsch Arch Klin Med *126:*329, 1918.
17. Short CL: Arthritis in Mediterranean theater of operations. N Engl J Med *236:*383, 1947.

18. Sharp JT: Reiter's syndrome. A review of current status and a hypothesis regarding its pathogenesis. Curr Probl Dermatol 5:157, 1973.
19. Davies NE, Haverty JR, Boatwright M: Reiter's disease associated with shigellosis. South Med J 62:1011, 1969.
20. Ravin JG: Reiter's syndrome in childhood. A sequel to traveler's diarrhea. J Pediatr Ophthalmol 9:87, 1972.
21. Good AE, Schultz JS: Reiter's syndrome following Shigella flexneri 2a: A sequel to traveler's diarrhea. Report of a case with hepatitis. Arthritis Rheum 20:100, 1977.
22. Hall WH, Finegold S: A study of 23 cases of Reiter's syndrome. Ann Intern Med 38:533, 1953.
23. Steinmetz PR, Green JP: Reiter's syndrome. US Armed Forces Med J 10:1185, 1959.
24. Levy B: Arthritis in venereal disease with particular reference to aetiology. Med J Malaya 5:42, 1950.
25. Corner BD: Reiter's syndrome in childhood. Arch Dis Child 25:398, 1950.
26. Jacobs AG: A case of Reiter's syndrome in childhood. Br Med J 2:155, 1961.
27. Moss I: Reiter's disease in childhood. Br J Vener Dis 40:166, 1964.
28. Lockie GN, Hunder GG: Reiter's syndrome in children. Arthritis Rheum 14:767, 1971.
29. Iveson JMI, Nanda BS, Hancock JAH, et al: Reiter's disease in three boys. Ann Rheum Dis 34:364, 1975.
30. Florman AL, Goldstein HM: Arthritis, conjunctivitis and urethritis (so-called Reiter's syndrome) in a four-year-old boy. J Pediatr 33:172, 1948.
31. King AJ: Arthritis and venereal urethritis. Excerpta Med 11:125, 1957.
32. Marche J: Spondylarthrite ankylosante et syndrome de Fiessinger-Leroy-Reiter. Deux aspects de la même maladie rhumatismale. France Medical 18:7, 1955.
33. Masbernard A: Le syndrome de Fiessinger-Leroy-Reiter; enseignements fournis par l'étude de 80 cas observées en Tunisie. Rev Rhum Mal Osteoartic 26:21, 1959.
34. Montgomery MM, Poske RM, Pilz CG, et al: Reiter's syndrome. GP 27:88, 1963.
35. Csonka G: Reiter's syndrome. Ergeb Inn Med Kinderheilkd 23:125, 1965.
36. Weinberger HW, Ropes MW, Kulka JP, et al: Reiter's syndrome: Clinical and pathological observations—a long term study of 16 cases. Medicine 41:35, 1962.
37. Popert AJ, Gill AJ, Laird SM: A prospective study of Reiter's syndrome—an interim report of the first 82 cases. Br J Vener Dis 40:160, 1964.
38. Catterall RD: Significance of non-specific genital infection in uveitis and arthritis. Lancet 2:739, 1961.
39. Oates JK, Hancock JAH: Neurological symptoms and lesions occurring in the course of Reiter's disease. Am J Med Sci 238:79, 1959.
40. Lindsay-Rea A: Un cas de maladie de Reiter. Congress of Ophthalmology SUK 67:241, 1947.
41. Lever WF, Crawford GM: Keratosis blennorrhagica without gonorrhea (Reiter's disease?). Arch Dermatol 49:389, 1944.
42. Wright V, Reed WB: The link between Reiter's syndrome and psoriatic arthritis. Ann Rheum Dis 23:12, 1964.
43. Good AE: Reiter's disease: A review with special attention to cardiovascular and neurologic sequelae. Semin Arthritis Rheum 3:253, 1974.
44. Lafon R, Pages P, Roux J, et al: Syndrome de Fiessinger-Leroy-Reiter, avec infiltrats pulmonaires labiles et hémiplégie régressive. Organismes L dans les sécrétions urétrales. Rev Neurol 92:611, 1955.
45. Bleehen SS, Everall JD, Tighe JR: Amyloidosis complicating Reiter's syndrome. Br J Vener Dis 42:88, 1966.
46. Caughey DE, Wakem CJ: A fatal case of Reiter's disease complicated by amyloidosis. Arthritis Rheum 16:695, 1973.
47. Shilet IE, Wilske KR, Decker JL: The occurrence of mucocutaneous lesions of Reiter's syndrome (keratosis blennorrhagica) in a patient with classical rheumatoid arthritis. Arthritis Rheum 7:177, 1964.
48. Good AE: Reiter's disease, ankylosing spondylitis and rheumatoid arthritis occurring within a single family. Arthritis Rheum 14:753, 1971.
49. Gray, RG, Altman RD: Classical rheumatoid arthritis in a patient with Reiter's syndrome. J Rheumatol 3:269, 1976.
50. Resnick D, Feingold ML, Curd J, et al: Calcaneal abnormalities in articular disorders. Rheumatoid arthritis, ankylosing spondylitis, psoriatic arthritis and Reiter's syndrome. Radiology 125:355, 1977.
51. Gerster JC, Saudan Y, Fallet GH: Talalgia. A review of 30 severe cases. J Rheumatol 5:210, 1978.
52. Csonka GW: Recurrent attacks in Reiter's disease. Arthritis Rheum 3:164, 1960.
53. Ellis FA, Bereston ES: Reiter's syndrome versus keratosis blennorrhagica sine blennorrhea. South Med J 52:828, 1959.
54. Peterson CC Jr, Silbiger ML: Reiter's syndrome and psoriatic arthritis. Their roentgen spectra and some interesting similarities. AJR 101:860, 1967.
55. Murray RS, Oates JK, Young AC: Radiologic changes in Reiter's syndrome and arthritis associated with urethritis. J Fac Radiologists 9:37, 1958.
56. Reynolds DF, Csonka GW: Radiological aspects of Reiter's syndrome ("venereal" arthritis). J Fac Radiologists 9:44, 1958.
57. Weldon WV, Scalettar R: Roentgen changes in Reiter's syndrome. AJR 86:344, 1961.
58. Sholkoff SD, Glickman MG, Steinback HL: Roentgenology of Reiter's syndrome. Radiology 97:497, 1970.
59. Mason RM, Murray RS, Oates JK, et al: A comparative radiological study of Reiter's disease, rheumatoid arthritis, and ankylosing spondylitis. J Bone Joint Surg [Br] 41:137, 1959.
60. Resnick D, Niwayama G: On the nature and significance of bony proliferation in "rheumatoid variant" disorders. AJR 129:275, 1977.
61. Resnick D: The interphalangeal joint of the great toe in rheumatoid arthritis. J Can Assoc Radiol 26:255, 1975.
62. Resnick D, Niwayama G, Feingold ML: The sesamoid bones of the hands and feet: Participators in arthritis. Radiology 123:57, 1977.
63. Bywaters EGL: Heel lesions of rheumatoid arthritis. Ann Rheum Dis 13:42, 1954.
64. Stadalnik RC, Dublin AB: Sesamoid periostitis in the thumb in Reiter's syndrome. J Bone Joint Surg [Am] 57:279, 1975.
65. Candardjis G, Saudan Y, DeBosset P: Etude radiologique de l'articulation manubrio-sternale dans la pelvispondylite rhumatismale et le syndrome de Reiter. J Radiol Electrol Med Nucl 59:93, 1978.
66. Russell AS, Davis P, Percy JS, et al: The sacroiliitis of acute Reiter's syndrome. J Rheumatol 4:293, 1977.
67. Oates JK, Young AC: Sacroiliitis in Reiter's disease. Br Med J 1:1013, 1959.
68. Cliff JM: Spinal bony bridging and carditis in Reiter's disease. Ann Rheum Dis 30:171, 1971.
69. Sundaram M, Patton JT: Paravertebral ossification in psoriasis and Reiter's disease. Br J Radiol 48:628, 1975.
70. McEwen C, Di Tata D, Lingg C, et al: Ankylosing spondylitis and spondylitis accompanying ulcerative colitis, regional enteritis, psoriasis and Reiter's disease. Arthritis Rheum 14:291, 1971.
71. Forestier J, Jacqueline F, Rotes-Querol J: Ankylosing Spondylitis. Translated by AU Desjardins. Springfield, IL, Charles C Thomas, 1956.
72. Ball J: Enthesopathy of rheumatoid and ankylosing spondylitis. The Heberden Oration. Ann Rheum Dis 30:213, 1970.
73. Bywaters EGL, Dixon AS: Paravertebral ossification in psoriatic arthritis. Ann Rheum Dis 23:313, 1965.
74. Ford DK: Natural history of arthritis following venereal urethritis. Ann Rheum Dis 12:177, 1953.
75. Latchaw, RE, Meyer GW: Reiter's disease with atlanto-axial subluxation. Radiology 126:303, 1978.
76. Weissberg D, Resnick D, Taylor A, et al: Rheumatoid arthritis and its variants: Analysis of scintiphotographic, radiographic, and clinical examination. AJR 131:665, 1978.
77. Rosenthall L, Hawkins D: Radionuclide joint imaging in the diagnosis of synovial disease. Semin Arthritis Rheum 7:49, 1977.
78. Khalkhali I, Stadalnik RC, Wiesner KB, et al: Bone imaging of the heel in Reiter's syndrome. AJR 132:110, 1979.
79. Russell AS, Lentle BC, Percy JS: Investigation of sacroiliac disease: Comparative evaluation of radiological and radionuclide techniques. J Rheumatol 2:45, 1975.
80. Ford DK, Rasmussen G: Relationships between genitourinary infection and complicating arthritis. Arthritis Rheum 7:220, 1964.
81. Schachter J, Barnes MG, Jones JP Jr, et al: Isolation of bedsoniae from the joints of patients with Reiter's syndrome. Proc Soc Exp Biol Med 122:283, 1966.
82. Grainger RG: Procto-colitis and other pelvic infections in relation to ankylosing spondylitis. J Fac Radiologists 10:138, 1959.
83. Batson OV: Role of vertebral veins in metastatic processes. Ann Intern Med 16:38, 1942.
84. Abel MS: Sacroiliac joint changes in traumatic paraplegics. Radiology 55:235, 1950.
85. Lévy JP, Ryckewaert A, Silvestre D, et al: Etude par microscopie électronique des inclusions des cellules synoviales dans un cas de syndrome oculo-uréthro-synovial (Fiessinger-Leroy-Reiter). Pathol Biol 14:216, 1966.
86. Bartholomew LE: Isolation and characterization of mycoplasmas (PPLO) from patients with rheumatoid arthritis, systemic lupus erythematosus and Reiter's syndrome. Arthritis Rheum 8:376, 1965.
87. Bluestone R: HL-AW 27 and the rheumatoid variants. Hosp Pract 10:131, 1975.
88. Brewerton DA, Caffrey M, Nicholls A, et al: Reiter's disease and HL-A 27. Lancet 2:996, 1973.
89. Arnett FC Jr, Hochberg MC, Bias WB: Cross-reactive HLA antigens in B-27 negative Reiter's syndrome and sacroiliitis. Johns Hopkins Med J 141:193, 1977.
90. Morris R, Metzger AL, Bluestone R, et al: HL-A W27—a clue to the diagnosis and pathogenesis of Reiter's syndrome. N Engl J Med 290:554, 1974.
91. Pekin TJ, Malinin TI, Zvaifler NJ: Unusual synovial fluid findings in Reiter's syndrome. Ann Intern Med 66:677, 1967.
92. Spriggs AI, Boddington MM, Mowat G: Joint fluid cytology in Reiter's disease. Ann Rheum Dis 37:557, 1978.
93. Martel W, Braunstein EM, Borlaza G, et al: Radiologic features of Reiter's disease. Radiology 132:1, 1979.
94. Smith DL, Bennett RM, Regan MG: Reiter's disease in women. Arthritis Rheum 23:335, 1980.
95. Morse HG, Rate RG, Bonnell MD, et al: Reiter's syndrome in a five-year-old girl. Arthritis Rheum 23:960, 1980.
96. Jacobs RP, Borenstein DG, Neuwelt CM: Reiter's syndrome: A male and female disease (Abstr). Arthritis Rheum 23:696, 1980.
97. Weiss JJ, Thompson GR, Good A: Reiter's disease after Salmonella typhimurium enteritis. J Rheumatol 7:211, 1980.
98. Leung FY-K, Littlejohn GO, Bombardier C: Reiter's syndrome after Campylobacter jejuni enteritis. Arthritis Rheum 23:948, 1980.
99. Benedek TG, Rodnan GP: A brief history of the rheumatic diseases. Bull Rheum Dis 32:59, 1982.

100. Morse HG, Rate RG, Bonnell MD, et al: Reiter's syndrome in a five-year-old girl. Arthritis Rheum 23:961, 1980.
101. Neuwelt CM, Borenstein DG, Jacobs RP: Reiter's syndrome: A male and female disease. J Rheumatol 9:268, 1982.
102. Ponka A, Martio J, Kosunen TU: Reiter's syndrome in association with enteritis due to *Campylobacter fetus* ssp. *jejuni.* Ann Rheum Dis 40:414, 1981.
103. Simon DG, Kaslow RA, Rosenbaum J, et al: Reiter's syndrome following epidemic shigellosis. J Rheumatol 8:969, 1981.
104. Willkens RF, Arnett FC, Bitter T, et al: Reiter's syndrome. Evaluation of preliminary criteria for definite disease. Arthritis Rheum 24:844, 1981.
105. Canoso JJ, Wohlgethan JR, Newberg AH, et al: Aspiration of the retrocalcaneal bursa. Ann Rheum Dis 43:308, 1984.
106. Stone, G, Wolfe F: Collateral ligament calcification complicating amyloidosis and Reiter's syndrome. J Rheumatol 11:248, 1984.
107. Doury P, Pattin S: Le calcaneum dans le syndrome de Fiessinger-Leroy-Reiter. Rev Rhum Mal Osteoartic 46:705, 1979.
108. Finder JG, Ellman MH, Jablon M: Massive synovial hypertrophy in Reiter's syndrome. J Bone Joint Surg [Am] 65:555, 1983.
109. Bomalaski JS, Jimenez SA: Erosive arthritis of the temporomandibular joint in Reiter's syndrome. J Rheumatol 11:400, 1984.
110. Leirisalo M, Skylv G, Kousa M, et al: Follow-up study on patients with Reiter's disease and reactive arthritis, with special reference to HLA-B27. Arthritis Rheum 25:249, 1982.
111. Keat A: Reiter's syndrome and reactive arthritis in perspective. N Engl J Med 309:1606, 1983.
112. Goldenberg DL: ''Postinfectious'' arthritis. Am J Med 74:925, 1983.
113. Yunus M, Calabro JJ, Miller KA, et al: Family studies with HLA typing in Reiter's syndrome. Am J Med 70:1210, 1981.
114. Baldassare AR, Weiss TD, Tsai CC, et al: Immunoprotein deposition in synovial tissue in Reiter's syndrome. Ann Rheum Dis 40:281, 1981.
115. Moilanen A, Yli-Kerrtula U, Vilppula A: Cervical spine involvements in Reiter's syndrome. ROFO 141:84, 1984.
116. Ishikawa H, Ohno O, Yamasaki K, et al: Arthritis presumably caused by Chlamydia in Reiter syndrome. Case report with electron microscopic studies. J Bone Joint Surg [Am] 68:777, 1986.
117. Bengtsson A, Lindström FD, Lindblom B: Reiter's syndrome—a comparative study of patients with the complete and the incomplete syndrome. Clin Rheumatol 5:70, 1986.
118. Cuttica RJ, Scheines EJ, Garay SM, et al: Juvenile onset Reiter's syndrome. A retrospective study of 26 patients. Clin Exp Rheumatol 10:285, 1992.
119. Weyand CM, Goronzy JJ: Immune responses to *Borrelia burgdorferi* in patients with reactive arthritis. Arthritis Rheum 32:1057, 1989.
120. Arnett FC: The Lyme spirochete: Another cause of Reiter's syndrome. Arthritis Rheum 32:1182, 1989.
121. Kransdorf MJ, Wehrle PA, Moser RP Jr: Atlantoaxial subluxation in Reiter's syndrome. A report of three cases and review of the literature. Spine 13:12, 1988.
122. Melsom RD, Benjamin JC, Barnes CG: Spontaneous atlantoaxial subluxation: An unusual presenting manifestation of Reiter's syndrome. Ann Rheum Dis 48:170, 1989.
123. Halla JT, Bliznak J, Hardin JG: Involvement of the craniocervical junction in Reiter's syndrome. J Rheumatol 15:1722, 1988.
124. Schumacher HR Jr, Magge S, Cherian PV, et al: Light and electron microscopic studies on the synovial membrane in Reiter's syndrome. Immunocytochemical identification of Chlamydial antigen in patients with early disease. Arthritis Rheum 31:937, 1988.
125. Linssen A, Feltkamp TEW: B27 positive diseases versus B27 negative diseases. Ann Rheum Dis 47:431, 1988.

31

Enteropathic Arthropathies

Donald Resnick, M.D.

The appearance of musculoskeletal abnormalities in patients with gastrointestinal disorders has been recognized with increasing frequency in recent years. These abnormalities have been designated enteropathic arthritis because of the close association of articular and intestinal findings. Ulcerative colitis, Crohn's disease (regional enteritis), and Whipple's disease are three intestinal diseases whose rheumatologic manifestations now are well known. In addition, musculoskeletal abnormalities can occur after certain intestinal infections, specifically those associated with Salmonella, Shigella, or Yersinia organisms, after intestinal by-pass surgery, and as a complication of extraintestinal disorders, including Laennec's and biliary cirrhosis, hepatitis, and pancreatic disease.

The relationship between inflammatory intestinal diseases and arthritis is not fully understood. Several theoretical possibilities exist to explain this relationship.[176] An infectious cause may be operational. Organisms originating in the gut could secondarily invade articular tissue, or both gastrointestinal tract and joint may be infected simultaneously. The arthritis complicating Salmonella, Shigella, or Yersinia enterocolitis is consistent with this etiologic basis. A second proposed cause implicates immune mechanisms. Cellular or humoral immune responses may be elaborated against a tissue antigen shared by the bowel and the joint; or, alternatively, immune complexes formed by the breakdown of the normal intestinal mucosal barrier incidentally may injure the joint as they circulate in the body. This mechanism may be important in the arthritis of ulcerative colitis, Crohn's disease, and intestinal bypass operations. Evidence also has indicated that genetic factors play an important role in the development of enteropathic arthropathies. Approximately 90 per cent of patients with ulcerative colitis and Crohn's disease who develop spondylitis or sacroiliitis demonstrate the genetically determined histocompatibility antigen HLA-B27 on their cells. This antigen may enhance a person's susceptibility to an infectious process, or it may be linked to an immune response gene that controls the generation of a particular pathogenetic immune response. Thus, articular disease might develop only in those patients possessing the HLA-B27–linked immune response gene.

This chapter summarizes the rheumatologic manifestations of the enteropathic arthropathies (Table 31–1). The arthritis associated with Reiter's syndrome and Behçet's syndrome is discussed elsewhere.

ULCERATIVE COLITIS

General Abnormalities

Ulcerative colitis is a chronic inflammatory disease of unknown cause with predilection for young adults, which

TABLE 31–1. Radiographic Manifestations of Enteropathic Arthropathies*

Disorders	Sacroiliitis	Spondylitis	Peripheral Joints	Other Manifestations
Ulcerative colitis	+	+	Soft tissue swelling Osteoporosis Joint space narrowing (r) Erosions, cysts (r)	Periostitis (r)
Crohn's disease	+	+	Soft tissue swelling Osteoporosis Joint space narrowing (r) Erosions, cysts (r) Septic arthritis (r)	Periostitis (r) Osseous granulomas (r) Osteomyelitis (r)
Whipple's disease	+	+	Soft tissue swelling Osteoporosis Joint space narrowing (r) Erosions, cysts (r)	Subcutaneous nodules (r)
Salmonella, Shigella, and Yersinia infections	+	+	Soft tissue swelling Osteoporosis Septic arthritis	
Intestinal bypass surgery	+	+	Soft tissue swelling Osteoporosis Gout (r)	Osteomalacia (r)
Laennec's cirrhosis			Soft tissue swelling Osteoporosis	Soft tissue calcification (r)
Biliary cirrhosis			Soft tissue swelling Joint space narrowing Erosions Destruction Chondrocalcinosis (r)	Osteomalacia Xanthoma Periostitis (r)
Viral hepatitis			Soft tissue swelling (r)	Subcutaneous nodules
Pancreatic disease			Soft tissue swelling (r) Osteoporosis Erosions, cysts (r) Osteonecrosis	Subcutaneous nodules Osteolysis Periostitis Metastasis

* + = present; r = rare.

involves predominantly the mucosa and submucosa of the colon. Clinical findings associated with colon involvement include malaise, anorexia, weight loss, and a change in consistency of the stools, which varies from constipation to incapacitating diarrhea. The severity of the disorder differs from one person to another, although significant complications may be encountered, including intestinal obstruction, perforation, fistulae, and perianal abnormalities. Systemic findings in ulcerative colitis may include erythema nodosum, pyoderma gangrenosum, uveitis, oral ulcerations, and arrest of normal skeletal development and growth.

Musculoskeletal abnormalities are the most common extraintestinal manifestation of the disease. The association between arthritis and colitis was first described by White[1] in the late nineteenth century and was later emphasized by Bargen in 1929.[2] Although Hench[3] in 1935 characterized the articular abnormalities of ulcerative colitis as distinct from rheumatoid arthritis, they still were described as coincident rheumatoid arthritis as recently as 1957.[4] Currently it is recognized that the arthritis of ulcerative colitis is a distinct entity whose manifestations have variously been termed colitic arthritis, intestinal arthritis, enteropathic arthritis, and acute toxic arthritis.[5, 6] The type of articular disease can be categorized as peripheral joint arthralgias and arthritis (50 to 60 per cent), sacroiliitis and spondylitis (20 to 30 per cent), and miscellaneous abnormalities (10 to 20 per cent).

Peripheral Joint Arthralgia and Arthritis

The reported frequency of abnormalities of the peripheral joints in ulcerative colitis has varied from 0 to 25 per cent, although a frequency of 10 to 12 per cent seems most typical.[5, 7–11, 294] Patients with ulcerative colitis and peripheral joint disease are similar in sex and age to patients with ulcerative colitis who do not have joint abnormalities. Adults usually are affected; however, children too may reveal ulcerative colitis and arthritis.[12] Although bowel disease usually is clinically evident prior to the onset of arthritis, articular abnormalities may appear before intestinal abnormalities in 10 to 15 per cent of patients. A close temporal association exists between exacerbations of intestinal and of joint findings.[239] Furthermore, articular manifestations appear more commonly with severe and widespread intestinal involvement and with bowel disease complicated by intestinal polyposis, perianal suppuration, massive hemorrhage, oral ulceration, and pyoderma gangrenosum; they are less frequent with intestinal alterations confined to the descending colon and rectosigmoid area.[9] The arthritis generally responds to conservative therapy directed at the joints or to aggressive treatment, including surgery of the diseased bowel segment.

The articular findings can be categorized as an acute synovitis that is predominantly monoarticular or pauciarticular in distribution, although it can be polyarticular.[10–12, 295]

The knees are involved most commonly, followed by the ankles, the elbows, the wrists, the shoulders, and the small joints of the hands and feet. Asymmetric inflammation of the proximal interphalangeal joints of the toes is suggestive of "colitic arthritis," although it also may be observed in other inflammatory joint disorders, particularly Reiter's syndrome. Joints in the lower extremity are affected more frequently than those in the upper extremity. The initial attack reaches a peak within 48 to 72 hours and consists of pain, swelling, erythema, and restriction of motion. Inflammation in one articulation may subside at the same time that other joints are being affected. The attacks usually are self-limited, frequently resolving within 1 to 3 months.[8] Fewer than 20 per cent of patients reveal joint inflammation that persists for longer than a year. Permanent joint abnormalities are infrequent even in the setting of recurrent clinical attacks of arthritis. Although cartilaginous and osseous changes can develop, joint deformities are exceedingly rare.[326]

Laboratory analysis reveals inflammatory synovial fluid on joint aspiration. Biopsy of the synovial membrane outlines chronic inflammatory changes with synovial cell hyperplasia, fibroblastic proliferation, and increased vascularity.[7, 13, 14] The cellularity of the tissue is less striking than in rheumatoid arthritis, and lymphoid follicles are not apparent.

The radiographic analysis is nonspecific. Soft tissue swelling and periarticular osteoporosis are the two most typical radiographic characteristics (Fig. 31–1). Joint space narrowing, osseous erosions and cysts, and periosteal proliferation also have been reported.[13, 14] Over a period of time, the erosions can reveal evidence of healing, and periostitis eventually can merge with the underlying bone.[7] It must be emphasized, however, that radiographic evidence of osseous and cartilaginous destruction indeed is unusual, although when present, the findings can simulate those of rheumatoid arthritis. The problem of differentiating between the peripheral arthritis of ulcerative colitis and rheumatoid arthritis is highlighted by some authors who emphasize the simultaneous occurrence of the two diseases[6, 7, 14]; however, other investigators conclude that the prevalence of rheumatoid arthritis in patients with ulcerative colitis is no different from that in the general population.

The cause and pathogenesis of peripheral joint disease in ulcerative colitis are not known. The close association of the presence, extent, and severity of the bowel disease with the clinical manifestations of the articular disease suggests that a common factor initiates inflammation in both structures. Antigenic release from the bowel into the circulation could conceivably lead to the formation of soluble antigen-antibody complexes that can enter the joint, producing a reactive synovitis.[15] The association of erythema nodosum with synovitis provides additional indirect evidence that a sensitivity reaction may be operational. Although no conclusive studies are available to document the role of antigen-antibody complexes in the pathogenesis of arthritis in ulcerative colitis, the absorption of antigenic material through damaged intestinal mucosa in this disease has been

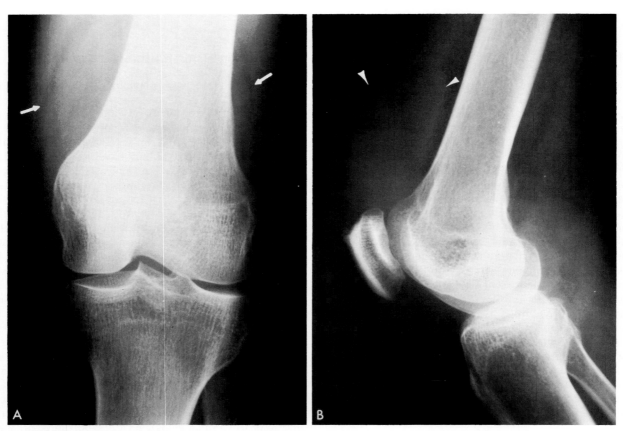

FIGURE 31–1. Ulcerative colitis: Peripheral joint abnormalities. Observe a large joint effusion of the knee with displacement of the fat pads (arrows) and prominence of the suprapatellar pouch (arrowheads).

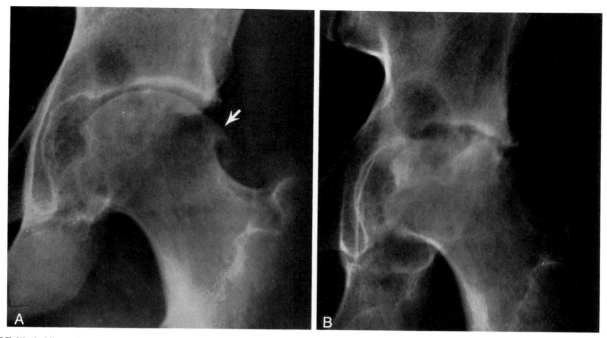

FIGURE 31–2. Ulcerative colitis and ankylosing spondylitis: Monoarthritis of the hip. A 25 year old man with well-established ulcerative colitis had a 5 year history of left hip pain and a limp that began as an acute episode after colectomy.

A The initial radiograph reveals diffuse loss of joint space, cystic changes, and osteophytosis, especially on the lateral aspect of the femoral head (arrow).

B Two years later, there is obvious progression of the hip abnormalities. In the interval, unilateral sacroiliitis developed. At the time of cup arthroplasty, 4 years after clinical presentation, a fibrous exudate, hyperemia, and cellular infiltration of the synovial membrane were evident. (Courtesy of M. Lequesne, M.D., Paris, France.)

demonstrated,[16] suggesting that deposition of immune complexes may cause some of the features of ulcerative colitis.[17]

Sacroiliitis and Spondylitis

An association between ulcerative colitis and ankylosing spondylitis has been confirmed by many investigators. The reported frequency of ankylosing spondylitis in patients with ulcerative colitis has varied from 1 to 26 per cent.[5, 6, 8, 9, 11, 18–24] Conversely, Jayson and his colleagues[25, 26] detected ulcerative colitis in 17.5 per cent of spondylitis patients. This increased prevalence has been confirmed by most other investigators (estimates of the frequency of chronic inflammatory bowel disease in ankylosing spondylitis varying from 2 to 18 per cent), although Green and coworkers[27] failed to document an increase in bowel disease in patients with ankylosing spondylitis. Similarly, data derived from other published series of such patients have raised questions about whether a meaningful association of inflammatory bowel disease and ankylosing spondylitis truly exists.[194, 195]

Spondylitis in ulcerative colitis is poorly correlated with activity of the bowel disease. Furthermore, spinal abnormalities may become manifest prior to, at the same time as, or after the onset of intestinal changes. In fact, spondylitis most commonly precedes the onset of colitis and may progress relentlessly without relation to exacerbation, remission, or treatment of the bowel disease.

The clinical features of ankylosing spondylitis in patients with ulcerative colitis are identical to those of classic ankylosing spondylitis, although the male predilection may be less striking (male-to-female ratio, 4 to 1). Findings include back pain and stiffness and restriction of chest and spinal movement. Peripheral joint abnormalities are detected in 50 to 70 per cent of patients, particularly in the hips and shoulders. Such abnormalities, especially in the hip, may occur as an early manifestation of the disease. In these instances, the radiographic features in the appendicular skeleton are those that are typical for ankylosing spondylitis, including the presence of joint space narrowing, osseous erosions, cysts, and bony proliferation, and the absence of osteoporosis (Fig. 31–2). Thus, the peripheral joint abnormalities are readily differentiated from the arthritis of ulcerative colitis.

Laboratory evaluation outlines the presence of a nonreactive serum rheumatoid factor and an increased frequency of the histocompatibility antigen HLA-B27,[28–31] although not so great as in classic ankylosing spondylitis.[196] This antigen is not commonly detected in patients with inflammatory bowel disease with or without peripheral joint disease who do not have spine or sacroiliac joint alterations.[28, 29] HLA-B27 antigen also is linked to inflammatory changes of the eye in patients with ulcerative colitis as well as to flare-ups of bowel disease. Thus, the detection of HLA-B27 antigen indicates an increased risk for the development of spondylitis and iritis in patients with inflammatory bowel disorders. A non–HLA-linked genetic predisposition both to inflammatory bowel disease and to spondylitis also has been reported.[196]

On radiographic examination, spinal and sacroiliac joint abnormalities in ulcerative colitis are virtually indistinguishable from those in classic ankylosing spondylitis.[23, 32–34] Sacroiliac joint involvement usually is bilateral and symmetric in distribution, although on rare occasions asymmetric changes are apparent (Fig. 31–3). Osseous erosion and sclerosis as well as joint space alterations are evident. Initially, the articular space may appear widened, although joint space narrowing and bony ankylosis are common in later stages of the disease. The ligamentous space above the true articulation frequently becomes indistinct or ossified. Additional pelvic abnormalities include bony erosion and sclerosis about the symphysis pubis and bony erosion and proliferation at the ischial tuberosities and iliac crests. In the spine, vertebral body erosions with alterations of vertebral shape (squaring) are seen (Fig. 31–4). Typical syndesmophytes also are evident. These appear as thin, vertical radiodense shadows extending from one vertebral body to the next across the intervertebral disc space, particularly at the thoracolumbar and lumbosacral junctions. With progression, these excrescences can involve a larger segment of the spine and a greater portion of the intervertebral disc. Eventually, a bamboo spine may be evident. In the apophyseal joints, articular space narrowing, erosion, sclerosis, and bony ankylosis are identical to changes in classic ankylosing spondylitis. Alterations in adjacent joints of the axial skeleton, such as the acromioclavicular, sternoclavicular, and manubriosternal joints, can include bony erosion and eburnation. In the hip and glenohumeral joints, typical joint manifestations of ankylosing spondylitis may appear (Fig. 31–5).

The sacroiliitis and spondylitis of classic ankylosing spondylitis and of ulcerative colitis (as well as Crohn's disease) are readily differentiated from the sacroiliitis and spondylitis of psoriatic arthritis and of Reiter's syndrome.[33] Bilateral symmetric sacroiliac joint changes with eventual intra-articular bony ankylosis are more common in classic ankylosing spondylitis and colitic disease than in psoriasis and Reiter's syndrome. In the spine, vertical syndesmophytes, significant apophyseal joint abnormalities, and vertebral squaring also are more typical of classic ankylosing spondylitis and colitic disorders than of psoriasis and Reiter's syndrome, as are increased vertebral osteoporosis and severe symphyseal changes.

It is apparent that the clinical and radiographic characteristics of spinal and sacroiliac joint abnormalities in ulcerative colitis are those of classic ankylosing spondylitis. Generally these two diseases are assumed to coexist in the same patient rather than being causally related. This assumption is reinforced by the observations that relatives of patients with ulcerative colitis have an increased prevalence of sacroiliitis and spondylitis[24, 35] and that the frequency of the histocompatibility antigen HLA-B27 is increased in patients with classic ankylosing spondylitis and in those with ulcerative colitis and spondylitis. The fact that this antigen is less common in patients with ulcerative colitis and spondylitis than in patients with classic ankylosing spondylitis, however, has led some investigators to speculate that the spine and sacroiliac joint changes in inflammatory bowel disease are not those of ankylosing spondylitis but rather represent manifestations of a different disorder.[31] It is possible that structural changes in the spine and sacroiliac joints in inflammatory intestinal processes are related to passage of an infectious agent through the diseased bowel wall into the pelvic veins, which anastomose with the vertebral plexus, or to transportation of antigenic substances by the adjacent lymphatics. If these factors indeed are operational, the spondylitis and sacroiliitis of ulcerative colitis might be attributed to classic ankylosing spondylitis (HLA-B27 positive) in some patients and to a "secondary" ankylosing spondylitis (HLA-B27 negative) in others.[31, 36]

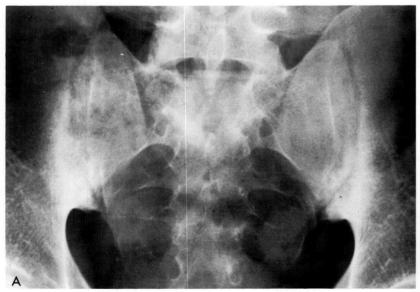
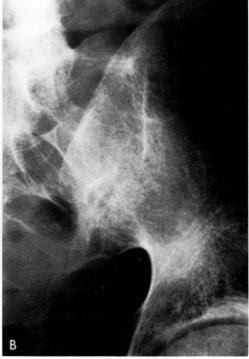

FIGURE 31–3. Ulcerative colitis and ankylosing spondylitis: Sacroiliac joint abnormalities.

A Bilateral and symmetric sacroiliac articular abnormalities are characterized by erosion and sclerosis, predominantly in the ilium.

B In another patient, segmental intra-articular osseous fusion has obliterated portions of the sacroiliac joint. The ligamentous space above the true joint also is ossified. The opposite side was involved similarly.

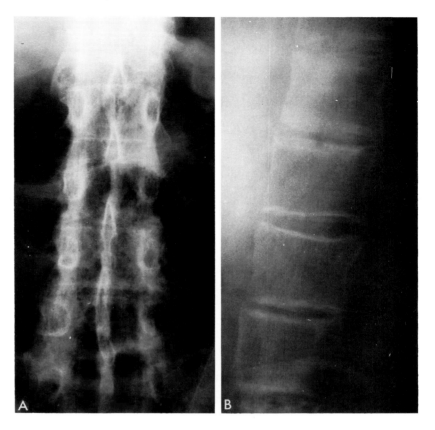

FIGURE 31–4. Ulcerative colitis and ankylosing spondylitis: Spinal abnormalities.

A, B Anteroposterior and lateral radiographs of the lumbar spine demonstrate typical findings of ankylosing spondylitis. Convexity and squaring of the anterior borders of the vertebral bodies, disc space loss, capsular ossification and ankylosis of apophyseal joints, and ossification of interspinous and supraspinous ligaments are evident. Note the dilated and diseased bowel.

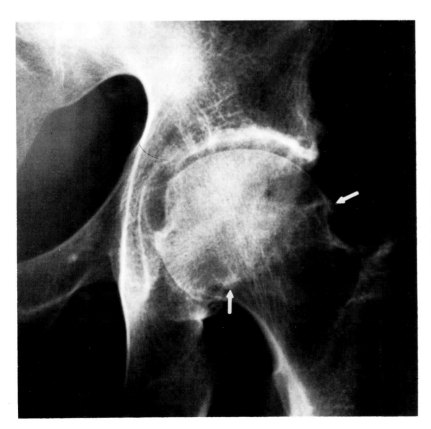

FIGURE 31–5. Ulcerative colitis and ankylosing spondylitis: Peripheral joint abnormalities. This radiograph reveals typical features of hip involvement in ankylosing spondylitis. Observe diffuse loss of joint space and osteophytes at the junction of the femoral head and neck (arrows). The sacroiliac joint is ankylosed.

Miscellaneous Abnormalities

Clubbing of the fingers is a recognized complication of ulcerative colitis. Young[37] reported clubbing in 4 per cent of 156 patients with this disease, confined to persons whose disease involved areas of the colon supplied by the vagus nerve. On rare occasions, hypertrophic osteoarthropathy also may be apparent, leading to periosteal bone formation in the tibia, fibula, radius, and ulna[38] (Fig. 31–6). Massive subperiosteal deposition of bone has been noted in these locations as well as in the femur, humerus, metacarpals, and clavicle.[197, 270] Such deposition apparently can occur during acute episodes of colitis, and the deposits can be incorporated into the underlying bone during remission of the bowel disease.[197]

Other rheumatologic conditions may accompany ulcerative colitis, although their frequency probably is no greater than that in the general population.[5–7, 14] Typical clinical and radiologic findings of rheumatoid arthritis may be observed in some patients with ulcerative colitis, which are easily differentiated from the peripheral joint abnormalities of the intestinal disease itself. Relapsing polychondritis is another disorder that has been reported in combination with ulcerative colitis.[198]

Differential Diagnosis

Radiographic features of peripheral joint arthritis in patients with ulcerative colitis are not specific. Soft tissue swelling and osteoporosis are the most common findings and are observed in association with synovial inflammation accompanying other disorders. Although the appearance of joint space narrowing, erosions, and cysts can simulate changes in rheumatoid arthritis, these abnormalities are not frequent in the arthritis of ulcerative colitis.

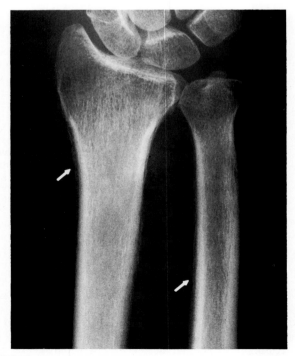

FIGURE 31–6. Ulcerative colitis: Hypertrophic osteoarthropathy: Note periostitis (arrows) of the diaphyses and metaphyses of the radius and ulna.

Spondylitis and sacroiliitis in ulcerative colitis are identical to the changes in classic ankylosing spondylitis. Bilateral and symmetric sacroiliac joint involvement and syndesmophytosis are seen in both disorders. These same changes also are evident in Crohn's disease. In psoriasis and Reiter's syndrome, sacroiliac joint abnormalities may be asymmetric or even unilateral in distribution, whereas spinal alterations include broad asymmetric bony excrescences that differ in appearance from typical syndesmophytes.

CROHN'S DISEASE

General Abnormalities

Crohn's disease is a chronic and recurrent granulomatous process of unknown cause that involves principally the terminal ileum and proximal portion of the colon, although it may localize in any segment of the gastrointestinal tract from esophagus to rectum. Crohn's disease is associated with a variety of clinical findings, including abdominal pain, tenderness, diarrhea, weight loss, and fever. Complications include intestinal hemorrhage, obstruction, draining sinuses, and fistulae. Additional systemic manifestations are ocular inflammation (uveitis, conjunctivitis, episcleritis), erythema nodosum, and musculoskeletal abnormalities. Crohn's disease is most frequent in young adults, although patients of all ages may be affected.

Musculoskeletal manifestations in Crohn's disease can take several forms: peripheral joint arthralgias and arthritis; sacroiliitis and spondylitis; and miscellaneous abnormalities.

Peripheral Joint Arthralgia and Arthritis

Enteropathic arthritis is a recognized finding in patients with Crohn's disease.[39, 40] The reported frequency of this complication has varied from less than 1 per cent to 22 per cent,[8, 18, 35, 39–52] much of the variation being related to methods of patient selection or clinical and radiographic examination. Some studies did not include patients with Crohn's disease who revealed colonic involvement, although arthritis is now known to be more common in patients with large bowel disease.[50, 52] It appears probable that enteropathic arthritis is more frequent in Crohn's disease than in ulcerative colitis.

Peripheral joint abnormalities in Crohn's disease are equally frequent in men and women. The pattern of articular involvement most typically is a mild, migratory synovitis of one or less commonly several joints, involving the lower extremity more frequently than the upper extremity. The knee is the most common site of abnormality, followed by the ankle, the shoulder, the wrist, the elbow, and the small joints of the hands and feet.[53] Clinical findings include pain, swelling, tenderness, and restricted motion; they generally are self-limited, resolving completely over a duration of 2 to 8 weeks, although they may recur. Arthritis, which may be associated with erythema nodosum, occurs simultaneously with the onset of bowel disease or at any time during its course. Rarely, it may precede intestinal alterations. The recrudescence of arthritis commonly is associated with an exacerbation of intestinal disease, and there appears to be a direct relationship between the activity of the articular and gastrointestinal manifestations. Surgical intervention on diseased bowel may not affect the course of the joint disease and, in fact, the onset of arthritis can occur in the postoperative period. This occurrence may relate to the widespread nature of bowel involvement in Crohn's disease and to the difficulty in excising the entire abnormal gut during surgical intervention.

Serum rheumatoid factor is not present in enteropathic arthritis accompanying Crohn's disease. Synovial fluid and synovial tissue examination demonstrates nonspecific inflammatory changes.[42, 49]

Radiographic abnormalities also are nondistinctive. Soft tissue swelling and regional osteoporosis may be observed. Permanent cartilaginous and osseous changes rarely are present, in contradistinction to their occurrence in patients with Crohn's disease who have granulomatous synovitis (see later discussion). In unusual circumstances synovial cysts may be encountered (Fig. 31–7).[184]

The cause of enteropathic arthritis accompanying Crohn's disease is not known. The close association of bowel and joint involvement in this disorder suggests that some unknown factor within the gut is responsible for joint inflammation, perhaps related to an immune response to the enteric lesion.[54, 296] This association, however, is not present uniformly, leading to interest in identifying additional factors that may be important in the initiation of enteropathic arthritis. In this regard, the finding of positive birefringent crystals, resembling calcium pyrophosphate dihydrate crystals, in some inflamed as well as in noninflamed joints,

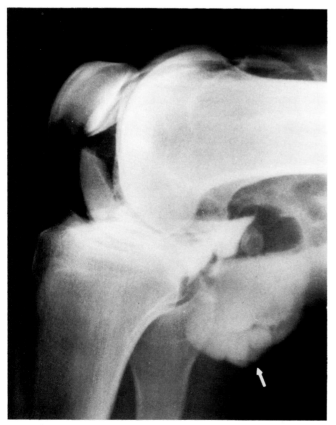

FIGURE 31–7. Crohn's disease: Peripheral joint abnormalities. Arthrography in a young patient with Crohn's disease and synovitis of the knee reveals evidence of a popliteal cyst (arrow).

could indicate another pathogenetic factor in the peripheral joint disorder associated with Crohn's disease.[203]

Sacroiliitis and Spondylitis

An association between Crohn's disease and ankylosing spondylitis has been widely popularized. A significant number of patients with Crohn's disease develop sacroiliac joint and spinal changes; conversely, a high frequency of Crohn's disease occurs in patients with ankylosing spondylitis. The reported prevalence of sacroiliac joint and spinal changes in patients with Crohn's disease has varied from 3 to 16 per cent.[20, 51, 55] The prevalence of clinical abnormalities is greater than that of routine radiographic abnormalities; however, the frequency of sacroiliac joint changes that are detectable with CT in patients with Crohn's disease has been reported to be as great as 29 per cent.[297] Men and women are affected with equal frequency. Symptoms and signs may antedate or follow the onset of bowel disease. Back pain, stiffness, restricted motion, and reduced chest expansion are observed. Exacerbation of these findings does not appear related to the activity of bowel disease, nor does the treatment of the intestinal disorder influence the progress of the arthritis. A definite relationship between the site of intestinal involvement and the presence and extent of articular abnormality has not been found. Specifically, axial skeletal joint alterations are equally frequent in patients with either large or small bowel involvement.[55]

Laboratory evaluation yields nonreactive serum rheumatoid factor test results. Serologic testing for the presence of HLA-B27 antigen in patients with Crohn's disease and sacroiliitis or spondylitis reveals an increased prevalence (approximately 50 per cent) of this histocompatibility antigen that is not found in those patients with gut disease alone or with enteropathic peripheral arthritis,[28, 56–58] although occasionally investigators fail to document this association.[59, 60] It has been suggested that the presence of HLA-B27 antigen in patients with Crohn's disease may not correlate with sacroiliac joint involvement alone but rather may indicate that severe sacroiliitis and spondylitis will both develop.[61] It also has been suggested that this antigen is found in those persons with Crohn's disease who first developed ankylosing spondylitis as opposed to those in whom the bowel disorder antedated the spondylitis or occurred at the same time.[204]

The radiographic features of spinal and sacroiliac articular abnormalities in Crohn's disease are identical to those of classic ankylosing spondylitis.[32, 33, 55] Bilateral sacroiliac joint narrowing and erosion and sclerosis of ilium and sacrum are evident (Fig. 31–8). Syndesmophytosis, vertebral erosion, sclerosis, and squaring, and apophyseal joint erosion, sclerosis, and narrowing can be noted in the spine. Progressive alterations can lead to intra-articular bony ankylosis of the sacroiliac joints and a bamboo spine, as well as to extensive discovertebral destruction.[298] In some patients, particularly women, the findings may remain isolated to the sacroiliac joints, revealing no tendency to involve the spine. The same distribution of disease has been noted in women with classic ankylosing spondylitis.[62] In those instances in which peripheral joint disease occurs during the course of sacroiliitis and spondylitis, findings are typical of ankylosing spondylitis (erosion, joint space narrowing, and

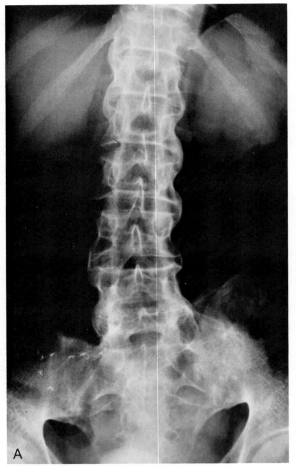

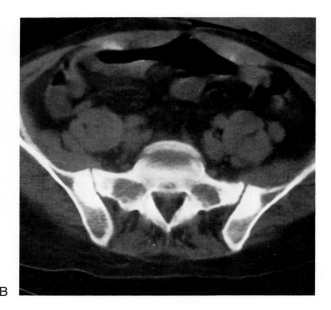

FIGURE 31–8. Crohn's disease and ankylosing spondylitis: Sacroiliac joint and spinal abnormalities.

A Frontal radiograph reveals bilateral symmetric sacroiliac joint changes with intra-articular bone fusion. Syndesmophytes are seen in the spine.

B In a different patient, transaxial CT scanning demonstrates bilateral and symmetric sacroiliitis, characterized by an extreme degree of bone sclerosis in both the ilium and the sacrum. (Courtesy of P. Ellenbogen, M.D., Dallas, Texas.)

FIGURE 31–9. Crohn's disease and ankylosing spondylitis: Peripheral joint abnormalities. Observe symmetric loss of joint space, cystic lesions, and osteophytosis of the femoral head (arrows), findings typical of the hip disease of ankylosing spondylitis.

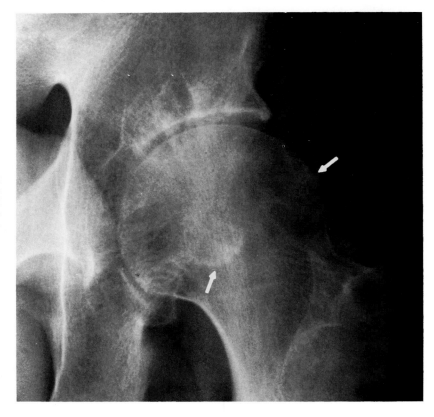

bone proliferation)[63] and are easily differentiated from those of enteropathic arthritis (Fig. 31–9).

Scintigraphy also has been employed to study the distribution of bone and joint involvement in Crohn's disease.[64] Use of bone-seeking radiopharmaceuticals, such as ^{99m}Tc-labeled pyrophosphate or polyphosphate, may show the frequency of sacroiliac joint inflammatory changes in this disease to be much greater than detected on radiographic examination. CT scanning also appears more sensitive than routine radiography in the detection of these inflammatory changes.[297]

The cause and pathogenesis of axial skeletal involvement in Crohn's disease are unclear, although it generally is assumed that factors similar to those in ulcerative colitis are responsible for the joint involvement. Spondylitis has been suggested to result from the passage of toxic substances from the site of pelvic inflammation into the pelvic veins and from there into the vertebral venous system, causing chronic recurrent inflammatory changes of the spine.[65] As this theory may implicate a diseased colon as the initial site of inflammation in patients with Crohn's disease, the lack of association between spondylitis and colonic involvement is noteworthy.[55] Furthermore, the appearance of spinal and sacroiliac joint disease prior to the onset of enteritis and colitis casts doubt on this causal relationship. Evidence that documents a relationship between the spondylitis and sacroiliitis of Crohn's disease and the presence of HLA-B27 antigen (and, perhaps, HLA-B44 antigen) supports the existence of a genetic linkage of a specific immune responsiveness gene to the disease or a strong immunologic cross reaction between the antigen and the involved etiologic

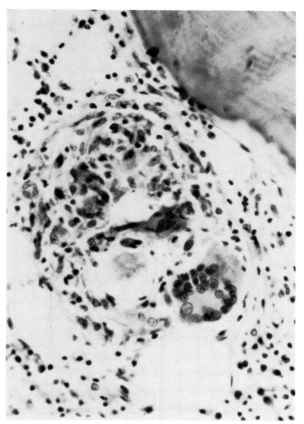

FIGURE 31–11. Crohn's disease: Granulomatous abnormalities of bone. In a 44 year old man with Crohn's disease, a biopsy of a femoral lesion (which had accumulated radionuclide on bone scintigraphy) outlines noncaseating granulomatous inflammation with giant cells. (From Nugent FW, et al: Reprinted by permission from The New England Journal of Medicine, *294*:262, 1976.)

agent.[299] The high rate of occurrence of sacroiliitis in families of patients with Crohn's disease lends further support for such a genetic factor.[66]

Miscellaneous Abnormalities

Digital clubbing has been detected in as many as 40 per cent of patients with Crohn's disease, particularly when the proximal small bowel is involved in the disease process or internal fistulae are present.[52, 67] Bilateral symmetric periostitis, which is a manifestation of hypertrophic osteoarthropathy, is an extremely rare complication of Crohn's disease[68, 69] (Fig. 31–10). It generally is unassociated with bone or joint pain.

Granulomatous and infectious processes of bone have been reported in association with Crohn's disease. Synovial, muscle, and bone biopsies in some patients with this disease have revealed pathologic findings similar to those in the gut[70, 71, 205, 271-273] (Fig. 31–11). These reports emphasize what may be a very rare manifestation of the disease, which can lead to joint space narrowing and to subchondral and distant osseous erosion.[199] In such cases, persistent monoarticular involvement is encountered more typically, which differs from the mild, migrating, asymmetric polyarthritis that is characteristic of enteropathic arthropathy in general. Osteomyelitis and septic arthritis in the hip, lumbar

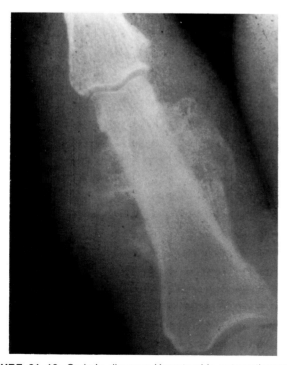

FIGURE 31–10. Crohn's disease: Hypertrophic osteoarthropathy. Striking periostitis and soft tissue swelling can be noted in the diaphyses of the proximal and middle phalanges of the second finger. The bones in other digits as well as the forearms and lower portions of the legs were affected. (Courtesy of M. Dalinka, M.D., Philadelphia, Pennsylvania.)

spine, sacrum, and hemipelvis (usually the right side) have been recorded in persons with Crohn's disease, perhaps related to spread of infection from a diseased gut into a psoas abscess and from there into the adjacent bones and joints.[72, 73, 300–302] Clinically, the diagnosis of septic arthritis of the hip in patients with Crohn's disease is difficult, although a persistent flexion deformity and a fluctuant mass in the inguinal region are important diagnostic signs.[303] Radiographic examination may reveal enlargement of the psoas muscle or adjacent soft tissue gas.

Although an abscess of the psoas muscle is an infrequent complication of Crohn's disease, its prevalence being approximately 3 to 5 per cent, reports have emphasized this occurrence,[200–202] and some investigators regard Crohn's disease as the leading cause of psoas abscesses. The proximity of a portion of the right psoas muscle to the terminal ileum and of the left psoas muscle to the sigmoid colon and jejunum provides the anatomic explanation for this complication. As plain films reveal only indirect findings of a psoas abscess, such as asymmetry of the musculature, radiolucent collections of gas, and calcification, CT is the diagnostic technique of choice.

Osteonecrosis in Crohn's disease probably is attributable to steroid medication.[74] This complication, however, is reported rarely. Atlantoaxial subluxation also has been noted.[293]

In children and adolescents, both Crohn's disease and ulcerative colitis can lead to retarded skeletal maturation and decreased linear growth.[75, 76] The reported frequency of retardation of stature in larger series of patients has ranged from 5 to 25 per cent.[75, 77, 78] Furthermore, skeletal osteopenia can be seen in patients with chronic inflammatory bowel disease.[79] In adolescents, mineralization indices that were less than 90 per cent of normal have been found in as many as 70 per cent of patients. The degree of osteopenia correlates well with retardation of both linear growth and skeletal maturation and is greater in patients with Crohn's disease than in those with other types of inflammatory bowel disease.[79] Factors that may be responsible for this exaggerated osteopenia are malnutrition, malabsorption, chronic inflammation, and administration of corticosteroids. Fractures of vertebral bodies, femora, tarsal bones, and ribs have been observed.[206]

Differential Diagnosis

The radiographic abnormalities in the peripheral joints in patients with Crohn's disease lack specificity. Soft tissue swelling and osteoporosis are observed, but permanent cartilaginous and osseous changes are indeed unusual. Thus, the findings can simulate the early changes of rheumatoid arthritis or other synovial diseases; however, the presence of joint space narrowing and erosions virtually eliminates the diagnosis of enteropathic arthritis.

The axial skeletal abnormalities in this disease cannot be differentiated from those of classic ankylosing spondylitis or the spondylitis of ulcerative colitis. The presence of bilateral and symmetric sacroiliac joint changes and syndesmophytosis of the spine is typical of these disorders. Although the prevalence of isolated or predominant articular abnormalities of the sacroiliac joints without spinal disease may be higher in Crohn's disease than in classic ankylosing spondylitis, the value of this sign is questionable. Asym-

metric or unilateral sacroiliac joint alterations and broad asymmetric spinal outgrowths are not features of enteropathic spondylitis but are apparent in psoriasis and Reiter's syndrome.

WHIPPLE'S DISEASE
General Abnormalities

Whipple's disease (intestinal lipodystrophy) is a rare progressive disorder affecting predominantly men in the fourth and fifth decades of life (male-to-female ratio is approximately 10 to 1) and leading to fever, weight loss, lymphadenopathy, peripheral edema, hypotension, brown pigmentation of the skin, polyserositis, and polyarthritis. It was described first by Whipple in 1907[80] and subsequently by a number of other investigators.[81–83] Pathologically, the major feature is the accumulation of periodic acid–Schiff (PAS)-positive inclusions in the macrophages of the lamina propria of the small intestine, lymph nodes, and other tissues. The cause of the disease appears to be related to a bacterial organism, as rod-shaped bacilli have been identified microscopically in these macrophages as well as in the synovial membranes.[294] The specific bacterium has not been identified, however, nor has the disease been reproduced in animals. In the past, Whipple's disease usually was fatal, although currently antibiotic therapy can effect a cure.

Musculoskeletal manifestations are an important feature of the disease. These manifestations can be divided into peripheral joint arthralgia and arthritis; sacroiliitis and spondylitis; and miscellaneous abnormalities.

Peripheral Joint Arthralgia and Arthritis

Acute migratory episodic arthralgia and arthritis are apparent in 60 to 90 per cent of patients with Whipple's disease.[81, 84–86] These findings may antedate other changes of Whipple's disease by 1 year to as many as 35 years,[81, 85] leading to difficulty in diagnosis. With the onset of gastrointestinal findings, the pattern of arthritis generally remains unaltered, although occasionally joint symptoms and signs may decrease in intensity.[87] Articular abnormalities usually are transient, lasting hours to days. The findings generally subside and subsequently recur after periods of remission of variable length. Residual joint deformities are rare.

Involvement of most joints in the appendicular skeleton has been described. Characteristically, the ankles, the knees, the shoulders, and the wrists are affected, although other sites that may be altered include the elbows, the hips, and the small joints of the hands and feet. Polyarthritis is more frequent than monoarthritis.

Clinical findings include mild to severe joint pain, swelling, warmth, and restrictive motion. Stiffness usually is not a prominent manifestation of the disease. Laboratory analysis reveals negative results for LE cell preparations and serologic tests for rheumatoid factor. Hypoalbuminemia, hypocalcemia, and anemia are nonspecific findings that are observed frequently. Synovial fluid is not markedly abnormal.[85] In addition, examination of the synovial membrane may demonstrate a mild nonspecific synovitis with hyperplasia of the synovial lining, increase in vascularity in the subendothelial tissues, and lymphocytic infiltration about small blood vessels.[85] In some cases, considerable inflammatory changes in the synovial membrane resemble the findings of septic arthritis.[88] Histiocytic infiltration within the membrane and PAS-positive granules may be apparent[85, 88] (Fig. 31–12). Synovial biopsy therefore has the potential to provide early and accurate diagnosis of Whipple's disease. Amyloid deposits also have been documented in Whipple's disease with this biopsy procedure.[214]

Autopsy data regarding joint disease are limited.[84, 89–91] Various descriptions of articular pathologic changes have included "degenerative changes,"[91] "nonspecific synovitis,"[85] and macrophages and cytoplasmic particles containing PAS-positive material.[92, 327]

Radiographic examination of involved peripheral joints may yield entirely normal results.[93–96] Soft tissue swelling, osteoporosis, and joint space narrowing occasionally are evident[81, 86, 97] (Fig. 31–12). These findings are most common in the metacarpophalangeal and metatarsophalangeal joints, the wrist, the ankle, the hip, and the knee. Although osseous erosion and osteophyte formation are indeed rare, several reports have documented significant radiographic abnormalities, especially in the hips.[207–209] Diffuse loss of joint space, osteophytosis, and large cystic lesions of bone are the observed alterations. As some of the patients with such hip involvement also have sacroiliitis and spondylitis,[207, 208] it should be noted that the abnormalities of the hip are not unlike those associated with classic ankylosing spondylitis. In one report, however, destruction of the hip occurred in the absence of spine and sacroiliac joint involvement, and eventually an arthroplasty was required.[209] Examination of the synovial membrane by electron microscopy in this patient revealed rod-shaped microorganisms similar in morphology to those known to occur in Whipple's disease. In another person with this disease, severe articular destruction in the wrist was observed.[210] In this case and in others,[207] resolution of the joint manifestations has been noted after the administration of tetracycline.

Sacroiliitis and Spondylitis

Sacroiliitis and spondylitis have been described in patients with Whipple's disease[81, 82, 86, 96, 98–100, 212] (Figs. 31–13 and 31–14). The exact frequency of these abnormalities is not known, although in their review of the literature, Kelly and Weisiger[86] noted spinal or sacroiliac joint changes in 18 of 94 patients with Whipple's disease. All of these 18 patients were men, and each had peripheral arthritis as well. In two patients, bilateral osseous fusion of the sacroiliac joints was observed, whereas one patient revealed unilateral ankylosis of this joint. Scintigraphy can confirm the involvement of the sacroiliac joint.[213] In most cases, spinal and sacroiliac joint alterations resemble those of classic ankylosing spondylitis. Syndesmophytes and narrowing, sclerosis, and osseous ankylosis of apophyseal joints have been noted.[101, 102] Test results for HLA-B27 antigen may be negative[96, 211] or positive.[102] Approximately one quarter to one third of patients with Whipple's disease have been reported to possess the HLA-B27 antigen.[211, 304] Data suggest that this antigen is associated with Whipple's disease even in the absence of spondylitis and sacroiliitis.[304]

Miscellaneous Abnormalities

Subcutaneous nodules, particularly on extensor surfaces of the extremities, have been evident in some patients with joint symptoms.[86, 103, 189] Additional manifestations that have been reported are clubbing of the fingers,[86] reflex sympathetic dystrophy syndrome,[100] and myalgias.[85, 104]

Etiology and Pathogenesis

The cause and pathogenesis of articular manifestations in Whipple's disease are not precisely known.[102] At present the most likely explanation relates the findings of the appendicular skeleton to bacterial colonization of the synovial membrane, a theory that is supported by the observation of PAS-positive macrophages[96, 105] and bacteria[105, 106] in synovial tissue. The cause of axial joint abnormalities in this disease is less clear.

Differential Diagnosis

The peripheral joint abnormalities in Whipple's disease are entirely nonspecific on radiographic evaluation. In the axial skeleton, sacroiliac joint and spinal changes, when present, are identical to those of classic ankylosing spondylitis and the spondylitis of ulcerative colitis and Crohn's disease. Although clinical features permit separation of these disorders, the radiographic changes do not allow accurate differential diagnosis.

INTESTINAL INFECTIONS AND REACTIVE ARTHRITIS

A variety of infectious agents can initiate or trigger a synovial reaction at one or more sites distant to the area of infection. The phenomenon, which is unrelated to direct contamination of the joint, is referred to as reactive arthritis and is a well-known occurrence in acute rheumatic fever. In this situation, a streptococcal throat infection initiates an arthritis (or even a carditis), but the bacteria cannot be recovered from the joint (or the heart).[215] The term reactive arthritis also can be applied to the articular manifestations in some patients with Reiter's syndrome[218] (see Chapter 30) as well as in patients with enteropathic arthritis complicating ulcerative colitis and Crohn's disease. Certain genetic factors, such as the presence of HLA-B27 antigen, appear to impart a susceptibility to reactive arthritis in some persons.[216, 329] As summarized by Goldenberg,[215] an immune-mediated response to an antigenic component of an infectious agent also may trigger the articular inflammation. The antigen might itself be localized to the joint or may circulate in immune complexes that subsequently are deposited in the synovial membrane, where they lead to inflammatory change. Viral hepatitis is an example of a disease in which the latter mechanism appears to be operational (see later discussion). Lyme arthritis may be an additional example in which an antigen-mediated immune response to an infectious agent (a spirochete) occurs (see Chapter 66).

Inman[294] outlined four possible mechanisms by which an enteric infectious agent could initiate or perpetuate articular inflammation: (1) altered bowel anatomy (example: the intestinal bypass syndrome); (2) autoimmunity due to molecular mimicry (examples: postdysenteric reactive arthritis and ankylosing spondylitis); (3) altered bowel permeability (examples: inflammatory bowel disorders, milk allergy, and celiac disease); and (4) toxin-mediated synovitis (example: pseudomembranous enterocolitis). In a more recent edito-

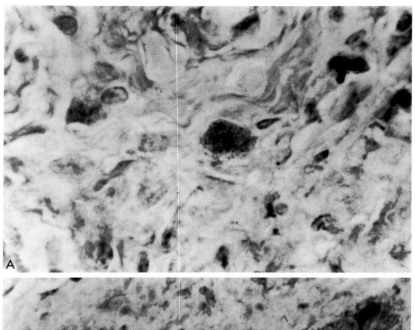

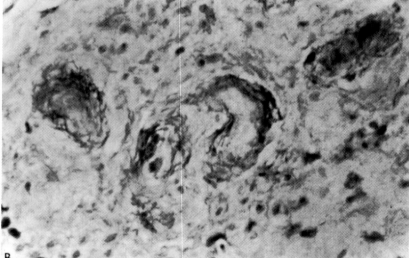

FIGURE 31–12. Whipple's disease: Peripheral joint abnormalities.

A A synovial biopsy in a patient with Whipple's disease reveals cellular infiltration with histiocytes containing periodic acid–Schiff-positive material.

B In a different area, perivascular fibrosis is observed.

(**A, B,** From Delcambre B, et al: Sem Hôp Paris *50:*847, 1974.)

C, D Observe bilateral joint space narrowing and osseous cysts.

(**C, D,** From LeChevallier P, et al: Rev Rhum Mal Osteoartic *43:*663, 1976.)

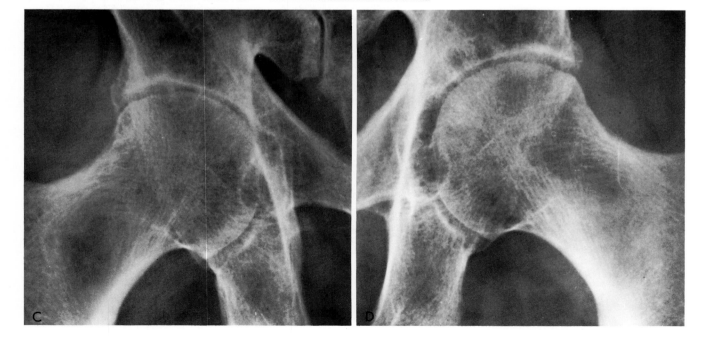

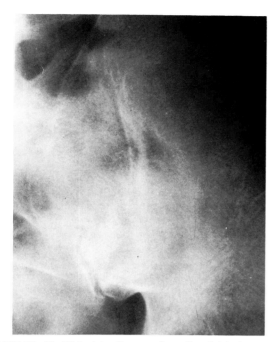

FIGURE 31–13. Whipple's disease: Sacroiliac joint abnormalities. This 50 year old man had a 10 year history of polyarthralgias and a 1 year history of steatorrhea. Lymph node and gastric biopsy confirmed the diagnosis of Whipple's disease. The sacroiliac joint reveals narrowing and sclerosis, predominantly in the ilium. The opposite side was affected similarly.

rial, Phillips[305] cited a number of investigations that supported the third of these possible mechanisms, altered bowel permeability. These investigations provided strong evidence that microbes do persist locally in joints of patients with reactive arthritis and Reiter's syndrome. The change in permeability of the bowel could allow direct in situ antigen deposition. Indeed, studies employing ileocolonoscopy in persons with reactive arthritis have confirmed a definite relationship between the extent of gut inflammation and that of articular inflammation.[306] Also, it has been reported that the presence of HLA-Bw62 could predispose to the clinical picture of reactive arthritis and that this histocompatibility antigen might serve as an indicator of chronic gut inflammation.[307]

General clinical characteristics of reactive arthritis include a symptom-free interval between the initiation of infection and the rheumatic reaction; a self-limited clinical course, usually associated with the acute onset of a migratory polyarthritis and fever; a tendency in some patients toward involvement of the heart; and a negative serologic test for rheumatoid factor.[217] Although the location of the inciting infection varies, three portals of entry are most typical: the oronasopharynx (e.g., tonsillitis, dental infection), the urogenital tract (e.g., urethritis), and the intestinal tract.[217]

Seronegative sterile arthritis may follow intestinal infections related to Salmonella, Shigella, Yersinia, or Campylobacter organisms. These enteric pathogens share the fea-

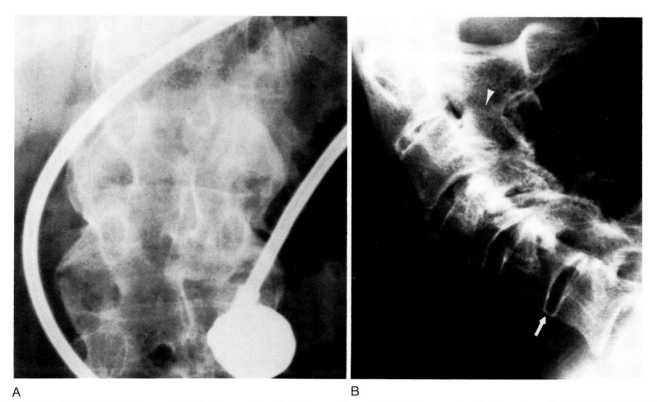

A   B

FIGURE 31–14. Whipple's disease: Spinal abnormalities. A 57 year old man had had recurrent arthritis and uveitis for 34 years, spinal symptoms for 10 years, and malabsorption for 4 months. HLA-B27 testing was positive.
  A A frontal radiograph of the upper lumbar spine confirms the presence of syndesmophytosis.
  B In the cervical spine, anterior syndesmophytes (arrow) and apophyseal joint ankylosis (arrowhead) are evident. (**B,** From Canuso JJ, Saini M: J Rheumatol *5:*79, 1978.)

tures of mucosal involvement[274] and, with the exception of Shigella, lymph node involvement and bacteremia.[219] The frequency of arthritis in patients following Salmonella or Shigella infection is 1 to 2 per cent[10, 107]; that following Yersinia infection may be as high as 30 per cent.[108] The reactive arthritis complicating Salmonella infection typically is an acute asymmetric or symmetric migratory polyarthritis that begins 1 to 2 weeks after the initial infection; it is self-limited, generally subsiding over a period of weeks to months.[109, 185, 310] The knee, the ankle, and the wrist are involved most commonly, although any articulation can be affected. Swelling and tenderness of the joints are characteristic, with erythema being less prominent. Malaise, intermittent fever, and weight loss often accompany the period of arthritis.[220] The articular fluid usually is serous, and cultures of it as well as of the blood are uniformly negative. Both *Salmonella typhimurium* and *Salmonella enteritidis* have been cultured from the stool.[220] Although these two microorganisms are implicated most frequently, many different causative Salmonella species may be recovered from the stool in patients with reactive arthritis, including *S. abony, S. blockley, S. haifa, S. heidelberg, S. manila, S. singapore, S. newport,* and *S. schwarzengrund.*[308, 309] As with the arthritis accompanying Yersinia and Shigella infection, patients with Salmonella-induced reactive arthritis frequently possess the HLA-B27 antigen. The frequency of the HLA-B7 antigen also may be increased in such patients.[310] Although the arthritis can simulate the findings in rheumatoid arthritis, its self-limited nature and its occurrence in patients with a history of abdominal pain, fever, and diarrhea are characteristic.

Shigella flexneri has been the inciting organism in virtually all patients with post-Shigella reactive arthritis,[219] although there is some evidence that implicates *S. sonnei* as a cause of reactive arthritis.[311]

In patients with Yersinia infection, recurrent and more prolonged arthritis occasionally may be apparent.[221–223, 275] This can be confused with rheumatic fever, particularly as carditis can accompany the arthritis of *Yersinia enterocolitica* infection.[108] Oligoarticular involvement of large and small joints, which occasionally persists for approximately 1 to 3 months, is typical of the self-limited acute phase.[221] In persistent arthritis, the knee is affected most frequently. Although adults typically are involved, reports exist of post-Yersinia arthritis in children.[224] *Yersinia enterocolitica* or, less commonly, *Yersinia pseudotuberculosis* is implicated.[312] Of interest, *Yersinia enterocolitica* has been demonstrated in the synovial membrane by indirect immunofluorescence in some patients with reactive arthritis and Yersinia infection of the gastrointestinal tract.[313] In other patients with such enteritis and arthritis, Yersinia-specific immune complexes have been demonstrated in the synovial fluid.[314, 315] Rarely, patients with articular involvement after Yersinia infection later develop seropositive rheumatoid arthritis,[222] although the existence of a definite association between the two diseases is debated.[223]

Reactive arthritis also is associated with *Campylobacter jejuni* infection.[226–231] Clinical manifestations resemble those associated with the other infectious diseases mentioned previously. The disorder affects predominantly males, and the ages of the patients vary widely. Asymmetrically distributed oligoarthritis affects the ankles, knees, wrists, and shoulders. Reiter's syndrome occasionally is noted after Campylobacter infection.[232, 233]

It is to be expected that additional infective processes of the gastrointestinal tract can be associated with reactive arthritis.[276–278] In this regard, patients with acute oligoarthritis associated with pseudomembranous colitis due to *Clostridium difficile* have been described.[234, 316] Arthritis also has been detected in patients with antibiotic-induced pseudomembranous colitis. In this situation, migratory articular inflammation is apparent at the time of severe diarrhea and subsides with resolution of the diarrhea.[240, 241] Chronic polyarthritis (as well as spondyloarthropathy) in patients with collagenous colitis also is reported.[269, 325, 330]

The various forms of sterile arthritis can be associated with soft tissue swelling and joint effusions, but other radiographic features generally are lacking. Rarely erosive bone changes are seen.[230] After bowel disease due to Yersinia, sacroiliitis and spondylitis have been noted.[110] In this regard, it is significant that approximately 90 per cent of patients in whom sterile arthritis develops after bowel infection with Salmonella, Shigella, or Yersinia organisms have the HLA-B27 antigen.[111, 225] Possibly, enteric infections also may lead to exacerbation of previously established spondyloarthropathies in patients who possess this antigen.[235]

A true septic arthritis is a definite and serious complication of Salmonella infection, particularly in children.[112] Monoarticular disease is apparent and can lead to cartilaginous and osseous destruction. The knee, shoulder, and hip are the joints involved most frequently.[220] Compared with staphylococcal arthritis, septic arthritis caused by Salmonella infection is less damaging and of brief duration.[220] *Yersinia enterocolitica* infection also has been associated with septic arthritis[236] as well as osteomyelitis[237] and psoas muscle abscess.[238]

ARTHROPATHY AFTER INTESTINAL BYPASS SURGERY

Intestinal bypass surgery has been performed for many years for the treatment of intractable obesity. Rheumatologic manifestations in the postoperative period include polymyalgia, polyarthralgia, acute or subacute arthritis, and tenosynovitis.[113–121, 183, 190, 317] The prevalence of these manifestations in patients undergoing such surgery is approximately 20 to 30 per cent. The symptoms and signs usually are transient, although occasionally they can persist and become incapacitating. They generally develop within 2 years after surgical intervention and resolve within 1 to 2 years. If severe, clinical manifestations of articular involvement may require that the normal anatomic sequence of the gut be restored surgically, a procedure that can relieve the arthritic complaints.[242] In this regard, it has been observed that simple revision of the length of the blind loop of bowel produces only a temporary relief of arthritic symptoms, whereas complete dismantlement of the blind loop by total anastomosis leads to complete and permanent disappearance of the arthritis.[245]

Symmetric polyarthritis is the rule. Articular involvement is most frequent in the knees, the ankles, the fingers, and the wrists. Radiographic evaluation demonstrates soft tissue swelling and osteoporosis. Rarely, osseous erosions can be evident.[282] More recently, sacroiliitis and spondylitis have been observed in patients undergoing jejunocolic type by-pass procedures who were followed up for a long period of time[115] (Fig. 31–15). Typical radiographic findings include erosions, sclerosis, and articular space narrowing at the sacroiliac joint and syndesmophytes of the spine. HLA-B27 antigen may be detected in patients with this axial joint involvement.

The cause and pathogenesis of arthropathy after intestinal bypass procedures have not been delineated clearly. Metabolic disturbances attributable simply to rapid weight reduction are unlikely to be a major factor, as articular symptoms and signs generally are absent in patients who lose weight rapidly in the absence of intestinal bypass surgery.[242] In some patients, cryoprecipitates containing antibodies to enteric organisms and complement components have been found to be associated temporarily with the arthritis.[113, 186, 187] This discovery led to the speculation that bacterial overgrowth in the bypassed loops of bowel caused absorption of bacterial antigens and the formation of circulating immune complexes. Some studies have failed to document specific immunologic abnormalities, however.[178, 244]

Apparently, the type of bowel surgery influences the pattern and distribution of arthritis. Initially, jejunocolic anastomoses were used, creating a large blind loop containing small bowel and ascending colon. Most reports of articular complaints after this type of anastomosis emphasized the role of colonic stasis. More recently, jejunoileal shunts have been advocated as a more physiologic type of operation. This type of surgery, too, can be associated with polyarthralgia and polyarthritis,[116, 242–244] confirming that colonic abnormalities are not necessary for the development of the rheumatologic manifestations. Articular changes occurring after the jejunoileal type of surgery may be different from those that follow jejunocolic anastomoses; in the former situation, large joints are affected more commonly, arthritis is of lesser duration, tenosynovitis generally is not apparent, and radiographic features usually are absent.

Additional radiographic findings seen after intestinal bypass surgery include gout,[10] osteomalacia, and osteoporosis.[118, 177, 191, 281]

Accompanying the musculoskeletal symptoms, a spectrum of cutaneous vasculitis, including urticaria and pustular necrosis affecting epidermis to subcutis, has been noted[243]; paresthesias, Raynaud's phenomenon, and pericarditis also may be evident. Immune complex deposits have been identified in biopsy samples of the skin lesions.[243] This latter finding supports the theory that emphasizes the importance of immune complexes in the pathogenesis of the arthritis, and it binds together the articular and cutaneous abnormalities in the form of an arthritis-dermatitis syndrome.[243, 244, 279] This same syndrome has been described in association with other gastrointestinal diseases, such as colitis and diverticulosis,[246] and other surgical procedures, such as gastric resection[280] and Roux-en-Y jejunostomy.[247] It appears, therefore, that bypass surgery is not an absolute prerequisite for the appearance of this syndrome, and that the disorder is similar or identical to others that accompany such diseases as ulcerative colitis and Crohn's disease. The term bowel-associated dermatosis–arthritis syndrome may be more appropriate.[246]

LAENNEC'S CIRRHOSIS

Inflammatory polyarthritis can occur in patients with Laennec's cirrhosis during the recovery period, when the liver function tests are showing improvement.[119] Most commonly, the shoulders, the elbows, and the knees are affected. Clinical findings include pain, swelling, tenderness, and limitation of motion. Radiographs reveal osteoporosis and a possible proclivity to develop calcific periarthritis. The condition appears self-limited, improvement usually occurring within 1 year. The pathogenesis of these arthritic alterations is unknown.

PRIMARY BILIARY CIRRHOSIS
General Abnormalities

Primary biliary cirrhosis is a rare disorder of unknown cause affecting women almost exclusively.[122–124] Clinical

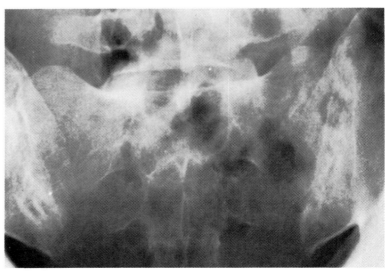

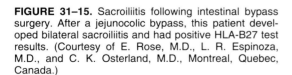

FIGURE 31–15. Sacroiliitis following intestinal bypass surgery. After a jejunocolic bypass, this patient developed bilateral sacroiliitis and had positive HLA-B27 test results. (Courtesy of E. Rose, M.D., L. R. Espinoza, M.D., and C. K. Osterland, M.D., Montreal, Quebec, Canada.)

findings include the insidious onset of jaundice, pruritus, hepatomegaly, and abnormal liver function. The diagnosis is confirmed by the presence of antimitochondrial antibodies and characteristic findings on liver biopsy.[125–127] Primary biliary cirrhosis has been associated with a number of other autoimmune diseases, including renal tubular acidosis,[128] scleroderma,[129] Sjögren's syndrome,[130] systemic lupus erythematosus,[127] and fibrosing alveolitis.[128]

Rheumatologic Manifestations

Osseous and articular manifestations are detected in some patients with biliary cirrhosis. Musculoskeletal complaints can relate to osteomalacia and osteoporosis, arthralgias or arthritis,[319, 320] hypertrophic osteoarthropathy, or the coexistence of a connective tissue disease such as scleroderma or Sjögren's syndrome. Osteomalacia and osteoporosis[123, 131–133, 253, 292] in this disorder probably are due to a combination of steatorrhea, cholestasis, and hepatic dysfunction. Hypercholesterolemia can lead to xanthoma formation. These cholesterol deposits can appear in soft tissues and in subperiosteal and intramedullary sites. Associated radiographic findings include nodular soft tissue masses, subperiosteal erosion of bone, and cystic lesions.[122, 133]

Of particular interest is the appearance of erosive arthritis of the hands and wrists in patients with primary biliary cirrhosis[133, 180, 251] (Fig. 31–16). Erosions are distributed predominantly in an asymmetric fashion in distal interphalangeal and proximal interphalangeal joints, with relative sparing of the metacarpophalangeal joints noted in some reports. The erosions are well defined, of varying size, and marginal in location. Articular cartilage loss with joint space narrowing also can be seen. Deformities are absent. Clinical findings generally are mild, perhaps related to the presence of jaundice, which may suppress the articular symptoms.[134] Serologic tests for rheumatoid factor generally yield negative results, although some studies have indicated that 25 per cent of patients have detectable circulating rheumatoid factor.[135] Rheumatoid arthritis itself has been reported in 5 to 10 per cent of patients.[179, 248]

The pathogenesis of these erosive changes is not known. It is attractive to attribute some of them to cholesterol deposition, but convincing pathologic documentation of such deposition is lacking. Chronic synovitis can be detected on synovial biopsy in some cases,[133] suggesting that erosive arthritis in this condition may be the result of a low grade inflammatory condition of the synovium analogous, perhaps, to the synovitis that occurs in some patients with chronic active hepatitis. In some respects, the osseous abnormalities of the hand in primary biliary cirrhosis resemble those in hyperparathyroidism,[136, 251] suggesting that parathyroid hyperfunction due to malabsorption could be a contributing factor. Calcium pyrophosphate dihydrate (CPPD) crystal deposition could be an additional factor in the production of synovitis in this condition, as chondrocalcinosis has been noted in patients with primary biliary cirrhosis.[133, 192]

A destructive arthropathy also has been reported in some patients with primary biliary cirrhosis[137, 252] (Fig. 31–17). Fragmentation, collapse, and disintegration of bone in the hips and glenohumeral joints resemble the findings of osteonecrosis, although steroid medication cannot be implicated in all cases. The association of liver disease and osteonecrosis has been reported previously, however, per-

haps explaining the appearance of destructive arthropathy in primary biliary cirrhosis.

The association of hypertrophic osteoarthropathy and primary biliary cirrhosis is debatable, although periostitis occasionally is recorded.[133] In fact, some reports have indicated that periosteal new bone occurs in 35 to 40 per cent of patients with this disease.[250, 251] The tibia, fibula, and metacarpal bones have been cited as areas revealing periostitis. Associated clinical findings generally are lacking,[251] although digital clubbing may be apparent.

The coexistence of scleroderma in some persons with primary biliary cirrhosis can lead to additional osteoarticular findings, including acro-osteolysis and periarticular calcification.[137] The reported prevalence of this collagen vascular disease in patients with primary biliary cirrhosis has varied from 0 to 17 per cent.[127, 137–140, 179, 188] The complete CRST syndrome (calcinosis cutis, Raynaud's phenomenon, sclerodactyly, and telangiectasia) has been noted in 2 to 5 per cent of patients with primary biliary cirrhosis.[249] Rarely, patients are described who have both primary biliary cirrhosis and systemic lupus erythematosus.[318]

VIRAL HEPATITIS

Articular manifestations can occur during the course of hepatitis B (serum hepatitis) and, less commonly, hepatitis A (infectious hepatitis).[141–143, 254, 255] A symmetric polyarticular pattern of joint disease is observed, which most commonly involves the hands, the wrists, the elbows, the knees, and the ankles. Spinal involvement is rare. Clinical findings include pain and stiffness, which may persist from a few days to more than 1 month, and which may decrease as jaundice develops. Joint tenderness and pain produced by palpation of bone prominences are observed. Transient low grade fever and skin rash are evident in approximately 25 per cent of patients. The skin lesions and joint symptoms resolve simultaneously.[255] Subcutaneous nodules have been recorded, particularly in the forearms and wrists.[141, 144] Joint destruction and deformity are not seen. The cause of articular findings in viral hepatitis has not been determined, although it may relate to circulating antigen-antibody complexes activating the complement system, resulting in a serum sickness syndrome. Inspection of joint fluid may reveal low complement levels, and viral antigen is detectable by immunoelectrophoresis. Deposits of immunoglobulins, complement, and certain antigens are demonstrated during histologic evaluation of synovial biopsy material.[255]

CHRONIC ACTIVE HEPATITIS

Chronic hepatitis, defined as liver disease that has persisted for longer than 6 months, can occur secondary to a variety of processes, such as hepatitis B virus infection, Wilson's disease, and drug therapy, or on an idiopathic basis, affecting predominantly young women (Fig. 31–18). In the latter situation, multisystem organ involvement is frequent.[256] Articular abnormalities in chronic active hepatitis typically consist of acute-onset, transient, or recurring migratory arthralgia affecting large joints such as the knees, ankles, wrists, and elbows.[249] Erythema, soft tissue swelling, and, rarely, joint effusions are seen. Serologic tests for rheumatoid factor and antinuclear factor commonly are positive, and results of radiologic examination usually are un-

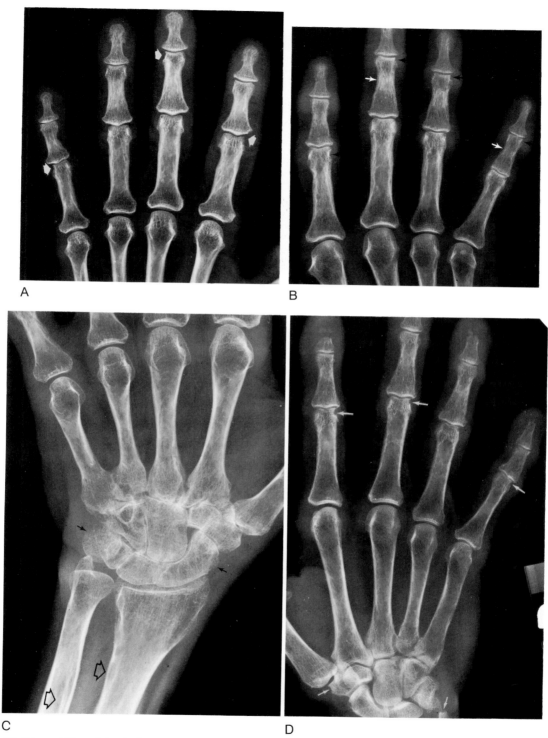

FIGURE 31–16. Primary biliary cirrhosis: Peripheral joint abnormalities.

A A 62 year old woman who had no arthritic symptoms. Note the small marginal erosions in the proximal interphalangeal and distal interphalangeal joints (arrows).

B A 58 year old woman who revealed symmetric soft tissue swelling adjacent to the proximal interphalangeal and distal interphalangeal joints. Note the small marginal erosions at both these locations (dark arrows). Also observe that the bones are osteopenic, with subperiosteal resorption (light arrows). Early acro-osteolysis of the index finger can be seen.

C A 42 year old woman with synovitis of the knees, metacarpophalangeal, and proximal interphalangeal joints. Joint space narrowing can be detected in the midcarpal and common carpometacarpal compartments of the wrist. Lytic defects are visible in the distal portions of the radius and ulna (open arrows). Soft tissue swelling about the metacarpophalangeal joints and osseous erosions of the scaphoid and pisiform (solid arrows) are observed.

D A 39 year old woman, whose examination revealed cutaneous xanthomatosis in periarticular regions. The radiograph of the hand indicates generalized osteopenia, subperiosteal resorption of bone, acro-osteolysis, and marginal erosions of the proximal interphalangeal joints and carpal bones (arrows). Soft tissue swelling about the metacarpophalangeal joints also is apparent.

(From O'Connell DJ, Marx WJ: Radiology *129*:31, 1978.)

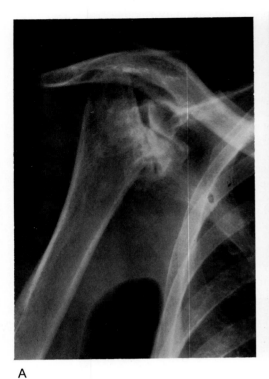

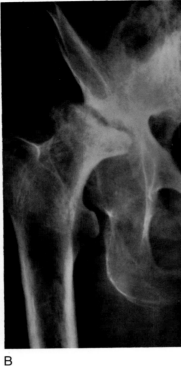

A

B

FIGURE 31–17. Primary biliary cirrhosis: Destructive arthropathy. Osseous collapse, flattening, sclerosis, and fragmentation associated with considerable narrowing of the interosseous space have been noted in patients with primary biliary cirrhosis. The changes are infrequent but can resemble osteonecrosis, calcium hydroxyapatite crystal deposition disease, or neuropathic osteoarthropathy. (From Clark AK, et al: Ann Rheum Dis *37*:42, 1978.)

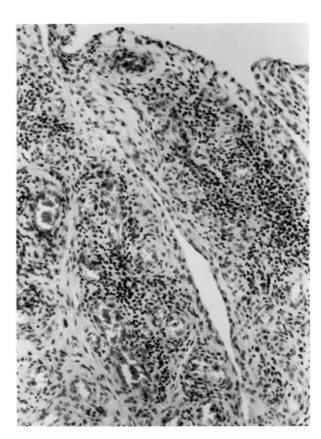

FIGURE 31–18. Chronic active hepatitis. This patient had a history of hepatitis B that had remained active. Progressive synovitis in the right shoulder became apparent. A synovial biopsy reveals hypervascularity and cellular infiltration, including plasma cells. Cultures were negative.

remarkable. In rare instances, bone erosion and periostitis are noted.[257]

PANCREATIC DISEASE

Fat Necrosis

Pancreatic disorders can be complicated by fat necrosis at multiple distant sites, resulting in subcutaneous nodular skin lesions, polyarthritis, and medullary fat necrosis.[145–149] These manifestations appear most frequently in older men in association with carcinoma of the pancreas,[150–154] although they also can occur with acute pancreatitis due to either abdominal trauma (including that related to the abused child syndrome)[155–158] or alcohol abuse,[159–161] pancreatic pseudocysts,[148, 151, 160] and pancreatic duct calculi.[149] The temporal relationship between the onset of articular findings and development of subcutaneous nodules and the onset of abdominal complaints is variable; in many patients, joint pain and nodules precede abdominal pain.[193, 321, 331] Such nodules and arthritis often occur together in a single patient; however, one finding may appear independent of the other.[332] Although the prognosis depends on the precise cause of the fat necrosis, for patients with pancreatic carcinoma and fat necrosis, it is dismal.[290]

The skin lesions resemble those of erythema nodosum[162] and frequently are tender. Nodules occur predominantly in the lower portions of the legs but may involve the upper extremities.[321] Articular abnormalities are characterized by a symmetric or asymmetric polyarthritis, which can be associated with pain, swelling, tenderness, warmth, and effusion. Predilection for the ankles, the elbows, the knees, the wrists, and the small joints of the hands and feet is seen. Reports of synovial fluid aspiration from involved joints or bursae[283] have described both inflammatory and noninflammatory changes. Fat globules may be apparent in the synovial fluid[148] or the periarticular tissue[158] (Fig. 31–19). One description of the synovial histologic features after biopsy of the membrane noted the presence of acute and chronic inflammatory cellular infiltration.[159] Another report has indicated that the synovial membrane also may be the site of fat necrosis and associated inflammatory reaction.[181] Radiographic findings related to joint disease are absent or minimal; osteoporosis and soft tissue swelling can be seen, but joint space narrowing and osseous erosion rarely are reported.[151]

Bone involvement can occur simultaneously with subcutaneous nodules and polyarthritis, or it can represent an isolated phenomenon. Osteolytic lesions with motheaten bone destruction and periostitis of the tubular bones of the extremities resemble findings of osteomyelitis or osteonecrosis (Figs. 31–20 and 31–21). These changes occur in the long bones of the extremities or in the small bones of the hands and feet, or in both locations. In the bones of the hands and feet, cystic defects and a coarsened trabecular

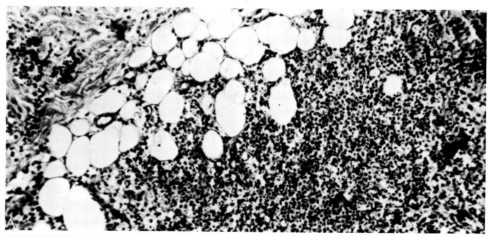

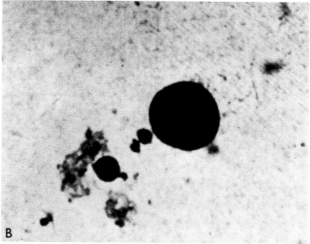

FIGURE 31–19. Pancreatic disease: Fat necrosis. Pathologic abnormalities.

A Subcutaneous fat. Observe cellular infiltration with polymorphonuclear leukocytes and lymphocytes (90×). (From Bennett RG, Petrozzi JW: Arch Derm *111:* 896, 1975. Copyright 1975, American Medical Association.)

B Synovial fluid. Fat globules are apparent (Sudan black, 800 ×). (From Gibson TJ, et al: J Rheumatol *2:*7, 1975.)

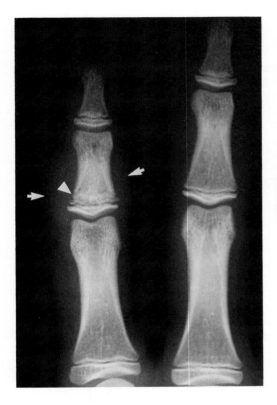

FIGURE 31–20. Pancreatic disease: Fat necrosis. Radiographic abnormalities. This child developed traumatic pancreatitis related to a karate injury. Observe soft tissue swelling (arrows) and metaphyseal destruction (arrowhead) in the middle phalanx of the second finger. The opposite hand was affected similarly.
(Courtesy of M. Alcarez, M.D., Madrid, Spain.)

pattern can be apparent, and the epiphyses may be unaffected. The lesions may heal, although residual periosteal reaction has been noted.[263] Scintigraphy using bone-seeking radiopharmaceutical agents sometimes documents more widespread involvement than is apparent on the radiographs.[264] In rare instances, severe and rapid osteolysis is seen.[265] MR imaging is sensitive to early changes of intraosseous fat necrosis, showing multiple foci of abnormal signal intensity[322] (Fig. 31–22).

Although the exact pathogenesis of the articular and osseous findings associated with pancreatic disorders has not been delineated accurately, it appears probable that widespread fat necrosis is responsible for these abnormalities.[148] Obstruction of pancreatic ducts by edema, calculi, or tumor or hormonal hypersecretion by acinar cell carcinomas[290] and functioning metastases can lead to release of excess circulating lipase into the bloodstream, which results in autodigestion of fat deposits at distant sites. A potential role of fat necrosis in inducing bone and joint abnormalities in patients with pancreatic disease is supported by observations that levels of lipase and amylase are elevated in these patients, that levels of these serum enzymes may correlate with clinical findings, that intra-articular free fatty acid concentration is elevated in patients with the pancreatitis-arthritis syndrome, that injection of free fatty acids into the knees of rabbits produces an inflammatory synovial response, and that widespread fat necrosis in dogs accompanies experimental pancreatitis.[148, 163, 261, 262] Furthermore, osseous and articular manifestations of Weber-Christian disease (relapsing nodular nonsuppurative panniculitis), a disorder characterized by widespread fat necrosis, resemble those of pancreatic disease, again emphasizing the importance of autodigestion of fat in the pathogenesis of bone

lysis and polyarthritis in carcinoma of the pancreas and pancreatitis.[164, 165, 266] In fact, some investigators speculate that Weber-Christian disease is a manifestation of pancreatic abnormality,[166] as many of the patients reported to have this disease have underlying pancreatitis or pancreatic carcinoma.

Osteonecrosis

Osteonecrosis is a recognized manifestation of pancreatic disease.[167] This complication most frequently is associated with chronic or inactive pancreatitis. Abnormalities of the femoral and humeral heads are typical, although diaphyseal and metaphyseal infarction in long tubular bones can simulate the changes in caisson workers (Fig. 31–23). Radiographically, epiphyseal involvement is characterized by mottled lysis and sclerosis, subchondral radiolucent areas, and partial or complete collapse of bone; diaphyseal and metaphyseal involvement, which is most frequent in the distal end of the femur and proximal portion of the tibia, is associated with radiolucency, calcification, and periosteal bone formation. Osteonecrosis also can be encountered in the small bones of the hands and feet[284] and in the axial skeleton in patients with pancreatic disorders.[182]

In patients with pancreatitis, a relationship of osteonecrosis to fat necrosis is not certain. Edema and increased pressure in the marrow cavity secondary to fat necrosis could lead to infarction by diminishing flow in small blood vessels; alternatively, pancreatic enzymes could damage vascular endothelium, producing thrombosis.[167] Embolization of fat globules to the medullary arterioles due to the hyperlipidemia that accompanies acute pancreatitis could be an additional contributing factor.

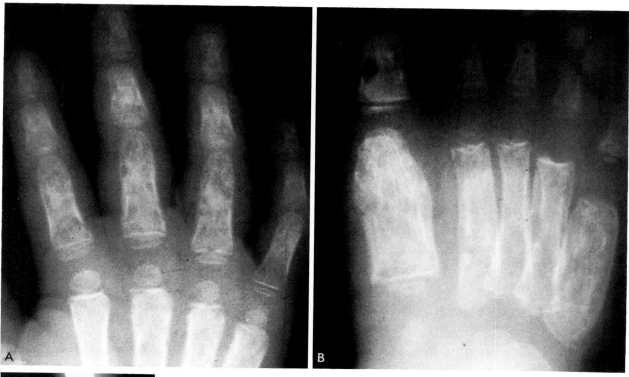

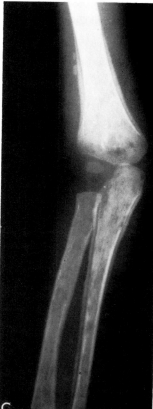

FIGURE 31–21. Pancreatic disease: Fat necrosis. Radiographic abnormalities. A 3 year old child fell off a moving truck and sustained a skull fracture and back trauma. Observe lytic defects of the metacarpals, phalanges, metatarsals, radius, ulna, and humerus with associated periostitis. Soft tissue swelling also is evident. (Courtesy of A. Brower, M.D., Norfolk, Virginia.)

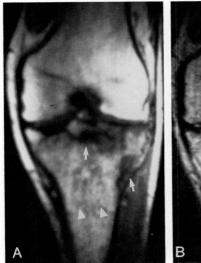
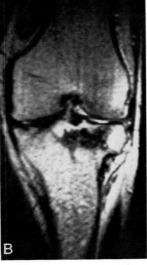

FIGURE 31–22. Pancreatic disease: Fat necrosis. MR imaging abnormalities. A 44 year old man with alcoholic pancreatitis developed joint swelling and subcutaneous nodules in the upper and lower extremities. Osteolysis was apparent at multiple sites, including the left tibia. A biopsy of a skin nodule confirmed the presence of fat necrosis.

A A coronal T1-weighted (TR/TE, 600/28) spin echo MR image shows inhomogeneous signal intensity in the metaphysis of the tibia (arrowheads). The adjacent epiphysis and a small portion of the metaphysis are characterized by decreased signal intensity (arrows).

B A coronal T2-weighted (TR/TE, 2025/120) spin echo MR image reveals considerable increase in signal intensity in the metaphysis and the epiphysis of the tibia, compatible with the presence of bone marrow edema and necrosis.

(Courtesy of G. Greenway, M.D., Dallas, Texas.)

Skeletal Metastasis

Osteolytic or osteoblastic lesions can occur in patients with skeletal metastasis from adenocarcinoma of the pancreas. The reported frequency of these changes has varied from 6 to 21 per cent.[168–171, 285] It has been suggested that carcinoma of the body and tail of the pancreas more commonly is associated with skeletal metastasis than carcinoma of the pancreatic head. Changes, particularly those that are osteoblastic in nature, are most common in the vertebral column.[172] Frequent involvement of the upper lumbar spine conceivably could indicate direct invasion of neoplasm rather than hematogenous spread in some patients with pancreatic carcinoma.[173–175]

Differential Diagnosis

The osseous changes of fat necrosis in patients with pancreatic disease simulate those of osteomyelitis and osteonecrosis. Lytic lesions and periostitis on radiographic examination and areas of increased radionuclide uptake on scintigraphic examination are common manifestations of these disorders. In fact, fat necrosis, osteonecrosis, and osteomyelitis can occur together in these patients. Although some reports have indicated the absence of periostitis in cases of intraosseous fat necrosis, the diagnostic value of this sign is questionable. The combination of osteolysis, periosteal bone formation, calcification of medullary bone, and epiphyseal osteonecrosis should stimulate a clinical investigation to exclude a pancreatic origin of these findings.

CARCINOID TUMORS

Intestinal and extraintestinal carcinoid tumors that are actively secreting serotonin produce widespread clinical abnormalities, including flushing, edema, and diarrhea. In unusual instances, arthralgias and arthritis are associated with peculiar radiographic alterations. In a report of five consecutive patients with the carcinoid syndrome, Plonk and Feldman[258] observed such alterations in four persons. Juxta-articular osteopenia, multiple cystic lesions in the phalan-

ges, and bone erosions were evident. In one patient, an equivocal region of subperiosteal resorption of bone was noted. These investigators suggested that serotonin may have directly affected the collagen in the small bones and joints of the hand. A more dramatic case of carcinoid arthropathy and osteopathy was described by Horwitz and Schachter.[259] Erosions of bone in juxta-articular locations in the hand and wrist were combined with osseous resorption and constriction of the phalangeal shafts (Fig. 31–24). The resulting radiographic image resembled that seen in hyperparathyroidism, although biochemical investigation made this latter diagnosis improbable. It is possible that the bone resorption evident in carcinoid osteopathy is mediated through the release of prostaglandins by the tumor or is related to inhibition of bone synthesis by histamine.[260]

OTHER DISEASES

Cystic fibrosis is associated with a transient arthritis that may involve one or more joints.[267, 324] Erythematous and purpuric skin rashes, erythema nodosum, and, in some cases, hypertrophic osteoarthropathy are additional abnormalities.[323, 324, 328] The clinical picture resembles that of the arthritis-dermatitis syndrome that follows jejunoileal bypass surgery.[268]

Juvenile gastrointestinal polyposis with or without pulmonary arteriovenous malformations may be associated with digital clubbing and hypertrophic osteoarthropathy[286] (Fig. 31–25). Digital clubbing also may relate to *laxative abuse.*[287]

Arthritis may accompany *celiac disease*[288, 291] and the *Cronkhite-Canada syndrome*[289] (Fig. 31–26).

SUMMARY

Musculoskeletal manifestations frequently are associated with disorders of the gastrointestinal system. Peripheral joint arthralgias and arthritis accompany ulcerative colitis, Crohn's disease, and Whipple's disease, although radiographic findings generally are minimal and nonspecific. In addition, these three disorders may be associated with sa-

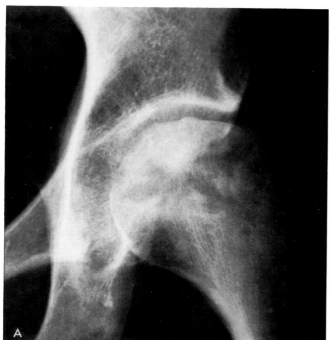

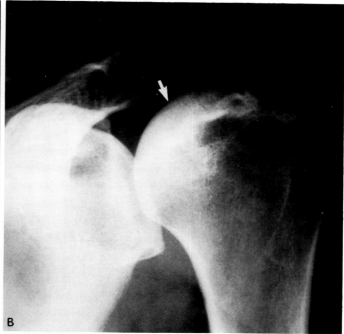

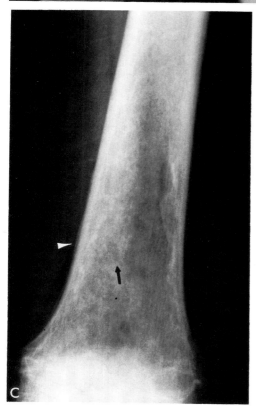

FIGURE 31–23. Pancreatic disease: Osteonecrosis.

A, B An alcoholic patient with a history of acute and chronic pancreatitis developed bone pain. Observe osteonecrosis of the femoral head with cystic lesions and bony collapse, and a typical "snow-cap" appearance (arrow) of the humeral head.

C In another patient with a similar history, obvious diaphyseal infarction of the distal portion of the femur is associated with calcification (arrow) and periostitis (arrowhead).

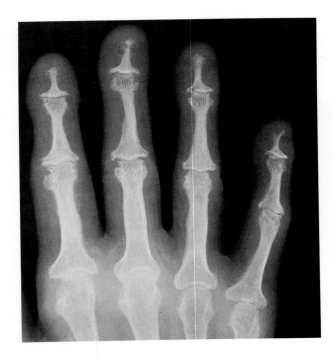

FIGURE 31–24. Carcinoid arthropathy. A 58 year old woman had a 10 year history of flushing and a 7 year history of diarrhea. An enlarged, nontender liver was palpable. Four years previously, a laparotomy had been performed with demonstration and excision of secondary carcinoid deposits in the liver. The site of the primary tumor was not identified. In recent years, the patient complained of increasing pain and stiffness in the metacarpophalangeal and interphalangeal joints of both hands. A radiograph shows resorption of the terminal tufts and marginal bone erosions about interphalangeal and metacarpophalangeal joints. Observe constriction of the shaft of middle and distal phalanges. The opposite hand was involved similarly, and less prominent abnormalities of the feet were evident. A skeletal survey was otherwise negative. (From Horwitz R, Schachter M: Br J Radiol *56*:131, 1983.)

croiliac and spinal abnormalities that are identical to those of classic ankylosing spondylitis. Intestinal infections related to Salmonella, Shigella, and Yersinia organisms can lead to polyarthritis and, in rare circumstances, sacroiliitis and spondylitis. Intestinal bypass surgery may provoke a similar response in joints of the appendicular and axial skeleton. Joint manifestations also accompany Laennec's cirrhosis, viral hepatitis, chronic active hepatitis, and biliary cirrhosis. In biliary cirrhosis, xanthomas and a peculiar type of erosive arthritis can be evident. Pancreatic disorders may become manifest as subcutaneous nodules, skin lesions, and polyarthritis, probably related to fat necrosis; epiphyseal and diametaphyseal infarction; and skeletal metastasis. Bone resorption in association with carcinoid tumors simulates the findings of hyperparathyroidism.

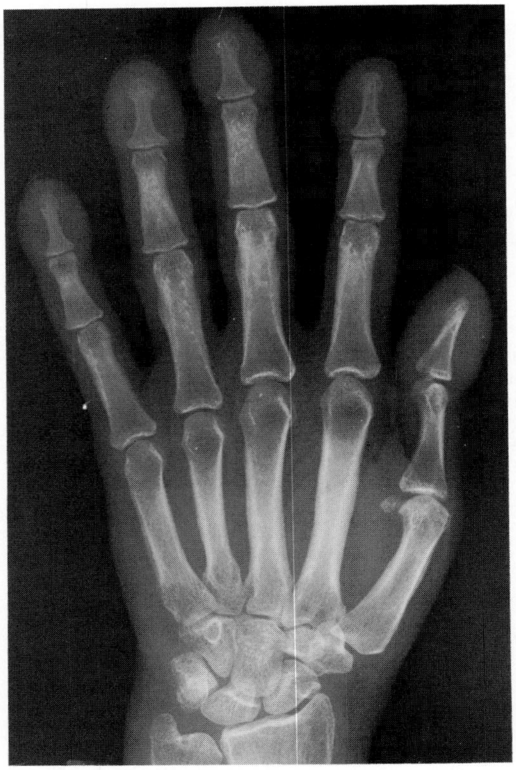

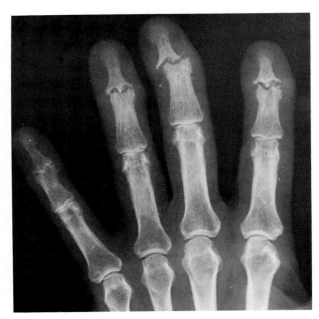

FIGURE 31–25. Juvenile gastrointestinal polyposis. This 14 year old girl, with histologic evidence of both juvenile and adenomatous polyps in the colon, developed digital clubbing. A radiograph of the hand shows extensive clubbing in all of the fingers and periostitis in the metacarpal bones and phalanges. Periosteal bone formation also was evident in other sites. (From Simpson EL, Dalinka MK: AJR *144*:983, 1985. Copyright 1985, American Roentgen Ray Society.)

FIGURE 31–26. Cronkhite-Canada syndrome. In a 72 year old man with hamartomatous gastrointestinal polyposis and alopecia, articular abnormalities correlated in clinical severity with that of his bowel disease. Extensive intra-articular bone erosions predominate in the distal interphalangeal joints. (From Sanders KM, et al: Radiology *156*:309, 1985.)

References

1. White WH: Colitis. Lancet *1:*537, 1895.
2. Bargen JA: Complications and sequelae of chronic ulcerative colitis. Ann Intern Med *3:*335, 1929.
3. Hench PS: Acute and Chronic Arthritis. Reprinted from Nelson's Loose-Leaf Surgery. New York, Thomas Nelson & Sons, 1935, p 104.
4. Short CL, Bauer W, Reynolds WE: Rheumatoid Arthritis. Cambridge, Harvard University Press, 1957, p 70.
5. Wright V, Watkinson G: The arthritis of ulcerative colitis. Br Med J *2:*670, 1965.
6. Fernandez-Herlihy L: The articular manifestations of chronic ulcerative colitis: An analysis of 555 cases. N Engl J Med *261:*259, 1959.
7. Bywaters EGL, Ansell BM: Arthritis associated with ulcerative colitis. A clinical and pathological study. Ann Rheum Dis *17:*169, 1958.
8. McEwen C, Lingg C, Kirsner JB: Arthritis accompanying ulcerative colitis. Am J Med *33:*923, 1962.
9. Wright V, Watkinson G: The arthritis of ulcerative colitis. Medicine *38:*243, 1959.
10. Ramer S, Bluestone R: Colitic arthropathies. Postgrad Med *61:*141, 1977.
11. Palumbo PJ, Ward LE, Sauer WG, et al: Musculoskeletal manifestations of inflammatory bowel disease. Ulcerative and granulomatous colitis and ulcerative proctitis. Mayo Clin Proc *48:*411, 1973.
12. Lindsley CB, Schaller JB: Arthritis associated with inflammatory bowel disease in children. J Pediatr *84:*16, 1974.
13. Clark RL, Muhletaler CA, Margulies SI: Colitic arthritis. Clinical and radiographic manifestations. Radiology *101:*585, 1971.
14. McEwen C: Arthritis accompanying ulcerative colitis. Clin Orthop *57:*9, 1968.
15. Haslock I: Enteropathic arthritis. *In* JT Scott (Ed): Copeman's Textbook of the Rheumatic Diseases. 5th Ed. Edinburgh, Churchill Livingstone, 1978, p 567.
16. Falchuck KR, Isselbacher KJ: Circulating antibodies to bovine albumin in ulcerative colitis and Crohn's disease. Gastroenterology *70:*5, 1976.
17. Thayer WR: Are the inflammatory bowel diseases immune complex diseases? Gastroenterology *70:*136, 1976.
18. Ford DK, Vallis DG: The clinical course of arthritis associated with ulcerative colitis and regional ileitis. Arthritis Rheum *2:*526, 1959.
19. Flood CA, Lepore MJ, Hiatt RB, et al: Prognosis in chronic ulcerative colitis. J Chron Dis *4:*267, 1956.
20. Acheson ED: An association between ulcerative colitis, regional enteritis and ankylosing spondylitis. Q J Med *29:*489, 1960.
21. Rotstein J, Entel I, Zeviner B: Arthritis associated with ulcerative colitis. Ann Rheum Dis *22:*194, 1963.
22. McBride JA, King MJ, Baikie AG, et al: Ankylosing spondylitis and chronic inflammatory diseases of the intestines. Br Med J *2:*483, 1963.
23. Zvaifler NJ, Martel W: Spondylitis in chronic ulcerative colitis. Arthritis Rheum *3:*76, 1960.
24. Macrae I, Wright V: A family study of ulcerative colitis, with particular reference to ankylosing spondylitis and sacro-iliitis. Ann Rheum Dis *32:*16, 1973.
25. Jayson MIV, Bouchier IAD: Ulcerative colitis with ankylosing spondylitis. Ann Rheum Dis *27:*219, 1968.
26. Jayson MIV, Salmon PR, Harrison WJ: Inflammatory bowel disease in ankylosing spondylitis. Gut *11:*506, 1970.
27. Green FA, Alea JA, McCluskey RT: The bowel in spondylitis—a controlled study (Abstr). Arthritis Rheum *16:*549, 1973.
28. Morris RI, Metzger AL, Bluestone R, et al: HL-A-W27—a useful discriminator in the arthropathies of inflammatory bowel disease. N Engl J Med *290:*1117, 1974.
29. Brewerton DA, Caffrey M, Nicholls A, et al: HL-A27 and arthropathies associated with ulcerative colitis and psoriasis. Lancet *1:*956, 1974.
30. Brewerton DA, James DCO: The histocompatibility antigen (HL-A27) and disease. Semin Arthritis Rheum *4:*191, 1975.
31. Dekker-Saeys BJ, Meuwissen SGM, Van Den Berg-Loonen EM, et al: Ankylosing spondylitis and inflammatory bowel disease. III. Clinical characteristics and results of histocompatibility typing (HLA B27) in 50 patients with both ankylosing spondylitis and inflammatory bowel disease. Ann Rheum Dis *37:*36, 1978.
32. Moll JMH, Haslock I, Macrae IF, et al: Associations between ankylosing spondylitis, psoriatic arthritis, Reiter's disease, the intestinal arthropathies, and Behçet's syndrome. Medicine *53:*343, 1974.
33. McEwen C, DiTata D, Lingg C, et al: Ankylosing spondylitis and spondylitis accompanying ulcerative colitis, regional enteritis, psoriasis and Reiter's disease. Arthritis Rheum *14:*291, 1971.
34. Dekker-Saeys BJ, Meuwissen SGM, Van Den Berg-Loonen EM, et al: Ankylosing spondylitis and inflammatory bowel disease. II. Prevalence of peripheral arthritis, sacroiliitis and ankylosing spondylitis in patients suffering from inflammatory bowel disease. Ann Rheum Dis *37:*33, 1978.
35. Hammer B, Ashurst P, Naish J: Diseases associated with ulcerative colitis and Crohn's disease. Gut *9:*17, 1968.
36. Hyla JF, Franck WA, Davis JS: Lack of association of HLA B27 with radiographic sacro-iliitis in inflammatory bowel disease. J Rheumatol *3:*196, 1976.
37. Young JR: Ulcerative colitis and finger clubbing. Br Med J *1:*278, 1966.
38. Farman J, Twersky J, Fierst S: Ulcerative colitis associated with hypertrophic osteoarthropathy. Am J Dig Dis (New Series) *21:*130, 1976.
39. Crohn BB, Yarnis H: Regional Ileitis. 2nd Ed. New York, Grune & Stratton, 1958, p 52.
40. Van Patter WN, Bargen JA, Dockerty MB, et al: Regional enteritis. Gastroenterology *26:*347, 1954.
41. Sprague PH, Anderson WS, Aaron TH: Longstanding fever due to regional ileocolitis. Am J Dig Dis (Old Series) *11:*295, 1944.
42. Austed WR, Thompson GR, Joseph RR: Regional enteritis presenting as acute arthritis. Mich Med *67:*324, 1968.
43. Wagner A: Arthralgien und Ileosakralarthritis bei Enteritis regionalis. Dtsch Med Wochenschr *94:*13, 1969.
44. Gronen LJ: A review of regional enteritis. J Am Osteop Assoc *60:*12, 1960.
45. Wilske KR, Decker JL: The articular manifestations of intestinal disease. Bull Rheum Dis *15:*362, 1965.
46. Daffner JE, Brown CH: Regional enteritis. Clinical aspects and diagnosis in 100 patients. Ann Intern Med *49:*580, 1958.
47. Clark RL: Regional enteritis. Symptomatology and review of cases. Proc Mayo Clin *13:*535, 1938.
48. Clark RL, Dixon CF: Regional enteritis. Surgery *5:*277, 1939.
49. Soren A: Joint affections in regional ileitis. Arch Intern Med *117:*78, 1966.
50. Cornes JS, Stecher M: Primary Crohn's disease of the colon and rectum. Gut *2:*189, 1961.
51. Ansell BM, Wigley RAD: Arthritic manifestations in regional enteritis. Ann Rheum Dis *23:*64, 1964.
52. Haslock I, Wright V: The musculoskeletal complications of Crohn's disease. Medicine *52:*217, 1973.
53. Wright V: Seronegative polyarthritis. A unified concept. Arthritis Rheum *21:*619, 1978.
54. Deshayes P, Geffroy Y, Houdent C, et al: Manifestations rhumatismales dans 80 cas de maladie de Crohn. Rev Rhum Mal Ostéoartic *43:*345, 1976.
55. Mueller CE, Seeger JF, Martel W: Ankylosing spondylitis and regional enteritis. Radiology *112:*579, 1974.
56. Bluestone R, Morris RI, Metzger AL, et al: HL-A W-27 and the spondylitis of chronic inflammatory bowel disease and psoriasis. Ann Rheum Dis *34*(Suppl 1):31, 1975.
57. Nicholls A, Brewerton DAB, Caffrey MFP, et al: HL-A27 in the arthropathies of inflammatory bowel disease (Abstr). Scand J Rheumatol Suppl *8:*30, 1975.
58. Russell AS, Percy JS, Schlaut J, et al: Transplantation antigens in Crohn's disease: Linkage of associated ankylosing spondylitis with HL-A27. Am J Dig Dis (New Series) *20:*359, 1975.
59. Jacoby RK, Jayson MIV: HL-A27 in Crohn's disease. Ann Rheum Dis *33:*422, 1974.
60. Gleeson MH, Walker JS, Wentzel J, et al: Human leukocyte antigens in Crohn's disease and ulcerative colitis. Gut *13:*438, 1972.
61. Hyla JF, Franck WA, Davis JS: Lack of association of HLA-B27 with radiographic sacro-iliitis in inflammatory bowel disease. J Rheumatol *3:*196, 1976.
62. Resnick D, Dwosh I, Goergen TG, et al: Clinical and radiographic abnormalities in ankylosing spondylitis. A comparison of men and women. Radiology *119:*293, 1976.
63. Resnick D: Patterns of peripheral joint disease in ankylosing spondylitis. Radiology *110:*523, 1974.
64. Davis P, Thomson ABR, Lentle BC: Quantitative sacro-iliac scintigraphy in patients with Crohn's disease. Arthritis Rheum *21:*234, 1978.
65. McBride JA, King MJ, Baikie AG, et al: Ankylosing spondylitis and chronic inflammatory diseases of the intestines. Br Med J *2:*483, 1963.
66. Haslock I, Macrae IF, Wright V: Arthritis and intestinal diseases: A comparison of two family studies. Rheumatol Rehabil *13:*135, 1973.
67. Anderson DO, Mullinger MA, Bagoch A: Regional enteritis involving the duodenum with clubbing of the fingers and steatorrhea. Gastroenterology *32:*917, 1957.
68. Neale G, Kelsall AR, Doyle FH: Crohn's disease and diffuse symmetrical periostitis. Gut *9:*383, 1968.
69. Farman J, Effmann EL, Grnja V: Crohn's disease and periosteal new bone formation. Gastroenterology *61:*513, 1971.
70. Nugent FW, Glaser D, Fernandez-Herlihy L: Crohn's colitis associated with granulomatous bone disease. N Engl J Med *294:*262, 1976.
71. Lindstrom C, Wramsby H, Ostberg G: Granulomatous arthritis in Crohn's disease. Gut *13:*257, 1972.
72. Kyle J: Psoas abscess in Crohn's disease. Gastroenterology *61:*149, 1971.
73. London D, Fitton JM: Acute septic arthritis complicating Crohn's disease. Br J Surg *57:*536, 1970.
74. Brom B, Bank S, Marks IN, et al: Periostitis, aseptic necrosis, and arthritis occurring in a patient with Crohn's disease. Gastroenterology *60:*1106, 1971.
75. McCaffery TD, Nasr K, Lawrence AM, et al: Severe growth retardation in children with inflammatory bowel disease. Pediatrics *45:*386, 1970.
76. Sobel EH, Silverman FN, Lee CM Jr: Chronic regional enteritis and growth retardation. Am J Dis Child *103:*569, 1962.
77. Frey CF, Weaver DK: Colectomy in children with ulcerative and granulomatous colitis. Arch Surg *104:*416, 1972.
78. Silverman FN: Regional enteritis in children. Aust Paediatr J *2:*207, 1966.
79. Genant HK, Mall JC, Wagonfeld JB, et al: Skeletal demineralization and growth retardation in inflammatory bowel disease. Invest Radiol *11:*541, 1976.
80. Whipple GH: A hitherto undescribed disease characterized anatomically by deposits of fat and fatty acids in the intestinal and mesenteric lymphatic tissues. Bull Johns Hopkins Hosp *18:*382, 1907.
81. Maizel H, Ruffin JM, Dobbins WO III: Whipple's disease: A review of 19 patients from one hospital and a review of the literature since 1950. Medicine *49:*175, 1970.

82. Puite RH, Tesluk H: Whipple's disease. Am J Med *19:*383, 1955.

83. Enzinger FM, Helwig EB: Whipple's disease: A review of the literature and report of fifteen patients. Virchows Arch (Pathol Anat) *336:*238, 1963.

84. Levine ME, Dobbins WO III: Joint changes in Whipple's disease. Semin Arthritis Rheum *3:*79, 1973.

85. Caughey DE, Bywaters EGL: The arthritis of Whipple's syndrome. Ann Rheum Dis *22:*327, 1963.

86. Kelly JJ III, Weisiger BB: The arthritis of Whipple's disease. Arthritis Rheum *6:*615, 1963.

87. Hargrove MD Jr, Verner JV, Smith AG, et al: Whipple's disease. Report of two cases with intestinal biopsy before and after treatment. Gastroenterology *39:*619, 1960.

88. Delcambre B, Luez J, Léonardelli J, et al: Les manifestations articulaires de la maladie de Whipple. A propos d'un cas avec étude histologique de la synoviale. Sem Hôp Paris *50:*847, 1974.

89. Farnan P: Whipple's disease: Clinical aspects. Q J Med *28:*163, 1959.

90. Jarcho S: Steatorrhea with unusual intestinal lesions. Bull Johns Hopkins Hosp *59:*275, 1936.

91. McDonald I: Whipple's disease (intestinal lipodystrophy). NZ Med J *59:*82, 1960.

92. Sieracki JC: Whipple's disease: Observations on systemic involvement. Arch Pathol *66:*464, 1958.

93. Triano GJ: Further roentgen observations of the small intestine in Whipple's disease. AJR *187:*717, 1962.

94. Schatzki SC: Whipple's disease—roentgenologic findings including those of an eight-year remission. Radiology *75:*908, 1960.

95. Jaffe IA: Whipple's intestinal lipodystrophy. Ann Intern Med *54:*776, 1961.

96. D'Eshougues JR, Delcambre B, Defrance D: Les manifestations articulaires de la maladie de Whipple. Rev Rhum Mal Ostéoartic *43:*565, 1976.

97. Chevallier PL, Vallat J-P, Luthier F, et al: Coxopathic bilaterale revelatrice d'une maladie de Whipple. A propos d'un cas. Rev Rhum Mal Osteoartic *43:*663, 1976.

98. Eyler WR, Doub HP: Extra-intestinal roentgen manifestations of intestinal lipodystrophy. JAMA *160:*534, 1956.

99. Houli J, Rezek J: Articular diseases in ulcerative colitis, regional ileitis, and Whipple's disease. Acta Rheumatol Scand *11:*291, 1965.

100. Katis J: Whipple's disease. McGill Med J *28:*66, 1959.

101. Elliott GB, Hill M, Howard DLG: Whipple's disease associated with benign thymoma. Can Med Assoc J *85:*1340, 1961.

102. Canoso JJ, Saini M, Hermos JA: Whipple's disease and ankylosing spondylitis: Simultaneous occurrence in HLA-B27 positive male. J Rheumatol *5:*79, 1978.

103. Fearrington EL, Monroe EW: Whipple's disease. Postgrad Med *44:*103, 1968.

104. Gross JB, Wollaeger EE, Sauer WG, et al: Whipple's disease: Report of four cases, including two in brothers, with observations on pathologic physiology, diagnosis, and treatment. Gastroenterology *36:*65, 1959.

105. Rubinow A, Canoso JJ, Goldenberg DL, et al: Synovial fluid and synovial membrane pathology in Whipple's disease (Abstr). Arthritis Rheum *19:*820, 1976.

106. Hawkins CF, Farr M, Morris CJ, et al: Detection by electron microscope of rod-shaped organisms in synovial membrane in a patient with the arthritis of Whipple's disease. Ann Rheum Dis *35:*502, 1976.

107. Warren CP: Arthritis associated with Salmonella infection. Ann Rheum Dis *29:*483, 1970.

108. Ahvonen P: Human yersiniosis in Finland. 2. Clinical features. Ann Clin Res *4:*39, 1972.

109. Vartiainen J, Hurri L: Arthritis due to *Salmonella typhimurium.* Acta Med Scand *175:*771, 1964.

110. Ahvonen P, Sievers K, Aho K: Arthritis associated with *Yersinia enterocolitica* infection. Acta Rheumatol Scand *15:*232, 1969.

111. Aho K, Ahvonen P, Lassus A, et al: HL-A27 in reactive arthritis: A study of yersinia arthritis and Reiter's disease. Arthritis Rheum *17:*521, 1974.

112. David JR, Black RL: Salmonella arthritis. Medicine *39:*385, 1960.

113. Wands JR, LaMont JL, Mann E, et al: Arthritis associated with intestinal bypass procedure for morbid obesity. Complement activation and characterization of circulating cryoproteins. N Engl J Med *294:*121, 1976.

114. Shagrin JW, Frame B, Duncan H: Polyarthritis in obese patients with intestinal bypass. Ann Intern Med *75:*377, 1971.

115. Rose E, Espinoza LR, Osterland CK: Intestinal bypass arthritis: Association with circulating immune complexes and HLA B27. J Rheumatol *4:*129, 1977.

116. Fernandez-Herlihy L: Arthritis after jejuno-ileostomy for intractable obesity. J Rheumatol *4:*135, 1977.

117. Utsinger PD, Farber N, Shapiro RF, et al: Clinical and immunologic study of the post-intestinal bypass arthritis-dermatitis syndrome (Abstr). Arthritis Rheum *21:*599, 1978.

118. Duncan H: Arthropathy and the intestinal bypass operation for obesity. J Rheumatol *4:*115, 1977.

119. Ferguson RH: Enteropathic arthritis. In JL Hollander, DJ McCarty Jr (Eds): Arthritis and Allied Conditions. 8th Ed. Philadelphia, Lea & Febiger, 1972, p 846.

120. Ginsburg JH, Quismorio FP, Mongan ES, et al: Articular complications after jejuno-ileal shunt. Clinical and immunologic studies. Arthritis Rheum *19:*797, 1976.

121. Mir-Madilessi SH, Mackenzie AH, Winkleman EI: Articular complications in obese patients after jejunocolic bypass. Cleve Clin Q *41:*119, 1974.

122. Ansell BM, Bywaters EGL: Histiocytic bone and joint disease. Ann Rheum Dis *16:*503, 1957.

123. Ahrens EH Jr, Payne MA, Kunkel HG, et al: Primary biliary cirrhosis. Medicine *29:*299, 1950.

124. Atkinson M, Nordin BE, Sherlock S: Malabsorption and bone disease in prolonged obstructive jaundice. Q J Med *25:*299, 1956.

125. Klatskin G, Kantor FS: Mitochondrial antibody in primary biliary cirrhosis and other diseases. Ann Intern Med *77:*533, 1972.

126. Hoffbauer FW: Primary biliary cirrhosis: Observations of the natural course of the disease in 25 women. Am J Dig Dis (New Series) *5:*348, 1960.

127. Sherlock S, Scheuer PJ: The presentation and diagnosis of 100 patients with primary biliary cirrhosis. N Engl J Med *289:*674, 1973.

128. Golding PL, Mason AS: Renal tubular acidosis and autoimmune liver disease. Gut *12:*153, 1971.

129. August PJ: Primary biliary cirrhosis and scleroderma. Proc R Soc Med *67:*1238, 1974.

130. Whaley K, Goudie RB, Williamson J, et al: Liver disease in Sjögren's syndrome and rheumatoid arthritis. Lancet *1:*861, 1970.

131. Kehayoglou AK, Holdsworth CD, Agnew JE, et al: Bone disease and calcium absorption in primary biliary cirrhosis with special reference to vitamin-D therapy. Lancet *1:*715, 1968.

132. Sherlock S: Primary biliary cirrhosis (chronic intrahepatic obstructive jaundice). Gastroenterology *37:*574, 1959.

133. O'Connell DJ, Marx WJ: Hand changes in primary biliary cirrhosis. Radiology *129:*31, 1978.

134. Whelton MJ: Arthropathy and liver disease. Br J Hosp Med *3:*243, 1970.

135. Bouchier IAD, Rhodes K, Sherlock S: Serological abnormalities in patients with liver disease. Br Med J *1:*592, 1964.

136. Resnick D: Erosive arthritis of the hand and wrist in hyperparathyroidism. Radiology *110:*263, 1974.

137. Clarke AK, Galbraith RM, Hamilton EBD, Williams R: Rheumatic disorders in primary biliary cirrhosis. Ann Rheum Dis *37:*42, 1978.

138. D'Angelo WA, Fries JF, Masi AT, et al: Pathologic observations in systemic sclerosis (scleroderma). Am J Med *46:*428, 1969.

139. Bartholomew LG, Cain JC, Winkelmann RK, et al: Chronic disease of the liver associated with systemic scleroderma. Am J Dig Dis (New Series) *9:*43, 1964.

140. Murray-Lyon IM, Thompson RPH, Ansell ID, et al: Scleroderma and primary biliary cirrhosis. Br Med J *3:*258, 1970.

141. Wenzel RP, McCormick DP, Busch HJ, et al: Arthritis and viral hepatitis. Arch Intern Med *130:*770, 1972.

142. Steigman AJ: Rashes and arthropathy in viral hepatitis. Mt Sinai J Med *40:*752, 1973.

143. McCarty DJ: Arthritis and HB Ag-positive hepatitis. Arch Intern Med *132:*264, 1973.

144. Koff RS: Immune-complex arthritis in viral hepatitis. N Engl J Med *285:*229, 1971.

145. Mullin GT, Caperton EM Jr, Crespin SR, et al: Arthritis and skin lesions resembling erythema nodosum in pancreatic disease. Ann Intern Med *68:*75, 1968.

146. Robertson JC, Eeles GH: Syndrome associated with pancreatic acinar cell carcinoma. Br Med J *2:*708, 1970.

147. Burns WA, Matthews MJ, Hamosh M, et al: Lipase-secreting acinar cell carcinoma of the pancreas with polyarthropathy. A light and electron microscopic, histochemical, and biochemical study. Cancer *33:*1002, 1974.

148. Gibson TJ, Schumacher HR, Pascual E, et al: Arthropathy, skin and bone lesions in pancreatic disease. J Rheumatol *2:*7, 1975.

149. Lucas PF, Gwen TK: Subcutaneous fat necrosis, "polyarthritis" and pancreatic disease. Gut *3:*146, 1962.

150. Osborne RR: Functioning acinous cell carcinoma of the pancreas accompanied with widespread focal fat necrosis. Arch Intern Med *85:*933, 1950.

151. Virshup AM, Sliwinski AJ: Polyarthritis and subcutaneous nodules associated with carcinoma of the pancreas. Arthritis Rheum *16:*388, 1973.

152. Belsky H, Cornell NW: Disseminated focal fat necrosis following radical pancreaticoduodenectomy for acinous carcinoma of head of pancreas. Ann Surg *141:*556, 1955.

153. Jackson SH, Savidge RS, Stein L, et al: Carcinoma of the pancreas associated with fat necrosis. Lancet *2:*962, 1952.

154. Hegler C, Wohlwill F: Fettgewebsnedrosen in Subcutis und Knochenmark durch Metastasen eines Carzinoms des Pankreasschwanzes. Virchows Arch (Pathol Anat) *274:*784, 1930.

155. Goluboff N, Cram R, Ramgotra B, et al: Polyarthritis and bone lesions complicating traumatic pancreatitis in two children. Can Med Assoc J *118:*924, 1978.

156. Keating JP, Shackelford GD, Shackelford PG, et al: Pancreatitis and osteolytic lesions. J Pediatr *81:*350, 1972.

157. Slovis TL, Berdon WE, Haller JO, et al: Pancreatitis and the battered child syndrome: Report of 2 cases with skeletal involvement. Am J Roentgenol *125:*456, 1975.

158. Leger L, Morin M, Fabiani P, et al: Nécrose sous-cutanée périphérique et toxémie pancréatique. Presse Med *74:*1403, 1966.

159. Kushner DS, Szanto PB: Fulminant polyarthritis, fever, and cutaneous nodules in an alcoholic patient. JAMA *167:*1625, 1958.

160. Szymanski FJ, Bluefarb SM: Nodular fat necrosis and pancreatic diseases. Arch Dermatol *83:*224, 1961.

161. Swerdlow AB, Berman ME, Gibbel MI, et al: Subcutaneous fat necrosis associated with acute pancreatitis. JAMA *173:*765, 1960.

162. Tannenbaum H, Anderson LG, Schur PH: Association of polyarthritis, subcutaneous nodules, and pancreatic disease. J Rheumatol 2:14, 1975.
163. Scarpelli DG: Fat necrosis of bone marrow in acute pancreatitis. Am J Pathol 32:1077, 1956.
164. Goldberg LM, Ritzmann LW: Unusual manifestations in a case of relapsing, nodular, febrile panniculitis (Weber-Christian disease). Am J Med 25:788, 1958.
165. Moore S: The relation of pancreatic disease to Weber-Christian disease. Can Med Assoc J 88:1238, 1963.
166. de Graciansky P: Weber-Christian syndrome of pancreatic origin. Br J Dermatol 79:278, 1967.
167. Gerle RD, Walker LA, Achord JL, et al: Osseous changes in chronic pancreatitis. Radiology 85:330, 1965.
168. Turner JW, Jaffe HL: Metastatic neoplasms. AJR 43:479, 1940.
169. Johnston AD: Pathology of metastatic tumors in bone. Clin Orthop 73:8, 1970.
170. Abrams HL, Spiro R, Goldstein N: Metastases in carcinoma. Analysis of 1000 autopsied cases. Cancer 3:74, 1950.
171. Grauer FW: Pancreatic carcinoma; a review of 34 autopsies. Arch Intern Med 63:884, 1939.
172. Joffe N, Antonioli DA: Osteoblastic bone metastases secondary to adenocarcinoma of the pancreas. Clin Radiol 29:41, 1978.
173. Borak J: Roentgen examination of pancreatic tumors. Radiology 41:170, 1943.
174. Mani JR, Zboralske FF, Margulis AR: Carcinoma of the body and tail of the pancreas. AJR 96:429, 1966.
175. Gillison EW, Grainger RG, Fernandez D: Osteoblastic metastasis in carcinoma of the pancreas. Br J Radiol 43:818, 1970.
176. Bluestein HG, Zvaifler NJ: Arthritis and the gastrointestinal tract. In HL Bockus (Ed): Gastroenterology. 3rd Ed. Vol 4. Philadelphia, WB Saunders Co, 1976, p 554.
177. Franck WA, Hoffman GS, Davis JS, et al: Osteomalacia and weakness complicating jejunoileal bypass. J Rheumatol 6:51, 1979.
178. Zapanta M, Aldo-Benson M, Biegel A, et al: Arthritis associated with jejunoilial bypass. Clinical and immunologic evaluation. Arthritis Rheum 22:711, 1979.
179. Mills PR, Rooney PJ, Watkinson G, et al: Hypercholesterolaemic arthropathy in primary biliary cirrhosis. Ann Rheum Dis 38:179, 1979.
180. Marx WJ, O'Connell DJ: Arthritis of primary biliary cirrhosis. Arch Intern Med 139:213, 1979.
181. Smukler NM, Schumacher HR, Pascual E, et al: Synovial fat necrosis associated with ischemic pancreatic disease. Arthritis Rheum 22:547, 1979.
182. Allen BL Jr, Jinkins WJ III: Vertebral osteonecrosis associated with pancreatitis in a child. A case report. J Bone Joint Surg [Am] 60:985, 1978.
183. Buchanan RF, Willkens RF: Arthritis after jejuno-ileostomy. Arthritis Rheum 15:644, 1972.
184. Reuler JB, Borthistle BK, Chang MK, et al: Pseudothrombophlebitis syndrome in the arthropathy of granulomatous colitis. Arch Intern Med 139:1178, 1979.
185. Stein HB, Abdullah A, Robinson HS, et al: Salmonella reactive arthritis in British Columbia. Arthritis Rheum 23:206, 1980.
186. Clegg DO, Samuelson CO Jr, Williams HJ, et al: Articular complications of jejunoileal bypass surgery. J Rheumatol 7:65, 1980.
187. Ginsberg J, Quismorio FP Jr, DeWind LT, et al: Musculoskeletal symptoms after jejunoileal shunt surgery for intractable obesity. Clinical and immunologic studies. Am J Med 67:443, 1979.
188. Miller F, Lane B, Soterakis J, et al: Primary biliary cirrhosis and scleroderma. The possibility of a common pathogenetic mechanism. Arch Pathol Lab Med 103:505, 1979.
189. Good AE, Beals TF, Simmons JL, et al: A subcutaneous nodule with Whipple's disease: Key to early diagnosis? Arthritis Rheum 23:856, 1980.
190. Utsinger PD: Bypass disease: A bacterial antigen-antibody systemic immune complex disease. Arthritis Rheum 23:758, 1980.
191. Mosekilde L, Melsen F: Dynamic differences in trabecular bone remodeling between patients after jejuno-ileal bypass for obesity and epileptic patients receiving anticonvulsant therapy. Metab Bone Dis Rel Res 2:77, 1980.
192. Akyol S, Macklon AF, Griffiths ID, et al: Rheumatological and serological features of primary biliary cirrhosis (Abstr). Ann Rheum Dis 39:186, 1980.
193. Phillips RM Jr, Sulser RE, Songcharoen S: Inflammatory arthritis and subcutaneous fat necrosis associated with acute and chronic pancreatitis. Arthritis Rheum 23:355, 1980.
194. Meuwissen SGM, Dekker-Sacys BJ, Agenant D, et al: Ankylosing spondylitis and inflammatory bowel disease. Ann Rheum Dis 37:30, 1978.
195. Costello PB, Alea JA, Kennedy AC, et al: Prevalence of occult inflammatory bowel disease in ankylosing spondylitis. Ann Rheum Dis 39:453, 1980.
196. Enlow RW, Bias WB, Arnett FC: The spondylitis of inflammatory bowel disease. Arthritis Rheum 23:1359, 1980.
197. Arlart IP, Maier W, Leupold D, et al: Massive periosteal new bone formation in ulcerative colitis. Radiology 144:507, 1982.
198. Ueno Y, Chia D, Barnett EV: Relapsing polychondritis associated with ulcerative colitis. J Rheumatol 8:456, 1981.
199. Tomlinson IW, Jayson MIV: Erosive Crohn's arthritis. J R Soc Med 74:540, 1981.
200. Van Dongen LM, Lubbers EJC: Psoas abscess in Crohn's disease. Br J Surg 69:589, 1982.
201. Pitt P, Goodwill CJ: Calcified psoas abscess causing limited hip movement in Crohn's disease. Clin Rheumatol 2:79, 1983.
202. Gray RR, St Louis EL, Grosman H, et al: Ilio-psoas abscess in Crohn's disease. J Can Assoc Radiol 34:36, 1983.

203. Heuman R, Boeryd B, Gillquist J, et al: Arthralgia and crystal deposits in Crohn's disease. Scand J Rheumatol 10:313, 1981.
204. Mulero J, Abreu L, Chantar C, et al: Enfermedad de Crohn, espondilitis anquilosante y HLA B27: A proposito de siete casos. Med Clin (Barcelona) 79:27, 1982.
205. Minard DB, Haddad H, Blain JG, et al: Granulomatous myositis and myopathy associated with Crohn's colitis. N Engl J Med 295:818, 1976.
206. Greenstein AJ, Janowitz HD, Sachar DB: The extra-intestinal complications of Crohn's disease and ulcerative colitis. A study of 700 patients. Medicine 55:401, 1976.
207. Koeger AC, Merlet CI, Prier A, et al: Manifestations articulaires de la maladie de Whipple. Sem Hop Paris 59:1237, 1983.
208. Bismuth JM, Arlet P, Dal Bianco C, et al: Hanche géodique au cours d'une maladie de Whipple. Nouv Rev Med Toulouse 11:15, 1984.
209. Farr M, Hollywell CA, Morris CJ, et al: Whipple's disease diagnosed at hip arthroplasty. Ann Rheum Dis 43:526, 1984.
210. Ayoub WT, Davis DE, Torretti D, et al: Bone destruction and ankylosis in Whipple's disease. J Rheumatol 9:930, 1982.
211. Khan MA: Axial arthropathy in Whipple's disease. J Rheumatol 9:928, 1982.
212. Bussiere JL, Epifanie JL, Leblanc B, et al: Maladie de Whipple et spondyloarthrite ankylosante. Rev Rhum Mal Osteoartic 47:577, 1980.
213. Ho G Jr, Claunch BC, Sadovnikoff N: Scintigraphic evidence of transient unilateral sacroiliitis in a case of Whipple's disease. Clin Nucl Med 5:548, 1980.
214. Farr M, Morris C, Hollywell CA, et al: Amyloidosis in Whipple's arthritis. J R Soc Med 76:963, 1983.
215. Goldenberg DL: "Postinfectious" arthritis. New look at an old concept with particular attention to disseminated gonococcal infection. Am J Med 74:925, 1983.
216. Keat A: Reiter's syndrome and reactive arthritis in perspective. N Engl J Med 309:1606, 1983.
217. Olhagen B: Diagnosis and treatment of reactive arthritis. IM 4:69, 1983.
218. Enlow RW, Bias WB, Bluestone R, et al: Human lymphocyte response to selected infectious agents in Reiter's syndrome and ankylosing spondylitis. Rheumatol Int 1:171, 1982.
219. Aho K: Pathogenesis of Reiter's syndrome and reactive arthritis. Scand J Rheumatol (Suppl) 52:30, 1984.
220. Carroll WL, Balistreri WF, Brilli R, et al: Spectrum of salmonella-associated arthritis. Pediatrics 68:717, 1981.
221. Luzar MJ, Caldwell JH, Mekhjian H, et al: Yersinia entercolitica infection presenting as chronic enteropathic arthritis. Arthritis Rheum 26:1163, 1983.
222. Marsal L, Winblad S, Wollhein FA: Yersinia enterocolitica arthritis in southern Sweden: A four-year follow-up study. Br Med J 283:101, 1981.
223. Aho K: Yersinia reactive arthritis. Br J Rheumatol 22 (Suppl 2):41, 1983.
224. Leino R, Makela A-L, Tiilikainen A, et al: Yersinia arthritis in children. Scand J Rheumatol 9:245, 1980.
225. Koivuranta-Vaara P, Repo H, Leirisalo M, et al: Enhanced neutrophil migration in vivo HLA B27 positive subjects. Ann Rheum Dis 43:181, 1984.
226. Schaad UB: Reactive arthritis associated with Campylobacter enteritis. Pediatr Infect Dis 1:328, 1982.
227. Short CD, Klouda PT, Smith L: Campylobacter jejuni enteritis and reactive arthritis. Ann Rheum Dis 41:287, 1982.
228. Kosunen TU, Ponka A, Kauranen O, et al: Arthritis associated with Campylobacter jejuni enteritis. Scand J Rheumatol 10:77, 1981.
229. Gumpel JM, Martin C, Sanderson PJ: Reactive arthritis associated with Campylobacter enteritis. Ann Rheum Dis 40:64, 1981.
230. Ebright JR, Ryan LM: Acute erosive reactive arthritis associated with Campylobacter jejuni-induced colitis. Am J Med 76:321, 1984.
231. Cowan R, Baig W, Lynch V, et al: Reactive arthritis—the need for diagnostic caution. J Rheumatol 9:645, 1982.
232. Urman JD, Zurier RB, Rothfield NF: Reiter's syndrome associated with Campylobacter fetus infection. Ann Intern Med 86:444, 1977.
233. Leung FYK, Littlejohn GO, Bonbardien C: Reiter's syndrome after Campylobacter jejuni enteritis. Arthritis Rheum 23:948, 1980.
234. Lofgren RP, Tadlock LM, Soltis RD: Acute oligoarthritis associated with Clostridium difficile pseudomembranous colitis. Arch Intern Med 144:617, 1984.
235. Rynes RI, Volastro PS, Bartholomew LF: Exacerbation of B27 positive spondyloarthropathy by enteric infection. J Rheumatol 11:96, 1984.
236. Spira TJ, Kabins SA: Yersinia enterocolitica septicemia with septic arthritis. Arch Intern Med 136:1305, 1976.
237. Sebes JI, Mabry EH, Rabinowitz JG: Lung abscess and osteomyelitis of ribs due to Yersinia enterocolitica. Chest 69:546, 1979.
238. Kahn FW, Glasser JE, Agger WA: Psoas muscle abscess due to Yersinia entercolitica. Am J Med 76:947, 1984.
239. Soren A: Joint inflammations as complications in intestinal inflammation. Z Rheumatol 40:1, 1981.
240. Rothschild BM, Masi AT, June PL: Arthritis associated with ampicillin colitis. Arch Intern Med 137:1605, 1977.
241. Rollins D, Moeller D: Acute migratory polyarthritis associated with antibiotic-induced pseudomembranous colitis. Am J Gastroenterol 65:353, 1976.
242. Delamere JP, Baddeley RM, Walton KW: Jejuno-ileal bypass arthropathy: Its clinical features and associations. Ann Rheum Dis 42:553, 1983.
243. Stein HB, Schlappner OLA, Boyko W, et al: The intestinal bypass arthritis-dermatitis syndrome. Arthritis Rheum 24:684, 1981.
244. Leff RD, Towles W, Aldo-Benson MA, et al: A prospective analysis of the

arthritis syndrome and immune function in jejunoileal bypass patients. J Rheumatol 10:612, 1983.

245. Leff RD, Aldo-Benson MA, Madura JA: The effect of revision of the intestinal bypass on post intestinal bypass arthritis. Arthritis Rheum 26:678, 1983.

246. Jorizzo JL, Apisarnthanarax P, Subrt P, et al: Bowel-bypass syndrome without bowel bypass: Bowel associated dermatosis-arthritis syndrome. Arch Intern Med 143:457, 1983.

247. Dicken CH: Bowel-associated dermatosis-arthritis syndrome: Bowel bypass syndrome without bowel bypass. Mayo Clin Proc 59:43, 1984.

248. James O, Macklon AF, Watson AJ: Primary biliary cirrhosis—a revised clinical spectrum. Lancet 1:1278, 1981.

249. Mills PR, Sturrock RD: Clinical associations between arthritis and liver disease. Ann Rheum Dis 41:295, 1982.

250. Epstein O, Dick R, Sherlock S: Prospective study of periostitis and finger clubbing in primary biliary cirrhosis and other forms of chronic liver disease. Gut 22:203, 1981.

251. Mills PR, Vallance R, Birnie G, et al: A prospective survey of radiological bone and joint changes in primary biliary cirrhosis. Clin Radiol 32:297, 1981.

252. Bourgeois P, Bocquet L, Grossin M, et al: Osteoarthropathie destructrice rapide de la hanche au cours d'une cirrhose biliaire primitive. Rev Rhum Mal Osteoartic 48:437, 1981.

253. Juttman JR: Bone disease and hepatobiliary disorders. Neth J Med 25:290, 1982.

254. Hyer FH, Gottlieb NL: Rheumatic syndromes associated with hepatitis-B antigenemia. IM 2:43, 1981.

255. Nath BJ, Isselbacher KJ: Joint symptoms as the presenting features of hepatitis. IM 3:82, 1982.

256. Sherlock S: Chronic hepatitis. Gut 15:581, 1974.

257. Barnardo DE, Vernon-Roberts B, Currey HL: A case of active chronic hepatitis with painless erosive arthritis. Gut 14:800, 1973.

258. Plonk JW, Feldman JM: Carcinoid arthropathy. Arch Intern Med 134:651, 1974.

259. Horwitz R, Schachter M: Carcinoid arthropathy—radiological features. Br J Radiol 56:131, 1983.

260. Crisp AJ: Carcinoid arthropathy. Br J Radiol 56:782, 1983.

261. Simkin PA, Brunzell JD, Wisner D, et al: Free fatty acids in the pancreatic arthritis syndrome. Arthritis Rheum 26:127, 1983.

262. Wilson HA, Askari AD, Neiderhiser DH, et al: Pancreatitis with arthropathy and subcutaneous fat necrosis. Evidence for the pathogenicity of lipolytic enzymes. Arthritis Rheum 26:121, 1983.

263. Schutte HE, Wackwitz JD: Case report 171. Skel Radiol 7:147, 1981.

264. Rao GM, Shadcher A, Poulose KP: Bone scan findings in pancreatitis. Clin Nucl Med 5:563, 1980.

265. Rittenberg GM, Korn JH, Schabel SI, et al: Rapid osteolysis in pancreatic carcinoma. West J Med 135:408, 1981.

266. Gombergh R, Blanchet-Bardon CI, Delmas PF, et al: Syndrome de Weber-Christian et pancreatite chronique. Ann Radiol 24:651, 1981.

267. Newman AJ, Ansell BM: Episodic arthritis in children with cystic fibrosis. J Pediatr 94:594, 1979.

268. Schidlow DV, Goldsmith DP, Palmer J, et al: Arthritis in cystic fibrosis. Arch Dis Child 59:377, 1984.

269. Erlendsson J, Fenger C, Meinicke J: Arthritis and collagenous colitis. Scand J Rheumatol 12:93, 1983.

270. Verbruggen LA, Buyck R, Handelberg F: Clavicular periosteal new bone formation in ulcerative colitis. Clin Exp Rheumatol 3:163, 1985.

271. Al-Hadidi S, Khatib G, Chhatwal P, et al: Granulomatous arthritis in Crohn's disease. Arthritis Rheum 27:1061, 1984.

272. Toubert A, Dougados M, Amor B: Erosive granulomatous arthritis in Crohn's disease. Arthritis Rheum 28:958, 1985.

273. Hermans PJ, Fievez ML, Descamps CL, et al: Granulomatous synovitis and Crohn's disease. J Rheumatol 11:710, 1984.

274. Mielants H, Veys EM, Cuvelier C, et al: HLA-B27 related arthritis and bowel inflammation. Part 2. Ileocolonoscopy and bowel histology in patients with HLA-B27 related arthritis. J Rheumatol 12:294, 1985.

275. Vilppula AH, Jussila TUA, Kokko AM-L: Atlanto-axial dislocation in an 18-year-old female with yersinia arthritis. Clin Rheum 3:239, 1984.

276. Woo P, Panayi GS: Reactive arthritis due to infestation with Giardia lamblia. J Rheumatol 11:719, 1984.

277. Lanham JG, Doyle DV: Reactive arthritis following psittacosis. Br J Rheumatol 23:225, 1984.

278. Valtonen VV, Leirisalo M, Pentikainen PJ, et al: Triggering infections in reactive arthritis. Ann Rheum Dis 44:399, 1985.

279. Clegg DO, Zone JJ, Samuelson CO Jr, et al: Circulatory immune complexes containing secretory IgA in jejunoileal bypass disease. Ann Rheum Dis 44:239, 1985.

280. Klinkhoff AV, Stein HB, Schlappner OLA, et al: Postgastrectomy blind loop syndrome and the arthritis-dermatitis syndrome. Arthritis Rheum 28:214, 1985.

281. Parfitt AM, Podenphant J, Villanueva AR, et al: Metabolic bone disease with and without osteomalacia after intestinal bypass surgery: A bone histomorphometric study. Bone 6:211, 1985.

282. Drenick EJ, Bassett LW, Stanley TM: Rheumatoid arthritis associated with jejunoileal bypass. Arthritis Rheum 27:1300, 1984.

283. Halla JT, Schumacher HR Jr, Trotter ME: Bursal fat necrosis as the presenting manifestation of pancreatic disease: Light and electron microscopic studies. J Rheumatol 12:359, 1985.

284. Baron M, Paltiel H, Lander P: Aseptic necrosis of the talus and calcaneal insufficiency fractures in a patient with pancreatitis, subcutaneous fat necrosis, and arthritis. Arthritis Rheum 27:1309, 1984.

285. Garcia JF: Rapid regional osteolysis from pancreatic carcinoma. J Can Assoc Radiol 36:150, 1985.

286. Simpson EL, Dalinka MK: Association of hypertrophic osteoarthropathy with gastrointestinal polyposis. AJR 144:983, 1985.

287. Malmquist J, Ericsson B, Hulten-Nosslin M-B, et al: Finger clubbing and aspartylglucosamine excretion in a laxative-abusing patient. Postgrad Med J 56:862, 1980.

288. Bourne JT, Kumar P, Huskisson EC, et al: Arthritis and coeliac disease. Ann Rheum Dis 44:592, 1985.

289. Sanders KM, Resnik CS, Owen DS: Erosive arthritis in Cronkhite-Canada syndrome. Radiology 156:309, 1985.

290. Radin DR, Colletti PM, Forrrester DM, et al: Pancreatic acinar carcinoma with subcutaneous and intraosseous fat necrosis. Radiology 158:67, 1986.

291. Pinals RS: Arthritis associated with gluten-sensitive enteropathy. J Rheumatol 13:201, 1986.

292. Hodgson SF, Dickson ER, Wahner HW, et al: Bone loss and reduced osteoblast function in primary biliary cirrhosis. Ann Intern Med 103:855, 1985.

293. Jordan JM, Obeid LM, Allen NB: Isolated atlantoaxial subluxation as the presenting manifestation of inflammatory bowel disease. Am J Med 80:517, 1986.

294. Inman RD: Arthritis and enteritis—an interface of protean manifestations. J Rheumatol 14:406, 1987.

295. Scarpa R, Del Puente A, D'Arienzo A, et al: The arthritis of ulcerative colitis: Clinical and genetic aspects. J Rheumatol 19:373, 1992.

296. van den Broek MF, van de Putte LBA, van den Berg WB: Crohn's disease associated with arthritis: A possible role for cross-reactivity between gut bacteria and cartilage in the pathogenesis of arthritis. Arthritis Rheum 31:1077, 1988.

297. Scott WW Jr, Fishman EK, Kuhlman JE, et al: Computed tomography evaluation of the sacroiliac joints in Crohn disease. Radiologic/clinical correlation. Skel Radiol 19:207, 1990.

298. Calin A, Robertson D: Spondylodiscitis and pseudoarthrosis in a patient with enteropathic spondyloarthropathy. Ann Rheum Dis 50:117, 1991.

299. Purrmann J, Zeidler H, Bertrams J, et al: HLA antigens in ankylosing spondylitis associated with Crohn's disease. Increased frequency of the HLA phenotypes B27, B44. J Rheumatol 15:1658, 1988.

300. Chandler JT, Riddle CD Jr: Osteomyelitis associated with Crohn's disease. A case report and literature review. Orthopedics 12:285, 1989.

301. Schwartz CM, Demos TC, Wehner JM: Osteomyelitis of the sacrum as the initial manifestation of Crohn's disease. Clin Orthop 222:181, 1987.

302. O'Malley BP, Minuk T, Castelli M: Buttock abscess complicating Crohn's disease. J Can Assoc Radiol 40:51, 1989.

303. Lucarotti ME, Cooper MJ, Ackroyd CE: Flexion deformity of the hip in Crohn's disease. J Bone Joint Surg [Br] 72:156, 1990.

304. Dobbins WO III: HLA antigens in Whipple's disease. Arthritis Rheum 30:102, 1987.

305. Phillips PE: How do bacteria cause chronic arthritis? J Rheumatol 16:1017, 1989.

306. Mielants H, Veys EM, Joos R, et al: Repeat ileocolonoscopy in reactive arthritis. J Rheumatol 14:456, 1987.

307. Mielants H, Veys EM, Joos R, et al: HLA antigens in the seronegative spondyloarthropathies. Reactive arthritis and arthritis in ankylosing spondylitis: Relation to gut inflammation. J Rheumatol 14:466, 1987.

308. Hannu TJ, Leirisalo-Repo M: Clinical picture of reactive salmonella arthritis. J Rheumatol 15:1668, 1988.

309. Cicuttini FM, Buchanan RRC: Reactive arthritis after infection with Salmonella singapore. J Rheumatol 16:1610, 1989.

310. Inman RD, Johnston MEA, Hodge M, et al: Postdysenteric reactive arthritis. A clinical and immunogenetic study following an outbreak of salmonellosis. Arthritis Rheum 31:1377, 1988.

311. Lauhio A, Lähdevirta J, Janes R, et al: Reactive arthritis associated with Shigella sonnei infection. Arthritis Rheum 31:1190, 1988.

312. Bignardi GE: Yersinia pseudotuberculosis and arthritis. Ann Rheum Dis 48:518, 1989.

313. Hammer M, Zeidler H, Klimsa S, et al: Yersinia enterocolitica in the synovial membrane of patients with Yersinia-induced arthritis. Arthritis Rheum 33:1795, 1990.

314. Lahesmaa-Rantala R, Granfors K, Isomäki H, et al: Yersinia specific immune complexes in the synovial fluid of patients with yersinia triggered reactive arthritis. Ann Rheum Dis 46:510, 1987.

315. Sieper J, Braun J, Brandt J, et al: Pathogenetic role of Chlamydia, Yersinia and Borrelia in undifferentiated oligoarthritis. J Rheumatol 19:1236, 1992.

316. Atkinson MH, McLeod BD: Reactive arthritis associated with Clostridium difficile enteritis. J Rheumatol 15:520, 1988.

317. Miller BH, McGuire MH: Non-infectious pyogenic arthritis after a blind-loop intestinal-bypass operation. A case report. J Bone Joint Surg [Am] 72:1409, 1990.

318. Clark M, Sack K: Deforming arthropathy complicating primary biliary cirrhosis. J Rheumatol 18:619, 1991.

319. Goldenstein C, Rabson AR, Kaplan MM, et al: Arthralgias as a presenting manifestation of primary biliary cirrhosis. J Rheumatol 16:681, 1989.

320. Llorente MJ, Martin-Mola E, Torrijos A, et al: Arthritis as an unusual presentation of primary biliary cirrhosis. J Rheumatol 18:1768, 1991.

321. Saag KG, Niemann TH, Warner CH, et al: Subcutaneous pancreatic fat necrosis associated with acute arthritis. J Rheumatol 19:630, 1992.

322. Haller J, Greenway G, Resnick D, et al: Intraosseous fat necrosis associated with acute pancreatitis: MR imaging. Radiology 173:193, 1989.

323. Lipnick RN, Glass RBJ: Bone changes associated with cystic fibrosis. Skel Radiol 21:115, 1992.

324. Dixey J, Redington AN, Butler RC, et al: The arthropathy of cystic fibrosis. Ann Rheum Dis 47:218, 1988.

325. Roubenoff R, Ratain J, Giardiello F: Collagenous colitis, enteropathic arthritis, and autoimmune diseases: Results of a patient survey. J Rheumatol 16:1229, 1989.

326. Maher JM, Strosberg JM, Rowley RF, et al: Jaccoud's arthropathy and inflammatory bowel disease. J Rheumatol 19:1637, 1992.

327. Rouillon A, Menkes CJ, Gerster J-C, et al: Sarcoid-like forms of Whipple's disease. Report of 2 cases. J Rheumatol 20:1070, 1993.

328. Lawrence JM III, Moore TL, Madson KL, et al: Arthropathies of cystic fibrosis: Case reports and review of the literature. J Rheumatol 20:12, 1993.

329. Kvien TK, Glennas A, Melby K, et al: Reactive arthritis: Incidence, triggering agents and clinical presentation. J Rheumatol 21:115, 1994.

330. Kingsmore SF, Kingsmore DB, Hall DB, et al: Cooccurrence of collagenous colitis with seronegative spondyloarthropathy: Report of a case and literature review. J Rheumatol 20:2153, 1993.

331. Watts RA, Kelly S, Hacking JC, et al: Fat necrosis: An unusual cause of polyarthritis. J Rheumatol 20:1432, 1993.

332. Ferrari R, Wendelboe M, Ford PM, et al: Pancreatic arthritis with periarticular fat necrosis. J Rheumatol 20:1436, 1993.

32

Periodic, Relapsing, and Recurrent Disorders

Donald Resnick, M.D.

Included in this chapter are three diseases that are characterized clinically by intermittent periods of activity separated by disease-free intercritical periods.[1] The grouping of these disorders into a single section does not imply that other diseases might not be associated with similar periodicity, nor does it indicate that they are related etiologically. In fact, their causes generally are unclear or unknown. The three diseases discussed in this chapter are relatively uncommon and are associated with nonspecific or unremarkable radiographic appearances.

FAMILIAL MEDITERRANEAN FEVER

Clinical Abnormalities

Familial Mediterranean fever (familial recurrent polyserositis) is an uncommon disease that affects predominantly Sephardic (non-Ashkenazi) Jews, Armenians, and Arabs.[2–6] It is inherited as an autosomal recessive trait with complete penetrance. Men are affected more commonly than women. Symptoms and signs of the disorder usually appear in childhood or adolescence and subsequently recur throughout the remainder of life.[127] The typical manifestations include episodes of fever with abdominal, thoracic, or joint pain due to inflammation of the peritoneum, pleura, and synovial membrane. Attacks occur at irregular intervals without periodicity, with widely varying breaks between episodes that may last for years. Amyloidosis, which is a recognized complication of the disease, is genetically determined and may affect as many as 35 to 45 per cent of Sephardic Jews who have familial Mediterranean fever. It is rare in other groups with the disease. Amyloidosis can produce the nephrotic syndrome and renal failure, resulting in early death.[74]

Attacks of familial Mediterranean fever usually are brief in duration. They are characterized by the rapid onset of fever, with or without abdominal or thoracic pain. The abdominal pain, which may be evident in 80 to 95 per cent of patients, varies in severity and persists for 12 to 24 hours or, rarely, longer. Chest discomfort is of short duration, may involve only one hemithorax, and is commonly accompanied by pleuritis or pericarditis, or both.

Musculoskeletal manifestations can occur in 30 to 70 per cent of patients.[7–13, 111] Arthritis may be the initial or sole feature of the disease in as many as 27 per cent of patients.[111] Asymmetric arthritis in the larger joints of the lower extremity is most typical; the affected articulations, in order of decreasing frequency, are the knees, ankles, hips, shoulders, feet, elbows, and hands and wrists.[1, 113] The sacroiliac, temporomandibular, and other articulations also can be involved. Monoarticular arthritis is more common than polyarticular arthritis. Joint attacks vary in severity, reach a peak in 1 to 2 days, and generally resolve in 1 to 2 weeks. Occasionally, more prolonged attacks are encountered.[74] Following repeated bouts, a chronic destructive arthritis may develop, especially in the hip.[11, 112] Once destructive alterations occur, the recurrent arthritic attacks are no longer separated by symptom-free intervals.[80]

Pain, tenderness, and swelling accompany the arthritis of familial Mediterranean fever. Muscle spasm, restriction of joint motion, and bursitis also are encountered. An effusion is present, and the synovial fluid may be noninflammatory in type, with a paucity of cells, or inflammatory, with cell counts greater than 100,000 cells per cu mm, predominantly polymorphonuclear leukocytes. Viscosity is poor, but the mucin clot is adequate. Glucose levels in the synovial fluid are normal or depressed, and bacteria are not found.

An erysipelas-like erythema frequently is evident on the lower extremities.[14] Histologically it is similar to that noted in the synovium or peritoneum during attacks, with acute inflammation characterized by edema, vasodilation, and perivascular collections of neutrophils.

Radiographic Abnormalities

Osteoporosis can develop rapidly and become profound.[9] In children, hyperemia can lead to epiphyseal overgrowth that, when combined with soft tissue swelling and an effusion, can simulate the findings in juvenile chronic arthritis or hemophilia. Chronicity leads to joint space narrowing and juxta-articular erosions. Rarely, more extensive alterations are encountered. These include bony ankylosis,[11, 15–17] productive osseous changes with sclerosis and osteophyto-

sis, and osteonecrosis. These productive and ischemic changes are most evident in the hip and the knee and may require arthroplasty (Fig. 32–1).[80, 112] Involvement in these locations has been observed in approximately 75 per cent of joints affected by protracted arthritis,[11] although significant destruction also has been reported in the ankle and in metatarsophalangeal and temporomandibular articulations.[80, 81] The pathogenesis of the femoral capital epiphyseal necrosis and collapse is not clear, although vascular compromise due to joint distention has been cited.[11]

Sacroiliac joint abnormalities also have been described in familial Mediterranean fever[18–20, 75] (Table 32–1), although the association of such abnormalities and familial Mediterranean fever is not accepted uniformly.[114] The reported frequency of these abnormalities has varied. Shahin and coworkers[19] observed sacroiliac joint changes in 1 of 40 cases (2.5 per cent), whereas Heller and colleagues[7] noted similar changes in 3 of 34 cases (9 per cent), and Brodey and Wolff[18] detected sacroiliac joint abnormalities in 6 of 43 patients (14 per cent). Widening of the articular space, loss of the normal subchondral bone definition, sclerosis with or without erosions, predominantly on the ilium, and bony ankylosis can appear in one or both sacroiliac

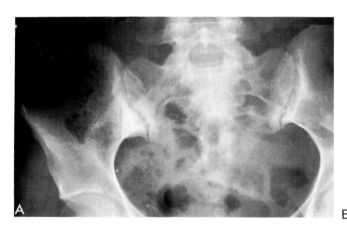

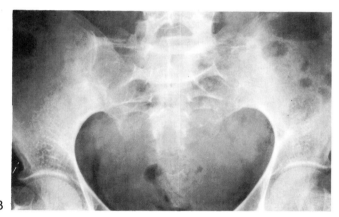

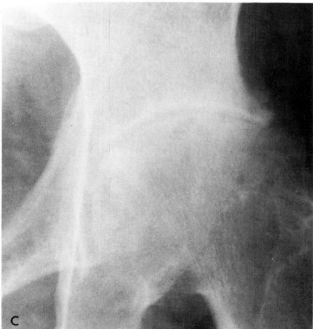

FIGURE 32–1. Familial Mediterranean fever: Sacroiliitis and hip involvement.

A Bilateral asymmetric sacroiliac joint disease is characterized by osseous erosions and reactive sclerosis, predominantly in the ilium.

B Bony ankylosis of the sacroiliac joint is seen.

C This 41 year old man with episodic hip and knee pain reveals symmetric loss of joint space and osteophytosis.

(**A, B,** From Brodey PA, Wolff SM: Radiology *114:* 331, 1975; **C,** Courtesy of D. Gershuni, M.D., San Diego, California.)

TABLE 32–1. Sacroiliac Joint Abnormalities

| | Distribution | | |
Disorder	Bilateral Symmetric	Bilateral Asymmetric	Unilateral
Familial Mediterranean fever	×	×*	×
Relapsing polychondritis	×	×*	×
Behçet's syndrome†	×	×	×

*Probably the predominant pattern of involvement.
†Questionable association with sacroiliitis.

joints; asymmetric abnormalities predominate (Fig. 32–1). The absence of HLA-B27 antigen in patients with familial Mediterranean fever and sacroiliitis[20–22] may indicate that the pathogenesis of the articular changes is different from that in classic ankylosing spondylitis, although it is of interest that patchy calcified and ossified bridges between lumbar vertebrae have been identified in persons with familial Mediterranean fever.[7] Furthermore, osseous fusion in the apophyseal joints of the cervical spine, similar to that occurring in ankylosing spondylitis, has been observed in familial Mediterranean fever.[104]

Pathologic Abnormalities

Nonspecific synovitis is evident in biopsy specimens of inflamed joints.[1] Perivascular round cell aggregates, increased vascularity, and the accumulation of stromal fibroblasts and polymorphonuclear leukocytes also are evident.[7, 81, 109] Fibrous tissue is contained within lytic lesions of bones.

Differential Diagnosis

The radiographic findings in familial Mediterranean fever are not diagnostic. In children, soft tissue swelling, osteoporosis, and epiphyseal overgrowth are evident in other articular disorders, such as juvenile chronic arthritis and hemophilia. In children and adults, joint space narrowing and osseous erosion can simulate the findings of arthritides associated with synovial inflammation, such as rheumatoid arthritis and septic arthritis. Sacroiliitis in familial Mediterranean fever simulates that of ankylosing spondylitis and other seronegative spondyloarthropathies; the absence of symmetry in the sacroiliac joint changes in some cases of familial Mediterranean fever may allow its differentiation from classic ankylosing spondylitis and the sacroiliitis of inflammatory bowel disease. Although a relatively specific pattern of femoral osteoporosis has been noted in some patients with familial Mediterranean fever,[7] further documentation of this finding is necessary.

RELAPSING POLYCHONDRITIS

Clinical Abnormalities

Relapsing polychondritis is an uncommon disorder characterized by episodic inflammation of cartilaginous tissue and special sense organs; abnormalities are especially prominent in the external ear, nose, trachea, larynx, sclera, ribs, and articular cartilage. The term "relapsing polychondritis" was introduced in 1960 by Pearson and associates,[23]

although the entity was recognized initially in 1923[24] and was known by such names as systemic chondromalacia, panchondritis, chronic atrophic polychondritis, rheumatic chondritis, and diffuse perichondritis.[25] In the last three decades, several reviews of relapsing polychondritis have appeared.[26–28, 83] McAdam and coworkers[29] established empirically the following diagnostic criteria: recurrent chondritis of both auricles; nonerosive inflammatory polyarthritis; chondritis of nasal cartilage; inflammation of ocular structures, including conjunctivitis, keratitis, scleritis, episcleritis, and uveitis; chondritis of the respiratory tract involving laryngeal or tracheal cartilages; and cochlear or vestibular damage manifested by neurosensory hearing loss, tinnitus, or vertigo.

Relapsing polychondritis appears in all age groups, with a maximal frequency in the fourth decade of life. Men and women are affected in equal numbers. The initial clinical findings usually are auricular chondritis and arthritis; less typically, respiratory tract involvement, nasal chondritis, and ocular involvement are evident at the outset of the disease. Auricular chondritis leads to painful erythematous swelling of one or both ears lasting from 5 to 10 days[29] (Fig. 32–2). This finding is limited to the cartilaginous portion of the external ears (helix, anthelix, tragus, and external auditory canal). Arthralgia and arthritis generally affect more than one joint, including the hips, knees, manubriosternal and sternoclavicular articulations, costochondral junctions, and small and large joints of the upper extremity. Less frequently, the feet, ankles, and spine are involved. Migratory polyarthritis can simulate rheumatoid arthritis or a seronegative spondyloarthropathy, although occasionally monoarticular arthritis appears that mimics infection or crystal-induced arthritis. Although commonly nonerosive in type, the arthritis may produce considerable deformity and mutilation in some persons. Tendinitis can appear. Relaps-

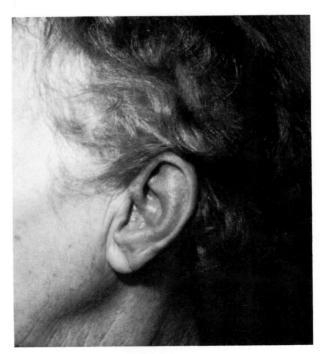

FIGURE 32–2. Relapsing polychondritis: Auricular chondritis. Observe the erythematous swelling on most of the external ear. (Courtesy of N. Zvaifler, M.D., San Diego, California.)

ing polychondritis also can be superimposed on a preexisting polyarthritis, such as rheumatoid arthritis,[115] juvenile chronic polyarthritis, collagen vascular disorders,[76, 84] ankylosing spondylitis,[116] or Reiter's syndrome.[29–31, 116] Because of this, some physicians regard relapsing polychondritis as a syndrome rather than a single disease entity.[116, 117]

Respiratory tract involvement is a potentially serious manifestation of the disease that may require tracheostomy. Laryngeal and tracheal tenderness, cough, hoarseness, and dyspnea secondary to collapse of the tracheal rings, edema, or granulomatous tissue proliferation within the respiratory tree can be evident. Nasal chondritis may be sudden in onset, painful, and associated with a feeling of fullness in the bridge of the nose and surrounding tissue.[29] Although these latter manifestations may disappear in a few days, chronic involvement can lead to characteristic saddle nose deformity. Episcleritis is the most common ocular abnormality, although any tissue in the eye can be affected in this disorder.

Additional manifestations include back pain due to spinal alterations, chest pain related to costochondritis, hearing loss attributable to obstruction of the external auditory meatus, fever, anorexia and weight loss, and cardiovascular abnormalities. McAdam and colleagues[29] have calculated the clinical manifestations in approximate order of frequency: auricular chondritis (89 per cent); polyarthritis (81 per cent); nasal chondritis (72 per cent); ocular inflammation (65 per cent); respiratory tract chondritis (56 per cent); audiovestibular damage (46 per cent); cardiovascular involvement (24 per cent); and cutaneous lesions (17 per cent).

Laboratory findings are not specific. During the active phases of the disease, anemia, leukocytosis, elevated erythrocyte sedimentation rate, moderate serum protein alterations, and, occasionally, a low serum titer positivity for rheumatoid factor may be detected. Synovial fluid usually is noninflammatory in type.

Radiographic Abnormalities

In most cases, radiographic features of joint involvement in relapsing polychondritis are not striking, although there may be extra-articular findings, such as tracheal narrowing or stenosis, calcification of the auricular cartilage, and aortic alterations after repeated attacks.[32, 33] Compromise of the tracheobronchial airways obviously is of great clinical importance and, although observed on routine radiographs, is best evaluated with CT.[105] Periarticular osteoporosis may or may not be evident.[34] Joint space narrowing and osseous erosions of the metacarpophalangeal and metatarsophalangeal articulations, identical to those of rheumatoid arthritis,[33, 118] and "arthritis mutilans"[28, 35, 36, 117] have been encountered (Fig. 32–3), but in some of these cases, changes may have been due to an underlying articular disorder. Typically, a nonerosive, nondeforming arthropathy appears.[37, 38, 120] The presence of joint space narrowing in the absence of bone erosions is reported to be characteristic of relapsing polychondritis[119] (Fig. 32–3).

Sacroiliitis has been evident in some patients with relapsing polychondritis,[38] although the prevalence probably is not high[29, 37] (see Table 32–1). Unilateral or bilateral abnormalities characterized by the presence of joint space loss,

erosion, and eburnation, and the absence of spinal alterations predominate[38] (Fig. 32–4). Of interest in this regard, HLA-B27 antigens do not appear to be associated with the arthropathy of relapsing polychondritis.[37] Rarely, radiographs of the spine reveal discovertebral erosions and severe kyphosis.[85]

Pathologic Abnormalities

Synovial membrane biopsy can reveal a synovitis characterized by chronic inflammation with preponderance of plasma cells[39] (Fig. 32–5). The lining layer of the synovium may have an increase of cells, not unlike that in rheumatoid arthritis or other types of chronic synovitis. An accumulation of lipid and lysosomes in all the superficial cells of the articular cartilage in this disease also is like that in rheumatoid arthritis. The findings in the middle and deeper layers of the cartilage may be unique, with large, perichondrocytic clear spaces containing one or more multivesicular bodies.[39]

Light microscopic and histochemical studies of involved cartilage at other sites, including the ear, suggest that there is a loss of acid mucopolysaccharide early in the process of cartilage destruction.[40, 41] In the ear, inflammatory reaction predominates in superficial areas of the cartilage[42] (Fig. 32–6). Deeper areas appear normal in most cases, although occasionally necrotic chondrocytes are seen. Typical pathologic changes also appear in vascular structures, including the aortic ring and ascending aorta, at which sites prominent abnormalities are seen in the media consisting of loss of elastic tissue, a decrease in basophilia, collagenous replacement, and focal accumulation of chronic inflammatory cells.

Etiology and Pathogenesis

The cause of relapsing polychondritis is unknown. It generally is considered a connective tissue disorder with an immunologic mediation.[43] The coexistence of relapsing polychondritis with other immune diseases, including systemic lupus erythematosus, rheumatoid arthritis, progressive systemic sclerosis, Sjögren's syndrome, and glomerulonephritis, is well known.[82] Immunoelectrophoretic anomalies are evident in approximately 60 per cent of cases; also seen are a positive serologic test for rheumatoid factor in 30 per cent, antinuclear antibodies (ANA) or LE cells in some instances, and antithyroglobulin, antiparietal cells, or antimuscle antibodies occasionally.[82] Despite the low antigenicity of cartilage proteoglycans, antibodies to cartilage and delayed hypersensitivity have been demonstrated in this disease. Hughes and coworkers,[27] Rogers and colleagues,[44] and Shaul and Schumacher[42] observed anticartilage antibodies using indirect immunofluorescent tests. Others could not confirm the presence of these antibodies but did detect delayed hypersensitivity to cartilage proteoglycan.[45, 46] The focal perichondrial chronic inflammatory collections that are observed during active phases of the disease, and that lead to matrix depletion of proteoglycans, could be caused by release of lysosomal enzymes from either chondrocytes or adjacent tissues.[42] Similar enzymatic release could be responsible for the aortic lesions that characterize relapsing polychondritis.

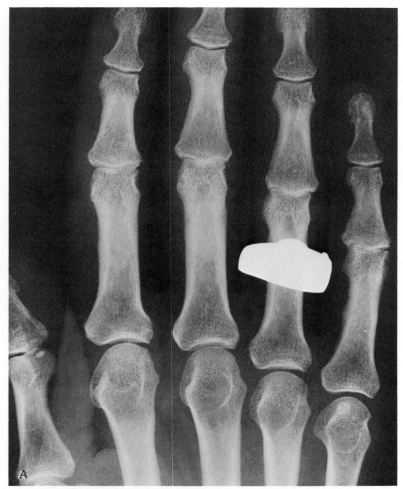

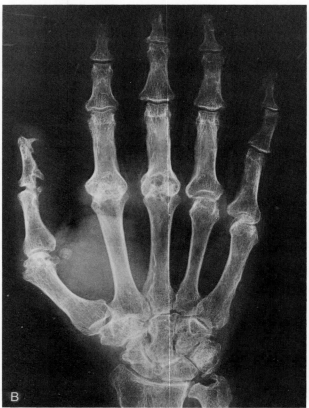

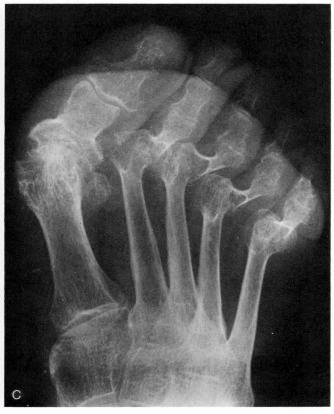

FIGURE 32–3. Relapsing polychondritis: Peripheral joint abnormalities.

A Note marked reduction in the joint spaces of the proximal interphalangeal joints and, to a lesser extent, the metacarpophalangeal joints.

(**A,** From Booth A, et al: Clin Radiol *40:*147, 1989.)

B, C In this woman, radiographic abnormalities in the hand and wrist (**B**) and in the foot (**C**) resemble those of rheumatoid arthritis. Osteopenia, erosive changes, joint space loss, and deformities are evident.

(**B, C,** From Schlapbach P, et al: Ann Rheum Dis *47:*1021, 1988.)

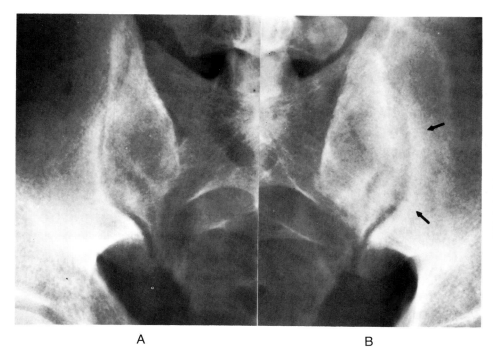

FIGURE 32–4. Relapsing polychondritis: Sacroiliac joint abnormalities. A 37 year old man with relapsing polychondritis of 4 years' duration reveals bilateral asymmetric abnormalities of the sacroiliac joints. On the right side **(A),** the changes are minimal: on the left side **(B),** moderate osseous erosions and reactive sclerosis are seen (arrows). (From Braunstein EM, et al: Clin Radiol *30:*444, 1979.)

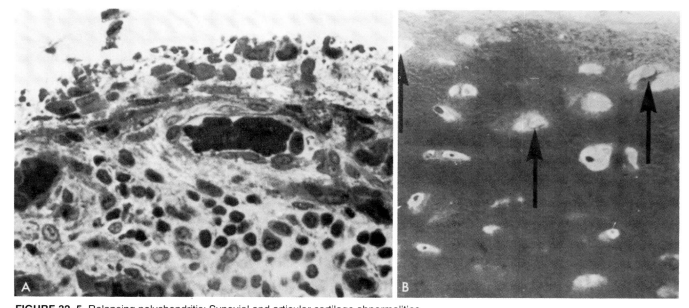

FIGURE 32–5. Relapsing polychondritis: Synovial and articular cartilage abnormalities.
 A A biopsy of a swollen, tender right third metacarpophalangeal joint in a 26 year old man with relapsing polychondritis reveals synovial inflammation with hypertrophy of the lining layer, cellular infiltration, and dilation of blood vessels (300×).
 B Evaluation of the articular cartilage from the same joint reveals an irregular chondral surface, decreased uptake of stain, and fat droplets (arrows) (340×).
 (From Mitchell N, Shepard N: J Bone Joint Surg [Am] *54:*1235, 1972.)

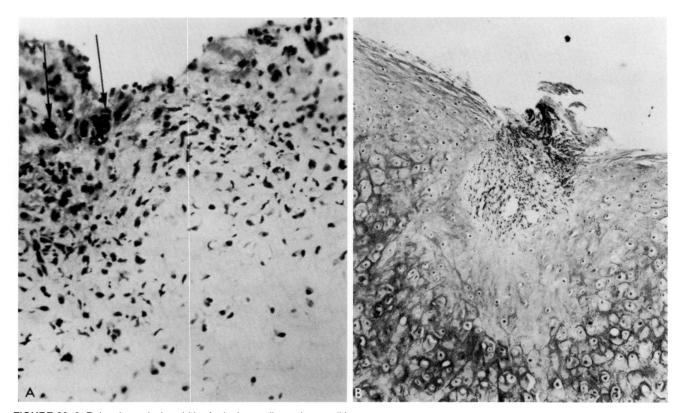

FIGURE 32–6. Relapsing polychondritis: Auricular cartilage abnormalities.
   A Superficial inflammatory cell reaction with infiltration of neutrophils and lymphocytes can be identified. Basophilic staining is lost. Blood vessels can be seen (arrows) (180×). (From Shaul SR, Schumacher HR: Arthritis Rheum 18:617, 1975.)
   B In another patient, an area of focal chondritis with a proliferative infiltrate is seen. There is significant damage of cartilage in the area of infiltrate (100×). (From McAdam LP, et al: Medicine 55:193, 1976. Copyright 1976, The Williams & Wilkins Co, Baltimore.)

Differential Diagnosis

The radiographic features of articular involvement in this disease lack specificity. Periarticular osteoporosis and soft tissue swelling about synovial articulations simulate changes in a variety of disorders. With the occurrence of diffuse joint space narrowing and osseous erosions in these sites, the radiographic picture is almost identical to that of rheumatoid arthritis, although symmetry and more extensive cartilaginous and osseous destruction with deformities are more characteristic of the latter disease. Sacroiliitis in relapsing polychondritis is similar to that in ankylosing spondylitis or other seronegative spondyloarthropathies. In some cases, the appearance also may resemble osteitis condensans ilii. Calcification of ear cartilage is seen not only in relapsing polychondritis but also in adrenal insufficiency, acromegaly, alkaptonuria, hyperparathyroidism, and diabetes mellitus and after injury.

BEHÇET'S SYNDROME

Clinical Abnormalities

Behçet's syndrome initially was described as a triad of painful, recurrent oral and genital ulcerations and ocular inflammation.[47] It now is recognized that many additional systems can be affected, including the skin, joints, and cardiovascular, neurologic, and gastrointestinal organs.[48–52] Original cases of Behçet's syndrome were evident in Med-

iterranean countries, but the disorder also has been noted in persons throughout Europe, the Middle East and Far East, and the United States. Of interest, Behçet's syndrome occurs most commonly between latitudes 30 and 45 degrees north in Asian and Eurasian populations; this area coincides with the old "Silk Road," opened during the Han Dynasty in the year 200 B.C.E., traveled by Marco Polo and Genghis Khan, and so named because it was the pathway for the Chinese traders whose caravans contained masses of silk.[121]

The age of onset of Behçet's syndrome varies from 5 to 70 years, with a mean age of approximately 25 to 30 years; men are affected more commonly than women. Neonatal Behçet's syndrome has been observed in an infant of a mother with the disease.[102] It has been suggested that the disease is more severe in male patients and in those with an earlier age of onset of the clinical manifestations.[106]

Over 90 per cent of patients reveal ulcerations in portions of the mouth or pharynx. The ulcerations, single or multiple and of varying size, appear rapidly, resolve in a period of 1 to 2 weeks, and recur. Biopsy of the mucosal lesions may reveal cellular infiltration, predominantly of mononuclear cells, and no vasculitis.

Ophthalmic lesions are evident in approximately 80 per cent of patients. Typically, iritis is seen, although episcleritis, conjunctivitis, keratitis, iridocyclitis, retinothrombophlebitis, optic neuritis and atrophy, and papilledema can be encountered. Late complications include glaucoma, cataracts, and blindness. Genital lesions appear in approximately 60 per cent of cases. In men, these include painful ulcerations of the penis and scrotum; in women, similar ulcerations of the vulva and vagina may produce few symptoms. Skin lesions may be observed in approximately 75 per cent of cases, consisting of pyoderma with pustules of varying size and erythema nodosum–like abnormalities of the lower extremity. Cutaneous induration at sites of trauma (e.g., needle puncture) is common. This response may relate to increased motility of polymorphonuclear leukocytes in Behçet's syndrome, leading to dense cellular infiltrates at sites of injury.[101]

Additional manifestations include venous thrombosis and thrombophlebitis; arterial occlusion and aneurysm; gastrointestinal inflammation leading to abdominal pain, distention, and diarrhea; and central nervous system findings, such as meningitis, transverse myelitis, and psychiatric disorders.[53, 122] Myositis also has been noted.[79] It may be diffuse[79] or focal[86] in distribution. Muscle fiber degeneration and cellular infiltration, especially in perivascular regions, are observed.[86, 87] Crista-like inclusions within the muscle fibers have been seen.[87]

Articular alterations appear in more than 50 per cent of patients. Monoarticular or oligoarticular involvement predominates,[97] affecting principally the knees but also other joints, including the ankles, wrists, and elbows.[123] With affliction in the feet, pseudopodagra can develop.[95] The sacroiliac and manubriosternal articulations[54] also may be involved. Findings in the spine, hips, and shoulders are rare.[97] An insidious onset, a variable duration, and recurrence after disappearance of the findings typify the bouts of arthralgia or arthritis. Joint effusion, stiffness, warmth, and tenderness are observed, but permanent changes are rare. Synovial cysts, particularly in the popliteal region, lead to periarticular masses and, with rupture, to symptoms and signs resembling those of thrombophlebitis.[89–91] Subcutaneous nodules, differing pathologically from rheumatoid nodules, are evident infrequently.[94]

Laboratory analysis may reveal an elevated erythrocyte sedimentation rate, a strongly positive C-reactive protein, and elevation of alpha-2 globulins during the acute phase of the disease.[1] Low grade anemia and mild leukocytosis also are observed. Many patients reveal high titers of serum antibodies directed against human oral mucosa, and some have peripheral lymphocytes that are stimulated by mucosal antigen, abnormalities that are not specific.[55]

An increased frequency of the tissue typing antigen HLA-B5 has been found in some series,[56, 96, 103] although this has not been confirmed by other investigators. A modest increase in prevalence of HLA-B27 also has been identified in some reports,[52] but this association, too, must await further documentation.

Evaluation of synovial fluid reveals inflammatory characteristics[97] with poor mucin clot, elevation in complement levels, and a polymorphonuclear leukocytosis.[57]

Radiographic Abnormalities

Radiographic findings in the skeleton usually are mild.[99] Osteoporosis and soft tissue swelling can be seen, but joint space narrowing and osseous erosions are encountered only rarely[58, 110] (Fig. 32–7). When present, these latter findings resemble changes in rheumatoid arthritis or other disorders

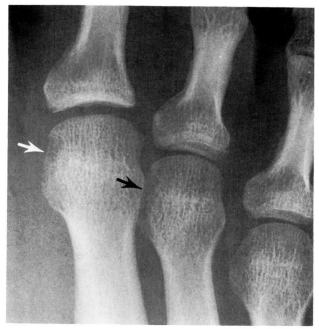

FIGURE 32–7. Behçet's syndrome: Peripheral joint abnormalities. Observe small osseous erosions of metatarsal heads (arrows) and osteoporosis. (Courtesy of A. Brower, M.D., Norfolk, Virginia.)

characterized by synovial inflammation.[107, 128] One report also has noted a patient with spontaneous atlantoaxial subluxation[77] (Fig. 32–8); others described subluxations and deformities in the hand, again simulating the abnormalities

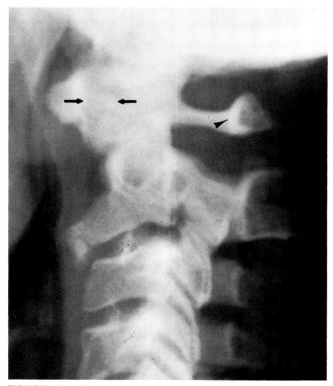

FIGURE 32–8. Behçet's syndrome: Atlantoaxial subluxation. Note the increased distance between the posterior surface of the anterior arch of the atlas and the odontoid process (between arrows), as well as an anterior position of the spinolaminar line (arrowhead). (Courtesy of M. Dalinka, M.D., Philadelphia, Pennsylvania.)

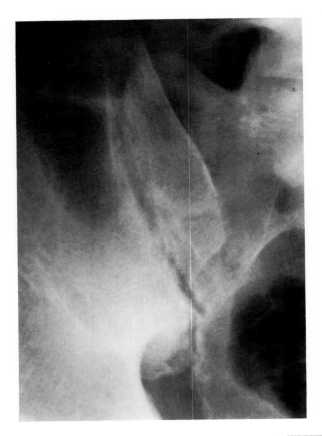

FIGURE 32–9. Behçet's syndrome: Sacroiliitis. In this patient, unilateral sacroiliitis is characterized by subchondral erosions and reactive sclerosis, predominantly in the ilium. (Courtesy of A. Brower, M.D., Norfolk, Virginia.)

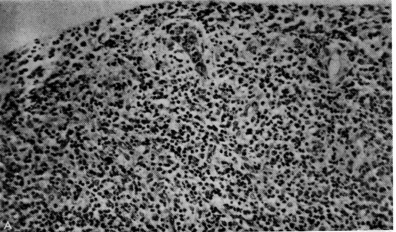

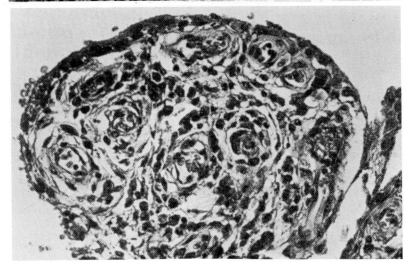

FIGURE 32–10. Behçet's syndrome: Pathologic abnormalities of synovial joints.

A Following a biopsy of the synovial membrane from an inflamed wrist joint, note the absence of lining cells and the presence of heavily inflamed granulation tissue (150×).

B A high-power view of a synovial villous process reveals numerous small vessels, some fibrosis, and a moderate plasma cell infiltrate (550×).

(From Vernon-Roberts B, et al: Ann Rheum Dis 37:139, 1978.)

B

in rheumatoid arthritis[92] or psoriatic arthritis.[124] Some reports have indicated the occurrence of sacroiliitis in Behçet's syndrome,[59, 60, 98, 108, 125] although others have failed to identify such an association[52, 93, 114] (Table 32–1, Fig. 32–9). When present, sacroiliac joint changes have included bone erosion, sclerosis, and joint space narrowing in a patchy or asymmetric distribution.[98] Bony ankylosis is unusual. It has been suggested that patients with Behçet's disease who are HLA-B27–positive are at risk of developing a mild sacroiliitis and spondylitis.[61] In addition, a possible relationship between Behçet's syndrome and ankylosing spondylitis or inflammatory bowel disorders such as ulcerative colitis and Crohn's disease could account for a link with sacroiliitis in Behçet's disease.[52, 62, 63, 126]

Pathologic Abnormalities

Histologic examination shows replacement of the superficial zones of the synovial membrane by dense, inflamed granulation tissue composed of lymphocytes, macrophages, fibroblasts, neutrophils, and vascular elements[58, 97, 100] (Fig. 32–10). Pannus, with erosion of cartilaginous and osseous surfaces, can be noted, and organisms cannot be recovered.

At sites of ulceration in the skin and mucosa, vasculitis generally is prominent. It also may be evident about ocular and gastrointestinal lesions, as well as in other locations. Aneurysms in the aorta and elsewhere may reveal acute and chronic cellular infiltration in the vessel walls, with an endarteritis of the vasa vasorum.[64, 65]

Etiology and Pathogenesis

The cause of Behçet's syndrome is unknown. Although there has been considerable speculation about the role of infection in this disorder,[47] particularly a viral disease[66, 67] or tuberculosis, this possibility has been discounted by some investigators.[68] Environmental pollutants have been stressed as etiologic factors in other reports.[61] The known geographic concentration of cases, the familial clustering,[69–71] and the recognition of the association of the disease with HLA-B5 in Japanese patients suggest that host factors are important.[55, 78] An immunologic disturbance is implicated by the detection of antibodies against buccal mucosa,[72, 73] lymphocytoxicity to oral epithelial cells, and the similarity of the histologic abnormalities to those of delayed hypersensitivity. The putative antigen leading to this disturbance has not been identified.

Differential Diagnosis

When they are evident, radiologic alterations of joints in Behçet's syndrome may resemble those of rheumatoid arthritis or related disorders. Sacroiliitis can simulate the changes in ankylosing spondylitis or other seronegative spondyloarthropathies.

SUMMARY

Familial Mediterranean fever, relapsing polychondritis, and Behçet's syndrome represent three uncommon disorders that may be associated with periodic, relapsing, or recurrent clinical manifestations. In each disease, synovitis

occasionally can lead to soft tissue swelling and periarticular osteoporosis, and in rare instances cartilaginous and osseous destruction can become evident. Furthermore, each of these three disorders has been associated with sacroiliitis, although this association is not frequent, nor is it without controversy in some cases.

References

1. Ehrlich GE: Intermittent and periodic arthritis syndromes. *In* JL Hollander, DJ McCarty Jr (Eds): Arthritis and Allied Conditions, 8th Ed. Philadelphia, Lea & Febiger, 1972, p 821.
2. Heller H, Sohar E, Sherf L: Familial Mediterranean fever. Arch Intern Med *102:*50, 1958.
3. Priest RJ, Nixon RK: Familial recurring polyserositis: A disease entity. Ann Intern Med *51:*1253, 1959.
4. Sohar E, Gafni J, Pras M, et al: Familial Mediterranean fever. A survey of 470 cases and review of the literature. Am J Med *43:*227, 1967.
5. Siegal S: Familial paroxysmal polyserositis. Analysis of 50 cases. Am J Med *36:*893, 1964.
6. Schwabe AD, Peters RS: Familial Mediterranean fever in Armenians. Analysis of 100 cases. Medicine *53:*453, 1974.
7. Heller H, Gafni J, Michaeli D, et al: The arthritis of familial Mediterranean fever. Arthritis Rheum *9:*1, 1966.
8. Makin M, Levin S: The articular manifestations of periodic disease (familial Mediterranean fever). J Bone Joint Surg [Am] *47:*1615, 1965.
9. Herness D, Makin M: Articular damage in familial Mediterranean fever. J Bone Joint Surg [Am] *57:*265, 1975.
10. Simon G, Marbach JJ: Familial Mediterranean fever with temporomandibular joint arthritis. Pediatrics *57:*810, 1976.
11. Sneh E, Pras M, Michaeli D, et al: Protracted arthritis in familial Mediterranean fever. Rheumatol Rehabil *16:*102, 1977.
12. Sohar E, Pras M, Gafni J: Familial Mediterranean fever and its articular manifestations. Clin Rheum Dis *1:*195, 1975.
13. Dinarello CA, Wolff SM, Goldfinger SE, et al: Colchicine therapy for familial Mediterranean fever. N Engl J Med *291:*934, 1974.
14. Azizi E, Fisher BK: Cutaneous manifestations of familial Mediterranean fever. Arch Dermatol *112:*364, 1976.
15. Mamou H, Cattan R: La maladie périodique (sur 14 cas personnels dont 8 compliqués de néphropathies). Sem Hôp Paris *28:*1062, 1952.
16. Siguier F: Maladies—Vedettes; Maladies d'Avenir, Maladies Quotidiennes, Maladies d'Exception. Paris, Masson, 1957, p 279.
17. Gumpel JM: Familial Mediterranean fever. Proc R Soc Med *65:*977, 1972.
18. Brodey PA, Wolff SM: Radiographic changes in the sacroiliac joints in familial Mediterranean fever. Radiology *114:*331, 1975.
19. Shahin N, Sohar E, Dalith F: Roentgenologic findings in familial Mediterranean fever. AJR *84:*269, 1960.
20. Lehman TJA, Hanson V, Kornreich H, et al: HLA-B27 negative sacroiliitis: A manifestation of familial Mediterranean fever in childhood. Pediatrics *61:*423, 1978.
21. Schwabe AD, Terasaki PI, Barnett EV, et al: Familial Mediterranean fever: Recent advances in pathogenesis and management. West J Med *127:*15, 1977.
22. Lehman TJA, Peters RS, Hanson V, et al: Diagnosis and treatment of familial Mediterranean fever (FMF) in childhood (Abstr). Arthritis Rheum *21:*573, 1978.
23. Pearson CM, Kline HM, Newcomer VD: Relapsing polychondritis. N Engl J Med *263:*51, 1960.
24. Jaksch-Wartenhorst R: Polychondropathia. Wien Arch Inn Med *6:*93, 1923.
25. Harders H: Panchondritis. Verh Dtsch Ges Rheumatol *3:*71, 1974.
26. Kaye RL, Sones DA: Relapsing polychondritis. Clinical and pathological features in fourteen cases. Ann Intern Med *60:*653, 1964.
27. Hughes RAC, Berry CL, Seifert M, et al: Relapsing polychondritis. Three cases with a clinico-pathologic study and literature review. Q J Med *41:*363, 1972.
28. Dolan DL, Lemmon GB, Teitelbaum SL: Relapsing polychondritis: Analytical literature review and studies on pathogenesis. Am J Med *41:*285, 1966.
29. McAdam LP, O'Hanlan MA, Bluestone R, et al: Relapsing polychondritis: Prospective study of 23 patients and a review of the literature. Medicine *55:*193, 1976.
30. Barth WF, Berson EL: Relapsing polychondritis, rheumatoid arthritis and blindness. Am J Ophthalmol *66:*890, 1969.
31. Anderson B Sr: Ocular lesions in relapsing polychondritis and other rheumatoid syndromes. Am J Ophthalmol *64:*35, 1967.
32. Rabuzzi DD: Relapsing polychondritis. Arch Otolaryngol *91:*188, 1970.
33. Owen DS Jr, Irby R, Toone E: Relapsing polychondritis with aortic involvement. Arthritis Rheum *13:*877, 1970.
34. Johnson TH, Mital N, Rodnan GP, et al: Relapsing polychondritis. Radiology *106:*313, 1973.
35. Butcher RB II, Tabb HG, Dunlap CE: Relapsing polychondritis. South Med J *67:*1443, 1974.
36. Rogers FB, Lansbury J: Atrophy of auricular and nasal cartilages following administration of chorionic gonadotrophins in a case of arthritis mutilans with the sicca syndrome. Am J Med Sci *229:*55, 1955.

37. O'Hanlan M, McAdam LP, Bluestone R, et al: The arthropathy of relapsing polychondritis. Arthritis Rheum *19:*191, 1976.
38. Braunstein EM, Martel W, Stillwell E, et al: Radiological aspects of the arthropathy of relapsing polychondritis. Clin Radiol *30:*441, 1979.
39. Mitchell N, Shepard N: Relapsing polychondritis. An electron microscopic study of synovium and articular cartilage. J Bone Joint Surg [Am] *54:*1235, 1972.
40. Verity MA, Larson WM, Madden SC: Relapsing polychondritis: Report of two necropsied cases with histochemical investigations of the cartilage lesion. Am J Pathol *42:*251, 1963.
41. Feinerman LK, Johnson WC, Weiner J, et al: Relapsing polychondritis: A histopathologic and histochemical study. Dermatologica *140:*369, 1970.
42. Shaul SR, Schumacher HR: Relapsing polychondritis. Electron microscopic study of ear cartilage. Arthritis Rheum *18:*617, 1975.
43. Tourtellotte CD: Relapsing polychondritis. *In* AS Cohen (Ed): The Science and Practice of Clinical Medicine. Vol 4, Rheumatology and Immunology. New York, Grune & Stratton, 1979, p 350.
44. Rogers PH, Boden G, Tourtellotte CD: Relapsing polychondritis with insulin resistance and antibodies to cartilage. Am J Med *55:*243, 1973.
45. Herman JH, Dennis MV: Immunopathologic studies in relapsing polychondritis. J Clin Invest *52:*549, 1973.
46. Rajapakse DA, Bywaters EGL: Cell mediated immunity to cartilage proteoglycan in relapsing polychondritis. Clin Exp Immunol *16:*497, 1974.
47. Behçet H: Some observations on the clinical picture of the so-called triple symptom complex. Dermatologica *81:*73, 1940.
48. Mason RM, Barnes CG: Behçet's syndrome with arthritis. Ann Rheum Dis *28:*95, 1969.
49. Chajek T, Fairnaru M: Behçet's disease. Report of 41 cases and review of the literature. Medicine *54:*179, 1975.
50. O'Duffy JD, Carney JA, Deodar S: Behçet's disease: Report of 10 cases, 3 with new manifestations. Ann Intern Med *75:*561, 1971.
51. Oshima Y, Shimizu T, Yokohari R, et al: Clinical studies on Behçet's syndrome. Ann Rheum Dis *22:*36, 1973.
52. Chamberlain MA: Behçet's syndrome in 32 patients in Yorkshire. Ann Rheum Dis *36:*491, 1977.
53. O'Duffy JD, Goldstein NP: Neurologic involvement in seven patients with Behçet's disease. Am J Med *61:*170, 1976.
54. Currey HLF, Elson RA, Mason RM: Surgical treatment of manubriosternal pain in Behçet's syndrome. Report of a case. J Bone Joint Surg [Br] *50:*836, 1968.
55. Medsger TA Jr: Behçet's disease. In AS Cohen (Ed): The Science and Practice of Clinical Medicine. Vol 4, Rheumatology and Immunology. New York, Grune & Stratton, 1979, p 233.
56. Ohno S, Aoki K, Sugiura S, et al: HL-A5 and Behçet's disease. Lancet *2:*1383, 1973.
57. Zizic TM, Stevens MB: The arthropathy of Behçet's disease. Johns Hopkins Med J *136:*243, 1975.
58. Vernon-Roberts B, Barnes CG, Revell PA: Synovial pathology in Behçet's syndrome. Ann Rheum Dis *37:*139, 1978.
59. Cooper DA, Penny R: Behçet's syndrome: Clinical, immunological and therapeutic evaluation of 17 patients. Aust NZ J Med *4:*585, 1974.
60. Dilsen AN: Sacroiliitis and ankylosing spondylitis in Behçet's disease (Abstr). Scand J Rheum Suppl 8:20–08, 1975.
61. O'Duffy JD: Summary of international symposium on Behçet's disease. Istanbul, September 29–30, 1977. J Rheumatol *5:*229, 1978.
62. Bøe J, Dalgaard JB, Scott D: Mucocutaneous-ocular syndrome with intestinal involvement. A clinical and pathological study of four fatal cases. Am J Med *25:*857, 1958.
63. Empey DW, Hale JE: Rectal and colonic ulceration in Behçet's disease. Proc R Soc Med *65:*163, 1972.
64. Enoch BA, Castillo-Olivares JL, Khoo TCL, et al: Major vascular complications in Behçet's syndrome. Postgrad Med J *44:*453, 1968.
65. Hills EA: Behçet's syndrome with aortic aneurysm. Br Med J *4:*152, 1967.
66. Sezer FN: The isolation of a virus as the cause of Behçet's disease. Am J Ophthalmol *36:*301, 1953.
67. Sezer FN: Further investigation on the virus of Behçet's disease. Am J Ophthalmol *41:*41, 1956.
68. Dugeon JA: Virological aspects of Behçet's disease. Proc R Soc Med *54:*104, 1961.
69. Goolamali SK, Comaish JS, Hassanyek F, et al: Familial Behçet's syndrome. Br J Dermatol *95:*637, 1976.
70. Fowler TJ, Humpston DJ, Nussey AM, et al: Behçet's syndrome with neurological manifestations in two sisters. Br Med J *2:*473, 1968.
71. Berman L, Trappler B, Jenkins T: Behçet's syndrome: A family study and the elucidation of a genetic role. Ann Rheum Dis *38:*118, 1979.
72. Jensen T: Rückfällige apthöse Geschwürsbildung an Mundscheleimhaut und Geschlechtsteilen nebst rückfälliger Regenbogenhautenzündung und Sehnervenschwund (Behçet's Syndrom) (Abstr). Zentralbl Ges Ophthalmol *46:*446, 1941.
73. Shimizu T, Katsuta Y, Oshimo Y: Immunological studies on Behçet's syndrome. Ann Rheum Dis *24:*494, 1965.
74. Meyerhoff J: Familial Mediterranean fever: Report of a large family, review of the literature, and discussion of the frequency of amyloidosis. Medicine *59:*66, 1980.
75. Gilsanz V, Stanley P: Pediatric case of the day. AJR *134:*1293, 1980.
76. Small P, Frenkiel S: Relapsing polychondritis. A feature of systemic lupus erythematosus. Arthritis Rheum *23:*361, 1980.
77. Koss JC, Dalinka MK: Atlantoaxial subluxation in Behçet's syndrome. Am J Roentgenol *134:*392, 1980.
78. Yazici H, Tuzun Y, Pazarli H, et al: The combined use of HLA-B5 and the pathergy test as diagnostic markers of Behçet's disease in Turkey. J Rheumatol *7:*206, 1980.
79. Arkin CR, Rothschild BM, Florendo NT, et al: Behçet's syndrome with myositis. A case report with pathologic findings. Arthritis Rheum *23:*600, 1980.
80. Kaushansky K, Finerman GAM, Schwabe AD: Chronic destructive arthritis in familial Mediterranean fever: The predominance of hip involvement and its management. Clin Orthop *155:*156, 1981.
81. Yagil Y, Mogle P, Ariel I: Case report 195. Skel Radiol *8:*157, 1982.
82. Giroux L, Paquin F, Guerard-Desjardins MJ, et al: Relapsing polychondritis: An autoimmune disease. Semin Arthritis Rheum *13:*182, 1983.
83. Lambrozo J, Brodaty Y: Polychondrite atrophiante chronique. Rev Med *5:*269, 1981.
84. Conn DL, Dickson ER, Carpenter HA: The association of Churg-Strauss vasculitis with temporal artery involvement, primary biliary cirrhosis, and polychondritis in a single patient. J Rheumatol *9:*744, 1982.
85. Spritzer HW, Weaver AL, Diamond HS, et al: Relapsing polychondritis. Report of a case with vertebral column involvement. JAMA *208:*355, 1969.
86. Yazici H, Tuzuner N, Tuzun Y, et al: Localized myositis in Behçet's disease. Arthritis Rheum *24:*636, 1981.
87. DiGiacomo B, Carmenini G, Meloni F, et al: Myositis in Behçet's disease. Arthritis Rheum *25:*1025, 1982.
88. Frayha R: Muscle involvement in Behçet's disease. Arthritis Rheum *24:*636, 1981.
89. Mulhern LM, Pollock BH: Pseudothrombophlebitis and Behçet's syndrome. Arthritis Rheum *25:*477, 1982.
90. Hamza M: Thrombophlebitis in Behçet's disease: Two causes of diagnostic error. Arthritis Rheum *27:*717, 1984.
91. Dawes PT, Raman D, Haslock I: Acute synovial rupture in Behçet's syndrome. Ann Rheum Dis *42:*591, 1983.
92. Ben-Dov I, Zimmerman J: Deforming arthritis of the hands in Behçet's disease. J Rheumatol *9:*617, 1982.
93. Yazici H, Tuzlaci M, Yurdakul S: A controlled survey of sacroiliitis in Behçet's disease. Ann Rheum Dis *40:*558, 1981.
94. Yurdakul S, Yazici H, Tuzuner N, et al: Olecranon nodules in a case of Behçet's disase. Ann Rheum Dis *40:*182, 1981.
95. Giacomello A, Sorgi ML, Zoppini A: Pseudopodagra in Behçet's syndrome. Arthritis Rheum *24:*750, 1981.
96. Yazici H, Chamberlain A, Schreuder I, et al: HLA antigens in Behçet's disease: A reappraisal by a comparative study of Turkish and British patients. Ann Rheum Dis *39:*344, 1980.
97. Yurakul S, Yazici H, Tuzun Y, et al: The arthritis of Behçet's disease: A prospective study. Ann Rheum Dis *42:*505, 1983.
98. Caporn N, Higgs ER, Dieppe PA, et al: Arthritis in Behçet's syndrome. Br J Radiol *56:*87, 1983.
99. Rosenberger A, Adler OB, Haim S: Radiological aspects of Behçet's disease. Radiology *144:*261, 1982.
100. Gibson T, Laurent R, Highton J, et al: Synovial histopathology of Behçet's syndrome. Ann Rheum Dis *40:*376, 1981.
101. Fordham JN, Davies PG, Kirk A, et al: Polymorphonuclear function in Behçet's syndrome. Ann Rheum Dis *41:*421, 1982.
102. Fam AG, Siminovitch KA, Carette S, et al: Neonatal Behçet's syndrome in an infant of a mother with Behçet's disease. Ann Rheum Dis *40:*509, 1981.
103. O'Duffy JD, Lehner T, Barnes CG: Summary of the third international conference on Behçet's disease. J Rheumatol *10:*154, 1983.
104. Sukenik S, Horowitz J, Boehm R, et al: Cervical spine involvement in familial Mediterranean fever. J Rheumatol *12:*603, 1985.
105. Mendelson DS, Som PM, Crane R, et al: Relapsing polychondritis studied by computed tomography. Radiology *157:*489, 1985.
106. Yazici H, Tuzun Y, Pazarli H, et al: Influence of age of onset and patient's sex on the prevalence and severity of manifestations of Behçet's syndrome. Ann Rheum Dis *43:*783, 1984.
107. Takeuchi A, Mori M, Hashimoto A: Radiographic abnormalities in patients with Behçet's disease. Clin Exp Rheumatol *2:*259, 1984.
108. Keysser M, Weber J: Wirbelsaulenbeteiligung beim Behçet-Syndrom (BS). Akt Rheumatol *9:*169, 1984.
109. Langer HE, Huth F, Behfar S, et al: Die synovitis des familiären Mittelmeerfiebers. Dtsch Med Wschr *110:*1695, 1985.
110. Jawad ASM, Goodwill CJ: Behçet's disease with erosive arthritis. Ann Rheum Dis *45:*961, 1986.
111. Barakat MH, Karnik AM, Majeed HWA, et al: Familial Mediterranean fever (recurrent hereditary polyserositis) in Arabs—a study of 175 patients and review of the literature. Q J Med *70:*837, 1986.
112. Goupille P, Burgot D, Soutif D, et al: Les coxites de la maladie périodique. Sem Hôp Paris *67:*232, 1991.
113. Hughes RA, Scott JT: Chronic synovitis of the shoulder in familial Mediterranean fever: A disease of symptoms not signs. Ann Rheum Dis *48:*163, 1989.
114. Yazici H, Turunc M, Özdogan H, et al: Observer variation in grading sacroiliac radiographs might be the cause of 'sacroiliitis' reported in certain disease states. Ann Rheum Dis *46:*139, 1987.

115. Rajaee A, Voossoghi AA: Classical rheumatoid arthritis associated with relapsing polychondritis. J Rheumatol *16:*1263, 1989.
116. Pazirandeh M, Ziran BH, Khandelwal BK, et al: Relapsing polychondritis and spondyloarthropathies. J Rheumatol *15:*630, 1988.
117. Hager MH, Moore ME: Relapsing polychondritis syndrome associated with pustular psoriasis, spondylitis and arthritis mutilans. J Rheumatol *14:*162, 1987.
118. Schlapbach P, Gerber NJ, Ramser P, et al: Relapsing polychondritis mimicking rheumatoid arthritis. Ann Rheum Dis *47:*1021, 1988.
119. Booth A, Dieppe PA, Goddard PL, et al: The radiological manifestations of relapsing polychondritis. Clin Radiol *40:*147, 1989.
120. Sartoris DJ, Resnick D: Radiologic vignette: Primary disorders of articular cartilage in childhood. J Rheumatol *15:*812, 1988.
121. James DG: "Silk Route disease" (Behçet's disease). West J Med *148:*433, 1988.
122. Hamza M'H: Large artery involvement in Behçet's disease. J Rheumatol *14:*554, 1987.
123. Al-Rawi ZS, Sharquie KE, Khalifa SJ, et al: Behçet's disease in Iraqi patients. Ann Rheum Dis *45:*987, 1986.
124. Takeuchi A, Hashimoto T: Arthropathy of Behçet's disease: A case with "pencil-in-cup" deformities. Arthritis Rheum *32:*1629, 1989.
125. Olivieri I, Gemignani G, Camerini E, et al: Computed tomography of the sacroiliac joints in four patients with Behçet's syndrome—confirmation of sacroiliitis. Br J Rheumatol *29:*264, 1990.
126. Olivieri I, Gemignani G, Busoni F, et al: Ankylosing spondylitis with predominant involvement of the cervical spine in a woman with Behçet's syndrome. Ann Rheum Dis *47:*780, 1988.
127. Gedalia A, Gorodischer R: Familial Mediterranean fever in children. J Rheumatol *19:*1, 1992.
128. Comesana NL, Rivera E, Rodriguez E, et al: Manifestaciones radiológicas osteoarticulares de la enfermedad de Behçet. Radiologia *34:*43, 1992.

SECTION

V

Connective Tissue Diseases

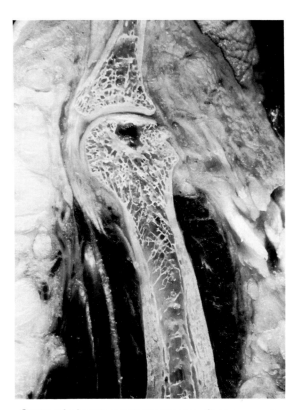

Systemic lupus erythematosus: Osteonecrosis of the head of the fifth metatarsal bone is seen. (From Resnick D, Pineda C, Trudell D: Skel Radiol *13*:33, 1985.)

33

Systemic Lupus Erythematosus

Donald Resnick, M.D.

Systemic lupus erythematosus is a relatively common connective tissue disorder characterized by significant immunologic abnormalities and involvement of multiple organ systems. The musculoskeletal system frequently is affected, leading to a variety of clinical, pathologic, and radiologic findings, which are delineated in this chapter. A complete discussion of the systemic manifestations of the disease is beyond the scope of this book.

HISTORICAL ASPECTS

Early reports considered lupus erythematosus to be an insignificant disorder of the skin. In 1872, Kaposi[1] first emphasized the systemic nature of the illness, and approximately 30 years later, Osler[2] delineated many of its clinical manifestations, suggesting a vascular cause for the disorder. During the ensuing years, the clinical and pathologic features of systemic lupus erythematosus were further outlined.[3, 4] The characteristic immunologic alterations in this disease were first noted in 1948 when Hargraves and his colleagues[5] discovered the lupus erythematosus (LE) cell. Subsequently, Miescher and collaborators[6] identified the LE cell factor as an antinuclear antibody, and additional antinuclear antibodies were found in association with this disease.[7, 8] As a direct result of these clinical and laboratory advances, an increased awareness of systemic lupus erythematosus became evident, leading to earlier diagnosis, particularly in mild and atypical forms of the disease, and to improved prognosis.[9]

It now is recognized that systemic lupus erythematosus is a chronic disease associated with acute exacerbations and a variable outlook. Furthermore, it is known that abnormalities in the immune mechanism are fundamental in the pathogenesis of this disorder; patients produce many autoantibodies that participate in tissue injury throughout the body. Although the exact cause of systemic lupus erythematosus remains unknown, a variety of precipitating events appear important, including genetic and infectious factors. In addition, exposure to sunlight or ultraviolet rays or to certain drugs (oral contraceptives, penicillin, and sulfonamides) or foreign proteins (tetanus antitoxin) may lead to exacerbations of this disease.

Considerable interest has been expressed in establishing reliable criteria for the diagnosis and classification of systemic lupus erythematosus. On two separate occasions, in 1971 and 1982, subcommittees of the American Rheumatism Association published reports dealing with and describing such criteria.[86, 87] In the interval between these reports[88-91] and subsequent to the second report,[92] the sensitivity and the reliability of the diagnostic criteria were tested, with variable results.[127, 128] With the addition of serologic tests (antinuclear antibody, anti-Sm, anti-DNA) to these criteria in 1982, some improvement in their sensitivity has been recorded.[92]

GENERAL CLINICAL ABNORMALITIES

Systemic lupus erythematosus is much more common in women than in men[10] and in blacks than in whites. Its familial nature also is well recognized.[97] Although onset may occur at any age, the disease is most frequent in women during the childbearing years. Children may be affected and, in general, the pattern of disease and its prognosis in childhood are similar to those in adults.[93] The disease is rare in persons over the age of 45 years. In this age group, clinical, serologic, and radiologic characteristics

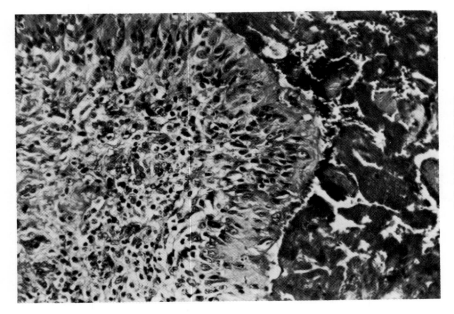

FIGURE 33–1. Systemic lupus erythematosus: Soft tissue nodule. Pathologic abnormalities. Soft tissue nodules may occur in systemic lupus erythematosus, particularly over the olecranon, on the extensor surface about the metacarpophalangeal joints, and in flexor tendon sheaths. Histologically, they resemble rheumatoid nodules with palisading and a basophil fibrinoid necrotic center (175×). (From Bywaters EGL: Clinics Rheum Dis *1:*125, 1975.)

have differed from those in younger patients, although reports have not agreed on these differences.[94–96] In the experience of some investigators, pleural and pericardial disease is more frequent in older patients with systemic lupus erythematosus, and the prevalence of arthritis also is higher. Soft tissue swelling in the hands and feet and hematologic malignancy are other reported characteristics of late-onset disease.[96]

Symptoms and signs are variable, related to the distribution and the extent of systemic alterations. In some persons, one or two organ systems are affected, whereas in others, multiple systems are involved. Initial clinical manifestations most frequently include constitutional symptoms and signs (malaise, weakness, fever, anorexia, and weight loss) and articular (polyarthritis) and cutaneous (skin rash) findings. Subsequently, major clinical abnormalities may relate to the musculoskeletal, cutaneous, neurologic, renal, pulmonary, and cardiac systems.

Skin manifestations are variable and include a typical butterfly eruption of the face; erythematous rashes on the eyelids, the forehead, and the neck; subungual erythema; urticaria; vasculitis with livedo reticularis; and alopecia. Skin nodules resembling those in rheumatoid arthritis may be observed in 5 to 10 per cent of patients with systemic lupus erythematosus (Fig. 33–1). These nodules also are seen in the synovial membrane and in extra-articular sites, such as the vocal cords.[98, 99]

Neurologic findings include personality changes, seizures, ataxia, hemiplegia, chorea, and peripheral neuropathy.[11] Ocular lesions include hemorrhage and exudation, although blindness is uncommon.[12]

Lupus nephritis can lead to hypertension, proteinuria, the nephrotic syndrome, and hematuria. Pulmonary manifestations are pleurisy with effusion, pneumonia, vasculitis, fibrosis, and atelectasis.[13] Cardiovascular abnormalities include cardiomyopathy, pericarditis, endocarditis, and vasculitis of the coronary arteries.

Additional clinical abnormalities may relate to the gastrointestinal system (peritonitis, pancreatitis, perihepatitis,

and intestinal arteritis), the reticuloendothelial system (splenomegaly, lymphadenopathy), and the peripheral vasculature (gangrene, thrombophlebitis). Patients with systemic lupus erythematosus may develop infections, perhaps related to lowered complement levels, impaired delayed hypersensitivity, and defective phagocytosis.

Laboratory analysis can reveal anemia (70 to 80 per cent of patients), leukopenia, and abnormalities of plasma proteins (hyperglobulinemia, hypoalbuminemia, false-positive serologic tests for syphilis, positive serum rheumatoid factor, positive Coombs' reaction, cryoglobulinemia, lowered serum complement activity, autoagglutination of red blood cells, and the formation of LE cells and other antinuclear factors).[9, 14] Investigations of the possible association of genetic markers of the major histocompatibility complex and systemic lupus erythematosus have been numerous and, in some, a significant association of the disease with certain histocompatibility antigens (DR 2, DR 3, and B 8) has been found.[129, 130]

MUSCULOSKELETAL ABNORMALITIES

Characteristic and significant musculoskeletal abnormalities are encountered in patients with systemic lupus erythematosus (Table 33–1). These may include myositis, symmetric polyarthritis, deforming nonerosive arthropathy,

TABLE 33–1. Musculoskeletal Manifestations of Systemic Lupus Erythematosus

Myositis
Polyarthritis
Deforming nonerosive arthropathy
Subchondral cysts
Tendon weakening and rupture
Osteonecrosis
Soft tissue calcification
Osteomyelitis and septic arthritis
Acrosclerosis
Tuftal resorption
Insufficiency fracture

subchondral cysts, spontaneous tendon weakening and rupture, osteonecrosis, soft tissue calcification, osteomyelitis and septic arthritis, and miscellaneous abnormalities.

Myositis

Clinical features suggesting muscle involvement have been observed in 30 to 50 per cent of persons with systemic lupus erythematosus.[100] Possible causes include pain referred to muscles from adjacent involved joints, a corticosteroid-induced myopathy, and myositis.

Myositis, which has been reported in 4 per cent of patients with systemic lupus erythematosus,[10] may be associated with diffuse muscular tenderness and weakness and elevation of serum levels of muscle enzymes. In addition, generalized or juxta-articular muscle atrophy may be evident. Some patients with this disease develop myasthenia gravis.[15, 16]

Symmetric Polyarthritis

Articular symptoms and signs are among the most common clinical manifestations of the disease, being present in 75 to 90 per cent of patients.[17, 18] The severity of the clinical findings varies widely; some patients have mild complaints, whereas in other patients, considerable pain with or without significant synovitis may be noted. The articular findings most frequently are bilateral and symmetric, involving particularly the small joints of the hand, the knee, the wrist, and the shoulder; they include morning stiffness, pain, tenderness, and soft tissue swelling. Joint effusions are detected but are not large, although a possible association of systemic lupus erythematosus with recurrent effusions in the knee (intermittent hydrarthrosis) has been suggested.[101] Analysis of synovial fluid reveals less intense inflammation compared with that in rheumatoid arthritis[18, 19]; the fluid varies in appearance from clear to cloudy and demonstrates good viscosity and low complement levels. LE cells may be detected in the synovial fluid.[18, 85]

Synovial membrane biopsy may reveal a thick layer of superficial fibrin-like material[20] and signs of synovial inflammation (Fig. 33–2). Lining cell proliferation and inflammation are of variable degree[18, 21–24] but frequently are less severe than in rheumatoid arthritis. Although vascular abnormalities have been reported in small arterioles and venules of the synovial membrane,[18, 24] the histologic findings generally are nondiagnostic. Hematoxyphil bodies and platelet-fibrin thrombi within the synovium occasionally are seen.[18]

Radiographic abnormalities accompanying uncomplicated synovitis in systemic lupus erythematosus consist of soft tissue swelling and periarticular osteoporosis[25, 96]; cartilaginous and osseous destruction is rare in the absence of coexistent osteonecrosis. In the hand, the findings of fusiform soft tissue prominence and regional osteoporosis about proximal interphalangeal and metacarpophalangeal joints simulate the abnormalities of rheumatoid arthritis. Although well-defined lytic lesions or cysts in periarticular bone occasionally have been recorded in patients with systemic lupus erythematosus,[25, 144] they do not resemble the marginal erosions of rheumatoid arthritis (Fig. 33–3). In addition, the joint space generally is not narrowed. Rarely, erosive arthritis in systemic lupus erythematosus simulating

rheumatoid arthritis has been reported,[17, 26] but it is not clear in some of these reports if overlap syndromes had been responsible for these changes (see discussion later in this chapter).

Deforming Nonerosive Arthropathy

A deforming nonerosive arthropathy is not uncommon in patients with systemic lupus erythematosus and may be evident in as many as 5 to 40 per cent of such patients with articular abnormalities.[18, 25, 27–33, 96, 102, 103, 137–140] The arthropathy often appears early in the disease course,[140] although it is more common and severe in patients with long-standing disease.[138, 139] Even children with systemic lupus erythematosus may reveal this deforming nonerosive arthropathy which, in this age group, can simulate juvenile chronic arthritis.[141] Characteristically, the deformities cause little functional disability and are completely reducible; in fact, they may disappear when the hand is placed firmly on the cassette during radiography. In some instances, chronic fixed deformities can appear.[34] Elbow contractures have been reported.[103]

The Jaccoud-like arthropathy has a variable appearance (Fig. 33–4). Symmetric involvement of interphalangeal joints of multiple digits of the hand is most typical. Hyperextension at the proximal interphalangeal joints and flexion at the distal interphalangeal joints create swan-neck deformities. Boutonnière deformities, with flexion at the proximal interphalangeal joints and hyperextension at the distal interphalangeal joints, also can be seen. Hyperextension at the interphalangeal joint of the thumb is characteristic. Additional deformities include subluxation with ulnar drift at the metacarpophalangeal joints and subluxation at the first carpometacarpal joint. Associated abnormalities in the foot include hallux valgus, subluxation at the metatarsophalangeal joints, and widening of the forefoot.[104, 105, 138] Instability in the knee or shoulder also has been encountered.[131, 142] Of further interest, atlantoaxial subluxation has been reported in approximately 10 per cent of patients with systemic lupus erythematosus, with a greater likelihood of occurrence in patients with deforming nonerosive arthropathy and articular hypermobility.[143]

It is important to stress that joint space narrowing and osseous erosion are not prominent in this deforming arthropathy, serving to distinguish it from the articular abnormalities of rheumatoid arthritis. Rarely, cartilaginous and osseous alterations do become evident in lupus arthropathy and may take several forms.[32]

Joint Space Narrowing (Fig. 33–5). Diminution of cartilage may be related either to atrophy of disuse or to pressure erosion from apposing bone in subluxed articulations. Histologically, in these situations, cartilaginous erosion is not accompanied by extensive synovial inflammation or pannus.

Hook Erosions (Fig. 33–6). Bilateral or unilateral defects on the metacarpal (and rarely the metatarsal) heads occasionally are evident; similar defects are seen in other disorders associated with long-standing deformities, particularly ulnar deviation, such as rheumatic fever, rheumatoid arthritis, and parkinsonism. The erosions, which predominate on the radial aspect of the bone, probably are produced by capsular pressure and deformity and may represent an adaptive change to altered stress across the involved artic-

Text continued on page 1174

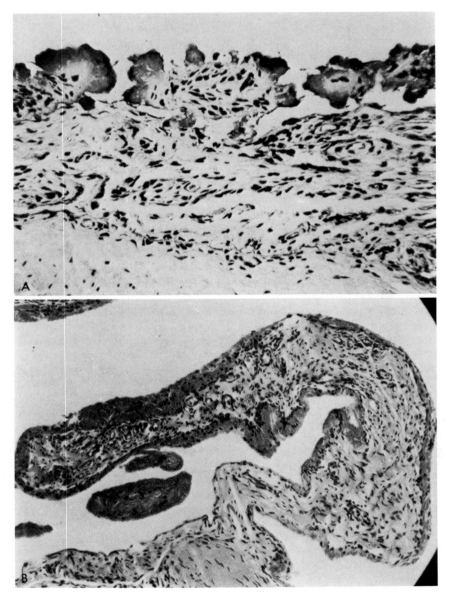

FIGURE 33–2. Polyarthritis: Pathologic abnormalities.

A A photomicrograph (210×) of the synovial membrane in a patient with acute polyarthritis demonstrates mild synovial inflammation with fibrinous deposits on the synovial cell surface and slight synovial cell hyperplasia.

B In a female patient with more chronic symptoms, the histologic findings are similar, with cellular hyperplasia and a fibrin-coated surface (105×).

(From Bywaters EGL: Clin Rheum Dis *1:*125, 1975.)

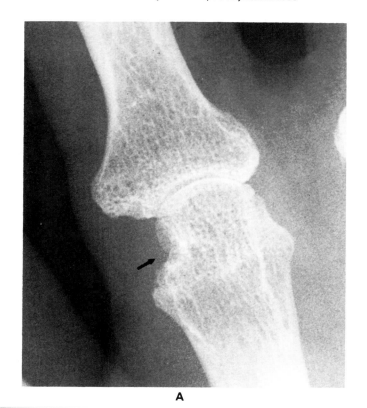

A

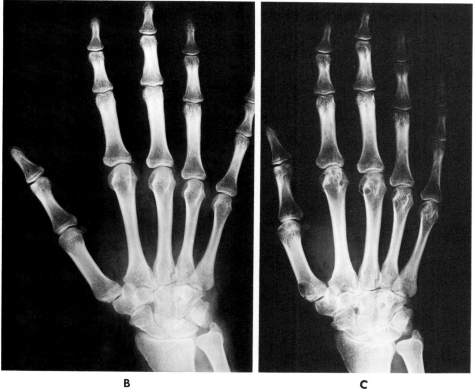

B   C

FIGURE 33–3. Polyarthritis: Radiographic abnormalities.

A Although soft tissue swelling and osteoporosis usually are the only radiographic manifestations of acute polyarthritis in systemic lupus erythematosus, joint space narrowing and erosions (arrow) that may simulate the appearance of rheumatoid arthritis occasionally are encountered.

B, C In this 23 year old woman, radiographs obtained 4 years apart reveal dramatic progression of the articular abnormalities with the development of multiple well-defined subchondral cysts.

(**B, C,** From Leskinen RH, et al: Radiology *153:* 349, 1984.)

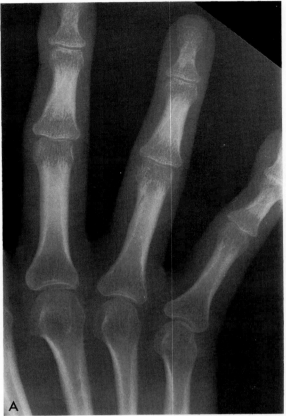

FIGURE 33–4. Lupus arthropathy: Varying appearance of deformities.

A In some patients, a Jaccoud-like distribution is seen with ulnar deviation at the metacarpophalangeal joints, predominantly in the fourth and fifth fingers. Osteoporosis is evident.

B In this person, severe (and reversible) swan-neck deformities of all the digits are characterized by hyperextension at the proximal interphalangeal joints and flexion at the distal interphalangeal joints.

C Flexion and ulnar deviation at the metacarpophalangeal and distal interphalangeal joints are most prominent in this person.

Illustration continued on opposite page

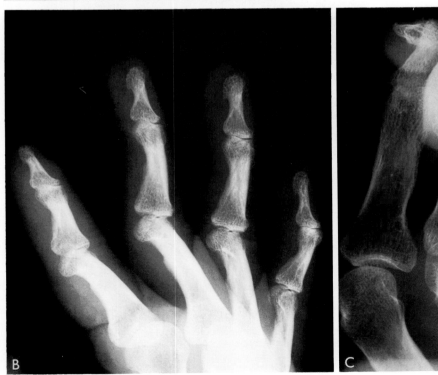

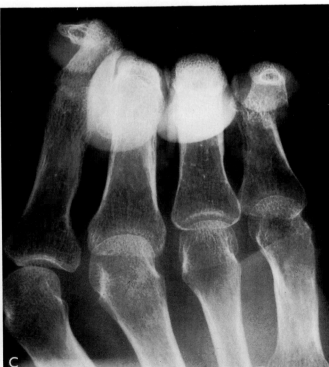

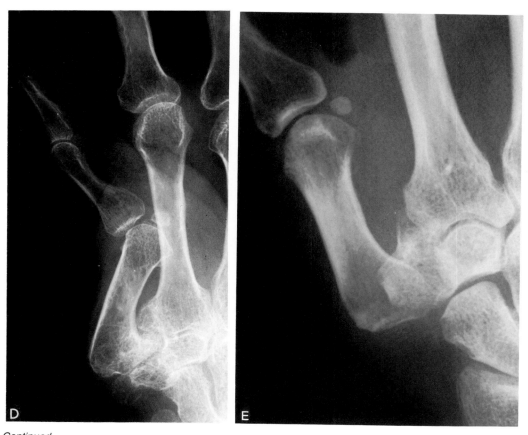

FIGURE 33–4 *Continued*
  D In the first ray, observe the considerable subluxation and flexion at the carpometacarpal joint associated with joint space narrowing, sclerosis, and osteophytosis, and hyperextension at the metacarpophalangeal joint.
  E Complete dislocation of the first carpometacarpal joint is evident.

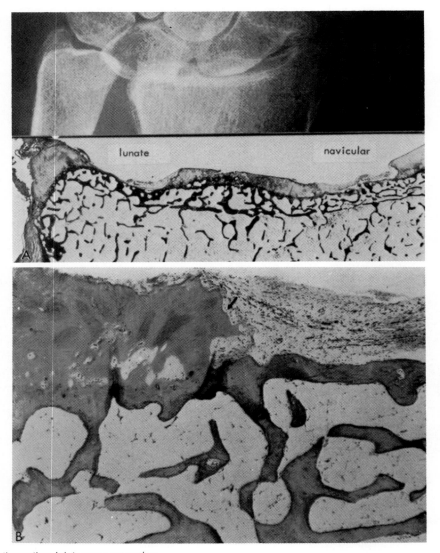

FIGURE 33–5. Lupus arthropathy: Joint space narrowing.
  A A radiograph and photomicrograph (4×) of the wrist indicate considerable narrowing of the radiocarpal joint. Pressure chondrolysis at the sites of radial articulation with the lunate and the navicular (scaphoid) is observed.
  B At higher magnification (45×), note marginal cartilage erosion and chondrolysis (arrow).
  (From Bywaters EGL: Clin Rheum Dis *1:*125, 1975.)

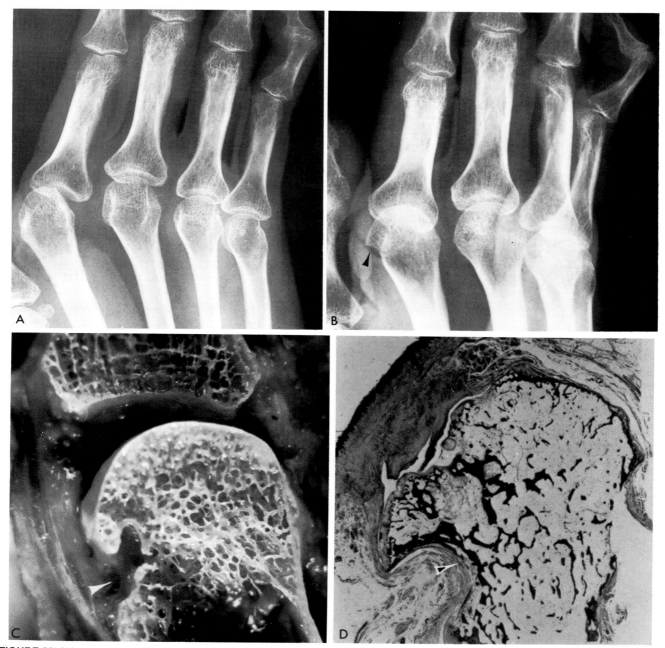

FIGURE 33–6. Lupus arthropathy: Hook erosions.

A, B Frontal and oblique radiographs outline ulnar deviation at metacarpophalangeal joints. Note the flexion deformity of the distal interphalangeal joint of the fifth finger and the considerable subluxation at the second metacarpophalangeal joint. Observe the hooklike erosion (arrowhead) on the radial and volar aspects of the second metacarpal head. This appearance and location are typical.

C A photograph of a macerated coronal section (in a slightly oblique attitude) through the second metacarpophalangeal joint in a cadaver with systemic lupus erythematosus reveals the hook erosion (arrowhead). Note its radial location.

D In a photomicrograph (10×) of a section of a metatarsophalangeal joint from a different patient with systemic lupus erythematosus, the hook erosion (arrowhead) is evident. The cartilage of the metatarsal head is irregular.

(**D,** From Bywaters EGL: Clin Rheum Dis *1:*125, 1975.)

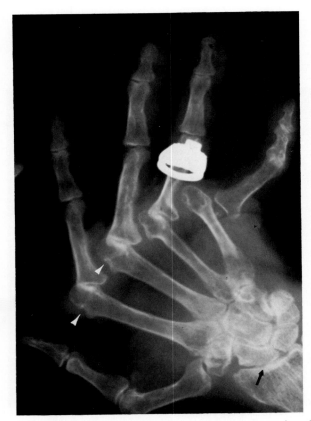

FIGURE 33–7. Lupus arthropathy: Severe manifestations. In a 55 year old woman with systemic lupus erythematosus, findings include radial deviation at the radiocarpal joint, ulnar deviation and subluxation at multiple metacarpophalangeal joints, and boutonnière and swan-neck deformities. Observe joint space narrowing in the radiocarpal compartment (arrow) and hook erosions of the metacarpal heads (arrowheads).

ulation. They are not associated with pannus erosion of bone and are different in appearance from the marginal erosions of rheumatoid arthritis.

The articular deformities of lupus arthropathy are related to capsular and ligamentous laxity and contracture and to muscular imbalance, perhaps occurring as a response to prolonged, recurrent low grade inflammation of intra-articular and periarticular structures (Fig. 33–7).[147] Indeed, this response may lead to fibrosis, a histologic finding that has been detected in the joint capsule and soft tissue of patients with systemic lupus erythematosus. Chronic renal disease with secondary hyperparathyroidism may contribute to the development of these deformities.[145, 146] Similar abnormalities occur in other deforming nonerosive arthropathies, particularly that which is apparent in patients with rheumatic fever.[35] The alterations are distinct from those of rheumatoid arthritis, in which severe intra-articular inflammatory changes produce permanent cartilaginous and osseous destruction, leading to instability and subluxation.

Subchondral Cysts

Osteoporosis and cyst formation within the subchondral bone can occur in systemic lupus erythematosus. The most common sites of involvement are the bones in the hand, wrist, and foot, particularly the carpus and metacarpal and metatarsal heads (Fig. 33–3).[144] The cystic lesions are of irregular shape and occur beneath cartilage that is relatively normal in appearance and in articulations in which the synovial membrane is not grossly inflamed. The cysts may occur as an isolated abnormality or in association with deforming nonerosive arthropathy. They appear to represent either a remodeling phenomenon that occurs in response to abnormal stress due to subluxation or a manifestation of ischemic necrosis of bone.[132]

Spontaneous Tendon Weakening and Rupture

Spontaneous rupture of tendons is observed in patients with systemic lupus erythematosus, almost invariably in association with systemically or locally administered steroids[36–43, 106–109, 134, 148–150] (Fig. 33–8). Because such tendon rupture also may occur in patients receiving steroids who do not have systemic lupus erythematosus, it is difficult to ascertain the role of this disease in the attenuation of tendons. Histologic evaluation of steroid-induced tendon tears reveals hemorrhage and degeneration without inflammation; similar abnormalities are encountered in involved tendons in systemic lupus erythematosus.[38, 39] In one report, however, histologic analysis of tissue about a ruptured patellar tendon in a patient with systemic lupus erythematosus revealed chalklike material containing hydroxyapatite and urate crystals, findings that implicate chronic renal disease and hyperparathyroidism as causative factors in such ruptures.[149] This is supported by documented changes in tendons and ligaments that occur in patients undergoing long-term hemodialysis.[146]

Single or multiple tendons at various sites may be torn in systemic lupus erythematosus. In general, tendons in weight-bearing locations are affected.[109] A tendency for older patients and for men to develop this complication has been suggested.[107] Weakening or rupture of the Achilles, quadriceps, and patellar tendons as well as the extensor tendons of the hand is encountered. Rarely, the triceps or biceps tendon is involved.[148] Ligamentous weakening and laxity also may contribute to atlantoaxial subluxation, which has been observed in patients with systemic lupus erythematosus.[44, 143]

Osteonecrosis

The association of osteonecrosis and systemic lupus erythematosus was first described in 1960 by Dubois and Cozen,[45] who noted the complication in 11 (3 per cent) of 400 patients with the disorder. Since that report, the appearance of bone necrosis in patients with systemic lupus erythematosus has been further documented in numerous publications,[18, 25, 29, 46–55, 78, 79, 110, 133, 135, 136] the most commonly reported frequency being approximately 5 to 6 per cent, with estimates as high as 40 per cent. Although the femoral head is the most typical site of abnormality, involvement of other and multiple sites has been confirmed.[151] Osteonecrosis in systemic lupus erythematosus is not uncommon in the humeral head, the femoral condyles, the tibial plateaus, and the talus and may even be apparent in the small bones of the hand, the wrist, and the foot. Symmetrically distributed osteonecrosis may be seen.[79, 82, 83, 152]

General clinical findings in patients with lupus erythe-

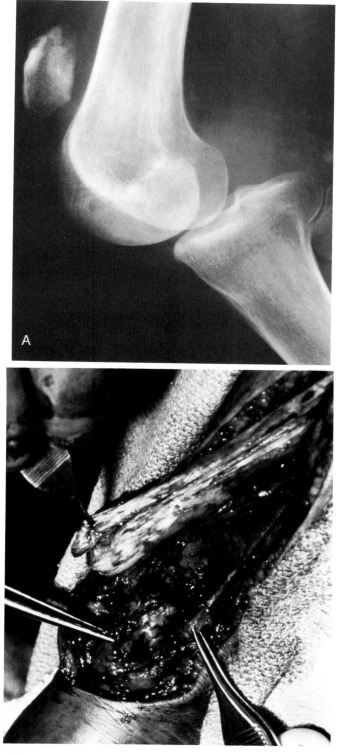

FIGURE 33–8. Tendon weakening and rupture: Radiographic and pathologic abnormalities.

A Spontaneous rupture of the patellar tendon and posterior subluxation of the tibia are evident. (Courtesy of A. G. Bergman, M.D., Stanford, California.)

B In another patient with systemic lupus erythematosus being treated with local steroid injections, spontaneous rupture of the Achilles tendon was observed. Note the torn tendon in this operative photograph.

matosus who develop osteonecrosis resemble the findings in lupus patients who do not develop osteonecrosis. Klipper and coworkers,[54] however, noted a high prevalence (61 per cent) of Raynaud's phenomenon as well as other signs of vasculitis in patients with both systemic lupus erythematosus and osteonecrosis, whereas Hurley and coworkers[51] and Smith and associates[52] have suggested that young patients with systemic lupus erythematosus are particularly susceptible to this complication. Additionally, it has been speculated that osteonecrosis in lupus erythematosus is more common in asymptomatic and physically active persons, in whom increased stress across weight-bearing joints leads to osseous collapse. The presence of persistent joint pain, particularly in a weight-bearing joint in patients with systemic lupus erythematosus whose disease is otherwise quiescent, should suggest the possibility of osteonecrosis,[78] although the infarcts may be unassociated with symptoms or signs.[79]

The pathogenesis of osteonecrosis in this disease has not been fully delineated. It has been popular to attribute bone necrosis in systemic lupus erythematosus to steroid administration.[153] Indeed, most of the affected patients have received corticosteroid medications, although, infrequently, patients with lupus erythematosus who have not received such medication may develop necrosis of bone.[46, 54] Various studies have appeared attributing osteonecrosis in patients with lupus erythematosus to duration,[51] total dose,[56] initial dose,[53] or highest daily dose[154] of corticosteroid therapy. It

also has been attractive to relate osteonecrosis in this disease to the presence and extent of vasculitis. In this regard, the observation of prominent clinical signs of vasculitis in patients with systemic lupus erythematosus who demonstrate this complication is of interest. However, histologic evidence of prominent vasculitis in necrotic bone in patients with systemic lupus erythematosus is unusual[57] (although this does not necessarily imply that vasculitis had not existed at some time). At this writing, a single inciting cause of osteonecrosis in this disorder has not been verified, and the pathogenesis of this complication may be multifactorial, related both to the basic disease process and to the prior administration of steroids.

The radiographic and pathologic features of osteonecrosis in patients with systemic lupus erythematosus are identical to those in patients who do not have this disease (Figs. 33–9 and 33–10). The occasional occurrence of bone necrosis in unusual sites such as the metacarpal heads,[25, 29, 50, 59] carpal bones,[18, 58, 59] tarsus, and metatarsal heads,[58, 59] however, should suggest systemic lupus erythematosus as a potential diagnosis (Figs. 33–11 to 33–13).

Soft Tissue Calcification

Soft tissue calcification occasionally is observed in systemic lupus erythematosus[25, 29, 60–62, 80] (Fig. 33–14). Budin and Feldman[63] described several patterns of calcification in

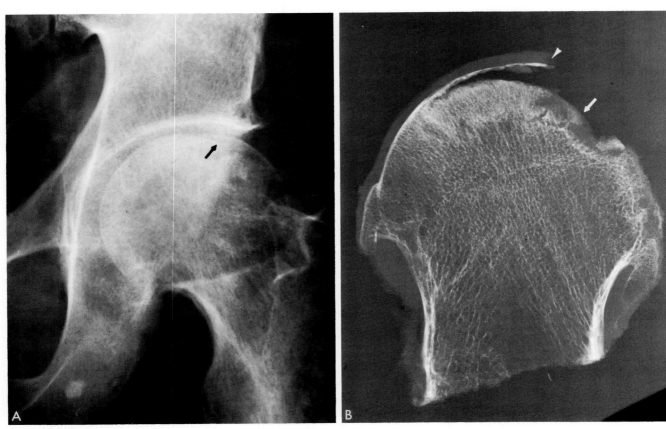

FIGURE 33–9. Osteonecrosis: Femoral head. A 31 year old man had received corticosteroid medication for systemic lupus erythematosus.

A The preoperative radiograph outlines depression of the outer surface of the femoral head (arrow), sclerosis, and mild narrowing of the joint space. Buttressing or thickening on the inner aspect of the femoral neck also is evident.

B On a radiograph of a coronal section of the femoral head after total hip arthroplasty, observe the displaced articular cartilage and subchondral bone plate (arrowhead), osseous necrosis and collapse (arrow), and surrounding new bone formation.

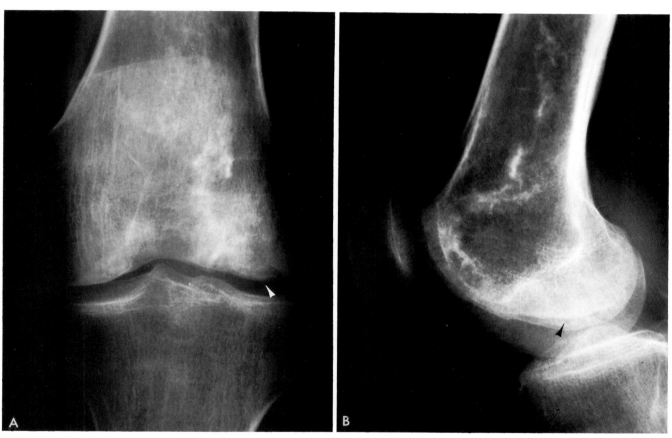

FIGURE 33–10. Osteonecrosis: Distal end of the femur. This 32 year old woman with systemic lupus erythematosus since age 19 years had been treated with corticosteroids. Radiographs of the distal end of the femur demonstrate calcified bony infarcts of the diaphysis and metaphysis with epiphyseal collapse of the lateral condylar surface (arrowheads). The femoral heads also were involved.

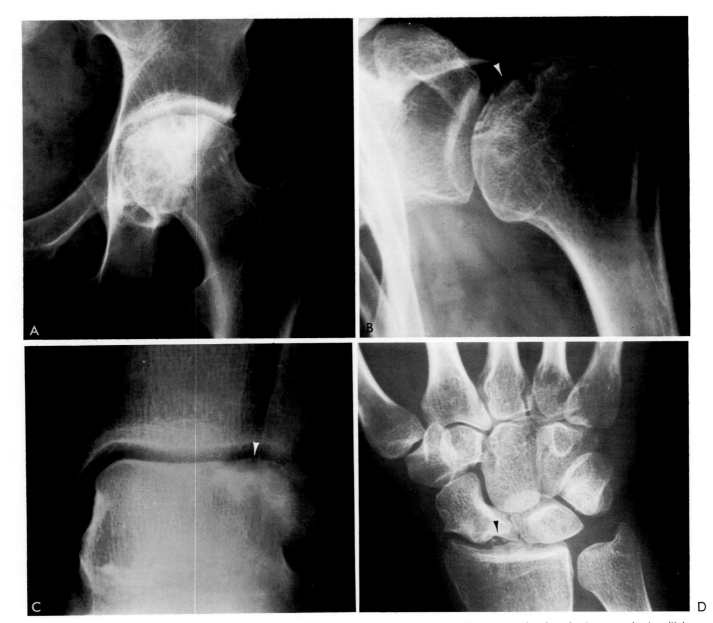

FIGURE 33–11. Osteonecrosis: Multiple sites. A young female patient with systemic lupus erythematosus developed osteonecrosis at multiple sites after corticosteroid therapy.

  A In the hip, typical changes in the femoral head are characterized by sclerosis, cyst formation, and collapse of the subchondral bone. The opposite side also was involved.

  B Observe the fragmentation of the humeral head with depression of the subchondral bone (arrowhead).

  C Collapse and irregularity of the lateral surface of the talus (arrowhead) are apparent.

  D Changes in this wrist related to osteonecrosis include fragmentation and collapse of the proximal portion of the scaphoid (arrowhead) and intra-articular debris.

  (Courtesy of I. Dwosh, M.D., Toronto, Ontario, Canada.)

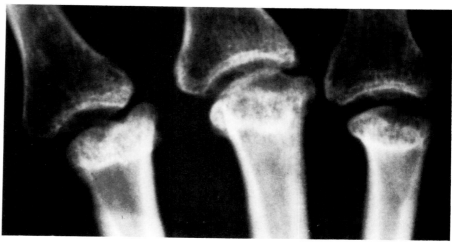

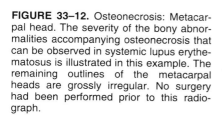

FIGURE 33–12. Osteonecrosis: Metacarpal head. The severity of the bony abnormalities accompanying osteonecrosis that can be observed in systemic lupus erythematosus is illustrated in this example. The remaining outlines of the metacarpal heads are grossly irregular. No surgery had been performed prior to this radiograph.

this disease: diffuse linear, streaky, or nodular calcification in the subcutaneous and deeper tissues, particularly in the lower extremities; focal or localized plaquelike calcification; periarticular calcification; and arterial calcification. Diffuse or focal calcific deposits are associated not infrequently with adjacent skin ulceration, inflammation, and necrosis,[63] although they may appear without concomitant skin lesions.[60] Juxta-articular calcifications appear as single or multiple deposits of varying size with or without adjacent joint disease[25, 29, 63]; these deposits usually are located in the soft tissues or, more rarely, the joint capsule. In the latter location, calcification may be related to concomitant calcium pyrophosphate dihydrate crystal deposition disease.[111] Vascular calcifications produce typical linear or tubular radiodense shadows.

The pathogenesis of soft tissue calcification in this disease has not been determined accurately, although local factors such as increased alkalinity and elevated levels of alkaline phosphatase in necrotic tissue may be important. The similarity of this calcification to that in other collagen vascular diseases should be noted.

Spontaneous resolution of soft tissue calcification in systemic lupus erythematosus rarely is observed.[80]

Osteomyelitis and Septic Arthritis

An unusually high frequency of bacterial and mycotic infections exists in patients with systemic lupus erythematosus.[64] Two major factors contribute to this susceptibility to infection—steroid administration and renal disease[65, 66]—although other factors, including leukopenia, defective phagocytosis,[67] decreased leukocyte chemotaxis, and impaired delayed hypersensitivity,[68, 69] also may be significant. The respiratory tract, the urinary tract, the skin, and the soft tissues are the commonly infected sites. The occurrence of bone and joint infection in systemic lupus erythematosus is less frequent[70–74, 155, 156] (Fig. 33–15). Monoarticular infection of the knee, the hip, and the ankle appears most typical, although simultaneous involvement of multiple joints and abnormalities of other articular sites may be evident. Implicated organisms have included *Neisseria gonorrheae, Neisseria meningitidis, Staphylococcus aureus,* gram-negative bacilli, atypical mycobacteria,[115] and *Mycobacterium*

tuberculosis.[84, 112] *Salmonella typhimurium* and *Salmonella enteritidis* represent other organisms responsible for septic arthritis in patients with systemic lupus erythematosus.[113, 114, 155, 156, 164] Indeed, owing to a potential risk for the development of salmonella arthritis, it has been suggested that a chronic Salmonella carrier state in a patient with systemic lupus erythematosus living in an endemic zone should be excluded before initiating immunosuppressive therapy.[156] Local factors such as preexisting lupus synovitis, osteonecrosis, and intra-articular steroid injections have been emphasized in some cases of septic arthritis. Radiographic findings of a large or increasing joint effusion and progressive cartilaginous and osseous destruction should raise the possibility of articular infection.

Sacroiliitis

Rarely, in systemic lupus erythematosus, imaging studies reveal alterations about the sacroiliac joints.[116, 117, 119, 165] On plain films, such abnormalities have included joint space narrowing, bone erosions, and reactive sclerosis in a unilateral or bilateral distribution. These changes are similar to those seen in osteoarthritis, so caution is required in assuming they are signs of sacroiliitis (Fig. 33–16). Furthermore, the asymptomatic nature of the sacroiliac joint abnormalities and their occurrence in patients with ischemic necrosis of the femoral heads may indicate that the changes are stress-related or, for that matter, secondary to avascularity in the ilium and sacrum. Reports of coexistent systemic lupus erythematosus and ankylosing spondylitis[118, 157] provide another potential cause of sacroiliac joint aberrations in systemic lupus erythematosus.

Abnormal accumulation of bone-seeking radiopharmaceutical agents in the sacroiliac region has been observed in 64 per cent of patients with systemic lupus erythematosus.[116] The disappearance of the abnormal radionuclide activity as the disease activity subsided and the presence of radiographically evident bone erosion were interpreted by the authors as evidence indicating synovitis in the sacroiliac joint. Other investigators also have observed scintigraphic abnormalities about the sacroiliac joints in patients with this disease; typically, the patients have little or no clinical or

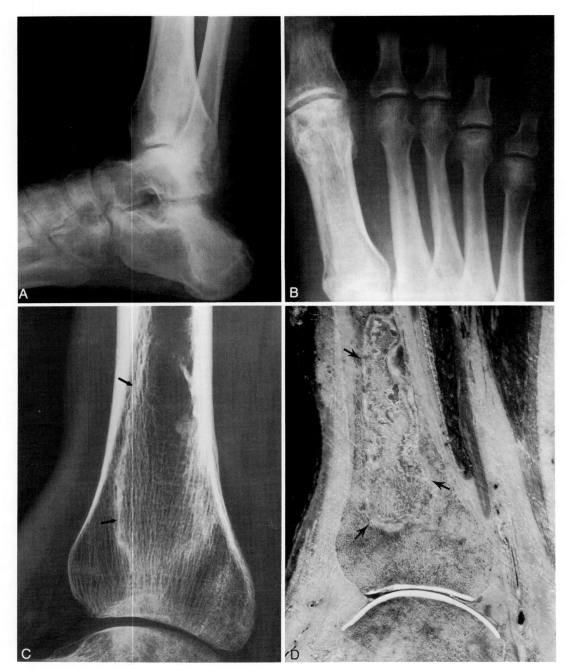

FIGURE 33–13. Osteonecrosis: Ankle and foot. This 33 year old man with systemic lupus erythematosus had clinical evidence of small-vessel disease as well as involvement of large vessels that resulted in occlusion of several major branches of the aorta, the carotid and the femoral arteries, retinal and cerebral vasculitis, and recurrent venous thrombosis. He had been treated with corticosteroids. Occlusion of the posterior and anterior right tibial arteries at the level of the foot and of the pedal arch necessitated an amputation of the leg.

A, B Lateral and frontal radiographs reveal evidence of ischemic necrosis of bone, manifested as serpentine calcification in the tibia, calcaneus, and first metatarsal bone. Increased radiodensity of the proximal and distal articular surfaces of the talus, navicular, and cuboid is evident. Subchondral sclerosis involves the heads of all of the metatarsals and is associated with flattening and collapse of the fourth and fifth metatarsal heads.

C, D A radiograph and photograph of a sagittal section of the distal end of the tibia demonstrate an extensive area of bone infarction (arrows), marked by a peripheral rim of calcification. Note that the talus contains a similar area of infarction.

Illustration continued on opposite page

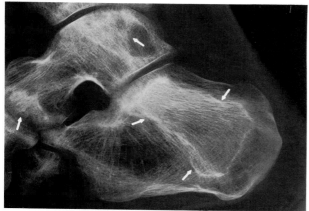

FIGURE 33–13 *Continued*

E A radiograph of a sagittal section of the hindfoot documents regions of bone infarction, associated with peripheral calcification, in the talus, calcaneus, and cuboid (arrows).

F A photograph of a sagittal section of the first metatarsal bone outlines an infarct in the subchondral region (arrowhead).

G In a photograph of a sagittal section of the fifth toe, note cystic degeneration, fracture, and collapse of the metatarsal head (arrow).

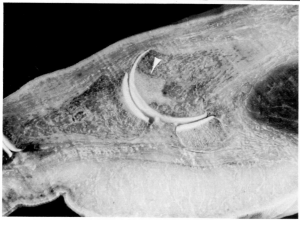

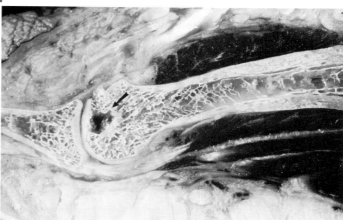

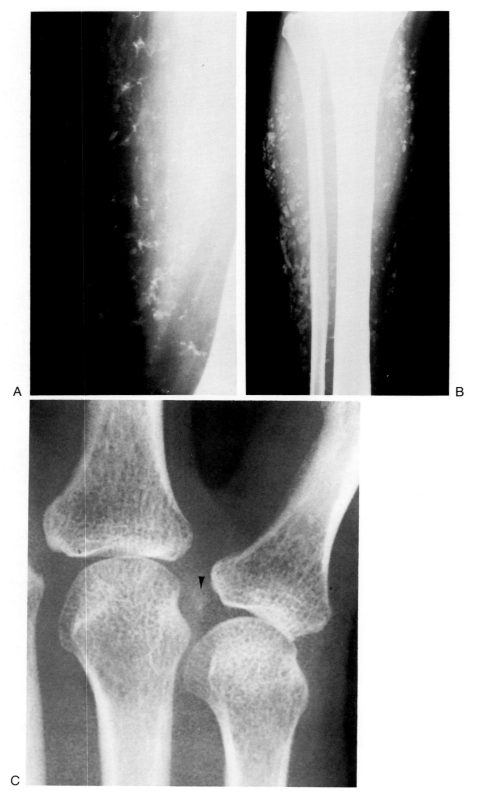

FIGURE 33–14. Soft tissue calcification. Three examples are shown that reveal the patterns of soft tissue calcification in systemic lupus erythematosus.
  A On a lateral radiograph of the distal end of the femur, focal collections of varying shape are seen.
  B Widespread soft tissue calcification is evident in the lower leg.
  C A periarticular calcific (or ossific) dense shadow is seen about the metacarpophalangeal joint (arrowhead).

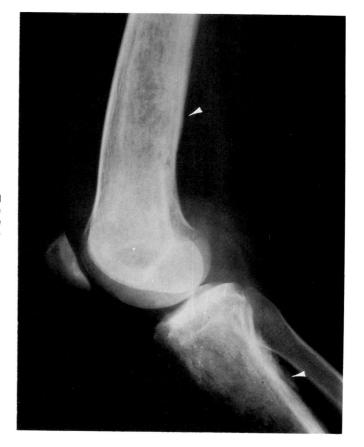

FIGURE 33–15. Osteomyelitis. A 22 year old woman developed *Escherichia coli* septicemia and osteomyelitis of multiple sites. In the distal end of the femur and proximal part of the tibia, changes include a motheaten pattern of bone destruction and periostitis (arrowheads).

radiographic evidence of sacroiliitis, and the ''scintigraphic sacroiliitis'' often is bilateral.[158]

Miscellaneous Abnormalities

Osteopenia, presumably representing osteoporosis, is observed in some patients with systemic lupus erythematosus.

Potential causes include debilitation and corticosteroid therapy. Insufficiency fractures relate to normal or abnormal forces on weakened bone, and their distribution in systemic lupus erythematosus is similar to that in rheumatoid arthritis (Fig. 33–17).

Reported alterations of the terminal tufts of the phalanges in systemic lupus erythematosus have included osteoscle-

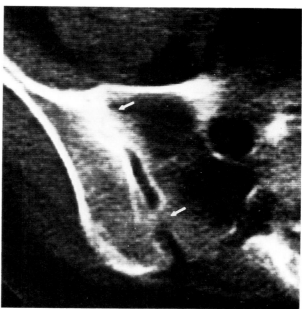

FIGURE 33–16. Sacroiliac joint abnormalities. With CT scanning, a transaxial section of the sacroiliac joint in a patient with systemic lupus erythematosus documents bone sclerosis and focal ankylosis (arrows). The nature of these changes is not clear. (Courtesy of R. Cope, M.D., Portland, Oregon.)

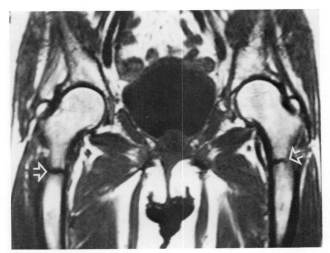

FIGURE 33–17. Insufficiency fractures. In this 48 year old woman with systemic lupus erythematosus, insufficiency fractures occurred in both femora. A coronal T1-weighted (TR/TE, 500/20) spin echo MR image reveals these fractures as linear areas of low signal intensity (arrows). More diffuse regions of decreased signal intensity about the fractures represent foci of bone marrow edema. (Courtesy of A. Motta, M.D., Cleveland, Ohio.)

rosis and resorption (Fig. 33–18). The appearance of sclerosis at this site (acral sclerosis) must be evaluated with caution, as focal sclerotic lesions of one or several phalanges may be an incidental finding, especially in women.[120] The detection of diffuse sclerosis of multiple digits may be more significant; this abnormality has been seen in a variety of collagen vascular disorders, including rheumatoid arthri-

tis,[75, 76, 120] and in sarcoidosis.[77] Reports indicate that this finding can be combined with tuftal resorption in systemic lupus erythematosus and may or may not be associated with Raynaud's phenomenon.[25, 81] The pattern of resorption of the phalangeal tufts in this disease is identical to that in scleroderma.

Temporomandibular joint involvement in systemic lupus erythematosus may be associated with clinical abnormalities, such as locking, tenderness, and pain, and with radiographic changes, including condylar flattening, erosion, sclerosis, and osteophytosis.[121–123] The abnormalities, which could relate to synovitis, osteoarthritis, or osteonecrosis, may occur in relative isolation or in combination with widespread articular alterations.

Periosteal new bone formation has been described as a manifestation of systemic lupus erythematosus.[159] It appears to be a rare manifestation of the disease, to involve the tubular bones of the lower extremity, and to be associated with signs of systemic vasculitis. The resultant periostitis resembles that seen in polyarteritis nodosa as well as in other conditions.

The occurrence of clinical and radiologic features of systemic lupus erythematosus in patients with other collagen vascular diseases has been documented in various overlap syndromes, as well as in mixed connective tissue disease. In patients with mixed connective tissue disease, high titers of antibodies to extractable nuclear antigen (ENA) are present in the serum. Additionally, renal disease is rare, and the prognosis is better than that for systemic lupus erythematosus. In both mixed connective tissue disease and overlap syndromes, musculoskeletal manifestations of systemic lupus erythematosus may be combined with those of sclero-

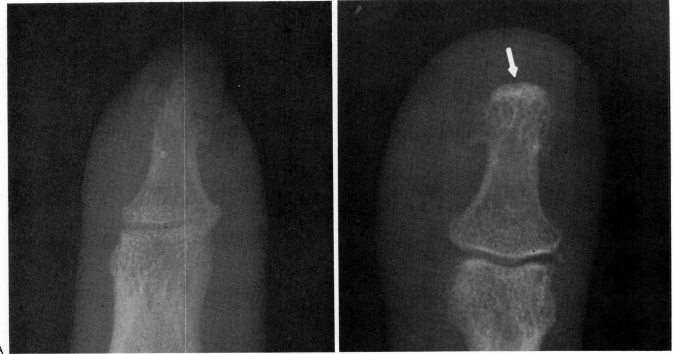

A   B

FIGURE 33–18. Tuftal sclerosis and resorption.
  A Severe abnormalities related to osseous and soft tissue resorption simulate the findings of scleroderma.
  B In a second patient, focal bone sclerosis is evident in the tuft (arrow). (Courtesy of A. Brower, M.D., Norfolk, Virginia.)

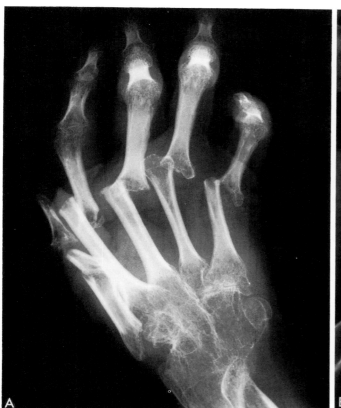

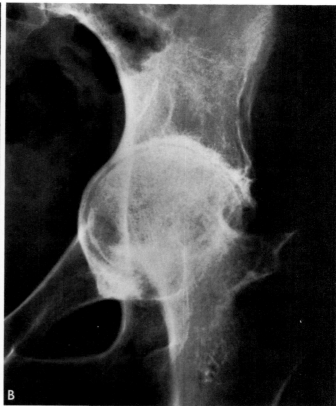

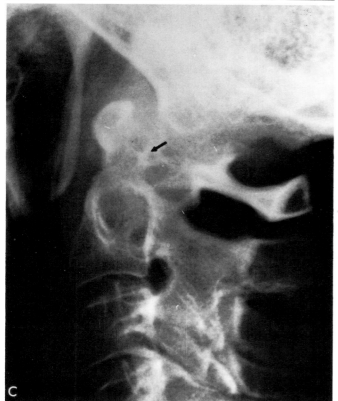

FIGURE 33–19. Overlap syndrome. This 30 year old woman initially had clinical manifestations of juvenile-onset rheumatoid arthritis and later developed the classic findings of systemic lupus erythematosus.

A In the hand, the findings are those of juvenile-onset rheumatoid arthritis with osteoporosis, bony ankylosis, and deformities. Surgical procedures had been accomplished on the metacarpal heads.

B Observe protrusion deformity of the hip with symmetric loss of joint space.

C On a lateral radiograph of the neck, the odontoid process is eroded, and only a small remnant can be seen (arrow).

(Courtesy of V. Vint, M.D., La Jolla, California.)

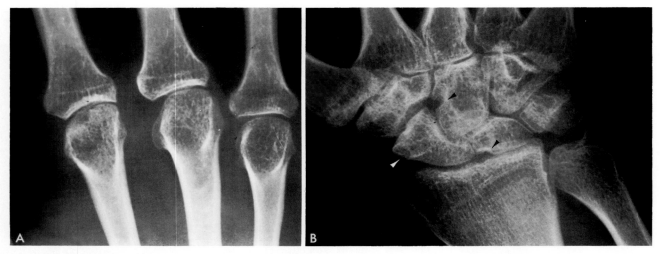

FIGURE 33–20. Overlap syndrome. This patient had overlapping clinical features of systemic lupus erythematosus and rheumatoid arthritis.
   A Joint space narrowing and collapse of bone can be seen at the metacarpophalangeal joints. The findings are reminiscent of those occurring in systemic lupus erythematosus alone.
   B Joint space diminution and osseous erosions (arrowheads) about the wrist may represent modified changes of rheumatoid arthritis. (Courtesy of P. Utsinger, M.D., Philadelphia, Pennsylvania.)

derma, dermatomyositis, or rheumatoid arthritis (Figs. 33–19 and 33–20). These manifestations are discussed in Chapter 37.
   Gout[111, 124–126] and calcium pyrophosphate dihydrate crystal deposition disease[111] have been described in association with systemic lupus erythematosus.

DIFFERENTIAL DIAGNOSIS

The symmetric polyarthritis that is associated with systemic lupus erythematosus produces nonspecific radiographic findings, including soft tissue swelling and osteoporosis. These same findings are encountered in other disorders that are characterized by synovial inflammation, such as rheumatoid arthritis.
   The deforming nonerosive arthropathy of the hands and wrists (and less commonly the feet) in systemic lupus erythematosus is similar to Jaccoud's arthropathy, which most typically follows rheumatic fever (Table 33–2). In the classic descriptions of Jaccoud's arthropathy, involvement of the ulnar digits (fourth and fifth fingers) is stressed, although a more extensive distribution may be encountered;

in the arthropathy of systemic lupus erythematosus, all the digits, including the thumb, frequently are affected, although a more limited distribution may be evident. A deforming arthropathy without significant erosive abnormality also may be seen as an articular manifestation of agammaglobulinemia (hypogammaglobulinemia). A similar arthropathy may accompany such rare disorders as the Ehlers-Danlos syndrome[160] and hypocomplementemic urticarial vasculitis syndrome.[161] In rheumatoid arthritis, joint space narrowing and bony erosion are characteristic, although, occasionally, digital deformity may occur in the absence of cartilaginous and osseous abnormalities (Fig. 33–21). In these instances, accurate differentiation of the joint disease of systemic lupus erythematosus from that of rheumatoid arthritis is difficult. Furthermore, the appearance of joint space narrowing, hook erosions, and cyst formation in some patients with lupus arthropathy complicates this differentiation.
   The thumb deformities in systemic lupus erythematosus can be extensive; hyperextension of the interphalangeal joint and subluxation at the first carpometacarpal joint are particularly characteristic. Significant thumb deformity (as

TABLE 37–2. Differential Diagnosis of Radiographic Abnormalities in the Hand

Diagnosis	Distribution*	Deformities	Erosions	Joint Space Narrowing
Lupus arthropathy	MCP and IP joints of all the digits; prominent abnormalities of the thumb	Initially reversible; subsequently may become fixed	Hook erosions on radial and volar aspects of metacarpal heads (uncommon)	Cartilage atrophy and pressure erosion in subluxed articulations (uncommon)
Classic Jaccoud's arthropathy	MCP and IP joints of ulnar digits, particularly the fourth and fifth fingers	Initially reversible; subsequently may become fixed	Hook erosions on radial and volar aspects of metacarpal heads (uncommon)	Cartilage atrophy and pressure erosion in subluxed articulations (uncommon)
Rheumatoid arthritis	MCP and PIP joints of all the digits; prominent abnormalities	Progressive	Widespread marginal and central erosions at involved sites (common)	"Pannus" destruction of cartilage in subluxed and nonsubluxed articulations (common)

*MCP, Metacarpophalangeal; IP, interphalangeal; PIP, proximal interphalangeal.

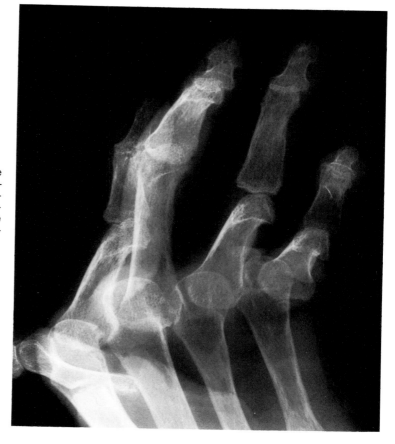

FIGURE 33–21. Rheumatoid arthritis. In this person, severe subluxation and deformities of multiple metacarpophalangeal joints overshadow the minor degree of erosive abnormality of the metacarpal heads. Because of this, the appearance is reminiscent of that in lupus arthropathy. More prominent erosions were present at the first metacarpophalangeal joint.

well as changes at the first carpometacarpal joint) is evident in other collagen vascular disorders, however, such as scleroderma.

Spontaneous tendon rupture, which has been noted in patients with systemic lupus erythematosus, also occurs without an obvious precipitating event in hyperparathyroidism and in patients who have received steroid medication for any reason.

Osteonecrosis complicating systemic lupus erythematosus generally cannot be differentiated from that accompanying a variety of disease processes. Involvement of the metacarpal and metatarsal heads and the tarsal and carpal bones, however, appears to be especially characteristic of systemic lupus erythematosus. At these sites, the occurrence of osteonecrosis should suggest this disease as one potential diagnosis, although osseous collapse, sclerosis, and fragmentation in these articulations of the hand and foot may indicate not the findings of osteonecrosis but rather the alterations of calcium pyrophosphate dihydrate crystal deposition disease or Wilson's disease. Osteonecrosis also has been reported as a complication of the antiphospholipid syndrome.[162] This syndrome shares many clinical manifestations with systemic lupus erythematosus, including arterial or venous thrombotic events, recurrent pregnancy loss, thrombocytopenia, leg ulcers, cutaneous changes, and hemolytic anemia, and it has received a great deal of attention in recent years (see Chapter 80).[163]

Soft tissue calcification, which is observed in systemic lupus erythematosus, accompanies other collagen vascular disorders, particularly scleroderma and dermatomyositis.

Differentiation among these disorders on the basis of the appearance of soft tissue calcific deposits is extremely difficult. Furthermore, phalangeal tuftal resorption or sclerosis has been identified in many collagen vascular diseases as well as in sarcoidosis.

SUMMARY

Musculoskeletal abnormalities represent a significant part of the clinical and radiologic picture of systemic lupus erythematosus. These abnormalities include myositis, symmetric polyarthritis, deforming nonerosive arthropathy, spontaneous rupture of tendons, osteonecrosis, soft tissue calcification, osteomyelitis and septic arthritis, and terminal phalangeal sclerosis and erosion. Many of these abnormalities are simulated by changes occurring in other collagen vascular disorders and rheumatoid arthritis. In addition, findings of systemic lupus erythematosus may be combined with these other collagen vascular diseases in various overlap syndromes and mixed connective tissue disease.

References

1. Kaposi MK: Kenntniss des Lupus erythematosus. Arch Dermatol Syphilol *4:*36, 1872.
2. Osler W: On the visceral manifestations of the erythema group of skin diseases. Am J Med Sci *127:*1, 1904.
3. Libman E, Sacks B: A hitherto undescribed form of valvular and mural endocarditis. Arch Intern Med *33:*701, 1924.
4. Baehr G, Klemperer P, Schifrin A: A diffuse disorder of the peripheral circulation (usually associated with lupus erythematosus and endocarditis). Trans Assoc Am Physicians *50:*139, 1935.

5. Hargraves MM, Richmond H, Morton R: Presentation of two bone marrow elements: The "tart" cell and the "LE" cell. Proc Mayo Clinic 23:25, 1948.

6. Miescher P, Fauconnet M, Bérund T: Immuno-nucléo-phagocytose expérimentale et phénomène L.E. Exp Med Surg 11:173, 1953.

7. Ceppellini R, Polli E, Celada F: A DNA-reacting factor in the serum of a patient with lupus erythematosus diffusus. Proc Soc Exp Biol Med 96:572, 1957.

8. Robbins WC, Holman HR, Deicher H, et al: Complement fixation with cell nuclei and DNA in lupus erythematosus. Proc Soc Exp Biol Med 96:575, 1957.

9. Hughes GRV: Systemic lupus erythematosus. In JT Scott (Ed): Copeman's Textbook of the Rheumatic Diseases. 5th Ed. Edinburgh, Churchill Livingstone, 1978, p 901.

10. Estes D, Christian CL: The natural history of systemic lupus erythematosus by prospective analysis. Medicine 50:85, 1971.

11. Johnson RT, Richardson EP: The neurological manifestations of systemic lupus erythematosus. A clinical-pathological study of 24 cases and review of the literature. Medicine 47:337, 1968.

12. Bishko F: Retinopathy in systemic lupus erythematosus. A case report and review of the literature. Arthritis Rheum 15:57, 1972.

13. Bulgrin JG, Dubois EL, Jacobson G: Chest roentgenographic changes in systemic lupus erythematosus. Radiology 74:42, 1960.

14. Cochrane CG, Koffler D: Immune complex disease in experimental animals and man. Adv Immunol 16:185, 1973.

15. Wolf SM, Barrows HS: Myasthenia gravis and systemic lupus erythematosus. Arch Neurol 14:254, 1966.

16. Alarcón-Segovia D, Galbraith RF, Maldonado JE, et al: Systemic lupus erythematosus following thymectomy for myasthenia gravis. Report of two cases. Lancet 2:662, 1963.

17. DuBois EL: Lupus Erythematosus. New York, McGraw-Hill Book Co, 1966, p 155.

18. Labowitz R, Schumacher HR Jr: Articular manifestations of systemic lupus erythematosus. Ann Intern Med 74:911, 1971.

19. Bywaters EGL: Anatomic changes in Jaccoud's syndrome (Abstr). Arthritis Rheum 14:153, 1971.

20. Cruickshank B: Lesions of joints and tendon sheaths in systemic lupus erythematosus. Ann Rheum Dis 18:111, 1959.

21. Phocas E, Andriotakis C, Kaklamanis P, et al: Joint involvement in systemic lupus erythematosus and in scleroderma (systemic sclerosis). Acta Rheumatol Scand 13:137, 1967.

22. Rodnan GP, Yunis EJ, Totten RS: Experience with punch biopsy of synovium in the study of joint disease. Ann Intern Med 53:319, 1960.

23. Schwartz S, Cooper N: Synovial membrane punch biopsy. Arch Intern Med 108:400, 1961.

24. Coste F, Delbarre F, Guiraudon C, et al: La synoviale du lupus érythémateux, de la périartérite noueuse et de la sclérodermie. Rev Rhum Mal Osteoartic 35:416, 1968.

25. Weissman BN, Rappoport AS, Sosman JL, et al: Radiographic findings in the hands in patients with systemic lupus erythematosus. Radiology 126:313, 1978.

26. Friedman HH, Schwartz S, Trubek M, et al: The "pararheumatic" arthropathies. Ann Intern Med 38:732, 1953.

27. Akizuki M, Wada H, Fujii T, et al: Deformity, nonerosive arthritis of the hands in a patient with systemic lupus erythematosus (SLE) (Abstr). J Jpn Rheum Assoc 11:375, 1971.

28. Kramer LS, Ruderman JE, Dubois EL, et al: Deforming nonerosive arthritis of the hands in chronic systemic lupus erythematosus (SLE) (Abstr). Arthritis Rheum 13:329, 1970.

29. Bleifeld CJ, Inglis AE: The hand in systemic lupus erythematosus. J Bone Joint Surg [Am] 56:1207, 1974.

30. Aptekar RG, Lawless OJ, Decker JL: Deforming non-erosive arthritis of the hand in systemic lupus erythematosus. Clin Orthop 100:120, 1974.

31. Russell AS, Percy JS, Rigal WM, et al: Deforming arthropathy in systemic lupus erythematosus. Ann Rheum Dis 33:204, 1974.

32. Bywaters EGL: Jaccoud's syndrome. A sequel to the joint involvement in systemic lupus erythematosus. Clin Rheum Dis 1:125, 1975.

33. Schumacher HR, Zweiman B, Bora FW Jr: Corrective surgery for the deforming hand arthropathy of systemic lupus erythematosus. Clin Orthop 117:292, 1976.

34. Evans JA, Hastings DE, Urowitz MB: The fixed lupus hand deformity and its surgical correction. J Rheumatol 4:170, 1977.

35. Bywaters EGL: The relation between heart and joint disease including "rheumatoid heart disease" and chronic post-rheumatic arthritis (type Jaccoud). Br Heart J 12:101, 1950.

36. Cowan MA, Alexander S: Simultaneous bilateral rupture of the Achilles tendon due to triamcinolone. Br Med J 1:1658, 1961.

37. Lee MLH: Bilateral rupture of the Achilles tendon. Letter to Editor. Br Med J 1:1829, 1961.

38. Twinning RH, Marcus WY, Garey JL: Tendon rupture in systemic lupus erythematosus. JAMA 189:377, 1964.

39. Lotem M, Maor P, Levi M: Rupture of the extensor tendons of the hand in lupus erythematosus disseminatus. Ann Rheum Dis 32:457, 1973.

40. Rascher JJ, Marcolin L, James P: Bilateral, sequential rupture of the patellar tendon in systemic lupus erythematosus. A case report. J Bone Joint Surg [Am] 56:821, 1974.

41. Wener JA, Schein AJ: Simultaneous bilateral rupture of the patellar tendon and quadriceps expansions in systemic lupus erythematosus. A case report. J Bone Joint Surg [Am] 56:823, 1974.

42. Martin JR, Wilson CL, Mathews WH: Bilateral rupture of the ligamenta patellae in a case of disseminated lupus erythematosus. Arthritis Rheum 1:548, 1958.

43. Strejcek J, Popelka S: Bilateral rupture of the patellar ligaments in systemic lupus erythematosus (Letter to Editor) Lancet 2:743, 1969.

44. Klemp P, Meyers OL, Keyzer C: Atlanto-axial subluxation in systemic lupus erythematosus. A case report. S Afr Med J 52:331, 1977.

45. Dubois EL, Cozen L: Avascular (aseptic) bone necrosis associated with systemic lupus erythematosus. JAMA 174:966, 1960.

46. Leventhal GH, Dorfman HD: Aseptic necrosis of bone in systemic lupus erythematosus. Semin Arthritis Rheum 4:73, 1974.

47. Siemsen JK, Brook J, Meister L: Lupus erythematosus and avascular bone necrosis: A clinical study of three cases and review of the literature. Arthritis Rheum 5:492, 1962.

48. Ruderman M, McCarty DJ Jr: Aseptic necrosis in systemic lupus erythematosus. Report of a case involving six joints. Arthritis Rheum 7:709, 1964.

49. Goldie I, Tibblin G, Scheller S: Systemic lupus erythematosus and aseptic bone necrosis. A discussion based on the presentation of one case treated with corticosteroids. Acta Med Scand 182:55, 1967.

50. Lightfoot RW Jr, Lotke PA: Osteonecrosis of metacarpal heads in systemic lupus erythematosus. Value of radiostrontium scintimetry in differential diagnosis. Arthritis Rheum 15:486, 1972.

51. Hurley RM, Steinberg RH, Patriquin H, et al: Avascular necrosis of the femoral head in childhood systemic lupus erythematosus. Can Med Assoc J 111:781, 1974.

52. Smith FE, Sweet DE, Brunner CM, et al: Avascular necrosis in SLE. An apparent predilection for young patients. Ann Rheum Dis 35:227, 1976.

53. Abeles M, Urman JD, Rothfield NF: Aseptic necrosis of bone in systemic lupus erythematosus. Relationship to corticosteroid therapy. Arch Intern Med 138:750, 1978.

54. Klipper AR, Stevens MB, Zizic TM, et al: Ischemic necrosis of bone in systemic lupus erythematosus. Medicine 55:251, 1976.

55. Urman JD, Abeles M, Houghton AN, et al: Aseptic necrosis presenting as wrist pain in SLE. Arthritis Rheum 20:825, 1977.

56. Bergstein JM, Wiens C, Fish AJ, et al: Avascular necrosis of bone in systemic lupus erythematosus. J Pediatr 85:31, 1974.

57. Velayos EE, Leidholt JD, Smyth CJ, et al: Arthropathy associated with steroid therapy. Ann Intern Med 64:759, 1966.

58. Aptekar RG, Klippel JH, Becker KE, et al: Avascular necrosis of the talus, scaphoid, and metatarsal head in systemic lupus erythematosus. Clin Orthop 101:127, 1974.

59. Green N, Osmer JC: Small bone changes secondary to systemic lupus erythematosus. Radiology 90:118, 1968.

60. Kabir DI, Malkinson FD: Lupus erythematosus and calcinosis cutis. Arch Dermatol 100:17, 1969.

61. Powell RJ: Systemic lupus erythematosus with widespread subcutaneous fat calcification. Proc R Soc Med 67:215, 1974.

62. Savin JA: Systemic lupus erythematosus with ectopic calcification. Br J Dermatol 84:191, 1971.

63. Budin JA, Feldman F: Soft tissue calcifications in systemic lupus erythematosus. AJR 124:358, 1975.

64. Staples PJ, Gerding DN, Decker JL, et al: Incidence of infection in systemic lupus erythematosus. Arthritis Rheum 17:1, 1974.

65. Ginzler E, Diamond H, Kaplan D, et al: Computer analysis of factors influencing frequency of infection in systemic lupus erythematosus. Arthritis Rheum 21:37, 1978.

66. Pillay VKG, Wilson DM, Ing TS, et al: Fungus infection in steroid-treated systemic lupus erythematosus. JAMA 205:261, 1968.

67. Orozco JH, Jasin HE, Ziff M: Defective phagocytosis in patients with systemic lupus erythematosus (Abstr). Arthritis Rheum 13:342, 1970.

68. Horwitz DA: Impaired delayed hypersensitivity in systemic lupus erythematosus. Arthritis Rheum 15:353, 1972.

69. Hahn BH, Bagby MK, Osterland CK: Abnormalities of delayed hypersensitivity in systemic lupus erythematosus. Am J Med 55:25, 1973.

70. Edelen JS, Lockshin MD, Leroy EC: Gonococcal arthritis in two patients with active systemic lupus erythematosus: A diagnostic problem. Arthritis Rheum 14:557, 1971.

71. Martin, CM, Merrill RH, Barrett O Jr: Arthritis due to serratia. J Bone Joint Surg [Am] 52:1450, 1970.

72. Quismorio FP, Dubois EL: Septic arthritis in systemic lupus erythematosus. J Rheumatol 2:73, 1975.

73. Hoffman WS, Myers RL, Stark FR, et al: Septic arthritis associated with Mycobacterium avium: A case report and literature review. J Rheumatol 5:199, 1978.

74. Mougeot-Martin M, Krulik M, Gintzburger S, et al: Arthrite septique spontanée au cours du lupus érythémateux disséminé. Sem Hôp Paris 52:883, 1976.

75. Goodman N: The significance of terminal phalangeal osteosclerosis. Radiology 89:709, 1966.

76. Halim W, VanDerKorst JK, Valkenburg HA, et al: Terminal phalangeal osteosclerosis. Ann Rheum Dis 34:82, 1975.

77. McBrine CS, Fisher MS: Acrosclerosis in sarcoidosis. Radiology 115:279, 1975.

78. Griffiths ID, Maini RN, Scott JT: Clinical and radiological features of osteonecrosis in systemic lupus erythematosus. Ann Rheum Dis 38:413, 1979.

79. Klippel JH, Gerber LH, Pollak L, et al: Avascular necroses in systemic lupus erythematosus. Silent symmetric osteonecrosis. Am J Med 67:83, 1979.

80. Weinberger A, Kaplan JG, Myers AR: Extensive soft tissue calcification (cal-

cinosis universalis) in systemic lupus erythematosus. Ann Rheum Dis 38:384, 1979.

81. Dimant J, Ginzler E, Schlesinger M, et al: The clinical significance of Raynaud's phenomenon in systemic lupus erythematosus. Arthritis Rheum 22:815, 1979.

82. Zizic TM, Hungerford DS, Stevens MB: Ischemic bone necrosis in systemic lupus erythematosus. I. The early diagnosis of ischemic necrosis of bone. Medicine 59:134, 1980.

83. Hungerford DS, Zizic TM: The treatment of ischemic necrosis of bone in systemic lupus erythematosus. Medicine 59:143, 1980.

84. Hunter T, Plummer FA: Infectious arthritis complicating systemic lupus erythematosus. Can Med Assoc J 122:791, 1980.

85. Seibold JR, Wechsler LR, Cammarata RJ: LE cells in intermittent hydrarthrosis. Arthritis Rheum 23:958, 1980.

86. Cohen AS, Reynolds WE, Franklin EC, et al: Preliminary criteria for the classification of systemic lupus erythematosus. Bull Rheum Dis 21:643, 1971.

87. Tan EM, Cohen AS, Fries JF, et al: The 1982 revised criteria for the classification of systemic lupus erythematosus. Arthritis Rheum 25:1271, 1982.

88. Davis P, Atkins B, Josse RG, et al: Criteria for classification of SLE. Br Med J 2:88, 1973.

89. Fries JF, Siegel RC: Testing the "preliminary criteria for classification of SLE." Ann Rheum Dis 32:171, 1973.

90. Trimble RB, Townes AS, Robinson H, et al: Preliminary criteria for the classification of systemic lupus erythematosus (SLE): Evaluation in early diagnosed SLE and rheumatoid arthritis. Arthritis Rheum 17:184, 1974.

91. Canoso JJ, Cohen AS: A review of the use, evaluations, and criticisms of the preliminary criteria for the classification of systemic lupus erythematosus. Arthritis Rheum 22:917, 1979.

92. Levin RE, Weinstein A, Peterson M, et al: A comparison of the sensitivity of the 1971 and 1982 American Rheumatism Association criteria for the classification of systemic lupus erythematosus. Arthritis Rheum 27:530, 1984.

93. Caeiro F, Michielson FMC, Bernstein R, et al: Systemic lupus erythematosus in childhood. Ann Rheum Dis 40:325, 1981.

94. Ballou SP, Khan MA, Kushner I: Clinical features of systemic lupus erythematosus. Differences related to race and age of onset. Arthritis Rheum 25:55, 1982.

95. Catoggio LJ, Skinner RP, Smith G, et al: Systemic lupus erythematosus in the elderly: Clinical and serological characteristics. J Rheumatol 11:175, 1984.

96. Braunstein EM, Weissman BN, Sosman JL, et al: Radiologic findings in late-onset systemic lupus erythematosus. AJR 140:587, 1983.

97. Lahita RG, Chiorazzi N, Gibofsky A, et al: Familial systemic lupus erythematosus in males. Arthritis Rheum 26:39, 1983.

98. Dubois EL, Friou GJ, Chandor S: Rheumatoid nodules and rheumatoid granulomas in systemic lupus erythematosus. JAMA 220:515, 1972.

99. Schwartz IS, Grishman E: Rheumatoid nodules of the vocal cords as the initial manifestation of systemic lupus erythematosus. JAMA 224:2751, 1980.

100. Isenberg DA, Snaith ML: Muscle disease in systemic lupus erythematosus: A study of its nature, frequency and cause. J Rheumatol 8:917, 1981.

101. Seibold JR, Wechsler LR, Cammarata RJ: LE cells in intermittent hydrarthrosis. Arthritis Rheum 23:958, 1980.

102. Winkler P, Baenkler H-W, Pfuhl E, et al: Die Bedeutung der Röntgendiagnostik der Hande beim Systemischen lupus erythematodes. Aus einer retrospektiven klinisch-röntgenologischen Studie von 124 Patienten mit Kollagenosen. Akt Rheumatol 5:255, 1980.

103. Esdaile JM, Danoff D, Rosenthall L, et al: Deforming arthritis in systemic lupus erythematosus. Ann Rheum Dis 40:124, 1981.

104. Morely KD, Leung A, Rynes RI: Lupus foot. Br Med J 284:557, 1982.

105. Mizutani W, Quismorio FP Jr: Lupus foot: Deforming arthropathy of the feet in systemic lupus erythematosus. J Rheumatol 11:80, 1984.

106. Cooney LM Jr, Aversa JM, Newman JH: Insidious bilateral infrapatellar rupture in a patient with systemic lupus erythematosus. Ann Rheum Dis 39:592, 1980.

107. Khan MA, Ballou SP: Tendon rupture in systemic lupus erythematosus. J Rheumatol 8:308, 1981.

108. Clement B, Vasey FB, Germain BF, et al: Subacute infrapatellar tendon rupture in systemic lupus erythematosus. J Rheumatol 10:164, 1983.

109. Potasman I, Bassan HM: Multiple tendon rupture in systemic lupus erythematosus: Case report and review of the literature. Ann Rheum Dis 43:347, 1984.

110. Arturi AS, Babini JC, Morteo OG, et al: Necrosis osea avascular en lupus eritematoso sistemico. Medicina 40:497, 1980.

111. Rodriguez MA, Paul H, Abadi I, et al: Multiple microcrystal deposition disease in a patient with systemic lupus erythematosus. Ann Rheum Dis 43:498, 1984.

112. Schenfeld L, Gray RG, Poppo MJ, et al: Bacterial monarthritis due to *Neisseria meningitidis* in systemic lupus erythematosus. J Rheumatol 8:145, 1981.

113. Shiota K, Miki F, Kanayama Y, et al: Suppurative coxitis due to *Salmonella typhimurium* in systemic lupus erythematosus. Ann Rheum Dis 42:312, 1981.

114. Lovy MR, Ryan PFJ, Hughes GRV: Concurrent systemic lupus erythematosus and salmonellosis. J Rheumatol 8:605, 1981.

115. Zvetina JR, Demos TC, Rubinstein H: *Mycobacterium intracellulare* infection of the shoulder and spine in a patient with steroid-treated systemic lupus erythematosus. Skel Radiol 8:111, 1982.

116. DeSmet AA, Mahmood T, Robinson RG, et al: Elevated sacroiliac joint uptake ratios in systemic lupus erythematosus. AJR 143:351, 1984.

117. Nassonova VA, Alekberova ZS, Folomeyer MY, et al: Sacroiliitis in male systemic lupus erythematosus. Scand J Rheumatol (Suppl) 52:23, 1984.

118. Naschel DJ, Leonard A, Mann DL, et al: Ankylosing spondylitis and systemic lupus erythematosus. Arch Intern Med 142:1227, 1982.

119. Kappes J, Schoepflin G, Barbana E: Lupoid sacroarthropathy. A previously undescribed association. Arthritis Rheum 23:699, 1980.

120. Williams M, Barton E: Terminal phalangeal sclerosis in rheumatoid arthritis. Clin Radiol 35:237, 1984.

121. Jonsson R, Lindvall A-M, Nyberg G: Temporomandibular joint involvement in systemic lupus erythematosus. Arthritis Rheum 26:1506, 1983.

122. Gerbracht D, Shapiro L: Temporomandibular joint erosions in systemic lupus erythematosus. Arthritis Rheum 25:597, 1982.

123. Liebling MR, Gold RH: Erosions of the temporomandibular joint in systemic lupus erythematosus. Arthritis Rheum 24:948, 1981.

124. Moidel RA, Good AE: Coexistent gout and systemic lupus erythematosus. Arthritis Rheum 24:969, 1981.

125. Wall BA, Agudelo CA, Weinblatt ME, et al: Acute gout and systemic lupus erythematosus: Report of 2 cases and literature review. J Rheumatol 9:305, 1982.

126. Lally EV, Parker VS, Kaplan SR: Acute gouty arthritis and systemic lupus erythematosus. J Rheumatol 9:308, 1982.

127. Passas CM, Wong RL, Peterson M, et al: A comparison of the specificity of the 1971 and 1982 American Rheumatism Association criteria for the classification of systemic lupus erythematosus. Arthritis Rheum 28:620, 1985.

128. Yokohari R, Tsunematsu T: Application, to Japanese patients, of the 1982 American Rheumatism Association revised criteria for the classification of systemic lupus erythematosus. Arthritis Rheum 28:693, 1985.

129. Kachru RB, Sequeira W, Mittal KK, et al: A significant increase of HLA-DR3 and DR2 in systemic lupus erythematosus among Blacks. J Rheumatol 11:471, 1984.

130. Bell DA, Rigby R, Stiller CR, et al: HLA antigens in systemic lupus erythematosus: Relationship to disease severity, age at onset, and sex. J Rheumatol 11:475, 1984.

131. De La Sota M, Garcia-Morteo O, Maldonado-Cocco JA: Jaccoud's arthropathy of the knees in systemic lupus erythematosus. Arthritis Rheum 28:825, 1985.

132. Leskinen RH, Skrifvars BV, Laasonen LS, et al: Bone lesions in systemic lupus erythematosus. Radiology 153:349, 1984.

133. Darlington LG: Osteonecrosis at multiple sites in a patient with systemic lupus erythematosus. Ann Rheum Dis 44:65, 1985.

134. Hanly JG, Urowitz MB: Tendon rupture in systemic lupus erythematosus. Ann Rheum Dis 45:349, 1986.

135. Ganczarczyk ML, Lee P, Furnasier VL: Early diagnosis of osteonecrosis in systemic lupus erythematosus with magnetic resonance imaging. Failure of core decompression. J Rheumatol 13:814, 1986.

136. Kalla AA, Learmonth ID, Klemp P: Early treatment of avascular necrosis in systemic lupus erythematosus. Ann Rheum Dis 45:649, 1986.

137. Alarcón-Segovia D, Abud-Mendoza C, Diaz-Jouanen E, et al: Deforming arthropathy of the hands in systemic lupus erythematosus. J Rheumatol 15:65, 1988.

138. Reilly PA, Evison G, McHugh NJ, et al: Arthropathy of the hands and feet in systemic lupus erythematosus. J Rheumatol 17:777, 1990.

139. Reilly PA, Evison G, Maddison PJ, et al: Reply. Deforming arthropathy of the hands in SLE and the growing pains of MCTD. J Rheumatol 18:632, 1991.

140. Alarcón-Segovia D: Deforming arthropathy of the hands in SLE and the growing pains of MCTD. J Rheumatol 18:632, 1991.

141. Martini A, Ravelli A, Viola S, et al: Systemic lupus erythematosus with Jaccoud's arthropathy mimicking juvenile rheumatoid arthritis. Arthritis Rheum 30:1062, 1987.

142. Siam ARM, Hammoudeh M: Jaccoud's arthropathy of the shoulders in systemic lupus erythematosus. J Rheumatol 19:980, 1992.

143. Babini SM, Cocco JAM, Babini JC, et al: Atlantoaxial subluxation in systemic lupus erythematosus: Further evidence of tendinous alterations. J Rheumatol 17:173, 1990.

144. Laasonen L, Gripenberg M, Leskinen R, et al: A subset of systemic lupus erythematosus with progressive cystic bone lesions. Ann Rheum Dis 49:118, 1990.

145. Babini SM, Cocco JAM, de la Sota M, et al: Tendinous laxity and Jaccoud's syndrome in patients with systemic lupus erythematosus. Possible role of secondary hyperparathyroidism. J Rheumatol 16:494, 1989.

146. Rillo OL, Babini SM, Basnak A, et al: Tendinous and ligamentous hyperlaxity in patients receiving longterm hemodialysis. J Rheumatol 18:1227, 1991.

147. Spronk PE, ter Borg EJ, Kallenberg CGM: Patients with systemic lupus erythematosus and Jaccoud's arthropathy: A clinical subset with an increased C reactive protein response? Ann Rheum Dis 51:358, 1992.

148. Furie RA, Chartash EK: Tendon rupture in systemic lupus erythematosus. Semin Arthritis Rheum 18:127, 1988.

149. Babini SM, Arturi A, Marcos JC, et al: Laxity and rupture of the patellar tendon in systemic lupus erythematosus. Association with secondary hyperparathyroidism. J Rheumatol 15:1162, 1988.

150. Pritchard CH, Berney S: Patellar tendon rupture in systemic lupus erythematosus. J Rheumatol 16:786, 1989.

151. Stolow J, Parikh S, Shybut G, et al: An atypical site of osteonecrosis in a patient with systemic lupus erythematosus. J Rheumatol 18:1623, 1991.

152. Fishel B, Caspi D, Eventov I, et al: Multiple osteonecrotic lesions in systemic lupus erythematosus. J Rheumatol 14:601, 1987.

153. Weiner ES, Abeles M: Aseptic necrosis and glucocorticosteroids in systemic lupus erythematosus: A reevaluation. J Rheumatol 16:604, 1989.

154. Nagasawa K, Ishii Y, Mayumi T, et al: Avascular necrosis of bone in systemic lupus erythematosus: Possible role of haemostatic abnormalities. Ann Rheum Dis 48:672, 1989.

155. van de Laar MHFJ, Meenhorst PL, van Soesbergen RM, et al: Polyarticular salmonella bacterial arthritis in a patient with systemic lupus erythematosus. J Rheumatol 16:231, 1989.

156. Medina F, Fraga A, Lavalle C: Salmonella septic arthritis in systemic lupus erythematosus. The importance of chronic carrier state. J Rheumatol 16:203, 1989.

157. Olivieri I, Gemignani G, Balagi M, et al: Concomitant systemic lupus erythematosus and ankylosing spondylitis. Ann Rheum Dis 49:323, 1990.

158. Gosset D, Foucher C, Lecouffe P, et al: Asymptomatic sacroiliitis in systemic lupus erythematosus. J Rheumatol 15:152, 1988.

159. Glickstein M, Neustadter L, Dalinka M, et al: Periosteal reaction in systemic lupus erythematosus. Skel Radiol 15:610, 1986.

160. Hoffman GS, Filie JD, Schumacher HR Jr, et al: Intractable vasculitis, resorptive osteolysis, and immunity to type I collagen in type VII Ehlers-Danlos syndrome. Arthritis Rheum 34:1466, 1991.

161. Sturgess AS, Littlejohn GO: Jaccoud's arthritis and panvasculitis in the hypocomplementemic urticarial vasculitis syndrome. J Rheumatol 15:858, 1988.

162. Seleznick MJ, Silveira LH, Espinoza LR: Avascular necrosis associated with anticardiolipin antibodies. J Rheumatol 18:1416, 1991.

163. Petri M: The clinical syndrome associated with antiphospholipid antibodies. J Rheumatol 19:505, 1992.

164. Bayahia R, Balafrej L, Ezaitouni F: Les arthrites septiques au cours du lupus érythémateux aigu disséminé. Sem Hôp Paris 68:421, 1992.

165. Kohli M, Bennett RM: Sacroiliitis in systemic lupus erythematosus. J Rheumatol 21:170, 1994.

34

Scleroderma (Progressive Systemic Sclerosis)

Donald Resnick, M.D.

Scleroderma is an uncommon generalized disorder of connective tissue that affects various organ systems, principally the skin, the lungs, the gastrointestinal tract, the heart, the kidneys, and the musculoskeletal system. Its pathologic characteristics include severe fibrosis and alterations of small blood vessels. The cause and pathogenesis of scleroderma are not known, although three potential mechanisms have been implicated: an abnormality of collagen metabolism, a vascular abnormality, and an immunologic process.[1-3]

This chapter describes musculoskeletal abnormalities associated with scleroderma, emphasizing their radiographic and pathologic characteristics. Although clinical findings of the disease also are summarized, the interested reader who wishes to learn the manifestations of multiorgan system involvement in scleroderma should consult standard textbooks.[4, 5, 118]

HISTORICAL ASPECTS AND NOMENCLATURE

Historical aspects of scleroderma are difficult to trace for a variety of reasons, including the facts that induration of the skin is a feature common to many disorders and that the original names of such disorders were, in large part, derived from the Greek root *skleros,* meaning "hard."[119] There seem to have been no clear descriptions of scleroderma prior to the middle of the nineteenth century, although reports of similar diseases such as sclerema neonatorum and scleroedema had appeared by that time. The earliest account of a patient with scleroedema is probably that of Curzio, a physician of Naples, in 1753[6] and, despite references that would suggest that this is actually a description of scleroderma, it appears not to be the case.[119] A French publication by Gintrac in 1847[7] led to the introduction of the term "scleroderma," although Gintrac may have falsely identified earlier reports of this disease. In the middle and latter parts of the nineteenth century, definite instances of scleroderma or progressive systemic sclerosis can be identified; however, the widespread nature of the illness was not fully appreciated until the twentieth century.

The many reports of scleroderma and the difficulty in differentiating it from other disorders associated with induration of the skin have led to a variety of descriptive terms and classification systems for the disease.[113] From 1817 to 1877, no fewer than 19 synonyms were used for diffuse scleroderma, including such names as sclerema adultorum, ichthyosis cornea, chorionitis, scleroma, sclerodermia, elephantiasis sclerosa, and dermatosklerosis.[119] Progressive systemic sclerosis was the term introduced by Goetz[120] in 1945, and it is widely used today. Additional nomenclature that is commonly encountered includes the following[4]:

Raynaud's Phenomenon or Syndrome: Paroxysmal occlusion of the digital arteries that is precipitated by cold or emotional stress and relieved by heat.[121] This syndrome, which is associated with local pallor, cyanosis, pain, burning, numbness, swelling, and hyperhidrosis, is caused by a change in the diameter of the digital, palmar, and plantar arteries. It can be further classified as primary or idiopathic and secondary. Diseases leading to secondary Raynaud's syndrome include collagen vascular disorders (progressive systemic sclerosis, systemic lupus erythematosus, rheumatoid arthritis, Sjögren's syndrome, dermatomyositis, and mixed connective tissue disease), other vasculitides (cryoglobulinemia, hepatitis B, and paroxysmal nocturnal hemoglobinuria), obstructive arterial disorders (arteriosclerosis, thromboses, and Buerger's disease), drug intoxications (ergot alkaloids, vinyl chloride, cytotoxic drugs, and heavy metals), neurologic and neoplastic processes, and thermal or occupational trauma (frostbite, physical injury, and vibration syndrome).[121, 122]

Acrosclerosis: Sclerosis of facial structures and fingers that is associated with Raynaud's phenomenon.

Diffuse Systemic Sclerosis: Involvement of the skin of the trunk that is commonly associated with systemic abnormalities and that may be associated with peripheral skin involvement.

CRST Syndrome: The association of subcutaneous calcinosis, Raynaud's phenomenon, sclerodactyly, and telangiectasia.

CREST Syndrome: The association of CRST syndrome with esophageal abnormalities.[106, 123]

Thibierge-Weissenbach Syndrome: The combination of calcinosis and digital ischemia.

Scleroderma Circumscriptum, Scleroderma Diffusum, Scleroderma Morphoea, Scleroderma en Bande: Dermatologic variants of the disease.

Shulman Syndrome: Scleroderma-like syndrome with eosinophilia and hypergammaglobulinemia but without systemic or vascular involvement.[8, 103–105] This syndrome, which also is called eosinophilic fasciitis, may follow an episode of physical exertion and is associated with painful swelling and induration of the skin and soft tissues in the upper and lower extremities, followed by a rapid progression to joint contracture owing to alterations in nearby tissues. Biopsy may indicate relative sparing of the epidermis and dermis, with marked thickening and fibrosis of the fascia between fat and muscle. Polyarthritis may be seen[116] (see discussion later in this chapter).

Scleroderma Adultorum: A benign, self-limited condition unrelated to true scleroderma, occurring after acute infections, characterized by nonpitting edema of the skin and spontaneous resolution within a few months.

A classification system for scleroderma and its variants has been proposed by Barnett and Coventry.[9, 10] This system divides scleroderma into two major types: progressive systemic sclerosis (scleroderma with systemic involvement), and localized scleroderma (scleroderma without systemic involvement). Progressive systemic sclerosis can be further divided into three groups. In the first group (Raynaud's phenomenon with sclerodactyly), patients first exhibit Raynaud's phenomenon and later develop skin abnormalities of the fingers and neck, dysphagia, and, in some cases, visceral abnormalities. In the second group (acrosclerosis), patients have Raynaud's phenomenon and widespread skin involvement of the hands, face, and forearms. Additional features include telangiectasia, calcinosis, and slowly progressive visceral involvement of the lung, the kidney, and the heart, which can lead to the patient's demise over a prolonged period of time. In the third group (systemic scleroderma with diffuse skin changes), the patient has widespread skin and visceral involvement, which progresses rapidly and which can result in death in a short period of time.

In localized scleroderma, skin changes, which may be related to trauma or a familial predisposition,[11–14] can be further divided into two groups.[5] In the first group (localized morphea), the changes are confined to the skin and subcutis and may occur at any age and affect any site. Initial discrete, erythematous, discolored patches or plaques subsequently are associated with softening of the skin and, at times, hemiatrophy, particularly of the face. In the second group (linear scleroderma), skin sclerosis of the extremities or head most frequently is apparent in childhood.[108, 192] Induration may extend into deep tissue, leading to fibrosis and fixation of para-articular structures, which can interfere with joint motion. Although these varieties of localized scleroderma generally are not accompanied by significant radiographic abnormalities, an association with melorheostosis has been reported,[15] leading to a characteristic "flowing" pattern of bone formation, distributed along one aspect of an involved bone.

This classification system has been modified by other investigators.[193] For example, Masi and collaborators,[124] while also recognizing systemic and localized forms of the disease, include three additional types: chemically induced scleroderma-like conditions (vinyl chloride disease, pentazocine-induced fibrosis, bleomycin-induced fibrosis); eosinophilic fasciitis; and pseudoscleroderma (edematous, indurative, and atrophic). These authors further identify major and minor diagnostic criteria. The single major criterion is proximal scleroderma, with a 91 per cent sensitivity and a greater than 99 per cent specificity. Minor criteria are sclerodactyly, digital pitting scars of fingertips or loss of substance of the finger pad, and bibasilar pulmonary fibrosis. One major or two or more minor criteria were found in 97 per cent of patients with definite systemic sclerosis but in only 2 per cent of comparison patients with closely related disorders.

Complicating any classification system in scleroderma is the occurrence of various overlap syndromes, in which features of scleroderma are combined with those of other collagen vascular diseases, including systemic lupus erythematosus and dermatomyositis.

CLINICAL ABNORMALITIES

General Features

Scleroderma affects women more frequently than men and usually becomes apparent in the third to fifth decades

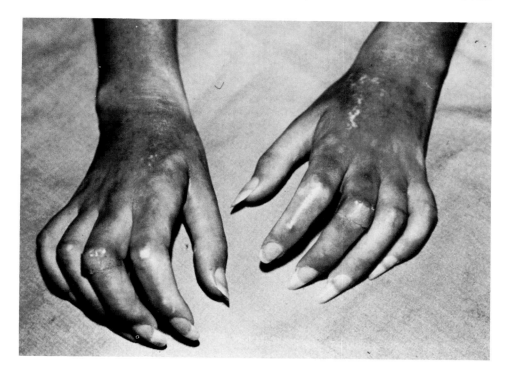

FIGURE 34–1. Scleroderma: Skin abnormalities. The skin is taut and shiny. Ulcerated subcutaneous calcific deposits are apparent, particularly at the proximal interphalangeal joints.

of life.[9, 10, 16, 17, 197] Occasionally the disease becomes manifest in patients over the age of 50 years,[243] but involvement of children is relatively rare.[18–20, 198, 244] The onset of the disease usually is insidious. A common presenting manifestation is intermittent pallor of the digits (fingers or toes) on exposure to cold (Raynaud's phenomenon). Additionally, initial symptoms may include gradual thickening of the skin and edema in the distal portion of the extremities and pain and stiffness arising in the small joints of the hands and knees. The last-mentioned findings resemble the early changes of rheumatoid arthritis. In some persons, the onset of scleroderma is characterized by severe muscular weakness or visceral involvement (dysphagia) without involvement of the skin.

The natural history of systemic sclerosis is variable.[197] Although a fulminant, rapidly progressive disorder occasionally is evident, a protracted disease course with survival for 20 years or more is most typical. As the disease advances, skin changes frequently represent its most characteristic clinical feature (Fig. 34–1). Edema is replaced by rigidity and thickening of the skin, particularly of the fingers, the face, and the dorsum of the hands and feet. These cutaneous findings become more widespread and extensive, with involvement of the entire limb, the trunk, and the perioral regions, and the skin becomes shiny, taut, and leathery. Melanotic hyperpigmentation, vitiligo, and telangiectasis can be observed. Small or large calcific collections in subcutaneous tissue develop, predominantly in women. Nodular lesions may ulcerate, extruding calcific material on the surface of the skin, particularly in the fingertips, the hands, and areas over bony protuberances. Secondary infection of the ulcerated lesions is common.

Systemic involvement in scleroderma can lead to a variety of symptoms and signs, depending on the site of abnormality. Gastrointestinal findings include dysphagia, heartburn, hematemesis, melena, abdominal distention, and perforation of the bowel. Pulmonary involvement, which generally occurs late in the course of the disease, can lead to dyspnea, coughing, and clinically detectable rales and rhonchi. Restrictive and obstructive pulmonary disease may be recognized. Renal abnormalities may progress rapidly, leading to renal failure, uremia, and hypertension. Cardiac alterations, which include pericarditis and myocardial fibrosis, may be associated with congestive heart failure. Additional clinical characteristics are jaundice, pruritus, and hepatomegaly (due to liver involvement); neuropathies and other neurologic abnormalities (due to involvement of nerve sheaths and arteritis)[186]; and anemia (due to renal failure, gastrointestinal bleeding, and malabsorption).

Rheumatologic Features

Articular involvement has been described as an initial manifestation in 12 to 65 per cent of patients with scleroderma and as an eventual manifestation in 46 to 97 per cent of patients.[17, 125, 197] The fingers, the wrists, and the ankles commonly are affected. The mode of onset can be acute or insidious, and the course generally is intermittent.[125] Oligoarticular and polyarticular patterns predominate. When symmetric in distribution, manifestations resemble those of rheumatoid arthritis. Clinical findings include soft tissue swelling, morning stiffness, tenderness, pain, redness, and warmth. A joint effusion may be detectable but typically is small. Tendon and tendon sheath involvement also is common, especially in the knees, the fingers, the wrists, the ankles, and the feet, and may lead to a coarse, palpable crepitus.[21] A similar finding can be evident over involved bursae in the olecranon and subscapular areas.[245] In these locations, the crepitus has been related to fibrinous deposits on the surface of tendon sheaths and fasciae. Additional findings attributable to tendon sheath abnormalities are distention and thickening of sheaths and nerve compression (e.g., median nerve compression within the carpal tunnel).[199, 200] Although rare, tendon rupture has been described.[126, 185] Flexion contractures are not uncommon, particularly in the digits of the hand, the wrist, and the elbow, although large joints such as the knee may be affected similarly.[201] Bowing of the fingers is reported to be a helpful diagnostic clue.[127]

Muscle involvement occurs in the majority of patients with scleroderma. On the basis of clinical, biochemical, and histologic evidence, Medsger and coworkers[22] detected such involvement in approximately 70 per cent of patients. Clements and associates[23] reported an even higher prevalence of muscle involvement in patients with this disease. These latter investigators noted three patterns of muscle alteration: a simple myopathy, which is stable or only mildly progressive (the most common variety); an inflammatory muscle disease that is indistinguishable from dermatomyositis; and muscle weakness associated with a generalized neuropathic process. Some of the patients who demonstrated the progressive inflammatory pattern of muscle disease revealed features of mixed connective tissue disease or overlap syndromes. Thus, the most characteristic variety of muscle abnormality in scleroderma is mild and nonincapacitating proximal muscle weakness, associated with mild serum elevations of muscle enzymes, and interstitial fibrosis and variation in diameter of muscle fibers without active inflammation on biopsy. In addition, some patients with scleroderma have weakness and wasting of skeletal muscle as a result of disuse and poor nutrition.

Laboratory Features

Laboratory analysis indicates elevation of the erythrocyte sedimentation rate in approximately 60 to 70 per cent of patients, positive serologic test results for rheumatoid factor in approximately 30 to 40 per cent of patients, and the presence of antinuclear antibodies in 35 to 96 per cent of patients.[4, 114] Analysis of aspirated synovial fluid may indicate a high protein content, a polymorphonuclear cellular exudate, and ragocytes.[24, 25]

Overlap Syndromes

Some patients with scleroderma demonstrate clinical patterns that suggest the presence of more than one collagen vascular disease; findings may indicate an overlap condition, consisting of scleroderma and dermatomyositis or scleroderma and systemic lupus erythematosus.[25–27] Furthermore, the demonstration of serum antibody to an extractable nuclear antigen (ENA) in patients with scleroderma-like clinical findings indicates the presence of mixed connective tissue disease.[28] This disease is discussed in Chapter 37.

RADIOGRAPHIC ABNORMALITIES

Bone and Soft Tissue Involvement

The radiographic abnormalities of bone and soft tissue in scleroderma are characteristic. These are best described in association with specific regions of the body.

Hand and Wrist (Fig. 34–2). Abnormalities of the hand

are characterized by resorption of soft tissue, subcutaneous calcification, and osseous destruction.[29–34] One or more of these changes were evident in 63 per cent of patients in a study of a large series of persons with scleroderma.[29] In this same study, similar changes were observed in only 5 per cent of patients with some other collagen vascular disease and in 41 per cent of patients with primary Raynaud's disease.

Soft tissue resorption of the fingertips is a common finding in scleroderma. Its frequency varies from 15 to 80 per cent according to previous reports[128] and increases dramatically in patients with accompanying Raynaud's phenomenon. Resorption of soft tissue produces a conical shape of the tips of the fingers. Its presence can be verified by measuring the vertical distance between the phalangeal tip and the skin surface on a frontal radiograph of the digit. If this distance is less than 20 per cent of the transverse diameter of the base of the same distal phalanx, soft tissue resorption indeed is present.[35] Soft tissue resorption can involve any digit of the hand, including the thumb. It frequently is accompanied by adjacent calcific deposits and bony abnormalities, including acrosclerosis.

Amorphous calcification in patients with scleroderma is common. This association was first established by Thibierge and Weissenbach in 1911.[36] Such calcification is most common in the hand; localization to this site has been recorded in 73 to 86 per cent of patients with calcinosis.[30, 37] The reported frequency of digital calcification in patients with scleroderma is approximately 10 to 30 per cent.[29, 30, 128, 129] This frequency increases with severe skin involvement but does not appear to be related to vascular abnormalities. It may occur early in the course of the disease. Soft tissue calcification in the fingers, along with tuftal resorption, is reported to be more common in children.[130]

Digital calcification can involve either the subcutaneous or the capsular tissues. The appearance includes small punctate deposits at the phalangeal tip, focal conglomerate deposits with a wider distribution, sheetlike or tumoral collections, and curvilinear deposits within the joint capsule.

The mechanism of soft tissue calcification in scleroderma (and other collagen vascular diseases) is not clear.[30] It generally is accepted that local tissue factors are more important than a systemic derangement in calcium and phosphorus metabolism; although some investigators have suggested that an abnormality of parathyroid function may contribute to soft tissue calcification in this disease, parathyroidectomy in patients with scleroderma does not lead to improvement in the calcinosis.[38, 39] The fact that calcification frequently involves sites of chronic stress, such as the radial aspect of the fingers that appose the thumb, the extensor surface of the elbow, and the soft tissues about bony prominences, suggests a role of trauma in the pathogenesis of these deposits.[40] This role is underscored by the presence of more severe calcification in the dominant hand[30] and by the absence of calcification (or bone resorption) in digits that are protected from the stress of normal activity because of a previous injury.[41] Of related interest, scleroderma skin changes have been reported to be absent in completely paretic limbs,[202] although the effect of paralysis on the distribution and extent of soft tissue calcification and osteolysis has not been documented.

Bony erosion of the phalanges in the hand occurs in 40 to 80 per cent of patients with scleroderma.[29, 35, 42] It com-

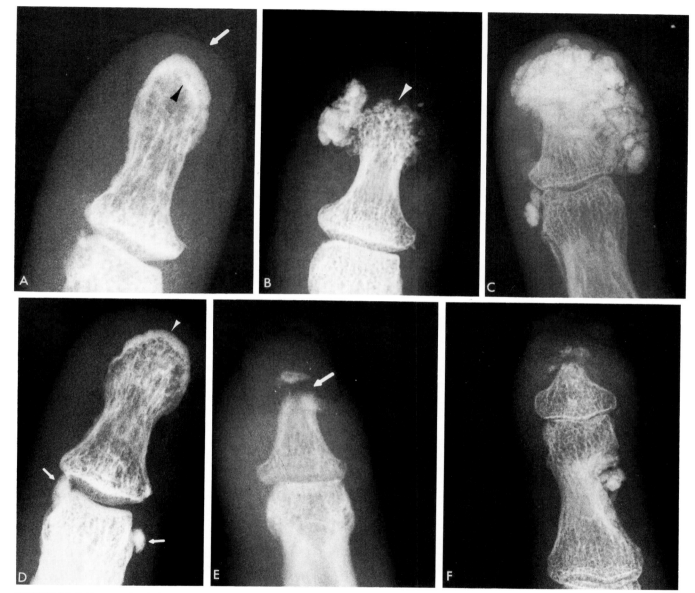

FIGURE 34–2. Bone and soft tissue abnormalities: Digits of the hand.

A Observe atrophy of the soft tissue (arrow) and hyperostosis of the phalangeal tuft (arrowhead).

B In this digit, findings include resorption of the tuft (arrowhead) and adjacent calcification.

C More extensive calcification is evident in another patient.

D In this example, note minimal hyperostosis of the phalangeal tuft (arrowhead) and periarticular calcifications, perhaps in the joint capsule (arrows).

E Bandlike resorption of the terminal phalanx (arrow) has isolated a small irregular fragment.

F Soft tissue swelling, tuftal resorption, and calcification are seen. Note the deformity of the nail.

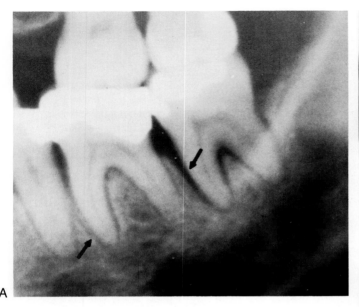

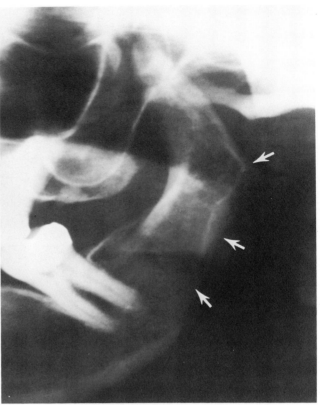

FIGURE 34–3. Bone and soft tissue abnormalities: Mandible.

A Observe the exaggerated radiolucent area between the teeth and the mandible (arrows) corresponding to the location of a thickened periodontal membrane.

B In another patient, resorption of the body of the mandible (arrows) is associated with complete osteolysis of the condylar process.

(**B**, Courtesy of L. Rogers, M.D., Chicago, Illinois.)

mences on the tuft, particularly on the palmar aspect of the bone. Continued resorption leads to "penciling" or sharpening of the phalanx and, in severe cases, much or all of the distal phalanx can be destroyed, leading to tapering of the entire digit. In rare instances, the middle phalanges also can be involved. Severe bony osteolysis has been reported more frequently in children with scleroderma.[43, 130]

Extradigital involvement of the hand and wrist may consist of more extensive soft tissue calcification, osteoporosis (related to chronic disuse and immobilization), and osseous destruction of portions of the carpal bones, distal portion of the radius, and ulna. These destructive changes are discussed later in this chapter.

Foot. Abnormalities of the bones and soft tissues of the foot are less frequent and less pronounced than those in the hand. Diffuse osteoporosis, soft tissue atrophy of the toes, and tuftal resorption occasionally are seen.

Mandible (Fig. 34–3). A relatively specific dental sign of scleroderma is thickening of the periodontal membrane[44]; the frequency of this radiographic finding in 30 patients with scleroderma was 21 per cent, compared with 5 per cent in controls.[102] The enlarged membrane creates an exaggerated radiolucent area between the tooth and the mandibular bone, which is best detected on dental films. The resulting radiolucent zone varies in size; it may be minute or extremely large. The abnormality usually is more evident about the posteriorly located teeth, although all teeth can be affected.[134] This mandibular alteration may lead to loss of the lamina dura and loosening of the teeth.

More extensive mandibular bone resorption has been noted in this disease. Seifert and collaborators[45] observed segmental resorption of bone at the angle of the mandible

in 5 of 16 patients with scleroderma. This finding was more frequent in black patients and appeared to be related to tightness of the facial skin, atrophy of the masseter and pterygoid muscles, and small size of the oral orifice. Extrinsic pressure and ischemia were suggested as etiologic factors. More recently, Caplan and Benny[100] described a patient with scleroderma who revealed osteolysis of both mandibular angles, a condyle, and the ipsilateral coronoid process. Adjacent soft tissue calcification also was evident. Other reports confirm the presence of mandibular resorption in scleroderma and indicate that although the loss of bone may be subtle, extensive osteolysis of the mandibular angle and coronoid and condylar processes is evident in some patients.[129, 131, 132, 134, 203]

Additional mandibular alterations in scleroderma include fracture of the rami,[46] and deformity and underdevelopment of the mandible in children with localized scleroderma of the linear type.[47, 48]

Ribs (Fig. 34–4). Symmetrically distributed erosions of the superior aspect of multiple ribs was first emphasized in scleroderma by Keats in 1967.[49] Similar abnormalities subsequently were noted by other investigators.[50, 51, 129] The changes predominate along the posterior aspects of the third to sixth ribs, and may occur in the absence of bone resorption at other sites.[129] With extensive rib destruction, pathologic fractures have been evident.

Although Haverbush and colleagues[51] suggested a vascular cause for these bony abnormalities, there is evidence to suggest that rib resorption in scleroderma is related to intercostal muscle atrophy with resultant loss of mechanical stress to the cortical bone at the muscle insertions, leading to osseous resorption.[52] Such evidence includes the demon-

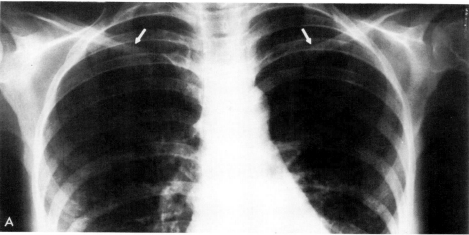

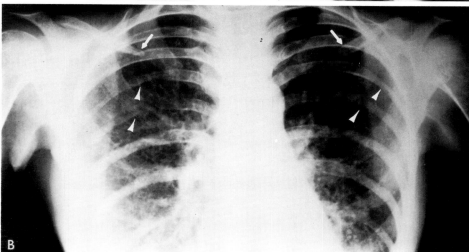

FIGURE 34–4. Bone and soft tissue abnormalities: Ribs and clavicle. Radiographs obtained 11 months apart reveal progressive resorption of the clavicles (arrows) and ribs (arrowheads). Observe peripheral abnormalities in the lower lobes of the lungs. (Courtesy of P. Kline, M.D., San Antonio, Texas.)

stration of osteoporosis alone in biopsy specimens of involved ribs[50] and the occurrence of identical changes in other disorders associated with muscle atrophy caused either by chest wall restriction or by loss of innervation, such as rheumatoid arthritis,[53] other collagen vascular diseases, poliomyelitis, and restrictive lung disease.[54]

Spine (Figs. 34–5 and 34–6). Paraspinal calcification recently has been emphasized as an additional manifestation of scleroderma. Such calcification, which may become massive, has been observed in the cervical,[205–207] thoracic,[208] and lumbar[209] segments. It may lead to local pain, discomfort, stiffness, dysphagia, and spinal cord or nerve root compression. The deposited material generally is calcium hydroxyapatite, identical to that occurring in other soft tissue sites in scleroderma. Transaxial images provided by CT scanning and MR imaging are ideally suited to analysis of the extent of the calcification, its effects on adjacent ligamentous and neurologic structures, and presence of associated osteolysis and subluxation.

Other Sites and Manifestations (Fig. 34–7). Soft tissue calcification in scleroderma occurs not only in the digits but also in the face, the axilla, the forearms, the lower legs, and pressure areas such as the ischial tuberosities.[37, 246] In addition, periarticular "tumoral" collections can appear at single or multiple sites, simulating the findings in milk-

alkali syndrome, hypervitaminosis D, and renal osteodystrophy.

Bone resorption in scleroderma also may be apparent at other sites, including portions of the acromion, radius, and ulna,[42, 129, 191, 203] distal end of the clavicle,[33] humerus,[133, 204] and cervical spine[51, 187] (Table 34–1) (Fig. 34–4).

An additional patient with scleroderma has been described who demonstrated periosteal bone formation in the diaphyseal portions of the femora and humeri.[55] The findings, which were associated with increased density of the tibial tuberosity and synostosis of the carpal bones, were reminiscent of the periostitis that may be observed in patients with vascular disorders such as systemic lupus erythe-

TABLE 34–1. Sites of Osteolysis in Scleroderma

Phalanges of hand and foot[29]
Carpal bones[62]
Distal portions of the radius and ulna[42, 129, 191]
Mandible[45, 100, 129, 131, 132, 134]
Ribs[49–51, 129]
Clavicle[33]
Humerus[133]
Acromion[42]
Cervical spine[51, 205]

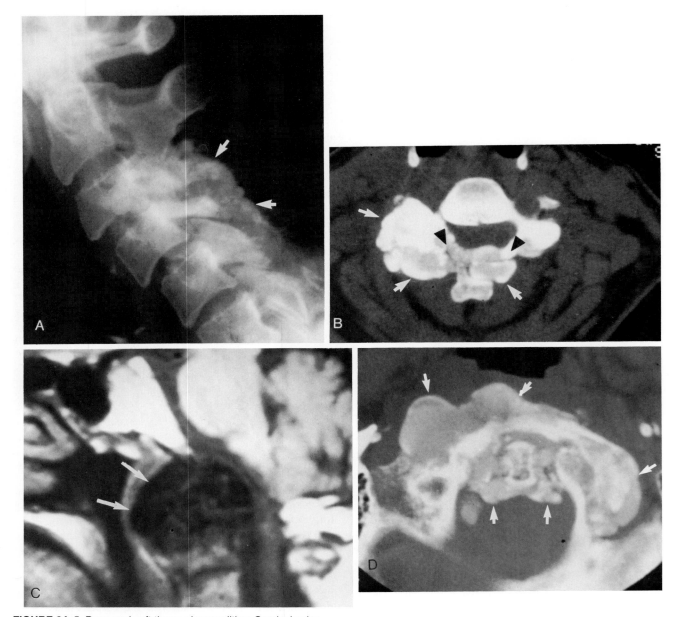

FIGURE 34–5. Bone and soft tissue abnormalities: Cervical spine.

A, B This 56 year old woman with progressive systemic sclerosis had a decreased range of motion in the cervical spine. A routine lateral radiograph **(A)** shows calcific masses about the apophyseal joints (arrows) between the third and sixth cervical levels. A transaxial CT scan **(B)** demonstrates the proximity of the calcifications (arrows) to the bone. Osteolysis (arrowheads) of the laminae is evident.

(Courtesy of W. Peck, M.D., Orange, California.)

C, D This 63 year old woman had an overlap syndrome consisting of scleroderma and systemic lupus erythematosus. A sagittal T1-weighted (TR/TE, 600/20) spin echo MR image **(C)** shows a large area of signal void (arrows) around the odontoid process. Transaxial CT scan **(D)** reveals an extensive lobulated, calcific mass (arrows) surrounding the dens and the atlas. Both of these structures are eroded.

(Courtesy of B. J. Manaster, M.D., Salt Lake City, Utah.)

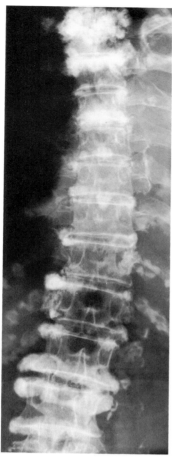

FIGURE 34–6. Bone and soft tissue abnormalities: Thoracolumbar spine. In a 77 year old man with a 40 year history of progressive systemic sclerosis, widespread paraspinal calcification is seen. (Courtesy of G. Harell, M.D., Metairie, Louisiana.)

matosus and polyarteritis nodosa.[56, 57] As peripheral arterial abnormalities can be evident on arteriograms in patients with scleroderma,[58] the changes in this patient indeed may have been related to vascular alterations.

Articular Involvement

In addition to the "articular" abnormalities that result from primary osseous resorption in scleroderma, several other articular manifestations occur in this disease (Table 34–2).[109] These latter joint changes in scleroderma must be evaluated critically because they may represent abnormalities related to overlap syndromes or coexistent rheumatoid arthritis. In fact, approximately 40 per cent of patients with scleroderma reveal a clinical picture compatible with rheumatoid arthritis and, on joint aspiration, some demonstrate an increase in protein levels and number of white blood cells indistinguishable from the findings of rheumatoid arthritis.[40] Over one third of patients with scleroderma have positive serologic test results for rheumatoid factor. Gout, also, has been described in patients with scleroderma,[210] perhaps related to renal insufficiency.

Distal Interphalangeal Joints (Fig. 34–8). Alterations at distal interphalangeal joints usually are confined to regional or periarticular osteoporosis and swelling and thick-

ening of adjacent soft tissues without evidence of joint space narrowing or osseous erosion.

Rabinowitz and coworkers[59] evaluated hand and wrist radiographs in 24 patients with "proved" scleroderma and emphasized the similarity of the bone and joint manifestations to those of rheumatoid arthritis. In addition to osteoporosis, joint space narrowing, and osseous erosion in typical "target" areas of rheumatoid arthritis, such as the ulnar styloid, all the compartments of the wrist, and the metacarpophalangeal and proximal interphalangeal joints, radiographic changes in some of their patients with scleroderma occurred at distal interphalangeal joints, articulations not commonly involved in rheumatoid arthritis. Although some of their patients may have had both scleroderma and rheumatoid arthritis (in fact, at least three had positive serologic test results for rheumatoid factor), the presence of distal interphalangeal joint abnormalities appears to represent a true manifestation of scleroderma joint disease.

The author has observed several patients with scleroderma without clinical or serologic evidence for rheumatoid arthritis who demonstrated mild to severe bilateral erosive abnormalities of distal interphalangeal and proximal interphalangeal joints, characterized by articular space narrowing, marginal and central osseous erosions, bony production with osteophytes, and intra-articular bony ankylosis. The findings resembled changes in psoriasis or inflammatory (erosive) osteoarthritis; unlike rheumatoid arthritis, the metacarpophalangeal and wrist articulations were relatively spared. Although the pathogenesis of the interphalangeal joint abnormalities and their relationship to scleroderma remain unclear, it is of interest that other investigators have described alterations of these joints in scleroderma.[125, 128, 129, 137] Findings resembling psoriatic arthritis[60] and neuropathic osteoarthropathy[61] have been recorded. Furthermore, intra-articular bony ankylosis has been described in interphalangeal and wrist joints in this disease.[55, 59] Erosive arthritis might be expected in some patients with scleroderma, as synovial biopsies outline initial inflammatory changes with cellular infiltration (lymphocytes, plasma cells), not unlike those in early rheumatoid arthritis, followed by synovial fibrosis.

Proximal Interphalangeal and Metacarpophalangeal Joints. Some reports of articular manifestations of scleroderma have described distinctive alterations in the proximal interphalangeal and metacarpophalangeal joints. An unusual pattern of focal resorption or erosion localized to the dorsal aspect of the metacarpal and proximal phalangeal heads is seen.[135] The abnormalities are best detected on steep oblique or lateral radiographic projections of the digits and are combined with erosions on the volar aspect of the bones. They lack specificity, being observed in some patients with rheumatoid arthritis. The pathogenesis of such peculiar osseous abnormalities is not clear. Additional articular changes at these sites resemble those typically apparent

TABLE 34–2. Sites of Erosive Articular Disease in Scleroderma

Metacarpophalangeal joints
Proximal and distal interphalangeal joints
First carpometacarpal joint
Inferior radioulnar joint
Metatarsophalangeal joints

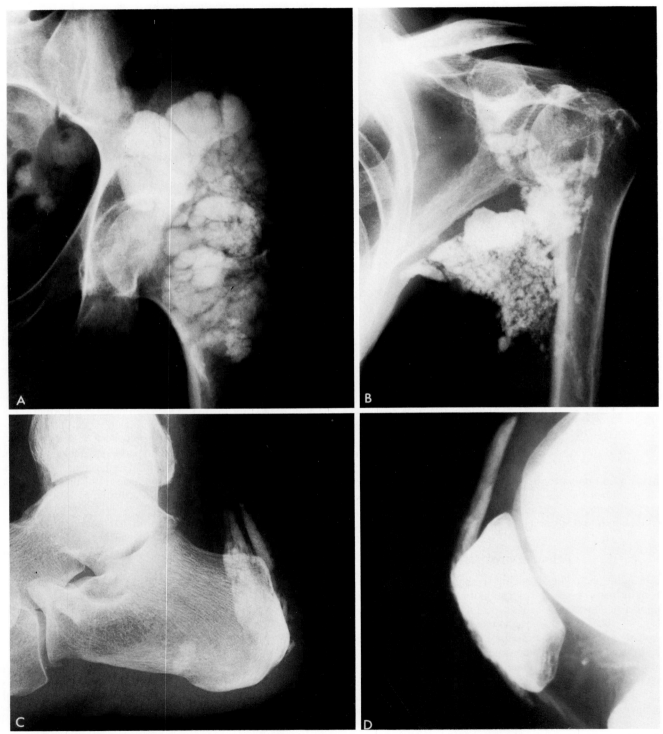

FIGURE 34–7. Bone and soft tissue abnormalities: Periarticular calcification. Periarticular deposits are evident about the hip, the shoulder, the heel, and the knee in different patients with scleroderma.

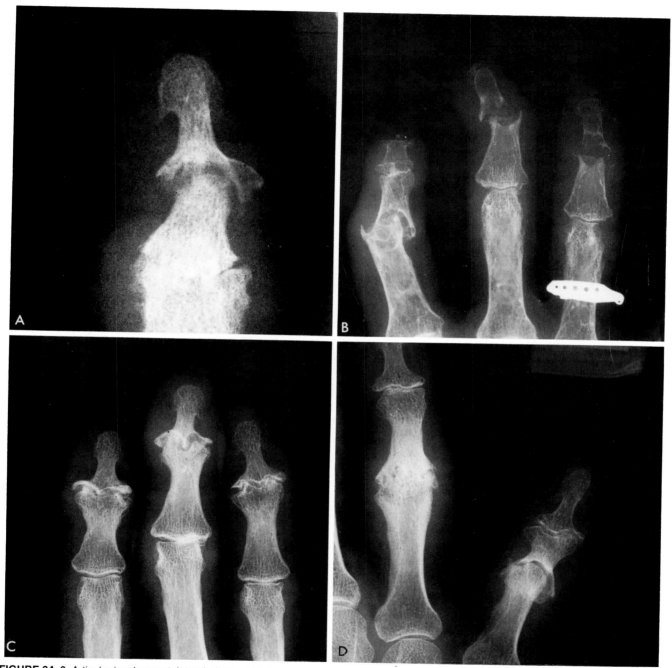

FIGURE 34–8. Articular involvement: Interphalangeal joints.

A Destructive osseous changes about the distal interphalangeal joint, which are associated with blunted and expanded bony surfaces (pencil-and-cup appearance), resemble the findings of psoriatic arthritis. Proliferative alterations are evident at the proximal interphalangeal joint.

B In another patient, extensive bony erosion about distal interphalangeal and proximal interphalangeal joints can be observed. Note the separation of the osseous margins and the sharply demarcated irregular surfaces. Subluxation also is apparent. The findings are reminiscent of psoriatic arthritis.

C In this person, expanded and closely applied bony surfaces with central irregularities at the distal interphalangeal joints resemble changes in inflammatory (erosive) osteoarthritis.

D Involvement of the fifth proximal interphalangeal joint with erosion and enlargement of the subchondral bone, and of the fourth proximal interphalangeal joint with intra-articular bony ankylosis, is identical to that occurring in psoriasis.

in rheumatoid arthritis or Jaccoud's arthropathy and, as such, may relate to synovial inflammation or capsular and ligamentous traction.[135, 136]

First Carpometacarpal Joints (Fig. 34–9). Selective involvement of the first carpometacarpal joint of the wrist can be apparent in scleroderma.[62, 188] Distinctive bilateral

resorption of the trapezium and adjacent metacarpal bone is observed with varying degrees of radial subluxation of the metacarpal base. Associated findings may include intra-articular calcification (discussed later in this chapter) and erosions at additional joints. The other joints of the wrist generally are spared, however.

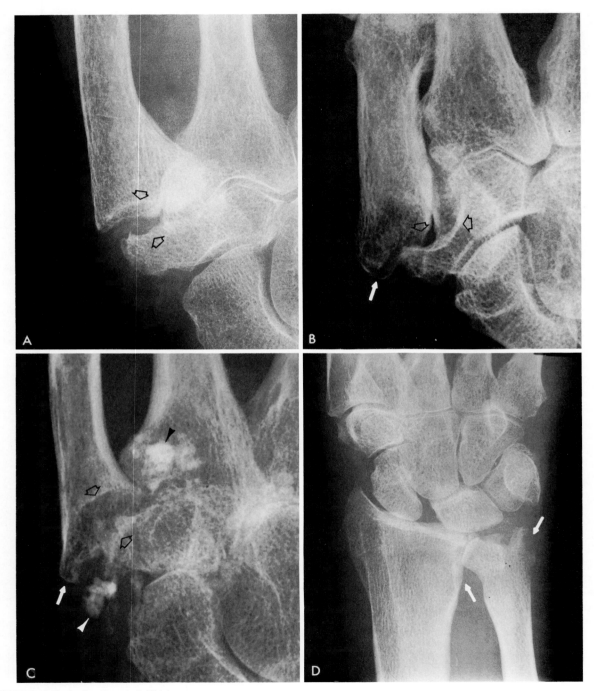

FIGURE 34–9. Articular involvement: Wrist.

A–C Three examples of selective involvement of the first carpometacarpal joint in scleroderma are shown. Observe scalloped erosions of the trapezium and base of the metacarpal (open arrows), radial and proximal subluxation of the metacarpal base (solid arrows), and intra-articular calcification (arrowheads).

D Observe erosions of the ulnar styloid process and of the distal aspect of the ulna and adjacent parts of the distal portions of the radius and ulna (arrows). These changes reflect synovial abnormalities of the extensor carpi ulnaris tendon sheath and inferior radioulnar compartment. Additional findings include separation (dissociation) of the scaphoid and lunate, and mild osteoporosis.

(B, C, From Resnick D, et al: AJR *131*:283, 1978. Copyright 1978, American Roentgen Ray Society.)

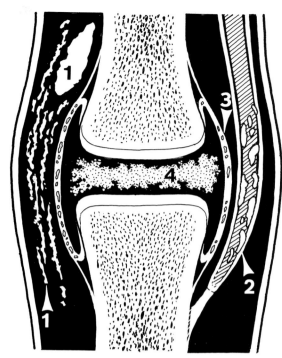

FIGURE 34–10. Sites of calcification in scleroderma. Deposits may occur in the soft tissues *(1)*, tendons and tendon sheaths *(2)*, and capsule *(3)*, as well as within the joint *(4)*.

Preferential involvement of the first carpometacarpal joint is the distinctive feature of this arthropathy. This pattern of articular disease has not been emphasized in the past, although a review of textbooks and articles dealing with scleroderma reveals additional cases with similar radiographic findings.[63, 64] The pathogenesis of the arthropathy is unknown. Its association with skin tightening, muscle atrophy of the hand and wrist, and contracture of the thumb in adduction may indicate that muscle and tendon imbalance produces joint subluxation at the first carpometacarpal joint, with subsequent pressure erosion of bone. In this regard, a similar arthropathy may be apparent in other disorders that alter muscle and tendon balance, such as systemic lupus erythematosus,[65, 66] Jaccoud's arthropathy,[35] dermatomyositis,[67] and Ehlers-Danlos syndrome.[63, 68] The possible role of synovial inflammation and intra-articular calcification in the production of this arthropathy must be evaluated.

Other Sites and Manifestations (Fig. 34–10). In addition to soft tissue and periarticular calcific deposition, intra-articular (free or intrasynovial) calcification also can become evident in scleroderma[69–72, 138, 139, 143] (Fig. 34–11). Radiographs reveal cloudlike radiodense regions conforming to a portion of the joint or the entire articulation. Although these dense areas probably can be observed in any joint, previous reports have indicated that intra-articular calcification is most frequent in the elbow, the inferior radioulnar and first carpometacarpal joints of the wrist, the metacarpophalangeal and metatarsophalangeal joints, the knee, and the hip. Additional radiographic findings in the involved joint include periarticular calcification and osseous resorption. In several reports,[69, 71, 138, 140] an associated destructive arthropathy of the first metatarsophalangeal joint could be demonstrated. Aspiration of joint contents outlines

chalky joint effusions[71, 72] containing hydroxyapatite crystals, the same substance found in the periarticular and paraspinal calcific deposits in this disease. The pathogenesis of crystal deposition and calcification within these joints is not known; although intra-articular extension of apatite deposits may occur from overlying soft tissue collections, the association of inflammatory synovial changes with this phenomenon may suggest that dystrophic calcification of a diseased synovium has taken place.

In addition to intra-articular localization, synovial calcification may be apparent within tendon sheaths or bursae in scleroderma (Fig. 34–12). The author has observed this most frequently about the heel, the elbow, the knee, and the shoulder. Extensive linear radiodense regions conforming to the location of the tendon sheath and cloudlike calcification conforming to the location of the bursa are seen.

In addition to the synostosis of the carpal bones that was mentioned earlier,[55] bony ankylosis of the hips has been observed in scleroderma.[141] The association of scleroderma and osteonecrosis of the femoral head also has been recorded.[73] This complication, which also has been described in the lunate bone in a patient with scleroderma,[211] apparently relates not only to administration of corticosteroids but also to the vasculitis that is part of the primary disease process.

A deforming nonerosive articular disease (Jaccoud's arthropathy) identical to that occurring after rheumatic fever occasionally is observed in patients with scleroderma (Fig. 34–13).

Synovial cysts[212] and sinus tracts[213] (identical to those occurring in ''fistulous'' rheumatoid arthritis) represent additional reported articular manifestations of scleroderma.

Vascular Involvement

Arteriography has been used to investigate manifestations of vasospasm in patients with scleroderma. Raynaud's phenomenon is one such manifestation, appearing as sudden pallor or cyanosis of the distal aspect of the digits. Associated findings include ischemic necrosis and gangrene of phalangeal soft tissue, in either the hand or the foot.[115] Clinical and laboratory tests in patients with Raynaud's phenomenon have revealed findings that apparently indicate a persistent structural defect in the blood vessels[5]; these findings include decreased capillary flow within the fingers in both warm and cold environments,[74] and an abnormally low digital pad temperature in the basal state.[75]

Arteriography confirms the presence of vascular abnormalities in patients with Raynaud's phenomenon.[76–80] Vasospasm, narrowing, and obstructive lesions of digital arteries are observed, although the extent and severity of the occlusive lesions do not always correlate with the clinical severity of digital ischemia, the duration of the disease, or the presence of Raynaud's phenomenon.[76, 80] Additional arteriographic findings have included incomplete, poorly formed, or absent palmar arterial arches and ulnar artery.[78, 80] These latter changes may be related to developmental or acquired factors.

Further confirmation of arterial lesions is supplied by histologic studies that reveal subintimal proliferation of connective tissue, subendothelial fibrin deposits, and thickening of the basement membrane[77, 81, 142] The abnormal tissue consists predominantly of collagen with little definable

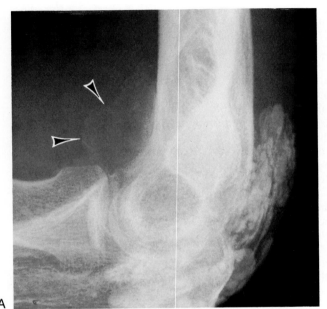

A

FIGURE 34–11. Articular involvement: Intra-articular calcification.

A–C This 37 year old man who had had scleroderma for 21 years developed severe pain in his elbow. A lateral radiograph **(A)** demonstrates periarticular calcification about the extensor surface of the elbow as well as faint homogeneous calcification with a curvilinear contour within the elbow joint (arrowheads). At surgery **(B)**, incision of the capsule is associated with extrusion of thick, cheesy material (arrow). A photomicrograph **(C)** shows cellular proliferation and calcium (arrowheads) within the synovial tissues (540×). The arrow indicates the articular lumen.

Illustration continued on opposite page

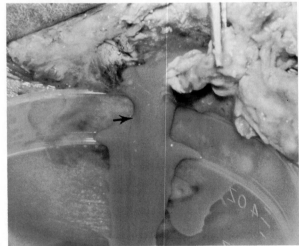

B

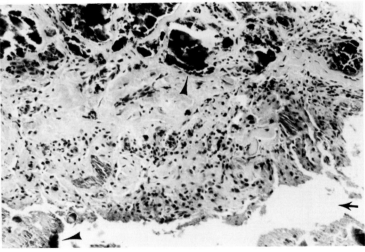

C

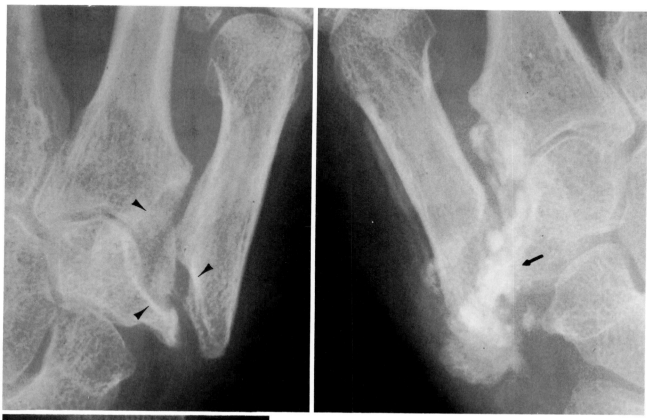

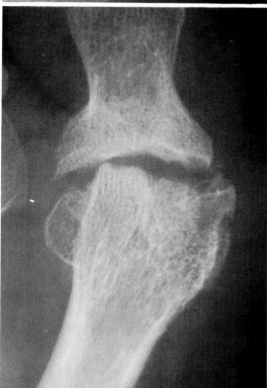

FIGURE 34–11 *Continued*

D–F A 53 year old woman with a 20 year history of scleroderma. Abnormalities of the first carpometacarpal joint are present on the right **(D)** and left **(E)** sides. Scalloped erosions at the bases of the first and second metacarpals and trapezium are well seen on the right (arrowheads). Bony debris may be present in this location. On the left side, note the extensive calcification, some of which is located within the first carpometacarpal joint (arrow). Flattening and irregularity of subchondral bone about the first metatarsophalangeal joint **(F)** are associated with soft tissue swelling and some bone formation.

Illustration continued on following page

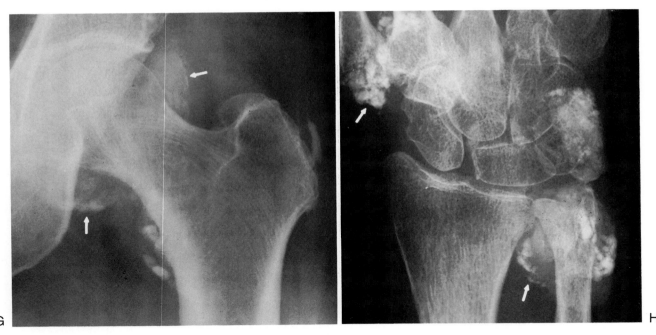

G   H

FIGURE 34–11 *Continued*
  G In a 50 year old patient with scleroderma, note periarticular calcification about both trochanters as well as a homogeneous dense area within the hip joint itself (arrows).
  H In another patient, intra-articular calcification is particularly evident at the first carpometacarpal and inferior radioulnar joints (arrows).
  (**A, C–G,** From Resnick D, et al: Radiology *124*:685, 1977.)

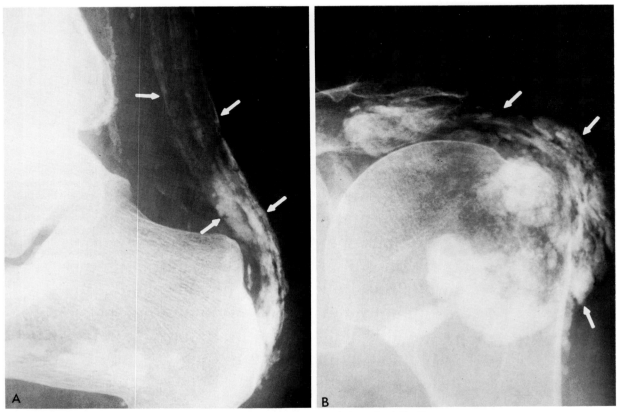

FIGURE 34–12. Articular involvement: Tendon and bursal calcification.
  A This is a striking example of diffuse calcification about the Achilles tendon (arrows).
  B Subacromial (subdeltoid) bursal calcification is obvious (arrows).

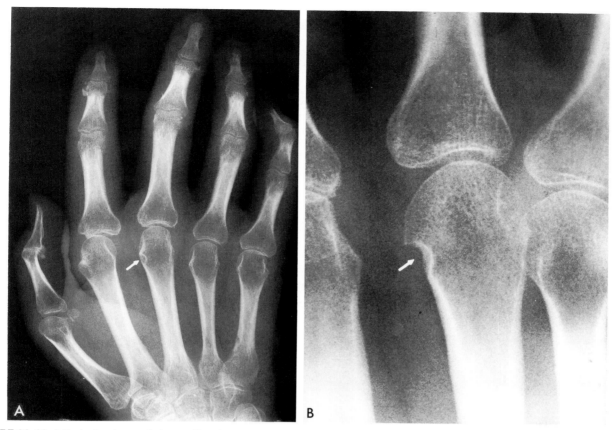

FIGURE 34–13. Articular involvement: Jaccoud's arthropathy. This patient with scleroderma developed deformity of the hands.

A In addition to soft tissue atrophy and bony atrophy of the phalangeal tufts and periarticular osteoporosis and calcification, observe slight ulnar deviation at the metacarpophalangeal joints and flexion at the distal interphalangeal joint of the fifth finger. A characteristic hooklike erosion of the metacarpal head (arrow), probably related to periarticular fibrosis, is seen.

B A close up of the third metacarpal head in an oblique attitude better delineates the erosion (arrow).

ground substance, and it is suggested that the vascular lesion may be related to a primary abnormality in collagen metabolism, which leads to thickening of the walls of the digital arteries in a manner analogous to the fibrosis and thickening that take place in the skin of patients with scleroderma[142] (Fig. 34–14).

PATHOLOGIC ABNORMALITIES

The pathologic changes in the skin of patients with scleroderma consist of a low grade inflammatory reaction characterized by perivascular cellular infiltration, predominantly of lymphocytes, plasma cells, and macrophages, and edema of the dermis[4, 82–84] (Fig. 34–14). Subsequently, progressive increase in compact collagen fibers in the dermis, thinning of the overlying epidermis, and atrophy of dermal appendages, as well as thickening of the intima, medial fibrosis, and thrombotic occlusion of arterioles, are evident.[82, 85, 107] A decrease in thickness of skin in clinically affected areas has been documented by ultrasonography[194, 195] and radiographic techniques,[86] although some investigators have noted a significant increase in skin thickness during the indurative phase of the disease, related to an increase in total dermal collagen content.[101] Subcutaneous nodules may develop,[87, 88] which can calcify. In striated muscle, degenerative changes of muscle cells and accumulation of inflam-

matory cells indicate the presence of myositis[4] (Fig. 34–15).

Abnormalities of the synovial membrane consist of inflammatory changes characterized by hyperemia, cellular infiltration with lymphocytes and plasma cells, vascular sclerosis, and surface fibrin deposition.[89] The abnormalities resemble those of early rheumatoid arthritis. Subsequently, intense fibrosis of superficial or all layers of the synovium becomes evident.

PATHOGENESIS

Although the exact pathogenesis of scleroderma is not known, it has been popular to link this disease with other collagen vascular disorders because of similar clinical, pathologic, and, in some instances, radiologic abnormalities. Vascular changes predominate in multiple tissues, suggesting that scleroderma is a disease of microvasculature.[90] Although this concept is strengthened by observations that have outlined distinctive microvascular patterns both in nail fold capillaries that correlated with the extent of organ involvement[91] and in skin capillaries,[92] the cause of these vascular abnormalities remains a mystery. Damage to the endothelial lining of small blood vessels or altered vasomotor control of the capillary circulation has been proposed as an initial or early lesion leading to vascular compromise,

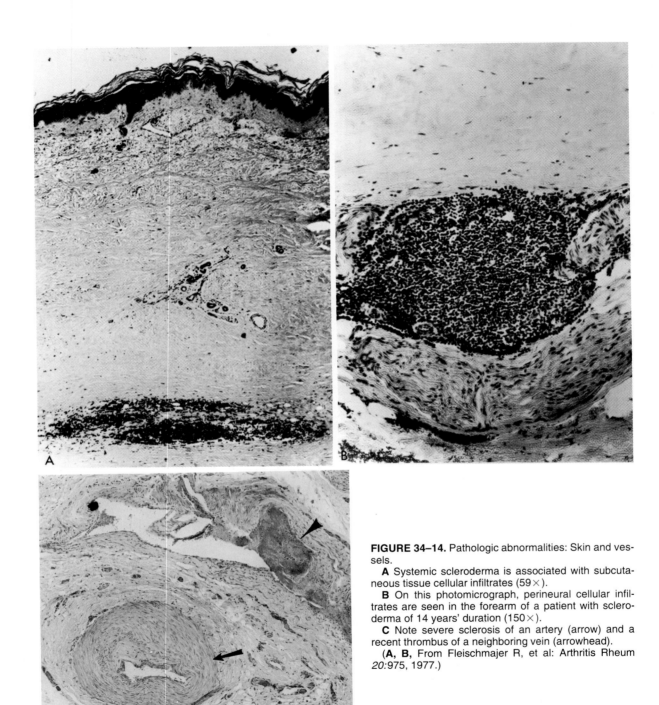

FIGURE 34–14. Pathologic abnormalities: Skin and vessels.

A Systemic scleroderma is associated with subcutaneous tissue cellular infiltrates (59×).

B On this photomicrograph, perineural cellular infiltrates are seen in the forearm of a patient with scleroderma of 14 years' duration (150×).

C Note severe sclerosis of an artery (arrow) and a recent thrombus of a neighboring vein (arrowhead).

(**A, B,** From Fleischmajer R, et al: Arthritis Rheum *20:*975, 1977.)

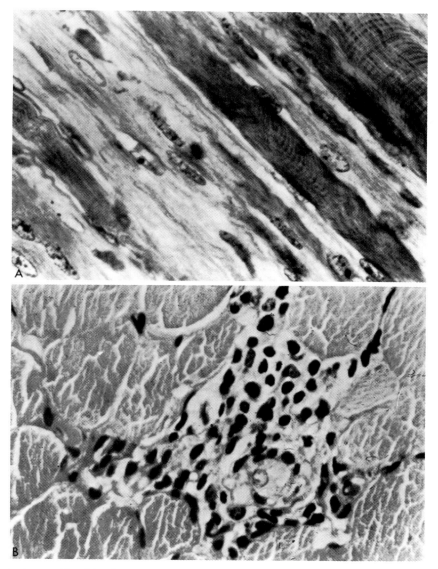

FIGURE 34–15. Pathologic abnormalities: Muscle.

A A biopsy specimen from a patient with scleroderma who demonstrated simple myopathy reveals muscle fibers of varying size with a marked increase in fibrocollagenous material and fibroblast-like cells (450×).

B A biopsy specimen from a patient with scleroderma who revealed inflammatory myositis demonstrates a typical perivascular inflammatory infiltrate (450×).

(From Clements PJ, et al: Arthritis Rheum *21*:62, 1978.)

tissue hypoxia, and widespread uncontrolled deposition of collagen and proteoglycan.[197] The cause of this damage remains elusive. The possibility of an underlying immunologic aberration must be considered. A variety of immunologic abnormalities in scleroderma have been reported but most lack specificity. Such abnormalities include defects in cell-mediated immunity, increases in serum immunoglobulins, antinuclear antibodies, and cryoglobulins.[144] A significant relationship exists between cell-mediated immunity to collagen and the appearance of scleroderma.

A few reports indicate a familial predisposition to the disease, although, despite preliminary data that show an increased prevalence of certain histocompatibility antigens (HLA-DRw3 and HLA-DR 5),[145, 146] a definitive genetic basis for progressive systemic sclerosis is lacking.[144]

ADDITIONAL SYNDROMES AND CONDITIONS ASSOCIATED WITH SCLERODERMA

Chemically Induced Scleroderma-like Conditions

Certain chemicals, including vinyl chloride, pentazocine, and bleomycin, can induce cutaneous abnormalities simulating those of scleroderma.[215, 216] With regard to the polymerizing agent vinyl chloride, Raynaud's phenomenon and pulmonary fibrosis along with a distinctive pattern of acro-osteolysis are evident in workers who clean reactor vessels and are exposed to this compound. This disorder is discussed further in Chapter 94.

Pentazocine was introduced in 1967 as a non-narcotic analgesic compound. Subsequently, cutaneous complications, including flat or nodular lesions of the dermis at sites of injection, were reported.[147] In descriptions of this complication, features have included a common history of diabetes mellitus, the onset of cutaneous induration weeks to years after the injections, diffuse sclerosis of the integument and subcutaneous tissue, and muscle abnormalities leading to contracture.[148] The histologic features are fibrosis affecting dermal, subcutaneous, and muscular tissues, thrombosis of small arteries and veins, and inflammatory cellular infiltration.[147]

Bleomycin, an antibiotic obtained from *Streptomyces verticillus,* in certain dosages is associated with pulmonary fibrosis and skin alterations that include hyperpigmentation, erythema, alopecia, ulceration, infiltrating plaques and nodules, and diffuse thickening.[149–151] Investigation of dermal fibroblasts in patients with thickened skin has revealed increased quantities of collagen resembling aberrations in progressive systemic sclerosis.[151] The fibrosis recedes after discontinuation of the drug[147] or the use of high dose steroid therapy.[217]

Scleroderma-like changes also are observed with other chemical agents, including solvents (trichloroethylene, benzene, toluene, xylene), paraffin and silicone implants, and cocaine.[152, 214, 251–253] Furthermore, a toxic epidemic syndrome (toxic oil syndrome; see later discussion) has been associated with the consumption of adulterated rapeseed oil, illegally marketed and sold cheaply as a cooking oil.[153, 189] Clinical findings include arthralgias and arthritis, muscle atrophy, neuropathy, and scleroderma-like skin involvement; radiologic abnormalities generally are confined to

osteopenia in the absence of joint space narrowing, bone erosions, and soft tissue calcification. Microscopic evaluation documents a non-necrotizing vasculitis and an increase in fibrous tissue.

Eosinophilic Fasciitis

Eosinophilic fasciitis, also known as Shulman syndrome, is seen predominantly in adults, although rarely it occurs in children.[154, 218, 219, 247] It is associated with inflammation and induration of the skin and subcutaneous tissues of the hands, forearms, feet, and legs occurring after, in most cases, an episode of physical exertion.[8, 103–105, 116, 157, 160, 164, 167, 218] Truncal areas also can be affected. Polyarthralgia, polyarthritis, muscle atrophy, and the carpal tunnel syndrome have been observed.[159, 165, 166] Arthritis is common in the joints of the hands and wrists and in the knees, and clinical findings resemble those of rheumatoid arthritis. Joint contractures, related to induration and sclerosis of subcutaneous tissues, are seen, especially in the elbows, wrists, ankles, knees, and hands.[218] The disorder is associated with peripheral blood eosinophilia, especially during the early stages, hypergammaglobulinemia (IgG), and an elevated erythrocyte sedimentation rate. Raynaud's phenomenon and visceral manifestations of progressive systemic sclerosis are conspicuously absent,[147, 155] although occasional reports indicate that additional findings, including Raynaud's phenomenon, Sjögren's syndrome, pulmonary changes, and myositis, rarely may be observed.[156, 161] Antinuclear antibodies typically are absent, and complement levels are normal. Improvement in clinical and laboratory parameters follows the systemic administration of corticosteroids, so that a complete or nearly complete recovery is expected in a period of a few years. Therapeutic failures have been reported.[166]

As the pathologic alterations involve the lower subcutaneous tissues and the fascia, a deep wedge biopsy that extends through these tissues as well as through muscle is required for diagnosis. Inflammation and fibrosis in all of these layers, but especially the fascia and muscles, are associated with infiltrates of lymphocytes, plasma cells, eosinophils, and histiocytes.[147, 161]

Radiographic abnormalities generally are confined to osteopenia, although additional findings have included bone erosions in the hands and wrists[158] and periostitis in the diaphyses of the tibia, fibula, radius, and ulna.[162, 163]

MR imaging has been used to study the soft tissue abnormalities of eosinophilic fasciitis.[221, 222] Findings have included thickening of the fascia and increased signal intensity in the superficial muscle fibers on proton density and T2*-weighted gradient echo images.[221] Increased attenuation values of superficial and deep fasciae have been evident with CT.[222]

Eosinophilic fasciitis has been described in association with a number of hematologic disorders, including aplastic anemia, thrombocytopenic purpura, leukemia, and Hodgkin's disease.[155, 159, 173, 174, 218]

The cause of eosinophilic fasciitis is unknown. Clues are provided by its common precipitation by physical exertion, although this feature is not uniform, and its clinical and radiologic resemblance to the reflex sympathetic dystrophy syndrome.[168] The association of eosinophilic fasciitis with anticonvulsant therapy[169] is interesting, as such agents also have been implicated in the development of the reflex sympathetic dystrophy syndrome.[168] Eosinophilic fasciitis most resembles scleroderma and, in the minds of some investigators, may not be a separate disorder at all. Although generally the disorder is self-limited and without systemic manifestations, these features too are not uniform. Vascular and connective tissue abnormalities in eosinophilic fasciitis are similar to those of scleroderma, accounting for the overlap in clinical and histologic findings in the two conditions.[170, 171] Scleroderma, however, is more common in women, and eosinophilic fasciitis is more frequent in men or of equal frequency in the two sexes.[218] Raynaud's phenomen is rare in eosinophilic fasciitis and common in scleroderma. Additional findings in eosinophilic fasciitis that are not characteristic of scleroderma are peripheral eosinophilia, hypergammaglobulinemia, elevated erythrocyte sedimentation rate, sparing of the epidermis and dermis as seen on skin biopsy, and precipitation by physical exercise. Eosinophilia, raised serum IgG levels, and the identification of immunoglobulin in the inflamed fascia suggest that a humoral or cellular immune mechanism is involved in Shulman syndrome.[147, 170] Genetic influences in this syndrome have been emphasized, and the disease has been reported in a pair of siblings.[220] In most reports, no statistically significant association of the disease with HLA-A or B antigens has been detected. Mast cells also have been implicated in the pathogenesis of eosinophilic fasciitis.[170, 172]

Another syndrome, the eosinophilia-myalgia syndrome, which has been related to the ingestion of L-tryptophan, bears a close resemblance to eosinophilic fasciitis (see subsequent discussion).

Eosinophilia-Myalgia Syndrome

In October, 1989, a group of physicians in New Mexico observed an unusual illness in three patients who had been ingesting the amino acid L-tryptophan.[223] The two prominent characteristics of the illness were incapacitating myalgia and marked eosinophilia. The New Mexico Department of Health notified the Centers for Disease Control (CDC) and, later, the Food and Drug Administration ordered a recall of all single-entity L-tryptophan–containing products owing to the identification of additional cases of this syndrome.[224] L-tryptophan is an essential amino acid that had been taken as an over the counter medication for insomnia, as a nutritional supplement, or as a treatment for anxiety, premenstrual syndrome, fibromyalgia, or depression.[224]

Initial reports of the eosinophilia-myalgia syndrome indicated a wide age range of affected patients (from childhood to the ninth decade of life) with a mean age of approximately 50 years, a marked female preponderance, and a geographic distribution that favored the western United States. Its serious nature also was emphasized, with deaths related to various causes including ascending paralysis from axonal polyneuropathy (Guillain-Barré syndrome).[224] Hospitalizations resulting from manifestations of the illness were common. The mean daily dosage of L-tryptophan taken by affected persons was 1500 mg, with considerable variation, and the duration of tryptophan ingestion prior to the onset of the syndrome ranged from 1 month to several years.[224]

Initial clinical abnormalities include fatigue, fever, and diffuse myalgia of the proximal muscles.[224–234] Additional early manifestations are related to pulmonary involvement leading to dyspnea and a cough, a maculopapular or urticarial skin rash, muscle weakness, cramps, and incapacitating pain and swelling of the extremities, with pitting or nonpitting edema. The disease continues to unfold over a period of several weeks or months, and eventually an impressive list of target organs may be involved, including the muscles, lungs, skin, nervous system, fasciae, joints, and heart, in rough chronologic order.[234] Nervous system changes may affect the brain, with altered mental status, acute dementia, or changes in coordination, but peripheral involvement is more frequent, leading to subacute peripheral neuropathy with paresthesias, hypesthesias, sensory loss, weakness, or paralysis.[234] Abnormalities on nerve conduction studies or electromyography have been observed. Arthralgias or, less commonly, arthritis is seen, usually involving large joints. Progressive contractures of knees and elbows may develop, and limited mobility of ankles and wrists has been evident in some cases.[234] Abnormalities of the heart include spasm of the coronary arteries and arrhythmias, which may relate to an unusual cardioneuropathy in which cuffs of lymphocytes surround nerves.[234]

Although a mild anemia and thrombocytosis may be evident with serologic analysis,[224] it is the impressive eosinophilia that, with rare exceptions,[235] most characterizes this disorder. Indeed, one of the criteria employed by the CDC in the diagnosis of the eosinophilia-myalgia syndrome is a peripheral eosinophil count greater than 1000 cells per cu mm. The median eosinophil count in this disease appears to be greater than 5000 cells per cu mm. In spite of this eosinophilia, immunoglobulin E levels usually are normal, as are the levels of immunoglobulins G, M, and A, and circulating immune complexes are not demonstrable.[224] Serum aldolase values may be elevated, but not those of creatine kinase.[224, 229]

The natural history of this syndrome is variable. Although cessation of ingestion of L-tryptophan occasionally leads to rapid subsidence of clinical manifestations, more typically slow clinical improvement, no improvement, or clinical deterioration results.[234] Corticosteroid therapy is not effective in most patients. The mortality rate varies from 2 to 6 per cent.[234]

With regard to pathologic findings, skin biopsies have shown fascial edema, inflammation, and perivascular infiltrates, whereas biopsies of the muscle have revealed perineural infiltrates and venulitis.[228] The infiltrate in the muscle consistently involves the perimysium and occasionally affects the epimysium.[229] Ultrastructural analysis indicates thickening and necrosis of endothelial cells in capillaries and arterioles,[236] underscoring the contribution of ischemia to the clinical manifestations of this syndrome.

The relationship of the eosinophilia-myalgia syndrome to other illnesses has been the subject of speculation.[224, 234, 237] It has been tempting to hypothesize that a unifying thread binds tryptophan or its metabolites to other conditions associated with tissue fibrosis.[237] Such fibrosis has been associated with use of a variety of drugs and chemical agents and the presence of a number of diseases, including progressive systemic sclerosis, eosinophilic fasciitis, morphea, and linear scleroderma. The clinical features of the eosinophilia-myalgia syndrome are remarkably similar to those of the toxic oil syndrome, in which an epidemic illness involving multiple organ systems follows the ingestion of illegally prepared and contaminated industrial-grade denatured rapeseed oil that was marketed as cooking oil.[224, 248] Acute findings of the toxic oil syndrome, including fever, dyspnea, pulmonary edema, myalgia, pruritus, rash, and eosinophilia, and chronic findings, including scleroderma-like skin lesions, joint contractures, Raynaud's phenomenon, neuromyopathy, and pulmonary hypertension, are similar to those of the eosinophilia-myalgia syndrome.[227] This similarity has led some investigators to implicate imperfect manufacturing of L-tryptophan–containing products as a causative factor in the latter syndrome.[249, 250] The explosive clinical onset and apparent epidemic nature of the eosinophilia-myalgia syndrome are consistent with this contaminant theory.[227]

Other investigators indicate that L-tryptophan or its metabolites themselves are important in the pathogenesis of this syndrome, a theory supported by the observation that the metabolism of biogenic amines derived from tryptophan may be abnormal in a variety of connective tissue disorders, including rheumatoid arthritis, systemic lupus erythematosus, scleroderma, dermatomyositis, and eosinophilic fasciitis.[227]

Although clinical and laboratory differences are observed when eosinophilic fasciitis and the eosinophilia-myalgia syndrome are compared,[224] ingestion of L-tryptophan has been documented in some patients with eosinophilic fasciitis.[238] Most investigators, however, believe they are unrelated. Patients with the eosinophilia-myalgia syndrome usually have a more acute clinical onset, more severe symptoms and signs, and a higher frequency of rash and of pulmonary, cardiac, neurologic, gastrointestinal, myopathic, and thyroid involvement than those with eosinophilic fasciitis.[239] Corticosteroid therapy is more effective in eosinophilic fasciitis. This evidence suggests that the two diseases are not identical and that the eosinophilia-myalgia syndrome is a more severe disorder.

Scleromyxedema (Papular Mucinosis)

Scleromyxedema, also known as papular mucinosis or lichen myxedematosus, is a rare connective tissue disorder characterized by diffuse thickening of the skin and nodular papules.[147, 196, 241] Sclerodactyly, stiff digits, and facial changes similar to those of scleroderma are evident. Myopathy also may be apparent.[240] Rarely, rheumatologic manifestations may dominate the clinical picture and lead to joint space narrowing and bone erosions resembling the changes of rheumatoid arthritis.[175, 190] An acid mucopolysaccharide is found between collagen bundles in the upper portion of the corium, and the presence of abnormal serum immunoglobulins (M-type globulin) suggests a link between this dermatologic condition and plasma cell dyscrasia.

Graft-Versus-Host Disease

Graft-versus-host disease occurs when immunologically competent cells engrafted onto a foreign host attack the tissues of that host. In current practice, this disease usually appears after allogeneic bone marrow transplantation,[110, 111,] [176–180, 182] although it also has been described after materno-fetal cell transfer in immunodeficient children and inadvertent transfusion of unirradiated blood products into immunodeficient patients, and it may be responsible for numerous other disorders, such as primary biliary cirrhosis.[176] The specific prerequisites for identifying graft-versus-host disease are the following: the graft must contain immunocompetent cells; the host must be sufficiently different genetically from the graft to be perceived as antigenically foreign; and the host must be unable to reject the graft effectively.[177, 178]

Graft-versus-host disease occurs in either an acute or a chronic form, the former appearing before 100 days after the transplantation and the latter generally later than 100 days. Compared with the chronic pattern, acute graft-versus-host disease is associated with limited organ involvement, principally of the skin, liver, and gastrointestinal tract, manifested clinically as a triad of dermatitis, diarrhea, and hepatic malfunction (jaundice, alterations in liver chemistry profiles).[176] In approximately 10 to 15 per cent of cases, the disease is mild and resolves spontaneously; in 30 to 40 per cent, death ensues, related to end-organ failure or, more commonly, sepsis.[178]

It is the chronic form of graft-versus-host disease that resembles a collagen vascular disease, specifically scleroderma.[242] This pattern is associated with more extensive abnormalities affecting a variety of organs, including the skin, gastrointestinal tract, liver, salivary glands, lymph nodes, mouth, eyes, lungs, and musculoskeletal system.[179] Chronic graft-versus-host disease, which develops in 10 to 30 per cent of patients undergoing bone marrow transplantation, can appear without previous evidence of the acute form of the disease, as a gradual progression from continuous active acute graft-versus-host disease, or after an interim of quiescence following the acute pattern of the disease.[178] Cutaneous abnormalities include erythematous or violaceous eruption, papulosquamous plaques, desquamation, periungual erythema, dystrophic nails, hyperpigmentation, alopecia, and, later, brawny induration.[178] In untreated cases, tightly bound skin, contractures, and tissue wasting are observed (Fig. 34–16). With involvement of other organ systems, additional clinical manifestations appear, which include the inability to open the mouth fully, xerostomia, xerophthalmia, chronic liver disease, dysphagia, regurgitation, malabsorption, diarrhea, pulmonary fibrosis, myositis, and arthralgias.[179, 181, 183] Laboratory aberrations include anemia, leukopenia, thrombocytopenia, eosinophilia, elevated serum levels of immunoglobulins, and the presence of circulating autoantibodies.[178]

The pathologic features of chronic graft-versus-host disease in a variety of organ systems have been well outlined.[178, 182] In some instances, such as in vascular lesions, they are remarkably similar to those of scleroderma.[111] Studies of the disease suggest a complex immunopathogenesis involving both cellular and humoral immunity.[179]

DIFFERENTIAL DIAGNOSIS

Individual radiographic features in scleroderma can resemble those in other disorders, although the combination of radiographic abnormalities usually is diagnostic.

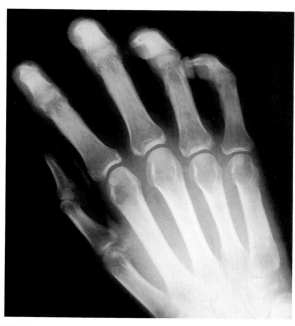

FIGURE 34–16. Graft-versus-host disease. The radiographic abnormalities, consisting of soft tissue atrophy, osteoporosis, and contractures of the fingers, simulate those of scleroderma. (Courtesy of A. Brower, M.D., Norfolk, Virginia.)

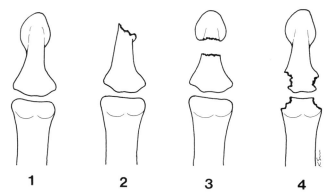

1   2   3   4

FIGURE 34–17. Phalangeal resorption: Differential diagnosis. The normal situation is depicted in diagram *1*. Resorption of the tuft *(2)* can be seen in scleroderma, other collagen vascular disorders, thermal injuries, hyperparathyroidism, psoriasis, and epidermolysis bullosa. Bandlike resorption of the terminal phalanx *(3)* is seen in familial and occupational acro-osteolysis, collagen vascular disorders, and hyperparathyroidism. Erosions about the distal interphalangeal joint *(4)* can be noted in psoriasis, multicentric reticulohistiocytosis, gout, thermal injuries, scleroderma, and hyperparathyroidism.

Bony Abnormalities

Generalized resorption of the terminal phalanges of the hand or foot, or both, in scleroderma is characterized by "penciling" of the tuft (Fig. 34–17). A similar finding can be seen in other disorders, such as Raynaud's disease without scleroderma, thermal injuries (burn, frostbite, electrical),[93, 94] trauma, other collagen vascular diseases (dermatomyositis),[95] neuropathic disease (congenital indifference to pain, leprosy, diabetes mellitus, meningomyelocele),[96] articular disorders (psoriasis, Lesch-Nyhan syndrome),[97] hyperparathyroidism, progeria, and epidermolysis bullosa.[98] In most of these diseases, the distribution of changes and the presence of additional abnormalities usually allow accurate diagnosis (Table 34–3). For example, sparing of the first digit in frostbite, destructive articular changes in psoriasis and Lesch-Nyhan syndrome, and subperiosteal resorption of phalanges in hyperparathyroidism are characteristic. Furthermore, the association of tuftal resorption, skin atrophy, and soft tissue calcification in scleroderma is of great diagnostic significance.

Tuftal resorption in scleroderma should not be confused with congenital disorders associated with hypoplasia of terminal phalanges. In these latter disorders, a small but otherwise normal bone is apparent. In addition, the type of bone resorption in scleroderma usually is easily differentiated from disorders characterized by bandlike resorption of the distal phalangeal shafts (polyvinyl chloride acro-osteolysis, familial acro-osteolysis, and hyperparathyroidism)[99] and from those characterized by intraosseous or eccentric destruction of the terminal phalanx (inclusion cyst, glomus tumor, enchondroma, osteomyelitis, and skeletal metastasis).[184] The combination of tuftal resorption and erosive arthritis of the distal interphalangeal joints may be apparent in scleroderma as well as in hyperparathyroidism,

psoriasis, thermal injuries, and multicentric reticulohistiocytosis.

Resorption of ribs is seen not only in scleroderma but also in other collagen vascular diseases, poliomyelitis, restrictive lung disease, hyperparathyroidism, and neurofibromatosis. In some cases, the distribution of bone destruction allows differentiation among these disorders (e.g., involvement of upper and lower surfaces in hyperparathyroidism; involvement of lower surfaces in neurofibromatosis).

Soft Tissue Abnormalities

Atrophy of the distal phalangeal soft tissue is a finding of scleroderma that can be observed in association with other collagen vascular diseases, thermal injuries, vascular disorders, Raynaud's disease, and epidermolysis bullosa, as

TABLE 34–3. Characteristic Sites of Distal Phalangeal Resorption in Various Disorders*

Disorder	Site		
	Tuft	Midportion or Waist	Periarticular
Scleroderma	+		+
Hyperparathyroidism	+	+	+
Thermal injury	+		+
Psoriasis	+		+
Epidermolysis bullosa	+		
Polyvinyl chloride acro-osteolysis		+	
Multicentric reticulohistiocytosis	+		+
Inflammatory (erosive) osteoarthritis			+
Lesch-Nyhan syndrome	+		
Progeria	+		

*Only the characteristic sites of bone resorption are indicated, although in any single disease, considerable variability in these sites may exist.

well as additional conditions. Furthermore, as already out-lined, scleroderma-like skin changes also can be evident in graft-versus-host disease after allogeneic bone marrow transplantation, in eosinophilic fasciitis, and after exposure to certain chemicals.

Widespread subcutaneous and periarticular calcification also is a finding that is not restricted to scleroderma. Calcification of the phalangeal soft tissues may be apparent in other collagen vascular diseases. More diffuse calcification in muscles and subcutaneous tissues is observed in many collagen vascular disorders, renal osteodystrophy, hypoparathyroidism, pseudohypoparathyroidism, pseudopseudohypoparathyroidism, fat necrosis, hypervitaminosis D, idiopathic hypercalcemia, milk-alkali syndrome, parasitic infections, Ehlers-Danlos syndrome, and idiopathic tumoral calcinosis. In many of these disorders, the pattern of calcification is distinctive, differing from the punctate or linear deposits that are observed in scleroderma. Scleroderma may be associated with "tumoral" periarticular calcifications, an appearance that also can be apparent in other collagen vascular diseases, renal osteodystrophy, milk-alkali syndrome, hypervitaminosis D, hydroxyapatite crystal deposition disease, and sarcoidosis, as well as after infections such as tuberculosis. Werner's syndrome, consisting of progeria, dwarfism, alopecia, skin thickening, cataract formation, and premature arteriosclerosis, can be accompanied by periarticular calcification simulating that in scleroderma, as well as by osteoporosis, osteomyelitis, and cardiovascular calcification.[112, 117]

Articular Abnormalities

An erosive arthritis of distal interphalangeal joints accompanies scleroderma, inflammatory (erosive) osteoarthritis, psoriasis, multicentric reticulohistiocytosis, gout, and thermal injuries. In most patients with scleroderma, erosions of these joints are mild, although, rarely, larger erosions with extensive phalangeal destruction and intra-articular bony ankylosis may be indistinguishable from psoriasis or inflammatory (erosive) osteoarthritis. Associated radiographic findings, including intra-articular calcification, allow accurate diagnosis of scleroderma in some cases.

Scalloped erosions of the first carpometacarpal joint can be seen in a variety of articular disorders, including scleroderma, dermatomyositis, Ehlers-Danlos syndrome, systemic lupus erythematosus, and rheumatoid arthritis. Isolated or predominant involvement of this joint without changes in the other wrist compartments eliminates rheumatoid arthritis as a diagnostic consideration, although any of the other disorders may be characterized by such a distribution. In scleroderma, the associated phalangeal abnormalities and the presence of intra- and extra-articular calcification at the first carpometacarpal joint allow a precise diagnosis.

Intra-articular cloudlike calcification in scleroderma differs in radiographic appearance from the appearance of calcium pyrophosphate dihydrate crystal deposition disease, idiopathic hydroxyapatite crystal deposition disease, idiopathic synovial osteochondromatosis, intra-articular osseous bodies, gout, and synovioma or hemangioma, although these other disorders are associated with calcific and ossific dense areas in and around joints.

SUMMARY

Scleroderma (progressive systemic sclerosis) leads to characteristic musculoskeletal abnormalities due to involvement of skin, subcutaneous tissues, muscles, bones, and joints. Many of the diverse clinical manifestations in this disease are represented on radiographs as soft tissue atrophy and calcification and bone resorption. Changes frequently predominate in the phalanges of the hand, although diffuse subcutaneous calcification, widespread periarticular calcification, and bone resorption at other sites, such as the mandible, the ribs, and the clavicles, are encountered. Major articular alterations consist of an erosive arthritis, particularly in the distal interphalangeal, proximal interphalangeal, metacarpophalangeal, first carpometacarpal, and inferior radioulnar joints, which may terminate as bony ankylosis, and intra-articular calcific collections.

References

1. Norton WL, Nardo JM: Vascular disease in progressive systemic sclerosis (scleroderma). Ann Intern Med 73:317, 1970.
2. LeRoy EC: Connective tissue synthesis by scleroderma skin fibroblasts in cell culture. J Exp Med 135:1351, 1972.
3. Alarcón-Segovia D, Fishbein E: Immunochemical characterization of the anti-RNA antibodies found in scleroderma and systemic lupus erythematosus. I. Differences in reactivity with Poly (U) and Poly (A)-Poly (U). J Immunol 115:28, 1975.
4. Grahame R: Scleroderma (progressive systemic sclerosis). In JT Scott (Ed): Copeman's Textbook of the Rheumatic Diseases. 5th Ed. Edinburgh, Churchill Livingstone, 1978, p 937.
5. Rodnan GP: Progressive systemic sclerosis (scleroderma). In JL Hollander, DJ McCarty Jr (Eds): Arthritis and Allied Conditions. 8th Ed. Philadelphia, Lea & Febiger, 1972, p 962.
6. Curzio C: Discussioni anatomio-pratiche di un raro e stravagante morbo cutaneo in una giovane donna felicemante curato in questo grande ospedale degl'incurabili. Napoli, G diSimione, 1753 (cited in Rodnan, 1972).
7. Gintrac E: Note sur la sclerodermie. Rev Med Chir (Paris) 2:263, 1847.
8. Shulman LE: Diffuse fasciitis with hypergammaglobulinemia and eosinophilia: A new syndrome? J Rheumatol 1(Suppl 1):46, 1974.
9. Barnett AJ, Coventry DA: Scleroderma. I. Clinical features, course of illness, and response to treatment in 61 cases. Med J Aust 1:992, 1969.
10. Barnett AJ: Scleroderma (Progressive Systemic Sclerosis). Springfield, Ill, Charles C Thomas, 1974, p 73.
11. Christianson HB, Dorsey CS, O'Leary PA, et al: Localized scleroderma: 235 cases. Arch Dermatol 74:629, 1956.
12. Burge KM, Perry HO, Stickler GB: Familial scleroderma. Arch Dermatol 99:681, 1969.
13. Chamberlain JL III, Bard JW: Localized scleroderma—en coup de sabre. South Med J 61:206, 1968.
14. Chazen EM, Cook CD, Cohen J: Focal scleroderma. Report of 19 cases in children. J Pediatr 60:385, 1962.
15. Murray-Lyon IM, Thompson RPH, Ansell ID, et al: Scleroderma and primary biliary cirrhosis. Br Med J 3:258, 1970.
16. Leinwand I, Duryee AW, Richter MN: Scleroderma (based on a study of over 150 cases). Ann Intern Med 41:1003, 1954.
17. Tuffanelli DL, Winkelmann RK: Systemic scleroderma: Clinical study of 727 cases. Arch Dermatol 84:359, 1961.
18. Dabich L, Sullivan DB, Cassidy JT: Scleroderma in the child. J Pediatr 85:770, 1974.
19. Kass H, Hanson V, Patrick J: Scleroderma in childhood. J Pediatr 68:243, 1966.
20. Velayos EE, Cohen BS: Progressive systemic sclerosis: Diagnosis at the age of 4 years. Am J Dis Child 123:57, 1972.
21. Shulman LE, Kurban AK, Harvey AM: Tendon friction rubs in progressive systemic sclerosis (scleroderma). Arthritis Rheum 4:438, 1961.
22. Medsger TA Jr, Rodnan GP, Moossy J, et al: Skeletal muscle involvement in progressive systemic sclerosis (scleroderma). Arthritis Rheum 11:554, 1968.
23. Clements PJ, Furst DE, Campion DS, et al: Muscle disease in progressive systemic sclerosis. Diagnostic and therapeutic considerations. Arthritis Rheum 21:62, 1978.
24. Rodnan GP, Medsger TA: Musculoskeletal involvement in progressive systemic sclerosis (scleroderma). Bull Rheum Dis 17:419, 1966.
25. Clark JA, Winkelman RK, Ward LE: Serologic alterations in scleroderma and sclerodermatomyositis. Mayo Clinic Proc 46:104, 1971.
26. Dubois EL, Chandor S, Friou GJ, et al: Progressive systemic sclerosis and localized scleroderma (morphea) with positive LE cell test and unusual manifestations compatible with SLE. Medicine 50:199, 1971.

27. Corson JK: Sclerodermatomyositis. Arch Dermatol 96:596, 1967.
28. Sharp GC, Irvin WS, Tan EM, et al: Mixed connective tissue disease: An apparently distinct rheumatic disease syndrome associated with a specific antibody to an extractable nuclear antigen (ENA). Am J Med 52:148, 1972.
29. Yune HY, Vix VA, Klatte EC: Early fingertip changes in scleroderma. JAMA 215:1113, 1971.
30. Schlenker JD, Clark DD, Weckesser EC: Calcinosis circumscripta of the hand in scleroderma. J Bone Joint Surg [Am] 55:1051, 1973.
31. Boyd JA, Patrick SI, Reeves RJ: Roentgen changes observed in generalized scleroderma: Report of 63 cases. Arch Intern Med 94:248, 1954.
32. Fraser GM: The radiological manifestations of scleroderma (diffuse systemic sclerosis). Br J Dermatol 78:1, 1966.
33. Meszaros WT: The regional manifestations of scleroderma. Radiology 70:313, 1958.
34. Scharer L, Smith DW: Resorption of the terminal phalanges in scleroderma. Arthritis Rheum 12:51, 1969.
35. Poznanski AK: The Hand in Radiologic Diagnosis. Philadelphia, WB Saunders Co, 1974, p 531.
36. Thibierge G, Weissenbach RJ: Concrétions calcaire sous-cutanées et sclérodermie. Ann Dermatol Syphiligr 2:129, 1911.
37. Muller SA, Brunsting LA, Winkelmann RK: Calcinosis cutis: Its relationship to scleroderma. Arch Dermatol 80:15, 1959.
38. Bernheim AR, Garlock JH: Parathyroidectomy in Raynaud's disease and scleroderma—late results. Arch Surg 38:543, 1939.
39. Kraus EJ: Zur Pathogenese der diffusen Sklerodermie. Zugleich ein Beitrag zur Pathologie der Epithelkörperchen. Virchows Arch (Pathol Anat) 253:710, 1924.
40. Rodnan GP, Medsger TA Jr: The rheumatic manifestations of progressive systemic sclerosis (scleroderma). Clin Orthop 57:81, 1968.
41. Scharer L, Smith DW: Resorption of the terminal phalanges in scleroderma. Arthritis Rheum 12:51, 1969.
42. Kemp Harper RA, Jackson DC: Progressive systemic sclerosis. Br J Radiol 38:825, 1965.
43. Szymanska-Jagiello W, Rondio H: Clinical picture of articular changes in progressive systemic sclerosis in children in the light of our own observations. Reumatologia 8:1, 1970.
44. Stafne EC, Austin LT: A characteristic dental finding in acrosclerosis and diffuse scleroderma. Am J Orthodontics 30:25, 1944.
45. Seifert MH, Steigerwald JC, Cliff MM: Bone resorption of the mandible in progressive systemic sclerosis. Arthritis Rheum 18:507, 1975.
46. Weber DD, Blunt MH, Caldwell JB: Fracture of mandibular rami complicated by scleroderma: Report of a case. J Oral Surg 28:860, 1970.
47. Foster TD, Fairburn FA: Dental involvement in scleroderma. Br Dent J 124:353, 1968.
48. Hoggins GS, Hamilton MC: Dentofacial defects associated with scleroderma. Oral Surg 27:734, 1969.
49. Keats TE: Rib erosions in scleroderma. AJR 100:530, 1967.
50. Elke M, Meier-Ruge W: Histologische Befunde an umschriebenen arrodierten Rippen bei Lungenfibrose im Verlaufe von Sklerodermie. Arch Klin Med 212:73, 1966.
51. Haverbush TJ, Wilde AH, Hawk WA Jr, et al: Osteolysis of the ribs and cervical spine in progressive systemic sclerosis (scleroderma), A case report. J Bone Joint Surg [Am] 56:637, 1974.
52. Sargent EN, Turner AF, Jacobson G: Superior marginal rib defects. AJR 106:491, 1969.
53. Alpert M, Feldman F: Rib lesions of rheumatoid arthritis. Radiology 82:872, 1964.
54. Keats TE: Superior marginal rib defects in restrictive lung disease. AJR 124:449, 1975.
55. Bjersand AJ: New bone formation and carpal synostosis in scleroderma. A case report. AJR 103:616, 1968.
56. Lovell RRH, Scott GBD: Hypertrophic osteo-arthropathy in polyarteritis. Ann Rheum Dis 15:46, 1956.
57. Saville PD: Polyarteritis nodosa with new bone formation. J Bone Joint Surg [Br] 38:327, 1956.
58. Schober R: Angiographische Befunde bei Sklerodermie. Roentgen-Bl 19:135, 1966.
59. Rabinowitz JG, Twersky J, Guttadauria M: Similar bone manifestations of scleroderma and rheumatoid arthritis. AJR 121:35, 1974.
60. Wild W, Beetham WP: Erosive arthropathy in systemic scleroderma. JAMA 232:511, 1975.
61. Karten I: CRST syndrome and "neuropathic" arthropathy. Arthritis Rheum 12:636, 1969.
62. Resnick D, Greenway G, Vint VC, et al: Selective involvement of the first carpometacarpal joint in scleroderma. AJR 131:283, 1978.
63. Jacobs P: Atlas of Hand Radiographs. Baltimore, University Park Press, 1973.
64. Reginato AJ, Schumacher HR: Synovial calcification in a patient with collagen-vascular disease: Light and electron microscopic studies. J Rheumatol 4:261, 1977.
65. Russell AS, Percy JS, Rigal WM, et al: Deforming arthropathy in systemic lupus erythematosus. Ann Rheum Dis 33:204, 1974.
66. Evans JA, Hasting DE, Urowitz MB: The fixed lupus hand deformity and its surgical correction. J Rheumatol 4:170, 1977.
67. Bunch TW, O'Duffy JD, McLeod RA: Deforming arthritis of the hands in polymyositis. Arthritis Rheum 19:243, 1976.
68. Murray RO, Jacobson HG: The Radiology of Skeletal Disorders. 2nd Ed. Edinburgh, Churchill Livingstone, 1977.

69. Winter H, Kammerhuber F: Seltene lokalisation von Knochenveränderungen bei progressiver (diffuser) Sklerodermie. ROFO 122:364, 1975.
70. Bard M, Djian A, Levi-Valensin G, et al: Synovite calcifiante diffuse dans la sclérodermie. J Radiol Electrol Med Nucl 55:321, 1974.
71. Resnick D, Scavulli JF, Goergen TG, et al: Intra-articular calcification in scleroderma. Radiology 124:685, 1977.
72. Brandt KD, Krey PR: Chalky joint effusion. The result of massive synovial deposition of calcium apatite in progressive systemic sclerosis. Arthritis Rheum 20:792, 1977.
73. Wilde AH, Mankin HJ, Rodnan GP: Avascular necrosis of the femoral head in scleroderma. Arthritis Rheum 13:445, 1970.
74. Coffman JD, Cohen AS: Total and capillary fingertip blood flow in Raynaud's phenomenon. N Engl J Med 285:259, 1971.
75. Fries JF: Physiologic studies in systemic sclerosis (scleroderma). Arch Intern Med 123:22, 1969.
76. Dabich L, Bookstein JJ, Zweifler A, et al: Digitial arteries in patients with scleroderma. Arteriographic and plethysmographic study. Arch Intern Med 130:708, 1972.
77. Laws JW, Lillie JG, Scott JT: Arteriographic appearances in rheumatoid arthritis and other disorders. Br J Radiol 36:477, 1963.
78. Higgins CB, Hayden WG: Palmar arteriography in acronecrosis. Radiology 119:85, 1976.
79. Tiedjen KU, Piaszek L: Durchströmungsuntersuchungen der Endstrombahn dei Gefässleiden des digitalen Lokalisationstyps (arterielles Verschlussleiden, Akrosklerose und Sklerodermia progressiva) mit Hilfe radioaktiver Spurensubstanzen. ROFO 123:56, 1975.
80. Scott JT, El Sallab RA, Laws JW: The digital artery design in rheumatoid arthritis—further observations. Br J Radiol 40:748, 1967.
81. Laws JW, El Sallab RA, Scott JT: An arteriographic and histological study of digital arteries. Br J Radiol 40:740, 1967.
82. Fisher ER, Rodnan GP: Pathologic observations concerning the cutaneous lesions of progressive systemic sclerosis: An electron microscopic, histochemical, and immunohistochemical study. Arthritis Rheum 3:536, 1960.
83. Fleischmajer R, Nedwich A: Generalized morphea. I. Histology of the dermis and subcutaneous tissue. Arch Dermatol 106:509, 1972.
84. Fleischmajer R, Perlish JS, Reeves JRT: Cellular infiltrates in scleroderma skin. Arthritis Rheum 20:975, 1977.
85. Hayes RL, Rodnan GP: The ultrastructure of skin in progressive systemic sclerosis (scleroderma). 1. Dermal collagen fibers. Am J Pathol 63:433, 1971.
86. Black MM, Bottoms E, Shuster S: Skin collagen content and thickness in systemic sclerosis. Br J Dermatol 83:552, 1970.
87. Bourgeois P, Cywiner-Golenzer CH, Lessana-Leibowitch M, et al: Les nodules sous-cutanés et tendineux dans la sclérodermie. A propos de 4 cas anatomo-cliniques. Rev Rhum Mal Ostéoartic 43:85, 1976.
88. Zuckner J, Baldassare A: The nonspecific rheumatoid subcutaneous nodule: Its presence in fibrositis and scleroderma. Am J Med Sci 271:69, 1976.
89. Rodnan GP: The nature of joint involvement in progressive systemic sclerosis (diffuse scleroderma). Clinical study and pathologic examination of synovium in 29 patients. Ann Intern Med 56:422, 1962.
90. Campbell PM, LeRoy EC: Pathogenesis of systemic sclerosis: A vascular hypothesis. Semin Arthritis Rheum 4:351, 1975.
91. Maricq HR, Spencer-Green G, LeRoy EC: Skin capillary abnormalities as indicators of organ involvement in scleroderma (systemic sclerosis), Raynaud's syndrome and dermatomyositis. Am J Med 61:862, 1976.
92. Fleischmajer R, Perlish JS, Shaw KV, et al: Skin capillary changes in early systemic scleroderma: Electron microscopy and "in vitro" autoradiography with tritiated thymidine. Arch Dermatol 112:1553, 1976.
93. Blair R, Schatzki R, Orr KD: Sequelae to cold injury in one hundred patients. JAMA 163:1203, 1957.
94. Rabinov D: Acromutilation of the fingers following severe burns. Radiology 77:968, 1961.
95. Sewell JR, Liyanage B, Ansell BM: Calcinosis in juvenile dermatomyositis. Skel Radiol 3:137, 1978.
96. Siegelman SS, Heimann WG, Manin MC: Congenital indifference to pain. AJR 97:242, 1966.
97. Becker MH, Wallin JK: Congenital hyperuricosuria. Associated radiologic features. Radiol Clin N Am 6:239, 1968.
98. Brinn LB, Khilnani MT: Epidermolysis bullosa with characteristic hand deformities. Radiology 89:272, 1967.
99. Wilson RH, McCormick WE, Tatum CF, et al: Occupational acroosteolysis. JAMA 201:577, 1967.
100. Caplan HI, Benny RA: Total osteolysis of the mandibular condyle in progressive systemic sclerosis. Oral Surg 46:362, 1978.
101. Rodnan GP, Lipinski E, Luksick J: Skin thickness and collagen content in progressive systemic sclerosis and localized scleroderma. Arthritis Rheum 22:130, 1979.
102. Rowell NR, Hopper FE: The periodontal membrane in systemic sclerosis. Br J Dermatol 93(Supp II):23, 1975.
103. Nassonova VA, Ivanova MM, Akhnazarova VD, et al: Eosinophilic fasciitis. Review and report of six cases. Scand J Rheumatol 8:225, 1979.
104. Gourvil J, Wechsler J, Revuz J, et al: Fasciite à éosinophiles (syndrome de Shulman) associée à un diabète insulino-dépendant. 1 observation. Nouv Presse Méd 50:4087, 1979.
105. Moore TL, Zuckner J: Eosinophilic fasciitis. Semin Arthritis Rheum 9:228, 1980.

106. Velayos EE, Masi AT, Stevens MB, et al: The "CREST" syndrome. Comparison with systemic sclerosis (scleroderma). Arch Intern Med *139:*1240, 1979.

107. Dorner RW: Scleroderma skin—conflicting mucopolysaccharide data reflect stages in connective tissue maturation. J Rheumatol *7:*128, 1980.

108. Buckingham RB, Prince RK, Rodnan GP, et al: Collagen accumulation by dermal fibroblast cultures of patients with linear localized scleroderma. J Rheumatol *7:*130, 1980.

109. Lovell CR, Jayson MIV: Joint involvement in systemic sclerosis. Scand J Rheumatol *8:*154, 1979.

110. Spielvogel RL, Goltz RW, Kersey JH: Scleroderma-like changes in chronic graft vs host disease. Arch Dermatol *113:*1424, 1977.

111. Herzog P, Clements PJ, Roberts NK, et al: Case report: Progressive systemic sclerosis-like syndrome after bone marrow transplantation. Clinical immunologic and pathologic findings. J Rheumatol *7:*56, 1980.

112. Jacobson HG, Rifkin H, Zucker FD: Werner's syndrome: A clinical roentgen entity. Radiology *74:*373, 1960.

113. Masi AT: Preliminary criteria for the classification of systemic sclerosis (scleroderma). Arthritis Rheum *23:*581, 1980.

114. Tan EM, Rodnan GP, Garcia I, et al: Diversity of antinuclear antibodies in progressive systemic sclerosis. Arthritis Rheum *23:*617, 1980.

115. Posner MA, Herness D, Green S: Severe peripheral vascular deterioration in scleroderma. A case report. Acta Orthop Scand *51:*239, 1980.

116. Rosenthal J, Benson MD: Diffuse fasciitis and eosinophilia with symmetric polyarthritis. Ann Intern Med *92:*507, 1980.

117. Zalla JA: Werner's syndrome. Cutis *25:*275, 1980.

118. LeRoy EC: Scleroderma (systemic Sclerosis). *In* WN Kelley, ED Harris Jr, S Ruddy, CB Sledge (Eds): Textbook of Rheumatology. Philadelphia, WB Saunders, 1981, p 1211.

119. Benedek TG, Rodnan GP: The early history and nomenclature of scleroderma and its differentiation from scleroderma neonatorum and scleroedema. Semin Arthritis Rheum *12:*52, 1982.

120. Goetz RH: Pathology of progressive systemic sclerosis (generalized scleroderma) with special reference to changes in the viscera. Clin Proc *4:*337, 1945.

121. McDonald CJ: Raynaud's syndrome. Dermatol Clin North Am *1:*493, 1983.

122. Spencer-Green G: Raynaud phenomenon. Bull Rheum Dis *33:*1, 1983.

123. Fritzler MJ, Kinsella TD, Garbutt E: The CREST syndrome: A distinct serologic entity with anticentromere antibodies. Am J Med *69:*520, 1980.

124. Masi AT, Rodnan GP, Medsger TA Jr, et al: Preliminary criteria for the classification of systemic sclerosis (scleroderma). Bull Rheum Dis *31:*1, 1981.

125. Baron M, Lee P, Keystone EC: The articular manifestations of progressive systemic sclerosis (scleroderma). Ann Rheum Dis *41:*147, 1982.

126. Horwitz HM, DiBeneditto JD Jr, Allegra SR, et al: Scleroderma, amyloidosis, and extensor tendon rupture. Arthritis Rheum *25:*1141, 1982.

127. Palmer DG, Hale GM, Grennan DM, et al: Bowed fingers: A helpful sign in the early diagnosis of systemic sclerosis. J Rheumatol *8:*266, 1981.

128. Brun B, Serup J, Hagdrup H: Radiological changes of the hands in systemic sclerosis. Acta Derm Venereol *63:*349, 1983.

129. Bassett LW, Blocka KLN, Furst DE, et al: Skeletal findings in progressive systemic sclerosis (scleroderma). AJR *136:*1121, 1981.

130. Shanks MJ, Blane CE, Adler DD, et al: Radiographic findings of scleroderma in childhood. AJR *141:*657, 1983.

131. White SC, Frey NW, Blaschke DD, et al: Oral radiographic changes in patients with systemic sclerosis. J Am Dent Assoc *94:*1178, 1977.

132. Osial TA Jr, Avakian A, Sassouni V, et al: Resorption of the mandibular condyles and coronoid processes in progressive systemic sclerosis (scleroderma). Arthritis Rheum *24:*729, 1981.

133. Quagliata F, Sebes J, Pinstein ML, et al: Long bone erosion and ascites in progressive systemic sclerosis (scleroderma). J Rheumatol *9:*641, 1982.

134. Marmary Y, Glaiss R, Pisanty S: Scleroderma: Oral manifestations. Oral Surg *52:*32, 1981.

135. Blocka KLN, Bassett LW, Furst DE, et al: The arthropathy of advanced progressive systemic sclerosis. A radiographic survey. Arthritis Rheum *24:*874, 1981.

136. Armstrong RD, Gibson T: Scleroderma and erosive polyarthritis: A disease entity? Ann Rheum Dis *41:*141, 1982.

137. Barry M, Katz L, Cooney L: An unusual articular presentation of progressive systemic sclerosis. Arthritis Rheum *26:*1041, 1983.

138. Hamza M, Moalla M, Hamza R, et al: Syndrome C.R.S.T. (syndrome de Thibierge-Weissenbach) avec calcification intra-articulaire. J Radiol *62:*267, 1981.

139. Albert J, Ott H: Association d'un syndrome de Gourgerot-Sjögren et d'un syndrome C.R.S.T. avec calcification intra-articulaires et lésions ostéolytiques inhabituelles. J Radiol *63:*757, 1982.

140. Rouzaud S, Katz AL: Joint changes with progressive systemic sclerosis. Arthritis Rheum *25:*1026, 1982.

141. Huyck CJ, Hoffman GS: Bony ankylosis of the hips in progressive systemic sclerosis. Arthritis Rheum *25:*1497, 1982.

142. Rodnan GP, Myerowitz RL, Justh GO: Morphologic changes in the digital arteries of patients with progressive systemic sclerosis (scleroderma) and Raynaud phenomenon. Medicine *59:*393, 1980.

143. Leroux J-L, Pernot F, Fedou P, et al: Ultrastructural and crystallographic study of calcifications from a patient with CREST syndrome. J Rheumatol *10:*242, 1983.

144. Haynes DC, Gershwin ME: The immunopathology of progressive systemic sclerosis (PSS). Semin Arthritis Rheum *11:*331, 1982.

145. Germain BF, Espinoza LR, Bergen LL, et al: Increased prevalence of DRw3 in the CREST syndrome. Arthritis Rheum *24:*857, 1981.

146. Gladman DD, Keystone EC, Baron M, et al: Increased frequency of HLA-DR5 in scleroderma. Arthritis Rheum *24:*854, 1981.

147. Rodnan GP: When is scleroderma not scleroderma? The differential diagnosis of progressive systemic sclerosis. Bull Rheum Dis *31:*7, 1981.

148. Palestine RF, Millns JL, Spigel GT, et al: Skin manifestations of pentazocine abuse. J Am Acad Dermatol *2:*47, 1980.

149. Ishizuka M, Takayama H, Takeuchi T: Activity and toxicity of bleomycin. J Antibiot (Tokyo) *20:*15, 1967.

150. Ichikawa T, Matsuda A, Miyamoto K: Biological studies on bleomycin. J Antibiot (Tokyo) *20:*149, 1967.

151. Finch WR, Rodnan GP, Buckingham RB, et al: Bleomycin-induced scleroderma. J Rheumatol *7:*651, 1980.

152. Rush PJ, Bell MJ, Fam AG: Toxic oil syndrome (Spanish oil disease) and chemically induced scleroderma-like conditions. J Rheumatol *11:*262, 1984.

153. Mateo IM, Izquierdo M, Fernandez-Dapica MP, et al: Toxic epidemic syndrome; musculoskeletal manifestations. J Rheumatol *11:*333, 1984.

154. Kaplinsky N, Bubus JJ, Pras M: Localized eosinophilic fasciitis in a child. J Rheumatol *7:*541, 1980.

155. Hoffman R, Young N, Ershler WB, et al: Diffuse fasciitis and aplastic anemia: A report of four cases revealing an unusual association between rheumatologic and hematologic disorders. Medicine *61:*373, 1982.

156. Kaplinsky N, Revach M, Katz WA: Eosinophilic fasciitis: Report of a case with features of connective tissue disease. J Rheumatol *7:*536, 1980.

157. Barraclough D, Begg MW: Diffuse fasciitis with eosinophilia. Aust NZ J Med *10:*333, 1980.

158. Fernandez-Herlihy L: Eosinophilic fasciitis: Report of a 22-year followup study. Arthritis Rheum *24:*97, 1981.

159. Michet CJ Jr, Doyle JA, Ginsburg WW: Eosinophilic fasciitis. Report of 15 cases. Mayo Clin Proc *56:*27, 1981.

160. Lee P: Eosinophilic fasciitis—new associations and current perspectives. J Rheumatol *8:*6, 1981.

161. Kent LT, Cramer SF, Moskowitz RW: Eosinophilic fasciitis. Clinical, laboratory, and microscopic considerations. Arthritis Rheum *24:*677, 1981.

162. Giordano M, Ara M, Cicala C, et al: Eosinophilic fasciitis. Ann Intern Med *93:*645, 1980.

163. Giordano M, Ara M, Rossiello R, et al: Die eosinophile Fasziitis. Eine Kürzlich heraugestellte oligotope Konnektivitis. Beschreiburg eines Falles. Z Rheumatol *39:*236, 1980.

164. Cohen JI: Eosinophilic fasciitis. Clinical conferences at The Johns Hopkins Hospital. Johns Hopkins Med J *148:*81, 1981.

165. Wollheim FA, Lindstrom CG, Eiken O: Eosinophilic fasciitis complicated by carpal tunnel syndrome. J Rheumatol *8:*856, 1981.

166. Berkten R, Shaller D: Chronic progressive eosinophilic fasciitis: Report of a 20-year failure to attain remission. Ann Rheum Dis *42:*103, 1983.

167. Avgerinos PC, Papadimitriou CS, Kokkini G, et al: Asymptomatic diffuse fasciitis with eosinophilia. Ann Rheum Dis *41:*621, 1982.

168. Itzkowitch DF, Famaey J-P, Appelboom T: Eosinophilic fasciitis and reflex sympathetic dystrophy syndrome. J Rheumatol *8:*528, 1981.

169. Buchanan RRC, Gordon DA, Muckle TJ, et al: The eosinophilic fasciitis syndrome after phenytoin (Dilantin) therapy. J Rheumatol *7:*733, 1980.

170. Cramer SF, Kent L, Abramowsky C, et al: Eosinophilic fasciitis. Immunopathology, ultra-structure, literature review, and consideration of its pathogenesis and relation to scleroderma. Arch Pathol Lab Med *106:*85, 1982.

171. Lewkonia RM, Marx LH, Atkinson MH: Granulomatous vasculitis in the syndrome of diffuse fasciitis with eosinophilia. Arch Intern Med *142:*73, 1982.

172. Gabrielli A, DeNictolis M, Campanati G, et al: Eosinophilic fasciitis: A mast cell disorder? Clin Exp Rheumatol *1:*75, 1983.

173. Littlejohn GO, Keystone EC: Eosinophilic fasciitis and aplastic anemia. J Rheumatol *7:*730, 1980.

174. Michaels RM: Eosinophilic fasciitis complicated by Hodgkin's disease. J Rheumatol *9:*473, 1982.

175. Frayha RA: Papular mucinosis, destructive arthropathy, median neuropathy, and sicca complex. Clin Rheumatol *2:*277, 1983.

176. Snover DC: Acute and chronic graft versus host disease: Histopathological evidence for two distinct pathogenetic mechanisms. Hum Pathol *15:*202, 1984.

177. Billignam RE: The biology of graft-v-host reaction. Harvey Lect *62:*21, 1966–1967.

178. James WD, Odom RB: Graft-v-host disease. Arch Dermatol *119:*683, 1983.

179. Shulman HM, Sullivan KM, Weiden PL, et al: Chronic graft-versus-host syndrome in man. A long-term clinicopathologic study of 20 Seattle patients. Am J Med *69:*204, 1980.

180. Seemayer TA, Gartner JG, Lapp WS: The graft-versus-host reaction. Hum Pathol *14:*3, 1983.

181. Reyes MG, Noronha P, Thomas W Jr, et al: Myositis of chronic graft versus host disease. Neurology *33:*1222, 1983.

182. Wick MR, Moore SB, Gastineau DA, et al: Immunologic, clinical, and pathologic aspects of human graft-versus-host disease. Mayo Clin Proc *58:*603, 1983.

183. Anderson BA, Young V, Kean WF, et al: Polymyositis in chronic graft versus host disease. A case report. Arch Neurol *39:*188, 1982.

184. Monsees B, Murphy WA: Distal phalangeal erosive lesions. Arthritis Rheum *27:*449, 1984.

185. Rosenbaum LH, Swartz WM, Rodnan GP, et al: Wrist drop in progressive systemic sclerosis (scleroderma): Complete rupture of the extensor tendon mechanism. Arthritis Rheum *28:*586, 1985.

186. Lee P, Bruni J, Sukenik S: Neurological manifestations in systemic sclerosis (scleroderma). J Rheumatol *11:*480, 1984.

187. Clement GB, Grizzard K, Vasey FB, et al: Neuropathic arthropathy (Charcot joints) due to cervical osteolysis: A complication of progressive systemic sclerosis. J Rheumatol *11:*545, 1984.

188. Albert J, Ott H: Unusual articular abnormalities in scleroderma. Clin Rheumatol *3:*323, 1984.

189. Izquierdo M, Mateo I, Rodrigo M, et al: Chronic juvenile toxic epidemic syndrome. Ann Rheum Dis *44:*98, 1985.

190. Jamieson TW, DeSmet AA, Stechschulte DJ: Erosive arthropathy associated with scleromyxedema. Skel Radiol *14:*286, 1985.

191. Olutola PS, Adelowo F: Osteolysis of the shaft of tubular bones in systemic scleroderma. Diagn Imaging Clin Med *54:*322, 1985.

192. Falanga V, Medsger TA Jr, Reichlin M, et al: Linear scleroderma. Clinical spectrum, prognosis, and laboratory abnormalities. Ann Int Med *104:*849, 1986.

193. Rocco VK, Hurd ER: Scleroderma and scleroderma-like disorders. Semin Arthritis Rheum *16:*22, 1986.

194. Myers SL, Cohen JS, Sheets PW, et al: B-mode ultrasound evaluation of skin thickness in progressive systemic sclerosis. J Rheumatol *13:*577, 1986.

195. Akesson A, Forsberg L, Wollheim F: Ultrasound examination of skin thickness in patients with progressive systemic sclerosis (scleroderma). Acta Radiol (Diagn) *27:*91, 1986.

196. Fudman EJ, Golbus J, Ike RW: Scleromyxedema with systemic involvement mimics rheumatic diseases. Arthritis Rheum *29:*913, 1986.

197. Lally EV, Jimenez SA, Kaplan SR: Progressive systemic sclerosis: Mode of presentation, rapidly progressive disease course, and mortality based on an analysis of 91 patients. Semin Arthritis Rheum *18:*1, 1988.

198. Lababidi HMS, Nasr FW, Khatib Z: Juvenile progressive systemic sclerosis: Report of five cases. J Rheumatol *18:*885, 1991.

199. Barr WG, Blair SJ: Carpal tunnel syndrome as the initial manifestation of scleroderma. J Hand Surg [Am] *13:*366, 1988.

200. Thurman RT, Jindal P, Wolff TW: Ulnar nerve compression in Guyon's canal caused by calcinosis in scleroderma. J Hand Surg [Am] *16:*739, 1991.

201. Kane-Wranger G, Ostrov BE, Freundlich B: Wrist contractures as the presenting manifestation of scleroderma. Ann Rheum Dis *51:*810, 1992.

202. Sethi S, Sequeira W: Sparing effect of hemiplegia on scleroderma. Ann Rheum Dis *49:*999, 1990.

203. Hendrix RW, Houk RW: Case 4. Scleroderma. AJR *150:*1435, 1988.

204. Khonstanteen I, Wright B, Russell ML: Localized bone resorption in systemic sclerosis. J Rheumatol *15:*1435, 1988.

205. Schweitzer ME, Cervilla V, Manaster BJ, et al: Cervical paraspinal calcification in collagen vascular diseases. AJR *157:*523, 1991.

206. Pinstein ML, Sebes JI, Leventhal M, et al: Case report 579. Skel Radiol *18:*603, 1989.

207. Petrocelli AR, Bassett LW, Mirra J, et al: Scleroderma: Dystrophic calcification with spinal cord compression. J Rheumatol *15:*1733, 1988.

208. Walden CA, Gilbert P, Rogers LF, et al: Case report 620. Skel Radiol *19:*377, 1990.

209. Meyer E, Kulenkampff H-A, Kortenhaus H: Ungewöhnliche, tumorartige Verkalkung bei Sklerodermie. Thibièrge-Weissenbach-Syndrom. Radiologe *27:*572, 1987.

210. Durback MA, Schumacher HR Jr: Acute gouty arthritis in 4 patients with systemic sclerosis. J Rheumatol *15:*1503, 1988.

211. Agus B: Bilateral aseptic necrosis of the lunate in systemic sclerosis. Clin Exp Rheumatol *5:*155, 1987.

212. Sattar MA, Al-Sughyer AA, Leven H: Acute synovial rupture in scleroderma. Scand J Rheumatol *17:*119, 1988.

213. Pile KD, Gendi NST, Mowat AG: Scleroderma with bilateral synovial fistulae. J Rheumatol *19:*1150, 1992.

214. Brasington RD Jr, Thorpe-Swenson AJ: Systemic sclerosis associated with cutaneous exposure to solvent: Case report and review of the literature. Arthritis Rheum *34:*631, 1991.

215. Black CM, Welsh KI: Occupationally and environmentally induced scleroderma-like illness: Etiology, pathogenesis, diagnosis, and treatment. IM *9:*135, 1988.

216. Straniero NR, Furst DE: Environmentally-induced systemic sclerosis-like illness. Ballieres Clin Rheumatol *3:*63, 1989.

217. Kerr LD, Spiera H: Scleroderma in association with the use of bleomycin: A report of 3 cases. J Rheumatol *19:*294, 1992.

218. Lakhanpal S, Ginsburg WW, Michet CJ, et al: Eosinophilic fasciitis: Clinical spectrum and therapeutic response in 52 cases. Semin Arthritis Rheum *17:*221, 1988.

219. Williams HJ, Ziter FA, Banta CA: Childhood eosinophilic fasciitis—progression to linear scleroderma. J Rheumatol *13:*961, 1986.

220. Thomson GTD, McDougall B, Watson PH, et al: Eosinophilic fasciitis in a pair of siblings. Arthritis Rheum *32:*96, 1989.

221. De Clerck LS, Degryse HR, Wouters E, et al: Magnetic resonance imaging in the evaluation of patients with eosinophilic fasciitis. J Rheumatol *16:*1270, 1989.

222. Tallec YL, Arlet P, de la Roque PM, et al: Magnetic resonance imaging in eosinophilic fasciitis. J Rheumatol *18:*636, 1991.

223. Blevins WL, Hertzman P, Ting M, et al: Eosinophilia-myalgia syndrome—New Mexico. MMWR *38:*765, 1989.

224. Shulman LE: The eosinophilia-myalgia syndrome associated with ingestion of L-tryptophan. Arthritis Rheum *33:*913, 1990.

225. Bulpitt KJ, Verity MA, Clements PJ, et al: Association of L-tryptophan and an illness resembling eosinophilic fasciitis. Arthritis Rheum *33:*918, 1990.

226. Roubenoff R, Coté T, Watson R, et al: Eosinophilia-myalgia syndrome due to L-tryptophan ingestion. Arthritis Rheum *33:*930, 1990.

227. Leblanc BAEW, Inman RD: Eosinophilia-myalgia syndrome—old questions for a new syndrome. J Rheumatol *17:*1435, 1990.

228. Chartash EK, Given WP, Vishnubhakat SM, et al: Tryptophan induced eosinophilia-myalgia syndrome. J Rheumatol *17:*1527, 1990.

229. Glickstein SL, Gertner E, Smith SA, et al: Eosinophilia-myalgia syndrome associated with L-tryptophan use. J Rheumatol *17:*1534, 1990.

230. Saag KG, Goldschmidt R, Vernof H, et al: An eosinophilia-myalgia syndrome associated with an L-tryptophan containing product. J Rheumatol *17:*1551, 1990.

231. Estrada CA, Harrington DW, Glasberg MR: Eosinophilic myositis—an expression of L-tryptophan toxicity? J Rheumatol *17:*1554, 1990.

232. Gresh JP, Vasey FB, Espinoza LR, et al: Eosinophilia-myalgia syndrome in association with L-tryptophan ingestion. J Rheumatol *17:*1557, 1990.

233. Katz JD, Wakem CJ, Parke AL: L-tryptophan associated eosinophilia-myalgia syndrome. J Rheumatol *17:*1559, 1990.

234. Hertzman PA, Falk H, Kilbourne EM, et al: The eosinophilia-myalgia syndrome: The Los Alamos conference. J Rheumatol *18:*867, 1991.

235. Schlessel K, Greenwald R, Hirschfield L: Scleroderma-like fasciitis without eosinophilia after L-tryptophan ingestion. J Rheumatol *18:*779, 1991.

236. Smith SA, Roelofs RI, Gertner E: Microangiopathy in the eosinophilia-myalgia syndrome. J Rheumatol *17:*1544, 1990.

237. Houpt JB: Tryptophan—new questions for an old amino acid. J Rheumatol *17:*1431, 1990.

238. Hamilton ME: Eosinophilic fasciitis associated with L-tryptophan ingestion. Ann Rheum Dis *50:*55, 1991.

239. Varga J, Griffin R, Newman JH, et al: Eosinophilic fasciitis is clinically distinguishable from the eosinophilia-myalgia syndrome and is not associated with L-tryptophan use. J Rheumatol *18:*259, 1991.

240. Helfrich DJ, Walker ER, Martinez J, et al: Scleromyxedema myopathy: Case report and review of the literature. Arthritis Rheum *31:*1437, 1988.

241. Gabriel SE, Perry HO, Oleson GB, et al: Scleromyxedema: A scleroderma-like disorder with systemic manifestations. Medicine *67:*58, 1988.

242. Ferrara JLM, Deeg HJ: Graft-versus-host disease. N Engl J Med *324:*667, 1991.

243. Czirjak L, Nagy Z, Szegedi G: Systemic sclerosis in the elderly. Clin Rheumatol *11:*483, 1992.

244. Goldenberg J, Pinto-Pessoa A, Odete-Hilario M, et al: Scleroderma in children. A report of eleven cases. Rev Rhum [Ed. Fr] *60:*131, 1993.

245. Lagana A, Canoso JJ: Subcutaneous bursitis in scleroderma. J Rheumatol *19:*1586, 1992.

246. Fam AG, Pritzker KPH: Acute calcific periarthritis in scleroderma. J Rheumatol *19:*1580, 1992.

247. Farrington ML, Haas JE, Nazar-Stewart V, et al: Eosinophilic fasciitis in children frequently progresses to scleroderma-like cutaneous fibrosis. J Rheumatol *20:*128, 1993.

248. Philen RM, Hill RH Jr: 3-(Phenylamino)alanine—a link between eosinophilia-myalgia syndrome and toxic oil syndrome? Mayo Clin Proc *68:*197, 1993.

249. Back EE, Henning KJ, Kallenbach LR, et al: Risk factors for developing eosinophilia myalgia syndrome among L-tryptophan users in New York. J Rheumatol *20:*666, 1993.

250. Henning KJ, Jean-Baptiste E, Singh T, et al: Eosinophilia-myalgia syndrome in patients ingesting a single source of L-tryptophan. J Rheumatol *20:*273, 1993.

251. Appleton BE, Lee P: The development of systemic sclerosis (scleroderma) following augmentation mammoplasty. J Rheumatol *20:*1052, 1993.

252. Spiera H, Kerr LD: Scleroderma following silicone implantation: A cumulative experience of 11 cases. J Rheumatol *20:*958, 1993.

253. Spiera RF, Gibofsky A, Spiera H: Silicone gel filled breast implants and connective tissue disease: An overview. J Rheumatol *21:*239, 1994.

35

Dermatomyositis and Polymyositis

Donald Resnick, M.D.

Dermatomyositis and polymyositis are disorders of striated muscle characterized by diffuse, nonsuppurative inflammation and degeneration. In dermatomyositis, both the skeletal muscle and the skin are involved, whereas in polymyositis, the skeletal muscle alone is affected. The disorders are of unknown cause and affect patients of all ages, although they are most frequent in middle-aged women. Dermatomyositis and polymyositis are grouped with other collagen vascular diseases because of similar clinical, pathologic, and radiologic features. Inflammation of skeletal muscle also can occur in a variety of viral and bacterial infections.

NOMENCLATURE AND CLASSIFICATION

Although the association of muscle and skin inflammation in dermatomyositis has been recognized since Unverricht's description in 1887,[1] not until recently has the occurrence of muscular inflammatory changes without typical skin abnormalities become fully appreciated. In fact, the variability in clinical and laboratory features of dermatomyositis and polymyositis has caused difficulty in classification of these diseases. The most satisfying classification systems have been proposed by Pearson[2] and Bohan and Peter,[66] and a modification of these is given in this chapter. Bohan and Peter have suggested five criteria in an attempt to better define the disorders: (1) proximal symmetric muscle weakness that progresses over a period of weeks to months; (2) elevated serum levels of muscle enzymes or an elevated level of urinary creatinine excretion; (3) an abnormal electromyogram; (4) abnormal muscle biopsy findings that are consistent with myositis; and (5) the presence of cutaneous disease typical of dermatomyositis.[66] Although strict application of these criteria is not without difficulty, the criteria are useful in excluding other causes of myopathy.

Type I: Typical Polymyositis

Type I is the most common type, constituting approximately 35 per cent of cases. It is most frequent in the third, fourth, and fifth decades of life and affects women more commonly than men, in a ratio of approximately 2 to 1. Cases generally are sporadic, although, on rare occasions, familial patterns emerge.[67] An antecedent febrile illness is not uncommon. Polymyositis is characterized by gradually increasing muscle weakness, first appearing in the musculature of the thighs and pelvic girdle and later affecting the upper extremity and the laryngeal and pharyngeal muscles. Dermal manifestations are inconstant; they are absent in some persons, whereas in others findings include an erythematous skin rash, Raynaud's phenomenon, or scleroderma. Joint manifestations include arthralgias and arthritis, which may be accompanied by a joint effusion and positive results in serologic tests for rheumatoid factor.

Type II: Typical Dermatomyositis

Present in approximately 25 per cent of patients, more frequently women, type II is characterized by muscular weakness and a diffuse erythematous skin rash on the face, the neck, the chest, the shoulders, and the arms. The age of disease onset is variable; adults in the fifth or sixth decade typically are affected. Dermal and muscular abnormalities may occur simultaneously, or the skin manifestations may precede the development of muscular weakness. Additional clinical features can include malaise and joint pain.

Type III: Typical Dermatomyositis with Malignancy

In patients over the age of 40 years, particularly men, type III dermatomyositis is characterized by the presence of skin rash, muscular weakness, and malignancy. Previous reports suggest that malignancy becomes evident in approximately 15 to 25 per cent of patients with dermatomyositis and that this prevalence increases with the age of the patient.[68, 69] Polymyositis without dermatologic abnormalities is associated less frequently with malignancy than is dermatomyositis. The temporal relationship of the findings is variable; most commonly, muscular and dermal manifestations antedate the appearance of malignancy by months to years. The neoplasm may originate from almost any site, although the most commonly associated tumors arise from the lungs, the prostate, the female pelvic organs, the breast, and the gastrointestinal tract. The prognosis in patients with type III dermatomyositis is guarded; progressive muscle involvement can lead to recurrent pulmonary infection, respiratory failure, and death. Myopathy may remit after resection of the accompanying tumor.[3]

Type IV: Childhood Dermatomyositis

Dermatomyositis or, less commonly, polymyositis affects children or adolescents in approximately 20 per cent of cases.[67] In this type, dermal and muscular alterations appear at any age in childhood, although they are most frequent between the ages of 5 and 10 years. Girls are affected more commonly than boys.[70, 71, 82] Proximal muscle weakness may either progress rapidly, leading to swallowing, phonation, and respiratory difficulties, or fluctuate, with periods of remission and exacerbation. Additional characteristics of childhood dermatomyositis are extensive edema and calcification of skin and subcutaneous tissues, vasculitis, and joint contractures.[4–7] Fever, loss of weight, and malaise also may be apparent. Dermatomyositis in childhood may be associated with other disorders, including hypogammaglobulinemia and leukemia.

The severity of dermatomyositis in children should be stressed; although the mortality in this disease is approximately the same in children and adults, the interval between the onset of myositis and death is shorter, and the degree of soft tissue calcification is more extensive in childhood dermatomyositis.[8, 82] With regard to prognosis, two types of dermatomyositis occurring in children have been identified: an acute fulminant pattern (Banker type) associated with vasculitis, little calcinosis, and poor prognosis; and a slowly progressive pattern (Brunsting type) accompanied by calcinosis without vasculitis, with a good prognosis.[68] Other investigators have confirmed the relationship between the severity of the vasculopathy and the clinical course of childhood dermatomyositis and polymyositis.[72] Distinctive vascular lesions included non-necrotizing lymphocytic vasculitis and a spectrum of endovascular injury leading to temporary or permanent occlusion of small arteries and capillaries. Zonal loss of the capillary bed, infarction of muscle, noninflammatory endarteropathy, and lymphocytic vasculitis were features associated with chronicity. Muscle morphology, determined from adequate biopsy material, appears to be the key in the identification of those children who are destined to have persistent morbidity.[72]

Type V: Acute Myolysis

Type V disease, which is present in approximately 3 per cent of patients, is characterized by the sudden onset of myolysis, particularly in patients in the first or second decade of life. Intermittent attacks, which may be initiated by a viral infection, are associated with clinical manifestations, such as diffuse muscular weakness involving facial, proximal, and distal musculature, and laboratory manifestations, such as myoglobinuria and elevation of serum muscle enzyme levels. A fatal outcome is not infrequent.

Type VI: Polymyositis in Sjögren's Syndrome and Other Connective Tissue Diseases

In some patients with Sjögren's syndrome (approximately 10 per cent) slowly progressive weakness of proximal musculature is evident.[9] This type of polymyositis, which represents approximately 5 per cent of all cases, generally is not accompanied by skin abnormalities.

Myositis accompanies other connective tissue diseases as well, including scleroderma, systemic lupus erythematosus, rheumatoid arthritis, and overlap syndromes.[81]

CLINICAL ABNORMALITIES

Although specific clinical abnormalities accompanying dermatomyositis and polymyositis depend on which type of disease is present, a few general characteristics deserve emphasis (Fig. 35–1). The most constant clinical finding is muscular weakness, which eventually appears in virtually all persons with the disease; this manifestation is the presenting symptom in approximately 50 per cent of patients.[10] Muscular weakness can occur rapidly or slowly, and it can affect any region of the body.[62] Symmetric involvement of proximal muscles is most characteristic. Fatigue, inability to walk or climb stairs, and aching are frequent, whereas tenderness to palpation is less prominent. Involvement of respiratory muscles may lead to the patient's demise.[11, 80] Physical findings associated with muscular inflammation include induration, contracture, and atrophy.

Typical or atypical skin rashes eventually occur in 40 to 60 per cent of patients and are an initial manifestation of the disease in 20 to 25 per cent.[10] In the face, dermal eruption usually is evident on the forehead and periorbital tissues. Elsewhere, skin abnormalities are frequent about the knuckles, the elbows, the knees, the ankles, the neck, the chest, and the shoulders. Elevated, violaceous to dusty-red lesions in these areas are called Gottron's papules. Associated findings include intradermal and subcutaneous edema as well as telangiectasia about the nails.

Raynaud's phenomenon occurs in about one third of patients with polymyositis. It appears more commonly in those persons who exhibit clinical features of scleroderma or acrosclerosis, and it generally is mild in nature.[12]

Arthralgias and arthritis are present in 20 to 50 per cent

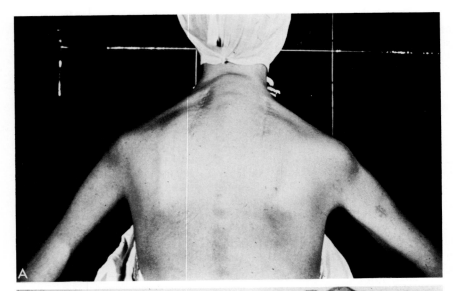

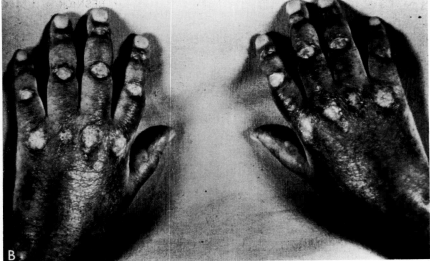

FIGURE 35–1. Dermatomyositis and polymyositis: Clinical abnormalities.

A Muscle atrophy of the neck, shoulders, and upper arms is evident.

B Note the skin lesions about the dorsum of the metacarpophalangeal, proximal interphalangeal, and distal interphalangeal joints.

of patients.[13–18] On rare occasions, joint manifestations may precede other clinical findings of the disease,[63] leading to an erroneous diagnosis of rheumatoid arthritis or systemic lupus erythematosus.[13] In some patients, serologic tests for rheumatoid factor yield positive results. Typically, the wrists, the knees, and the small joints of the fingers are affected symmetrically. Permanent joint damage is unusual (see discussion later in this chapter).

Clinical manifestations of visceral involvement in dermatomyositis and polymyositis include cardiac (arrhythmia, pericarditis), pulmonary (pneumonitis, fibrosis), gastrointestinal (dysphagia, abdominal pain, constipation), renal, neurologic, and ocular abnormalities.[19–24]

The association of neoplasm and dermatomyositis (and to a lesser extent, polymyositis) is well known[3, 25] and accepted by most investigators,[83, 84] but not all.[85] As indicated previously, the prevalence of tumor in patients with myositis is approximately 15 to 25 per cent. The more advanced the age of onset of dermatomyositis, the more likely is the occurrence of an associated neoplasm; the reported frequency of this complication in men who develop myositis

after the age of 50 years is 71 per cent.[26] The tumor most commonly is a carcinoma, although myeloma, leukemia, lymphoma, thymoma, sarcoma, and reticulosis also have been recorded. The clinical features associated with myositis in patients with coexistent neoplasm generally are severe, whereas those associated with the neoplasm itself usually are mild. Of interest, articular abnormalities are rare in those patients with malignant disease.[68]

Laboratory tests reveal characteristic abnormalities in many but not all patients with dermatomyositis and polymyositis.[81] Serum levels of one muscle enzyme, creatine kinase, usually are elevated during periods of active myositis, fall during remissions and after therapy, and may be normal during the chronic fibrotic stages of the disease. Elevation of levels of alanine aminotransferase (ALT), aspartate aminotransferase (AST), and aldolase in the serum also may be evident.[27, 28]

Electromyographic alterations in polymyositis have been reported by Marinacci[29]: spontaneous fibrillation and positive or sawtooth potentials, which occur at complete rest; polyphasic or short duration potentials, which appear on voluntary contraction; and salvos of repetitive potentials or "pseudomotic-myotonic" chains of oscillations of high frequency, which are evoked by mechanical stimulation of the nerve or movement of the electrode.[27]

RADIOGRAPHIC ABNORMALITIES

Radiographic abnormalities of the musculoskeletal system in dermatomyositis and polymyositis can be divided into two types: soft tissue abnormalities and articular abnormalities.

Soft Tissue Abnormalities

Although soft tissue abnormalities occur in both children and adults, most reports emphasize alterations in children because of the greater frequency and severity of the findings in the younger age groups.[30–33]

The initial soft tissue manifestation is edema of the subcutaneous tissue and muscle, producing increased muscular bulk and radiodensity, thickening of subcutaneous septa, and poor delineation of the subcutaneous tissue–muscle interface[30] (Fig. 35–2). The changes are more prominent in the proximal musculature, the axillae, the chest wall, the forearms, the thighs, and the calves[34]; correlate well with clinical symptoms; and require high quality radiographs using soft tissue technique. After effective treatment, tissue edema can decrease or disappear entirely, although in many patients, fibrosis and muscle atrophy and contracture become apparent in the later stages of the disease. In these stages, decreased soft tissue and muscular bulk, increased soft tissue lucency, contractures, and associated osteoporosis are evident.[30]

The most characteristic soft tissue abnormality in dermatomyositis and polymyositis is calcification. The frequency of this finding in children is high,[74] particularly in large series of patients in whom long-term follow-up examinations are available.[33] This does not indicate that calcification is confined to persons with long-standing disease; it may occur within the first year of illness. The extent of calcification, particularly that within musculature, appears to increase with the severity of the disease.

The radiographic pattern of calcification is variable. Small or large calcareous intermuscular fascial plane calcification is distinctive (Fig. 35–3), although it may not be so common as subcutaneous calcification.[33] The favorite sites of intermuscular calcification are the large muscles in the proximal portion of the limbs. Tendon and fat calcification occasionally is encountered. The appearance and distribution of subcutaneous calcification in dermatomyositis and polymyositis simulate those in scleroderma; linear and curvilinear deposits demonstrate predilection for the knees, the elbows, and the fingers (Fig. 35–4). Fingertip calcification can be associated with terminal phalangeal erosion, further complicating the radiographic differentiation of these two disorders (Fig. 35–5). Subcutaneous calcification may be accompanied by cutaneous ulceration and soft tissue infection.

Blane and associates[73] delineated four distinct patterns of soft tissue calcification in childhood dermatomyositis: deep calcareal masses, superficial calcareal masses, deep linear deposits, and lacy, reticular, subcutaneous collections encasing the torso. Of these, the first and third patterns, evi-

dent in deeper tissues, were more common, and the fourth, although infrequent, appeared to identify a subgroup of children in whom the disorder had a severe clinical course.

Soft tissue calcification may progress with increasing duration of the disease. Occasionally, spontaneous regression and resolution of calcinosis become apparent at puberty,[6, 32, 33, 35–37] associated with an improvement in clinical findings. This clinical and radiologic remission can occur in the absence of specific drug therapy, although more commonly it is recorded in patients who are receiving various anticalcinotic therapeutic regimens.[38–41]

On rare occasions, ossification rather than calcification has been observed in the soft tissues of patients with dermatomyositis and, in one such instance, an osteosarcoma developed in the area of ossification.[75]

Articular Abnormalities

The arthralgia and arthritis of dermatomyositis and polymyositis usually are unaccompanied by radiographic abnormalities or are associated with transient radiographic features, which include soft tissue swelling and periarticular osteoporosis. Destructive joint changes occasionally have been noted,[15, 16, 63] although details of these changes rarely have been presented. An exception to this is the report of Bunch and associates,[42] who found that arthritis of the hands was accompanied by osseous erosion, calcification, and joint instability in six patients with polymyositis. Although overlap features, such as Raynaud's phenomenon and positive results of LE clot test and antinuclear antibody tests, were present in these patients, the primary disease clearly was polymyositis. One patient had a positive serologic test result (1:160) for rheumatoid factor. Reported radiographic changes included soft tissue swelling (particularly in the metacarpophalangeal and interphalangeal joints), periosteal and soft tissue calcification in the form of flecks or small clumps in these same joints, bony erosions (inferior radioulnar, metacarpophalangeal, proximal interphalangeal, and distal interphalangeal joints as well as the ulnar styloid), and alignment abnormalities (flexion deformities of metacarpophalangeal joints; swan-neck deformities). Particularly characteristic was radial subluxation or dislocation at the interphalangeal joint of the thumb ("floppy thumb" sign), which was evident in five of the six patients (Fig. 35–6). Electromyography and muscle biopsies revealed typical findings of inflammatory myopathies. A synovial biopsy of the interphalangeal joint of the thumb outlined inflammatory changes and calcification.

Although Bunch and coworkers[42] included an addendum that described an additional patient with similar articular findings, the specificity and significance of these changes are not yet clear. Oddis and coworkers[86] described four patients with polymyositis or dermatomyositis associated with the anti-Jo-1 antibody who developed deforming, predominantly nonerosive arthropathy with subluxations of the distal interphalangeal joints in the hand. The interphalangeal joint of the thumb showed dramatic subluxation in these patients. The author of this chapter has observed one additional patient with polymyositis who demonstrated considerable deformity in both hands, characterized by lateral subluxation of the interphalangeal joint of the thumb, interphalangeal joint erosions, and periarticular soft tissue calcifications[76] (Fig. 35–7). The possibility that the disorders

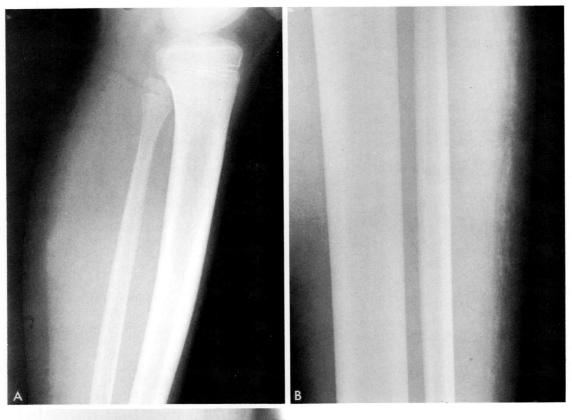

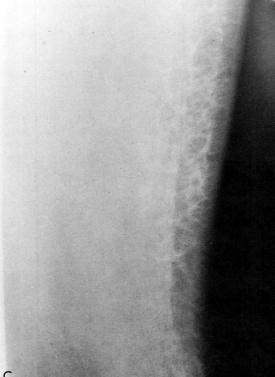

FIGURE 35–2. Dermatomyositis and polymyositis: Early soft tissue edema.

A Note the increased bulk and density of the muscles. Edema has produced poor delineation of the muscle edge.

B In an 11 year old girl with muscle weakness of 5 months' duration, the muscle-subcutaneous tissue interface is blurred by edema.

C Observe extensive edema of the subcutaneous tissue septa.

(From Ozonoff MB, Flynn FJ Jr: AJR *118:*206, 1973. Copyright 1973, American Roentgen Ray Society.)

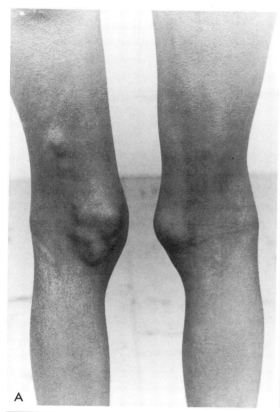
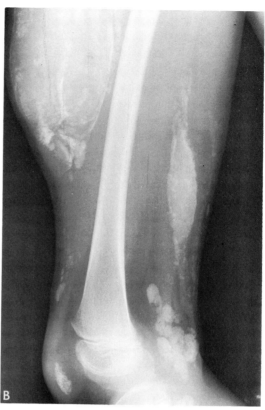
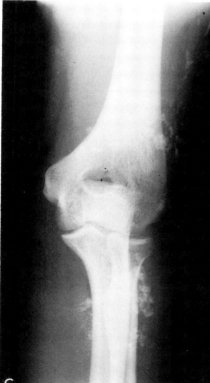

FIGURE 35–3. Dermatomyositis and polymyositis: Intermuscular fascial plane calcification.

A, B In a 10 year old boy with disease of 4 years' duration, large calcareous muscular masses have produced nodular deformity of the overlying skin. Note the "tumoral" nature of the calcifications.

C In a different patient, intermuscular fascial plane calcification has resulted in focal circular radiodense areas.

(**A, B,** From Ozonoff MB, Flynn FJ Jr: AJR *118:*206, 1973. Copyright 1973, American Roentgen Ray Society.)

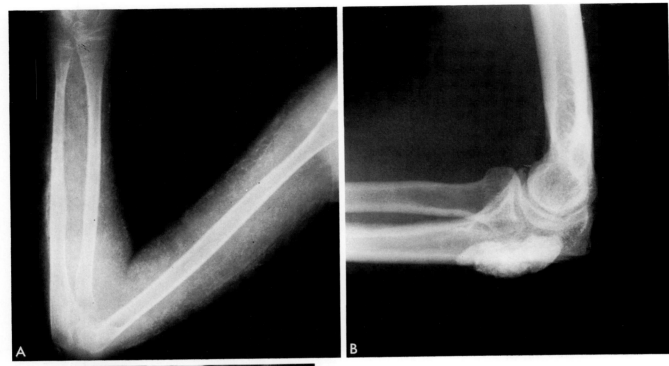

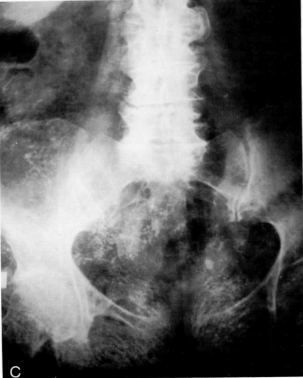

FIGURE 35–4. Dermatomyositis and polymyositis: Subcutaneous calcification.

A In this child, diffuse linear subcutaneous calcinosis is evident.

B In an older patient, a well-circumscribed calcified focus about the elbow is apparent.

C In an elderly woman, a lacy, reticular subcutaneous pattern of calcification is seen.

(Courtesy of L. Goldberger, M.D., San Diego, California.)

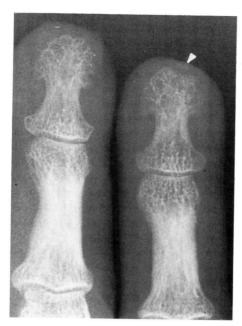

FIGURE 35–5. Dermatomyositis and polymyositis. Tuftal calcification and erosion. Observe soft tissue and tuftal resorption of the third and fourth fingers associated with small calcifications (arrowhead).

in some of these patients were representative of an overlap of several collagen vascular diseases[43] is underscored by the similarities of the floppy thumb sign to thumb abnormalities in systemic lupus erythematosus[44, 45] and of the calcification to that seen in scleroderma or systemic lupus erythematosus.[46] Indeed, in some patients with polymyositis, extensive erosions about the interphalangeal joints of the hands has been accompanied by periarticular and intra-articular calcification related to hydroxyapatite crystal deposition.[87, 106] Thus, it is possible that some of the joint manifestations of polymyositis or dermatomyositis are related to crystal accumulation. The detailed report by Schumacher and collaborators,[63] however, describing nine patients with polymyo-

sitis or dermatomyositis, in some of whom were observed radiographic evidence of joint erosions and pathologic evidence of synovial inflammation and fibrin deposition, may indicate that destructive articular alterations indeed are a distinctive subset of these diseases.

SCINTIGRAPHIC ABNORMALITIES

Although the role of radionuclide examination in the early detection of osseous and articular disorders is well known, its role in the detection and grading of muscular inflammation is less well recognized. Technetium polyphosphate and similar agents may accumulate in abnormal muscle in patients with dermatomyositis and polymyositis.[47, 58–60] This abnormal accumulation demonstrates some correlation with the severity of muscle weakness and may improve after corticosteroid therapy. Gallium also may be used in this clinical situation.[61]

MAGNETIC RESONANCE IMAGING ABNORMALITIES

Magnetic resonance (MR) imaging is well suited to the analysis of a variety of muscle disorders, including dermatomyositis and polymyositis. Kaufman and associates[88] provided one of the early descriptions of the role of MR imaging in this regard. They examined five patients with polymyositis and eight with dermatomyositis; 8 of these 13 patients had clinically active disease. Using standard spin echo techniques, these investigators observed muscle atrophy, fatty replacement of muscles, and intramuscular regions of decreased signal intensity that correlated in extent with the activity of the disease processes. Keim and coworkers[89] and Hernandez and collaborators[90] studied patients with juvenile dermatomyositis using both T1- and T2-weighted spin echo imaging. At the outset of the disease, a significant increase in signal intensity on the T2-weighted MR images occurred in the involved muscle groups. With clinical improvement, this signal intensity returned to normal and, with the recurrence of clinically evi-

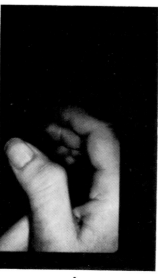

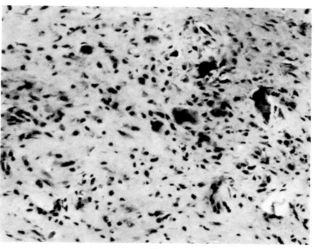

FIGURE 35–6. Dermatomyositis and polymyositis: "Floppy thumb sign."

A This deformity is characterized by radial subluxation at the interphalangeal joint of the first digit.

B Synovial biopsy of the interphalangeal joint of the right thumb in a 69 year old man reveals inflammatory changes of a nodular type with calcification (250×).

(From Bunch TW, et al: Arthritis Rheum 19:243, 1976.)

A

B

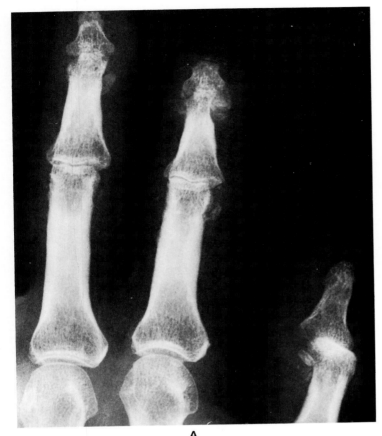

A

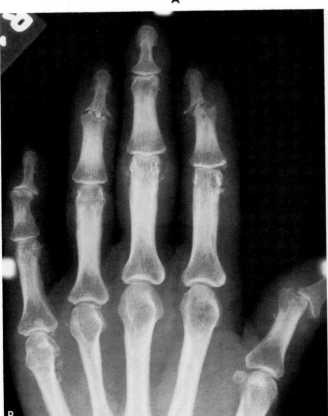

B

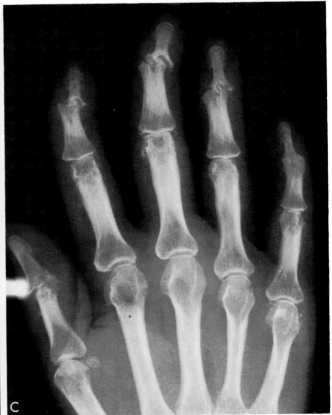

C

FIGURE 35–7. Dermatomyositis and polymyositis: Destructive articular abnormalities.

A Observe tuftal destruction and erosion at several distal interphalangeal joints, bony fragmentation, and periarticular calcification in a 52 year old man with severe muscular and articular abnormalities.

B, C In a 50 year old woman with well-documented polymyositis, note bilateral articular abnormalities consisting of erosions of multiple distal interphalangeal joints, periarticular calcifications, and subluxation of the interphalangeal joint of the right thumb.

dent disease activity, an increase in signal intensity at sites of muscle involvement again was noted on the T2-weighted images. The authors postulated that shifts in the distribution of water owing to muscle inflammation and infarction were responsible for the imaging abnormalities. They also indicated that similar alterations in signal intensity could occur in muscles affected by infection, infarction, trauma, and rhabdomyolysis. The investigators discounted the effect of steroid-induced myopathy in the production of the MR imaging abnormalities.

Other studies generally have confirmed the usefulness of this imaging method in the assessment of the degree, activity, and distribution of muscle involvement in dermatomyositis and polymyositis. Differences have been found in the patterns of muscle abnormalities in these inflammatory disorders when compared with congenital myopathies and muscular dystrophies,[91] although in all disease categories, certain muscles appear to be less affected than others, perhaps related to specific anatomic and functional characteristics.[91] In some investigations, predominant involvement of the vastus lateralis muscle and, to a lesser extent, the vastus intermedius and vastus medialis muscles, with relative sparing of the rectus femoris and biceps femoris muscles, has been noted in patients with dermatomyositis.[92] T1 and T2 values in affected muscles have been higher than those in normal controls.[92] P-31 spectra of the diseased muscles have shown decreased concentrations of adenosine triphosphate and phosphocreatine, and these metabolic data have correlated with clinical assessment.[92] Preliminary evidence also has suggested that a correlation exists between histopathologic findings and the degree of abnormality revealed by MR spectroscopy.[88, 93]

Although most of the reported investigations of the value of MR imaging in the assessment of inflammatory muscle disease have stressed standard spin echo sequences, some of the more recent ones have employed modified imaging parameters. One of these, fat suppression, has shown promise in this regard.[107] As an example, Fraser and colleagues[94] compared quantitative and qualitative indices of signal intensity in muscle in patients with myositis to two measures of disease activity: a subjective global impression of disease activity and a quantitative measure of such activity based on level of muscle enzymes and strength. Seventeen patients had polymyositis, 10 had dermatomyositis, and 13 had inclusion body myositis (see later discussion in this chapter). These investigators used T1- and T2-weighted spin echo sequences and a short tau (inversion time) inversion recovery (STIR) sequence. The last, characterized by a 180 degree inversion pulse prior to a standard spin echo technique, can be designed to suppress the signal of fat. T2-weighted images were found useful in identifying abnormally high signal intensity in muscle, particularly in patients with acute or newly diagnosed disease; however, in those with chronic disease, differentiation of areas of myositis and of fatty infiltration was difficult. STIR imaging improved diagnostic accuracy, with areas of muscle inflammation displaying high signal intensity on a background of depressed signal of fat. Both transaxial and coronal images provided useful information, and the signal intensity of affected muscles on the STIR sequences was higher in patients with clinically active disease than in those with inactive disease. Of interest, differences in the distribution patterns of disease were seen with MR imaging in

dermatomyositis and polymyositis versus inclusion body myositis. In polymyositis, involvement was greater in the anterior than in the posterior compartment in the leg and a more focal pattern of increased signal intensity was seen.

Hernandez and coworkers[95] confirmed the value of fat suppressed MR imaging in the evaluation of muscle disease in a small group of children with dermatomyositis or similar disorders. In their study, a hybrid fat suppression technique was employed.[96] This hybrid method uses two distinct techniques to suppress the signal of fat. In the first, a 180 degree refocusing radiofrequency pulse is shifted temporarily to render the water and fat components of the signal in and out of phase on alternate acquisitions. Subtraction of these echoes during signal averaging ideally yields only the desired water signal.[95] In the second technique, a frequency-selected binomial pulse precedes the spin echo segment of the sequences to saturate the fat signal selectively with little effect on the water signal.[95] In a direct comparison of conventional T2-weighted spin echo images and T2-weighted fat suppressed images, Hernandez and coworkers found that the latter method improved the detection of muscle abnormalities owing to the greater contrast provided by the suppression of the fat signal (Fig 35–8). The signal intensity in unaffected muscles was decreased to a greater extent than that in involved muscles, presumably related to a greater concentration of fat in normal musculature. Abnormal muscles demonstrated higher signal intensity owing to prolongation of the T2 relaxation time, which likely is due to accumulation of extracellular water.

These fat suppression methods have been employed increasingly in the analysis of disorders of the musculoskele-

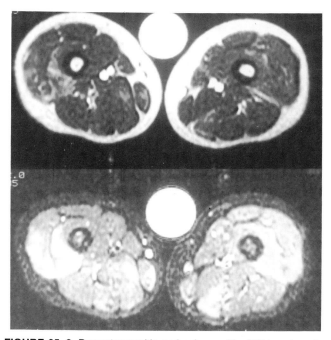

FIGURE 35–8. Dermatomyositis and polymyositis: MR imaging abnormalities. This 7 year old girl had clinical and serologic evidence of dermatomyositis. In the top image, a T2-weighted (TR/TE, 2500/80) spin echo MR image of the thighs, in the transverse plane, reveals subtle abnormalities in signal intensity of the vastus lateralis muscle on the right side. In the bottom image, a fat-suppressed T2-weighted (TR/TE, 2500/80) spin echo MR image delineates more extensive muscle abnormalities in both thighs. (Reproduced with permission from Hernandez RJ, et al: Radiology 182:217, 1992.)

tal system. Basically, by reducing the masking effect of fat, these techniques accentuate the visibility of alterations in tissue water.[95] The resulting regions of high signal intensity are not diagnostic of any particular pathologic condition (i.e., tumor, infection, edema), but in the clinical setting of myositis, edematous tissue clearly can be distinguished from fat when such techniques are used. An advantage of the STIR method is that contrast for T1 and T2 effects is additive, making it extremely sensitive for the detection of changes in water content; disadvantages include a poor signal to noise ratio, a limited number of available sections, and supression that is not specific for fat.[97–99] Furthermore, enhancement techniques using intravenous administration of gadolinium compounds are not compatible with STIR imaging. Hybrid methods of chemical shift imaging produce fat suppression while maintaining images with high contrast and a good signal to noise ratio.[95]

On analysis of reported experience with MR imaging in patients with polymyositis and dermatomyositis, it becomes evident that this method shows great promise in several respects: it reveals signal intensity alterations in muscle that correlate with disease activity; changes in signal patterns can be used to monitor response to therapy; muscle sites suitable for biopsy can be ascertained; and specific findings on MR imaging studies may allow differentiation of these muscle diseases and others. Furthermore, signal intensity of involved muscles appears to correlate with muscle strength, although abnormal MR imaging findings and serum levels of muscle enzymes may have different sensitivities.[107]

PATHOLOGIC ABNORMALITIES

On gross examination, involved skeletal muscles in dermatomyositis and polymyositis frequently are pale red, grayish red, or yellowish in color. They feel soft and friable or rubbery and firm. The microscopic aberrations in involved musculature have been well delineated[10, 48] (Fig. 35–9). As outlined by Pearson,[12] these findings include focal or extensive degeneration of muscle fibers; regenerative activity characterized by basophilia of fibers and prominent nuclei; muscle necrosis; infiltration with chronic inflammatory cells, particularly lymphocytes and plasma cells; interstitial fibrosis; phagocytosis of necrotic fibers; and variation in cross-sectional diameter of adjacent muscle fibers. These histologic aberrations vary little among the various subgroups of the disease.[77] In children with dermatomyositis, angiitis frequently is a prominent feature in the abnormal musculature,[4] suggesting that muscle lesions are ischemic

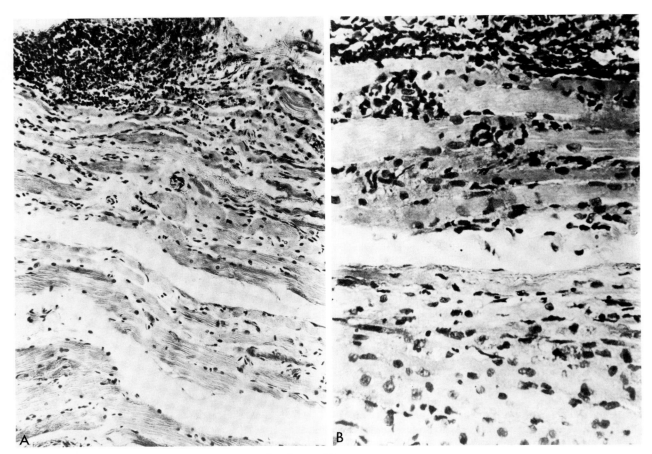

FIGURE 35–9. Dermatomyositis and polymyositis: Muscular abnormalities.
   A A biopsy specimen of an involved muscle demonstrates marked inflammatory infiltration. Fibers show variation in size with degeneration, some regeneration, and fibrosis.
   B In the same muscle, perivascular cuffing with inflammatory cells, particularly mononuclear cells, is evident. There is variation in nuclear size in the muscles. At the bottom, regenerating fibers with large nuclei are apparent.
   (From Ansell BM: Dermatomyositis and polymyositis. *In* JT Scott [Ed]: Copeman's Textbook of the Rheumatic Diseases. 5th Ed. Edinburgh, Churchill-Livingstone, 1978.)

in origin. Ultrastructural studies confirm the microscopic muscular abnormalities.[49] After treatment, some improvement in the microscopic appearance of involved muscles is seen, although precise correlation between any of the morphologic features and specific clinical parameters generally is lacking.[77]

ETIOLOGY AND PATHOGENESIS

Although the cause of dermatomyositis and polymyositis is unknown, several mechanisms have been suggested as the primary cause of the muscle damage. Considerable evidence exists that a cell-mediated immune mechanism is responsible for this damage by affecting either the muscle or the adjacent blood vessels.[50–53, 65] A genetic predisposition to such immunologic mechanisms has been suggested, as an abnormal circulating antinuclear antibody (anti-Jo-1) has been identified in 23 per cent of patients with dermatomyositis or polymyositis.[78] Furthermore, an association of this finding with the histocompatibility antigen HLA-DR 3 has been observed.[70, 78] The prevalence of this antigen, as well as the combination of HLA antigens A7, B8, and CW7, reportedly is increased in childhood dermatomyositis.[68] Autoallergic myositis can be produced experimentally when an animal is immunized with its own muscle and Freund's adjuvant.[79]

An infectious cause also is plausible.[64] Virus-like inclusions in endothelial cells have been recorded in dermatomyositis, although viruses have not been isolated. The possibility of a viral cause for this disorder is strengthened by the observation that a clinical picture resembling dermatomyositis may occur in some patients with disseminated viral infections (see later discussion).[54–57] The association of dermatomyositis and neoplasm has raised the additional possibility that tumor may precipitate inflammatory muscle disease, perhaps by provoking a cross sensitization to a muscle component or combining with a component of muscle to form a complex allergen.[27]

OTHER DISEASES OF MUSCLE

Inclusion Body Myositis

It was Chou's report in 1967[100] that initially called attention to an inflammatory process of muscle characterized by the presence of intranuclear and cytoplasmic inclusions within cells derived from muscle biopsy. Electron microscopic study of these inclusions showed structures that resembled paramyxovirus nucleocapsid. Other reports subsequently appeared of cases of myositis in which similar histopathologic findings were evident.[101, 102]

Inclusion body myositis is a rare disease occurring predominantly in men. The age of onset is variable, with the disease appearing from the second through the eighth decades of life.[103–105] Clinical findings resemble those of polymyositis, although some patients also have distal or asymmetric weakness and neuropathic changes on electromyography.[105] The course of the disease is variable; muscle weakness may progress slowly or reach a plateau.[105] Laboratory analysis indicates mild or minimal elevation of muscle enzyme levels.[103] In contrast to polymyositis, there is little or no association with malignancy or connective tissue disease (although inclusion body myositis has been reported in

association with rheumatoid arthritis[108]), and patients with inclusion body myositis show resistence to high-dose corticosteroid therapy.[103] Also, as outlined earlier, MR imaging may reveal distinctive changes in this disease.[94] Most important, however, in the differentiation of inclusion body myositis from polymyositis are the distinctive pathologic features of the former disease, with identification of large intranuclear and intracytoplasmic inclusions with light microscopy and of characteristic microtubular elements with electron microscopy.

DIFFERENTIAL DIAGNOSIS

Soft Tissue Abnormalities

Soft tissue calcification is a common feature of various collagen vascular diseases, particularly dermatomyositis (polymyositis) and scleroderma. In dermatomyositis and polymyositis, calcific deposits may appear in intermuscular fascial planes, providing distinctive radiographic features, which are seen more rarely in other collagen vascular diseases. Occasionally this pattern of calcification may be simulated by findings in scleroderma, systemic lupus erythematosus, mixed collagen vascular disease, or overlap syndromes. A second pattern of calcification in dermatomyositis and polymyositis relates to deposition in subcutaneous tissue. This appearance has not been emphasized in these disorders, although it is well recognized in scleroderma. Its occurrence in dermatomyositis and polymyositis again emphasizes the similar radiographic features that may be apparent in the various collagen vascular diseases. Subcutaneous calcification also can be evident in systemic lupus erythematosus, mixed collagen vascular disease, and overlap syndromes.

Periarticular calcific deposits in dermatomyositis and polymyositis generally are linear or punctate in appearance, allowing differentiation in most instances from the ''tumoral'' deposits that are associated with hyperparathyroidism, hypervitaminosis D, and the milk-alkali syndrome.

Articular Abnormalities

If the erosive and deforming arthritis of the hands that has been reported in patients with polymyositis[42, 76] is further documented in future reports, it will require differentiation from abnormalities accompanying other diseases. In particular, severe deformity of the interphalangeal joint of the thumb may be apparent in additional collagen vascular disorders, especially systemic lupus erythematosus. Interphalangeal joint erosions (with or without metacarpophalangeal joint and wrist abnormalities), which were noted in these previous reports,[42, 76] also may occur in scleroderma, rheumatoid arthritis, psoriasis, multicentric reticulohistiocytosis, and gout, and after thermal injuries.

SUMMARY

Dermatomyositis and polymyositis are disorders of unknown cause characterized by inflammation and degeneration of muscle. A variety of clinical patterns may be observed in both children and adults affected by these disorders. The radiographic features of musculoskeletal involvement consist of soft tissue edema, atrophy, contracture, and calcification; bony resorption (phalangeal tufts); and, possibly, articular erosion and subluxation. These features most resemble abnormalities accompanying other collagen vascular diseases, including scleroderma and systemic lupus erythematosus.

References

1. Unverricht H: Polymyositis acuta progressiva. Zeitschr Klin Med 12:533, 1887.
2. Pearson CM: Polymyositis. Annu Rev Med 17:63, 1966.
3. Williams RC Jr: Dermatomyositis and malignancy: A review of the literature. Ann Intern Med 50:1174, 1959.
4. Banker BQ, Victor M: Dermatomyositis (systemic angiopathy) of childhood. Medicine 45:261, 1966.
5. Sullivan DB, Cassidy JT, Petty RE, et al: Prognosis in childhood dermatomyositis. J Pediatr 80:555, 1972.
6. Wedgwood RIP, Cook CD, Cohen J: Dermatomyositis: Report of 26 cases in children with discussion of endocrine therapy in 13. Pediatrics 12:447, 1953.
7. Everett MA, Curtis AC: Dermatomyositis. A review of nineteen cases in adolescents and children. Arch Intern Med 100:70, 1957.
8. Muller SA, Winkelmann RK, Brunsting LA: Calcinosis in dermatomyositis. Observations on course of disease in children and adults. Arch Dermatol 79:669, 1959.
9. Bunim JJ: A broader spectrum of Sjögren's syndrome and its pathogenetic implications. Ann Rheum Dis 20:1, 1961.
10. Walton JN, Adams RD: Polymyositis. Baltimore, Williams & Wilkins, 1958.
11. Medsger TA, Robinson H, Masi AT: Factors affecting survivorship in polymyositis: A life-table study of 124 patients. Arthritis Rheum 14:249, 1971.
12. Pearson CM: Polymyositis and dermatomyositis. In JL Hollander, DJ McCarty Jr (Eds): Arthritis and Allied Conditions. 8th Ed. Philadelphia, Lea & Febiger, 1972, p 940.
13. Pearson CM: Rheumatic manifestations of polymyositis and dermatomyositis. Arthritis Rheum 2:127, 1959.
14. Barwick DO, Walton JN: Polymyositis. Am J Med 35:646, 1963.
15. Sheard C Jr: Dermatomyositis. Arch Intern Med 88:640, 1951.
16. Logan RG, Bandera JM, Mikkelsen WM, et al: Polymyositis: A clinical study. Ann Intern Med 65:996, 1966.
17. O'Leary PA, Waisman M: Dermatomyositis: A study of forty cases. Arch Dermatol 41:1001, 1940.
18. Eaton LM: The perspective of neurology in regard to polymyositis: A study of 41 cases. Neurology 4:245, 1954.
19. Schaumburg HH, Nielson SL, Yurchak PM: Heart block in polymyositis. N Engl J Med 284:480, 1971.
20. Fernandez-Herlihy L: Heart block in polymyositis. N Engl J Med 284:1101, 1971.
21. Lynch PG: Cardiac involvement in chronic polymyositis. Br Heart J 33:416, 1971.
22. Duncan PE, Griffin JP, Garcia A, et al: Fibrosing alveolitis in polymyositis. A review of histologically confirmed cases. Am J Med 57:621, 1974.
23. Kagen LJ: Myoglobulinemia and myoglobinuria in patients with myositis. Arthritis Rheum 14:457, 1971.
24. Susac J, Garcia-Mullin R, Glaser JS: Ophthalmoplegia in dermatomyositis. Neurology 23:305, 1973.
25. Arundell F, Wilkinson RD, Haserick JR: Dermatomyositis and malignant neoplasms in adults. Arch Dermatol 82:772, 1960.
26. Shy GM: The late onset myopathy. World Neurology 3:149, 1962.
27. Ansell BM: Dermatomyositis and polymyositis. In JT Scott (Ed): Copeman's Textbook of the Rheumatic Diseases. 5th Ed. Edinburgh, Churchill Livingstone, 1978, p 923.
28. Vignos PJ, Goldwyn J: Evaluation of laboratory tests in the diagnosis and management of polymyositis. Am J Med Sci 263:291, 1972.
29. Marinacci AA: Electromyography in the diagnosis of polymyositis. Electromyography 5:255, 1965.
30. Ozonoff MB, Flynn FJ Jr: Roentgenologic features of dermatomyositis of childhood. AJR 118:206, 1973.
31. Wheeler CE, Curtis AC, Cawley EP, et al: Soft tissue calcification with special reference to its occurrence in "collagen diseases." Ann Intern Med 36:1050, 1952.
32. Steiner RM, Glassman L, Schwartz MW, et al: The radiological findings in dermatomyositis of childhood. Radiology 111:385, 1974.
33. Sewell JR, Liyanage B, Ansell BM: Calcinosis in juvenile dermatomyositis. Skel Radiol 3:137, 1978.
34. Dubowitz LMS, Dubowitz V: Acute dermatomyositis presenting with pulmonary manifestations. Arch Dis Child 39:293, 1964.
35. Bitnum S, Daeschner CW Jr, Travis LB, et al: Dermatomyositis. J Pediatr 64:101, 1964.
36. Spahr A, Brenn H: Die Calcinosis interstitialis bei Dermatomyositis. Helv Paediatr Acta 12:48, 1957.
37. Vanace PW: Chronic state treatment of dermatomyositis. Arthritis Rheum 20(Suppl 2):342, 1977.
38. Cram RL, Barnada R, Geho WB, et al: Diphosphonate treatment of calcinosis universalis. N Engl J Med 285:1012, 1971.
39. Dent CE, Stamp TCB: Treatment of calcinosis circumscripta with probenecid. Br Med J 1:216, 1972.
40. Herd JK, Vaughan JH: Calcinosis universalis complicating dermatomyositis—its treatment with disodium EDTA. Arthritis Rheum 7:259, 1964.
41. Nassim JR, Connolly CK: Treatment of calcinosis universalis with aluminum hydroxide. Arch Dis Child 45:118, 1970.
42. Bunch TW, O'Duffy JD, McLeod RA: Deforming arthritis of the hands in polymyositis. Arthritis Rheum 19:243, 1976.
43. Lockshin MD: Discussion. Arthritis Rheum 19:247, 1976.
44. Bleifeld CJ, Inglis AE: The hand in systemic lupus erythematosus. J Bone Joint Surg [Am] 56:1207, 1974.
45. Aptekar RG, Lawless OJ, Decker JL: Deforming non-erosive arthritis of the hand in systemic lupus erythematosus. Clin Orthop 100:120, 1974.
46. Kabir DI, Malkinson FD: Lupus erythematosus and calcinosis cutis. Arch Dermatol 100:17, 1969.
47. Brown M, Swift TR, Spies SM: Radioisotope scanning in inflammatory muscle disease. Neurology 26:517, 1976.
48. Adams RD, Denny-Brown D, Pearson CM: Diseases of Muscle: A Study in Pathology. 2nd Ed. New York, Hoeber, 1962.
49. Hughes JT, Esiri MM: Ultrastructural studies in human polymyositis. J Neurol Sci 25:347, 1975.
50. Dawkins RL, Zilko PJ: Polymyositis and myasthenia gravis: Immunodeficiency disorders involving skeletal muscle. Lancet 1:200, 1975.
51. Dawkins RL: Experimental autoallergic myositis, polymyositis and myasthenia gravis. Autoimmune muscle disease associated with immunodeficiency and neoplasia. Clin Exp Immunol 21:185, 1975.
52. Johnson RI, Fink CW, Ziff M: Lymphotoxin formation by lymphocytes and muscle in polymyositis. J Clin Invest 51:2435, 1972.
53. Whitaker JN, Engel WK: Vascular deposits of immunoglobulin and complement in idiopathic inflammatory myopathy. N Engl J Med 286:333, 1972.
54. Middleton PJ, Alexander RM, Szymanski MT: Severe myositis during recovery from influenza. Lancet 2:533, 1970.
55. Dietzman DE, Schaller J, Ray CG, et al: Myositis associated with influenza infections (Abstr). Pediatr Res 8:423, 1974.
56. Chou SM: Myxovirus-like structures and accompanying nuclear changes in chronic polymyositis. Arch Pathol 86:649, 1968.
57. Sato T, Walker DL, Peters HA, et al: Chronic polymyositis and myxovirus-like inclusions. Electron microscopic and viral studies. Arch Neurol 24:409, 1971.
58. Spies SM, Swift TR, Brown M: Increased ^{99m}Tc polyphosphate muscle uptake in a patient with polymyositis: Case report. J Nucl Med 16:1125, 1975.
59. Steinfeld JR, Thorne NA, Kennedy TF: Positive ^{99m}Tc pyrophosphate bone scan in polymyositis. Radiology 122:168, 1977.
60. Siegel BA, Engel WK, Derrer EC: ^{99m}Tc diphosphonate uptake in skeletal muscle: A quantitative index of acute damage. Neurology 25:1055, 1975.
61. Smith WP, Robinson RG, Gobuty AH: Positive whole-body ^{67}Ga scintigraphy in dermatomyositis. AJR 133:126, 1979.
62. Dietz F, Logeman JA, Sahgal V, et al: Cricopharyngeal muscle dysfunction in the differential diagnosis of dysphagia in polymyositis. Arthritis Rheum 23:491, 1980.
63. Schumacher HR, Schimmer B, Gordon GV, et al: Articular manifestations of polymyositis and dermatomyositis. Am J Med 67:287, 1979.
64. Chaouat D: Pathogénie des polymyosites. Nouv Presse Med 9:1435, 1980.
65. Nishikai M, Reichlin M: Heterogeneity of precipitating antibodies in polymyositis and dermatomyositis. Arthritis Rheum 23:881, 1980.
66. Bohan A, Peter JB: Polymyositis and dermatomyositis. N Engl J Med 292:344, 1982.
67. Bradley WG: Inflammatory disease of muscle. In WN Kelley, ED Harris Jr, S Ruddy, CB Sledge (Eds): Textbook of Rheumatology. Philadelphia, WB Saunders, 1981, p 1255.
68. Callen JP: Dermatomyositis. Dermatol Clin 1:461, 1983.
69. Black KA, Zilko PJ, Dawkins RL, et al: Cancer in connective tissue disease. Arthritis Rheum 25:1130, 1982.
70. Pachman LM, Maryjowski MC: Juvenile dermatomyositis and polymyositis. Clin Rheum Dis 10:95, 1984.
71. Hanissian AS, Masi AT, Pitner SE, et al: Polymyositis and dermatomyositis in children: An epidemiologic and clinical comparative analysis. J Rheumatol 9:390, 1982.
72. Crowe WE, Bove KE, Levinson JE, et al: Clinical and pathogenetic implications of histopathology in childhood polydermatomyositis. Arthritis Rheum 25:126, 1982.
73. Blane CE, White SJ, Braunstein EM, et al: Patterns of calcification in childhood dermatomyositis. AJR 142:397, 1984.
74. Bruguier A, Texier P, Sluzewski W, et al: Les calcinoses des dermatomyositis infantiles. A propos de 10 cas. Helv Paediatr Acta 39:47, 1984.
75. Eckardt JJ, Ivins JC, Perry HO, et al: Osteosarcoma arising in heterotopic ossification of dermatomyositis. Cancer 48:1256, 1981.
76. Greenway G, Weisman MH, Resnick D, et al: Deforming arthritis of the hands: An unusual manifestation of polymyositis. AJR 136:611, 1981.
77. Schwarz HA, Slavin G, Ward P, et al: Muscle biopsy in polymyositis and dermatomyositis: A clinicopathological study. Ann Rheum Dis 39:500, 1980.
78. Arnett FC, Hirsch TJ, Bias WB, et al: The Jo-1 antibody system in myositis: Relationships to clinical features and HLA. J Rheumatol 8:925, 1981.
79. Dawkins RL: Experimental autoallergic myositis, polymyositis, and myasthenia gravis-autoimmune muscle disease associated with immunodeficiency and neoplasia. Clin Exp Immunol 21:185, 1975.
80. Benbassat J, Gefel D, Larholt KL, et al: Prognostic factors in polymyositis/dermatomyositis. Arthritis Rheum 28:249, 1985.
81. Tymms KE, Webb J: Dermatomyositis and other connective tissue diseases: A review of 105 cases. J. Rheumatol 12:1140, 1985.

82. Pachman LN: Juvenile dermatomyositis. Pediatr Clin North Am *33:*1097, 1986.

83. Schulman P, Kerr LD, Spiera H: A reexamination of the relationship between myositis and malignancy. J Rheumatol *18:*1689, 1991.

84. Manchul LA, Jin A, Pritchard KI, et al: The frequency of malignant neoplasms in patients with polymyositis-dermatomyositis. Arch Intern Med *145:*1835, 1985.

85. Lakhanpal S, Bunch TW, Ilstrup DM, et al: Polymyositis-dermatomyositis and malignant lesions: Does an association exist? Mayo Clin Proc *61:*645, 1986.

86. Oddis CV, Medsger TA Jr, Cooperstein LA: A subluxing arthropathy associated with the anti-Jo-1 antibody in polymyositis/dermatomyositis. Arthritis Rheum *33:*1640, 1990.

87. Kazmers IS, Scoville CD, Schumacher HR: Polymyositis associated apatite arthritis. J Rheumatol *15:*1019, 1988.

88. Kaufman LD, Gruber BL, Gersten DP, et al: Preliminary observations on the role of magnetic resonance imaging for polymyositis and dermatomyositis. Ann Rheum Dis *46:*569, 1987.

89. Keim DR, Hernandez RJ, Sullivan DB: Serial magnetic resonance imaging in juvenile dermatomyositis. Arthritis Rheum *34:*1580, 1991.

90. Hernandez RJ, Keim DR, Sullivan DB, et al: Magnetic resonance imaging appearance of the muscles in childhood dermatomyositis. J Pediatr *117:*546, 1990.

91. Lamminen AE: Magnetic resonance imaging of primary skeletal muscle diseases: Patterns of distribution and severity of involvement. Br J Radiol *63:*946, 1990.

92. Park JH, Vansant JP, Kumar NG, et al: Dermatomyositis: Correlative MR imaging and P-31 MR spectroscopy for quantitative characterization of inflammatory disease. Radiology *177:*473, 1990.

93. Borghi L, Savoldi F, Scelsi R, et al: Nuclear magnetic resonance response of protons in normal and pathological human muscles. Exp Neurol *81:*89, 1983.

94. Fraser DD, Frank JA, Dalakas M, et al: Magnetic resonance imaging in the idiopathic inflammatory myopathies. J Rheumatol *18:*1693, 1991.

95. Hernandez RJ, Keim DR, Chenevert TL, et al: Fat-suppressed MR imaging of myositis. Radiology *182:*217, 1992.

96. Szumowski J, Eisen JK, Vinitski S, et al: Hybrid methods of chemical-shift imaging. Magn Reson Med *9:*379, 1989.

97. Dousset M, Weissleder R, Hendrick RE, et al: Short T1 inversion-recovery imaging of the liver: Pulse-sequence optimization and comparison with spin-echo imaging. Radiology *171:*327, 1989.

98. Bydder GM, Young IR: MR imaging: Clinical use of the inversion recovery sequence. J Comput Assist Tomogr *9:*659, 1985.

99. Shuman WP, Baron RL, Peters MJ, et al: Comparison of STIR and spin-echo MR imaging at 1.5 T in 90 lesions of the chest, liver, and pelvis. AJR *152:*852, 1989.

100. Chou SM: Myxovirus-like structure in a case of human polymyositis. Science *158:*1453, 1967.

101. Yunis EJ, Samaha FJ: Inclusion body myositis. Lab Invest *25:*240, 1971.

102. Carpenter S, Karpati G, Heller I, et al: Inclusion body myositis: A distinct variety of inflammatory myopathy. Neurology *28:*8, 1978.

103. Calabrese LH, Mitsumoto H, Chou SM: Inclusion body myositis presenting as treatment-resistant polymyositis. Arthritis Rheum *30:*397, 1987.

104. Sayers ME, Chou SM, Calabrese LH: Inclusion body myositis: Analysis of 32 cases. J Rheumatol *19:*1385, 1992.

105. Wortmann RL: The dilemma of treating patients with inclusion body myositis. J Rheumatol *19:*1327, 1992.

106. Schultz E, Barland P: Erosive arthritis with dermatomyositis without elevated anti-Jo-1 antibodies and not associated with pain. J Rheumatol *20:*597, 1993.

107. Hernandez RJ, Sullivan DB, Chenevert TL, et al: MR imaging in children with dermatomyositis: Musculoskeletal findings and correlation with clinical and laboratory findings. AJR *161:*359, 1993.

108. Soden M, Boundy K, Burrow D, et al: Inclusion body myositis in association with rheumatoid arthritis. J Rheumatol *21:*344, 1994.

Polyarteritis Nodosa and Other Vasculitides

Donald Resnick, M.D.

A variety of disorders are characterized by inflammation of blood vessels. Clinical symptoms and signs in these disorders are protean, depending on the distribution, the extent, and the severity of the vascular lesions; although musculoskeletal abnormalities may be encountered, these usually are overshadowed by findings related to involvement of other organ systems. Characteristic radiographic findings are detected most reliably by arteriography. Abnormalities on plain films related to articular and osseous involvement generally are infrequent and nonspecific.

In this chapter, the major vasculitides are discussed. Radiographic features are delineated without emphasis on angiographic abnormalities, which are discussed elsewhere in the book (Chapter 14). The discussion, by design, is brief, as the role of plain film radiography in the evaluation of musculoskeletal alterations in these disorders is limited.

HISTORICAL ASPECTS AND CLASSIFICATION OF VASCULITIDES

In 1866, Kussmaul and Maier[1] used the term "periarteritis nodosa" to describe an inflammatory necrotizing disease of medium-sized blood vessels causing nodular aneurysms at sites of vascular necrosis. With the appearance of subsequent reports describing additional patients with this disease, a problem in terminology became evident. The designation "nodosa" was discarded by some observers because of the lack of nodular lesions in many cases. Furthermore, because inflammation of the entire thickness of the arterial wall was evident in this disorder, the terms "panarteritis" and "polyarteritis" were substituted as more appropriate than "periarteritis."

In 1952, Zeek[2] used the generic term "necrotizing angiitis" to describe five forms of vasculitis: periarteritis nodosa; angiitis associated with hypersensitivity to serum and drugs (hypersensitivity angiitis); angiitis in patients with a long history of asthma who abruptly developed a fatal illness accompanied by fever and eosinophilia (allergic granulomatous angiitis); arteritis occurring in the hearts and lungs of patients with fulminant rheumatic fever (rheumatic arteritis); and temporal (giant cell) arteritis. The separation of cases into one of these five groups was based on the distribution, the type, the size, and the pathologic features of vascular involvement, a separation that, according to some investigators, was not always feasible.[3]

The limitations of the classification systems for the vasculitides became increasingly obvious in the last 30 years because of the enlarging spectrum of these disorders.[4] The term "hypersensitivity angiitis" was expanded to include several cutaneous and visceral syndromes characterized by necrotizing or allergic angiitis.[5, 6] Inflammatory vascular complications became well known in rheumatoid arthritis and systemic lupus erythematosus. Wegener's granulomatosis, a disease that is associated with necrotizing granulomas of the respiratory tract, generalized necrotizing vasculitis, and focal glomerulonephritis,[7] also became well recognized. Less inflammatory types of systemic vascular diseases were identified, such as a nonspecific arteritis of the aorta and its branches (Takayasu arteritis)[8] and the vascular changes that accompany scleroderma.[9]

The histologic characteristics of the vascular lesions have

been used as guidelines for classification of the various systemic vascular disorders[4] despite overlapping of certain clinical and pathologic characteristics. Three groups of diseases were recognized: inflammatory vascular lesions (necrotizing angiitis), including polyarteritis nodosa, hypersensitivity angiitis, granulomatous angiitis, and Wegener's granulomatosis; vasculitides accompanied by granuloma formation, including granulomatous angiitis, Wegener's granulomatosis, temporal arteritis, and Takayasu arteritis; and vasculitides associated with intimal hyperplasia, necrosis of the media and elastic lamina, and varying degrees of inflammation in the adventitia and vasa vasorum, including temporal arteritis, Takayasu arteritis, and scleroderma.

In 1980, Alarcón-Segovia[45] identified three major groups of vasculitides that, he believed, were distinct, on the bases of both pathologic characteristics and size of the affected vessels: polyarteritis nodosa group, small vessel vasculitides, and giant cell arteritides. Characteristics of the first group were involvement of medium-sized and, to a lesser extent, small-sized arteries, the presence of microaneurysms, the sequential initiation of the arterial damage, and histologic findings varying from acute inflammation to necrosis to scarring. Included in the polyarteritis nodosa group were generalized or classic disease, localized (to pulmonary, mesenteric, or other vessels) disease, and Kawasaki's disease (with prominent coronary artery involvement). Small vessel vasculitides, the second group, were characterized by involvement of arterioles and venules and, commonly, by prominent or exclusive skin involvement. Disorders in this group were numerous and diverse; some produced granulomatous reaction (Churg-Strauss syndrome, Wegener's granulomatosis), whereas others did not. Giant cell arteritides affected large arteries and consisted principally of two diseases: cranial (temporal) arteritis, which occurs in elderly Caucasian subjects; and Takayasu arteritis, which affects the aorta, especially in young Oriental people and American Indians.

Classification of vascular disorders not on histopathology but on pathogenesis also had been attempted.[4] Hypersensitivity appeared to be important in the development of disorders in the necrotizing angiitis group. The pathogenesis of granulomatous lesions was not clear, although a delayed type of hypersensitivity was considered important. The pathogenesis of disorders characterized by intimal hypertrophy was not defined.

The preceding historical review underscores the difficulty encountered in attempting to classify the diverse group of disorders that lead to inflammation of the walls of blood vessels. Involvement of vascular channels of varying size and of different organ systems, a spectrum of histologic aberrations, and incomplete understanding of causative mechanisms have contributed to this difficulty. Recognizing the problems created by the lack of a uniformly accepted classification system, the American College of Rheumatology appointed a subcommittee to investigate the possibility of developing a standard classification of vasculitis.[80] Only seven forms of vasculitis that usually are considered clinically distinct syndromes were considered by the committee: polyarteritis nodosa, Churg-Strauss syndrome, Wegener's granulomatosis, hypersensitivity vasculitis, Henoch-Schönlein purpura, giant cell (temporal) arteritis, and Takayasu arteritis. The report of this subcommittee was published in

1990, in a series of articles, some of which are referenced in this chapter. Eight hundred and seven patients gathered from 48 medical centers served as the study sample. Classification rules for each of the seven disorders were developed by comparing patients who had a particular vasculitis with the remaining group of vasculitis patients.[81] Final criteria were presented in a traditional format and as a classification tree, the latter serving as a diagnostic algorithm.

POLYARTERITIS NODOSA

General Features

Polyarteritis nodosa is a disorder of unknown cause characterized by inflammation and necrosis in the walls of medium-sized and small arteries. It affects men more frequently than women and occurs predominantly in young and middle-aged adults (20 to 50 years of age).[3] Occasionally, it may become evident in older and younger persons, including infants.[10]

Ten diagnostic criteria for polyarteritis nodosa were chosen by the subcommittee of the American College of Rheumatology.[82] These were weight loss of 4 kg of more; livedo reticularis (mottled reticular pattern in the skin of portions of the extremities or torso); testicular pain or tenderness (not due to infection, trauma, or other causes); myalgias, weakness, or leg tenderness; mononeuropathy or polyneuropathy; diastolic blood pressure greater than 90 mm Hg; elevated levels of blood urea nitrogen or creatinine; the presence of hepatitis B surface antigen or antibody in serum; arteriographic abnormality (characterized by aneurysms or occlusions of the visceral arteries, not due to arteriosclerosis, fibromuscular dysplasia, or other noninflammatory causes); and histologic changes (as obtained from a biopsy of a small or medium-sized artery) showing the presence of granulocytes or granulocytes and mononuclear leukocytes in the arterial wall. A patient is considered likely to have polyarteritis nodosa if at least three of these 10 criteria are met.

Clinical Abnormalities

The clinical manifestations of polyarteritis nodosa, which are extremely variable, relate to the distribution and extent of the vascular lesions. The spectrum of disease varies from a mild and limited form to a fulminating and rapidly fatal process.[46] Fever, weight loss, tachycardia, anemia, and leukocytosis are frequent. Renal involvement, which occurs in approximately 75 to 80 per cent of patients, can lead to blood and protein in the urine, hypertension, and renal failure with uremia. Acute vascular episodes involving other abdominal viscera can produce severe abdominal pain and gastrointestinal hemorrhage or perforation. Cardiac manifestations due to coronary artery involvement include myocardial infarction, arrhythmia, and congestive heart failure. Peripheral vascular involvement can lead to gangrene. Pulmonary arteritis and granulomas can be associated with clinical findings, such as asthma, bronchitis, or pneumonia, and radiographic findings, such as infiltration, cavitation, atelectasis, and pleural effusion. Cutaneous manifestations are common and include ulceration, subcutaneous nodules, maculopapules, purpura, and necrotic lesions. Vascular changes in the peripheral and central nervous systems can lead to peripheral neuropathy, convulsions, dementia, cranial nerve palsies, hemiplegia, cerebellar abnormalities, and transverse myelopathy.

Symptoms and signs of muscular involvement include pain, tenderness, and atrophy (related to peripheral neuropathy or ischemic lesions).[11] These clinical findings may be accentuated by activity and relieved by rest. Swelling in the lower extremities, including the feet, has been described in association with periostitis (discussed later in this chapter).[12, 13, 83]

The most prominent articular manifestation in polyarteritis nodosa is pain, which frequently occurs simultaneously with muscular tenderness.[14] Migratory polyarthralgia is characteristic. Larger joints in the lower extremity typically are affected. Actual synovitis with joint effusion is rare, appearing in 10 to 15 per cent of patients who have articular symptoms.[11, 14] Synovial fluid analysis reveals findings indicative of mild inflammation with a moderate increase in the leukocyte count.[46]

An association between polyarteritis and rheumatoid arthritis has been emphasized in recent years.[47] Typically, patients with this combination of disorders reveal high titer seropositive rheumatoid arthritis, antinuclear factor in the serum, and nodules. Widespread necrotizing arteritis is observed with neuropathy, mesenteric vascular occlusion, renal abnormalities, cutaneous ulceration, and scleritis. A relationship between this entity and previous corticosteroid administration has been suggested, although some patients with rheumatoid arthritis and vasculitis have not received such medication.[15, 16] The cause and pathogenesis of arteritis in patients with rheumatoid arthritis, therefore, are not certain, although many types of vascular lesions are well known in rheumatoid disease.[17, 18, 47, 77]

Radiographic Abnormalities

Plain film radiographic manifestations of polyarteritis nodosa are unusual. Soft tissue swelling may accompany arthritis, but cartilaginous and osseous destruction is not apparent. Articular abnormalities are observed not only in the generalized form of the disease but in the localized varieties as well. In this regard, Mekori and associates[48] identified a young Thai man with cutaneous polyarteritis nodosa who developed rapidly progressive arthritis, which first affected his ankles and subsequently involved multiple joints. Radiographs revealed soft tissue swelling, and histologic evaluation of the synovial membrane showed hypertrophic, erythematous tissue with an inflammatory cellular infiltrate (Fig. 36–1). The nonspecific nature of the pathologic aberrations in this case is consistent with those mentioned in other reports[49] and underscores the nondestructive pattern of articular disease that is evident in polyarteritis nodosa.

Periosteal bone formation has been observed in some patients with this disease. Saville[19] described a middle-aged man with pain and swelling of the proximal portion of the lower limbs. Periostitis on both tibiae and fibulae was evident on the radiographs. Although a muscle biopsy revealed arteritis, the periosteum did not show inflammatory changes. Similar cases with pain and swelling of the lower extremity combined with periostitis of the tibia and fibula were observed by Ball and Grayzel (three patients)[12] and by Murray and Jacobson (one patient).[20] In one of Ball and Grayzel's patients, periosteal biopsy revealed focal lesions of the arterioles, whereas synovial biopsy in another patient outlined hyperemia and cellular infiltration. More extensive periosteal bone formation in patients with polyarteritis nodosa was found by Serre and collaborators (tibia, fibula, and metatarsals),[21] by Lovell and Scott (tibia, fibula, radius, and ulna),[22] by Woodward and Andreini (tibia, fibula, and metatarsals),[13] by Meijers and collaborators (femur, tibia, and fibula),[50] and by Short and Webley (fibula and ulna).[51]

It is obvious from these reports and others[83] that periosteal bone formation in patients with polyarteritis nodosa (and other types of arteritis) has predilection for men and for the lower extremities, particularly the tibia and fibula, may be bilateral or unilateral, and is associated with pain and swelling, elevated erythrocyte sedimentation rate, and cutaneous abnormalities (Fig. 36–2). Digital clubbing is uncommon, and symptoms and signs may improve dramatically with corticosteroid therapy. Upper extremity involvement is unusual (Fig. 36–3). Periostitis in this disease gen-

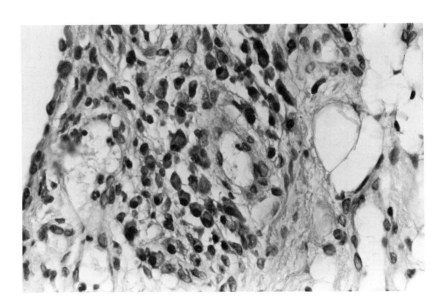

FIGURE 36–1. Polyarteritis nodosa: Articular abnormalities. In this young Thai man with cutaneous polyarteritis nodosa and polyarthritis, histologic evaluation of the synovial membrane obtained during arthroscopy of the knee documents inflammatory cellular infiltration. (From Mekori YA, et al: Arthritis Rheum 27:574, 1984.)

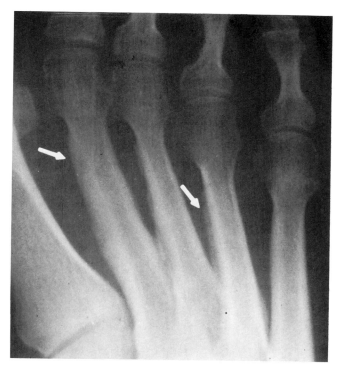

FIGURE 36–2. Polyarteritis nodosa: Periostitis in lower extremity. Observe periosteal new bone formation, predominating on the medial aspect of multiple metatarsals (arrows). (Courtesy of M. Dalinka, M.D., Philadelphia, Pennsylvania.)

erally is identical to that in hypertrophic osteoarthropathy, although more extensive undulating new bone formation has been observed in a few instances (Fig. 36–4).[50, 51]

Ischemic necrosis of bone, leading to osteolysis and osteosclerosis, rarely is recorded in polyarteritis nodosa. Such lesions have been identified in the ribs,[52] tibia, and femur.[53]

Pathologic Abnormalities

Medium and small caliber arteries from involved tissues (kidneys, heart, lungs, liver, spleen, adrenal glands, intestinal tract, testes, nerves, skin) reveal characteristic abnormalities (Fig. 36–5). Initial changes are most common in the tunica media, with subsequent extension into the intima and adventitia and disruption of the internal elastic lamina. Necrosis, fibrinoid change, and cellular infiltration are observed. Polymorphonuclear neutrophils, eosinophils, and mononuclear cells may be evident. Weakening of the vessel wall can lead to aneurysm formation, rupture, and hemorrhage. Abnormalities in later stages of the disease include intimal proliferation leading to thrombosis and infarction, recanalization, dissection, and scarring.

Lie and coworkers[84] have emphasized the focal and segmental character of the vascular lesions. A normal artery may be found adjacent to one that is severely affected, only a segment of the artery along its length may be affected, or only a portion of the circumference of the arterial wall may be involved.

COGAN'S SYNDROME

Nonsyphilitic keratitis with vestibuloauditory dysfunction was described by Cogan in 1945.[54] Young adults of either sex are affected. Additional manifestations include fever, cardiac involvement, lymphadenopathy, and myalgias.[55, 56] In approximately 70 per cent of cases, a vasculitis involving predominantly small vessels is evident.[55] Although arthralgias are not infrequent, frank arthritis is rare. When present, polyarticular involvement resembling that of rheumatoid arthritis[55] or monoarticular involvement resembling septic arthritis[57] is seen. Accumulation of synovial fluid is accompanied by radiographically evident soft tissue swelling; bone erosions and loss of cartilage are not apparent. Biopsy of the synovial membrane reveals a nonspecific synovitis.

FIGURE 36–3. Polyarteritis nodosa: Periostitis in upper extremity. In this patient with diffuse vasculitis and prominent clinical findings in the thenar eminence in both hands, note periosteal new bone formation along the diaphyseal portion of the first metacarpals (arrows).

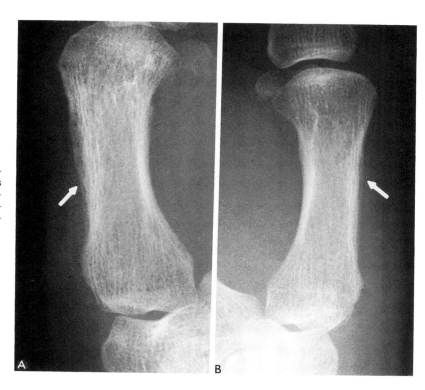

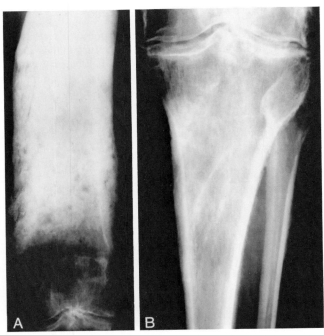

FIGURE 36–4. Polyarteritis nodosa: Extensive periostitis in lower extremity. In this 40 year old man who had had dull leg pain for many years, radiographs of the femur **(A)** and lower leg **(B)** show dramatic periosteal new bone formation involving predominantly the diaphyses of the femur and tibia. The fibula is affected to lesser extent. (Courtesy of H. Kroon, M.D., Leiden, The Netherlands.)

Cogan's syndrome should be considered in the differential diagnosis of a process characterized by aortic insufficiency and arthritis; other diagnostic possibilities include rheumatic fever, ankylosing spondylitis, Reiter's syndrome, systemic lupus erythematosus, relapsing polychondritis, and rheumatoid arthritis.[57]

CHURG-STRAUSS SYNDROME

Churg-Strauss syndrome, also designated allergic granulomatosis and angiitis, is characterized by the combination of asthma, eosinophilia, vasculitis, and extravascular granulomas.[58] It is a disease more frequent in men than in women and affects patients of different ages. The basic pathologic lesion is a necrotizing vasculitis involving small arteries and veins, resulting in granulomas.[78] Regardless of which organs are involved, the two essential findings in this syndrome are angiitis and extravascular necrotizing granulomas, usually with eosinophilic infiltrates.[84] Respiratory symptoms dominate the initial stages of the disease, although other organs or organ systems, including the kidney, spleen, heart, gastrointestinal tract, and skin, subsequently are affected. Subcutaneous nodules may be observed. Polyarthralgias are uncommon, and arthritis is rare.[46] Diagnostic criteria emphasize six findings: asthma, eosinophilia, mononeuropathy or polyneuropathy, pulmonary infiltrates, abnormalities of the paranasal sinuses, and a biopsy specimen containing a blood vessel with extravascular eosinophils.[85]

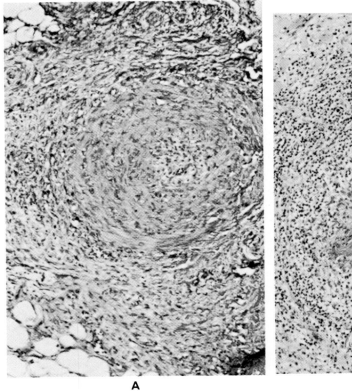
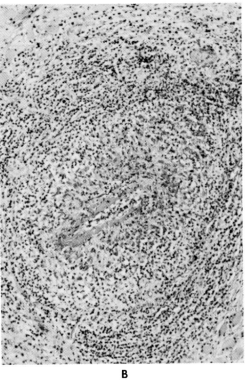

A **B**

FIGURE 36–5. Polyarteritis nodosa: Pathologic abnormalities.
 A Histologic section (65×) of skin demonstrates fibrinoid necrosis and inflammation around an arteriole.
 B Histologic section (100×) of a skin nodule in a patient with polyarteritis nodosa indicates acute and subacute vasculitis with fibrinoid necrosis and eosinophilic infiltration.
 (From Woodward AH, Andreini PH: Arthritis Rheum *17*:1017, 1974.)

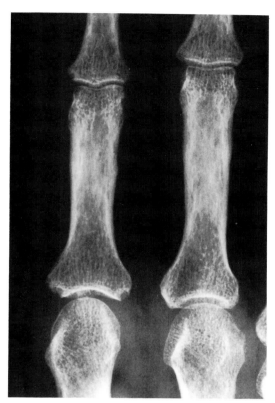

FIGURE 36–6. Wegener's granulomatosis: Articular abnormalities. In this patient with well-established disease, osteoporosis and subtle periarticular bone erosions are present about the interphalangeal and metacarpophalangeal joints. The nature and significance of these findings are unknown. (Courtesy of A. Brower, M.D., Norfolk, Virginia.)

WEGENER'S GRANULOMATOSIS

Wegener's granulomatosis is associated with necrotizing granulomatous lesions of the respiratory tract, vasculitis, and glomerulonephritis.[59] The age of onset in patients may range from the very young to the aged; the disease is slightly more common in men than in women. Clinical features include acute or chronic sinusitis, chronic rhinitis, nasal ulceration, anorexia, weight loss, and fever. More widespread manifestations accompany involvement of other organ systems, such as the lungs and kidneys. Purpura and optic and orbital alterations also are apparent in some cases. With regard to articular abnormalities, arthralgias and arthritis are evident in approximately one half of cases.[97] They generally are unassociated with significant radiographic changes. Rarely, bone erosions are seen,[86, 96] although they may be related to chronic renal disease (Fig. 36–6). The precise cause of Wegener's granulomatosis is unknown, but hypersensitivity is a leading candidate.[46]

Pathologically, the classic triad of Wegener's granulomatosis consists of necrotizing granulomas of the upper or lower respiratory tract, or both; necrotizing or granulomatous vasculitis, usually of small arteries and veins, almost always in the lung and, more selectively, in other organs; and focal, segmental, necrotizing glomerulitis.[84] Diagnostic criteria, as proposed by the American College of Rheumatology, include abnormal urinary sediment; abnormal findings on chest radiograph (nodules, cavities, or fixed infil-

trates); oral ulcers or nasal discharge; and granulomatous inflammation on biopsy.[87]

MIDLINE GRANULOMA

Midline granuloma is a disease associated with destructive lesions of the nose, midface, and upper airways. Pulmonary and renal involvement typically is lacking.[60] Soft tissues and adjacent bones are affected by a pathologic process that is associated with dense cellular infiltrates consisting of lymphocytes, plasma cells, histiocytes, and immunoblasts in an angiocentric distribution.[46] Symptoms and signs relate to abnormalities in the mouth, nose, and upper airways.

GIANT CELL (TEMPORAL) ARTERITIS AND POLYMYALGIA RHEUMATICA

Giant cell (temporal) arteritis is characterized by granulomatous inflammation of large arteries, particularly the internal and the external carotid, the occipital, the temporal, and the ophthalmic arteries, although other branches of the abdominal and thoracic aorta can be involved.[23] Typically, patients over the age of 50 years are affected. The arteritis is more frequent in women than in men, in a ratio of approximately 2 to 1. The onset of disease is either abrupt or insidious, and constitutional symptoms, such as fatigue, anorexia, and weight loss, may dominate the initial clinical manifestations.[61] Clinical findings include painful swelling of the temporal arteries, headaches, visual disturbances, and peripheral neuropathy.[23–26, 88] The diagnosis is supported by characteristic findings on temporal artery biopsy[25, 27, 43, 64, 98, 100] or angiogram.[28–32] Diagnostic criteria recommended by the American College of Rheumatology include age of onset of disease at 50 years or later; new onset of localized headache; tenderness of the temporal artery or decreased temporal artery pulse; elevation of the erythrocyte sedimentation rate (Westergren) to a value equal to or greater than 50 mm per hour; and biopsy sample including an artery showing necrotizing arteritis, characterized by a predominance of mononuclear cell infiltrates or a granulomatous process with multinucleated giant cells.[90]

Synovitis is detected in approximately 15 per cent of biopsy-proved cases of giant cell arteritis. Clinical findings related to articular involvement usually are confined to soft tissue swelling, although an erosive, seronegative polyarthritis may appear before or after the onset of arteritis.[62, 76] Coexistent rheumatoid arthritis also has been documented.[63]

An association has been suggested between giant cell arteritis and polymyalgia rheumatica. This latter condition is encountered most frequently in elderly patients, particularly women, and is associated with progressive pain of the back, the thighs, the neck, and the shoulders. Morning stiffness without joint swelling is particularly characteristic of polymyalgia rheumatica.[44] The clinical resemblance of this disorder to rheumatoid arthritis is accentuated by the occasional presence in polymyalgia rheumatica of a transient inflammatory synovitis of the knee, the shoulder, the hip, the wrist, and, rarely, the small joints of the fingers.[33, 34] This synovitis can result in soft tissue swelling and osteoporosis on radiographs.[79] A carpal tunnel syndrome, due to compression of the median nerve by adjacent synovial tissue, is encountered.[64] Chronic inflammatory changes are evident when the synovial membrane is examined.[66] Significant cartilaginous and bony abnormalities generally are not encountered, although sacroiliac joint sclerosis has been reported.[33, 35] In some cases, resulting radiographic abnormalities resemble those of sacroiliitis[67] and are associated with alterations in the symphysis pubis[67] and sternoclavicular[68] joints. The involvement of the axial skeleton, the sternoclavicular and sternomanubrial joints, and the shoulder region is consistent with a "central" synovitis in this disease.[67] Technetium scintigraphy may reveal increased accumulation of radioisotope in involved articulations.[36, 67]

Approximately 50 per cent of patients with giant cell arteritis demonstrate a prodromal phase with features of polymyalgia rheumatica, and approximately 30 per cent of patients with polymyalgia rheumatica reveal symptoms and signs of giant cell arteritis. In fact, giant cell arteritis may occur in some patients with polymyalgia rheumatica in the absence of symptoms referable to the temporal artery.[25, 29] In these patients, blind biopsy of the proximal portion of the temporal artery can reveal such clinically silent disease.[25, 37, 38] A normal biopsy specimen in this situation does not exclude arteritis, as it may indicate sampling of an uninvolved section of the artery. Some investigators recommend biopsy of the contralateral temporal artery when results of the first biopsy are negative.[84, 89]

HENOCH-SCHÖNLEIN (ANAPHYLACTOID) PURPURA

This syndrome, which consists of nonthrombocytopenic purpura, arthralgia or arthritis, abdominal pain, and renal disease, is related to a generalized angiitis involving arterioles and capillaries. Increased vascular permeability is associated with edema and hemorrhage. The cause of this condition is unknown, although an allergic phenomenon has been suggested. The disease is more frequent in children than in adults, with a peak age incidence of 3 years. Many tissues may be affected, including the synovial membrane.[39] Diagnostic criteria proposed by the American College of Rheumatology were age of onset of disease at 20 years or younger; palpable purpura; acute abdominal pain; and biopsy specimen showing granulocytes in the walls of small arterioles or venules.[91] Immunofluorescence microscopy may reveal Ig A deposits in the skin and renal glomeruli.[84]

The onset of the disease frequently follows an infection of the upper respiratory tract. The classic triad of findings, observed in 70 to 80 per cent of cases, consists of purpura, abdominal pain, and arthritis.[84] Soft tissue edema is evident in the lower extremities, feet, and, to a lesser extent, face, scalp, and hands.[46] Gastrointestinal abnormalities include pain, hemorrhage, and even visceral perforation. Renal involvement occasionally is seen and varies in severity.

Approximately 60 to 70 per cent of patients with Henoch-Schönlein purpura develop articular manifestations with pain, tenderness, and swelling.[40] The joints involved most commonly are the knees, the ankles, the hips, the wrists, and the small joints of the hand. Periarticular soft tissue swelling, the only radiographic abnormality, is related to synovial effusion (Fig. 36–7). Complete resolution of clinical and radiographic joint abnormalities is characteristic.

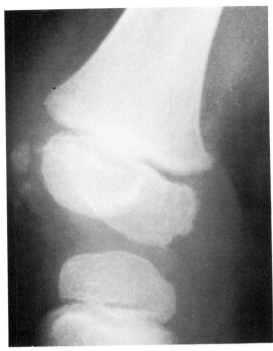

FIGURE 36–7. Henoch-Schönlein (anaphylactoid) purpura: Joint effusion. In this 4 year old child, observe soft tissue swelling and joint effusion of the knee.

CRYOGLOBULINEMIA

Cryoproteins represent molecules that possess a unique property of reversible precipitation at low temperatures. Two classes of cryoproteins are identified: cryofibrinogens, which are detected rarely and generally are unassociated with clinical manifestations; and cryoglobulins (cryoimmunoglobulins), which are much more frequent in occurrence, accompanying a variety of diseases and producing significant clinical abnormalities.

Two types of cryoglobulins are encountered: the monoclonal type and the mixed type. Monoclonal cryoglobulins, present in approximately one third of persons with cryoglobulinemia, are evident in a number of myeloproliferative disorders, such as multiple myeloma, macroglobulinemia, and leukemias. Mixed cryoglobulins, representing two thirds of the entire group of cryoglobulinemias, are immune complexes that produce symptoms and signs attributable to vasculitis, which may appear in various organ systems. These cryoglobulins are seen in certain infectious diseases (viral, bacterial, and parasitic infections), autoimmune states (rheumatoid arthritis, systemic lupus erythematosus, polyarteritis nodosa, scleroderma, Sjögren's syndrome), lymphoproliferative disorders (lymphomas, leukemias, macroglobulinemias), renal and hepatic processes (glomerulonephritis, hepatitis, cirrhosis), and familial and essential forms.

In all of the disorders associated with mixed cryoglobulinemia, clinical manifestations relate to the site and the severity of the accompanying vasculitis. Purpura, arthralgia, Raynaud's phenomenon, cutaneous ulceration, cold urticaria, pericarditis, thyroiditis, renal failure, hepatosplenomegaly, lymphadenopathy, and peripheral neuropathy occur in variable combinations. As would be expected, the course

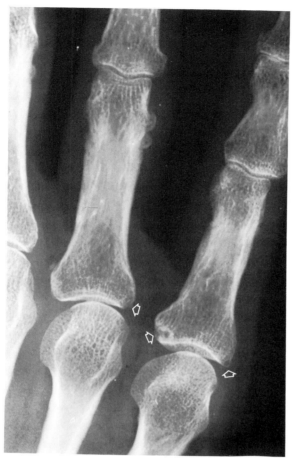

FIGURE 36–8. Cryoglobulinemia: Articular abnormalities. In this 55 year old man, small, discrete osteolytic foci (arrows) are seen in the phalanges. Bone proliferation involves the proximal phalanx of the fourth finger. (Courtesy of V. Vint, M.D., San Diego, California.)

and the prognosis of the disease also depend on the pattern of the vasculitis; although the course of the disease frequently is protracted, renal involvement is associated with higher morbidity and mortality.

Essential cryoglobulinemia is a distinct type of disease that is manifested as arthralgia or arthritis; the skin, lungs, kidneys, nervous system, and gastrointestinal tract are involved[69-71] The disorder may follow a chronic course, with minimal symptoms, or result in death from renal abnormalities.[72] Intermittent arthralgia is observed in 20 to 75 per cent of patients, whereas arthritis is less frequent, being evident in 5 to 25 per cent of cases.[73] The joints involved most commonly are those in the hands, knees,[99] ankles, and elbows. Although the radiographic features in these locations are not dramatic (Fig. 36–8), well-defined subchondral cystic lesions have been identified.[72] Furthermore, abnormalities of the spine have been reported in 25 per cent of patients.[74] Bone erosions and cyst formation in the articular facets of the cervical spine and vertebral bodies, which are evident in this disease, appear to lack specificity.

HYPOCOMPLEMENTEMIC VASCULITIS

Originally described in 1973 by McDuffie and collaborators,[75] this uncommon condition affects young adults, especially women. Urticaria, involving the skin on the face,

upper extremities, and trunk, purpura, fever, and abdominal and joint pain are evident. Symmetric articular disease, especially in small joints, resembles that seen in systemic lupus erythematosus, and deforming nonerosive arthropathy may be apparent.[92] A similar deforming arthropathy may accompany other types of necrotizing vasculitis.[93] Residual deformity is reported to be uncommon in cases of hypo-complementemic vasculitis.[46] As its name implies, hypo-complementemia is characteristic, and it may be associated with low serum levels of cryoglobulins.

TAKAYASU ARTERITIS

Takayasu arteritis is a chronic, nonarteriosclerotic, inflammatory disease of the aorta and its main branches and of the elastic pulmonary arteries.[84] It is observed most commonly in young women between the ages of 15 and 45 years and shows greatest prevalence in the Orient.[84] Initial symptoms are not specific and include weight loss, fever, arthralgias, myalgias, and anemia. The disorder progresses at a variable rate with gradual obliteration of the involved vessels. Aortic arch syndrome, pulseless disease, renovascular hypertension, and claudication are among its later manifestations. Diagnostic criteria include age of disease onset at 40 years or younger; claudication of an extremity; decreased pulse in the brachial artery; a difference in systolic pressure between arms that is greater than 10 mm Hg; a bruit over the subclavian arteries or the aorta; and arteriographic evidence of narrowing or occlusion of the entire aorta, its primary branches, or large arteries in the proximal portion of the upper or lower extremities.[94]

Although arthralgias may be observed in more than 50 per cent of patients, radiographic findings of joint disease are lacking. One report, however, has described the association of Takayasu arteritis and secondary hypertrophic osteoarthropathy.[95]

ERYTHEMA NODOSUM

Erythema nodosum is a disorder characterized by red, tender, and warm nodular cutaneous lesions (particularly in the lower legs), which, on biopsy, demonstrate vasculitis and cellular infiltration.[41] The disorder may be an allergic or hypersensitivity response to a number of precipitating factors, such as infection and drugs. Erythema nodosum occurs in some patients with ulcerative colitis, Crohn's disease, sarcoidosis, and Behçet's syndrome.

Approximately three fourths of patients with erythema nodosum develop recurrent episodes of arthralgia and arthritis. Joint findings usually are symmetric in distribution, with predilection for the knees, the ankles, the elbows, the wrists, and the small joints of the hands. Soft tissue swelling related to a joint effusion is the only prominent radiographic abnormality.[42]

SUMMARY

Vasculitis occurs in a number of disorders and may be associated with musculoskeletal manifestations. Although arteriography can reveal characteristic alterations in these disorders, plain film radiographic abnormalities are unimpressive. In polyarteritis nodosa, periosteal bone formation may be seen, particularly in the lower extremity. The appearance, which also has been described in Takayasu arteritis, is similar to that of hypertrophic osteoarthropathy. Articular abnormalities in giant cell (temporal) arteritis relate to its association with polymyalgia rheumatica and include soft tissue swelling and osteoporosis. Sacroiliitis and other abnormalities in central joints have been observed. In Henoch-Schönlein purpura and erythema nodosum, joint effusions are the only characteristic radiographic abnormality. Cryoglobulinemia occasionally is accompanied by cystic and erosive lesions of bone in both the axial and the appendicular skeleton.

References

1. Kussmaul A, Maier R: Über eine Bisher nicht beschriebene eigenthümliche Arterienerkrankung (Periarteritis nodosa), die mit Morbus Brightii und rapid fortschreitender allgemeiner Muskellähmung einhergeht. Dtsch Arch Klin Med 1:484, 1866.
2. Zeek PM: Periarteritis nodosa; a critical review. Am J Clin Pathol 22:777, 1952.
3. Rose GA, Spencer H: Polyarteritis nodosa. Q J Med 26:43, 1957.
4. Zvaifler NJ: Vasculitides: Classification and pathogenesis. Aust NZ J Med 8(Suppl 1):134, 1978.
5. Winkelmann RK, Ditto WB: Cutaneous and visceral syndromes of necrotizing or "allergic" angiitis. A study of 38 cases. Medicine 43:59, 1964.
6. Soter NA, Mihm MC, Gigli I, et al: Two distinct cellular patterns in cutaneous necrotizing angiitis. J Invest Dermatol 66:344, 1976.
7. Fauci AS, Wolff SM: Wegener's granulomatosis: Studies in 18 patients and a review of the literature. Medicine 52:535, 1973.
8. Sen PK, Kinare SG, Kelkar MD, et al: Non-specific stenosing arteritis of the aorta and its branches: A study of a possible etiology. Mt Sinai J Med 39:221, 1972.
9. D'Angelo WA, Fries JF, Masi AT, et al: Pathologic observations in systemic sclerosis (scleroderma). A study of 58 autopsy cases and 58 matched controls. Am J Med 46:428, 1969.
10. Benyo RB, Perrin EV: Periarteritis nodosa in infancy. Am J Dis Child 116:539, 1968.
11. Lowman EW: Joint and neuromuscular manifestations of periarteritis nodosa. Ann Rheum Dis 11:146, 1952.
12. Ball J, Grayzel AI: Arteritis and localized periosteal new bone formation. J Bone Joint Surg [Br] 46:244, 1964.
13. Woodward AH, Andreini PH: Periosteal new bone formation in polyarteritis nodosa. A syndrome involving the lower extremities. Arthritis Rheum 17:1017, 1974.
14. McCall M, Pennock JW: Periarteritis nodosa: Our present knowledge of the disease. Ann Intern Med 21:628, 1944.
15. Ball J: Rheumatoid arthritis and polyarteritis nodosa. Ann Rheum Dis 13:277, 1954.
16. Bywaters EGL: Peripheral vascular obstruction in rheumatoid arthritis and its relationship to other vascular lesions. Ann Rheum Dis 16:84, 1957.
17. Sokoloff L, Wilens SL, Bunim JJ: Arteritis of striated muscle in rheumatoid arthritis. Am J Pathol 27:157, 1951.
18. Scott JT, El Sallab RA, Laws JW: The digital artery design in rheumatoid arthritis—further observations. Br J Radiol 40:748, 1967.
19. Saville PD: Polyarteritis nodosa with new bone formation. J Bone Joint Surg [Br] 38:327, 1956.
20. Murray RO, Jacobson HG: The Radiology of Skeletal Disorders: Exercises in Diagnosis. Baltimore, Williams & Wilkins Co, 1971.
21. Serre H, Simon L, Mion C: Reaction periostée avec neo-formation osseous révélatrice d'une periarterite noueuse. Rev Rhum Mal Osteoartic 28:120, 1961.
22. Lovell RRH, Scott GBD: Hypertrophic osteo-arthropathy in polyarteritis. Ann Rheum Dis 15:46, 1956.
23. Hamilton CR Jr, Shelley WM, Tumulty PA: Giant cell arteritis: Including temporal arteritis and polymyalgia rheumatica. Medicine 50:1, 1970.
24. Warrell DA, Godfrey S, Olsen EGJ: Giant-cell arteritis with peripheral neuropathy. Lancet 1:1010, 1968.
25. Fauchald P, Rygvold O, Oystese B: Temporal arteritis and polymyalgia rheumatica—clinical and biopsy findings. Ann Intern Med 77:845, 1972.
26. Andrews JM: Giant cell ("temporal") arteritis: A disease with variable clinical manifestations. Neurology 16:963, 1966.
27. Ainsworth RW, Gresham GA, Balmforth GV: Pathological changes in temporal arteries removed from unselected cadavers. J Clin Pathol 14:115, 1961.
28. Layfer LF, Banner BF, Huckman MS, et al: Temporal arteriography. Analysis of 21 cases and a review of the literature. Arthritis Rheum 21:780, 1978.
29. Hunder GG, Baker HL, Rhoton AL, et al: Superficial temporal arteriography in patients suspected of having temporal arteritis. Arthritis Rheum 15:561, 1972.
30. Gillanders LA: Temporal arteriography. Clin Radiol 20:149, 1969.
31. Moncada R, Baker D, Rubinstein H, et al: Selective temporal arteriography and biopsy in giant cell arteritis: Polymyalgia rheumatica. AJR 122:580, 1974.
32. Elliott PD, Baker HL, Brown AL: The superficial temporal angiogram. Radiology 102:635, 1972.
33. Henderson D, Tribe A, Dixon AS: Synovitis in polymyalgia rheumatica. Rheumatol Rehabil 14:244, 1975.
34. Gordon I: Polymyalgia rheumatica. Q J Med 29:473, 1960.
35. Andrews FM: Polymyalgia rheumatica. Ann Rheum Dis 24:432, 1965.
36. O'Duffy JD, Wahner HW, Hunder GG: Joint imaging in polymyalgia rheumatica. Mayo Clin Proc 51:519, 1976.
37. Dixon AS, Beardwell C, Kay A, et al: Polymyalgia rheumatica and temporal arteritis. Ann Rheum Dis 25:203, 1966.
38. Hamrin B, Jonsson N, Landberg T: Arteritis in polymyalgia rheumatica. Lancet 1:397, 1964.
39. Norkin S, Wiener J: Henoch-Schoenlein syndrome. Review of pathology and report of two cases. Am J Clin Pathol 33:55, 1960.
40. Gairdner D: The Schönlein-Henoch syndrome (anaphylactoid purpura). Q J Med 17:95, 1948.
41. Blomgren SE: Erythema nodosum. Semin Arthritis Rheum 4:1, 1974.
42. Truelove LH: Articular manifestations of erythema nodosum. Ann Rheum Dis 19:174, 1960.
43. Sewell JR, Allison DJ, Tarin D, et al: Combined temporal arteriography and selective biopsy in suspected giant cell arteritis. Ann Rheum Dis 39:124, 1980.
44. Papaioannou CC, Gupta RC, Hunder GG, et al: Circulating immune complexes in giant cell arteritis and polymyalgia rheumatica. Arthritis Rheum 23:1021, 1980.
45. Alarcón-Segovia D: Classification of the necrotizing vasculitides in man. Clin Rheum Dis 6:223, 1980.
46. Hunder GG, Conn DL: Necrotizing vasculitis. In WN Kelley, ED Harris Jr, S Ruddy, et al (Eds): Textbook of Rheumatology. Philadelphia, WB Saunders, 1981, p 1165.
47. Weisman MH, Zvaifler NJ: Vasculitis in connective tissue diseases. Clin Rheum Dis 6:351, 1980.
48. Mekori YA, Awai LE, Wiedel JD, et al: Cutaneous polyarteritis nodosa associated with rapidly progressive arthritis. Arthritis Rheum 27:574, 1984.
49. Smukler NM, Schumacher HR Jr: Chronic nondestructive arthritis associated with cutaneous polyarteritis. Arthritis Rheum 20:1114, 1977.
50. Meijers KAE, Paré DM, Loose H, et al: Periarteritis nodosa and subperiosteal new bone formation. J Bone Joint Surg [Br] 64:592, 1982.
51. Short DJ, Webley M: Periosteal new bone formation complicating juvenile polyarteritis nodosa. J R Soc Med 77:325, 1984.
52. Gaucher A, Wiederkehr P, Raul P, et al: Nécrose osseuse au cours d'une periartérite noueuse. Nouv Presse Med 11:604, 1982.
53. Bucknall RC: Polyarteritis with symmetrical bone cysts. Proc R Soc Med 69:578, 1976.
54. Cogan DG: Syndrome of nonsyphilitic interstitial keratitis and vestibulo-auditory symptoms. Arch Ophthalmol 33:144, 1945.
55. Cheson BD, Bluming AZ, Alroy J: Cogan's syndrome: A systemic vasculitis. Am J Med 60:549, 1976.
56. Gelfand ML, Kantor T, Gorstein F: Cogan's syndrome with cardiovascular involvement: Aortic insufficiency. NY Acad Med 48:647, 1972.
57. Pinals RS: Cogan's syndrome with arthritis and aortic insufficiency. J Rheumatol 5:294, 1978.
58. Churg J, Strauss L: Allergic granulomatosis, allergic angiitis, and periarteritis nodosa. Am J Pathol 27:277, 1951.
59. Godman GC, Churg J: Wegener's granulomatosis: Pathology and review of the literature. Arch Pathol 58:533, 1954.
60. Schechter SL, Bole GG, Walker SE: Midline granuloma and Wegener's granulomatosis: Clinical and therapeutic considerations. J Rheumatol 3:241, 1976.
61. Hunder GG, Hazleman BL: Giant cell arteritis and polymyalgia rheumatica. In WN Kelley, ED Harris Jr, S Ruddy, et al (Eds): Textbook of Rheumatology. Philadelphia, WB Saunders, 1981, p 1189.
62. Ginsburg WW, Cohen MD, Randall S, et al: Chronic seronegative polyarthritis in patients with temporal arteritis (Abstr). Arthritis Rheum 25:S31, 1982.
63. Hall S, Ginsburg WW, Vollersten RS, et al: The coexistence of rheumatoid arthritis and giant cell arteritis. J Rheumatol 10:995, 1983.
64. Allison MC, Gallagher PJ: Temporal artery biopsy and corticosteroid treatment. Ann Rheum Dis 43:416, 1984.
65. Healey LA: Polymyalgia rheumatica and the American Rheumatism Association criteria for rheumatoid arthritis. Arthritis Rheum 26:1417, 1983.
66. Douglas WAC, Martin BA, Morris JH: Polymyalgia rheumatica: An arthroscopic study of the shoulder joint. Ann Rheum Dis 42:311, 1983.
67. O'Duffy JD, Hunder GG, Wahner HW: A follow-up study of polymyalgia rheumatica: Evidence of chronic axial synovitis. J Rheumatol 7:685, 1980.
68. Paice EW, Wright FW, Hill AGS: Sternoclavicular erosions in polymyalgia rheumatica. Ann Rheum Dis 42:379, 1983.
69. Abrambsky O, Slavin S: Neurologic manifestations in patients with mixed cryoglobulinemia. Neurology 24:245, 1974.
70. Ellis FA: The cutaneous manifestations of cryoglobulinemia. Arch Dermatol 89:690, 1964.
71. Reza MJ, Roth BE, Pops MA, et al: Intestinal vasculitis in essential mixed cryoglobulinemia. Ann Intern Med 81:632, 1974.
72. Weinberger A, Berliner S, Pinkhas J: Articular manifestations of essential cryoglobulinemia. Semin Arthritis Rheum 10:224, 1981.
73. Meltzer M, Franklin EL, Elias K: Cryoglobulinemia—a clinical and laboratory study. II. Cryoglobulins with rheumatoid factor activity. Am J Med 40:837, 1966.
74. Weinberger A, Berliner S, Pinkhas J: Spine manifestations in essential cryoglobulinemia. Rheumatol Rehabil 21:27, 1982.
75. McDuffie FC, Sams WM Jr, Maldonado JE, et al: Hypocomplementemia with

cutaneous vasculitis and arthritis: Possible immune complex syndrome. Mayo Clin Proc 48:340, 1973.

76. Ginsburg WW, Cohen MD, Hall SB, et al: Seronegative polyarthritis in giant cell arteritis. Arthritis Rheum 28:1362, 1985.

77. Rush PJ, Inman R, Reynolds J: Rheumatoid arthritis after Takayasu's arteritis. J Rheumatol 13:427, 1986.

78. Henochowicz S, Eggensperger D, Pierce L, et al: Necrotizing systemic vasculitis with features of both Wegener's granulomatosis and Churg-Strauss vasculitis. Arthritis Rheum 29:565, 1986.

79. Chou C-T, Schumacher HR Jr: Clinical and pathologic studies of synovitis in polymyalgia rheumatica. Arthritis Rheum 27:1107, 1984.

80. Hunder GG, Arend WP, Bloch DA, et al: The American College of Rheumatology 1990 criteria for the classification of vasculitis. Introduction. Arthritis Rheum 33:1065, 1990.

81. Bloch DA, Michel BA, Hunder GG: The American College of Rheumatology 1990 criteria for the classification of vasculitis. Patients and methods. Arthritis Rheum 33:1068, 1990.

82. Lightfoot RW Jr, Michel BA, Bloch DA, et al: The American College of Rheumatology 1990 criteria for the classification of polyarteritis nodosa. Arthritis Rheum 33:1088, 1990.

83. Nash P, Fryer J, Webb J: Vasculitis presenting as chronic unilateral painful leg swelling. J Rheumatol 15:1022, 1988.

84. Lie JT, Hunder GG, Arend WP, et al: Illustrated histopathologic classification criteria for selected vasculitis syndromes. Arthritis Rheum 33:1074, 1990.

85. Masi AT, Hunder GG, Lie JT, et al: The American College of Rheumatology 1990 criteria for the classification of Churg-Strauss syndrome (allergic granulomatosis and angiitis). Arthritis Rheum 33:1094, 1990.

86. Othmani S, Bahri M, Louzir B, et al: Les manifestations articulaires au cours de la granulomatose de Wegener. Sem Hôp Paris 67:1679, 1991.

87. Leavitt RY, Fauci AS, Bloch DA, et al: The American College of Rheumatology 1990 criteria for the classification of Wegener's granulomatosis. Arthritis Rheum 33:1101, 1990.

88. Golbus J, McCune WJ: Giant cell arteritis and peripheral neuropathy: A report of 2 cases and review of the literature. J Rheumatol 14:129, 1987.

89. Fernandez-Herlihy L: Temporal arteritis: Clinical aids to diagnosis. J Rheumatol 15:1797, 1988.

90. Hunder GG, Bloch DA, Michel BA, et al: The American College of Rheumatology 1990 criteria for the classification of giant cell arteritis. Arthritis Rheum 33:1122, 1990.

91. Mills JA, Michel BA, Bloch DA, et al: The American College of Rheumatology 1990 criteria for the classification of Henoch-Schönlein purpura. Arthritis Rheum 33:1114, 1990.

92. Sturgess AS, Littlejohn GO: Jaccoud's arthritis and panvasculitis in the hypocomplementemic urticarial vasculitis syndrome. J Rheumatol 15:858, 1988.

93. de la Sota M, Cocco JAM: Jaccoud's arthropathy in a patient with necrotizing vasculitis. J Rheumatol 19:998, 1992.

94. Arend WP, Michel BA, Bloch DA: The American College of Rheumatology 1990 criteria for the classification of Takayasu arteritis. Arthritis Rheum 33:1129, 1990.

95. Sanders ME, Fischbein LC: Hypertrophic osteoarthropathy with Takayasu's arteritis. Clin Exp Rheumatol 5:71, 1987.

96. Jacobs RP, Moore M, Brower A: Wegener's granulomatosis presenting with erosive arthritis. Arthritis Rheum 30:943, 1987.

97. Noritake DT, Weiner SR, Bassett LW, et al: Rheumatic manifestations of Wegener's granulomatosis. J Rheumatol 14:949, 1987.

98. Ponge T, Barrier JH, Grolleau J-Y, et al: The efficacy of selected unilateral temporal artery biopsy versus bilateral biopsies for diagnosis of giant cell arteritis. J Rheumatol 15:997, 1988.

99. An HS, Namey TC, Kim K: Essential cryoglobulinemia associated with intense and persistent synovitis of the knee. Clin Orthop 215:173, 1987.

100. Disdier P, Pellissier J-F, Harle J-R, et al: Significance of isolated vasculitis of the vasa vasorum on temporal artery biopsy. J Rheumatol 21:258, 1994.

37

Mixed Connective Tissue Disease and Collagen Vascular Overlap Syndromes

Donald Resnick, M.D.

Mixed Connective Tissue Disease
    Clinical Abnormalities
    Radiographic Abnormalities
    Pathologic Abnormalities
Collagen Vascular Overlap Syndromes
Summary

Diagnosis of the collagen vascular disorders that are described in Chapters 33 to 36 is based on the composite evaluation of clinical, laboratory, radiologic, and pathologic data and the application of a variety of selective and non-selective disease criteria. In many patients, this diagnostic exercise provides a single answer, a specific disease into which the constellation of findings can be placed comfortably. In other patients, however, this is not the case. Rather, difficulty is encountered because the manifestations of the disease process appear incompatible with a single diagnosis using traditional classification systems. Some examples of this diagnostic dilemma are provided by the patient with rheumatoid arthritis who also demonstrates antinuclear antibodies and a positive serologic test for LE cells or who may develop the skin alterations of scleroderma, or the person with lupus erythematosus who also has sclerodactyly or whose radiographs reveal an erosive arthritis.[49] These patients, as well as many others, appear to have more than one collagen vascular disease, and the diagnosis of an overlap syndrome is offered as an explanation for the diversity of the clinical, radiologic, and laboratory aberrations. Indeed, it has been suggested that as many as 25 per cent of cases of connective tissue disease fall into the category of an overlap syndrome.[69] In these situations, it generally is unclear whether classic definitions of the "pure" collagen vascular diseases are too limited, two or more pure collagen vascular disorders coexist at the same time, or a new and distinct clinical entity has emerged. Proponents of the last possibility offer mixed connective tissue disease as evidence of a new disorder that can be segregated effectively from the other collagen vascular diseases primarily on the basis of laboratory data. Others would debate the accuracy or appropriateness of such segregation, and the occurrence of "overlap" features, such as pulmonary disease, Sjögren's syndrome, and renal and cerebral abnormalities in some patients with mixed connective disease provides fuel for this debate.[69]

In this chapter, the features commonly ascribed to mixed connective tissue disease as well as those associated with some of the more commonly encountered collagen vascular overlap syndromes are presented.

MIXED CONNECTIVE TISSUE DISEASE

Mixed connective tissue disease (MCTD) first was described as a distinct syndrome by Sharp and his colleagues[1] in 1972. This syndrome, which has been further defined in other investigations,[2–9] is characterized by clinical features that suggest an overlap of systemic lupus erythematosus, scleroderma, dermatomyositis, and, more recently, rheumatoid arthritis.[7] The initially described unifying laboratory feature of MCTD was the presence of antibodies to a saline-soluble extractable nuclear antigen (ENA), which was ribonuclease (RNase) sensitive. Subsequently, ENA has been shown to consist of two distinct substances: a soluble ribonucleoprotein (RNP) and a glycoprotein termed Sm antigen.[10] Ribonuclease-sensitive ENA is synonymous with RNP.[2] The presence of antibodies to RNP is fundamental to the diagnosis of MCTD, although the antibodies also may be found in a small percentage of patients with systemic lupus erythematosus or scleroderma.[11–13] Anti-Sm antibodies may be restricted to patients with systemic lupus erythematosus.[14]

As indicated previously, the existence of MCTD as a definite entity is not accepted universally despite the recent emphasis placed on its clinical and radiologic features.[51] Reichlin and Mattioli[15] and Gilliam and Prystowsky[16] have suggested that MCTD represents systemic lupus erythematosus that has been altered or modified by the presence of RNP antibodies; the frequency of serious renal involvement appears to be less in these patients than in those with systemic lupus erythematosus,[47] and they demonstrate a more predictable response to corticosteroid therapy. Other investigators favor the concept that MCTD is a relatively undifferentiated rheumatic disease that has the potential to develop features consistent with systemic lupus erythematosus, scleroderma, dermatomyositis, and rheumatoid arthritis.[2, 46]

Clinical Abnormalities

MCTD is characterized by overlapping clinical features of scleroderma, systemic lupus erythematosus, dermatomyositis, and rheumatoid arthritis and by the presence in the serum of high titers of antibodies to RNP. Adults or children can be affected.[1, 44] Multiple cases in a single family[52] and involvement of twins[53] have been described. In a given patient, the clinical abnormalities of any one or a combination of these collagen vascular diseases may predominate. Changing stages of the disease may occur, in which the clinical and laboratory parameters at one time are those of one collagen vascular disorder, whereas at another time a second disease process becomes evident.[50] Thus, the variable clinical alterations of MCTD include fatigue, weight loss, fever, myalgia and myositis, lymphadenopathy, sclerodactyly, digital swelling, Raynaud's phenomenon, dyspnea, dysphagia, diarrhea, skin rash, and neuralgia. Trigeminal neuropathy and the carpal tunnel and cauda equina syndromes also are among the clinical manifestations of the disorder.[55, 70, 79] In general, the prognosis of the disease is regarded as good,[6] although serious gastrointestinal,[17] neurologic,[18, 71] or renal[48] manifestations can become apparent. Sharp[6] noted a mortality rate of 4 per cent in 100 patients with a mean disease duration of 6 years.

Clinically detectable joint abnormalities in MCTD are common, and some authors report arthritis in as many as 90 to 100 per cent of patients with this disease.[2–4, 54] Any joint may be affected, although involvement of the small joints of the hand and foot as well as the wrist is most typical. Knee, elbow, shoulder, and ankle abnormalities also are relatively common. Even the temporomandibular joint can be involved.[3] Intermittent arthralgia may progress to arthritis with considerable pain, stiffness, and swelling. Synovitis of joints, tendon sheaths, and bursae can be detected on clinical examination, although the degree of synovial abnormality may be less striking than that in rheumatoid arthritis.[2] Subcutaneous and peritendinous nodules also can be evident, particularly in the forearms and on the dorsum of the hands,[67] which, on biopsy, may demonstrate the characteristic features of a rheumatoid nodule.[4] Joint deformities simulating those of rheumatoid arthritis can appear in MCTD, with ulnar deviation and subluxation at the metacarpophalangeal joints, flexion contractures of the fingers, claw toes, and even arthritis mutilans.[45] As in rheumatoid arthritis and systemic lupus erythematosus, septic arthritis, even that related to tuberculosis, may become evident in patients with MCTD.[72]

The most important laboratory finding is the presence of RNP antibodies in the serum. High titers of these antibodies generally are detected, although these titers may change during the course of the disease.[50, 69] In addition, patients may reveal positive serologic test results for rheumatoid factor, elevation of erythrocyte sedimentation rate, and anemia. Noninflammatory fluid generally is recovered on joint aspiration.

Radiographic Abnormalities

On radiographs, osseous, articular, and soft tissue abnormalities confirm the overlapping nature of MCTD; bone and soft tissue findings may be identical to those in scleroderma, whereas articular abnormalities are more variable. Initially, the joint changes in this disease were considered nonerosive and nondeforming,[1] although more recent reports have indicated a broader spectrum of joint disease, which may include osseous erosion and joint deformity.[2–4, 19, 20, 45, 73]

Previous reports have described in detail the radiographic alterations that are present in patients with MCTD.[2–4, 19, 20] In most of these reports, radiographic evaluation of the hands, the wrists, and the feet was emphasized (Figs. 37–1 to 37–3). There is general agreement regarding the types of abnormality that may be encountered in these areas of the skeleton, although the reported prevalence of the findings has varied considerably. Radiographic alterations in the hands, wrists, and feet can include the following characteristics.

Joint Distribution. Radiographic abnormalities are most frequent in the proximal interphalangeal and metacarpophalangeal joints of the hands, midcarpal and radiocarpal compartments of the wrist, and metatarsophalangeal and interphalangeal joints of the feet. Distal interphalangeal joint changes also are encountered. A symmetric or asymmetric distribution of abnormalities has been reported, and, in fact, asymmetry has been stressed as one way in which this arthritis differs from rheumatoid arthritis.[2]

Osteoporosis (10 to 100 per cent of patients). Diffuse or periarticular osteoporosis is common. In this regard, the findings simulate those of rheumatoid arthritis.

Soft Tissue Swelling (65 to 75 per cent of patients). Symmetric soft tissue swelling is common about involved articulations. Asymmetric swelling may indicate the presence of a rheumatoid nodule. Diffuse swelling of the hand also is apparent, related to widespread edema.

Joint Space Narrowing (10 to 100 per cent of patients). Diffuse narrowing of the articular space also is common. Intra-articular bony ankylosis likewise has been noted.[2, 3] Ankylosis between the capitate and trapezoid bones could possibly have diagnostic significance.[3]

Erosions (25 to 75 per cent of patients). The osseous erosions in MCTD are similar to those in rheumatoid arthritis; well-delineated marginal defects and abnormalities of the ulnar styloid are features common to both disorders.[57] Erosions of distal interphalangeal joints of the fingers can be observed in MCTD, however, and are not prominent in rheumatoid arthritis.[19] In addition, severe destructive arthritis (Fig. 37–4) in an occasional patient with MCTD can simulate the appearance of psoriatic arthritis.[2, 45, 73]

Changes in the Phalangeal Tips (25 to 70 per cent of patients). Soft tissue atrophy, soft tissue calcification, and resorption of the terminal tufts of the phalanges simulate the findings of scleroderma. The tuftal calcific deposits

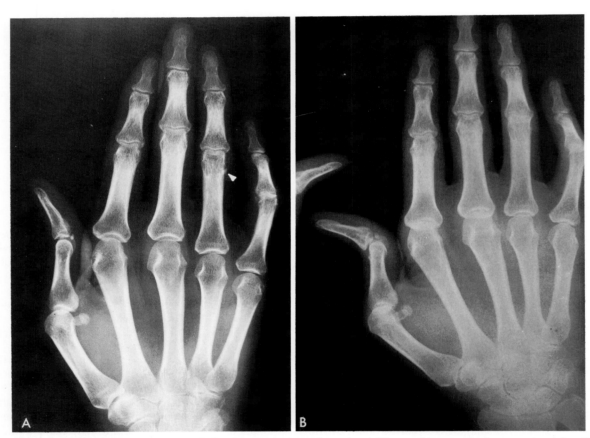

FIGURE 37–1. Mixed connective tissue disease: Deforming nonerosive arthropathy. A 32 year old woman had progressive deformities of the hand.

  A The initial radiograph outlines periarticular osteoporosis, capsular calcification (arrowhead), and a minor degree of ulnar deviation at the metacarpophalangeal joints.

  B Nine years later, joint deformities have progressed. Observe flexion at the first metacarpophalangeal joint and hyperextension of the interphalangeal joint of the same digit. Also note radial deviation at the wrist, ulnar deviation and flexion at the metacarpophalangeal joints, and flexion at the proximal interphalangeal joints. The width of the joint spaces is difficult to evaluate because of the associated deformities.

  (Courtesy of M. Dalinka, M.D., Philadelphia, Pennsylvania.)

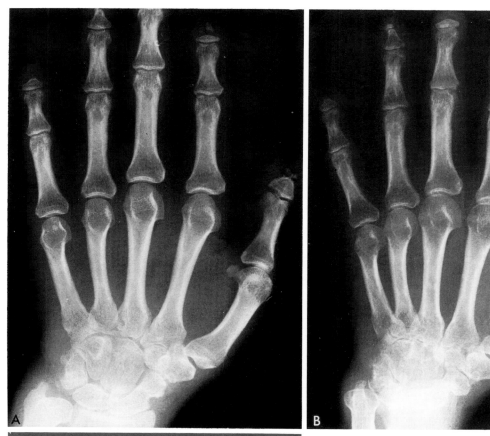

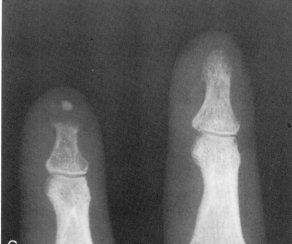

FIGURE 37–2. Mixed connective tissue disease: Bony erosions and phalangeal tuftal resorption.

A The initial radiograph reveals destruction with disappearance of several phalangeal tufts, soft tissue swelling and marginal erosions in the wrist, and periarticular osteoporosis.

B Six years later, the phalangeal abnormalities are relatively unchanged, although joint destruction throughout the wrist has progressed considerably.

C In a different patient, observe osteolysis of the terminal phalangeal tuft of the second finger and, to a lesser extent, the third finger. Punctate calcification is evident in the second digit.

(**A, B,** Courtesy of M. Dalinka, M.D., Philadelphia, Pennsylvania; **C,** Courtesy of D. Alarcón-Segovia, M.D., Mexico City, Mexico.)

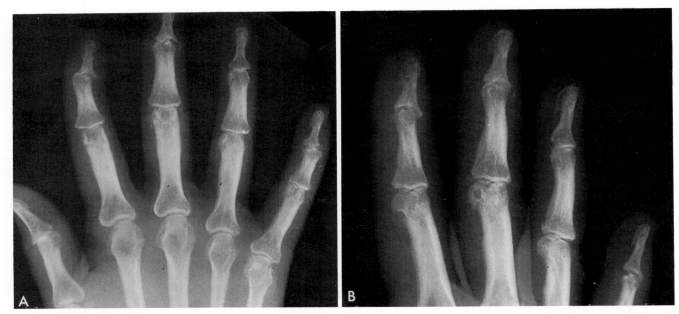

FIGURE 37–3. Mixed connective tissue disease: Distal interphalangeal joint erosions. A 48 year old woman complained of pain and deformity of her hands.

A The frontal radiograph outlines periarticular osteoporosis, capsular calcification, and a destructive arthritis of multiple distal interphalangeal joints.

B In the oblique projection, the erosions of the distal interphalangeal joints in all of the digits can be recognized. Note the cystic changes and calcification at the proximal interphalangeal joints.

(Courtesy of M. Dalinka, M.D., Philadelphia, Pennsylvania.)

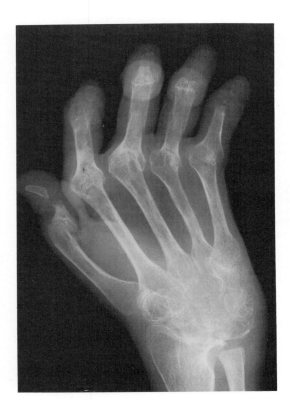

FIGURE 37–4. Mixed connective tissue disease: Arthritis mutilans. Severe destructive arthropathy involving multiple locations in the hand and wrist resembles psoriatic arthritis. The opposite side (not shown) was involved similarly. (Courtesy of D. Alarcón-Segovia, M.D., Mexico City, Mexico.)

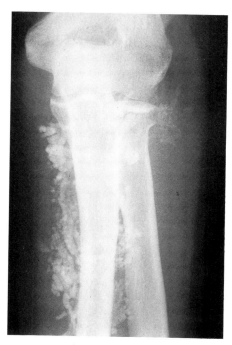

FIGURE 37–5. Mixed connective tissue disease: Periarticular calcification. A 38 year old woman complained of elbow pain. A frontal radiograph delineates extensive circular and linear collections of calcification about the elbow. (Courtesy of M. Dalinka, M.D., Philadelphia, Pennsylvania.)

skeleton in MCTD, it is apparent that features of scleroderma (soft tissue atrophy, soft tissue calcification, tuftal resorption, distal interphalangeal joint erosions), rheumatoid arthritis (periarticular osteoporosis, marginal erosions, joint space narrowing), and systemic lupus erythematosus (joint deformities without erosions, osteonecrosis) are encountered (Table 37–1). The severity of any one group of radiographic abnormalities varies, just as the clinical similarities to any one collagen vascular disease may vary.

The erosive arthritis of MCTD generally is indistinguishable from rheumatoid arthritis. Although some investigators stress an asymmetric distribution and sharply marginated defects as findings allowing accurate diagnosis of MCTD, these abnormalities are not constant, and similar findings occasionally are encountered in rheumatoid arthritis. In patients with MCTD who demonstrate erosive arthritis, serologic testing for rheumatoid factor may yield positive or negative results.

The soft tissue calcifications that are detected in patients with MCTD generally are indistinguishable from those in scleroderma. Although some investigators suggest that linear calcification overlying or within the joint capsule is of diagnostic significance in MCTD,[4] similar calcification can appear in scleroderma and other collagen vascular diseases, as well as in hyperparathyroidism and calcium pyrophosphate dihydrate crystal deposition disease. Intra-articular calcifications, related to hydroxyapatite crystal deposition, also have been observed in the hands and wrists of patients with MCTD.[74]

Soft tissue swelling in periarticular locations in MCTD also is nonspecific. Diffuse swelling in the hands corresponding to edema is a sign that is suggestive of MCTD.

The diagnosis of MCTD can be suggested when radiographic examination of the skeleton reveals features typical of more than one collagen vascular disease. A variety of overlap syndromes can have a similar radiographic appearance, however (see later discussion).

often are small and punctate, although larger collections may be apparent in adjacent areas of the same or different digits.[56] Osseous resorption leads to typical ''penciling'' of the phalanges.

Subluxation (12 to 100 per cent of patients). When present, joint subluxation is identical to that in rheumatoid arthritis or systemic lupus erythematosus.

Although clinical involvement of other joints is not uncommon, radiographic changes in these locations rarely are recorded. Periarticular osteoporosis and, rarely, calcification may be seen about the knee, the elbow, or the hip (Fig. 37–5)[57]; additionally, in the hip, diffuse loss of joint space has been noted.[4] Osteonecrosis of the femoral head, the femoral condyles, the diaphyses of the femur, and even the carpal bones has been found in MCTD,[2] although the relationship of these abnormalities to the administration of corticosteroids has not been determined. Other reported abnormalities have included rib resorption[73] and atlantoaxial subluxation.[75]

From this summary of radiographic abnormalities of the

Pathologic Abnormalities

Pathologic data in cases of MCTD are lacking. In children and adults, proliferative vascular lesions with intimal and medial thickening and luminal narrowing but without fibrinoid or inflammatory change are evident in large vessels and small arterioles of many organs.[21] Distinctive lesions of the esophagus (atrophy of the inner muscle area), thymus (hyperplasia), kidney (membranous change), liver, lung, and salivary glands also are noted.[21]

Histologic examination of skeletal muscle frequently delineates focal inflammatory lesions[1, 21, 22] that simulate the findings of idiopathic polymyositis and the inflammatory myopathy associated with systemic lupus erythematosus.[23]

TABLE 37–1. Radiographic Features of Mixed Connective Tissue Disease

Scleroderma–like Features	Lupus Erythematosus–like Features	Rheumatoid Arthritis–like Features	Dermatomyositis–like Features
Soft tissue atrophy	Deforming nonerosive arthropathy	Symmetric soft tissue swelling	Soft tissue calcification
Soft tissue or capsular calcification	Osteonecrosis	Periarticular osteoporosis	
Phalangeal tuftal erosion		Diffuse joint space narrowing	
Distal interphalangeal joint erosion		Marginal erosion	
		Soft tissue nodule	

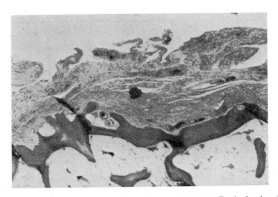

FIGURE 37–6. Mixed connective tissue disease: Pathologic abnormalities in the synovial membrane and cartilage. In a patient with arthritis mutilans characterized by extensive destruction of carpal bones, a specimen from a synovial biopsy during an arthrodesis of the wrist demonstrates synovial membrane covering bone. The cartilage has been completely destroyed, and the membrane itself is greatly hypertrophied and shows increased vascularity and mononuclear cellular infiltration. (From Bennett RM, O'Connell DJ: Ann Rheum Dis 37:397, 1978.)

Biopsy may outline mild inflammatory proliferation of the synovial membrane[2] or typical features of a rheumatoid nodule (Fig. 37–6).

COLLAGEN VASCULAR OVERLAP SYNDROMES

As indicated previously, the clinical features in many patients with collagen vascular disorders cannot be classified precisely as those of a specific disease but rather are consistent with more than one disease. Such overlap syndromes have been summarized by several investigators[2, 49, 58] and include dermatomyositis and scleroderma[24, 25]; rheumatoid arthritis and scleroderma[24, 26]; systemic lupus erythematosus and dermatomyositis[27, 28]; rheumatoid arthritis and systemic lupus erythematosus[29–32, 76]; scleroderma and systemic lupus erythematosus[24, 26, 33–38, 77]; and scleroderma and Sjögren's syndrome. Additional overlap syndromes include the combinations of subacute cutaneous lupus erythematosus (florid cutaneous lesions that are serpentine) and Sjögren's syndrome, pericarditis, and arthritis; antiphospholipid syndrome (characterized by venous and arterial thromboses, thrombocytopenia, and recurrent fetal loss) with other connective tissue diseases such as systemic lupus erythematosus; and polymyositis, pulmonary fibrosis, anti-Jo-1 antibodies, Raynaud's phenomenon, and Sjögren's syndrome.[69, 78] The fact that the clinical manifestations of the overlap syndromes do not fall into a single disease category does not clarify whether a single rheumatic disease syndrome with wide clinical expression or two coexistent disorders are present. MCTD is but one of the overlap syndromes, which is differentiated from the remainder by the presence of RNP antibodies.

Clinical and radiographic features of other overlap syndromes simulate the findings of MCTD. In scleroderma–systemic lupus erythematosus overlap syndrome, radiographic changes of both diseases may be evident; Silver and coworkers[20] were unable to differentiate these changes from those of MCTD (Fig. 37–7). In addition to clinical manifestations typical of scleroderma, alopecia, fever, pleural effusions, pericarditis, hemolytic anemia, and arthritis may be evident in this overlap syndrome. Renal abnormalities are infrequent, and familial clustering of cases has been observed.[61]

In patients with rheumatoid arthritis–scleroderma overlap syndrome, findings of the latter disease include typical skin abnormalities, nailfold changes, telangiectasia, and subcutaneous calcification; abnormalities of rheumatoid arthritis include prolonged morning stiffness and the presence of a symmetric deforming polyarthritis with cartilage loss, bone erosions, and a positive serologic test for rheumatoid factor (Fig. 37–8).[59, 60]

An overlap syndrome consisting of rheumatoid arthritis and systemic lupus erythematosus has been identified.[62] Serologic overlap of the two disorders is documented by the occurrence of LE cells in patients who appear to have rheumatoid arthritis. Subsequently, some of these patients develop additional features of systemic lupus erythematosus, including cutaneous and visceral manifestations; however, the association of erosive rheumatoid arthritis and classic clinical and serologic findings of systemic lupus erythematosus is rare. Of interest, reports have appeared that document an additional overlap syndrome of juvenile rheumatoid arthritis and systemic lupus erythematosus.[63] Furthermore, patients with both rheumatoid arthritis and subacute cutaneous lupus erythematosus have been described.[68]

These descriptions of overlap syndromes have been confined to only a few of the more characteristic patterns. Others have been defined and will continue to be identified, including some in which a collagen vascular disorder is combined with a related condition, such as Reiter's syndrome.[64–66] It should be kept in mind, while reviewing these descriptions, that heterogeneous and confusing clinical manifestations are more likely an expanded expression of a single collagen vascular disease than an indication of a second process.[49]

Although differentiation of various overlap syndromes and MCTD on the basis of radiographic alterations is not possible in many patients, it appears that distinguishing MCTD from a single or pure collagen vascular disease usually can be accomplished because each of the major collagen vascular diseases is characterized by relatively distinctive abnormalities. In some situations, however, radiographic abnormalities that are considered typical of one collagen vascular disease may be seen in another without implying that clinical features of the second disorder are evident. Thus, erosive arthritis not too dissimilar from rheumatoid arthritis can be seen in scleroderma,[39, 40] systemic lupus erythematosus, and dermatomyositis; deforming nonerosive arthropathy simulating systemic lupus erythematosus also can be apparent in scleroderma and rheumatoid arthritis; and soft tissue atrophy and calcification with tuftal resorption, findings typical of scleroderma, occasionally are observed in systemic lupus erythematosus and dermatomyositis.[41–43]

SUMMARY

MCTD is an overlap syndrome defined serologically by the presence of a ribonuclease-sensitive extractable nuclear

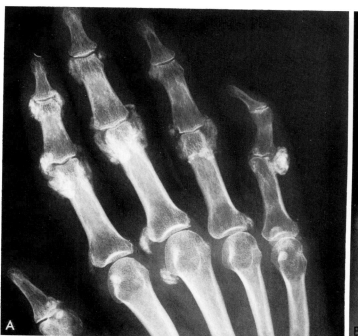

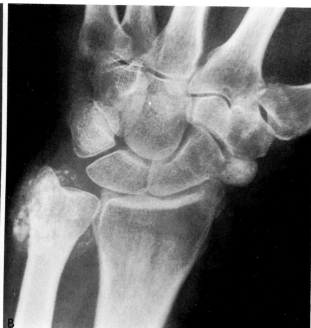

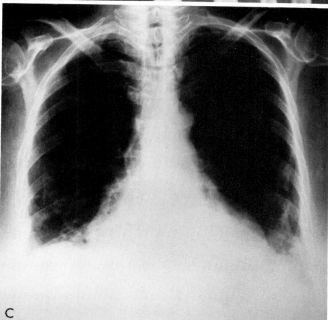

FIGURE 37–7. Scleroderma-systemic lupus erythematosus overlap syndrome. A 55 year old woman had clinical features of both scleroderma and systemic lupus erythematosus.

A Extensive calcification can be seen about metacarpophalangeal and interphalangeal joints. Deformity of the fifth finger also is evident.

B In the wrist, calcific deposits are apparent about the radial styloid and inferior radioulnar joint.

C Pleural and pericardial effusions are present.

(Courtesy of J. Scavulli, M.D., San Diego, California.)

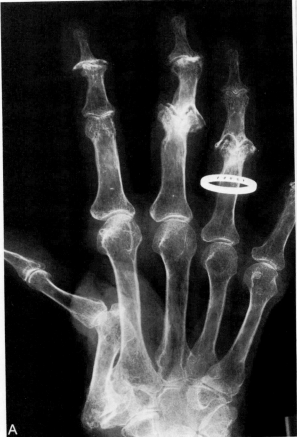

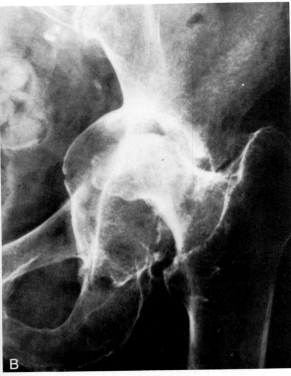

FIGURE 37–8. Rheumatoid arthritis–scleroderma overlap syndrome. This 81 year old woman had an 8 year history of arthritis with clinical and radiologic features consistent with both rheumatoid arthritis and scleroderma.

A Articular abnormalities in the hand reveal peculiar bone erosions and osteophytes about several proximal interphalangeal joints, characteristic of changes observed in scleroderma. Furthermore, the findings in the first digit, including the hyperextension at the metacarpophalangeal joint and the deformity and subluxation at the carpometacarpal joint, have been described in scleroderma.

B Acetabular protrusion and fracture and erosion of the femoral head are abnormalities consistent with rheumatoid arthritis. (Courtesy of R. Cavanagh, M.D., Boynton Beach, Florida.)

antigen. It demonstrates clinical features of several collagen vascular diseases, including systemic lupus erythematosus, scleroderma, dermatomyositis, and rheumatoid arthritis, and, in fact, patients with this syndrome may fulfill diagnostic criteria for any or all of these disorders.

The radiographic characteristics of MCTD also underscore the mixed character of the disease. Changes compatible with rheumatoid arthritis (articular erosion, joint space narrowing, periarticular osteoporosis), scleroderma (tuftal resorption, soft tissue calcification), and systemic lupus erythematosus (deforming nonerosive arthropathy) can be observed. The detection on radiographs of skeletal abnormalities characteristic of more than one collagen vascular disease should raise the possibility of MCTD, although other overlap syndromes may reveal similar findings.

References

1. Sharp GC, Irvin WS, Tan EM, et al: Mixed connective tissue disease—an apparently distinct rheumatic disease syndrome associated with a specific antibody to an extractable nuclear antigen (ENA). Am J Med 52:148, 1972.
2. Bennett RM, O'Connell DJ: The arthritis of mixed connective tissue disease. Ann Rheum Dis 37:397, 1978.
3. Halla JT, Hardin JG: Clinical features of the arthritis of mixed connective tissue disease. Arthritis Rheum 21:497, 1978.
4. Ramos-Niembro F, Alarcón-Segovia D, Hernandez-Ortiz J: Articular manifestations of mixed connective tissue disease. Arthritis Rheum 22:43, 1979.
5. Sharp GC, Irvin W, LaRoque RL, et al: Association of autoantibodies to different nuclear antigens with clinical patterns of rheumatoid disease and responsiveness to therapy. J Clin Invest 50:350, 1971.
6. Sharp GC: Mixed connective tissue disease. Bull Rheum Dis 25:828, 1975.
7. Hench PK, Edgington TS, Tan EM: The evolving clinical spectrum of mixed connective tissue disease (MCTD) (Abstr). Arthritis Rheum 18:404, 1975.
8. Minkin W, Rabhan N: Mixed connective tissue disease. Arch Dermatol 112:1535, 1976.
9. Farber SJ, Bole GG: Antibodies to components of extractable nuclear antigen. Arch Intern Med 136:425, 1976.
10. Mattioli M, Reichlin M: Physical association of two nuclear antigens and the mutual occurrence of their antibodies; the relationship of Sm and RNA protein (Mo) systems in SLE sera. J Immunol 110:1318, 1977.
11. Reichlin M, Mattioli M: Correlation of a precipitin reaction to RNA protein antigen and a low prevalence of nephritis in patients with systemic lupus erythematosus. N Engl J Med 286:908, 1972.
12. Sharp GC, Irvin WS, May CM, et al: Association of antibodies to ribonucleoprotein and Sm antigens with mixed connective tissue disease, systemic lupus erythematosus, and other rheumatic diseases. N Engl J Med 295:1149, 1976.
13. Parker MD: Ribonucleoprotein antibodies: Frequency and clinical significance in systemic lupus erythematosus, scleroderma, and mixed connective tissue disease. J Lab Clin Med 82:769, 1973.
14. Notman DD, Kurata N, Tan EM: Profile of antinuclear antibodies in systemic rheumatic disease. Ann Intern Med 83:464, 1975.
15. Reichlin M, Mattioli M: Antigens and antibodies characteristic of systemic lupus erythematosus. Bull Rheum Dis 24:756, 1973.
16. Gilliam JN, Prystowsky SD: Conversion of discoid lupus erythematosus to mixed connective tissue disease. J Rheumatol 4:165, 1977.
17. Norman DA, Fleischmann RM: Gastrointestinal systemic sclerosis in serologic mixed connective tissue disease. Arthritis Rheum 21:811, 1978.
18. Weiss TD, Nelson JS, Woolsey RM, et al: Transverse myelitis in mixed connective tissue disease. Arthritis Rheum 21:982, 1978.
19. Udoff EJ, Genant HK, Kozin F, et al: Mixed connective tissue disease: The spectrum of radiographic manifestations. Radiology 124:613, 1977.

20. Silver TM, Farber SJ, Bole GG, et al: Radiological features of mixed connective tissue disease and scleroderma-systemic lupus erythematosus overlap. Radiology 120:269, 1976.
21. Singsen BH, Landing B, Wolfe JF, et al: Histologic evaluation of mixed connective tissue disease in children and adults (Abstr). Arthritis Rheum 21:593, 1978.
22. Oxenhandler R, Hart M, Corman L, et al: Pathology of skeletal muscle connective tissue disease. Arthritis Rheum 20:985, 1977.
23. Brooke MH, Kaplan H: Muscle pathology in rheumatoid arthritis, polymyalgia rheumatica, and polymyositis. Arch Pathol 94:101, 1972.
24. Tuffanelli DL, Winkelmann RK: Systemic scleroderma: A clinical study of 727 cases. Arch Dermatol 84:359, 1961.
25. Clark JA, Winkelmann RK, Ward LE: Serological alterations in scleroderma and sclerodermatomyositis. Mayo Clin Proc 46:104, 1971.
26. Poirier TJ, Rankin GB: Gastrointestinal manifestations of progressive systemic scleroderma based on a review of 364 cases. Am J Gastroenterol 58:30, 1972.
27. Keil H: Dermatomyositis and systemic lupus erythematosus. A clinical report of transitional cases with consideration of lead as a possible etiologic factor. Arch Intern Med 66:109, 1940.
28. Estes D, Christian CL: The natural history of systemic lupus erythematosus by prospective analysis. Medicine 50:85, 1971.
29. Dubois EL: Lupus erythematosus, lupoid syndromes, and their relation to collagen diseases, part 2. Postgrad Med 32:568, 1962.
30. Toone EC, Irby R, Pierce EL: The LE cell in rheumatoid arthritis. Am J Med Sci 240:599, 1960.
31. Sigler JW, Monto RW, Ensign DC, et al: The incidence of the LE cell phenomenon in patients with rheumatoid arthritis (a two-year study). Arthritis Rheum 1:115, 1958.
32. Haserick JR: Modern concepts of systemic lupus erythematosus: A review of 126 cases. J Chronic Dis 1:317, 1955.
33. Dubois EL, Chandor S, Friou GJ, et al: Progressive systemic sclerosis and localized scleroderma with positive LE cell test and unusual systemic manifestations compatible with systemic lupus erythematosus. Medicine 50:199, 1971.
34. D'Angelo WA, Fries JF, Masi AT, et al: Pathologic observations in systemic sclerosis (scleroderma). A study of 58 autopsy cases and 58 matched controls. Am J Med 46:428, 1969.
35. Rowell NR: Lupus erythematosus cells in systemic sclerosis. Ann Rheum Dis 21:70, 1962.
36. Bianchi FA, Bistue AR, Wendt VE, et al: Analysis of twenty-seven cases of progressive systemic sclerosis (including two with combined systemic lupus erythematosus) and a review of the literature. J Chronic Dis 19:953, 1966.
37. Chorzelski T, Jablónska S: Coexistence of lupus erythematosus and scleroderma in light of immunopathological investigations. Acta Derm-Venereol 50:81, 1970.
38. Tuffanelli DL: Scleroderma and its relationship to the "collagenoses": Dermatomyositis, lupus erythematosus, rheumatoid arthritis, and Sjögren's syndrome. Am J Med Sci 243:133, 1962.
39. Resnick D, Greenway G, Vint VC, et al: Selective involvement of the first carpometacarpal joint in scleroderma. AJR 131:283, 1978.
40. Rabinowitz JG, Twersky J, Guttadauria M: Similar bone manifestations of scleroderma and rheumatoid arthritis. AJR 121:35, 1974.
41. Budin JA, Feldman F: Soft tissue calcifications in systemic lupus erythematosus. AJR 124:358, 1975.
42. Kabir DI, Malkinson FD: Lupus erythematosus and calcinosis cutis. Arch Dermatol 100:17, 1969.
43. Quismorio FP, Dubois EL, Chandor SB: Soft-tissue calcification in systemic lupus erythematosus. Arch Dermatol 111:352, 1975.
44. Peskett SA, Ansell BM, Fizzman AP, et al: Mixed connective tissue disease in children. Rheumatol Rehabil 17:245, 1978.
45. Alarcón-Segovia D, Uribe-Uribe O: Mutilans-like arthropathy in mixed connective tissue disease. Arthritis Rheum 22:1013, 1979.
46. LeRoy EC, Maricq HR, Kahalch MB: Undifferentiated connective tissue syndromes. Arthritis Rheum 23:341, 1980.
47. Prystowsky SD: Mixed connective tissue disease. West J Med 132:288, 1980.
48. Manthorpe R, Elling H, Van der Meulen JT, et al: Two fatal cases of mixed connective tissue disease. Scand J Rheumatol 9:7, 1980.
49. LeRoy EC: Overlap features of connective tissue disease. Arthritis Rheum 25:889, 1982.
50. Grant KD, Adams LE, Hess EV: Mixed connective tissue disease—a subset with sequential clinical and laboratory features. J Rheumatol 8:587, 1981.
51. Alarcón-Segovia D: Mixed connective tissue disease—a decade of growing pains. J Rheumatol 8:535, 1981.
52. Horn JR, Kapur JJ, Walker SE: Mixed connective tissue disease in siblings. Arthritis Rheum 21:709, 1978.
53. Kish LS, Steck WD: Mixed connective tissue disease in identical twins. Cleve Clin Q 50:205, 1983.
54. Bennett RM: The differential diagnosis of mixed connective-tissue disease. IM 3:40, 1982.
55. Kappes J, Bennett RM: Cauda equina syndrome in a patient with high titer anti-RNP antibodies. Arthritis Rheum 25:349, 1982.
56. Szanto D: MCTD-syndrome (mixed connective tissue disease). ROFO 133:445, 1980.
57. Lacombe P, Zenny JC, Benhamou L, et al: Signes radiologiques des connectivités "mixtes" avec anticorps anti-RNP. J Radiol 62:417, 1981.
58. Sharp GC: Mixed connective tissue diseases and overlap syndromes. In WN Kelley, ED Harris Jr, S Ruddy, et al (Eds): Textbook of Rheumatology. Philadelphia, WB Saunders, 1981, p 1151.
59. Cohen MJ, Persellin RH: Coexistence of rheumatoid arthritis and systemic sclerosis in four patients. Scand J Rheumatol 11:241, 1982.
60. Baron M, Srolovitz H, Lander P, et al: The coexistence of rheumatoid arthritis and scleroderma: A case report and review of the literature. J Rheumatol 9:947, 1982.
61. Flores RH, Stevens MB, Arnett FC: Familial occurrence of progressive systemic sclerosis and systemic lupus erythematosus. J Rheumatol 11:321, 1984.
62. Fischman AS, Abeles M, Zanetti M, et al: The coexistence of rheumatoid arthritis and systemic lupus erythematosus. A case report and review of the literature. J Rheumatol 8:405, 1981.
63. Saulsbury FT, Kesler RW, Kennaugh JM, et al: Overlap syndrome of juvenile rheumatoid arthritis and systemic lupus erythematosus. J Rheumatol 9:610, 1982.
64. Fallahi S, Miller RK, Halla JT: Coexistence of Reiter's syndrome and rheumatoid arthritis in a genetically susceptible individual. Ann Rheum Dis 42:210, 1983.
65. Aisen PS, Cornstein BN, Kramer SB: Systemic lupus erythematosus in a patient with Reiter's syndrome. Arthritis Rheum 26:1405, 1983.
66. Jalava S, Paljarvi L, Isomaki H: Keratodermia blenorrhagica, arthritis, and polymyositis with cardiopulmonary complications. Ann Rheum Dis 42:455, 1983.
67. Babini SM, Maldonado-Cocco JA, Barcello HA, et al: Peritendinous nodules in overlap syndrome. J Rheumatol 12:160, 1985.
68. Cohen S, Stastny P, Sontheimer RD: Concurrence of subacute cutaneous lupus erythematosus and rheumatoid arthritis. Arthritis Rheum 29:421, 1986.
69. Cervera R, Khamashta MA, Hughes GRV: "Overlap" syndromes. Ann Rheum Dis 49:947, 1990.
70. Neau JPh, Larrard G, Boissonnot L, et al: Syndrome bilatéral du canal carpien au cours d'une connectivite mixte (syndrome de Sharp). Semin Hôp Paris 63:2137, 1987.
71. Martyn JB, Wong MJ, Huang SHK: Pulmonary and neuromuscular complications of mixed connective tissue disease: A report and review of the literature. J Rheumatol 15:703, 1988.
72. Stecher DR, Gusis SE, Cocco JAM: Tuberculous arthritis in the course of connective tissue disease: Report of 4 cases. J Rheumatol 19:1418, 1992.
73. Martínez-Cordero E, López-Zepeda J: Resorptive arthropathy and rib erosions in mixed connective tissue disease. J Rheumatol 17:719, 1990.
74. Hutton CW, Maddison PJ, Collins AJ, et al: Intra-articular apatite deposition in mixed connective tissue disease: Crystallographic and technetium scanning characteristics. Ann Rheum Dis 47:1027, 1988.
75. Stuart RA, Maddison PJ: Atlantoaxial subluxation in a patient with mixed connective tissue disease. J Rheumatol 18:1617, 1991.
76. Cohen MG, Webb J: Concurrence of rheumatoid arthritis and systemic lupus erythematosus: Report of 11 cases. Ann Rheum Dis 46:853, 1987.
77. Asherson RA, Angus H, Mathews JA, et al: The progressive systemic sclerosis/systemic lupus overlap: An unusual clinical progression. Ann Rheum Dis 50:323, 1991.
78. Cohen MG, Ho KK, Webb J: Finger joint calcinosis followed by osteolysis in a patient with multisystem connective tissue disease and anti-Jo-1 antibody. J Rheumatol 14:605, 1987.
79. Shiokawa S, Yasuda M, Kikuchi M, et al: Mixed connective tissue disease associated with lupus lymphadenitis. J Rheumatol 20:147, 1993.

Rheumatic Fever

Donald Resnick, M.D.

Rheumatic fever is a disorder characterized clinically by fever, carditis, and polyarthritis; historically there has been a previous episode of group A beta-hemolytic streptococcal infection. Although rheumatic fever affects many tissues of the body, it is the cardiac involvement that is most significant to the patient and that has received considerable attention through the years. In 1864, Lasègue[1] emphasized the cardiac abnormalities in this disorder when he noted that "acute rheumatism licks the joints but bites the heart." This investigator's appraisal of the potential severity of cardiac manifestations in rheumatic fever subsequently has been verified in numerous accounts of the disease. Rheumatic fever, however, also can "bite" other organs of the body, including the joints.

This chapter discusses only the articular abnormalities of rheumatic fever; the interested reader who wishes to learn about involvement of other organ systems should consult additional sources.

HISTORICAL ASPECTS

The relationship among rheumatic fever, valvular disease of the heart, and rheumatoid arthritis has interested many investigators. In 1950, Bywaters[2] traced the historical aspects of this relationship, noting that three major schools of thought had developed: that rheumatic fever and rheumatoid arthritis were separate disorders that occasionally occurred in the same person; that rheumatic fever and rheumatoid arthritis were closely allied or identical disorders; and that certain types of rheumatic fever were associated with a chronic rheumatic syndrome that could be distinguished from rheumatoid arthritis, whereas certain types of

rheumatoid arthritis were associated with cardiac lesions that were different from those of rheumatic fever. It was the third theory that received the support of Bywaters and that since has gained further support owing to the documentation by additional investigators of the occurrence of a distinct chronic arthropathy in some patients with rheumatic fever.

A report of post–rheumatic fever arthropathy first appeared in 1867 when Jaccoud[3] described a young man with rheumatic fever and recurrent bouts of polyarthritis who developed a chronic deforming arthropathy. The arthropathy was characterized by muscle atrophy, ulnar deviation with flexion and subluxation at multiple metacarpophalangeal joints, and hyperextension of distal interphalangeal joints. Subsequent reports of Jaccoud's arthropathy have indicated that it also may involve the feet, that it is correctable initially but later may become fixed, and that it is not confined to patients with rheumatic fever but also may appear in patients with collagen vascular disorders, such as systemic lupus erythematosus. Although other articular manifestations accompany bouts of rheumatic fever, it is Jaccoud's arthropathy that has received the most emphasis.

ARTICULAR ABNORMALITIES

Classically, an attack of rheumatic fever occurs from several days to several weeks after a streptococcal throat infection. The average latent period between the two events is 16 to 18 days; rarely it is less than 7 days or longer than 5 weeks.[32] Symptoms and signs of the clinical attack are variable; an acute onset may be characterized by fever, night sweats, headaches, and joint pains, whereas an insidious onset may be accompanied by pallor, fatigue, anorexia, weight loss, and muscular pain.

Polyarthritis

Joint involvement is the most common clinical manifestation of rheumatic fever and frequently appears early during the course of a rheumatic attack. It occurs in approximately 75 per cent of patients and is more frequent with increasing patient age.[32] The involvement varies in severity

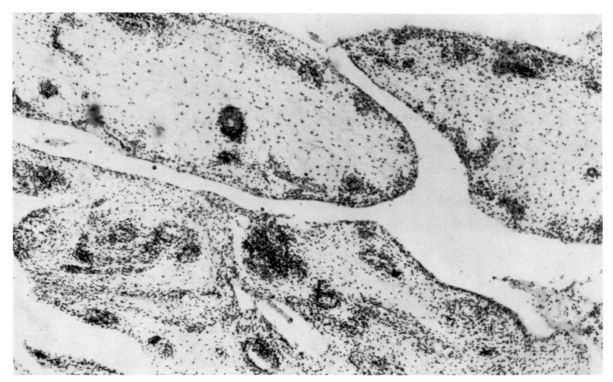

FIGURE 38–1. Rheumatic fever: Acute polyarthritis. A low-grade proliferation of synovial lining cells with edema of the stroma is evident. Lymphocytes surround the small vessels. (From Fassbender HG: Pathology of Rheumatic Diseases. New York, Springer-Verlag, 1975.)

from arthralgia (joint pain without inflammation) to arthritis (joint pain with inflammation). In the latter case, swelling, redness, and heat are additional articular abnormalities, although these inflammatory changes may be mild compared to the severity of the joint pain. Multiple joints usually are affected, particularly large joints, such as the knees and the ankles, although involvement of the elbows, the wrists, the hips, and the small joints of the hands and wrists is common.[4, 29] Many joints may be affected simultaneously or in quick succession, leading to the designation of a "migratory polyarthritis." Without treatment, joint inflammation may persist for several days to a week, subsequently diminishing and eventually disappearing completely. Joint effusions seldom are large. Aspiration of joint fluid reveals approximately 30,000 to 40,000 cells per cu mm, 60 to 90 per cent of which are polymorphonuclear leukocytes. If the disease persists for a few weeks, lymphocytes also may appear. Radiographs reveal soft tissue swelling without evidence of cartilaginous or osseous destruction. Mild osteoporosis may be apparent.

In a few patients, swelling and stiffness of the metacarpophalangeal and proximal interphalangeal joints persist up to 6 months, associated with inflammation of the adjacent tendon sheaths.[5] In these patients, interosseous muscle wasting and osteoporosis can be prominent, simulating the findings of rheumatoid arthritis.[6]

Pathologic characteristics in the acute polyarticular phase of rheumatic fever confirm the mild nature of the synovitis (Fig. 38–1). Macroscopic inspection of involved joints reveals only slightly edematous synovial villi; the articular cartilage and bone appear unremarkable. Microscopically, fibrin deposition on the synovial surface is associated with

mild hyperemia, loss of synoviocytes, and proliferation of surface cells.[7, 8] The inflammatory changes are limited to the superficial layers of the synovial membrane and, unlike the case with rheumatoid arthritis, are not associated with prominent lymphocytic or plasma cellular infiltration. More deeply, fibrinoid change of collagen fibers can be observed in the synovium and joint capsule of patients with rheumatic fever.

After the acute episode, regression of synovitis, regeneration of surface synovial cells, and decrease in fibroblasts underscore the temporary nature of the joint affliction. Although vascular sclerosis and synovial stromal fibrosis may remain, these residual abnormalities are not prominent. The cartilage, which is normal in the acute phase, can reveal some loss of chondrocytes and the presence of fibrinoid foci.[8] Such foci also may be evident in the periosteal membrane, tendons, and fascia.[8, 9]

Deforming Nonerosive (Jaccoud's) Arthropathy

The deforming arthropathy that may appear after repeated attacks of arthritis in patients with rheumatic fever has received considerable attention.[10–20] This arthropathy, which Jaccoud originally described as "rheumatisme chronique fibreux," also has been referred to as Jaccoud's syndrome, Jaccoud's arthropathy, Jaccoud's arthritis, and chronic post–rheumatic fever arthropathy. Although its pathogenesis is not clear, Jaccoud's arthropathy appears to result from capsular inflammation and fibrosis, and it is not confined to patients with rheumatic fever but also may

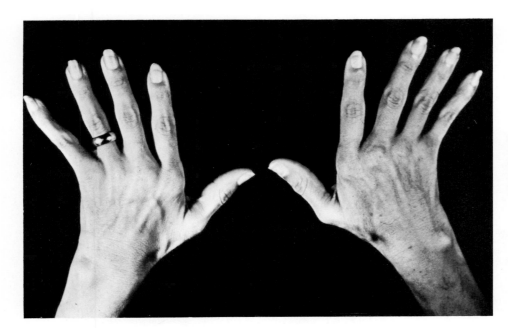

FIGURE 38–2. Rheumatic fever: Jaccoud's arthropathy. Clinical abnormalities. Observe ulnar deviation at all of the metacarpophalangeal joints of both hands. (Courtesy of N. Zvaifler, M.D., San Diego, California.)

occur in association with systemic lupus erythematosus and scleroderma.[30]

The clinical findings are characteristic, although superficial evaluation may lead to an erroneous diagnosis of rheumatoid arthritis. A history of previous attacks of rheumatic fever is combined with symptoms and signs of residual heart lesions. Symptomless and reversible joint deformities appear, particularly in the hands, but also in the feet.[33] Typically, ulnar deviation and flexion deformities are evident at the metacarpophalangeal joints, predominantly in the fourth and fifth digits, and may be combined with hyperextension at interphalangeal joints (Fig. 38–2). In the foot, fibular deviation and subluxation at metatarsophalangeal joints, especially those in the first and second toes, can be observed.[33] In the hands and feet, the reversible nature of the articular deformity is striking. On physical examination, the clinician may easily reduce the joint subluxations with only mild pressure. During radiography, pressing the hand against the cassette may result in an entirely normal posteroanterior radiograph; placing the hand in an oblique projection with the fingers lifted from the cassette will reveal the striking deformities (Fig. 38–3). Eventually, fixed deformities may appear that cannot be corrected on clinical or radiographic examination.

These clinical manifestations have been summarized as specific criteria that are necessary for the diagnosis of Jaccoud's arthropathy[12]:

1. A history of recurrent attacks of acute rheumatic fever.

2. A delayed recovery after joint inflammation with initial stiffness and subsequent deformity, particularly in the metacarpophalangeal joints.

3. A characteristic articular deformity that is associated with periarticular, fascial, and tendon fibrosis rather than synovitis, which consists of flexion and ulnar deviation at the metacarpophalangeal joints, particularly in the fourth and fifth digits, in association with soft tissue swelling.

4. The elicitation of tendon crepitus.

5. Joint disease that generally is asymptomatic, with little evidence of active synovitis and with good functional capacity.

On radiographic evaluation, joint deformities may be apparent (Fig. 38–4) (Table 38–1). In most patients, articular space narrowing and osseous erosions are not evident, allowing differentiation of Jaccoud's arthropathy from rheumatoid arthritis and other inflammatory synovial processes. Occasionally, however, articular space diminution is encountered, probably representing cartilaginous atrophy due to disuse and cartilaginous erosion due to closely applied subluxed osseous surfaces (Fig. 38–5). Furthermore, hook erosions on the radial and palmar aspects of the metacarpal heads, which can appear in Jaccoud's arthropathy, superficially resemble the marginal erosions of rheumatoid arthritis (Fig. 38–6).[31]

The arthropathy is not related to synovitis. Rather, capsular and periarticular fibrosis is important in the evolution of the joint disease, and the fibrotic lesion is similar to that occurring in the heart in patients with rheumatic fever.[28] It has been suggested that capsular abnormality results in ulnar displacement of extensor tendons, phalangeal deviation, and progressive periarticular fibrosis. The hook erosion of the metacarpal heads may be produced by pressure erosion beneath the distorted capsule in the deformed articulations, a process that is identical to that occurring in lupus arthropathy (see Chapter 33).

TABLE 38–1. Radiographic Characteristics of Jaccoud's Arthropathy

Flexion and ulnar deviation of metacarpophalangeal joints, particularly fourth and fifth
Flexion and fibular deviation of metatarsophalangeal joints
Periarticular osteoporosis
Joint space narrowing (rare)
Hook erosions on radial and palmar aspect of metacarpal heads (rare)

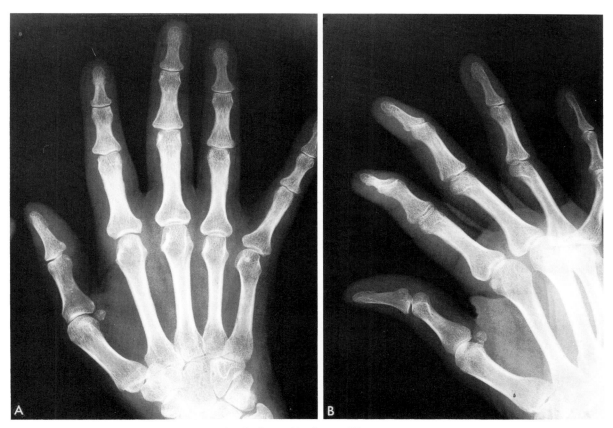

FIGURE 38–3. Rheumatic fever: Jaccoud's arthropathy. Radiographic abnormalities.

A On a posteroanterior radiograph with the hand pressed firmly against the cassette, the only striking deformity is ulnar deviation of the fifth finger at the metacarpophalangeal joint. Mild periarticular osteoporosis is seen. There is no evidence of osseous erosion.

B On the oblique radiograph, the hand has been lifted from the cassette. Boutonnière and swan-neck deformities of all the digits can be seen.

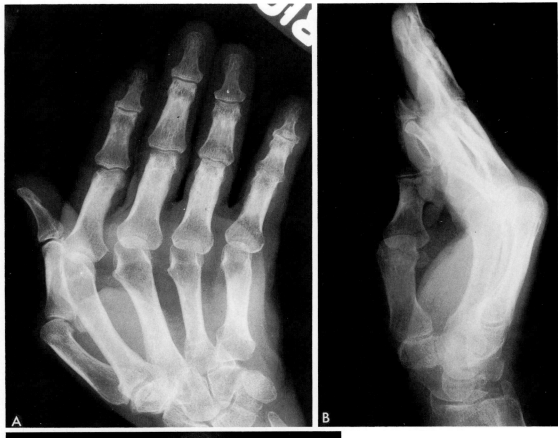

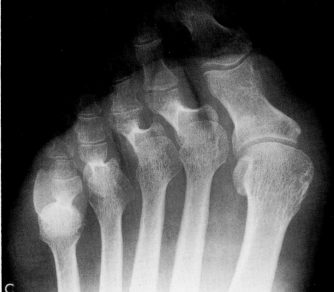

FIGURE 38–4. Rheumatic fever: Jaccoud's arthropathy. Radiographic abnormalities. A 76 year old man with a history of rheumatic fever as a teenager had long-standing deformities of his hands and feet.

A, B The frontal and lateral radiographs reveal typical deformities, particularly flexion and ulnar deviation at the metacarpophalangeal joints. Note periarticular osteoporosis and the absence of osseous erosions.

C, Deformities of the foot consist of fibular deviation at the first to fourth metatarsophalangeal joints with associated dorsiflexion of all of the digits. No erosions are apparent. The opposite foot was involved similarly.

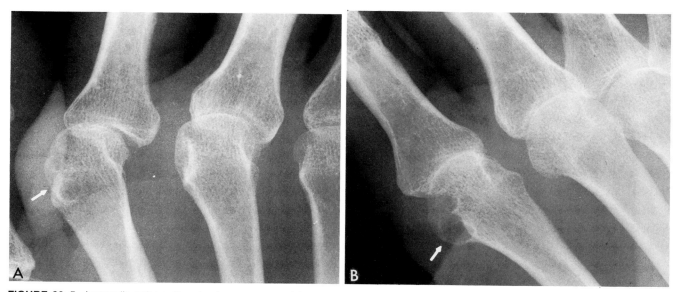

FIGURE 38–5. Jaccoud's arthropathy of unknown cause—joint space narrowing and osseous erosion. A 45 year old man had had long-standing articular deformities of the hands without significant symptoms. Extensive work-up failed to document the cause of the abnormalities. Rheumatoid factor was not present in the serum. Frontal and oblique radiographs reveal ulnar deviation of the second to fourth metacarpophalangeal joints with articular space narrowing. A cystic lesion (arrows) can be seen on the radial aspect of the second metacarpal head. Associated soft tissue swelling and osteoporosis are evident.

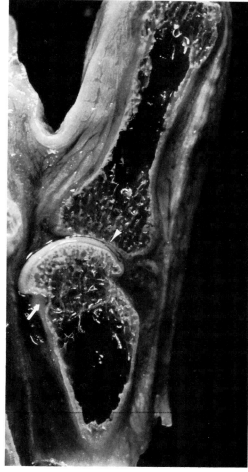

FIGURE 38–6. Rheumatic fever: Jaccoud's arthropathy. Osseous erosion. A coronal section of the fifth metacarpophalangeal joint in a cadaver with rheumatic fever demonstrates typical ulnar deviation of the digit. Note a hooklike erosion on the radial aspect of the metacarpal head (arrow). A similar defect of unknown cause is present on the ulnar aspect of the bone. The cartilage on the metacarpal head appears preserved. Some diminution of the cartilaginous surface on the proximal phalanx (arrowhead) may be present, perhaps related to pressure or disuse.

Other Abnormalities

Not surprisingly, Jaccoud's arthropathy often is misdiagnosed as rheumatoid arthritis on the basis of the hand and foot deformities.[34] Confusion between the two entities is accentuated by the occasional occurrence of soft tissue nodules in patients with rheumatic fever.[17] Such nodules are round, firm, painless, freely movable, and 0.5 to 2.0 cm in size; they are located over bony prominences and tendons, especially those in the hands and feet.[32] Nodules are evanescent, rarely lasting more than a few weeks, and are smaller, more discrete, and less persistent than rheumatoid nodules.[32] Furthermore, serologic tests for rheumatoid factor characteristically are negative in patients with rheumatic fever.

Atlantoaxial subluxation has been associated with acute rheumatic fever.[35, 36] The mechanism of such subluxation appears to relate to the hyperemia associated with the throat and neck inflammation (Grisel's syndrome) rather than to diffuse ligamentous laxity. Anterior subluxation of the atlas is the dominant pattern of displacement.

DIFFERENTIAL DIAGNOSIS

Syndromes of Cardiac and Articular Disease

The relationships between articular and cardiac disease are complex. Several "syndromes" may be encountered: rheumatoid arthritis and *rheumatoid* heart disease; rheumatoid arthritis and *rheumatic* heart disease; and rheumatic heart disease and Jaccoud's arthropathy. In addition, ankylosing spondylitis may be associated with aortic insufficiency.

Cardiac damage may occur during the course of rheumatoid arthritis,[21, 22] although the prevalence of clinically manifest valvular heart disease in patients with rheumatoid arthritis probably is less than 10 per cent.[13] Pathologic changes in the heart may include vasculitis, pericarditis, and cardiomyopathy. Granulomatous inflammation in the epicardium, myocardium, and valves may resemble rheumatoid subcutaneous nodules histologically.[22–24] In general, rheumatoid cardiac involvement is accompanied by other manifestations of systemic rheumatoid disease.

At the opposite end of the spectrum is the association of Jaccoud's arthropathy and rheumatic heart disease. This arthropathy is distinct from rheumatoid arthritis; the absence of significant symptoms and signs of synovitis, the presence of relatively normal functional capacity, and the absence of elevated erythrocyte sedimentation rate and serum rheumatoid factor on laboratory analysis are characteristic of Jaccoud's arthropathy.

Between these two extremes are cases in which both rheumatoid arthritis and rheumatic heart disease appear to be present. According to Weintraub and Zvaifler,[13] the occurrence of rheumatic heart disease in patients with rheumatoid arthritis[22] may be explained by unusual selection factors, a common etiologic or pathogenetic mechanism, or a predisposition of one disease for the development of the other. The clinical and radiographic features of rheumatoid arthritis in these cases are typical.

The association of ankylosing spondylitis and aortic insufficiency is well known.[25–27] Valvular involvement is more frequent in patients with long-standing spondylitis and in those with peripheral joint involvement. Occasion-

TABLE 38–2. Diseases That May Lead to Deforming Nonerosive Arthropathy

Rheumatic fever
Collagen vascular disorders, particularly systemic lupus erythematosus
Rheumatoid arthritis (rare)
Agammaglobulinemia (rare)
Ehlers-Danlos syndrome (rare)

ally patients with rheumatoid arthritis develop similar clinical and pathologic abnormalities of the aortic valve.[13]

Jaccoud's Arthropathy

Jaccoud's deforming arthropathy is not diagnostic of rheumatic fever (Table 38–2). Rather, it is a descriptive term for characteristic joint subluxation and malalignment in the hands (and feet), which frequently occur without clinical findings of synovial disease and without radiographic findings of joint space narrowing and osseous erosion. The deforming nonerosive arthropathy of rheumatic fever is similar to that of systemic lupus erythematosus and, more rarely, other collagen vascular diseases and vasculitides. Although classically the ulnar digits are more commonly affected in rheumatic fever and all the digits, including the thumb, are affected in systemic lupus erythematosus, the patterns of distribution are variable and may be identical in

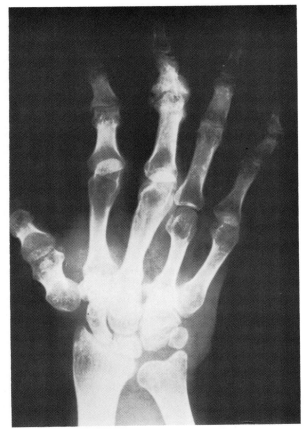

FIGURE 38–7. Ehlers-Danlos syndrome. A radiograph from a patient with this rare syndrome reveals deformities of multiple digits, particularly the thumb. Abnormalities of bone growth and osseous hypertrophy at the third proximal interphalangeal joint, probably traumatic and degenerative in nature, are observed.

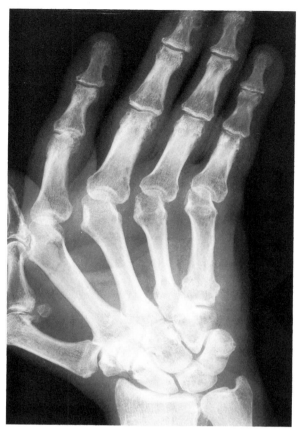

FIGURE 38–8. Rheumatoid arthritis. In this patient with classic seropositive rheumatoid arthritis, radial deviation at the radiocarpal joint and ulnar deviation at the metacarpophalangeal joints have occurred without significant osseous erosion. Periarticular osteoporosis can be noted.

SUMMARY

Articular involvement in rheumatic fever typically appears as polyarthritis, particularly in large joints, and as Jaccoud's arthropathy. Polyarthritis is associated with nonspecific radiographic features, including soft tissue swelling and mild osteoporosis. Jaccoud's arthropathy is associated with typical radiographic abnormalities, which are best classified as deforming nonerosive articular changes. Jaccoud's arthropathy shows predilection for the ulnar digits of the hand, leading to deviation and subluxation at the metacarpophalangeal joints, which may be accompanied by deformities of interphalangeal joints of the fingers and of metatarsophalangeal joints of the feet. The hand abnormalities, which resemble changes in systemic lupus erythematosus and other collagen vascular diseases, usually can be differentiated from rheumatoid arthritis, in which early and significant cartilaginous and osseous destruction is apparent.

References

1. Lasègue C: Considérations sur la sciatique. Arch Gen Med 2:558, 1864.
2. Bywaters EGL: The relation between heart and joint disease including "rheumatoid heart disease" and chronic post-rheumatic arthritis (type Jaccoud). Br Heart J 12:101, 1950.
3. Jaccoud S: Leçons de Clinique Medicale faites a l'Hôpital de la Charité. Vingt-troisième leçon, sur une forme de rhumatisme chronique. Paris, Adrien Delahaye, 1867, p 598.
4. Feinstein AR, Spagnuolo M: The clinical patterns of acute rheumatic fever: A reappraisal. Medicine 41:279, 1962.
5. Bywaters EGL: Rheumatic fever (including chorea). In JT Scott (Ed): Copeman's Textbook of the Rheumatic Diseases. 5th Ed. Edinburgh, Churchill Livingstone, 1978, p 763.
6. Bywaters EGL: A variant of rheumatoid arthritis characterized by recurrent digital pad nodules and palmar fasciitis, closely resembling palindromic rheumatism. Ann Rheum Dis 8:1, 1949.
7. Klinge F: Der Rheumatismus. Pathologische-anatomische und experimentell pathologische Tatsachen ihre und Auswertung für das ärztliche Rheumaproblem. In W Hueck, W Frei (Eds): Ergebnisse der allgemeinen Pathologie und pathologischen Anatomie. Vol. 27. Munchen, Bergmann, 1933.
8. Fassbender HG: Pathology of Rheumatic Diseases. New York, Springer-Verlag, 1975, p 62.
9. Tilp A: Nodi rheumatici galeae aponeuroticae. Verh Dtsch Ges Pathol 17:469, 1914.
10. Thomas AE: Chronic arthritis after recurrent rheumatic fever. Ann Rheum Dis 14:259, 1955.
11. Twigg H, Smith BF: Jaccoud's arthritis. Radiology 80:417, 1963.
12. Zvaifler NJ: Chronic postrheumatic-fever (Jaccoud's) arthritis. N Engl J Med 267:10, 1962.
13. Weintraub AM, Zvaifler NJ: The occurrence of valvular and myocardial disease in patients with chronic joint deformity. A spectrum. Am J Med 35:145, 1963.
14. Beausang E, Barnett EV, Goldstein S: Jaccoud's arthritis. A case report. Ann Rheum Dis 26:239, 1967.
15. Burda CD, Sanders CV: Chronic postrheumatic-fever (Jaccoud's) arthritis. Arch Intern Med 120:712, 1967.
16. Rabkin SW, Fiedotin A: Chronic postrheumatic arthropathy (type Jaccoud): Report of two cases and a review of the American literature. South Med J 66:645, 1973.
17. Ruderman JE, Abruzzo JL: Chronic postrheumatic fever arthritis (Jaccoud's): Report of a case with subcutaneous nodules. Arthritis Rheum 9:640, 1966.
18. Levin EB: Jaccoud's arthritis: Postrheumatic fever complication—not rheumatoid arthritis. Calif Med 112:19, 1970.
19. Murphy WA, Staple TW: Jaccoud's arthropathy reviewed. AJR 118:300, 1973.
20. Grahame R, Mitchell ABS, Scott JT: Chronic postrheumatic fever (Jaccoud's) arthropathy. Ann Rheum Dis 29:622, 1970.
21. Baggenstoss AH, Rosenberg EF: Cardiac lesions associated with chronic infectious arthritis. Arch Intern Med 67:241, 1941.
22. Sokoloff L: The heart in rheumatoid arthritis. Am Heart J 45:635, 1953.
23. Goehrs HR, Baggenstoss AH, Slocumb CH: Cardiac lesions in rheumatoid arthritis. Arthritis Rheum 3:298, 1960.
24. Cruickshank B: Heart lesions in rheumatoid disease. J Pathol Bacteriol 76:223, 1958.
25. Schilder DP, Harvey WP, Hufnagel CA: Rheumatoid spondylitis and aortic insufficiency. N Engl J Med 255:11, 1956.
26. Clark WS, Kulka JP, Bauer W: Rheumatoid aortitis with aortic regurgitation. Am J Med 21:580, 1957.

both disorders. Deforming nonerosive arthropathies also may be encountered in agammaglobulinemia (hypogammaglobulinemia), Ehlers-Danlos syndrome (Fig. 38–7), sarcoidosis,[37] and, rarely, rheumatoid arthritis (Fig. 38–8).

The deformities that occur in association with Jaccoud's arthropathy resemble those in rheumatoid arthritis. In some patients with Jaccoud's arthropathy, the appearance of joint space narrowing and osseous erosion complicates the differentiation between these two disorders. The distribution and extent of articular space loss, however, are less widespread and severe in Jaccoud's arthropathy than in rheumatoid arthritis. In addition, diminution of joint space is an early manifestation of rheumatoid arthritis, and, when present, a late manifestation of Jaccoud's arthropathy. The hook erosions of this latter disorder also differ in appearance from erosions in rheumatoid arthritis. They involve the volar and radial aspects of the metacarpal heads, are located further from the articular margin, and usually are unassociated with joint space narrowing or erosive changes on the ulnar aspect. In rheumatoid arthritis, erosions on the radial aspect of the metacarpal head are closer to the articular margin, are quickly accompanied by erosive changes on the ulnar aspect of the bone as well as by joint space narrowing, and are associated with interphalangeal joint and wrist alterations.

27. Graham DC, Smythe HA: The carditis and aortitis of ankylosing spondylitis. Bull Rheum Dis *9:*171, 1958.

28. Girgis FL, Popple AW, Bruckner FE: Jaccoud's arthropathy. A case report and necropsy study. Ann Rheum Dis *37:*561, 1978.

29. McDanald EC, Weisman MH: Articular manifestations of rheumatic fever in adults. Ann Intern Med *89:*917, 1978.

30. Manthorpe R, Bendixen G, Schiøler H, et al: Jaccoud's syndrome. A nosographic entity associated with systemic lupus erythematosus. J Rheumatol *7:*169, 1980.

31. Pastershank SP, Resnick D: "Hook" erosions in Jaccoud's arthropathy. J Can Assoc Radiol *31:*174, 1980.

32. Stollerman GH: Rheumatic fever. *In* WN Kelley, ED Harris Jr, S Ruddy, et al (Eds): Textbook of Rheumatology. Philadelphia, WB Saunders, 1981, p 1306.

33. Joseph B, Chacko V: Chronic post-rheumatic-fever arthritis (Jaccoud's arthritis) involving the feet. A case report. J Bone Joint Surg [Am] *66:*1124, 1984.

34. Selby CL: Review and differential diagnosis of Jaccoud's arthropathy. IM *6:*55, 1985.

35. Bicknell JM, Kirsch WM, Seigel R, et al: Atlanto-axial dislocation in acute rheumatic fever. Case report. J Neurosurg *66:*286, 1987.

36. De Coster TA, Cole HC: Atlanto-axial dislocation in association with rheumatic fever. Spine *15:*591, 1990.

37. Sukenik S, Hendler N, Yerushalmi B, et al: Jaccoud's-type arthropathy: An association with sarcoidosis. J Rheumatol *18:*915, 1991.

INDEX

Note: Page numbers in *italics* refer to illustrations; page numbers followed by (t) refer to tables.

I

Clavicle (*Continued*)
  resorption of, in hyperparathyroidism, 2026,
    2028
    in rheumatoid arthritis, 905, *905*
    in scleroderma, *1197*
  rhomboid ligament insertion at, 43
  rotatory subluxation of, radical neck dissec-
    tion and, 1312–1313
  sclerosis of, *140*
  sternal end of, *697, 699, 700*
  stress injury to, activity and, 3232t
  synovial cysts of, in rheumatoid arthritis,
    903
  tumors of, 3626
  wavy, 4323
Clavicular facet, *694, 2952*
Claw hallux, 3183
Claw osteophyte, vs. traction osteophyte,
  1410, *1411*
Claw toe, 1355
Clay-shoveler's fracture, 2861, *2863*
Clear cell chondrosarcoma, 3759–3762. See
  also *Chondrosarcoma, clear cell.*
Clear cell sarcoma, 4554, 4558, *4562*
Cleavage lesion, of meniscus, 3075–3076
Cleft(s), neural arch, 2602, *2603*
  vertebral, coronal, 4187, *4187*, 4245
    paraspinous, *2603*
    pars interarticularis, *2603*. See also *Spon-*
      dylolysis.
    pediculate, *2603*
    retroisthmic, *2603*
    retrosomatic, *2603*
    spinous, *2603*
Cleidocranial dysplasia, 610, *610*, 4194,
  4195, 4196
Clinodactyly, 4593
  electrical burns and, 3274
  in Down's syndrome, 4226, *4227*
  in macrodystrophia lipomatosa, 4152
  in myositis ossificans progressiva, 4126
Clipping injury, 2649, *2653*, 3100
  vs. epiphyseal fracture, 3237
Cloaca (cloacae), 2326
  in humeral osteomyelitis, *2346*
  in osteomyelitis, *2346*
Clonorchis sinensis, 2536(t)
Closing zone, of cortical remodeling unit, 623,
  624
Clostridia, in arthritis, 1134
Clostridium difficile, in oligoarthritis, 1134
Clostridium novyi, 2459–2460
Clostridium perfringens, 2459–2460
  in myonecrosis, 2387, *2388*
  in septic arthritis, 2371
Clostridium septicum, 2459–2460
Clostridium tetani, 2459–2460
Cloverleaf skull, in thanatophoric dysplasia,
  4165
Clubbing, digital, differential diagnosis of,
  4434
    in bronchogenic carcinoma, 4427
    in chronic leukemia, 2253
    in Crohn's disease, 1129
    in hemodialysis, 2058
    in juvenile gastrointestinal polyposis,
      1142, *1144*
    in laxative abuse, 1142
    in paralysis, 3382
    in polyarteritis nodosa, 1234
    in secondary hypertrophic osteoarthropa-
      thy, 4427
    in thyroid acropachy, 1999, 1999(t), *2000*
    in ulcerative colitis, 1126
    in Whipple's disease, 1131
Clubfoot, 4313–4314, *4313*
  flattop talus in, 4314, *4314*

Clubfoot (*Continued*)
  in diastrophic dysplasia, 4178
  in Larsen's syndrome, 4197
  talocalcaneonavicular joint arthrography in,
    396
Clutton's joints, 2496, 2499
Coagulation, heritable disorders of, 2315t
Coalition. See also *Ankylosis; Arthrodesis;*
  Fusion.
  calcaneocuboid, 4301
  calcaneonavicular, 4294, *4295*, 4296
    computed tomography of, *4296*
    fracture with, *4296*, *4296*
    magnetic resonance imaging of, *4297*
    reinforcement lines in, *4296*
    talar beaking in, *4296*
  carpal, 4290–4291, *4292*
    congenital, 46, *47*
    in rheumatoid arthritis, *881*
  cubonavicular, 4301
  familial, *3585*
  lunotriquetral, 4290–4291, *4292*
  naviculocuneiform, 4301
  of toes, 64, *66*
  subtalar, scintigraphy in, 463
  talocalcaneal, *110*, 4296, *4297–4301*
    anterior facet, 4296, *4298*
    arthrography of, 4300, *4300*
    ball-and-socket ankle joint in, 4299–4300,
      4299, 4300
    computed tomography of, 4300, *4300,
      4301*
    concave talar neck in, 4299
    Harris-Beath view in, 4296, *4298*
    lateral talar process widening in, *4298,
      4298–4299*
    middle facet, 4296, *4297, 4298*
    middle subtalar joint in, 4299
    posterior facet, 4296, *4298*
    scintigraphy of, 4300, *4300*
    subtalar joint narrowing in, 4299
    talar beaking in, 4298–4299, *4298*
  talonavicular, 4300–4301, *4301*
  tarsal, *110*, 4294–4301, *4295–4301*
    arthrography in, 396
    ball-and-socket ankle joint in, 4299–4300,
      4299, 4300
    computed tomography in, 155, *156*
    scintigraphy in, 463
Cobalamin metabolism, disorders of, 4102
Cobalt, deficiency of, 3361
Cobalt-chromium, stress-strain curve for, *793*
Cocaine, scleroderma-like changes and, 1210
Coccidioides immitis, 2508, 2510, *2511–2516*
  histology of, 2510, *2516*
  in infective spondylitis, 2510, *2512–2514*
  in osteomyelitis, 2510, *2511, 2512*
  in septic arthritis, 2510, *2514, 2515*
  in tenosynovitis, 2510, *2515*
Coccidioidomycosis, 2508, 2510, *2511–2516*
  bone marrow lesion of, *2516*
  disseminated, *2512, 2514*
  granuloma of, *2516*
  parasynovial tissue in, *2516*
  pathology of, *2516*
  psoas abscess in, *2513*
  spinal, *2438*
  vs. tumor, 2510
Coccygeal cornua, 717
Coccygodynia, coccygeal segment angulation
  and, 717
  glomus tumors and, 3834
Coccyx, 25, *27, 28*, 717. See also
  Sacrococcygeal joint.
  agenesis of, 4287–4288, *4289*
  fracture of, 2804, *2805*
Cock spur disease, 1402

Cocktail sausage digit. See *Digit(s), sausage.*
Cock-up toe, in rheumatoid arthritis, 906
Codman's triangle, *4435*
  in osteosarcoma, 3663, *3668, 3673, 3676*
  radiation therapy and, *3297*
  tumor in, 3617, *3621, 3622*
Codman's tumor. See *Chondroblastoma.*
Coffin-Lowry syndrome, calcium
  pyrophosphate dihydrate crystals in, 1563
Cogan's syndrome, 1235–1236
Coherent scatter densitometry, 1862
Coils, of nuclear magnetic resonance, 172–
  173, *173*
Cold injury, phalangeal microgeodic
  syndrome from, 3265, 3268
Cold lesion, scintigraphic, in bone infection,
  2397
  in Ewing's sarcoma, 3887
  in ischemic necrosis, 457, *458*
  in Legg-Calvé-Perthes disease, *3562,
    3573*
  in osteomyelitis, 442–443
  in osteonecrosis, 3502
  in plasma cell myeloma, *2157*
  in sickle cell crisis, 2120, *2121*
  in skeletal metastases, 436, *439*
Coliform bacterial infection, 2454. See also
  Enterobacter (Aerobacter) aerogenes;
  Escherichia coli.
Colitic arthritis. See *Ulcerative colitis.*
Colitis, arthritis-dermatitis syndrome with,
  1135
  arthropathies associated with, 1120–1144
  collagenous, polyarthritis in, 1134
  pseudomembranous, arthritis in, 1134
  ulcerative. See *Ulcerative colitis.*
Collagen, 631, 770–777
  alpha chains of, 774, *774*
  armor plate layer of, 771
  bovine, 776
  chemistry of, 772–775, *773, 774*, 775(t)
  coils of, 631
  cross links of, 775–777, *776*
  digestion of, 785
  enzymatic degradation of, 815
  fibers of, 631
  fibrillar, 774, 775(t), 4105
    cross-links of, 4105
    in Ehlers-Danlos syndrome, 4102
  glycine of, 774
  hydroxyproline of, 774
  in chondromalacia patellae, 1347
  in degenerative joint disease, 1268
  in desmoplastic fibroma, *3781*
  in fibrogenesis imperfecta ossium, 4131
  in malignant fibrous histiocytoma, 3809
  in Paget's disease, 1924
  in renal osteodystrophy, 1905
  in traumatic neuroma, *4558*
  layers of, 770–771, *770, 771*
  molecular structure of, 772–774, *773, 774*
  morphology of, 770–772, *770–773*
  non–fibril-forming, 774, 775(t)
  of fibrous histiocytoma, *4532*
  of menisci, 3069–3070
  polarized light examination of, 772, *772,
    773*
  proline of, 774
  quarter stagger assembly of, 772, *773, 774*
  synthesis of, *774*, 776–777
    1,25–dihydroxyvitamin D effects on, 641
    in Ehlers-Danlos syndrome, 4105, 4106
    in homocystinuria, 4100
    in psoriatic arthritis, 1094
  type I, in Ehlers-Danlos syndrome, 4106
    in osteogenesis imperfecta, 4111

Hip (*Continued*)
vs. diffuse idiopathic skeletal hyperostosis, 1485–1486
destruction of, in pyrophosphate arthropathy,
1584, *1587*
developmental dysplasia of, 4067–4091
acetabula in, 4070, *4071*
acetabular anteversion in, 4083
acetabular depth in, 4072, *4073*
acetabular dysplasia in, 4072, 4081
acetabular index in, 4070, *4071, 4072*
acetabular labrum in, 3026, *3028,* 4068,
4069
acetabular measurements in, 4072, *4073*
acetabular slope in, 4072, *4073*
acetabular variation in, 4068
arthrography of, 339, *340*
arthrogryposis multiplex congenita with,
4091, *4091*
canine model of, 4067, *4068*
caudal regression syndrome with, *4091*
center-edge angle in, 4072, *4073*
Chiari osteotomy for, 4087, 4089
classification system for, 4068, *4069*
clinical tests of, 4068–4069
computed tomography in, 155, *155,* 4083,
4083, 4084
contrast arthrography in, 4074–4075,
4075
conventional tomography in, 4072, 4074
coxa magna deformity in, 4090
diagnostic imaging of, 155, *155,* 223–224,
225, 4069–4084
differential diagnosis of, 4090–4091, *4091*
dislocation in, 4068–4069, *4069*
radiography of, 4069–4070
ultrasonography of, 4078, 4081, *4081,
4082*
epidemiology of, 4068
etiology of, 4067–4068, *4068*
femoral anteversion in, 4083, *4086*
femoral head dislocation in, 4072, *4073*
ultrasonography of, 4078, 4081, *4081,
4082*
femoral head ossification in, 4070, *4071,
4084*
femoral head position in, 4070, *4071*
femoral head subluxation in, 4078, *4080,*
4083
femoral neck variation in, 4068
femoral varus osteotomy for, 4087
femur in, 4070, *4071*
Frejka pillow in, 4084, 4087
ganglion in, *4526*
heritable factors in, 4067–4068
Hilgenreiner's line in, 4070, *4071, 4072*
intraosseous ganglion in, 1275
magnetic resonance imaging of, 213,
4083–4084, *4084–4087, 4086*
ossification in, 4077–4078, *4079*
osteoarthritis and, 1321, *1323*
osteonecrosis and, 3519
osteotomies for, 4084, 4087, *4088,* 4089,
4089
acetabular dysplasia in, 4090
complications of, 4089–4090
coxa vara deformity after, 4090
degenerative arthritis after, 4090
femoral head osteonecrosis after, 4089–
4090
growth plate fusion in, 4090
growth recovery lines in, 4090
trochanteric overgrowth after, 4090
pathogenesis of, 4067–4068, *4068*
Pavlik harness in, 4081–4082, 4084, 4087
pelvic/femoral osteotomies for, 4087,
4088

Hip (*Continued*)
Pemberton osteotomy for, 4087, *4088,*
4089
Perkin's line in, 4070, *4071, 4072*
radiographic measurements in, 4072,
4073–4075
radiography of, 4069–4070, *4070–4075*
abduction-internal rotation view in,
4070, *4070*
childhood, 4070, 4071, *4071–4075*
neonatal, 4069–4070, *4070, 4071*
Ortolani position in, 4069, *4070*
von Rosen view in, 4070, *4070*
radiologic lines in, 4070, *4071, 4072,
4072*
real-time ultrasonography of, 4082–4083
recurrent, after pelvic osteotomy, 4089,
4089
reduction of, computed tomography of,
4083, *4083*
sagging rope sign in, 4090
Salter osteotomy for, 4087, *4089*
Shenton's line in, 4070, *4071, 4072*
subluxation in, 4068–4069, *4069*
ultrasonography of, 4078–4081, *4079–
4081*
total hip arthroplasty in, 4089
treatment of, 4084, 4087–4089, *4088,
4089*
complications of, 4089–4090
type I, *4070, 4071, 4086*
untreated, 4072, *4074*
type II, *4071, 4085*
Salter osteotomy in, *4089*
untreated, 4083, *4083*
type III, pseudoacetabulum in, 4072,
4074, 4075
types of, 4068, *4069*
ultrasonography of, 223–224, *225,* 4075–
4082, *4076–4082, 4081*
coronal image in, 4077, *4077*
femoral head dislocation in, 4078,
4081, *4081, 4082*
femoral head subluxation in, 4078,
4080
hip dislocation in, 4078, 4081, *4081,
4082*
ossification in, 4077–4078, *4079*
Pavlik harness in, 4076
reliability of, 4081–4083
stress maneuvers in, 4078, *4080*
subluxation in, 4078, *4079–4081,* 4081
technical aspects in, 4076
transaxial image in, 4077, *4078*
untreated, degenerative joint disease and,
4072, *4074*
von Rosen splint, 4084, 4087
vs. abnormal joint laxity, 4091
vs. congenital coxa vara, 4091
vs. inflammatory disease, 4090–4091
vs. traumatic epiphyseal slip, 4091
Y line in, 4070, *4072*
disease distribution in, 1774–1777
dislocation of, 2752, 2755, *2756, 2757.* See
also *Dislocation(s); hip; Hip, developmental dysplasia of.*
displacement of, congenital. See *Hip, developmental dysplasia of.*
dual x-ray absorptiometry of, *1865*
dysplasia epiphysealis hemimelica of, 4212,
4213
dysplasia of. See also *Hip, developmental
dysplasia of.*
femoral head subluxation and, 797
ectopic ossification of, in hemophilia, 2302,
2307
effusion of, 223

Hip (*Continued*)
percutaneous needle aspiration of, 223
epiphysis of, dysplasia of, 339
in multiple epiphyseal dysplasia, *4136*
erosion of, in rheumatoid arthritis, 921, 923,
923
fat planes of, 725, 728, *732, 734–735*
fibrocartilage of, calcium pyrophosphate dihydrate crystal deposition in, 1566,
1568
fibrous capsule of, 725, 3023, *3024*
bulging of, 54, *56*
fibrous dysplasia of, *4385*
fluid in, magnetic resonance imaging of,
198–199, *199*
plain film radiography of, 28, 54
ultrasonography of, 223
forces on, 796
in monopedal stance, *519*
fracture of, 142, *143*
occult, in femoral shaft fracture, 2766
fracture-dislocation about, *3040*
fusion of. See *Hip, ankylosis of; Hip, arthrodesis of.*
ganglion of, 4519, *4526, 4527*
gluteal fat plane of, 725, 728, *732, 734–735*
gluteal insertions of, calcification of, 1627,
1628
gonococcal arthritis of, 2451, *2453*
gout of, 1535–1536, *1536,* 1775
growth disturbances of, in sickle cell anemia, 2114
heterotopic ossification of, central nervous
system disorders and, 3375, *3375*
scintigraphy in, *470*
hyaline cartilage of, calcium pyrophosphate
dihydrate crystal deposition in, 1566,
1568
idiopathic chondrolysis of, 1776
idiopathic synovial (osteo)chondromatosis
of, 1777, 3029, *3031, 3032, 3961–
3963,* 4540, *4546*
iliopsoas fat plane of, 725, 728, *732, 734–
735*
in acromegaly, 1973, *1977*
in alkaptonuria, 1777
in chondrodysplasia punctata, *4147*
in Crohn's disease, 1127, *1128*
in degenerative joint disease. See *Hip, osteoarthritis of.*
in diffuse idiopathic skeletal hyperostosis,
1485–1486
in familial Mediterranean fever, 1150, 1151,
1151
in hemochromatosis, 1658, *1659*
in hemophilia, 2300, 2302, *2305, 2307*
in hypoparathyroidism, 2062
in Meyer's dysplasia, 4148, *4148, 4149*
in multiple epiphyseal dysplasia, *4136*
in osteoarthritis. See *Osteoarthritis, hip.*
in osteonecrosis. See *Hip, osteonecrosis of.*
in primary biliary cirrhosis, *1138*
in Reiter's syndrome, 1105, *1105,* 1775
in rheumatoid arthritis, 921, 923, *923*
in sickle cell anemia, 2114
in sickle cell hemoglobinopathy, 2127
in slipped capital femoral epiphysis, 2647
in systemic lupus erythematosus, *1185*
in ulcerative colitis, 1124, *1125*
in Whipple's disease, 1131, *1132*
infant, magnetic resonance imaging of,
4083, *4084*
ultrasonography of, 4076–4077, *4077,
4079*
coronal image in, 4077, *4077*
reliability of, 4081–4083
transaxial image in, 4077, *4078*

Humerus (*Continued*)
pigmentation of, in alkaptonuria, *1673*
plain film radiography of, 12
posterolateral, compression fracture of, 3245–3246, *3246*
in anterior glenohumeral joint dislocation, 2694, *2697, 2698*
proximal, exostosis of, radiation therapy and, *3300*
fracture of, 2710, 2710(t), *2711–2714, 2712–2715.* See also *Fracture(s), humerus, proximal.*
fracture-dislocation of, 2713, *2713*
brachial plexus injury in, 2715
heterotopic bone formation in, 2714, *2714*
growth plate of, injury to, 2641, 2654, *2656, 2657*
notches of, plain film radiography of, 44, *45*
osteolysis of, *847*
in Hodgkin's disease, *2267*
osteosclerosis of, in non-Hodgkin's lymphoma, *2261*
pitching stress injury to, 3237–3238, *3239*
separation of, birth and, 2654
slipped epiphysis of, radiation therapy and, 3290
tumors of, 3626
pseudarthrosis of, 2575
in osteogenesis imperfecta, *4118*
pseudocyst of, *4270*
psoriatic arthritis of, *1084*
rheumatoid arthritis of, *901*
rotator cuff rupture and, *833*
Salmonella infection of, in sickle cell anemia, *2117,* 2117–2118
sarcoma of, *3551*
radiation therapy and, *3301*
sequestra of, in osteomyelitis, *2343*
spiral groove of, radial nerve entrapment in, 3395
streptococcal infection of, in neonate, 2449
stress fracture of, 2597
stress injuries to, activity and, 3232t
pitching and, 3237–3238, *3239*
subluxation of, in drooping shoulder, 3382
supracondylar (supracondyloid) process of, 3745–3746, *3745*
synovial cyst of, in rheumatoid arthritis, *903*
torsion of, angle of, 695
trabeculae of, *1837*
trochlea of, fracture of, 2728, *2729*
ossification center of, 2657, *2658*
trough fracture of, in posterior glenohumeral joint dislocation, 2700, *2702, 2703*
tuberculosis of, 2474–2475, *2475, 2477*
tuberosity of, 692, *693*
greater, 692, *693, 2951, 2952, 2954, 2996*
avulsion fracture of, 2695
cysts of, in rotator cuff tears, 2969
fracture of, *2711,* 2712–2713, *2713, 3022*
in anterior glenohumeral joint dislocation, 2695
simulated destruction of, 44, *45*
in acromegaly, 1985
lesser, 692, *693, 2951, 2952, 2954, 2996*
avulsion fracture of, 2700, *2703*
fracture of, *2711,* 2712, 2713
in posterior glenohumeral joint dislocation, 2700, *2703*
tumor of, *3616*
varus deformity of, in thalassemia, 2132–2133
Wilson's disease of, 1665, *1665*
Hunter's syndrome (MPS II), 4232

Hunter's syndrome (MPS II) (*Continued*)
characteristics of, 4230t
hand in, 4232, *4232*
pelvis in, 4229, *4231*
spine in, 4232, *4232*
upper extremity in, 4229, *4232*
Hurler's syndrome (MPS I), 4229, 4231, *4231, 4232*
arylsulfatase B in, 786
characteristics of, 4230t
osteopenia in, 4229, *4232*
skull in, 4229, *4231*
spine in, 4229, *4231*
vertebral body scalloping in, 1991
Hurler-Scheie syndrome (MPS I-H-S), 4230t, 4232
Hutchinsonian triad, in congenital syphilis, 2493
Hutchinson's fracture, 2733, 2734, *2735*
characteristics of, 2733t
complications of, 2733t
mechanism of injury in, 2733t
Hutchinson's teeth, 2495
in congenital syphilis, 2493
Hyaline fibromatosis, juvenile, 4513, 4516(t)
Hyaluronan, 777–778, *778*
structure of, *777*
Hyaluronidase, 785
Hydatid cysts, 2537(t), 2539–2542, *2540, 2541*
Hydrarthrosis, intermittent, in systemic lupus erythematosus, 1167
magnetic resonance imaging of, 248
Hydrocephalus, in hypervitaminosis A, 3343, 3344
Hydrogen density, in nuclear magnetic resonance imaging, 176
Hydrogen spectroscopy, 214–215
Hydromyelia, magnetic resonance imaging in, 29, 265, 271, *271*
Hydrops fetalis, 2129
Hydroxyapatite crystal deposition disease. See *Calcium hydroxyapatite crystal deposition disease.*
Hydroxyapatite crystals. See *Calcium hydroxyapatite crystal(s).*
Hydroxyapatite grafts, in spinal fusion, 533, *533*
Hydroxyproline, serum, in bone matrix turnover, 630
urinary, in bone matrix turnover, 630
in Paget's disease, 1924, 1925
25–Hydroxyvitamin D₃ (25–OH-D₃), 1886
anticonvulsant drugs and, 1901–1902
enterohepatic circulation of, 1899
hydroxylation of, 1887–1888
in liver disease, 1900–1901
in renal osteodystrophy, 1903
Hygroma, cystic, 4531
Hymenolepis nana, 2536(t)
Hypaque Sodium 50%, for arthrography, 278–279, *280*
Hyperalimentation, intravenous, rickets and, 1792, *1792*
Hypercalcemia, bone mineralization and, 634
differential diagnosis of, 2013t
familial, 2034–2035, 2034t. See also *Multiple endocrine neoplasia syndrome.*
benign, 2035
hypocalciuric, 2034t, 2035
idiopathic, 1214, 3350
in aluminum toxicity, 1905
in congenital primary hyperthyroidism, 2033
in disuse osteoporosis, 1797
in hyperthyroidism, 1995
in lymphoma, 1887
in primary hyperparathyroidism, 2013

Hypercalcemia (*Continued*)
in rheumatoid arthritis, 869
infantile, 3350
of malignancy, 2013, 2013t, 3996, 4058
renal transplantation and, 2059
Hypercalciuria, in disuse osteoporosis, 1797
in hyperthyroidism, 1995
Hypercholesterolemia, familial. See also *Hyperlipoproteinemia.*
xanthomas of, of Achilles tendon, 228
in primary biliary cirrhosis, 1136
xanthoma formation in, 228, 1136
Hypercortisolism, exogenous, osteonecrosis in, 2077, *2079*
osteoporosis in, 1788, *1788*
Hyperemia, 3463
in hemophilia, 2311
synovial inflammation and, 815
thermal burns and, 3269
Hyperextension, axial dislocation from, 2855
in hangman's fracture, 2853
knee, congenital subluxation with, 4307–4308, *4308, 4309*
of cervical spine, 2826(t), 2856–2857, *2857*
spinal fracture from, in ankylosing spondylitis, 1023
Hyperflexion, of cervical spine, 2826(t), 2859–2865, *2862–2864*
Hyperglycemia, maternal, fetal hyperinsulinemia from, 2088
Hyperlipidemia, osteonecrosis and, 3454, 3456
Hyperlipoproteinemia, 2232–2238
Achilles tendon in, 100
arthralgia in, 2232(t), 2235
arthritis in, 2232(t), 2235
broad-beta, 2232–2233, 2232(t)
cerebrotendinous xanthomatosis in, 2235, 2238, *2239*
cholesterol in, 2232
chylomicrons in, 2232, 2232(t)
classification of, 2232–2233, 2232(t)
differential diagnosis of, 2238
erosions in, 2238
familial, 2232, 2232(t)
features of, 2232–2233
gout in, 2235, *2238*
heredity in, 2232–2233, 2232(t)
hyperuricemia in, 2232(t)
β-lipoproteins in, 2232, 2232(t)
low density lipoproteins in, 2233
musculoskeletal abnormalities in, 2233, 2234–2237
pre-β-lipoproteins in, 2232–2233, 2232(t)
secondary forms of, 2232(t)
synovitis in, 2235, 2238
triglycerides in, 2232
types of, 2232–2233, 2232(t)
vs. gout, 2238
xanthoma in, 2232, 2232(t), 2233, *2234–2237*
Hyperlordosis. See *Lordosis.*
Hypermobility, joint. See also *Laxity, joint.*
degenerative joint disease and, 1293
differential diagnosis of, 4091
in cerebrotendinous xanthomatosis, 2238
in Ehlers-Danlos syndrome, 4107, *4107*
meniscal, 365, *365*
Hyperostosis. See also *Periostitis.*
ankylosing, of Forestier and Rotes-Querol. See *Diffuse idiopathic skeletal hyperostosis (DISH).*
spinal, diabetes mellitus and, 2081–2082, *2082*
calvarial, 1962, *1962*
clavicular, in chronic recurrent multifocal osteomyelitis, 2389, *2389*

Magnetic resonance imaging *(Continued)*
in postmeniscectomy osteonecrosis, *3099*
in postoperative discitis, 555
in postoperative intervertebral disc infection, 2435
in posttraumatic bone marrow alterations, 210, *210*
in posttraumatic radial cyst, *2605*
in preachilles fat body, *3175*
in precocious osteopetrosis, 4201
in prepatellar bursitis, 3155–3156, *3156*
in prepatellar hematoma, 3155–3156, *3156*
in prepatellar varicosities, 3156, *3156*
in prevertebral hematoma, 2839, 2859
in primitive neuroectodermal tumors, 2271
in proximal tibial avulsion fracture, 2767, *2774*
in pseudarthrosis, 554
in pseudomeningocele, 530
in psoas abscess, 2386, *2386*
in psoas tuberculous abscess, 2467, *2468*
in pubic rami stress fracture, *2597*
in pyomyositis, *2394*
in quadriceps tendon rupture, *2665*
in quadriceps tendon tear, *3321*
in quadrilateral space syndrome, *3020*
in radial desmoplastic fibroma, *3778*
in radiation bone changes, *3303,* 3305, *3305*
in radiation fibrosis vs. recurrent tumor, 3305, *3305*
in recurrent carpal tunnel syndrome, 3394, *3394*
in reflex sympathetic dystrophy, 1844
in renal cell carcinoma metastases, *3999*
in retrocalcaneal bursitis, *827*
in rhabdomyolysis, 2676
in rhabdomyosarcoma, 4523, *4524*
in rheumatoid arthritis, 213, *213,* 948–953, *949–953,* 2932–2933, *2933*
  of knee, 3051–3052, *3051*
in rheumatoid nodules, 836, *837*
in rotator cuff tears, 211, *211,* 951, 2970, 2973–2984, *2976–2981*
in rotator cuff tendinopathy, 2985–2986, *2985–2987*
in rotator cuff tendon scar, *2986*
in sacral insufficiency fracture, 2593, *2598*
in sacral neurofibroma, *4376*
in sacrococcygeal chordoma, *3850*
in sacroiliac joint infection, 2441, *2442, 2443*
in sacroiliitis, 1060, *1063*
in Salter-Harris fracture, 2948, 3237, *3238*
in sarcoidosis, 4344, *4346, 4347,* 4348
in scaphocapitate syndrome, *2927*
in scaphoid osteonecrosis, 2925, *2928,* 3524, *3526*
in scapholunate interosseous ligament defect, 2921–2925, *2922–2924*
in sciatic neurofibroma, *4376*
in scleroderma, *1198*
in scoliosis, 4253–4254
in segmental vertebral sclerosis, 1436
in Segond fracture, 3108, *3108, 3109, 3240*
in semimembranosus tendon injury, 3103
in septic arthritis, *2370,* 2408(t), 3029, *3032*
in shoulder impingement syndrome, 2965, *3250*
in sickle cell anemia, 2120, 2122–2126, *2122, 2124–2126, 3507*
in silicone synovitis, 601, *601*
in Sinding-Larsen-Johansson disease, *3602*
in sinus tarsi syndrome, 3200, *3201*
in skeletal muscle infarction, 2084
in skip metastases, 205
in SLAP (superior labral, anterior and posterior) lesion, 3011–3012, *3012*

Magnetic resonance imaging *(Continued)*
in sleeve fracture, *2672*
in slipped capital femoral epiphysis, 2647, *2649*
in soft tissue chondrosarcoma, 4548, *4548*
in soft tissue injury, 209
in soft tissue lipoma, *4502*
in soft tissue liposarcoma, *4502*
in soft tissue mass, 207–209, *207–209,* 4500–4503, *4502*
in soft tissue tumors, 3941, 4500–4503, *4502*
in spinal coccidioidomycosis, 2513, *2514*
in spinal cord compression, 952–953, *952,* 2133
in spinal cord hemorrhage, 2835, *2835*
in spinal cord infection, 2435
in spinal cord injury, 2831, 2834–2835, *2835*
in spinal cord masses, 267–272, *269–272*
in spinal cord trauma, 29, *30*
in spinal fracture, 265, *266*
in spinal hemangioma, 28–29, *3823*
in spinal infection, 2431–2435, *2432–2434*
in spinal injury, 2830–2832, *2831, 2832*
in spinal large cell lymphoma, 2274
in spinal ligament injury, 2831, *2831*
in spinal metastases, 4020, 4049, *4049, 4050*
in spinal schwannoma, *33*
in spinal stenosis, 260, *261*
in spinal tuberculosis, 2432, *2434*
in spinal tumors, 264–265
in spinal vacuum phenomenon, *1382*
in spondylodiscitis, 1057, *1062*
in spondylolysis, 2602–2603
in spontaneous osteonecrosis, 3541, *3543, 3544*
in spontaneous quadriceps tendon rupture, *2034*
in Stener lesion, 2936, *2936*
in sternocostoclavicular hyperostosis, *4457*
in stress fractures, 210, 951, 2585, *2587*
in stress injuries, 3231, *3233*
in subacromial bursitis, 951, 2687
in subacromial enthesophyte, *1311*
in subchondral cysts, 819, 2311
in subdeltoid bursa calcification, *1633*
in subdeltoid bursitis, 4569
in subscapularis tendon calcification, *1633*
in subungual glomus tumor, *4536*
in suprascapular nerve entrapment, 3017, *3019*
in supraspinatus tendon rupture, *2665*
in supraspinatus tendon scar, 2985, *2986*
in supraspinatus tendon tear, 211, *211*
in synovial chondrosarcoma, 3067, *3069,* 4547, *4547*
in synovial cysts, 838, *839,* 897, *903,* 951, 3976
  of knee, *3059*
in synovial hemangioma, 3067
in synovial hemosiderin deposition, 2632, 2634
in synovial inflammation, 213, *213*
in synovial sarcoma, *3060,* 3965, 4549, *4552*
in synovitis, of hip, 3573
  of knee, 3051–3052, *3051*
in syringomyelia, 35, *36,* 271, *272,* 2836, *2837*
in systemic mastocytosis, *2280*
in talar osteonecrosis, 3513, *3514*
in talofibular ligament tears, 3197, *3197*
in tarsal navicular osteonecrosis, *3546*
in tarsal navicular stress fracture, 3235
in tarsal tunnel syndrome, 3400, *3401, 3402*
in telangiectatic osteosarcoma, *3681*

Magnetic resonance imaging *(Continued)*
in temporomandibular joint arthritis, 953
in temporomandibular joint foreign body giant cell reaction, 1751, *1751*
in temporomandibular joint locking, *1747, 1748*
in temporomandibular meniscus dislocation, *1745*
in tendinitis, 3173
in tendo Achillis bursitis, *3255*
in tendon sheath giant cell tumor, *34,* 2932, *4535,* 4566
in tendon tears, 2663, *2665*
in tenosynovitis, 2930, 3173
in thalassemia, 2136
in thoracic sagittal slice fracture, 2875
in thoracolumbar fracture-dislocation, *2884,* 2885
in thoracolumbar spinal stenosis, 2879, *2881*
in tibial aneurysmal bone cyst, *3877*
in tibial avulsion fracture, 2666
in tibial cartilage abnormalities, 3143–3144, *3143, 3144*
in tibial chondrosarcoma, *3709*
in tibial epidermoid carcinoma, *2363*
in tibial fracture, 2787
in tibial ganglion cyst, *3880*
in tibial giant cell tumor, *3797*
in tibial hemangioma, *3826*
in tibial hereditary multiple exostoses, *3741*
in tibial infarct, *3489*
in tibial non-Hodgkin's lymphoma, *2264, 2271,* 2271
in tibial nonossifying fibroma, *3771*
in tibial osteochondroma, *3731*
in tibial osteoid osteoma, *3644*
in tibial osteonecrosis, 3513, *3514*
in tibial osteosarcoma, *3673*
in tibial plateau fracture, 2610, 2611, *2612,* 2767, *2772*
in tibial stress fracture, 210
in tibial triplane fracture, *2656*
in tibialis anterior tendon tears, 3183, *3184*
in tibialis posterior tendinitis, *3170*
in tibialis posterior tendon injury, 212
in tibialis posterior tendon tears, *194,* 3180, 3182, *3182*
in tibiofibular ganglion, *3403*
in trauma, 209–210, *209, 210,* 2567, *2568*
in triangular fibrocartilage complex degeneration, 2912–2913, *2913–2915*
in triangular fibrocartilage complex lesions, 2912–2916, *2912–2917*
in triangular fibrocartilage complex tear, *2914, 2915*
in triceps tendon tear, *2945*
in trochanteric bursitis, *3034,* 4569
in tuberculous arthritis, 2483
in tuberculous bursitis, 2484
in tuberculous psoas abscess, 2469
in tuberculous spondylitis, *2469, 2470, 2472*
in tuberous sclerosis, 4355–4356, *4357*
in tumorous vs. nontumorous vertebral body compression fracture, 4050–4051, *4053, 4054*
in ulnar erosion, *213*
in ulnar impaction syndrome, *2917, 2918*
in ulnar nerve entrapment, 3394, *3395*
in ulnar tunnel syndrome, 2931
in ulnocarpal abutment syndrome, *1301*
in unilateral facet lock, 2866, *2866*
in vertebral body collapse, 4009, *4010*
in vertebral body fractures, 1837–1839, *1838, 1839*
in vertebral body plasmacytoma, *2168*
in vertebral osteonecrosis, 3527, *3530*
in vertebral pathologic fracture, 4051

Par interarticularis, in spondylolysis, 2597, *2600*
Parachuting injuries, 3230
Paracoccidioidomycosis, 2508, *2508*
Paraffin, scleroderma-like changes from, 1210
Paragonimiasis, 2542
Paragonimus westermani, 2536(t), 2542
Parahemophilia, heredity in, 2315t
Parallel track sign, in secondary hypertrophic osteoarthropathy, 4432, *4433*
Paralysis. See also *Immobilization; Paraplegia; Quadriplegia.*
    arthritis in, 3381, *3382*
    atlantoaxial subluxation and, 932
    bone shortening in, 3374
    cartilage atrophy and, *4483*
    cartilaginous nutrition in, 3378, *3378*
    digital clubbing in, 3382
    drooping shoulder in, 3382
    Erb-Duchenne, obstetric trauma and, 3373–3374, *3374*
    heterotopic ossification in, 466, 470, 471, 3375, *3375–3377*, 3377
    hip dislocation in, *3372*
    hip, in cartilage atrophy in, 3378, *3379*
        disuse atrophy of, *729*
    HLA antigen testing in, 3380
    in arthritis, 3381, *3382*
    in fibrous dysplasia, 4382
    in rheumatoid arthritis, 868
    insufficiency fracture in, 3366, *3368*
    joint space narrowing in, 3378, *3379*
    Klumpke's, obstetric trauma and, 3373
    lipoma in, 3942
    musculoskeletal abnormalities in, 3406, 3406t. See also *Neuromuscular disorders.*
    neuropathic osteoarthropathy in, 3436
    osteoporosis of, 1795–1797, 3365
    paravertebral ossification in, 3380, *3381*
    periosteal lipoma in, 3947
    protective effect of, in arthritis, 3381, *3382*
    reflex sympathetic dystrophy in, 3382
    sacroiliac joint in, 1065, 3378, 3380, *3380*
        pelvic sepsis and, 3375
        vs. ankylosing spondylitis, 3378, 3380
    spastic, triangular femoral head in, 3372–3373
    spondylopathy in, 3380–3381, *3381*
    synovitis in, 3381, *3382*
    tophaceous nodules and, 1515
    vs. thermal burns, 3270
Paramyxovirus, in subacute sclerosing panencephalitis, 1925
Paramyxovirus-like filamentous intranuclear inclusions, in giant cell tumors, 3787
Paraosteoarthropathy, 466, *470*, 471
Paraplegia. See also *Paralysis; Quadriplegia.*
    acute, after needle biopsy, 483
    decubitus ulcers in, *2423*
    epidural lipomatosis and, 3321
    fracture in, 3366, *3367*
    heterotopic ossification in, 466, 470, 471, 3375
    hip dislocation in, 3371, *3372*
    HLA antigen testing in, 3380
    in lumbar spine infection, *2423*
    in neurofibromatosis, 4370
    in plasmacytoma, 2162
    in spondylitis, 2425
    in thoracic fracture-dislocation, 2874
    in tuberculous spondylitis, 2467
    neuromuscular scoliosis in, 4260
    neuropathic osteoarthropathy in, 3436
    physical therapy in, fracture from, 3366, *3367*
    sacroiliac joint alterations in, 3378

Paraplegia *(Continued)*
    scintigraphy in, 456
    spinal abnormalities in, 3380–3381, *3381*
    spinal cord injury and, 2833, 3375
    teardrop fracture and, 2864
Paraproteinemia, in rheumatoid arthritis, 939
Paraproteins, in POEMS syndrome, 2172
Paraspinal ligaments, ossification of, in myositis ossificans progressiva, 4128, *4128*
Paraspinal muscles, atrophy of, in ankylosing spondylitis, 1057, *1061*
    fat infiltration of, 3366, *3369*
    infection of, *2394*
    ossification of, in myositis ossificans progressiva, 4128
Parasymphyseal bone, fracture of, *452*, 2804, *2805*, 2807, *2808*
Paratendinitis, 3168
    of Achilles tendon, 3174, *3175*
Paratenonitis, rheumatoid, 100
Paratenonitis (crepitans) achillea, 100–102, *100, 101.* See also *Achilles tendon.*
Paratenosynovitis, definition of, 3168
Parathormone. See *Parathyroid hormone.*
Parathyroid gland(s). See also *Hyperparathyroidism; Hypoparathyroidism; Osteodystrophy, renal; Pseudohypoparathyroidism; Pseudopseudohypoparathyroidism.*
    adenoma of, 232, *232*
    1,25–dihydroxyvitamin D_3 effect on, 1889
    disorders of, 2012–2036, 2061–2065
    hyperplasia of, 232, *232*
    in familial hypocalciuric hypercalcemia, 2035
    in multiple endocrine neoplasia syndrome type IIB, 2034
    in scleroderma, 1194
    ultrasonography of, 232
    vitamin D–dependent calcium-binding protein of, 1888
Parathyroid hormone, 638–639, 638(t), *639.* See also *Hyperparathyroidism; Hypoparathyroidism; Osteodystrophy, renal; Pseudohypoparathyroidism; Pseudopseudohypoparathyroidism.*
    aluminum toxicity and, 3361
    heparin effect on, 1788
    in bone mineralization, 635
    in 1,25–dihydroxyvitamin D_3 regulation, 1890
    in familial hypocalciuric hypercalcemia, 2035
    in fluorosis, 3324
    in hyperparathyroidism, 2013
    in hypoparathyroidism, 2061
    in Paget's disease, 1925
    in postmenopausal bone loss, 1787
    in pseudohypoparathyroidism, 2064
    in renal transplantation, 2059
    intestinal effects of, 639
    osseous effects of, 630, *630*, 638–639, *639*
    osteosclerosis and, 2030
    renal effects of, 639
    secretion of, 638, 639
    structure of, 638
Parathyroidectomy, apatite-induced periarthritis after, 2046
    joint laxity after, 2033
Paravertebral ligaments, calcification of, in X-linked hypophosphatemia, 1908, *1908, 1909*
Paravertebral ossification. See *Ossification, paravertebral.*
Paravertebral venous plexus. See *Batson's paravertebral venous plexus.*

Parenteral hyperalimentation, Candida infection and, 2519
Parenteral nutrition, aluminum toxicity in, 3360
    rickets and, 1899
Paresthesias, after intestinal bypass surgery, 1135
    in OPLL, 1498
Parietal bone, convexity of, 617, *623*
Park, lines of, 3353, 3354(t), 3355, *3355, 3356.* See also *Growth recovery lines.*
Parke-Weber syndrome, 2314, 4153. See also *Arteriovenous malformation; Klippel-Trenaunay-Weber syndrome.*
Paronychia, 2350, *2351*
Parosteal osteosarcoma. See *Osteosarcoma, parosteal.*
Parotid gland, calcification of, in hypothyroidism, 2007
Pars interarticularis. See also *Spondylolysis.*
    axial, traumatic spondylolisthesis of, 2853, *2854*
        classification systems for, 2853–2854
        hyperextension in, 2853
        mechanism of injury in, 2853
        neurologic deficits in, 2854–2855
        prevertebral hematoma in, 2854
        retrolisthesis in, 2854
        types of, 2853–2854
        vertebral body extension of, 2853, *2854*
    C5, fracture of, 264, *264*
    fracture of, in failed back syndrome, 529
    in spondylolysis, 2597, *2600*
    lumbar, defect of, 2886, 2887–2888, *2887*
        computed tomography of, *2889*, 2889–2890
        magnetic resonance imaging of, 2890
        malalignment in, 2889
        nerve root entrapment in, 2890
        radiographic abnormalities in, 2888–2889, *2888*
        radiographic grading system for, 2890
        scintigraphy in, 2890
    elongated, 2887
    fracture of, 2886–2887
    scintigraphy of, 2602
    spondylolisthesis of, 2886–2887
    radiography of, 2890
    single photon emission computed tomography of, 245
    spondylolytic defects in, 265, *266, 267, 267*
    stress injury to, 2890
    stresses on, 2598
Partial transient osteoporosis. See *Osteoporosis, transient.*
Particles, wear, 349, 2634
Parvovirus, arthritis with, 2534
Pasteurella, in rheumatoid arthritis, 939
Pasteurella hemolytica, 2459
Pasteurella multocida, 2459, *2459*
    in cat bites, 2359, *2359*
Pasteurella pneumotropica, 2459
Pasteurella ureae, 2459
Patella, 3041, *3109.* See also *Knee.*
    anatomy of, 728, 733, *737, 740, 742*
    aneurysmal bone cyst of, 3871
    aplasia of, in osteo-onychodysostosis, 4317
    articular surface of, 733, *740*, 3042–3043
    artificial. See *Patellar prosthetic component.*
    bipartite, 59, *59*, 4276, *4279*, 4279–4280
    Brodie's abscess of, *2341*
    chondromalacia of, 3117–3118, *3118.* See also *Chondromalacia patellae.*
    chondrosarcoma of, *3751*
    classification of, *740*
    configurations of, *740*
    cysts of, in gout, 1531, *1534*

ISBN 0-7216-5068-6

9 780721 650685

90038